Endocrinology and Diabetes

Francisco Bandeira • Hossein Gharib
Luiz Griz • Manuel Faria
Editors

Endocrinology and Diabetes

A Problem Oriented Approach

Second Edition

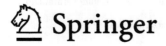 Springer

Editors
Francisco Bandeira
Division of Endocrinology
Agamenon Magalhães Hospital
University of Pernambuco Medical School
Recife, PE, Brazil

Luiz Griz
School of Medicine
University of Pernambuco
Recife, Brazil

Hossein Gharib
Division of Endocrinology
Mayo Clinic College of Medicine
Rochester, MN, USA

Manuel Faria
School of Medicine
University of Maranhao
Sao Luis, Brazil

ISBN 978-3-030-90686-3   ISBN 978-3-030-90684-9   (eBook)
https://doi.org/10.1007/978-3-030-90684-9

This Springer imprint is published by the registered company Springer Nature Switzerland AG
The registered company address is: Gewerbestrasse 11, 6330 Cham, Switzerland

This task was a labor of love. We dedicate this book to our families without whose support and patience, we could not have finished this project; to our patients whose care and concerns remain our focus and priority; and to our younger colleagues and students who continue to inspire us.

Preface to Second Edition

The enthusiastic reception and warm welcome of the first edition of this book was overwhelming and gratifying. Despite many standard texts that cover physiology and clinical aspects of endocrinology, this book found a special place because it focused on patient care and practical aspects of endocrine practice. In the current volume, we were fortunate to again have the honor of collaboration by international authors who pride themselves foremost as clinical endocrinologists. We hope our readers will find this updated, improved edition worthwhile, and use it for the benefit of their patients.

Our heartfelt thanks to our contributing authors and to our publisher.

Recife, Brazil	Francisco Bandeira
Rochester, MN, USA	Hossein Gharib
Recife, Brazil	Luiz Griz
Sao Luis, Brazil	Manuel Faria

Contents

Contributors

Krystallenia I. Alexandraki, PhD, MSc, MSc, MD 2nd Department of Surgery, Aretaieion Hospital, Kapodistrian and National University of Athens, Athens, Greece

Lívia Amaral, MD Universidade Federal de Alagoas (UFAL), Tabuleiro do Martins Maceió - Algoas, AL, Brazil

Paula Aragão, MD Division of Endocrinology and Diabetes, Agamenon Magalhães Hospital, University of Pernambuco Medical School, Recife, Pernambuco, Brazil

Ambika P. Ashraf, MD Department of Pediatrics/Division of Pediatric Endocrinology and Metabolism, Children's of Alabama, University of Alabama at Birmingham, Birmingham, AL, USA

Children's Hospital, UAB, Birmingham, AL, USA

Antonio Balsamo, MD Pediatric Unit, Department of Medical and Surgical Sciences, St. Orsola-Malpighi Hospital, University of Bologna, Bologna, Italy

Francisco Bandeira, MD, PhD Agamenon Maghalhaes Hospital, University of Pernambuco Medical School, Recife, Pernambuco, Brazil

John P. Bilezikian, MD Metabolic Bone Diseases Unit, Division of Endocrinology, Department of Medicine, College of Physicians and Surgeons, Columbia University, New York, NY, USA

Marcello D. Bronstein, MD, PhD Hospital das Clinicas, University of Sao Paulo, Neuroendocrine Unit, Division of Endocrinology and Metabolism, Sao Paulo, SP, Brazil

Bruno Cesar Caldas Fellowship of Endocrinology of Agamenon Magalhães Hospital – Division of Endocrinology and Diabetes, Recife, PE, Brazil

Ana P. M. Canton, MD, PhD Unidade de Endocrinologia Genetica, Laboratorio de Endocrinologia Celular e Molecular LIM/25, Disciplina de Endocrinologia, Hospital das Clinicas da Faculdade de Medicina da Universidade de São Paulo, São Paulo, SP, Brazil

Nara N. C. Carvalho, MD Department of Endocrinology, Federal University of Paraíba, João Pessoa, Brazil

Elaine Y. K. Chow, BSc, MBChB, MSc, PhD, MRCP Phase 1 Clinical Trial Centre, Department of Medicine and Therapeutics, Prince of Wales Hospital, The Chinese University of Hong Kong, Hong Kong, SAR, China

Bart L. Clarke, MD Mayo Clinic E18-A, Rochester, MN, USA

Department of Medicine, Division of Endocrinology, Diabetes, Metabolism, and Nutrition, Mayo Clinic College of Medicine, Rochester, MN, USA

Maria L. Collazo-Clavell, MD Division of Endocrinology, Diabetes, Metabolism, and Nutrition, Mayo Clinic, Rochester, MN, USA

Caroline Colvin, MD Department of Pediatrics/Division of Pediatric Endocrinology and Metabolism, Children's of Alabama, University of Alabama at Birmingham, Birmingham, AL, USA

Aline G. Costa, MD Metabolic Bone Diseases Unit, Division of Endocrinology, Department of Medicine, College of Physicians and Surgeons, Columbia University, New York, NY, USA

Bruna Burkhardt Costi, MD Endocrinology, Agamenon Magalhaes Hospital, Jaboatao dos Guararapes, Recife, PE, Brazil

Natalie E. Cusano, MD, MS Division of Endocrinology, Lenox Hill Hospital, Department of Medicine, New York, NY, USA

Maria da Conceição Chaves de Lemos, PhD Federal University of Pernambuco, Nutrition Department, Recife, Pernambuco, Brazil

Ana Maíra Quental Da Nóbrega, MD Division of Endocrinology, Diabetes and Metabolic Bone Diseases, Agamenon Magalhães Hospital, University of Pernambuco Medical School, Recife, PE, Brazil

Natália Rocha da Silva, MD Department of Endocrinology, Agamenon Magalhães Hospital, Division of Endocrinology, Recife, Pernambuco, Brazil

Ricardo Oliveira, MD State University of Rio de Janeiro, Rio de Janeiro, RJ, Brazil

Department of Internal Medicine, Avenida Padre Leonel Franca 116/104. Gavea, Rio de Janeiro, RJ, Brazil

Maria Elba Bandeira de Farias, MD, MSc Division of Endocrinology and Diabetes, University of Pernambuco Medical School, Agamenon Magalhães Hospital, State Department of Health/SUS/UPE, Recife, Pernambuco, Brazil

Narriane C. P. Holanda, MD Federal University of Paraíba – Ufpb, João Pessoa, Brazil

Lauro Wanderley University Hospital, Department of Endocrinology, João Pessoa, PB, Brazil

Deborah Cristina de Lemos Araújo Queiroz, MD Endocrinology, Agamenon Magalhães, Recife, Pernambuco, Brazil

Josivan Gomes de Lima, MD Departamento de Medicina Clinica, Hospital Universitaro Onofre Lopes, Natal, RN, Brazil

Natalia Nobrega de Lima, MD Departamento de Medicina Clinica, Hospital Universitaro Onofre Lopes, Natal, RN, Brazil

Sérgio Ricardo de Lima Andrade, MD Agamenon Magalhães Hospital, Division of Endocrinology and Diabetes, University of Pernambuco Medical School, Recife, Pernambuco, Brazil

Vanessa Leão de Medeiros Fabrino, MD Instituto de Medicina Professor Fernando Figueira (IMIP), Department of Pediatric Endocrinology, Recife, Pernambuco, Brazil

Bruna Lúcia de Mendonça Soares, Me Federal University of Pernambuco, Nutrition Department, Recife, Pernambuco, Brazil

Ana Carolina S. M. Cardoso, MD Agamenon Magalhaes Hospital, Department of Endocrinology and Metabolism, Recife, PE, Brazil

Amanda R. L. Oliveira Professor of Internal Medicine of University Center (UNIPE), Lauro Wanderley University Hospital (UFPB), Department of Hepatology, João Pessoa, Paraiba, Brazil

Bruno L. Souza, MD Professor of Pediatrics of Unipê University Center Hospital and of the Nova Esperança Medical School, Department of Pediatrics, João Pessoa, Paraíba, Brazil

Gayathri Devineni, MD EndoHealth Atlanta, Pediatric Endocrinologist, Department of Endocrinology, Kennesaw, GA, USA

Erik T. Diniz, MD Universidade Federal de Campina Grande, Paraiba, Brazil

Felipe Gaia Duarte, PhD AC Camargo Cancer Center and Clinical Hospital of the University of São Paulo Medical School, São Paulo, Brazil
Endocrinology Service, of the AC Camargo Cancer Center, São Paulo, Brazil
Neuroendocrine Unit in the Department of Endocrinology and Metabology of the Clinical Hospital of the University of São Paulo Medical School, R. Professor Antônio Prudente, Sao Paulo, SP, Brazil

Morgana Barbosa Duarte, MD Division of Endocrinology, Diabetes and Metabolic Bone Diseases, Agamenon Magalhães Hospital, University of Pernambuco Medical School, Recife, PE, Brazil

Paulo Escarião, MD, MBA, PhD H.Olhos Piedade - Recife, PE, Brazil
Hospital de Olhos de Pernambuco - Recife, PE, Brazil

André M. Faria, MD, PhD Hospital das Clínicas da Faculdade de Medicina de São Paulo, Neurofunctional Surgery Division, Neuroendocrine Unit, São Paulo, SP, Brazil

Manuel Faria, MD, PhD Department of Internal Medicine I, Service of Endocrinology and Metabolism, Hospital Universitário Presidente Dutra, Federal University of Maranhão, São Luís, MA, Brazil

Leonardo Bandeira, MD Federal University of Sao Paulo, Department of Endocrinology, Sao Paulo, SP, Brazil

Maria Paula Costa Bandeira E. Farias Faculdade Pernambucana de Saúde, Recife, PE, Brazil

Vahab Fatourechi, MD Endocrinology, Metabolism and Nutrition, Mayo Clinic College of Medicine, Rochester, MN, USA

Daniel Araujo Ferraz, MD, PhD Department of Ophthalmology, Universidade Federal de São Paulo, São Paulo, SP, Brazil
NIHR Biomedical Research Centre for Ophthalmology, Moorfields Eye Hospital, NHS Foundation Trust and UCL, Institute of Ophthalmology, London, UK

Manoel Aderson Soares Filho, MD Division of Endocrinology, Agamenon Magalhães Hospital, University of Pernambuco Medical School, Recife, PE, Brazil

Daniele Fontan, MD Agamenon Magalhães Hospital, Department of Endocrinology and Diabetes, Recife, Pernambuco, Brazil

Thyciara Fontenelle, MS Endocrinology and Metabolism, Hospital Agamenom Magalhães, Recife, PE, Brazil

Elizabeth Fudge, MD University of Florida, Department of Pediatrics, Gainesville, FL, USA

Yuri Galeno, MD State Institute of Endocrinology and Diabetes, Rio de Janeiro, Brazil

Alessandra Gambineri, MD, PhD Division of Endocrinology, Department of Medical and Surgical Sciences, St. Orsola-Malpighi Hospital, University of Bologna, Bologna, Italy

Luigi Gennari, MD Department of Medicine, Surgery and Neurosciences, University of Siena, Siena, Italy

Hossein Gharib, MD Division of Endocrinology, Mayo Clinic College of Medicine, Rochester, MN, USA

Andrea Glezer, MD, PhD Hospital das Clinicas, University of Sao Paulo, Neuroendocrine Unit, Division of Endocrinology and Metabolism, Sao Paulo, SP, Brazil

Marcio Longhi Griebeler, MD Cleveland Clinic Lerner College of Medicine, Endocrinology and Metabolism Institute, Cleveland, OH, USA

Luiz Griz, MD, PhD, FACE School of Medicine, University of Pernambuco, Recife, Brazil

Ashley B. Grossman, BA BSC MD FRCP FMedSci Oxford Centre for Diabetes, Endocrinology and Metabolism, Churchill Hospital, University of Oxford, Oxford, UK

Kavinga Gunawardane, MBBS (Col), MD (Col), MRCP (UK) Provincial General Hospital – Ratnapura, Diabetes and Endocrinology Unit, Ratnapura, Sri Lanka

Matthew J. L. Hare, MB BS Department of Endocrinology and Diabetes, The Alfred, Melbourne, VIC, Australia

Simon Heller, DM, FRCP Academic Unit of Diabetes, Endocrinology and Metabolism, School of Medicine and Biomedical Sciences, Sheffield, UK

Alexandre Hohl, MD, MSc, PhD University Hospital (Federal University of Santa Catarina), Endocrinology and Metabolism Department, Florianópolis, Santa Catarina, Brazil

Maria Daniela Hurtado, MD, PhD Division of Endocrinology, Diabetes, Metabolism & Nutrition, Mayo Clinic, Rochester, MN, USA

Alexander A. L. Jorge, MD, PhD Unidade de Endocrinologia Genetica, Laboratorio de Endocrinologia Celular e Molecular LIM/25, Disciplina de Endocrinologia, Hospital das Clinicas da Faculdade de Medicina da Universidade de São Paulo, São Paulo, SP, Brazil

Faculdade de Medicina da USP (LIM-25), São Paulo, SP, Brazil

Mark Kilbane, PhD Department of Clinical Chemistry, St. Vincent's University Hospital, Elm Park, Dublin 4, Ireland

Alyne Layane Pereira Lemos, MD Agamenon Magalhães Hospital, Division of Endocrinology and Diabetes, University of Pernambuco Medical School, Recife, Pernambuco, Brazil

E. Michael Lewiecki, MD New Mexico Clinical Research & Osteoporosis Center, Albuquerque, NM, USA

Vivien Lim, MBBS Gleneagles Hospital, Singapore, Singapore

Aline Alves Lopes Fellowship of Endocrinology of Agamenon Magalhães Hospital – Division of Endocrinology and Diabetes, Recife, PE, Brazil

Juliana Maria Coelho Maia, MD Department of Endocrinology, Agamenon Magalhães Hospital, Recife, Pernambuco, Brazil

Manoel R. A. Martins, MD, PhD Department of Clinical Medicine, Hospital Universitário Walter Cantídio, Federal University of Ceará, Fortaleza, Ceará, Brazil

H. David McIntyre, MD FRACP Department of Obstetric Medicine, Mater Health Services and Mater Clinical Unit, University of Queensland, South Brisbane, QLD, Australia

Malachi J. McKenna, MD Department of Endocrinology, St. Vincent's University Hospital, Dublin, Ireland

UCD School of Medicine and Medical Sciences, University College Dublin, Dublin, Ireland

Patrícia Nunes Mesquita, MD Department of Endocrinology, Agamenon Magalhães Hospital, Recife, Pernambuco, Brazil

Ana Carla Montenegro, PhD Internal Medicine and Endocrinology, IMIP—Instituto de Medicina Integral de Pernambuco, Recife, Pernambuco, Brazil

Fábio Moura, MD Endocrinology and Metabolism, Osvaldo Cruz Hospital— University of Pernambuco, Recife, PE, Brazil

Manpreet S. Mundi, MD Division of Endocrinology, Diabetes, Metabolism, and Nutrition, Mayo Clinic, Rochester, MN, USA

Gilvan Cortês Nascimento, MD Department of Internal Medicine I, Service of Endocrinology and Metabolism, Hospital Universitário Presidente Dutra, Federal University of Maranhão, São Luís, MA, Brazil

Todd B. Nippoldt, MD Department of Endocrinology, Diabetes and Nutrition, Mayo Clinic College of Medicine, Rochester, MN, USA

Lúcia Helena Coelho Nóbrega, MD Departamento de Medicina Clinica, Hospital Universitaro Onofre Lopes, Natal, RN, Brazil

Jeremy J. N. Oats, MB BS DM School of Population and Global Health, University of Melbourne, Carlton, VIC, Australia

Renato Pasquali, MD Department of Medicine, University of Bologna, Bologna, Italy

Marcia Puñales, MD, PhD Instituto da Criança com Diabetes and Hospital Criança Conceição, Grupo Hospitalar Conceição, Porto Alegre, RS, Brazil

Crystal L. Ramanujam, DPM, MSc Division of Podiatric Medicine and Surgery, Department of Orthopaedics, University of Texas Health San Antonio Long School of Medicine, San Antonio, TX, USA

Marcelo Fernando Ronsoni, MD, MSc, PhD University Hospital (Federal University of Santa Catarina), Endocrinology and Metabolism Department, Florianópolis, Santa Catarina, Brazil

Jad G. Sfeir, MD Division of Endocrinology, Metabolism, Diabetes and Nutrition, Mayo Clinic College of Medicine, Rochester, MN, USA

Barbara C. Silva, MD Division of Endocrinology, Felicio Rocho and Santa Casa Hospital, Belo Horizonte, Brazil

John J. Stapleton, DPM LVPG Orthopaedics, Allentown, PA, USA

Division of Podiatric Surgery, Lehigh Valley Hospital, Allentown, PA, USA

Penn State College of Medicine, Hershey, PA, USA

Mary O. Stevenson, MD Division of Endocrinology, Metabolism and Lipids, Emory University, Department of Medicine, Atlanta, GA, USA

Bhuvana Sunil, MD Department of Pediatrics/Division of Pediatric Endocrinology and Metabolism, Children's of Alabama, University of Alabama at Birmingham, Birmingham, AL, USA

Vin Tangpricha, MD, PhD Division of Endocrinology, Metabolism and Lipids, Emory University Department of Medicine, Atlanta, GA, USA

Duncan J. Topliss, MB, BS, MD, FRACP, FACE Department of Endocrinology and Diabetes, The Alfred, Melbourne, VIC, Australia

Department of Medicine, Monash University, Clayton, VIC, Australia

Balduino Tschiedel, MD, MSc Instituto da Criança com Diabetes, Grupo Hospitalar Conceição, Porto Alegre, RS, Brazil

Adrian Vella, MD Division of Endocrinology, Diabetes, Metabolism & Nutrition, Mayo Clinic, Rochester, MN, USA

Fernanda Moura Victor, MD Agamenon Magalhães Hospital, Division of Endocrinology and Diabetes, University of Pernambuco Medical School, Recife, Pernambuco, Brazil

Endocrinology, Agamenon Magalhães, Recife, Pernambuco, Brazil

Roberto Zagury, MD Laboratório de Performance Humana da Casa de Saúde São José (Rio de Janeiro), Rio de Janeiro, RJ, Brazil

Thomas Zgonis, DPM Division of Podiatric Medicine and Surgery, Department of Orthopaedics, University of Texas Health San Antonio Long School of Medicine, San Antonio, TX, USA

Part I

Endocrinology

Hyperthyroidism and Thyrotoxicosis

Vahab Fatourechi

Introduction

The term thyrotoxicosis applies to a clinical condition resulting from increased thyroid hormone concentration and action. When the clinical condition is diagnosed by appropriate laboratory tests, the etiology should be determined. A high radioiodine uptake of thyroid will usually indicate either a very common condition called Graves' hyperthyroidism or a very uncommon TSH-secreting pituitary adenoma. A very low uptake or no uptake will indicate destructive thyroiditis, iodine-induced hyperthyroidism, or very rare cases of extra-thyroidal thyroid hormone production or exogenous thyroid hormone intake. Normal radioactive thyroid uptake can occur in mild Graves' hyperthyroidism or in multinodular toxic goiter and toxic adenoma. Management should be problem oriented and should depend on the etiology. Antithyroid medications, surgery, or radioactive iodine therapy can be used for high uptake types, and symptomatic therapy can be used for destructive thyroiditis. Iodine-induced hyperthyroidism will respond to antithyroid medications and elimination of exogenous iodine.

When the etiology is related to increased rate of thyroid hormone synthesis, the term hyperthyroidism is applicable. Thyrotoxicosis can also result from a destructive process in the thyroid resulting in unregulated excess release of stored thyroid hormones without increased production [1, 2]. The thyrotoxicosis syndrome may also be due to exogenous source either iatrogenic or factitious. Hyperthyroidism is considered subclinical if TSH is low with normal FT4 and FreeT3. In this case hypothalamus–pituitary axis senses the excess, and the negative feedback mechanism results in suppressed or abnormally low thyrotrophic hormone (TSH). Thus it can be argued that this is a biochemical definition rather than a clinical one. Subclinical hyperthyroidism may be symptomatic or asymptomatic but in either case could have adverse effects [3]. In the United States, subclinical hyperthyroidism is more common (0.7%) than clinical hyperthyroidism (0.5%), however much less common than subclinical hypothyroidism (3–10%). If biologic activity of thyroid hormones is reduced such as in thyroid hormone resistance [4], increased peripheral thyroid levels do not result in thyrotoxicosis syndrome.

Thyrotoxicosis is a syndrome with many diverse etiologies [1]. When clinical symptomatology along with biochemical findings establishes excess thyroid hormone effect, diagnostic measures should be directed at finding the specific etiology, since management and therapy will depend on the etiology. Graves' hyperthyroidism is the most common cause of hyperthyroidism in the United States. Toxic multinodular goiter and toxic adenomas are the next common causes. Nodular toxic goiter is more common in older individuals and in geographic areas with historical iodine deficiency [5]. Inappropriate excess thyroxine (T4) therapy or T4 suppressive therapies for follicular cell-derived thyroid cancer are also common causes of subclinical hyperthyroidism.

The first step after establishing the diagnosis of thyrotoxicosis syndrome, if not contraindicated because of pregnancy or lactation, is to obtain a radioactive iodine uptake of thyroid. High radioactive iodine uptake (RAIU) in iodine-sufficient areas is consistent with Graves' hyperthyroidism and very rarely TSH-producing pituitary adenoma or trophoblastic disease. Occasionally toxic nodular goiter may have mildly elevated uptake, but usually uptake is normal and sometimes low [6]. In Graves' disease degree of elevated uptake is usually proportional to the severity of Graves' disease; subclinical cases may have normal uptake. Very low and near-zero RAIU is consistent with silent thyroiditis, subacute thyroiditis, postpartum thyroiditis, iodine-induced hyperthyroidism, drug-induced hyperthyroidism, or any cause of hyperthyroidism after iodine contrast studies or excess exogenous iodine consumption. Normal RAI uptake can be associated with mild or subclinical hyperthyroidism of Graves' disease or nodular toxic goiter.

V. Fatourechi (✉)
Endocrinology, Metabolism and Nutrition, Mayo Clinic College of Medicine, Rochester, MN, USA
e-mail: Fatourechi.vahab@mayo.edu

© Springer Nature Switzerland AG 2022
F. Bandeira et al. (eds.), *Endocrinology and Diabetes*, https://doi.org/10.1007/978-3-030-90684-9_1

Hyperthyroidism associated with Graves' disease is an autoimmune condition in which the pathogenesis of hyperthyroidism is stimulation of TSH receptors by TSH receptor antibodies (TRAB) [7]. Pathogenesis of extra-thyroidal manifestations such as ophthalmopathy and dermopathy is less clear. Interaction of TRAB with TSH receptors in non-thyroidal tissues is important in the pathogenic process [7, 8].

Recently published 2016 American Thyroid Association (ATA) guidelines for the management of various types of thyrotoxicosis conditions are an excellent source since recommendations are problem oriented [2].

Presentation of Thyrotoxicosis State

Thyrotoxicosis usually presents with weight loss despite an increased appetite. Common symptoms are also palpitations, decreased exercise tolerance and dyspnea, nervousness, heat intolerance and excessive sweating, tremor, irritability, sleep disorder, and muscle weakness of varying degrees. In older individuals hyper-stimulation and adrenergic symptoms are less marked, and patients may be apathetic and complain of fatigue, weight loss, and muscle weakness, or the disease may present with cardiac findings such as atrial fibrillation or heart failure. Increased appetite may be absent in the older patients who often have anorexia. In younger patients occasionally increased appetite may prevent weight loss, and in a few cases, even weight gain is reported [9]. Pedal edema can be present without heart failure because of vasodilation. Gynecomastia may be present in severe cases. Diarrhea is a feature but most patients may have only more frequent bowel movements. In the case of Graves' disease, an enlarged firm thyroid may be present, but some patients have normal size thyroid. In Graves' disease continuous bruits over thyroid may be audible, and flow murmur of carotid or venous hum may also be present [10]. Onset of symptoms in Graves' disease is subacute over weeks, or months, whereas in multinodular toxic goiter, it is slow and subtle over a longer period of time [10]. In the latter a palpable nodular goiter is present or may become visible after weight loss. Graves' disease may present with extra-thyroidal manifestations such as ophthalmopathy and dermopathy. Thyrotoxicosis may precede extra-thyroidal manifestations, occur simultaneously, or in some cases may develop later [7, 11]. Mild stare of the eyes may be present in severely thyrotoxic patients who do not have ophthalmopathy but is not a prominent sign in my experience. Thyroid dermapathy in Graves' disease is usually a later manifestation and is associated with ophthalmopathy and high level of autoimmunity [12].

Clinical Presentations of Thyrotoxicosis Mimicking Other Conditions

Severe proximal muscle weakness in individuals older than age 50 may result in neurology referral before diagnosis is made. Also, in the same age group, atrial fibrillation or congestive heart failure may result in cardiology consultation. Symptoms of thyrotoxicosis are similar to anxiety disorder, and diagnosis is missed if thyroid dysfunction is not considered. In cases of postpartum thyroiditis 2–3 months after childbirth, symptoms in the mother can be attributed to poor sleep and newborn care, and thyroid diagnosis is often overlooked. Elderly patients commonly present with apathetic form and do not have the usual hyper-stimulated features. Thus diagnosis may be missed and malignancy or depression may be suspected. In patients presenting with diarrhea and weight loss, malabsorption or gastrointestinal conditions will be in the differential diagnosis. Some patients may have hypercalcemia, and differential diagnosis of hypercalcemia initially may be a consideration before correct diagnosis [6, 10].

Laboratory studies may also be misleading. Suppressed TSH can be seen in pituitary problems, in euthyroid sick syndrome, and with medications such as high-dose corticosteroids. Elevated peripheral thyroid hormone levels can be seen in thyroid hormone resistance. In cases with increased thyroxine binding capacity, if only total T3 and T4 levels are measured, T4 and T3 levels will be high, but TSH will be normal [10].

A hypokalemic periodic paralysis syndrome can occur with thyrotoxicosis [13]. It is more common in Asian patients and much less common in other ethnic groups [14]. A genetic predisposition is needed, and attacks of paralysis are precipitated by high carbohydrate intake and exercise. Acute attacks should be treated with parenteral potassium administration. Management of hyperthyroidism should be urgent and definitive for achievement of euthyroidism by RAI or surgery [13]. To achieve immediate euthyroidism, surgical thyroidectomy may be the best management in some cases of thyrotoxic hypokalemic periodic paralysis.

Thyrotoxicosis Syndromes (Table 1.1)

Hyperthyroidism Associated with High Thyroid RAIU [5]

These conditions include Graves' disease, TSH-secreting pituitary adenoma, and trophoblastic disease because of stimulation of thyroid by HCG, TSH receptor-activating mutations, and hyperthyroidism in pituitary thyroid hormone resistance and occasional cases of nodular goiter.

Table 1.1 Causes of thyrotoxicosis

Hyperthyroidism associated with elevated or normal thyroid radioactive iodine uptake
Graves' hyperthyroidism[a]
Multinodular goiter or toxic adenoma
TSH-producing pituitary adenoma[b]
Some cases of thyroid hormone resistance
Hyperthyroidism associated with trophoblastic disease
TSH receptor-activating mutations
Hyperthyroidism in some cases of McCune–Albright syndrome

[a]In mild cases RAI uptake may be normal
[b]Usually uptake is normal or occasionally low

Table 1.2 Causes of thyrotoxicosis

Thyrotoxicosis associated with near-zero thyroid radioactive iodine uptake
Silent thyroiditis
Postpartum thyroiditis
Surgery induced manipulation for non-thyroid neck surgery such as neck malignancy or parathyroid surgery
Granulomatous (subacute thyroiditis or de Quervain's)
Acute infectious thyroiditis
External beam radiation-induced thyroiditis
Extensive metastatic follicular cancer encountered after thyroidectomy
Iatrogenic or factitious
Struma ovarii
Bleeding into functioning thyroid nodule
Amiodarone-induced thyroiditis
Drug-induced and biotherapy-induced thyroiditis
Thyrotoxicosis from meat or sausage with high thyroid tissue contamination
Iodine-induced hyperthyroidism
Any hyperthyroid cause associated with exogenous iodine ingestion or iodinated radiologic contrast (depending on the cause uptake may be low but not near zero)

Table 1.3 Medications commonly used in management of thyrotoxicosis

Symptomatic therapy		
Short-acting propranolol[a]	10–40 mg	TID–QID
Slow-release propranolol	70–240 mg	QD–BID
Atenolol[b]	25–100 mg	QD–BID
Nadolol[c]	40–160 mg	QD
Antithyroid medications		
Methimazole, starting dose[d]	10–40 mg/day	QD–BID
Methimazole, maintenance dose	5–20 mg/day	QD
Propylthiouracil (PTU), starting dose[e]	100–400 mg/day	TID
Propylthiouracil (PTU), maintenance dose	50–200 mg/day	BID–TID
Saturated solution of potassium iodide[f] 5 drops (0.25 cc or 250 mg) BID alternative is lugol solution		

[a]Propranolol is a nonselective beta-blocker and has the potential of reducing T4 to T3 conversion at high doses. It is contraindicated in asthma. Should be stopped when thyroxine levels normalize
[b]Atenolol is a selective beta-1 adrenergic blocker
[c]Nadolol is a nonselective beta-blocker and also has possibility of inhibiting T4–T3 conversion
[d]Methimazole has lower side effect profile than PTU and can be given once a day. It is the drug of choice except for first trimester of pregnancy
[e]PTU has higher rate of hepatic side effects and has to be given divided. Is the only antithyroid used in first trimester of pregnancy
[f]Potassium iodide is mostly used for preoperative preparation of Graves' disease or management of thyroid storm. Although it has been reported for chronic use, ATA has no recommendations for or against its chronic use for therapy of mild Graves' hyperthyroidism [2]

Hyperthyroidism Associated with Normal RAIU

In all of the above conditions of mild degree, in particular if hyperthyroidism is subclinical, radioiodine thyroid uptake may be normal [5]. RAI uptake is usually normal in toxic multinodular goiter and toxic adenoma. Some cases of multinodular goiter may have low radioactive iodine uptake [6].

Thyrotoxicosis Associated with Very Low or Near-Zero (Table 1.2) Neck RAIU [2, 5]

These include iodine-induced hyperthyroidism, silent thyroiditis, granulomatous thyroiditis [15, 16], postpartum thyroiditis [17], and any form of thyrotoxicosis associated with exogenous iodine. One rare cause is struma ovarii [18] when thyroid RAIU is very low and pelvic ultrasound followed by pelvic radioactive iodine scan will be diagnostic. Silent and postpartum thyroiditis has a similar course as subacute gran-

ulomatous thyroiditis, but pain is not present and etiologies are either autoimmune [17] or drugs. Sedimentation rate will be normal and antithyroid antibodies will be positive. Palpation and surgical manipulation of thyroid may also cause transient thyrotoxicosis [19]. For diagnosis of silent thyroiditis, absence of history of iodine intake and iodinated contrast studies are needed, and for confirmation urinary iodine measurement is helpful. Transient thyrotoxicosis states are treated with nonselective beta-blockers such as propranolol (Table 1.3).

Thyrotoxicosis with Low Thyroid RAIU and Low Serum Thyroglobulin

Iatrogenic and factitious thyrotoxicosis is associated with low RAIU [1]. In the presence of small thyroid size and thyrotoxicosis associated with very low thyroid RAI uptake and absence of iodine contamination, if factitious thyrotoxicosis is suspected, a very low serum thyroglobulin should suggest exogenous factitious or inadvertent thyroid hormone intake, even if patient does not volunteer the history. If thyroglobulin antibodies are positive, they interfere with the assay, and low thyroglobulin is not reliable. It should be noted that serum thyroglobulin may be normal if patient has preexisting nodular goiter concurrent with excess thyroid hormone intake. Herbal supplements for weight loss presumably containing thyroid hormone have been reported with thyrotoxicosis [20]. Consumption of hamburger and sausages containing thyroid tissue has also been associated with exogenous thyrotoxicosis in some reported cases [21].

Thyrotoxicosis Presenting with Neck Pain

Three conditions may present with thyroid pain and thyrotoxicosis: the most common is granulomatous thyroiditis or de Quervain's thyroiditis [22], most likely a viral condition. It usually follows an upper respiratory infection, is associated with a febrile illness, and presents with exquisite thyroid pain and tenderness radiating to ears and very firm and irregular thyroid. One lobe can be involved first followed by the other. Thyroid hormone levels are elevated, TSH is suppressed, RAIU is close to zero, sedimentation rate is high, blood count is normal, and serum thyroglobulin level is elevated [22]. Hyperthyroid phase is followed by a transient hypothyroid phase and less commonly (in 5–15%) by permanent hypothyroidism. The process lasts few months. Management of thyrotoxicosis is by nonselective beta-blockers (Table 1.3) and nonsteroidal anti-inflammatory agents (NSAIDS) and in severe cases with a short course of glucocorticoids. Recurrence may occur in 2–5% after several years [22].

The second cause of painful transient thyrotoxicosis is bleeding into a functioning nodule resulting in release of stored hormones. This will be unilateral with distinct palpable nodule. ESR is normal, radioactive iodine uptake is low, and serum thyroglobulin levels are extremely high. Diagnosis is by thyroid ultrasound showing cystic development in a nodule as a result of bleeding. Symptoms are usually mild; pain has a short duration. Duration of hyperthyroidism is also shorter than subacute thyroiditis [23].

The third cause is rare association of thyrotoxicosis with suppurative thyroiditis. Bacterial infection of thyroid and abscess formation are rare. Infection may occur after procedures or spontaneously and also from infected piriform sinus fistula [24]. It is associated with fever and local inflammatory signs and symptoms and abnormal blood count. Diagnosis is with neck ultrasound showing abscess formation. Fine needle aspiration (FNA) and culture establish the infectious etiology. Thyrotoxicosis is usually short-lived and may be masked by inflammatory and systemic symptoms [24, 25]. Management is management of infection and beta-blocker for thyrotoxicosis symptoms.

Drug-Induced Thyrotoxicosis and Hyperthyroidism

Iodine-containing contrast media can cause iodine-induced hyperthyroidism particularly in iodine-deficient areas and in patients with nodular goiter. The duration depends on the half-life of clearance of exogenous iodine. In the case of radiologic contrast media, usually it will be a few weeks or months; in the case of amiodarone, it may be months to a year. Lithium [26, 27], denileukin diftitox [28], interferon gamma, pembrolizumab anti-PD-1 monoclonal antibodies (an immune checkpoint blocker) [29], pegylated interferon alfa-2b [30], and anti-cytokine therapies and biotherapies can cause transient painless thyroiditis that lasts weeks to few months and should be managed with beta-blockers and supportive care. Sometimes thyroid autoimmunity such as Graves' disease is induced by these medications. Tyrosine kinase inhibitors such as sunitinib and cabozantinib [31, 32] and thalidomide derivatives may cause thyroid dysfunction and sometimes thyroiditis with transient hyperthyroidism [31–33].

Amiodarone-Induced Thyrotoxicosis

This is one of the most difficult management problems in thyroid practice [34–36]. Patients usually have a critical and sometimes life-threatening cardiac arrhythmia. Amiodarone has high concentration of iodine and after discontinuation of therapy may stay in the body up to 6–12 months. Obtaining thyroid RAIU is not helpful for diagnosis because it is low due to a high iodine pool. Two types of thyrotoxicosis are recognized with amiodarone: Type I is iodine induced and is more common in iodine-deficient areas. Type II, a toxic destructive thyroiditis, is the more common type. Type I occurs usually in the background of nodular goiter [34, 35]. It is essential to differentiate these two types since therapies are quite different. Therapy of type I includes antithyroid drugs plus discontinuation of amiodarone if it is considered safe. Therapy of type II is with glucocorticoids. Ultrasound of thyroid is helpful in differentiation of these two: In type II, thyroid size is usually normal and gland is distinctly hypovascular [35]. The problem is that although most likely majority of the cases in the United States are type II, many cases are mixed and thyrotoxicosis develops as a result of both increased release and increased production of hormones. Although pure type II should respond to corticosteroids within 2–5 weeks, sometimes combination empiric therapy with methimazole along with corticosteroids is used. In this situation early response to corticosteroids and normalization of thyroid function within 2–5 weeks favor type II diagnosis. Amiodarone therapy should only be stopped if possible and safe, since iodine-induced type will continue and type II thyroiditis may recur. Some cases may not respond to medical therapy, and in those surgery is a good option for rapid cure [36, 37].

Subclinical Hyperthyroidism

Subclinical hyperthyroidism is defined by lower than normal serum TSH, not explained by other causes such as pituitary disease, medications and acute illness, and normal levels of T3 and T4 [3]. This condition is more common than overt symptomatic hyperthyroidism. Etiologies are similar to clinical hyperthyroidism and thyrotoxicosis. It is present in mild Graves' disease or in early-stage toxic nodular goiter. Approximately 50% of subclinical hyperthyroidism cases have subtle symptoms such as increased pulse rate. Symptoms are usually absent if TSH is >0.1 mIU. Younger individuals may tolerate the condition without adverse effects, but in postmenopausal women increased bone loss is the consequence. Individuals older than 60 years have three times higher likelihood of atrial fibrillation [38]. There is some epidemiologic evidence suggesting increased mortality with persistent serum TSH levels <0.5 in this age group. Thus confirmed subclinical hyperthyroidism should be treated in this group [39, 40]. Therapy depends on etiology. In cases of toxic adenoma or multinodular goiter, resolution of subclinical hyperthyroidism is unlikely, and definitive therapy with radioactive iodine or surgery should be recommended. More than one abnormal test over time is needed before intervention.

Transient causes such as silent and subacute thyroiditis can be managed by beta-blockers while waiting for resolution. In subclinical Graves' disease, antithyroid and RAI therapy are equally effective. In younger age group, betablocker therapy alone or observation is acceptable [39].

Hyperthyroidism Associated with Pregnancy

Differentiation of physiologic gestational thyrotoxicosis from hyperthyroidism in the first 3 months of pregnancy is important and often difficult [41]. Thyroid is stimulated by human chorionic gonadotropin (HCG). TSH may be low or even suppressed, and symptoms may also be misleading. Very high levels of free T4, presence of goiter, and positive TRAB are helpful for diagnosis. Preexisting Graves' disease may improve during pregnancy and may relapse after childbirth. Treatment of hyperthyroidism is PTU in the first 3 months because of teratogenic effect of methimazole [2, 42], but after the first trimester, PTU can be switched to methimazole because of its lower side effect profile. Total T4 should be kept 1.5 times above the upper limit of normal and free T4 at the upper limit of normal to prevent fetal hypothy-

roidism. Surgery can be done in the second trimester if there are adverse reactions to antithyroid therapies, or large doses of antithyroids are required for control of hyperthyroidism [43]. In mild cases of Graves' disease under antithyroid therapy, discontinuation of antithyroid therapy and observation in the onset of pregnancy may be a consideration (2).

There is no evidence that subclinical hyperthyroidism has adverse effect in pregnancy for the fetus or the mother; thus therapy is not recommended [43].

Fetal and Neonatal Hyperthyroidism

Because TRAB crosses the placenta and can affect fetal thyroid, these antibodies should be checked at weeks 18–22 in pregnant patients with current or previous history of Graves' disease or a history of neonatal Graves' or previous elevated TRAB [2]. If TRAB is positive at 2–3 times above normal, fetal thyroid should be monitored by ultrasound at 18–22 weeks and repeated every 4–6 weeks. Evidence of fetal hyperthyroidism is goiter, hydrops, advanced fetal bone age, increased pulse, and cardiac failure. In this case even if the mother is euthyroid on thyroxine therapy, antithyroids should be given with close monitoring. Neonatal hyperthyroidism is fortunately temporary, but short-term antithyroid therapy for the newborn may be needed [2].

Hyperthyroidism in Pediatric Age Group

In this age group, the cause is usually Graves' disease, and The American Thyroid Association guidelines recommends avoidance of RAI therapy in children younger than age 5, and in this group methimazol therapy or surgery in the hands of high volume surgeons is recommended.

ATA guidelines allow RAI therapy as an acceptable therapy in some older children with certain conditions [2]. However, most clinicians prefer long-term antithyroid therapy and (avoiding PTU) in some persistent cases thyroidectomy.

Hyperthyroidism in Trophoblastic Disease

HCG and TSH have similarities in their structure and receptors. Thus in the first trimester of pregnancy, TSH levels are low and have inverse relationship with HCG levels. Mild physiologic thyrotoxicosis by HCG stimulation may be present that may be more pronounced in hyperemesis gravidarum [44]. Very high levels of HCG in hydatidiform mole and choriocarcinoma can present with significant hyperthyroidism and even thyroid storm [44, 45]. Treatment is management of the trophoblastic condition and antithyroid therapy.

Hyperthyroidism with Inappropriately Normal Serum TSH in TSH-Producing Pituitary Adenoma

In the presence of inappropriately normal serum TSH with elevated thyroid hormone levels and symptoms of hyperthyroidism, laboratory artifacts such as heterophile antibodies and abnormal binding to proteins should be excluded, as should thyroid hormone resistance. An MRI of pituitary should follow. Elevated beta-subunit will be in favor of TSH-secreting pituitary adenoma causing hyperthyroidism. These cases are very rare [2].

Hyperthyroidism in Thyroid Hormone Resistance

Most adult patients with generalized thyroid hormone resistance have elevated peripheral thyroid hormone levels and inappropriately normal serum TSH and have clinical thyroid [46]. If there is pituitary thyroid hormone resistance or if the degree of resistance is higher in the pituitary than in the peripheral tissues, hyperthyroidism may occur [47]. Diagnosis of this rare condition is difficult and should be guided by clinical evaluation surrogates of excess thyroxine effects such as sex hormone-binding globulin (SHBG) may be useful.

Thyrotoxicosis Associated with "Café au Lait" Pigmentation and Fibrous Dysplasia (McCune–Albright Syndrome)

In this syndrome associated with polyostotic fibrous dysplasia and "café au lait" pigmentation, because of constitutive activation of G(s) alpha by inhibition of its GTPase, non-autoimmune hyperthyroidism may develop and may be associated with nodular goiter. In this rare syndrome, treatment is surgery or RAI ablation. Remission with antithyroid medications does not occur [2].

Non-autoimmune Hyperthyroidism Caused by Genetic Mutation of TSH Receptor

Germline-activating mutation of TSH receptor is a rare cause of hyperthyroidism in infancy and childhood. Best treatment after preparation with antithyroid medications is surgery at appropriate age. In adult patients RAI therapy can also be considered [48]. Activating mutations can also result in toxic adenoma that may present in adulthood.

Metastatic Follicular Cancer and Hyperthyroidism

Thyrotoxicosis is rarely a presenting picture in widespread metastatic follicular cancer. Occasionally it may present after excision of the primary tumor and may resolve with radioactive iodine therapy or excision of bulky tumors or tyrosine kinase inhibitor therapy [49]. It also can present with T3 toxicosis because of high rate of conversion of exogenous T4 to T3 of the therapeutic administered T4 by tumor that expresses high di-iodinase [50].

Hyperthyroidism Associated with Normal T4 but Elevated T3 (T3 Toxicosis)

It is doubtful that T3 toxicosis is a distinct entity [2]. In the early phase of hyperthyroidism, only T3 elevation may be present, and T4 elevation occurs later. It is conceivable that in iodine-deficient areas and in certain conditions, more T3 than T4 may be produced. Patients with hyperthyroidism on antithyroid therapy and after failure of RAI therapy may have normal free T4 and elevated free T3.

Patients on excess thyroid extract therapy also have T3 toxicosis which can be associated with normal or low free T4, suppressed TSH, and elevated free T3 levels. This is due to excess T3-to-T4 ratio in the commercial thyroid extract products. Thus in patients with thyroid extract therapy, measurement of peripheral hormones does not correlate with thyroid function status, and TSH measurement is the definitive test for assessment of therapy.

Laboratory Investigation of Thyrotoxicosis and Hyperthyroidism

Although the first and most sensitive test in the presence of normal pituitary function is serum TSH, it is only an indirect measure of thyroid function, and when thyrotoxicosis is suspected, circulating hormone levels such as free T4 and free T3 should be measured [2]. First, free T4 should be measured, and, if normal, measurement of free T3 should follow. To differentiate between the two main categories of high and low RAIU thyrotoxicosis, thyroid RAIU should be measured next [2]. Thyroid scan usually is not needed except for cases of nodular disease with hyperthyroidism [2]. Ultrasound is sometimes helpful in the differential diagnosis. Ultrasound identifies nodule size, number of nodules, and vascularity. Increased vascularity in a diffuse goiter suggests Graves' disease, whereas low vascularity is seen in cases of destructive thyroiditis such as type 2 amiodarone-induced hyperthyroidism [34]. Also in cases of Graves' disease, associated significant conditions such as occult malignancy change the management. When there is doubt about the etiology and also for prognostic assessment and monitoring of antithyroid therapy effectiveness, measurement of TRAB is helpful [2, 8]. Thyroid-stimulating immunoglobulin assay (TSI), a bio-assay, is more expensive and is being replaced by immunoassay of TRAB.

Management of Thyrotoxicosis and Hyperthyroidism

For transient conditions such as silent, subacute, and post-partum thyroiditis and all conditions associated with the release of stored thyroid hormones, symptomatic therapy with nonselective beta-blocker medications (Table 1.3) is adequate as noted previously [2]. Two major and common causes of hyperthyroidism, Graves' disease and multinodular toxic goiter, require more detailed discussion.

Management of Graves' Hyperthyroidism

Nonselective beta-blockers, if not contraindicated, will improve most symptoms and can be continued until hormone levels are normalized by specific therapy [2]. Hyperthyroid patients may require relatively high doses, and 120–240 mg/day of propranolol and equivalent other beta-blockers may be needed (Table 1.3). If beta-blockers are contraindicated, calcium channel blockers can be used [2].

Choice of modality of definitive therapy for Graves' hyperthyroidism should be based on severity of hyperthyroidism, patient preference, and age of the patient.

Pediatric patients deserve a 1.5–2-year course of antithyroid medication [2, 51]. Longer-term antithyroid therapies are also a possibility. Methimazole is the drug of choice for all patients especially for pediatric age due to recent reports of life-threatening liver toxicity with (propylthiouracil) PTU [2, 51]. In pediatric patients if antithyroid medications are not tolerated, thyroidectomy would be an option. However, despite hesitancy to use in children, it should be noted that RAI therapy in pediatric group has not been associated with long-term adverse effects [2, 52].

In adults, one of these three choices should be presented to the patient: antithyroid drugs, radioactive iodine, or surgery [2]. None of these modalities addresses the basic autoimmune process in Graves' disease, although a mild immunosuppressive action is suggested for antithyroid medications. Theoretically, and based on some studies, a near-total thyroidectomy eliminates the source of thyroid antigen the fastest. RAI therapy increases the release of antigen hence TRAB levels in the first few months, but if total thy-roid ablation is done eventually, the antigen source will be decreased, hence resulting in decreased antibodies later on, and there may be long-term benefit.

Pros and Cons of Antithyroid Therapy

Antithyroid therapy for 18 months results in only a 50% remission rate. This is an argument in favor of thyroid-ablative modalities such as RAI, in particular in older individuals and in patients with comorbidities [2]. Patient should also be counseled about possible side effects of antithyroid therapy, such as skin allergy and a 1/1000 likelihood of agranulocytosis and pancytopenia [53], liver toxicity particularly with PTU [54], and rare cases of ANCA-positive vasculitis and lupus-like syndrome [55]. However some patients who want to avoid lifelong thyroxine therapy after ablative therapies prefer to use antithyroid drugs. The majority of endocrinologists in the United States traditionally have chosen RAI therapy as the preferred definitive therapy in adults [2]. However the trend is changing to some degree in favor of antithyroid therapy [2].

If antithyroid therapy is chosen, drug of choice is methimazole with a starting dose of 20–30 mg daily which can be given in once-a-day program [2, 55]. Prior to initiation of therapy, a blood count and white count with differential and liver function tests such as transaminase and bilirubin should be obtained [2]. When thyroid functions normalize with therapy, which is usually in 5–8 weeks, maintenance dose of 5–10 mg will be usually adequate. Therapy should be continued for 18 months, and, at that point if thyroid function is normal; it can be stopped [2]. Under certain conditions and for patients with reduced life expectancy, nursing home patients, in pediatric age group, and if patient does not accept ablative therapy, antithyroid therapy can be continued for a longer period of time [2]. TRAB measurement 6 months after antithyroid therapy may predict the rate of remission or relapse and is recommended by ATA [2].

Monitoring of antithyroid therapy is by measurement of free T4, and T3 and liver function tests initially, and TSH, free T4, and liver function tests thereafter periodically. Blood count does not seem to predict impending agranulocytosis since it can happen in between tests. Advising patient to stop medication in case of complications, fever, and sore throat and obtaining a complete blood count with differential at that point are more helpful [2]. It should be noted that hyperthyroidism can cause mild leukopenia and also abnormal liver function tests, hence the need for baseline studies. If initial transaminases are more than five times, normal antithyroid therapy should not be initiated [2]. Measurement of TRAb levels prior to stopping ATD therapy is suggested because it aids in predicting which patients can be weaned from the medication, with normal levels indicating greater chance for remission [2]. Minor skin reactions can be transient, but significant skin allergies should result in discontinuing medications. At that point alternate therapies or switching to PTU should be considered. However because of cross-reactivity in the case of minor skin reactions, it may be best to choose RAI or surgery.

How to Manage Recurrence of Hyperthyroidism After 18 Months of Antithyroid Therapy?

In adults, ablative therapy, preferably RAI therapy, is usually recommended. For women with pregnancy planned in the next 6 months, surgery may be a better choice. Surgery, with the availability of a high-volume experienced surgeon, may be suitable for patients with large goiter who are at good surgical risk or have moderate-to-severe ophthalmopathy, because of concern about worsening of eye disease after RAI [2]. Long-term antithyroid therapy may be considered in very old patients or in children. Recent guidelines of ATA consider long-term antithyroid therapy as an acceptable option for patients [2]. This recommendation is based on recent studies providing evidence for safety and effectiveness of long-term antithyroid therapy. A recent meta-analysis of six studies with duration of therapy of 41–98 months showed remission rate of 57% [56]. Patient preference also should be a factor in decision [2].

Radioactive Iodine Therapy (RAI) for Graves' Hyperthyroidism

In some clinics this is the first choice for initial management of nonpregnant adults with Graves' disease who accept post-RAI hypothyroidism. RAI should be avoided in women who plan pregnancy in the next 6–9 months. But women who have no intention of pregnancy for 9 months but wish to have pregnancy after definitive management are also candidates for RAI therapy. Unavailability of a high-volume thyroid surgeon and failure of or intolerance to antithyroid therapy are also good indications for ablative radioactive iodine therapy. Obviously, pregnancy and lactation are absolute contraindications. If RAI is given, it should be with the intention of making the patient hypothyroid within 3–6 months and to be followed by lifelong thyroxine therapy. The dose of RAI must be proportional to the size of thyroid and degree of thyroid RAI uptake. The weight of thyroid estimated by palpation, or volume measured by ultrasound, can be used. In our clinic, we usually give 200 micro-Curie (uCi) per estimated gram of thyroid weight adjusted for 24-hr RAIU. Some authors suggest a fixed dose of 370 MBq for smaller thyroids and 555 MBq for larger goiters; however hypothyroidism

rate in a 12-month follow-up was 56% for the lower dose and 71% for the higher dose [57]. If same-day treatment is desired, a 4- or 3-hr [58] uptake can be obtained, and 24-hr uptake calculated. Prior PTU therapy reduces sensitivity to RAI, and for this group we give 250 uCi per estimated gram of thyroid weight. Methimazole may not reduce sensitivity to RAI. RAI dose should not be underestimated since the desirable hypothyroidism will be achieved sooner with higher doses. In our clinic with the above program, 90% of patients will be hypothyroid within 3 months. TSH and free thyroxine should be obtained in 2 months and 3 months.

Management Before and Immediately After RAI Therapy

Beta-blockers given before and for 4 weeks after RAI therapy are usually adequate [2]. Patients with severe thyrotoxicosis and patients with cardiac failure or with fragile health can be prepared with 3–4 weeks of methimazole therapy to reduce thyroxine levels to a safe range [59]. Antithyroid drug therapy should be stopped 3–5 days before RAI and can be restarted 3–5 days after RAI and continued for 4 weeks. Thyroid storm is rare after RAI, but worsening of symptoms if significant should be reported and approbate measures such as adjustment of beta-blockers, stable iodine, or short course corticosteroids be given.

Surgical Management of Graves' Hyperthyroidism

Surgery with near-total thyroidectomy, rendering patients hypothyroid and placing patients immediately on thyroxine therapy in the hands of experienced thyroid surgeon, is a safe and effective treatment for Graves' disease [60]. It is an option for patients with very large goiters or with associated nodular disease, for patients with suspicious nodules in the thyroid, and for patients not responding to antithyroid therapy that do not want or are not candidates for RAI therapy. Pediatric age group patients with failure or intolerance to antithyroid therapy [61, 62] are also candidates. Pregnant women with poor response to antithyroid therapy are also candidate for surgery in the second trimester of pregnancy. Patients with significant ophthalmopathy may also be candidates for surgery since it has been shown that after surgery TRAB decreases, whereas they increase with RAI therapy alone in the first year [2]. There is also 15% possibility of worsening of ophthalmopathy, 5% being permanent, if corticosteroid therapy is not given for 2–3 months concurrently [63]. Thyroidectomy for Graves' hyperthyroidism should be done only by a high-volume endocrine surgeon.

Preparing Patients with Graves' Hyperthyroidism for Surgery

Although mild cases can be prepared with beta-blockers and iodide (few drops of Lugol's solution or SSKI in water or juice three times a day for 10 days prior to surgery) [2, 64], usually it is best to normalize or significantly improve thyroid function with methimazole prior to surgery. With these precautions postoperative thyroid storm can be avoided. Iodine reduces vascularity as well as release of thyroid hormones from the gland.

To reduce the rate of post-surgical significant hypocalcemia, ATA suggests that calcium and 25-hydroxy vitamin D should be assessed preoperatively and repleted if necessary or given prophylactically. Calcitriol supplementation should be considered preoperatively in patients at increased risk for transient or permanent hypoparathyroidism [2].

Management of Severe Hyperthyroidism and Thyroid Storm

Severe life-threatening thyrotoxicosis can occur in patients with associated non-thyroid-related acute conditions such as infection, rarely after radioactive iodine therapy, abrupt cessation of antithyroid therapy in severe cases, thyroid or non-thyroid surgery, and in unrecognized and untreated patients [2, 64]. Thyroid storm manifests by arrhythmia, heart failure, hyperpyrexia, dehydration, hypotension, vomiting, diarrhea, confusion, agitation, stupor, and occasionally coma [65]. This is a true endocrine emergency and should be managed in intensive care setting [2] with hydration, cooling, respiratory support, and management of arrhythmia and cardiac complications. Thyroid hormone synthesis should be blocked by high-dose antithyroids (60 mg of methimazole or 600 mg of PTU) followed by inorganic iodide drops to stop release of thyroid hormones. Intravenous corticosteroid therapy is usually needed. Plasmapheresis has been used effectively in some cases [66]. Some cases of severe hyperthyroidism at risk of thyroid storm, but not yet in crisis, can be treated with combination of above modalities in outpatient setting with close observation.

Management of Toxic Adenoma and Toxic Multinodular Goiter

Comprehensive guidelines for management of toxic adenoma and toxic multinodular goiter are well outlined elsewhere [2].

In single toxic adenoma, surgery is more appropriate for larger toxic nodules, younger patients, patient desire for a rapid cure, desirability of less than 1% incidence of postsur-

gical hypothyroidism as opposed to 3–20% for radioactive iodine therapy, and 100% rate of cure of hyperthyroidism as opposed to 80% for radioactive iodine [2]. Availability of experienced thyroid surgeon, absence of comorbid conditions, and increased risk of surgery should be taken into account. RAI on the opposite is more appropriate for older patients, smaller nodules in younger individuals [2].

For toxic multinodular goiter (Plummer's disease), same factors should be considered. However, in multinodular disease the rate of hypothyroidism after thyroidectomy is 100% and is low after radioactive iodine therapy [2]. Compressive symptoms and presence of nodules with risk of malignancy will be an indication for surgery. Antithyroid medications are not appropriate for long-term therapy of nodular toxic disease except for individuals with decreased life expectancy or increased risk factors for other modalities. In general antithyroids are not recommended except for preparation for surgery or in some cases prior to radioactive iodine therapy. Beta-blockers are usually adequate pre-therapy and post-therapy for radioactive iodine and pre-therapy for surgery. For patients receiving RAI therapy, isotopic thyroid scan should be available since nonfunctioning nodule will need FNA for confirmation of benign nature prior decision for RAI therapy [2]. ATA suggests that alternative therapies such as ethanol or radiofrequency ablation of TA and TMNG can be considered in select patients in whom RAI, surgery, and long-term ATD are inappropriate, contraindicated, or refused and expertise in these procedures is available [2].

Management of Hyperthyroidism Associated with Ophthalmopathy and Thyroid Dermopathy

Management of hyperthyroidism in the presence of ophthalmopathy is a matter of debate [67]. Surgery, and to a lesser degree antithyroids, reduces the receptor antibody levels, whereas RAI if not given with concomitant corticosteroids may increase the TRAB in the first year. Tobacco cessation in smokers and rapid achievement of euthyroidism are essential [67, 68]. In the absence of ophthalmopathy and in non-smokers, ATA guidelines recommend RAI therapy without concurrent corticosteroids. For mild ophthalmopathy and no risk factors for thyroid eye disease, ATA accepts all three modalities of therapy, but if radioactive iodine is chosen, concurrent corticosteroid treatment is recommended. However, ATA recommends antithyroid therapy or surgery for moderate-to-severe and sight-threatening ophthalmopathy [2]. Ablative therapy by radioactive iodine or surgery eliminates source of thyroid antigen and may have theoretical long-term benefit on the course of extra-thyroidal manifestations, but evidence is lacking.

Conclusions

Thyrotoxicosis is the general term for excess thyroid hormone action. Hyperthyroidism is when thyroid is producing and releasing excess hormones. The most common cause is Graves' hyperthyroidism, the next being toxic nodular goiter (Plummer's disease). There are also several rare causes of overproduction of thyroid hormones. In conditions when destructive process in the thyroid results in release of stored hormones, the term thyrotoxicosis is a better term, since thyroid is not overproducing hormones. In these conditions only symptomatic therapy is needed. For hyperthyroid overproduction category, either antithyroid medication or ablative therapies such as surgery and radioactive iodine are needed. Recent ATA guidelines recommend long-term antithyroid therapy as an option for some patients with Graves' disease and emphasize the importance of periodic TRAB measurement during antithyroid therapy as a guide for prediction of remission. Management of thyrotoxicosis syndromes should be tailored to the cause associated with autoimmune manifestations, age of the patient, and other clinical considerations and patient preferences.

References

1. Franklyn JA, Boelaert K. Thyrotoxicosis. Lancet. 2012;379:1155–66.
2. Ross DS, Burch HB, Cooper DS, Greenlee MC, Laurberg P, Maia AL, Rivkees SA, Samuels M, Sosa JA, Stan MN, Walter MA. 2016 American Thyroid Association guidelines for diagnosis and management of hyperthyroidism and other causes of thyrotoxicosis. Thyroid. 2016 Oct;26(10):1343–421.
3. Cooper DS, Biondi B. Subclinical thyroid disease. Lancet. 2012;379:1142–54.
4. Kim TJ, Travers S. Case report: thyroid hormone resistance and its therapeutic challenges. Curr Opin Pediatr. 2008;20:490–3.
5. Seigel SC, Hodak SP. Thyrotoxicosis. Med Clin North Am. 2012;96:175–201.
6. Kahara T, Shimizu A, Uchiyama A, Terahata S, Tajiri J, Nishihara E, et al. Toxic multinodular goiter with low radioactive iodine uptake. Intern Med. 2011;50:1709–14.
7. Bahn RS. Autoimmunity and Graves disease. Clin Pharmacol Ther. 2012;91:577–9.
8. Matthews DC, Syed AA. The role of TSH receptor antibodies in the management of Graves' disease. Eur J Intern Med. 2011;22:213–6.
9. van Veenendaal NR, Rivkees SA. Treatment of pediatric Graves' disease is associated with excessive weight gain. J Clin Endocrinol Metab. 2011;96:3257–63.
10. Weetman AP. Thyrotoxicosis. Medicine. 2009;37:430–5.
11. Lazarus JH. Epidemiology of Graves' orbitopathy (GO) and relationship with thyroid disease. Best Pract Res Clin Endocrinol Metab. 2012;26:273–9.
12. Bartalena L, Fatourechi V. Extrathyroidal manifestation of Graves' disease a 2014 update. J Endocrinol Investig. 2014;37:691.
13. Pothiwala P, Levine SN. Analytic review: thyrotoxic periodic paralysis: a review. J Intensive Care Med. 2010;25:71–7.
14. Sinharay R. Thyrotoxic periodic paralysis amongst the ethnic Asians living in the west - an important entity to consider in the hospital setting. QJM. 2009;102:361–2.
15. Mittra ES, McDougall IR. Recurrent silent thyroiditis: a report of four patients and review of the literature. Thyroid. 2007;17:671–5.
16. Samuels MH. Subacute, silent, and postpartum thyroiditis. Med Clin North Am. 2012;96:223–33.
17. Stagnaro-Green A. Approach to the patient with postpartum thyroiditis. J Clin Endocrinol Metab. 2012;97:334–42.
18. Kim D, Cho HC, Park JW, Lee WA, Kim YM, Chung PS, et al. Struma ovarii and peritoneal strumosis with thyrotoxicosis. Thyroid. 2009;19:305–8.
19. Espiritu RP, Dean DS. Parathyroidectomy- induced thyroiditis. Endocr Pract. 2010;16:656–9.
20. Poon WT, Ng SW, Lai CK, Chan YW, Mak WL. Factitious thyrotoxicosis and herbal dietary supplement for weight reduction. Clin Toxicol (Phila). 2008;46:290–2.
21. Hendriks LE, Looij BJ. Hyperthyroidism caused by excessive consumption of sausages. Neth J Med. 2010;68:135–7.
22. Erdem N, Erdogan M, Ozbek M, Karadeniz M, Cetinkalp S, Ozgen AG, et al. Demographic and clinical features of patients with subacute thyroiditis: results of 169 patients from a single university center in Turkey. J Endocrinol Investig. 2007;30:546–50.
23. Onal IK, Dagdelen S, Atmaca A, Karadag O, Adalar N. Hemorrhage into a thyroid nodule as a cause of thyrotoxicosis. Endocr Pract. 2006;3:299–301.
24. Paes JE, Burman KD, Cohen J, Franklyn J, McHenry CR, Shoham S, et al. Acute bacterial suppurative thyroiditis: a clinical review and expert opinion. Thyroid. 2010;20:247–55.
25. Spitzer M, Alexanian S, Farwell AP. Thyrotoxicosis with post-treatment hypothyroidism in a patient with acute suppurative thyroiditis due to porphyromonas. Thyroid. 2012;22:97–100.
26. Bandyopadhyay D, Nielsen C. Lithium-induced hyperthyroidism, thyrotoxicosis and mania: a case report. QJM. 2012;105:83–5.
27. Brownlie BEW, Turner JG. Lithium associated thyrotoxicosis. Clin Endocrinol. 2011;75:402–3.
28. Ghori F, Polder KD, Pinterr-Brown LC, Hoff AO, Gagel RF, Sherman SI, Duvic M. Thyrotoxicosis after denileukin diftitox therapy in patients with mycosis fungoides. J Clin Endocrinol Metab. 2006;91:2205–8.
29. de Fillete J, Jensen Y, Schreuer M, EvEraert H, Vrselkenie B, Neyns B, Brafvenboer B. Incidence of thyroid-related adverse events in melanoma patients treated with pembrolizumab. J Clin Endocrinol Metab. 2016;101:4431–9.
30. Minelli R, Valli MA, Di Secli C, Finardi L, Chiodera P, Bdertoni R, Ferrari C, et al. Is steroid therapy needed in the treatment of destructive thyrotoxicosis induced by alpha- interferon in chronic hepatitis C? Horm Res. 2005;63:194–9.
31. Jazvic M, Propic M, Jukic T, Murgic J, Jaksic B, KusRest D, et al. Sunitinib-induced thyrotoxicosis – a not so rare entity. Anticancer Res. 2015;35:481–5.
32. Yavuz S, Apolo AB, Kummar S, del Rivero J, Madan RA, Shawker T, Celi FS. Cabozantinib-induced thyroid dysfunction: a review of two ongoing trials for metastatic bladder cancer and sarcoma. Thyroid. 2014;24:1223–31.
33. van Doorn L, Eskens FA, Visser TJ, van der Lugt A, Mathijssen RH, Peeters RP. Sorafenib induced thyroiditis in two patients with hepatocellular carcinoma. Thyroid. 2011;21:197–202.
34. Bogazzi F, Tomisti L, Bartalena L, Aghini-Lombardi F, Martino E. Amiodarone and the thyroid: a 2012 update. J Endocrinol Investig. 2012;35:340–8.
35. Piga M, Serra A, Boi F, Tanda ML, Martino E, Mariotti S. Amiodarone-induced thyrotoxicosis. A review. Minerva Endocrinol. 2008;33:213–28.
36. Pratap R, Qayyum A, Ahmad N, Jani P. Surgical management of amiodarone-induced thyrotoxicosis in a patient with Eisenmenger's syndrome: literature review and case report. J Laryngol Otol. 2009;123:1276–9.
37. Pierret C, Tourtier JP, Pons Y, Merat S, Duverger V, Perrier E. Total thyroidectomy for amiodarone-associated thyrotoxicosis: should

surgery always be delayed for pre-operative medical preparation? J Laryngol Otol. 2012;126:701–5.

38. Biondi B, Kahaly GJ. Cardiovascular involvement in patients with different causes of hyperthyroidism. Nat Rev Endocrinol. 2010;6:431–43.

39. Wiersinga WM. Should we treat mild subclinical/mild hyperthyroidism? Yes. Eur J Intern Med. 2011;22:324–9.

40. Yapar AF, Reyhan M, Aydin M, Sukan A. Efficacy of radioiodine treatment in subclinical hyperthyroidism. Acta Endocrinol. 2012;8:77–85.

41. Negro R, Beck-Peccoz P, Chiovato L, Garofalo P, Guglielmi R, Papini E, et al. Hyperthyroidism and pregnancy. An Italian Thyroid Association (AIT) and Italian Association of Clinical Endocrinologists (AME) joint statement for clinical practice. J Endocrinol Investig. 2011;34:225–31.

42. Yoshihara A, Noh JY, Yamaguchi T, Ohye H, Sato S, Sekiya K, et al. Treatment of Graves' disease with antithyroid drugs in the first trimester of pregnancy and the prevalence of congenital malformation. J Clin Endocrinol Metab. 2012;97:2396–403.

43. Stagnaro-Green A, Abalovich M, Alexander E, Azizi F, Mestman J, Negro R, et al. Guidelines of the American Thyroid Association for the diagnosis and management of thyroid disease during pregnancy and postpartum. Thyroid. 2011;21:1081–125.

44. Chiniwala NU, Woolf PD, Bruno CP, Kaur S, Spector H, Yacono K. Thyroid storm caused by a partial hydatidiform mole. Thyroid. 2008;18:479–81.

45. Walkington L, Webster J, Hancock BW, Everard J, Coleman RE. Hyperthyroidism and human chorionic gonadotrophin production in gestational trophoblastic disease. Br J Cancer. 2011;104:1665–9.

46. Persani L, Gelmini G, Marelli F, Beck-Peccoz P, Bonomi M. Syndromes of resistance to TSH. Ann Endocrinol. 2011;72:60–3.

47. Lee S, Young BM, Wan W, Chan IH, Privalsky ML. A mechanism for pituitary-resistance to thyroid hormone (PRTH) syndrome: a loss in cooperative coactivator contacts by thyroid hormone receptor (TR)beta2. Mol Endocrinol. 2011;25:1111–25.

48. Bertalan R, Sallai A, Solyom J, Lotz G, Szabo I, Kovacs B, et al. Hyperthyroidism caused by a germline activating mutation of the thyrotropin receptor gene: difficulties in diagnosis and therapy. Thyroid. 2010;20:327–32.

49. Denilovic DL, de Camargo RY, Castro G Jr, Papadia C, Marius S, Hoff AO. Rapid control of T3 thyrotoxicosis in patients with metastatic follicular thyroid cancer treated with lenvatinib. Thyroid. 2015;25:1262–4.

50. Rosario F, Marques AR, Roque L, Rodrigues R, Ferreira TC, Limbert E, Sobrinho L, Leite V. Metastatic follicular cancer associated with hyperthyroidism. Clinc Nuc Med. 2005;30:79–82.

51. Karras S, Tzotzas T, Krassas GE. Toxicological considerations for antithyroid drugs in children. Expert Opin Drug Metab Toxicol. 2011;7:399–410.

52. Lubin E. Radioactive iodine 1311 (RAI) treatment. The nearest to the "magic bullet" but should always be preceded by a risk assess-

ment, especially in the pediatric patient. Pediatr Endocrinol Rev. 2011;9:415–6.

53. Watanabe N, Narimatsu H, Noh JY, Yamaguchi T, Kobayashi K, Kami M, et al. Antithyroid drug-induced hematopoietic damage: a retrospective cohort study of agranulocytosis and pancytopenia involving 50,385 patients with Graves' disease. J Clin Endocrinol Metab. 2012;97:E49–53.

54. Bahn RS, Burch HS, Cooper DS, Garber JR, Greenlee CM, Klein IL, et al. The role of propylthiouracil in the management of Graves' disease in adults: report of a meeting jointly sponsored by the American thyroid association and the food and drug administration. Thyroid. 2009;19:673–4.

55. Cooper DS, Rivkees SA. Putting propylthiouracil in perspective. J Clin Endocrinol Metab. 2009;94:1881–2.

56. Azizi F, Kalnoubaf R. Long-term antithyroid drug treatment. A systemic review and meta-analysis. Throid. 2017;27:1223–31.

57. Santos RB, Romaldini JH, Ward LS. A randomized controlled trial to evaluate the effectiveness of 2 regimens of fixed iodine (1-131) doses for Graves disease treatment. Clin Nucl Med. 2012;37:241–4.

58. Osaki Y, Sakurai K, Arihara Z, Hata M, Fukazawa H. Prediction of late (24-hour) radioactive iodine uptake using early (3-hour) uptake values in Japanese patients with Graves' disease. Endocr J. 2012;59:173–7.

59. Westphal SA. Warfarin toxicity and exacerbation of thyrotoxicosis induced by radioactive iodine therapy for Graves' disease. Endocrinologist. 2008;18:35–8.

60. Liu J, Bargren A, Schaefer S, Chen H, Sippel RS. Total thyroidectomy: a safe and effective treatment for Graves' disease. J Surg Res. 2011;168:1–4.

61. Peroni E, Angiolini MR, Vigone MC, Mari G, Chiumello G, Beretta E, et al. Surgical management of pediatric Graves' disease: an effective definitive treatment. Pediatr Surg Int. 2012;28:609–14.

62. Chiapponi C, Stocker U, Mussack T, Gallwas J, Hallfeldt K, Ladurner R. The surgical treatment of Graves' disease in children and adolescents. World J Surg. 2011;35:2428–31.

63. Bartalena L. The dilemma of how to manage Graves' hyperthyroidism in patients with associated orbitopathy. J Clin Endocrinol Metab. 2011;96:592–9.

64. Bahn RS, Burch HB, Cooper DS, Garber JR, Greenlee MC, Klein I, et al. Hyperthyroidism and other causes of thyrotoxicosis: management guidelines of the American Thyroid Association and American Association of Clinical Endocrinologists. Endocr Pract. 2011;17:456–520.

65. Carroll R, Matfin G. Endocrine and metabolic emergencies: thyroid storm. Ther Adv Endocrinol Metab. 2010;1:139–45.

66. Koball S, Hickstein H, Gloger M, Hinz M, Henschel J, Stange J, et al. Treatment of thyrotoxic crisis with plasmapheresis and single pass albumin dialysis: a case report. Artif Organs. 2010;34:E55–8.

67. Hegedus L, Bonnema SJ, Smith TJ, Brix TH. Treating the thyroid in the presence of Graves' ophthalmopathy. Best Pract Res Clin Endocrinol Metab. 2012;26:313–24.

68. Bartalena L. Prevention of Graves' ophthalmopathy. Best Pract Res Clin Endocrinol Metab. 2012;26:371–9.

Hypothyroidism

Jad G. Sfeir and Hossein Gharib

Introduction

Hypothyroidism is the clinical state which results from either inadequate production of thyroid hormone or impaired action of thyroid hormone at the tissue level. It is defined by the laboratory parameters of a low free thyroxine (FT4), associated with an elevated thyroid-stimulating hormone (TSH) in primary hypothyroidism or, less commonly, a low to low-normal TSH in central hypothyroidism.

Primary hypothyroidism, where the defect is at the level of the thyroid gland itself, accounts for over 95% of cases of overt hypothyroidism. The remaining 5% are caused by secondary or tertiary hypothyroidism (defect at the level of the pituitary gland or the hypothalamus) or thyroid hormone resistance.

Subclinical hypothyroidism (SCH), defined as an elevation in TSH but with a corresponding normal FT4 level, assumes that there is an intact hypothalamic-pituitary-thyroid axis and an absence of intercurrent illness. The values should also be reproducible over a 4–6-week period.

Given vague symptomatology that overlaps with other endocrine and non-endocrine disorders, hypothyroidism is commonly tested in clinical practice. It thus becomes important to differentiate overt hypothyroidism that thyroid hormone replacement, from non-thyroidal cause of such symptoms as fatigue, weight gain, or impaired cognitive function.

J. G. Sfeir
Division of Endocrinology, Metabolism, Diabetes and Nutrition, Mayo Clinic College of Medicine, Rochester, MN, USA
e-mail: sfeir.jad@mayo.edu

H. Gharib (✉)
Division of Endocrinology, Mayo Clinic College of Medicine, Rochester, MN, USA
e-mail: gharib.hossein@mayo.edu

Epidemiology

The prevalence of overt hypothyroidism in the United States has been reported to range between 0.3% and 0.8% and in Europe between 0.2% and 5.3% [1–3]. Worldwide, its prevalence is between 0.6 and 12 per 1000 women and between 1.3 and 4.0 per 1000 men [4]. The variation in reported prevalence is due to both differences in case detection and availability of dietary iodine, whereby a lower prevalence is seen in areas of iodine deficiency [5]. Subclinical hypothyroidism is more prevalent with an estimation of 0.7–13% in US adults [1].

There are significant ethnic and sex differences in thyroid disease prevalence. It is ten times more common in women than men, and its incidence rises with age [6]. White and Mexican Americans are at approximately three times higher risk compared to Black Americans [1]. Pregnant women also seem to be at higher risk, with gestational hypothyroidism, defined as both overt and subclinical hypothyroidism, reported at 15.5% based on large laboratory-based datasets [7].

Clinical Presentation and Physical Examination

Common clinical presentation of hypothyroidism is generally related to decrease in metabolism and consequent symptoms of fatigue, weight gain, cold intolerance, constipation, and less commonly in extreme situations myxedema and hypothermia. Other symptoms include decline in cognitive function, dry skin, and muscle weakness. However all of these symptoms are nonspecific to thyroid disease and overlap with other endocrine diseases such as abnormal glucose metabolism or pituitary or adrenal dysfunction.

Associated biochemical and laboratory abnormalities include dyslipidemia, elevation in creatinine phosphokinase, prolactinemia, hyponatremia, and mild anemia.

Table 2.1 Common physical examination findings in hypothyroidism

Skin	Puffiness of the periorbital tissues, hands, and feet and supraclavicular fossae secondary to myxedema; pallor from anemia; dry, coarse skin secondary to reduced sebaceous gland secretions; easy bruising; dry brittle hair and nails
Cardiovascular	Narrow pulse pressure; reduction in cutaneous blood flow leading to cool, pale skin; distant heart sounds (if pericardial effusion is present)
Gastrointestinal	Weight gain from fluid retention, abdominal gaseous distension (myxedema ileus)
Nervous system	Slowing of higher mental function including speech, slowing of the relaxation phase of tendon reflexes
Muscular	Slightly increased muscle mass due to interstitial myxedema, myoclonus

Physical signs of hypothyroidism are notoriously nonspecific and vary according to the severity of the disorder. The use of sensitive thyroid assays has largely superseded the value of physical examination findings in making the diagnosis of thyroid dysfunction (Table 2.1).

A firm, moderate-sized goiter that moves freely on swallowing is the most common physical feature of Hashimoto's thyroiditis. A large goiter can also be found in patients with severe iodine deficiency. Rarely, an atrophic gland is present, the end result of autoimmune destruction of the gland. The natural history of the untreated goiter is a slow enlargement over many years. When there is rapid, painful enlargement of the gland, thyroid lymphoma should be suspected, and an expedient work-up performed.

Etiology

Primary Hypothyroidism

Primary hypothyroidism has several causes, all resulting in a decreased output of thyroid hormone from the thyroid gland. The most common cause in the United States and other iodine-sufficient areas is chronic autoimmune thyroiditis, known as Hashimoto's thyroiditis. The hallmark of the disease is the presence of circulating antithyroid peroxidase (TPO) antibodies. Histopathologic examination of the thyroid gland, if performed, reveals diffuse lymphocytic infiltration, follicular destruction, and Hürthle cells. There is a polygenic susceptibility, with a known association between Hashimoto's thyroiditis and HLA-DR3 [8]. Other factors such as pregnancy, radiation exposure, and, as evidenced by animal studies, viral infections can also predispose to developing the condition [9].

Worldwide, the most common cause of primary hypothyroidism is iodine deficiency with approximately two billion people at risk, particularly those living in mountainous areas due to persistent glacial runoff depleting iodine stores. Large geographic areas of Africa and Asia also remain iodine-deficient. Consumption of cassava which contains compounds metabolized to thiocyanate enhances the iodine-deficient state by inhibiting thyroid iodine transport. Iodine is required for thyroid hormone production and an essential mineral component of the hormone. The World Health Organization recommends a daily iodine intake of 150 μg for the general adult population and 200 μg for pregnant or lactating women.

Other forms of thyroiditis may also cause primary hypothyroidism. Subacute or granulomatous thyroiditis that initially presents with neck pain and biochemical hyperthyroidism may progress to transient or permanent hypothyroidism. In one study, about 10% of patients developed permanent hypothyroidism, defined as an elevation in TSH lasting beyond 1 year [10]. Postpartum thyroiditis (PPT) may present with hyperthyroidism followed by transient hypothyroidism, hyperthyroidism alone, or hypothyroidism alone in about 50% of cases, usually within 2–6 months after delivery. It is more common in women with elevated titers of TPO antibodies, which confers up to a 50% chance of developing PPT [11]. Most patients are euthyroid within the first postpartum year, although permanent hypothyroidism is more likely to develop in women with higher TSH values and higher antibody titers [12].

Iatrogenic hypothyroidism includes surgical thyroidectomy and post-ablative hypothyroidism. Hypothyroidism occurs up to 4 weeks following total thyroidectomy owing to thyroxine's half-life of 7 days. Data from patients undergoing radioactive iodine therapy for Graves' disease indicate that the rate of subsequent hypothyroidism is largely dependent on the dose of radioiodine used; in the United States, most patients are hypothyroid within the first year of treatment [13]. External beam radiation which exceeds 25 Gy also causes hypothyroidism, which may be gradual in onset.

Infiltrative processes including hemochromatosis, lymphoma, amyloidosis, and sarcoidosis are rare causes of primary hypothyroidism. They tend to present as progressive, painless bilateral enlargement of the thyroid gland and are usually part of more widespread systemic involvement of the underlying condition. Infection of the thyroid is rare as the gland is encapsulated and has good blood flow and a high iodine content. However *Pneumocystis jiroveci* infection in immune-compromised patients has been reported to cause enough destruction of the thyroid gland leading to inadequate thyroid hormone production [14].

Consumptive hypothyroidism is a rare disorder that was initially identified in infants with visceral hemangiomas. There is a marked elevation in deiodinase type 3 enzyme activity which results in the conversion of T4 to reverse T3 and conversion of T3 to T2. The condition is treatable medically with glucocorticoids and interferon-α.

Congenital hypothyroidism affects 1:2000 to 1:4000 live births internationally. In the United States, data from the National Newborn Screening and Global Resource Center (NNSGRC) reveals an incidence of 0.04% [15]. It is more frequent in iodine-deficient regions; the prevalence of elevated TSH can be greater than 40 percent in severely iodine-deficient regions but less than 3 percent in iodine-sufficient populations [16]. Infants with the disorder have little to no clinical features of hypothyroidism, and they are detected largely through universal newborn screening programs in place since the 1970s. Thyroid dysgenesis is responsible for 85% of these cases, with the remaining being caused by defects in thyroid hormone production at every level. Worldwide, the commonest cause is thyroid ectopy which accounts for about two-thirds of patients with thyroid dysgenesis. Central congenital hypothyroidism is much rarer and may be missed by screening programs that utilize TSH only. These infants usually have other pituitary hormone deficiencies [17]. Transient hypothyroidism in infants can occur as a result of maternal iodine insufficiency, maternal TSH receptor-blocking antibodies, or exposure to antithyroid drugs; infants are rendered euthyroid once the offending agent (antibody or drug) is naturally cleared over several weeks following birth.

Medication-Induced Thyroid Dysfunction

Medications can affect thyroid function in several ways; these are summarized in Table 2.2.

Drugs that affect thyroid hormone synthesis and secretion include amiodarone and other iodine-containing drugs and radiographic agents, lithium, perchlorate, and others. Other drugs increase thyroxine requirements by either binding to exogenous thyroid hormone, e.g., calcium salts, sucralfate, and cholestyramine, or increasing its metabolism, e.g., rifampicin, carbamazepine, and phenytoin. Tyrosine kinase inhibitors such as sorafenib and sunitinib have been shown to cause hypothyroidism in up to 70% of patients, a side effect directly related to length of therapy [18]. The proposed mechanisms vary slightly between the different agents and include destructive thyroiditis with a reduction in thyroid hormone synthesis by inhibition of thyroid peroxidase activity. In patients already on thyroxine therapy, requirements increase, an effect thought to be mediated by type 3 deiodinase activity which increases the metabolism of T4 and T3 [19].

Medications that cause a reduction in TSH secretion, such as glucocorticoids, opiates, and dopamine agonists, are also implicated in causing hypothyroidism.

Immune checkpoint inhibitors have emerged as effective antitumor treatment for an increasing number of solid and hematologic tumors. The reported incidence of thyroid immune-related adverse effects varies based on medication type (anti-PD-1 vs. anti-CTLA-4) and seems to be more common when these drugs are used in combination as opposed to monotherapy. Overall, it is estimated between 5 and 10% and more commonly presents as thyrotoxicosis followed by hypothyroidism (62%) or overt hypothyroidism (22%) [20].

Table 2.2 Common medications that affect thyroid function

Drug	Mechanism
Inhibition of thyroid hormone synthesis and secretion	
Amiodarone	Inhibits type I and type II 5′ deiodinase, leading to decreased T3 generation from T4
Iodinated contrast agents	Inhibit type I and type II 5′ deiodinase, leading to decreased T3 generation from T4
	Decrease hepatic uptake of T4
	Inhibit T3 binding to its nuclear receptor
Thiocyanate, perchlorate	Inhibit iodide transport into the thyroid gland
Propylthiouracil, methimazole	Inhibit thyroid peroxidase; propylthiouracil additionally inhibits peripheral conversion of T4 to T3
Lithium	Inhibits iodide binding and thyroid hormone release
Decreased absorption of exogenous thyroid hormone	
Calcium compounds, sucralfate, aluminum hydroxide, ferrous compounds, cholestyramine, colesevelam, proton pump inhibitors, H2 blockers	Bind to levothyroxine and reduce its absorption
Increased T4 clearance	
Rifampin	Induces hepatic microsomal enzymes
Phenobarbital, carbamazepine	Induce hepatic microsomal enzymes
	Compete with thyroid hormone binding to TBG
	Accelerate the conjugation and hepatic clearance of T4/T3
Decreased TSH secretion	
Dopamine, L-dopa, bromocriptine	Increase T3 synthesis from T4 in the brain
Opiates	Block the breakdown of T3 in the brain
Others	
Estrogens, SERMs	Increase thyroid-binding globulin
Steroids	Influenced by dose, type, and route of administration of glucocorticoid. Inhibit deiodination of T4; suppress TSH secretion; increase in renal iodide clearance
Salicylates	Compete for thyroid hormone-binding sites on binding proteins
Thalidomide	Immune-mediated subacute destructive thyroiditis
Immune checkpoint inhibitors	Suggested to be immune-mediated thyroiditis

Central (Secondary and Tertiary) Hypothyroidism

Central hypothyroidism is caused by TSH deficiency from disorders of the pituitary gland or hypothalamus. It is usually accompanied by deficiencies of other pituitary hormones and can vary in severity. About 15% of the function of the thyroid gland is independent of TSH, and therefore central hypothyroidism may be milder clinically than primary hypothyroidism. Central hypothyroidism may be caused by tumors, surgery, and infiltrative, inflammatory, or infective processes and medications.

Generalized Thyroid Hormone Resistance

Thyroid hormone resistance is a rare, autosomal dominant disorder in which the majority of patients have a mutation in the thyroid receptor TR-beta gene. This results in reduced T3-binding affinity at the level of the thyroid hormone receptor and a reduced response to thyroid hormone. Two-thirds of patients have goiters, but their symptoms may be a mix of hypo- and hyperthyroid complaints. There is an increased prevalence of attention-deficit disorder which is present in about 10% of patients [21]. Laboratory testing shows an elevated free thyroxine with normal or slightly increased TSH levels; the disorder therefore has to be differentiated from a TSH-secreting pituitary tumor. Treatment with T4 or T3 may be beneficial in patients with symptoms of hypothyroidism.

Evaluation

Given the lack of sensitivity and specificity of clinical findings, laboratory testing is essential to confirm the diagnosis and identify the cause of hypothyroidism.

The most sensitive, "gold standard" test is measurement of TSH levels using a third-generation chemiluminescent immunoassay, which has the advantage of being more sensitive at the lower range than the second-generation test. The FT4 level will differentiate between overt and SCH. Equilibrium dialysis is the gold standard for the measurement of FT4; however, direct measurement via ultrafiltration is the most widely available method. It can also be measured indirectly through the FT4 index. Total thyroxine levels are affected by conditions that increase binding protein (e.g., pregnancy and illness) and must therefore be interpreted with caution. There is considerable debate about the upper limit of normal for the TSH reference range. There is also suggestion of differences in reference range by sex, age, and ethnicity [22]. Data from the NHANES studies has shown an age-specific distribution of TSH, with higher normal values being seen in the elderly [23].

There is possibility for laboratory interference with human anti-animal antibodies or high levels of drugs and supplements such as heparin or biotin. Consequently, interpretation of thyroid function testing should be interpreted carefully with consideration to the clinical presentation.

The diagnosis of Hashimoto's thyroiditis is confirmed by the presence of circulating TPO antibodies, but antibodies to thyroglobulin (TG) and the TSH receptor antibody (TRAb) may also be present. The presence of TPO antibodies is 92% sensitive and 93% specific for the diagnosis of Hashimoto's thyroiditis in the correct clinical setting [24]. Elevated titers of TPO antibodies can, however, be present in up to 11% of the general disease-free population [16]. In patients with SCH, the measurement of TPO antibodies is helpful in predicting the likelihood of progression to overt hypothyroidism.

Ultrasound of the thyroid gland is not routinely recommended but may confirm the diagnosis of Hashimoto's thyroiditis if the characteristic heterogeneous echotexture is seen.

Treatment

Thyroid hormone replacement is the mainstay of treatment of hypothyroidism. Levothyroxine (LT4) is the preferred agent as it allows for normal physiologic mechanisms to maintain T3 production in peripheral tissues. It has a half-life of 7 days, and therefore dose titration should be done after about 6 weeks, allowing for equilibration to be achieved. A TSH goal should be used to adjust the dose of therapy, except in patients without an intact hypothalamic-pituitary-thyroid axis, in which case FT4 is used. Patients with suspected glucocorticoid deficiency should be evaluated and treated prior to initiation of levothyroxine, as the latter may precipitate an adrenal crisis in untreated individuals.

The typical daily dose of LT4 in a patient without endogenous thyroid function is about 1.6 µg/kg body weight per day. Care should be taken when initiating treatment in elderly patients with angina, as thyroid hormone can increase myocardial oxygen demand. Therefore, a recommended starting dose of 25–50 µg/day is preferred with titration by 12.5–25 µg every few weeks in this population. Patients with SCH also require a lower starting dose of levothyroxine, if treatment is initiated.

Levothyroxine should be taken on an empty stomach, ideally separated from food by at least 1 hour. Several medications may affect the absorption of thyroid hormone (Table 2.2), and patients should be educated to allow at least 4 hours to pass after a meal prior to taking thyroid hormone. Gastric acid is required for complete absorption of thyroid hormone; in patients on acid-reducing medication, one strategy may be to administer the dose at night when there is higher basal secretion of acid in combination with a slower intestinal transit time [25]. In patients who are unable to adhere to a daily dosing regimen, once-weekly dosing of levothyroxine with a dose slightly higher than seven times the daily dose has been shown to achieve biochemical euthyroidism without significant side effects [26].

Monitoring of therapy should be performed every 6 weeks after any change in treatment is made, be it to the dose or the brand of medication [27]. Among generic LT4 formulations, there is some variation in bioequivalence despite adherence to FDA standards. Therefore, in the athyreotic patient particularly, many practitioners advocate using brand name medication only. Once the ideal dose is achieved, monitoring can be done on an annual basis. Certain circumstances should prompt reassessment of thyroid function sooner, for example, pregnancy which can increase requirements by up to 50% [28]. Conversely, women on androgen therapy for breast cancer require less levothyroxine, as do hypothyroid patients in general as they get older. Medications can also interfere with thyroid hormone metabolism (Table 2.2), and these potential interactions should be kept in mind.

Therapeutic Target

The goal of treatment of hypothyroidism is to restore both biochemical and clinical euthyroidisms. Most patients achieve normal TSH levels within the first year of treatment. One study estimated this at 75% in patients with spontaneous hypothyroidism and 68% in those with hypothyroidism following surgery or RAI therapy. There should be avoidance of undertreatment and overtreatment. The same study observed overtreatment with LT4 in 4% to 6% of patients [29].

Given the fact that TSH normal level rises with the age, some groups have proposed targeting a lower TSH level within the reference range, particularly in younger individuals. There is however mixed evidence regarding benefit of such practices [30]. Controversy also continues regarding the benefits of thyroxine therapy in SCH, with some recommending treatment [31, 32] and others arguing against replacement therapy, particularly in the elderly [33].

Persistent Complaints Despite Normal TSH

In some patients, despite achieving biochemical euthyroidism, hypothyroid symptoms such as fatigue and weight gain persist. Many factors have been suggested as an explanation to this observation, including the presence of concomitant autoimmune diseases, other hormonal changes such as menopause, or genetic deiodinase polymorphism. Further, levothyroxine monotherapy does not restore physiologic ratios of T4 and T3 that are seen in euthyroid individuals.

Combination Therapy

The thyroid gland is responsible for 20% of the body's T3 secretion with the remainder derived from peripheral conversion of T4 to T3. The theory of, therefore, supplementing the athyreotic patient with T3 in order to restore "physiologic balance" is an appealing one. Several studies have looked at whether a replacement strategy with both LT4 and triiodothyronine (LT3) results in better outcomes. Overall, the majority of clinical studies did not demonstrate benefit of use of combination therapy to treat hypothyroid patients with regard to quality of life, fatigue, body weight, cognition, and mood [34, 35]. An early positive study showed improvement in mood and neuropsychological parameters in these patients but was criticized for its small number of patients, excessive use of thyroid hormone, and short follow-up [36]. Several subsequent, more rigorous studies and a large meta-analysis failed to replicate those results [37–42]. In addition, most of these trials have used once or twice daily dosing of T3, which is a short-acting preparation, and thus provided surges of free T3 rather than normalization of the steady-state levels.

The European Thyroid Association (ETA) and the Italian Association of Clinical Endocrinologists (AME) have suggested consideration of combination therapy on a trial basis to address patient well-being, with avoidance of such therapy in the pregnant and elderly population [34, 35]. The Italian Guide tabulated a possible approach for the combination therapy [35]. Additionally, the use of "non-solid" LT4 formulations may be considered in hypothyroid patients with gastroenteric diseases due to improved GI absorption of these products [35].

Commercially available desiccated animal thyroid preparations, usually porcine in origin, contain both T3 and T4. The ratio of T3 to T4 in these preparations tends to be higher than the ratio found in humans, thereby leading to supraphysiologic T3 levels. Additionally, due to the nature of the product, monitoring and standardization of desiccated thyroid preparations are lacking, leading to difficulty in dose adjustment. There is also insufficient information about the safety or benefit of the surge of free T3 that is seen shortly after the ingestion of such thyroid extracts [43].

Special Populations

Subclinical Hypothyroidism (SCH)

SCH is a biochemical diagnosis made in a patient with an elevated serum TSH level and normal serum free T4. Symptoms may be vague and nonspecific or similar to those with overt hypothyroidism. Its prevalence increases with age, and it is more common in women and in iodine-sufficient areas [44].

Some conditions need to be excluded prior to making this diagnosis. In a patient recovering from a non-thyroidal illness, there may be a transient increase in TSH. Similarly, often after the hyperthyroid phase of thyroiditis, there can be a transient period of hypothyroidism. There is also a diurnal variation and a nocturnal surge in TSH with the highest values being seen in the morning. Hence, the diagnosis of subclinical hypothyroidism should only be made in a patient in whom the biochemical abnormalities are reproducible after about 6 weeks and in whom there is an intact hypothalamic-pituitary-thyroid axis with no intercurrent illness.

The risk of progression from SCH to overt hypothyroidism is determined by the magnitude of TSH elevation and the presence of TPO antibodies [45]. In women with both high TSH values and high antibody concentrations, the cumulative incidence of hypothyroidism has been reported to be as high as 55% [46]. Conversely, normalization of TSH values occurs more frequently in people with concentrations of 4–6 mU/L [47]. The underlying etiology for SCH also influences the rate of progression to overt hypothyroidism. For example, patients who recently received radioiodine therapy or external beam radiation are more likely to progress to overt hypothyroidism than patients who received external beam radiation as children.

There is inconsistent data regarding the risk of cardiovascular disease, neuropsychiatric symptoms, and mortality rates in patients with SCH with studies demonstrating both an increased and decreased risk of each outcome measure.

Current guidelines recommend treating all patients with a TSH >10 mIU/L and those with positive TPO antibodies, because of a higher risk of progression to overt hypothyroidism [48]. Additionally pregnant women or women contemplating pregnancy should also be treated [49]. More unclear is the benefit of treating patients with TSH between 5 and 9 mIU/L. SCH might be associated with greater cardiovascular risk in young and middle-aged people than in those older than 65 years, and therefore treatment may be justifiable in this group [50]. Levothyroxine therapy has been shown to improve cholesterol levels as well as surrogate cardiovascular endpoints such as carotid intimal thickness, endothelial function, and left ventricular function in several studies, but the mortality benefit may only be seen after prolonged therapy [51, 52]. Symptomatic patients with TSH values between 5 and 9 mIU/L may benefit from treatment, although studies show the effects to be greatest in patients with TSH >10 mIU/L [53].

The goal of therapy should be to bring TSH to the lower range of normal (0.5–3.0 mIU/L) in patients <65 years of age and between 3 and 4.5 mIU/L in patients >65 years of age. In patients who do not clearly qualify for therapy, monitoring thyroid function every 6–12 months is a reasonable strategy.

Hypothyroidism and Pregnancy

Pregnancy results in a twofold increase in thyroid-binding globulin and stimulation of the TSH receptor by β-HCG, an effect that wanes with decreasing production of β-HCG as the pregnancy progresses. Therefore the recommendation by the American Thyroid Association that there should be trimester-specific reference ranges for TSH in pregnancy has a sound physiologic basis, but is not widely practiced by commercial laboratories [54].

This phenomenon has impacted the definitions of overt and subclinical hypothyroidism in pregnancy. Overt hypothyroidism is defined as having a TSH of >2.5 mIU/L with a corresponding trimester-specific low FT4 or a TSH of >10 mIU/L regardless of FT4 levels. SCH is defined as having TSH between 2.5 and 10 mIU/L with a normal FT4 level. About 10–20% of all pregnant women are TPO antibody positive and biochemically euthyroid. These women are more likely to have a TSH level that is >4.0 mIU/L by the third trimester, and up to half will develop PPT [55]. SCH can also persist postpartum, particularly in women with TPO antibodies.

Overt hypothyroidism in pregnancy, if left untreated, may result in adverse maternal and fetal outcomes including preterm delivery, low birth weight, miscarriage, increased risk of fetal loss, and gestational hypertension [56, 57]. The data in women with SCH with or without thyroid autoantibodies also shows an increase in adverse pregnancy outcomes, including preeclampsia, placental abruption, and neonatal mortality [58, 59]. However, there is less clear evidence that the neurocognitive development of the fetus is affected in women with untreated SCH [54, 60].

Thyroid autoimmunity itself may predispose to adverse fetal outcomes. In recent meta-analyses looking at euthyroid women with thyroid autoantibodies, there was a twofold increase in the rate of both spontaneous miscarriage and preterm delivery [61, 62].

There is currently insufficient evidence for universal TSH screening of all pregnant women in the first trimester of pregnancy. Clinical practice guidelines instead advocate a "case-finding" approach and recommend certain high-risk groups of women have their serum TSH checked at the confirmation of pregnancy (Table 2.3) [54, 63].

The current ATA recommendation is to treat all pregnant women with overt hypothyroidism as well as those with SCH and positive TPO antibodies and to consider treatment in pregnant women with negative TPO antibodies and a TSH ranging between the upper limit of normal and 10 mU/L [54]. If the decision is made not to treat women with SCH or thyroid autoimmunity, then monitoring thyroid function every 4 weeks during the first half of pregnancy and at least once between 26 and 32 weeks gestation is a reasonable strategy.

Table 2.3 Target populations for TSH screening during pregnancy

Women at high risk for overt hypothyroidism during pregnancy
History of thyroid dysfunction, postpartum thyroiditis, or prior thyroid surgery
Age >30 years
Symptoms of thyroid dysfunction or biochemical features suggestive of thyroid dysfunction including anemia, hypercholesterolemia, or hyponatremia
Presence of goiter
TPO antibody positivity
Type 1 diabetes or other autoimmune disorders
History of infertility, miscarriage, or preterm delivery
Multiple prior pregnancies (≥2)
History of head or neck radiation
Family history of autoimmune thyroid disease or thyroid dysfunction
Use of amiodarone or lithium or recent administration of iodinated radiologic contrast
Residing in an area of known moderate-to-severe iodine insufficiency
Body mass index ≥40 kg/m^2

Women with preexisting hypothyroidism will likely require an increase in their dose of hormone replacement by up to 50% until delivery [64]. The dose of levothyroxine should be increased by about 30% as soon as pregnancy is confirmed and titrated to maintain a trimester-specific normal TSH. Practically speaking, this can be achieved by adding two extra doses of levothyroxine a week, i.e., nine doses, from seven. Ideally, preconception TSH should be <2.5 mIU/L to achieve the most favorable outcomes during pregnancy. Serum TSH should be monitored every 4 weeks in the first half of pregnancy and at least once between 26 and 32 weeks gestation. In the absence of laboratory-specific ranges, it is reasonable to use the following upper limits of normal for TSH: 2.5 mIU/L in the first trimester, 3.0 mIU/L in the second trimester, and 3.5 mIU/L in the third trimester [49, 54]. Postpartum, the patient should return to her prepregnancy dose of levothyroxine, and a serum TSH should be checked about 6 weeks later.

Myxedema Coma

Myxedema coma is the result of severe untreated hypothyroidism and manifests with hypothermia, generalized slowing of all organ functions, and decreased cognition. It is a medical emergency with a high mortality rate if left unrecognized and untreated. It can be a result of long-standing untreated hypothyroidism or may be precipitated by exposure to cold, infection, trauma, or central nervous system depressants particularly in the elderly population.

The typical patient presents with a history of known hypothyroidism and slowly worsening mental status changes. It is usually accompanied by a variety of clinical features which, in its most severe form, can include hypothermia, hypotension, bradycardia, hyponatremia, hypoglycemia, and hypoventilation. The myxedema is a result of abnormal mucin deposition in the tissues and manifests as non-pitting edema of the face, tongue, and peripheries. Pleural, pericardial, and peritoneal effusions are not uncommon. Seizures may be present, partially due to hyponatremia which is present in about 50% of patients [65].

The diagnosis should be considered in the hypothyroid patient who presents with typical clinical features and confirmed biochemically. Serum TSH, free T4, and cortisol levels should be drawn prior to administering any therapy. The majority of patients will have primary hypothyroidism, but an inappropriately normal TSH in the setting of a low free T4 would indicate a pituitary or a hypothalamic etiology.

Treatment should be initiated based on clinical suspicion, even before biochemical confirmation, due to the high mortality rate of this condition. Severe hypometabolism can impair drug absorption from the gut, and thus medications should be administered intravenously. Thyroid hormone replacement with both T4 and T3 is widely practiced as T3 has a faster onset of action and there is unpredictable T4-to-T3 conversion in the setting of severe hypothyroidism and concurrent non-thyroidal illness. A single loading dose of 400–500 μg of levothyroxine intravenously is initially given to replete the peripheral pool; this is converted to a daily dose of 1.6 μg/kg thereafter. The loading dose should be lowered in the elderly and in patients with cardiovascular disease. T3 may be administered simultaneously, with or without a loading dose, at a dose of 2.5–10 μg every 8 hours. Care must be taken to ensure that T3 levels are monitored appropriately as high levels have been shown to increase mortality [66]. Once the patient is able to tolerate oral medications, thyroid hormone replacement can be done orally at a dose of about three-quarters of the intravenous dose.

Glucocorticoids at stress doses should also be given until the diagnosis of adrenal insufficiency can be excluded. Additionally, supportive treatment, electrolyte monitoring, and treatment of any precipitating illness must be instituted. Hypothermia is best managed with passive warming as active warming may cause redistribution of blood flow to subcutaneous tissues and cardiovascular collapse. Hypotension generally resolves with thyroid hormone replacement over hours to days, but vasopressor support may be required temporarily.

Poor prognostic factors include increased age, reduced consciousness, persistent hypothermia, and sepsis. However, with expedient treatment, the mortality rate approaches that due to sepsis alone [67]. The key to successfully managing myxedema coma remains having a keen clinical suspicion for the condition and the prompt institution of thyroid hormone replacement.

References

1. Hollowell JG, Staehling NW, Flanders WD, et al. Serum TSH, T (4), and thyroid antibodies in the United States population (1988–1994): National Health and Nutrition Examination Survey (NHANES III). J Clin Endocrinol Metab. 2002;87(2):489–99.
2. Canaris GJ, Manowitz NR, Mayor G, et al. The Colorado thyroid disease prevalence study. Arch Intern Med. 2000;160(4):526–34.
3. Garmendia Madariaga A, Santos Palacios S, Guillén-Grima F, et al. The incidence and prevalence of thyroid dysfunction in Europe: a meta-analysis. J Clin Endocrinol Metab. 2014;99:923–31.
4. Vanderpump MP. The epidemiology of thyroid disease. Br Med Bull. 2011;99:39–51.
5. Aghini-Lombardi F, Antonangeli L, Martino E, et al. The spectrum of thyroid disorders in an iodine-deficient community: the Pescopagano Survey. J Clin Endocrinol Metab. 1999;84:561–6.
6. McLeod DS, Caturegli P, Cooper DS, et al. Variation in rates of autoimmune thyroid disease by race/ethnicity in US military personnel. J Am Med Assoc. 2014;311(15):1563–5.
7. Blatt AJ, Nakamoto JM, Kaufman HW. National status of testing for hypothyroidism during pregnancy and postpartum. J Clin Endocrinol Metab. 2012;97(3):777–84.
8. Tandon N, Zhang L, Weetman AP. HLA associations with Hashimoto's thyroiditis. Clin Endocrinol. 1991;34:383–6.
9. Tomer Y, Davies TF. Infection, thyroid disease and autoimmunity. Endocr Rev. 1993;14:107–20.
10. Fatourechi V, Aniszewski JP, Fatourechi GZ, et al. Clinical features and outcome of subacute thyroiditis in an incidence cohort: Olmsted County, Minnesota, study. J Clin Endocrinol Metab. 2003;88:2100–5.
11. Muller AF, Drexhage HA, Berghout A. Postpartum thyroiditis and autoimmune thyroiditis in women of childbearing age: recent insights and consequences for antenatal and postnatal care. Endocr Rev. 2001;22:605–30.
12. Stagnaro-Green A. Clinical review 152: postpartum thyroiditis. J Clin Endocrinol Metab. 2002;87(9):4042–7.
13. Franklyn JA, Daykin J, Drolc Z, Farmer M, Sheppard MC. Long-term follow-up of treatment of thyrotoxicosis by three different methods. Clin Endocrinol (Oxf). 1991;34(1):71.
14. Pearce EN, Farwell AP, Braverman LE. Thyroiditis. N Engl J Med. 2003;348:2646–55.
15. Hinton CF, Harris KB, Borgfeld L, et al. Trends in incidence rates of congenital hypothyroidism related to select demographic factors: data from the United States, California, Massachusetts, New York, and Texas. Pediatrics. 2010;125(Suppl 2):S37–47.
16. Endocrine Society. Endocrine Facts and Figures: Thyroid. 1st ed. Washington, DC, USA: Endocrine Society; 2015.
17. van Tijn DA, de Vijlder J, Vulsma T. Role of the thyrotropin-releasing hormone stimulation test in diagnosis of congenital central hypothyroidism in infants. J Clin Endocrinol Metab. 2008;93(2):410.
18. Torino F, Corsello SM, Longo R, et al. Hypothyroidism related to tyrosine kinase inhibitors: an emerging toxic effect of targeted therapy. Nat Rev Clin Oncol. 2009;6(4):219–28.
19. Abdulrahman RM, Verloop H, Hoftijzer H, et al. Sorafenib-induced hypothyroidism is associated with increased type 3 deiodination. J Clin Endocrinol Metab. 2010;95(8):3758.
20. Lee H, Hodi FS, Giobbie-Hurder A, et al. Characterization of Thyroid Disorders in Patients Receiving Immune Checkpoint Inhibition Therap. Cancer Immunol Res. 2017;5(12):1133–40.
21. Hauser PH, Zametkin AJ, Martinez P, et al. Attention deficit hyperactivity disorder in people with generalized resistance to thyroid hormone. N Engl J Med. 1993;328:997–1001.
22. Chaker L, Bianco AC, Jonklaas J, et al. Hypothyroidism. Lancet. 2017;390(10101):1550–62.
23. Surks MI, Hollowell JG. Age-specific distribution of serum thyrotropin and anti-thyroid antibodies in the US population: implications for the prevalence of subclinical hypothyroidism. J Clin Endocrinol Metab. 2007;92(12):4575–82.
24. Tozzoli R, Villalta D, Kodermaz G, Bagnasco M, Tonutti E, Bizzaro N. Autoantibody profiling of patients with autoimmune thyroid disease using a new multiplexed immunoassay method. Clin Chem Lab Med. 2006;44(7):837–42.
25. Vanderpump M. Pharmacotherapy: hypothyroidism—should levothyroxine be taken at bedtime? Nat Rev Endocrinol. 2011;7(4):195–6.
26. Grebe SK, Cooke RR, Ford HC, et al. Treatment of hypothyroidism with once weekly thyroxine. J Clin Endocrinol Metab. 1997;82(3):870–5.
27. American Thyroid Association; Endocrine Society; American Association of Clinical Endocrinologists. Joint Statement on the US Food and Drug Administration's decision regarding bioequivalence of levothyroxine sodium. Thyroid. 2004;14(7):486.
28. Mandel SJ, Larsen PR, Seely EW, et al. Increased need for thyroxine during pregnancy in women with primary hypothyroidism. N Engl J Med. 1990;323:91–6.
29. Solter D, Solter M. Do we treat hypothyroidism properly? A survey of 2488 patients from University Hospital Center. Zagreb, Croatia. Ann Endocrinol. 2013;74(1):27–9.
30. Fatourechi V. Upper limit of normal serum thyroid-stimulating hormone: a moving and now an aging target? J Clin Endocrinol Metab. 2007;92:4560–2.
31. Razvi S, Ingoe L, Keeka G, et al. The beneficial effect of l-thyroxine on cardiovascular risk factors, endothelial function, and quality of life in subclinical hypothyroidism: randomized, crossover trial. J Clin Endocrinol Metab. 2007;92:1715–23.
32. Gharib H. Subclinical hypothyroidism—the treatment controversy. US Endocrinol. 2008;4(1):92–4.
33. Fatourechi V, Klee GG, Grebe SK, et al. Effects of reducing the upper limit of normal TSH values. JAMA. 2003;290(24):3195–6.
34. Wiersinga WM, Duntas L, Fadeyev V, et al. 2012 ETA Guidelines: The Use of L-T4 + L-T3 in the Treatment of Hypothyroidism. Eur Thyroid J. 2012;1(2):55–71.
35. Guglielmi R, Frasoldati A, Zini M, et al. Italian Association of Clinical Endocrinologists Statement-Replacement Therapy for Primary Hypothyroidism: A Brief Guide for Clinical Practice. Endocr Pract. 2016;22(11):1319–26.
36. Bunevicius R, Kazanavicius G, Zalinkevicius R, et al. Effects of thyroxine as compared with thyroxine plus triiodothyronine in patients with hypothyroidism. N Engl J Med. 1999;340:424–9.
37. Cooper DS. Combined T4 and T3 therapy—back to the drawing board. JAMA. 2003;290:3002–4.
38. Grozinsky-Glasberg S, Fraser A, Nahshoni E, et al. Thyroxine-triiodothyronine combination therapy versus thyroxine monotherapy for clinical hypothyroidism: meta-analysis of randomized controlled trials. J Clin Endocrinol Metab. 2006;91(7):2592.
39. Celi FS, Zemskova M, Linderman JD, et al. Metabolic effects of liothyronine therapy in hypothyroidism: a randomized, double-blind, crossover trial of liothyronine versus levothyroxine. J Clin Endocrinol Metab. 2011;96(11):3466–74.
40. Saravanan P, Simmons DJ, Greenwood R, et al. Partial substitution of thyroxine (T4) with triiodothyronine in patients on T4 replacement therapy: results of a large community-based randomized controlled trial. J Clin Endocrinol Metab. 2005;90:805–12.
41. Appelhof BC, Fliers E, Wekking EM, et al. Combined therapy with levothyroxine and liothyronine in two ratios, compared with levothyroxine monotherapy in primary hypothyroidism: a double-blind, randomized, controlled clinical trial. J Clin Endocrinol Metab. 2005;90:2666–74.
42. Walsh JP, Shiels L, Lim EM, et al. Combined thyroxine/liothyronine treatment does not improve well-being, quality of life or cogni-

tive function compared to thyroxine alone: a randomized controlled trial in patients with primary hypothyroidism. J Clin Endocrinol Metab. 2003;88:4543–50.

43. Hoang TD, Olsen CH, Mai VQ, et al. Dessicated thyroid extract compared with levothyroxine in the treatment of hypothyroidism: a randomized, double-blind, crossover study. J Clin Endocrinol Metab. 2013;98:1982–90.

44. Szabolcs I, Podoba J, Feldkamp J, et al. Comparative screening for thyroid disorders in old age in areas of iodine deficiency, long-term iodine prophylaxis and abundant iodine intake. Clin Endocrinol (Oxf). 1997;47:87–92.

45. Huber G, Staub JJ, Meier C, et al. Prospective study of the spontaneous course of subclinical hypothyroidism: prognostic value of thyrotropin, thyroid reserve, and thyroid antibodies. J Clin Endocrinol Metab. 2002;87(7):3221.

46. Vanderpump MP, Tunbridge WM, French JM, et al. The incidence of thyroid disorders in the community: a twenty-year follow-up of the Whickham Survey. Clin Endocrinol (Oxf). 1995;43(1):55–68.

47. Diez JJ, Iglesias P, Burman KD. Spontaneous normalization of thyrotropin concentrations in patients with subclinical hypothyroidism. J Clin Endocrinol Metab. 2005;90:4124–7.

48. Surks MI, Ortiz E, Daniels GH, et al. Subclinical thyroid disease: scientific review and guidelines for diagnosis and management. JAMA. 2004;291(2):228.

49. Garber JR, et al. Clinical practice guidelines for hypothyroidism in adults: Co-sponsored by the American Association of Clinical Endocrinologists and the American Thyroid Association. Endocr Pract. 2012;18(6):988–1028.

50. Cooper DS, Biondi B. Subclinical thyroid disease. Lancet. 2012;379(9821):1142–54.

51. Zhao M, Liu L, Wang F, et al. A Worthy Finding: Decrease in Total Cholesterol and Low-Density Lipoprotein Cholesterol in Treated Mild Subclinical Hypothyroidism. Thyroid. 2016;26(8):1019–29.

52. Razvi S, Weaver JU, Vanderpump MP, Pearce SH. The incidence of ischemic heart disease and mortality in people with subclinical hypothyroidism: reanalysis of the Whickham Survey cohort. J Clin Endocrinol Metab. 2010;95:1734–40.

53. Meier C, Staub JJ, Roth CB, et al. TSH-controlled L-thyroxine therapy reduces cholesterol levels and clinical symptoms in subclinical hypothyroidism: a double blind, placebo-controlled trial (Basel Thyroid Study). J Clin Endocrinol Metab. 2001;86(10):4860.

54. Alexander EK, Pearce EN, Brent GA, et al. 2017 Guidelines of the American Thyroid Association for the Diagnosis and Management of Thyroid Disease During Pregnancy and the Postpartum. Thyroid. 2017;27(3):315–89.

55. Negro R, Formoso G, Mangieri T, Pezzarossa A, et al. Levothyroxine treatment in euthyroid pregnant women with autoimmune thyroid disease: effects on obstetrical complications. J Clin Endocrinol Metab. 2006;91:2587–91.

56. Haddow JE, Garbe PL, Allan WC, et al. Maternal thyroid deficiency during pregnancy and subsequent neuropsychological development of the child. N Engl J Med. 1999;341:549–55.

57. Leung AS, Millar LK, Koonings PP, et al. Perinatal outcome in hypothyroid pregnancies. Obstet Gynecol. 1993;81:349–53.

58. Mannisto T, Vääräsmäki M, Pouta A, et al. Thyroid dysfunction and autoantibodies during pregnancy as predictive factors of pregnancy complications and maternal morbidity in later life. J Clin Endocrinol Metab. 2010;95:1084–94.

59. Negro R, Schwartz A, Gismondi R, et al. Increased pregnancy loss rate in thyroid antibody negative women with TSH levels between 2.5 and 5.0 in the first trimester of pregnancy. J Clin Endocrinol Metab. 2010;95:E44–8.

60. Lazarus JH, Bestwick JP, Channon S, et al. Antenatal thyroid screening and childhood cognitive function. N Engl J Med. 2012;366:493–501.

61. Chen L, Hu R. Thyroid autoimmunity and miscarriage. Clin Endocrinol. 2011;74:513–9.

62. Thangaratinam S, Tan A, Knox E. Association between thyroid autoantibodies and miscarriage and preterm birth: meta-analysis of evidence. BMJ. 2011;342:d2616.

63. Abalovich M, Amino N, Barbour LA, et al. Management of thyroid dysfunction during pregnancy and post-partum: an endocrine society clinical practice guideline. J Clin Endocrinol Metab. 2007;92(Suppl 8):S1–47.

64. Alexander EK, Marqusee E, Lawrence J, et al. Timing and magnitude of increases in levothyroxine requirements during pregnancy in women with hypothyroidism. N Engl J Med. 2004;351(3):241.

65. Iwasaki Y, Oiso Y, Yamauchi K, et al. Osmoregulation of plasma vasopressin in myxedema. J Clin Endocrinol Metab. 1990;70(2):534.

66. Hylander B, Rosenqvist U. Treatment of myxoedema coma—factors associated with fatal outcome. Acta Endocrinol (Copenh). 1985;108(1):65.

67. Gardner DG. Chapter 24: Endocrine emergencies. New York: McGraw-Hill; 2011.

Thyroid Nodules and Cancer

Marcio L. Griebeler and Hossein Gharib

Introduction and Clinical Importance

Thyroid nodules are very common in clinical practice with a prevalence ranging from 2% to 6% by palpation [1] and up to 19–68% by ultrasound [2–4]. Most patients with a palpable thyroid nodule on physical examination have additional nodules on US investigation [5, 6]. The main clinical importance of these nodules is to rule out malignancy.

The majority of nodules are benign; approximately 6% are malignant [1, 3]. The incidence of thyroid cancer has been increasing due to the use of neck ultrasonography and other imaging leading to early diagnosis of occult and incidental cancer with unclear clinical significance [7]. The incidence of thyroid cancer has tripled from 4.9 per 100,000 in 1975 to 14.3 per 100,000 in 2009 [8, 9]. The estimated annual incidence of thyroid nodules is 0.1% per year, suggesting that approximately 350,000 new nodules will be detected this year, conferring a 10% lifetime probability for developing a thyroid nodule [3, 10]. Thyroid nodules are more common in elderly persons, in women, and in areas with iodine deficiency and with a history of childhood radiation exposure [6, 11]. The prevalence of nodular thyroid disease is high so the main purpose of thyroid nodule evaluation is to determine which nodules are malignant or require surgical intervention.

History and Physical Examination

Clinical evaluation begins with a complete medical history and thyroid palpation. Both benign and malignant disorders can cause thyroid nodules (Table 3.1). Attention should be directed to information on prior history of radiation treatment of the head and neck, rate of growth of the mass (location, size, and consistency), associated cervical lymphadenopathy, local symptoms (pain, dysphonia, dyspnea, or dysphagia), and other associated symptoms of hypothyroidism or hyperthyroidism. Most patients will have no symptoms during evaluation as the majority of thyroid nodules will be discovered incidentally. Malignancy rate in younger and older patients is increased three- to four-fold when compared to adults [12, 13].

Family history should be obtained, paying special attention to a history of medullary thyroid carcinoma (MTC), papillary thyroid carcinoma, multiple endocrine neoplasia types 2A and 2B, familial polyposis disease, Cowden disease, Carney complex, Gardner syndrome, and other rare diseases [14–17]. Table 3.2 shows findings suggestive of increased risk of malignancy potential.

Table 3.1 Common causes of thyroid nodules

Common causes of thyroid nodules
Benign nodular goiter
Thyroiditis
Cysts
Primary thyroid cancer
Papillary carcinoma
Follicular carcinoma
Hurtle cell carcinoma
C cell-derived carcinoma, medullary carcinoma
Anaplastic carcinoma
Metastatic cancer
Lymphoma

M. L. Griebeler
Cleveland Clinic Lerner College of Medicine, Endocrinology and Metabolism Institute, Cleveland, OH, USA
e-mail: griebem@ccf.org

H. Gharib (✉)
Division of Endocrinology, Mayo Clinic College of Medicine, Rochester, MN, USA
e-mail: gharib.hossein@mayo.edu

Table 3.2 Findings of increased malignancy potential

Findings of increased malignancy potential
Prior history of head and neck irradiation
Family history of MTC, MEN type 2, PTC, or other syndromes
Age <14 or >70 years
Male sex
Growing nodule, firm or hard consistency, fixed
Cervical adenopathy
Persistent dysphonia, dysphagia, dyspnea, or vocal cord paralysis

Diagnostic Evaluation

Serum Markers

Besides a complete history and physical exam, all patients should have a serum TSH measurement [8, 18]. If the TSH is low, a thyroid scintigraphy should be performed to determine the functional status of the nodule as low TSH suggests overt or subclinical hyperthyroidism, hyperfunctioning ("hot"), and autonomous functioning adenoma. If indeed the nodule is found to be "hot," it is unlikely to be malignant, and FNA should be deferred [19].

TSH levels are independent predictors of malignancy in patients with thyroid nodules: the risk of malignancy increases as the TSH levels also increase [20, 21]. Routine measurement of serum thyroglobulin (Tg) for initial evaluation of thyroid nodules is not recommended [8].

Calcitonin is a marker for detection of C-cell hyperplasia and MTC, and levels >10 pg/mL have high sensitivity for the detection of MTC. Calcitonin should be measured in high-risk patients, such as in those with a family history of MTC, with high clinical suspicion of MTC by US or cytology, or with MEN 2 syndromes. Overall, the prevalence of MTC is low enough in the United States that both the recent ATA and AACE Guidelines recommend "neither for or against routine calcitonin measurement" [8, 22].

Thyroid Ultrasound and Indication for Fine-Needle Aspiration (FNA)

Ultrasonography, more sensitive than palpation, is the imaging of choice to detect a thyroid nodule. Thyroid ultrasound (US) with survey of the cervical lymph nodes should be performed in all patients with a suspected thyroid nodule, a goiter, or after an incidentally found nodule by other imaging modalities [8]. Thyroid US is noninvasive and inexpensive, has a sensitivity of 95%, and can identify nodules usually not palpated on the physical exam. Ultrasound provides a very good evaluation of nodule size, dimensions, structure, and any possible suspicious features. It can also differentiate solid from cystic nodules [8, 22, 23].

Ultrasound-guided fine-needle aspiration (FNA) is the procedure of choice (gold standard) in the evaluation of thyroid nodules and is the most accurate test for determining malignancy [8, 22]. It is safe, cost-effective, and preferred over palpation-guided leading to much lower rates of non-diagnostic and false-negative cytology results [24]. When performed by experienced physicians, adequate sample can be obtained from solid nodules in 90–97% of aspirations [24]. There is no single ultrasound characteristic of malignancy but instead a combination of features that need to be evaluated as predictors of malignancy [10].

The most recent American Thyroid Association guidelines classify nodules into five risk groups based on a constellation of sonographic pattern [8], while the current AACE guidelines offer a more practical, three-tier risk analysis, including low (<1%), intermediate (5–15%), and high risk (50–90%) [22]. Per ATA guidelines, the recommendations for diagnostic FNA are the following:

- Nodules ≥1 cm in greatest dimension with high suspicious sonographic pattern.
- Nodules ≥1 cm in greatest dimension with intermediate suspicion sonographic pattern.
- Nodules ≥1.5 cm in greatest dimension with low suspicion sonographic pattern.
- FNA may be considered in nodules ≥2 cm in greatest dimension with very low suspicion sonographic pattern (spongiform). Observation is an option.
- Cystic nodules are considered to have very low suspicion sonographic pattern and don't require FNA.

The nodular characteristics mostly associated with being predictive of malignancy include shape that is taller than wide in the transverse dimension, hypoechogenicity, irregular margins, microcalcifications, and absent halo. These characteristics have high specificity, but the positive predictive value is lowered by their relatively low sensitivity. None of these features alone is enough to differentiate a benign from malignant lesion [25–28]. Findings such as isoechogenicity and spongiform appearance are features of benignity [29]. Complex nodules with solid and cystic components often with a dominant cystic part are frequently benign.

Numbers of nodules and size are not predictive of malignancy. In a gland with multiple nodules, the selection for FNA should be based on the US features rather than size alone. Cancer is not less frequent in small nodules so diameter cutoff alone to evaluate cancer risk is not recommended [30, 31]. Ultrasound should only be performed in patients with known or suspected thyroid nodules or the presence of risk factors [8]. Advances in diagnostic imaging have improved the management of thyroid nodules, but it also increased the discovery of incidentalomas (small thyroid nodules with <1 cm in diameter).

Other Imaging

Other techniques like MRI and CT scan are not recommended as routine tests as they are expensive and rarely diagnostic. CT scan and MRI have more value to assess goiter size, substernal extension, or extension to surround structures. Iodine contrast should be avoided as it decreases subsequent iodine 131 uptake [22]. Thyroid scintigraphy should be performed when there is suspicion of autonomy of the nodule (low TSH) suggesting overt subclinical hyperthyroidism.

Cytology

Thyroid FNA slides should be reviewed by a cytopathologist with experience in thyroid. FNA has reduced the number of surgical procedures in patients with nodules by more than 50% and substantially increased the malignancy yield at thyroidectomy [32]. An adequate sample is highly accurate for diagnosing thyroid cancer. Biopsy results may be classified as satisfactory or unsatisfactory (non-diagnostic). To be considered diagnostic or satisfactory, the aspirate needs to contain no less than six groups of well-preserved thyroid epithelial cells consisting of at least ten cells in each group [33].

The *Bethesda System for Reporting Thyroid Cytopathology* is the most commonly used. Currently there are six diagnostic categories: benign; malignant; suspicious for malignancy; follicular neoplasm or suspicious for a follicular neoplasm (FN/SFN); follicular lesion or atypia of undetermined significance (FLUS or AUS); non-diagnostic (Table 3.3) [33] [34]. The expertise of the cytopathologist is crucial in correct and clear interpretation of FNA slides and classification of the cytology [35].

Overall, 6–11% of the FNAs will be unsatisfactory (non-diagnostic), usually because of sampling error, bloody smears, or poor technique [36–38]. Biopsy should be repeated, but ultimately, about 5% of nodules will still be unsatisfactory [8, 39–42]. The false-negative rates range from 1 to 11% but usually will be less than 5% in most clinics with enough FNA experience [41, 43].

Management, Therapy, and Follow-Up

Benign Thyroid Nodule

The most common benign lesions include colloid nodule, macrofollicular adenoma, benign cyst, and lymphocytic thyroiditis. The majority of these nodules do not need specific treatment once malignancy and abnormal thyroid function are excluded [1, 8, 22]. If patient reports local symptoms including dysphagia, choking, dysphonia, dyspnea, or pain, surgical treatment may be warranted. The clinician should make sure that the symptoms are caused by the thyroid mass or enlargement, and not due to other processes such as pulmonary, cardiac, or esophageal disorders [10]. Patients with a single toxic nodule or a toxic multinodular goiter may be treated with surgery or radioiodine. Treatment with 131 I for large toxic nodules is not preferred as these nodules usually require high doses and are associated with more side effects [18].

Routine use of T4 suppressive therapy has no role in the management of benign thyroid nodules [8, 22]. Therapy with levothyroxine may be associated with increased risk of atrial fibrillation, other cardiac abnormalities, and reduced bone density, so therapy should be avoided in patients with large nodules, long-standing goiters, low TSH levels, postmenopausal women, and men older than 60 years [44–46].

The chance of a false-negative FNA (malignancy rate) is reported around 1–2% only [47, 48], and an initial benign FNA has negligible mortality risk in long-term follow-up [49]. Some studies report an increased risk of malignancy in nodules greater than 4 cm due to decreased FNA accuracy and recommend surgery [50–52], but based on current evi-

Table 3.3 Bethesda system; data compiled from Baloch et al. [33]

The Bethesda system for reporting thyroid cytopathology: implied risk of malignancy and recommended clinical management			
Diagnostic category	Risk of malignancy (%)	Actual risk of malignancy	Management
Non-diagnostic	1–4	20 (9–32)	Repeat FNA with ultrasound guidance
Benign	0–3	2.5 (1–10)	Clinical follow-up
Atypia of undetermined significance/follicular lesion of undetermined significance	5–15	14 (6–48)	Repeat FNA
Follicular neoplasm/ suspicious for a follicular neoplasm	15–30	25 (14–34)	Surgical lobectomy
Suspicious for malignancy	60–75	70 (53–97)	Near-total thyroidectomy or surgical lobectomy
Malignancy	97–99	99 (94–100)	Near-total thyroidectomy

dence, it is still unclear if patients with nodules with greater than 4 cm and benign cytology carry higher risk of malignancy [8].

The follow-up of thyroid nodules with benign cytology should be determined by risk stratification according to ultrasonography pattern [8]. The current guidelines of the American Thyroid Association published recommend that nodules with high suspicion US pattern should undergo repeat US and US-guided FNA within 12 months. Nodules with low to intermediate suspicion US pattern should have repeat US at 12–24 months; in nodules with very low suspicion US pattern, the utility of surveillance US and assessment of nodule growth as an indication to consider repetition of FNA are limited. If US is considered, it should be done at >24 months. If the nodule has undergone repeat US-guided FNA with a second benign cytology results, US surveillance for evaluation of malignancy is no longer warranted [8].

Malignant Thyroid Nodule

If cytologic results are positive for thyroid malignancy, surgery is almost always indicated [8] [22]. Consultation with an experienced endocrine surgeon is preferred and should be done as soon as possible. This category includes papillary cancer, follicular carcinoma, Hurthle cell (oncocytic) carcinoma, medullary cancer, thyroid lymphoma, anaplastic cancer, and metastatic cancer to the thyroid. Metastatic disease to the thyroid is rare [53] and usually precludes immediate surgery until further investigation for the primary site is completed. Full workup should also be performed for anaplastic carcinoma and lymphoma [18].

An active surveillance approach may be considered in a small subgroup of patients including those with a very low-risk tumors (papillary thyroid microcarcinoma without evident metastasis or local invasion), high surgical risk patients due to comorbid conditions, and patients with short remaining life spans [8]. Most patients with papillary thyroid carcinoma have an indolent course, and a few prospective studies have reported very good outcomes with very low rate of loco-regional recurrence and distant metastasis, and this approach may be considered in thyroid micro-carcinoma (tumors <1 cm in diameter) [54].

Suspicious for Malignancy

This category represents the cytologic results with strong suspicious for malignancy but lacking clear diagnostic criteria, with an estimated cancer risk of 60–75% [34]. Usually surgical management is similar to a malignant cytology, depending on clinical risk factors, sonographic features,

patient preference, and possible mutation testing. As more data become available from the molecular testing field, management of this category may change in the future. Mutation testing could improve risk stratification prior to surgery, including possibly BRAF mutations and seven-gene panel of mutations (including BRAF, RAS< RET/PTC, with or without PAX9/PPARy) [55, 56].

Indeterminate Thyroid Nodule (AUS/FLUS and FN/SFN)

This group carries the most challenging diagnostic dilemma. In this category a clear cytologic diagnosis cannot be made, and examples include follicular neoplasms, Hurthle cell neoplasm, atypical PTC, or lymphoma. Indeterminate cytology also includes AUS/FLUS (atypia of undetermined significance/follicular lesion of undetermined significance) and FN/SFN (follicular neoplasm/suspicious for follicular neoplasm).

According to the Bethesda system, AUS/FLUS compromises specimens that contain cells with architectural and/or nuclear atypia that is more pronounced than expected for benign changes but not sufficient to be placed on the higher-risk categories [57]. Frequency range is around 7% of reports, and the risk of cancer is between 6 and 48%, with a mean risk of 16% [58].

Treatment options for AUS/FLUS include a repeat FNA, molecular testing, observation, and surgical intervention. Providers should take into consideration clinical and ultrasound risk factors and patient preferences when making management decisions. Of repeated FNAs 10–30% yield again AUS/FLUS [59–61]. Thyroid core needle biopsy could also be considered [62]. Molecular testing is another option commonly used in this subset of patients. Mutation testing for BRAF has a high specificity but low sensitivity [63, 64], while a panel of mutations (BRAF, NRAS, HRAS, KRAS, RET/PTC1, RET/PTC3, PAX8/PPARy) has a higher sensitivity [55] [65]. Recent studies are also using sonographic features to estimate risk of malignancy [66].

FN/SFN cytology compromises follicular cells arranged in an altered architectural pattern characterized by cell crowding and/or microfollicle formation and lacking nuclear features of papillary carcinoma or compromised almost exclusively of oncocytic (Hurthle) cells [33]. This category carries a 14–33% risk of malignancy (mean 26%), with a frequency of 1–25% (mean 10%) of all thyroid FNA samples [58].

For this category usually surgical excision for diagnosis had been an established practice. Again, with the introduction and availability of molecular testing, this can be used to supplement malignancy risk assessment after considering the clinical and ultrasound risk factors and patient preferences [8]. Risk stratification with molecular testing including seven-gene panel shows a sensitivity of 57–75% and specificity of 97–100%, PPV of 87–100%, and NMPV of 79–86% [55, 65].

Non-diagnostic

Patients with non-diagnostic biopsies are those that do not meet specified criteria (the presence of at least six follicular cell groups, each containing 10–15 cells derived from at least two aspirates of a nodule) [33]. If initial FNA biopsy is non-diagnostic, it should be repeated with possible onsite cytological assessment [8, 22, 67]. If the results are again non-diagnostic, core needle biopsy, close observation, or surgery should be considered, the latter especially if there are suspicious pattern on ultrasound, clinical risk factors, and growth of the nodule. A repeat FNA after initial non-diagnostic cytology may yield a 75% diagnostic cytology in solid nodules and 50% in cystic nodules [68].

Figure 3.1 shows an algorithm with a summary for the diagnosis and management of palpable thyroid nodules.

Special Situations

Thyroid Nodule During Pregnancy

The majority of the thyroid nodules during pregnancy are pre-existing, but in some cases they can be initially diagnosed. Overall they should be managed exactly the same way in non-pregnant women except that radioactive agents should be avoided [22] [69]. If the clinical and imaging features are suspicious for malignancy, patient will require a FNA biopsy, regardless of the gestational age [70]. Some studies showed that the cancer behavior during pregnancy is the same when compared to the general population, without any differences in survival rates or recurrence. Suppressive therapy with levothyroxine for thyroid nodules is not recommended.

Patient's preferences should always be considered, and a multi-disciplinary approach including an endocrinologist, pathologist, obstetrician, surgeon, and anesthesiologist is recommended. Women with no evidence of aggressive thyroid cancer may be reassured, and surgical treatment can be

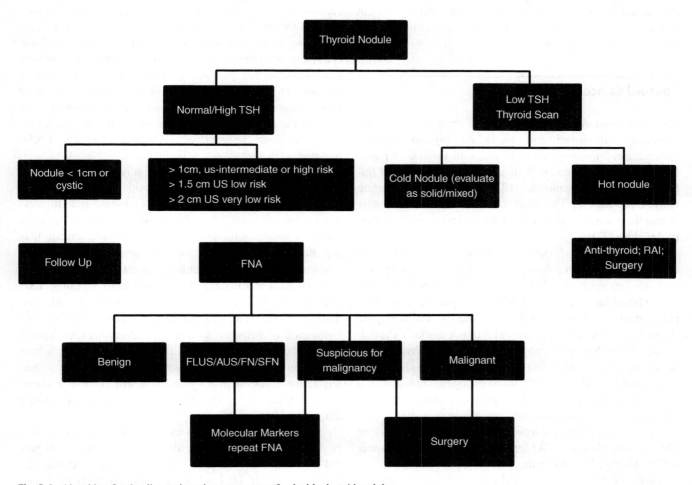

Fig. 3.1 Algorithm for the diagnosis and management of palpable thyroid nodules

performed after delivery [71]. The cytologic suspicious nodule is the most challenging situation during pregnancy. The malignancy rate is similar between pregnant women and non-pregnant women, so deferring surgical treatment to the postpartum is reasonable [72]. Some may recommend postponing FNA until delivery unless worrisome features are seen in the ultrasound as this may lead to possible thyroidectomy during pregnancy depending of the FNA results. If the outcome of the results will be unchanged, meaning that surgical treatment will be postponed, this will just expose the patient to anxiety regarding diagnosis and except management [73].

Thyroid Nodules in Children

The prevalence of thyroid nodules in children is up to 1.8%, and some cohort studies showed higher malignancy rates [74, 75]. These findings suggest that the surgical approach for thyroid nodules in children is more common than that in adults. The evaluation of nodular disease in children is similar to adults. Overall the prognosis of thyroid cancer in children remains good despite the increase prevalence of local metastatic disease [76]. As in adults, the most common thyroid cancer is the papillary.

Thyroid Cancer

The most common histologic types of thyroid cancers are follicular cell-derived and medullary thyroid cancers. *Follicular cell-derived cancer* includes all variants of papillary thyroid carcinoma (85% of all thyroid cancers) and follicular thyroid carcinoma (10–15% lesions, including Hürthle cell cancer). The other follicular cell-derived cancer is anaplastic carcinoma that accounts for less than 5% of thyroid tumors [77].

Medullary thyroid cancer originates in C cells and accounts for less than 5% of thyroid malignancies. While the majority has sporadic MTC, around 25% of patients may have a hereditary form as part of the multiple endocrine neoplasia type 2 syndromes (MEN 2). They will also require thyroidectomy and are followed with tumor markers like calcitonin. Even though the majority of medullary thyroid cancer is sporadic, genetic testing is recommended to all patients for evaluation including RET proto-oncogene mutation. If a mutation is found, all family members should undergo screening for the same mutation as early as possible.

The recently published recommendations of the American Thyroid Association (ATA) for differentiated thyroid cancer will be reviewed briefly in the following [8].

Goals of thyroidectomy include removing the tumor, improving overall disease-specific survival, and decreasing the rate of recurrence and morbidity. All patients should undergo pre-operative neck ultrasound for evaluation of lymphadenopathy. *Risk stratification* after surgery is paramount to outline a strategy for radioiodine treatment, follow-up plan, and TSH suppression.

For tumors <1 cm, without extra-thyroidal extension or regional lymph node metastasis, a thyroid lobectomy may be sufficient. For tumors 1–4 cm, without extra-thyroidal extension or lymph nodes, total thyroidectomy or, in selected patients, a lobectomy may be considered. Tumors greater or equal to 4 cm, with extra-thyroidal extension or metastases, should always undergo total thyroidectomy.

American Thyroid Association Risk Stratification System

ATA Low Risk

Patients with *papillary thyroid cancer* with no local or distant metastasis; all macroscopic tumor has been resected, no tumor invasion of loco-regional tissues or structures, no aggressive histology (tall cell, hobnail variant, columnar cell carcinoma); if I131 is given, no RAI avid metastatic foci outside the thyroid bed on the first post-treatment whole body RAI scan, no vascular invasion, clinical N0 or <5 pathologic N1 micro metastases (<0.2 cm in the largest dimension); *intrathyroidal, encapsulated follicular variant of papillary thyroid cancer; intrathyroidal, well-differentiated follicular thyroid cancer* with capsular invasion and no or minimal (<4 foci) vascular invasion; *intrathyroidal, papillary microcarcinoma, unifocal or multifocal, including V600E BRAF mutated.*

For this group of patients, especially in tumors <1 cm (unifocal or multifocal), there is no evidence suggesting that radioactive iodine (RAI) improves disease-specific and disease-free survival. Overall post-surgical RAI is not indicated. In patients with tumor size 1–4 cm, there are conflicting data that RAI improves disease-free survival and post-surgical RAI is not routinely indicated.

In patients that undergo total thyroidectomy, initial TSH goal is 0.5–2 mU/L if non-stimulated TG <0.2 ng/mL, and TSH goal is 0.1–0.5 mU/L if non-stimulated Tg >0.2 ng/mL. Evaluation of response to therapy includes at least annual thyroglobulin testing and neck ultrasound. Diagnostic whole body scan is not routinely recommended. Follow-up is usually annually for the first 5 years. If serum TG level is rising or neck ultrasound is abnormal, patient may require further diagnostic tests.

In patients undergoing lobectomy, post-op serum TG may be considered as well as neck ultrasound. Although after partial thyroidectomy serum TG will be undetectable, an increase in stable TG levels should give rise to suspicion of recurrent disease warranting further evaluation. RAI remnant ablation is not recommended and initial TSH goal should be 0.5–2 mU/L. Evaluation for response to therapy includes annual ultrasound and consideration for thyroglobulin testing.

ATA Intermediate Risk

Patients with microscopic invasion of tumor into the peri-thyroidal soft tissues, RAI avid metastatic foci in the neck on the first post-treatment whole body RAI scan, aggressive histology, papillary thyroid cancer with vascular invasion, clinical N1 or ≥5 pathologic N1 with all involved lymph nodes <3 cm in largest dimension, intrathyroid, papillary thyroid cancer, primary tumor 1–4 cm, V600E BRAF mutated, multifocal papillary micro-carcinoma with extra-thyroidal extension and V600E BRAF mutated.

In patients with tumor size >4 cm, post-surgical RAI may be considered, especially in patients with adverse features. In patients with microscopic extra-thyroidal extension (any size tumors), post-surgical RAI is usually favored based on risk of recurrence of disease.

In patients with central compartment neck lymph node metastasis, post-surgical RAI is usually favored, mainly due to higher risk of persistent and recurrent disease, especially in larger tumors (>2 cm) or clinical evidence of lymph nodes or extra-nodal extension.

Initial therapy for these patients includes total thyroidectomy, neck dissection for clinical N1 disease, and possible prophylactic central neck dissection. Diagnostic RAI scanning may be considered. Surveillance includes serum thyroglobulin and ultrasound of the neck.

RAI scanning should be considered in patients with intermediate risk. For remnant ablation 30 mCI may be considered. For adjuvant therapy, usually up to 150 mCi is given. Initial TSH goal is 0.1–0.5 mU/L, and evaluation for response to therapy includes thyroglobulin testing, neck ultrasound, and consideration for diagnostic whole body scan. Again, periodic (annual) evaluation with thyroglobulin (non-stimulated) and ultrasound of the neck are recommended.

ATA High Risk

This group of patients includes macroscopic invasion of tumor into the peri-thyroidal soft tissues (gross extra-thyroidal extension), incomplete tumor resection, distant metastases, and post-operative serum thyroglobulin suggestive of distant metastases.

In patients with ATA high risk, the body of evidence suggests that RAI improves disease-specific survival and disease-free survival; therefore routine RAI use is recommended. Initial therapy includes total thyroidectomy, therapeutic neck dissection, and possible prophylactic central neck dissection. Post-operatively, monitoring with thyroglobulin, ultrasound, and RAI scanning are recommended.

RAI therapy is routinely recommended with up to 150 mCI as adjuvant therapy. For known structural disease, empiric 100–200 mCI or dosimetry-guided dosing is recommended. Initial TSH goal is <0.1 mU/L. This group of patients is at increased risk for recurrence, and follow-up should include thyroglobulin testing, neck ultrasound, whole body scan, and CT/MRI or FDG/PET scanning.

Summary

Thyroid nodules are very common and are usually benign; only around 5% carry the risk of malignancy. The challenge in the management of thyroid nodules is to reliably identify benign nodules and diagnose malignant thyroid disease as early as possible. Thyroid evaluation starts with a careful history and physical exam followed by thyroid function tests and ultrasound exam. An initial low TSH requires additional tests for evaluation of hyperthyroidism. When TSH is normal and US shows an indeterminate or suspicious nodule, an US-FNA should follow as it remains the single most important procedure for differentiating benign from malignant thyroid nodules. When cytology is suspicious for malignancy, surgery is usually recommended. Benign thyroid nodules can be followed clinically and with serial ultrasound images. An indeterminate nodule poses a clinical challenge; treatment may include observation, molecular markers, or surgery. The most common type of thyroid cancer is papillary thyroid cancer. Treatment usually entails total thyroidectomy with or without lymph node dissection. Depending on risk stratification, some patients may benefit from radioactive iodine therapy. Long-term follow-up includes ultrasound of the neck, TSH, and thyroglobulin. The overall prognosis of thyroid cancer remains good.

Appendix

References

1. Hegedus L. Clinical practice. The thyroid nodule. N Engl J Med. 2004;351(17):1764–71.
2. Dean DS, Gharib H. Epidemiology of thyroid nodules. Best practice & research. Clin Endocrinol Metab. 2008;22(6):901–11.
3. Tan GH, Gharib H. Thyroid incidentalomas: management approaches to nonpalpable nodules discovered incidentally on thyroid imaging. Ann Intern Med. 1997;126(3):226–31.
4. Guth S, Theune U, Aberle J, Galach A, Bamberger CM. Very high prevalence of thyroid nodules detected by high frequency (13 MHz) ultrasound examination. Eur J Clin Investig. 2009;39(8):699–706.
5. Ezzat S, Sarti DA, Cain DR, Braunstein GD. Thyroid incidentalomas. Prevalence by palpation and ultrasonography. Arch Intern Med. 1994;154(16):1838–40.

6. Mazzaferri EL. Management of a solitary thyroid nodule. N Engl J Med. 1993;328(8):553–9.

7. Brito JP, Al Nofal A, Montori VM, Hay ID, Morris JC. The impact of subclinical disease and mechanism of detection on the rise in thyroid cancer incidence: a population-based study in Olmsted County, Minnesota during 1935 through 2012. Thyroid. 2015;25(9):999–1007.

8. Haugen BR, Alexander EK, Bible KC, Doherty GM, Mandel SJ, Nikiforov YE, et al. 2015 American Thyroid Association management guidelines for adult patients with thyroid nodules and differentiated thyroid cancer: the American Thyroid Association guidelines task force on thyroid nodules and differentiated thyroid cancer. Thyroid. 2016;26(1):1–133.

9. Davies L, Welch HG. Current thyroid cancer trends in the United States. JAMA Otolaryngol Head Neck Surg. 2014;140(4):317–22.

10. Gharib H, Papini E. Thyroid nodules: clinical importance, assessment, and treatment. Endocrinol Metab Clin N Am. 2007;36(3):707–35. vi

11. Volzke H, Ludemann J, Robinson DM, Spieker KW, Schwahn C, Kramer A, et al. The prevalence of undiagnosed thyroid disorders in a previously iodine-deficient area. Thyroid. 2003;13(8):803–10.

12. Corrias A, Einaudi S, Chiorboli E, Weber G, Crino A, Andreo M, et al. Accuracy of fine needle aspiration biopsy of thyroid nodules in detecting malignancy in childhood: comparison with conventional clinical, laboratory, and imaging approaches. J Clin Endocrinol Metab. 2001;86(10):4644–8.

13. Rosai J, Carcangiu ML. Pathology of thyroid tumors: some recent and old questions. Hum Pathol. 1984;15(11):1008–12.

14. Heshmati HM, Gharib H, van Heerden JA, Sizemore GW. Advances and controversies in the diagnosis and management of medullary thyroid carcinoma. Am J Med. 1997;103(1):60–9.

15. Loh KC. Familial nonmedullary thyroid carcinoma: a meta-review of case series. Thyroid. 1997;7(1):107–13.

16. Punales MK, da Rocha AP, Meotti C, Gross JL, Maia AL. Clinical and oncological features of children and young adults with multiple endocrine neoplasia type 2A. Thyroid. 2008;18(12):1261–8.

17. Farooq A, Walker LJ, Bowling J, Audisio RA. Cowden syndrome. Cancer Treat Rev. 2010;36(8):577–83.

18. Gharib H, Papini E, Paschke R, Duick DS, Valcavi R, Hegedus L, et al. American Association of Clinical Endocrinologists, Associazione Medici Endocrinologi, and European Thyroid Association medical guidelines for clinical practice for the diagnosis and management of thyroid nodules. Endocr Pract. 2010;16(Suppl 1):1–43.

19. Fiore E, Rago T, Provenzale MA, Scutari M, Ugolini C, Basolo F, et al. Lower levels of TSH are associated with a lower risk of papillary thyroid cancer in patients with thyroid nodular disease: thyroid autonomy may play a protective role. Endocr Relat Cancer. 2009;16(4):1251–60.

20. Boelaert K, Horacek J, Holder RL, Watkinson JC, Sheppard MC, Franklyn JA. Serum thyrotropin concentration as a novel predictor of malignancy in thyroid nodules investigated by fine-needle aspiration. J Clin Endocrinol Metab. 2006;91(11):4295–301.

21. Haymart MR, Repplinger DJ, Leverson GE, Elson DF, Sippel RS, Jaume JC, et al. Higher serum thyroid stimulating hormone level in thyroid nodule patients is associated with greater risks of differentiated thyroid cancer and advanced tumor stage. J Clin Endocrinol Metab. 2008;93(3):809–14.

22. Gharib H, Papini E, Garber JR, Duick DS, Harrell RM, Hegedus L, et al. American Association of Clinical Endocrinologists, American College of Endocrinology, and Associazione Medici Endocrinologi medical guidelines for clinical practice for the diagnosis and management of thyroid nodules--2016 update. Endocr Pract. 2016;22(5):622–39.

23. Solbiati L, Osti V, Cova L, Tonolini M. Ultrasound of thyroid, parathyroid glands and neck lymph nodes. Eur Radiol. 2001;11(12):2411–24.

24. Danese D, Sciacchitano S, Farsetti A, Andreoli M, Pontecorvi A. Diagnostic accuracy of conventional versus sonography-guided fine-needle aspiration biopsy of thyroid nodules. Thyroid. 1998;8(1):15–21.

25. Leenhardt L, Erdogan MF, Hegedus L, Mandel SJ, Paschke R, Rago T, et al. 2013 European thyroid association guidelines for cervical ultrasound scan and ultrasound-guided techniques in the postoperative management of patients with thyroid cancer. Eur Thyroid J. 2013;2(3):147–59.

26. Cappelli C, Castellano M, Pirola I, Cumetti D, Agosti B, Gandossi E, et al. The predictive value of ultrasound findings in the management of thyroid nodules. QJM. 2007;100(1):29–35.

27. Remonti LR, Kramer CK, Leitao CB, Pinto LC, Gross JL. Thyroid ultrasound features and risk of carcinoma: a systematic review and meta-analysis of observational studies. Thyroid. 2015;25(5):538–50.

28. Papini E. The dilemma of non-palpable thyroid nodules. J Endocrinol Investig. 2003;26(1):3–4.

29. Moon WJ, Jung SL, Lee JH, Na DG, Baek JH, Lee YH, et al. Benign and malignant thyroid nodules: US differentiation--multicenter retrospective study. Radiology. 2008;247(3):762–70.

30. Kim EK, Park CS, Chung WY, Oh KK, Kim DI, Lee JT, et al. New sonographic criteria for recommending fine-needle aspiration biopsy of nonpalpable solid nodules of the thyroid. AJR. Am J Roentgenol. 2002;178(3):687–91.

31. Papini E, Guglielmi R, Bianchini A, Crescenzi A, Taccogna S, Nardi F, et al. Risk of malignancy in nonpalpable thyroid nodules: predictive value of ultrasound and color-Doppler features. J Clin Endocrinol Metab. 2002;87(5):1941–6.

32. Werk EE Jr, Vernon BM, Gonzalez JJ, Ungaro PC, McCoy RC. Cancer in thyroid nodules. A community hospital survey. Arch Intern Med. 1984;144(3):474–6.

33. Baloch ZW, LiVolsi VA, Asa SL, Rosai J, Merino MJ, Randolph G, et al. Diagnostic terminology and morphologic criteria for cytologic diagnosis of thyroid lesions: a synopsis of the National Cancer Institute Thyroid Fine-Needle Aspiration State of the Science Conference. Diagn Cytopathol. 2008;36(6):425–37.

34. Cibas ES, Ali SZ. The Bethesda system for reporting thyroid cytopathology. Thyroid. 2009;19(11):1159–65.

35. Cibas ES, Baloch ZW, Fellegara G, LiVolsi VA, Raab SS, Rosai J, et al. A prospective assessment defining the limitations of thyroid nodule pathologic evaluation. Ann Intern Med. 2013;159(5):325–32.

36. Bongiovanni M, Spitale A, Faquin WC, Mazzucchelli L, Baloch ZW. The Bethesda system for reporting thyroid cytopathology: a meta-analysis. Acta Cytol. 2012;56(4):333–9.

37. Theoharis CG, Schofield KM, Hammers L, Udelsman R, Chhieng DC. The Bethesda thyroid fine-needle aspiration classification system: year 1 at an academic institution. Thyroid. 2009;19(11):1215–23.

38. Bohacek L, Milas M, Mitchell J, Siperstein A, Berber E. Diagnostic accuracy of surgeon-performed ultrasound-guided fine-needle aspiration of thyroid nodules. Ann Surg Oncol. 2012;19(1):45–51.

39. Gharib H. Fine-needle aspiration biopsy of thyroid nodules: advantages, limitations, and effect. Mayo Clinic Proc Mayo Clinic. 1994;69(1):44–9.

40. Gharib H, Goellner JR. Fine-needle aspiration biopsy of thyroid nodules. Endocr Pract. 1995;1(6):410–7.

41. Gharib H, Goellner JR, Zinsmeister AR, Grant CS, Van Heerden JA. Fine-needle aspiration biopsy of the thyroid. The problem of suspicious cytologic findings. Ann Intern Med. 1984;101(1):25–8.

42. Yeh MW, Demircan O, Ituarte P, Clark OH. False-negative fine-needle aspiration cytology results delay treatment and adversely

affect outcome in patients with thyroid carcinoma. Thyroid. 2004;14(3):207–15.

43. Castro MR, Gharib H. Thyroid fine-needle aspiration biopsy: progress, practice, and pitfalls. Endocr Pract. 2003;9(2):128–36.

44. Uzzan B, Campos J, Cucherat M, Nony P, Boissel JP, Perret GY. Effects on bone mass of long term treatment with thyroid hormones: a meta-analysis. J Clin Endocrinol Metab. 1996;81(12):4278–89.

45. Sawin CT, Geller A, Wolf PA, Belanger AJ, Baker E, Bacharach P, et al. Low serum thyrotropin concentrations as a risk factor for atrial fibrillation in older persons. N Engl J Med. 1994;331(19):1249–52.

46. Parle JV, Maisonneuve P, Sheppard MC, Boyle P, Franklyn JA. Prediction of all-cause and cardiovascular mortality in elderly people from one low serum thyrotropin result: a 10-year cohort study. Lancet. 2001;358(9285):861–5.

47. Tee YY, Lowe AJ, Brand CA, Judson RT. Fine-needle aspiration may miss a third of all malignancy in palpable thyroid nodules: a comprehensive literature review. Ann Surg. 2007;246(5):714–20.

48. Orlandi A, Puscar A, Capriata E, Fideleff H. Repeated fine-needle aspiration of the thyroid in benign nodular thyroid disease: critical evaluation of long-term follow-up. Thyroid. 2005;15(3):274–8.

49. Nou E, Kwong N, Alexander LK, Cibas ES, Marqusee E, Alexander EK. Determination of the optimal time interval for repeat evaluation after a benign thyroid nodule aspiration. J Clin Endocrinol Metab. 2014;99(2):510–6.

50. Pinchot SN, Al-Wagih H, Schaefer S, Sippel R, Chen H. Accuracy of fine-needle aspiration biopsy for predicting neoplasm or carcinoma in thyroid nodules 4 cm or larger. Arch Surg. 2009;144(7):649–55.

51. Kuru B, Gulcelik NE, Gulcelik MA, Dincer H. The false-negative rate of fine-needle aspiration cytology for diagnosing thyroid carcinoma in thyroid nodules. Langenbeck's Arch Surg. 2010;395(2):127–32.

52. Wharry LI, McCoy KL, Stang MT, Armstrong MJ, LeBeau SO, Tublin ME, et al. Thyroid nodules (>/=4 cm): can ultrasound and cytology reliably exclude cancer? World J Surg. 2014;38(3):614–21.

53. Hegerova L, Griebeler ML, Reynolds JP, Henry MR, Gharib H. Metastasis to the thyroid gland: report of a large series from the Mayo Clinic. Am J Clin Oncol. 2015;38(4):338–42.

54. Ito Y, Miyauchi A, Kihara M, Higashiyama T, Kobayashi K, Miya A. Patient age is significantly related to the progression of papillary microcarcinoma of the thyroid under observation. Thyroid. 2014;24(1):27–34.

55. Nikiforov YE, Ohori NP, Hodak SP, Carty SE, LeBeau SO, Ferris RL, et al. Impact of mutational testing on the diagnosis and management of patients with cytologically indeterminate thyroid nodules: a prospective analysis of 1056 FNA samples. J Clin Endocrinol Metab. 2011;96(11):3390–7.

56. Moon HJ, Kwak JY, Kim EK, Choi JR, Hong SW, Kim MJ, et al. The role of BRAFV600E mutation and ultrasonography for the surgical management of a thyroid nodule suspicious for papillary thyroid carcinoma on cytology. Ann Surg Oncol. 2009;16(11):3125–31.

57. Krane JF, Vanderlaan PA, Faquin WC, Renshaw AA. The atypia of undetermined significance/follicular lesion of undetermined significance:malignant ratio: a proposed performance measure for reporting in the Bethesda System for thyroid cytopathology. Cancer Cytopathol. 2012;120(2):111–6.

58. Bongiovanni M, Crippa S, Baloch Z, Piana S, Spitale A, Pagni F, et al. Comparison of 5-tiered and 6-tiered diagnostic systems for the reporting of thyroid cytopathology: a multi-institutional study. Cancer Cytopathol. 2012;120(2):117–25.

59. Nayar R, Ivanovic M. The indeterminate thyroid fine-needle aspiration: experience from an academic center using terminology similar to that proposed in the 2007 National Cancer Institute Thyroid Fine Needle Aspiration State of the Science Conference. Cancer. 2009;117(3):195–202.

60. Baloch Z, LiVolsi VA, Jain P, Jain R, Aljada I, Mandel S, et al. Role of repeat fine-needle aspiration biopsy (FNAB) in the management of thyroid nodules. Diagn Cytopathol. 2003;29(4):203–6.

61. Yang J, Schnadig V, Logrono R, Wasserman PG. Fine-needle aspiration of thyroid nodules: a study of 4703 patients with histologic and clinical correlations. Cancer. 2007;111(5):306–15.

62. Na DG, Baek JH, Jung SL, Kim JH, Sung JY, Kim KS, et al. Core needle biopsy of the thyroid: 2016 consensus statement and recommendations from Korean Society of Thyroid Radiology. Korean J Radiol. 2017;18(1):217–37.

63. Kim SK, Hwang TS, Yoo YB, Han HS, Kim DL, Song KH, et al. Surgical results of thyroid nodules according to a management guideline based on the BRAF(V600E) mutation status. J Clin Endocrinol Metab. 2011;96(3):658–64.

64. Adeniran AJ, Hui P, Chhieng DC, Prasad ML, Schofield K, Theoharis C. BRAF mutation testing of thyroid fine-needle aspiration specimens enhances the predictability of malignancy in thyroid follicular lesions of undetermined significance. Acta Cytol. 2011;55(6):570–5.

65. Nikiforov YE, Steward DL, Robinson-Smith TM, Haugen BR, Klopper JP, Zhu Z, et al. Molecular testing for mutations in improving the fine-needle aspiration diagnosis of thyroid nodules. J Clin Endocrinol Metab. 2009;94(6):2092–8.

66. Yoo WS, Choi HS, Cho SW, Moon JH, Kim KW, Park HJ, et al. The role of ultrasound findings in the management of thyroid nodules with atypia or follicular lesions of undetermined significance. Clin Endocrinol (Oxf). 2014;80(5):735–42.

67. Orija IB, Pineyro M, Biscotti C, Reddy SS, Hamrahian AH. Value of repeating a nondiagnostic thyroid fine-needle aspiration biopsy. Endocr Pract. 2007;13(7):735–42.

68. Alexander EK, Heering JP, Benson CB, Frates MC, Doubilet PM, Cibas ES, et al. Assessment of nondiagnostic ultrasound-guided fine needle aspirations of thyroid nodules. J Clin Endocrinol Metab. 2002;87(11):4924–7.

69. Meier DA, Brill DR, Becker DV, Clarke SE, Silberstein EB, Royal HD, et al. Procedure guideline for therapy of thyroid disease with (131)iodine. J Nucl Med. 2002;43(6):856–61.

70. Abalovich M, Amino N, Barbour LA, Cobin RH, De Groot LJ, Glinoer D, et al. Management of thyroid dysfunction during pregnancy and postpartum: an Endocrine Society Clinical Practice Guideline. J Clin Endocrinol Metab. 2007;92(8 Suppl):S1–47.

71. Moosa M, Mazzaferri EL. Outcome of differentiated thyroid cancer diagnosed in pregnant women. J Clin Endocrinol Metab. 1997;82(9):2862–6.

72. Marley EF, Oertel YC. Fine-needle aspiration of thyroid lesions in 57 pregnant and postpartum women. Diagn Cytopathol. 1997;16(2):122–5.

73. Popoveniuc G, Jonklaas J. Thyroid nodules. Med Clin North Am. 2012;96(2):329–49.

74. Rallison ML, Dobyns BM, Keating FR Jr, Rall JE, Tyler FH. Thyroid nodularity in children. JAMA. 1975;233(10):1069–72.

75. Raab SS, Silverman JF, Elsheikh TM, Thomas PA, Wakely PE. Pediatric thyroid nodules: disease demographics and clinical management as determined by fine needle aspiration biopsy. Pediatrics. 1995;95(1):46–9.

76. Feinmesser R, Lubin E, Segal K, Noyek A. Carcinoma of the thyroid in children--a review. J Pediatr Endocrinol Metab. 1997;10(6):561–8.

77. Hundahl SA, Fleming ID, Fremgen AM, Menck HR. A National Cancer Data Base report on 53,856 cases of thyroid carcinoma treated in the U.S., 1985-1995 [see comments]. Cancer. 1998;83(12):2638–48.

Evaluation of Sellar Masses

Todd B. Nippoldt

Introduction

The clinical presentation of a patient with a sellar mass can include signs and symptoms of hormonal excess, hormonal deficiency, or of the mass itself such as vision loss or headache. Alternatively a sellar mass may be discovered incidentally on brain imaging performed for an unrelated reason. Autopsy and radiology studies suggest the prevalence of incidentally found pituitary masses to be approximately 10% of the population [1]. Clinically significant pituitary lesions are diagnosed in 1 in 1000 people [2]. Although a wide variety of diseases can manifest as sellar or parasellar masses (Table 4.1), the vast majority of clinically apparent and incidentally found lesions are pituitary adenomas or Rathke's cleft cyst [3]. The effects of excess hormonal secretion (prolactin (PRL), growth hormone (GH), corticotrophin (ACTH), thyrotropin (TSH)) from functioning pituitary adenomas can lead to significant morbidity and increased mortality. Hypopituitarism can be a consequence of any mass lesion in the sellar or parasellar region.

In this chapter the clinical, radiologic, and laboratory evaluation of patients with a sellar mass will be discussed. As over 94% of sellar masses are either pituitary adenomas or Rathke's cleft cysts [4], management of these lesions will be emphasized. A limited discussion of the less common lesions is included emphasizing those characteristics that help differentiate them from adenomas and Rathke's cleft cysts.

T. B. Nippoldt (✉)
Department of Endocrinology, Diabetes and Nutrition, Mayo Clinic College of Medicine, Rochester, MN, USA
e-mail: nippoldt.todd@mayo.edu

Key Points to the Diagnosis

Radiologic Findings

Sellar, parasellar, and pituitary stalk pathology (Table 4.1) can be identified by abnormalities on plain X-rays, computed tomography (CT), or magnetic resonance imaging (MRI). Enlargement of the boney sella turcica, erosion of the clinoid processes, and intra- or supra-sellar calcifications are findings of pituitary lesions on skull X-ray. Cross-sectional imaging defines the size of the mass, degree of parasellar extension, and relationship with other intracranial structures and provides imaging characteristics that suggest the etiology of the lesion (Table 4.2). MRI scanning is superior to CT scanning in defining sellar masses and should be obtained in all patients if possible [11]. Clinical decisions regarding further evaluation and management depend on findings that are most accurately demonstrated by MRI imaging.

Pituitary adenomas are arbitrarily categorized by size as microadenomas (<10 mm) or macroadenomas (≥10 mm). On high-resolution CT, pituitary adenomas are typically hypodense compared with the normal gland on both unenhanced and contrast-enhanced images. On MRI imaging [12, 13], 80–90% of microadenomas appear as a focal hypointense lesion compared with the normal gland (Fig. 4.1) on unenhanced T1-weighted images. After gadolinium, an adenoma typically enhances less avidly than the rest of the gland (Fig. 4.2a). On T2-weighted images, up to 50% of microadenomas are hyperintense. Other findings that can be seen with pituitary adenomas are focal erosion of the sella floor or focal convexity of the superior surface of the gland. Deviation of the pituitary stalk can be seen with microadenomas but may simply represent normal variation. Macroadenomas have similar signal characteristics as microadenomas. Comparing the pre- and post-contrast signal to the normal pituitary may not be possible as the normal pituitary may be compressed and totally obscured by the macroadenoma. Macroadenomas may grow and extend outside of the confines

© Springer Nature Switzerland AG 2022
F. Bandeira et al. (eds.), *Endocrinology and Diabetes*, https://doi.org/10.1007/978-3-030-90684-9_4

Table 4.1 Sellar, parasellar, and pituitary stalk lesions [3–10]

Neoplastic	Cysts	Inflammatory/infiltrative	Vascular
Pituitary adenoma	Rathke's cleft cyst	Lymphocytic hypophysitis	Carotid aneurysm
Craniopharyingioma	Arachnoid cyst	Granulomatous hypophysitis	
Chordoma	Epidermoid cyst	Drug induced hypophysitis	
Metastasis		Sarcoidosis	
Meningioma		Langerhans cell histiocytosis	
Germ cell tumor		Eosinophilic infiltration (Churg–Strauss)	
Glioma		Infection: bacterial, mycobacterial, fungal, protozoal	
Granular cell tumor (pituicytoma)			
Hypothalamic neuronal hamartoma			
Dermoid			
Primary plasmacytoma			
Primary lymphoma			
Cavernous sinus hemangioma			
Pituitary carcinoma			

Table 4.2 Imaging characteristics of selected sellar masses

	MRI			CT		
	T1	T2	+ GAD	No contrast	Contrast	Clinical hints
Pituitary adenoma	Hypointense[a] (80–90%)	Hyperintense[a] (50%)	Hypointense[a]	Hypodense[a]	Hypodense[a]	Hormonal excess syndrome
Rathke's cleft cyst	Hyperintense[a] (50%) Hypointense[a] (50%)	Hyperintense[a] (70%) Iso- or hypointense[a] (30%)	Non-enhancing	Homogenous hypodense[a]	Non-enhancing	Location: often central between anterior and posterior lobes Cyst contains non-enhancing nodule (77%)
Craniopharyingioma (Adamantinomatous)	Cystic portion: Iso- to hyperintense[b]	Cystic portion: hyperintense[b] (80%)	Enhancing	Calcifications (90%) Cystic portion: CSF density	Solid portion: enhancing (90%)	Mixed solid and cystic components
(Papillary)	Cystic portion: hypointense[b] (85%) Solid portion: iso- to hypointense[b]	Variable or mixed signal	Enhancing	Calcifications are uncommon Cystic portion: CSF density	Solid portion: enhancing	
Lymphocytic hypophysitis	Isointense[b] Thickened infundibulum Posterior pituitary bright spot may be absent	Parasellar hypointensity[b]	Enhancing Dural enhancement may be present	Soft tissue density	Enhancing	Female predominance F:M ~ 9:1 Often occurs during pregnancy or postpartum
Metastasis	Intrasellar or infundibulum May have dural thickening or bone destruction Signal characteristics as in primary tumor	Signal characteristics as in primary tumor	Enhancing	Soft tissue density	Enhancing	Known primary malignancy
Meningioma	Isointense[b] (60–90%)	Isointense[b] (50%) Hyperintense[b] (35–40%) Hypointense[b] (10–15%)	Intense homogeneous enhancing	Calcification (20–30%) Slightly hyperdense[b] (60%)	Homogeneously enhancing (72%)	
Chordoma	Iso- to hypointense[b] May have foci of hyperintensity	Hyperintense[b]	Heterogeneous enhancing	Involves clivus Usually mid-line posterior Lytic bone destruction	Moderate to marked enhancing	

GAD gadolinium contrast, *CSF* cerebral spinal fluid
[a]Compared to normal pituitary gland
[b]Compared to brain

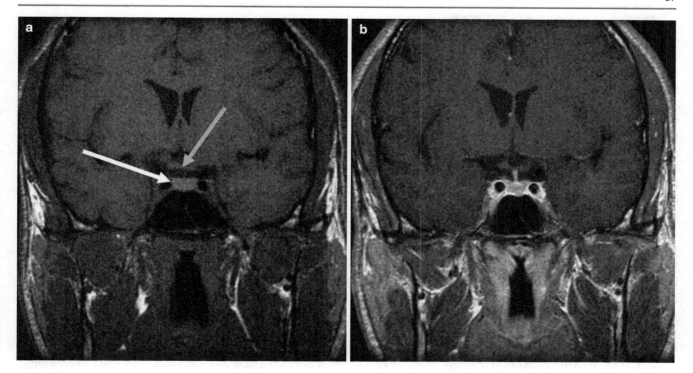

Fig. 4.1 Normal pituitary gland on MRI T1-weighted image in the coronal plane prior to contrast (**a**) showing the normal pituitary gland (*white arrow*) and the relationship to the optic chiasm (*gray arrow*).

T1-weighted image after gadolinium (**b**) demonstrates uniform enhancement of the normal pituitary gland and infundibulum

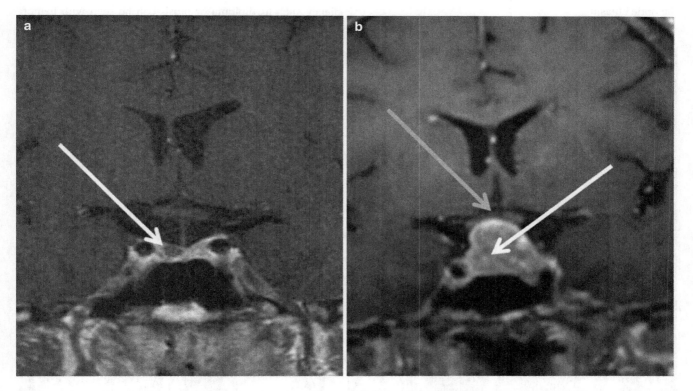

Fig. 4.2 MRI T1-weighted images in the coronal plane after gadolinium showing (**a**) a pituitary microadenoma (*white arrow*) located in the right side of the gland that enhances less than the normal pituitary tissue

and (**b**) a pituitary macroadenoma (*white arrow*) with suprasellar extension displacing and deforming the optic chiasm (*gray arrow*) of the sella turcica. Superior extension of the tumor can cause displacement or compression of the optic nerves and chiasm (Fig. 4.2b). Some adenomas may grow inferiorly, erode through the floor of the sella, and fill the sphenoid sinus. Adenomas that invade laterally into the cavernous sinus are unlikely to be cured surgically. Unfortunately both CT and MRI are not highly accurate in predicting cavernous sinus invasion. Encasement of the internal carotid artery is conclusive evidence. A tumor extending beyond the lateral aspect of the internal carotid artery on coronal MRI images is highly suggestive of cavernous sinus involvement. There are cystic variants of pituitary adenomas, and cystic degeneration and hemorrhage may also be present.

The imaging characteristics of Rathke's cleft cysts [12, 13] reflect their etiology. These non-neoplastic cysts arise from remnants of epithelium from Rathke's pouch (tiny intrasellar cysts in this area may be referred to as pars intermedia cysts). They are typically seen in the center of the gland, although they can be laterally located or present in the suprasellar space (Fig. 4.3). Many of these cysts are isointense with cerebral spinal fluid (CSF) on MRI imaging; however, if they contain proteinaceous fluid, they may be hyperintense on T1- and T2-weighted sequences. They lack contrast enhancement and do not contain calcifications. A small intracystic nodule is present in 77% of cases [14]. Occasionally a Rathke's cleft cyst can enlarge and compress the optic chiasm.

History, Physical Examination, and Laboratory Findings

Symptoms, findings on physical examination, and laboratory abnormalities associated with pituitary tumors are due to the effects of hormonal excess, hormonal deficiency, or local effects of the mass on surrounding tissues. Detailed questioning regarding the symptoms and examination for the physical signs associated with excess and deficiency of each hormonal axis should be obtained. Symptoms related to mass effect include vision loss that is classically loss of peripheral vision from compression of the optic chiasm. Other patterns of visual loss can occur due to anatomic variation in the anatomy of the optic nerves and chiasm. As vision loss can occur very slowly over years, some patients may not be aware of vision loss even in the presence of significant visual field deficits. Although loss of peripheral vision may be demonstrable on physical examination, automated perimetry should be obtained with masses that approach or contact the optic apparatus. Headaches are unlikely to occur with small masses that are confined to the sella. Larger masses with extrasellar extension can cause headaches. Interestingly, likely due to slow growth and tissue adaptation, many patients with huge sellar-based masses do not have headaches. The sudden onset of a severe headache, acute onset of symptoms of pituitary insufficiency, and cranial nerve deficiency such as diplopia or ptosis can be seen with hemor-

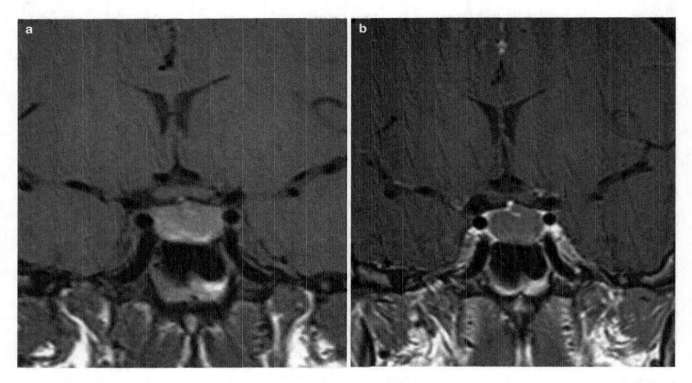

Fig. 4.3 MRI T1-weighted images in the coronal plane showing an intrasellar Rathke's cleft cyst. Prior to contrast (**a**) the cyst shows mild increased intensity compared to normal brain. After gadolinium (**b**) the cyst does not enhance

rhage in a pituitary adenoma (pituitary apoplexy). Polyuria and polydipsia will be present in lesions affecting the posterior pituitary, pituitary stalk, or hypothalamus that cause deficiency of antidiuretic hormone (diabetes insipidus). Although it is uncommon, many different systemic illnesses can involve the pituitary and parasellar area, and a thorough review of systems should be completed. If the history or physical exam suggests hormonal excess or deficiency, the appropriate hormonal laboratory evaluation should be obtained including dynamic testing if necessary. The laboratory evaluation for asymptomatic patients with a pituitary mass is discussed below.

Evaluation of the Incidentally Found Pituitary Mass

Clinicians are commonly presented with patients who have had a pituitary mass incidentally discovered. The "pituitary incidentaloma" is defined as an asymptomatic mass in the pituitary, found on imaging done for an unrelated reason. The majority of these lesions are small, usually less than 1 cm in diameter, and represent either pituitary adenomas or Rathke's cleft cysts. To decide what tests, if any, should be obtained and if treatment or observation is indicated, one needs to confirm the patient is asymptomatic and also consider the potential for, and the clinical impact of, hormone deficiency, hormone excess, and tumor growth.

Incidentally found macroadenomas are commonly associated with hormone deficiencies with a reported prevalence of hypopituitarism ranging between 15 and 57% [15, 16]. The presence of hormone deficiencies in incidentally found microadenomas is controversial, likely reflecting the arbitrary size cutoff of greater or less than 1 cm and the fact that subtle deficiencies may be present despite normal baseline hormonal levels. Retrospective studies suggest that incidentally found microadenomas have a very low chance of being associated with hormonal hypofunction with most studies reporting a 0% incidence. However, this needs to be interpreted in light of a study [17] involving 38 patients with microadenomas (55% incidentally found, 45% found on imagining done to evaluate abnormal laboratory tests suggesting pituitary dysfunction). GH releasing hormone (GHRH)/arginine stimulation found 50% of these patients to be GH deficient. In addition, basal hormone levels and/or 1 µg Cortrosyn stimulation identified at least one deficiency of gonadotropins, TSH, and/or ACTH in 50% of the patients. This led the Endocrine Society task force that developed the clinical guidelines for pituitary incidentalomas to favor screening for hormone deficiency in tumors greater than 5 mm [11].

Recommendations vary widely as to the specific laboratory tests that should be obtained. Given the current litera-

Table 4.3 Recommended hormonal tests for asymptomatic patients with an incidentally found pituitary mass

	To rule out subclinical hormone excess	To rule out subclinical hormone deficiency	
	All sizes	Size ≤5 mm	Size >5 mm
Prolactin[a]	X		
IGF-1[b]	X		X
FT4, TSH			X
Testosterone (men)			X
Menstrual history (premenopausal women)			
AM Cortisol[b]			X

[a]Measure after dilutions in macroadenomas to rule out high-dose hook effect
[b]IGF-1 and AM cortisol levels may not be sufficient to indicate normalcy or deficiency, and dynamic studies may be necessary

ture, laboratory testing to identify subclinical hypopituitarism in asymptomatic patients with an incidentally found pituitary mass should be obtained when the mass is greater than 5 mm in size (Table 4.3). It is reasonable to obtain TSH and free thyroxine to rule out secondary hypothyroidism, IGF-1 to screen for GH deficiency, and a morning cortisol level to screen for secondary adrenal insufficiency, realizing that basal levels of IGF-1 and morning cortisol may not be adequate to determine normalcy or deficiency, and dynamic testing may be required. Obtaining a testosterone level in men and a menstrual history in women will determine if hypogonadism is present. Measuring LH and FSH may be helpful in some instances, for example, if there is concern about coincidental primary hypogonadism.

Clinically non-functioning adenomas are most commonly found. Classification of non-functioning adenomas using mitotic count, Ki-67 proliferation index, the density and pattern of granules, and immunohistochemical assessment of certain receptors, enzymes, proteins, and hormones may be helpful in identifying those tumors that are more aggressive [18].

The most common hormone overproduced in incidentally found pituitary masses is PRL with an incidence of 12–28% [16, 19, 20]. Prolactin measurement should be done after serial dilutions of the serum in macroadenomas as falsely low values may be present when prolactin concentration is in fact very high due to the high-dose hook effect of the assay [21]. Prolactinomas have potential for morbidity, testing is easy, and safe and effective treatment is available.

The incidence of GH overproduction by an incidentally found mass is between 2 and 8% [16]. In early cases symptoms and physical findings may be quite subtle, but there is potential for serious morbidity and mortality if GH excess is not detected. There is also a high likelihood of surgical cure when the tumor is small.

No instances of ACTH excess have been reported in clinical studies of pituitary incidentaloma. Autopsy studies report between 1 and 13.8% of the adenomas stained for ACTH [22]. The screening tests for ACTH excess are cumbersome to perform and, particularly in asymptomatic patients, have high false-positive rates [23]. Although Cushing's disease is serious, screening for ACTH excess in patients with no clinical suspicion of glucocorticoid excess is not recommended due to the low prevalence and the high false-positive rate of the screening tests [11].

Although autopsy studies indicate 4% of incidentally found adenomas stain for gonadotropins, LH and FSH are usually in the normal range and are often biologically inactive in surgically proven gonadotropin adenomas. Rare cases of elevated testosterone levels in men and ovarian hyperstimulation in women due to gonadotropin-secreting pituitary adenomas have been reported [24, 25]. If a clinical syndrome is present with a gonadotropin producing adenoma, it is usually hypogonadism associated with a macroadenoma.

TSH-secreting pituitary adenomas are exceedingly rare, and none has been reported in clinical or autopsy series of incidentally found masses. These usually present clinically as macroadenomas with symptoms of hyperthyroidism [26]. Routine screening in the setting of a pituitary incidentaloma is not recommended.

Given the frequency and the clinical impact of overproduction of the various hormones, and the sensitivity and specificity of the screening tests, it is reasonable to obtain levels of PRL and IGF-1 to rule out subclinical excess secretion for all truly asymptomatic patients with incidentally found pituitary masses (Table 4.2).

An automated visual field examination should also be obtained at baseline if a macroadenoma is approaching or contacting the optic chiasm on MRI images [11]. This serves to determine if there is subclinical vision loss and also to serve as a baseline to determine if future growth, or surgical or radiation treatment, caused new vision loss.

Both microadenomas and macroadenomas have the potential to increase in size over time. Growth may occur after several years of stability. Macroadenomas likely grow more often (7–51%) than microadenomas (0–14%) [3]. Any increase in size of a macroadenoma has a higher chance of causing clinically significant mass effects.

Observation is appropriate if there is no hormonal over- or underproduction and the mass is not causing or threatening vision loss. If the decision is made to observe, repeat imaging with MRI scanning should be done initially at 6–12 months, and then annually for 2–4 years, and periodically thereafter. Doubling the interval since the last scan if no change is noted is appropriate. With macroadenomas, follow-up should include hormonal assessment for hypopituitarism, assessment for symptoms of mass effect, and imaging

with MRI. Since the decision to do surgery on a non-functioning macroadenoma is going to rest primarily on the development of vision loss, formal visual fields (if the mass is in proximity to the optic chiasm) should be obtained at these same intervals. All follow-up scans should be compared to the baseline scan in addition to the prior scan, since minor consecutive increases in size may not be appreciated.

Differential Diagnosis

A wide spectrum of lesions with various etiologies can manifest as masses in the sellar or parasellar region (Table 4.1). Excluding pituitary adenomas and Rathke's cleft cysts, they represent only about 6% of clinically apparent lesions [4]. Brief discussions of some of these lesions follow.

Craniopharyngiomas are tumors of epithelial origin that can affect both children and adults. Craniopharyngiomas are often located in the suprasellar space but can be within the sella. They can appear solid on imaging but often contain both solid and cystic components. Calcifications, seen on plain X-ray or CT, may be present. These tumors commonly present with vision loss, anterior pituitary hormone deficiencies, and diabetes insipidus [27].

Chordoma is an aggressive, rare bone cancer that is locally invasive and has a predilection for the axial skeleton, with the most common sites being the sacrum, skull base, and spine. Parasellar chordomas usually involve the dorsum sella, clivus, or nasopharynx and cause local bone destruction (best seen on CT). Symptoms of headache or neck pain are common, and diplopia or facial numbness can occur if cavernous sinus invasion is present [28].

Germ cell tumors can affect the central nervous system. The pineal gland is the most common site for intracranial germ cell tumors. These tumors can also be located in the suprasellar region, basal ganglia, posterior fossa, pituitary gland, or medulla. They may manifest as multiple discreet lesions, and leptomeningeal spread occurs in 10–15% of cases. Common symptoms include headache, diplopia, hypopituitarism, and diabetes insipidus [29]. They typically present in teenagers or young adults (peak incidence age 10–14 years) and rarely present in patients greater than 30 years old. The diagnosis is facilitated by measuring the tumor markers beta-human chorionic gonadotropin (βHCG) and alpha-fetoprotein (AFP), which may be present in blood or CSF.

Metastatic tumors to the sellar area are usually asymptomatic from the pituitary standpoint and typically are found in patients with known metastatic disease. The posterior lobe of the pituitary or the hypothalamus are more commonly involved making diabetes insipidus the most common pituitary-related symptom. Metastases may also cause anterior pituitary dysfunction, vision loss, diplopia, and retro-orbital pain. The most common primary sites are the breast, lung, gastrointestinal tract, kidney, prostate, and melanoma [30].

Primary brain tumors may present in or around the sella. Parasellar meningiomas are often located by dorsum sella or clivus [31]. Radiologically meningiomas are typically isointense to hypointense to gray matter on T1-weighted MRI sequences and isointense to hyperintense on T2-weighted MRI sequences. They typically display intense homogeneous enhancement and may show calcification. Gliomas located in the parasellar region often arise from the optic nerves or optic chiasm and have an unpredictable clinical course [32].

Lymphocytic hypophysitis is a presumed autoimmune inflammation of the pituitary that is more common in premenopausal women (80–90%), often presenting during pregnancy or postpartum, but can occur in men, children, and the elderly [33]. Symptoms commonly include headache that is often intense. Pituitary insufficiency may involve only one hormone axis, including diabetes insipidus, or multiple hormone deficiencies may be present. Imaging can be variable showing diffuse pituitary enlargement, enlargement of both the pituitary and pituitary stalk, and stalk enlargement only that may appear as a suprasellar mass. Usually homogeneous contrast enhancement is present. Occasionally a presumptive diagnosis of lymphocytic hypophysitis is made with a normal appearance of the pituitary on imaging.

Hypophysitis can occur in patients being treated with immune checkpoint inhibitors for solid tumor malignancies. These monoclonal antibodies have different mechanisms of action, and hypophysitis is usually seen with the CTLA-4 (cytotoxic T-lymphocyte associated protein-4) preparation ipilimumab and the PD-1 (programmed cell death-1) preparations nivolumab and pembrolizumab. The predicted incidence of hypophysitis with ipilumimab is 3.8% and 1.1% with nivolumab and pembrolizumab. Combination therapy with ipilimumab and nivolumab has an 8% predictive incidence of hypophysitis [34, 35].

Neurosarcoidosis can affect the parasellar region and often involves the hypothalamus and/or pituitary stalk [36]. Angiotensin-converting enzyme (ACE) levels usually are elevated in the blood or CSF. Other organs are typically affected at some point in the course of the disease, but parasellar neurosarcoidosis can be the only manifestation.

Present and Future Therapies

Transsphenoidal Surgery

Since the 1970s, the standard surgical approach for most pituitary tumors has been via the sublabial transsphenoidal route [37]. This approach to the sphenoid sinus involves making a sublabial incision for access to the nasal cavity and then removing the nasal septum. The sphenoid sinus is then entered allowing access to the sella turcica. After resection of the tumor, the nasal septum is replaced requiring nasal packing postoperatively. In the mid-1990s, surgeons began using a modification of the standard surgical technique utilizing the nasal endoscope [38]. With this endoscopic transnasal transsphenoidal approach, there is no external incision. The nasal endoscope is placed through one nostril and advanced to the anterior wall of the sphenoid sinus. The sphenoid ostium is identified and enlarged, and the posterior portion of the vomer is removed allowing access to the sphenoid sinus. After placement of a self-retaining nasal speculum, the sella turcica is entered, and the neurosurgical portion of the procedure is undertaken as with the sublabial transseptal approach. After resection of the tumor, the nasal speculum is withdrawn, the nasal septum is adjusted to midline if necessary, and a mustache nasal dressing is applied. The main difference in the two procedures from the surgeon's standpoint is that with the endoscopic transnasal approach, the surgical field is smaller and is angled approximately 10° off-center [39]. The disadvantages this may present to the surgeon can be overcome with experience [40].

For the patient, the absence of the sublabial incision eliminates the possibility of developing lip numbness postoperatively, and leaving the nasal septum intact decreases postoperative discomfort from nasal packs and decreases the chance for complications related to the nasal septum. Additionally, the length of hospitalization, anesthesia time, and blood loss are reportedly less with the endoscopic approach [41, 42].

Operative success regarding extent of tumor resection, normalization of visual deficits, and normalization of hormonal hypersecretion are similar or better using the transnasal endoscopic technique. Surgical complications, including mortality, vision loss, new pituitary hormonal deficits, CSF leak, and infections are comparable between the two procedures [39, 43–49].

Radiation

Radiation therapy of pituitary adenomas has been used as primary therapy for pituitary adenomas as well as for treatment of residual or recurrent tumors after surgery. The major limiting factor for radiation therapy is damage to the normal surrounding tissues. For pituitary adenomas the radiation must pass through normal brain tissue, and the tumors are often adjacent to radiation-sensitive structures such as the optic nerves and normal pituitary gland.

The state of the art for fractionated X-ray radiotherapy is termed fractionated stereotactic radiation therapy (FRST) and is an improvement over conventional radiation therapy (CRT) in that it uses techniques to increase the radiation dose to the tumor while limiting the exposure of normal tissues. Control of non-functioning pituitary adenoma growth appears to be better with FRST compared to CRT [50].

Stereotactic radiosurgery is a technique using multiple lower-dose X-ray radiation beams conformationally focused on the tumor and delivered in a single session. It has proven to be effective with both non-functioning and hormone-secreting pituitary adenomas for patients with recurrent or residual tumors after surgery or if medical therapy has failed. Inhibition of further tumor growth occurs in greater than 95% of patients treated with radiosurgery for non-functioning adenomas [51].

Patients with hormone-secreting pituitary adenomas treated with radiosurgery have a very wide range of reported biochemical remission, varying from 17 to 82% [52]. This variation in published reports on remission rates following radiosurgery for hormone-producing pituitary adenomas likely is due to advances in the technique over time, varied definitions of endocrine cure, and relatively short follow-up periods after radiosurgery.

It remains controversial whether pituitary-suppressive medications (somatostatin analogues or dopamine agonists) at the time of radiosurgery have any impact on remission of hormone hypersecretion. Several studies have noted that patients using either somatostatin or dopamine agonists at the time of radiosurgery for GH- or PRL-secreting tumors less frequently achieved biochemical remission [53, 54]. A study of 46 acromegalic patients who underwent radiosurgery found that patients who did not receive pituitary-suppressive medications at the time of radiosurgery were four times more likely to reach normal GH and IGF-1 levels than those who had [52]. Conversely, some studies have failed to find any association between biochemical remission rates for acromegalic patients who received somatostatin analogues at the time of radiosurgery and those who did not [55, 56].

The primary adverse effect of pituitary radiosurgery is the development of new anterior pituitary hormone deficits. The development of new pituitary hormone deficits ranges between 7 and 41% in studies with mean follow-up intervals of 4–5 years. The different rates of hypopituitarism reported likely relate to variation in the patient characteristics including history of prior surgery or fractionated radiation therapy, radiation dose prescribed, treatment volume, follow-up intervals, and the completeness of the patients' endocrine evaluation [57].

An alternative to X-ray radiation is using proton therapy as the radiation source. Proton therapy exposes normal tissue closer to the surface of the body to lower radiation doses than the tumor receives and is effective in treating functioning and non-functioning pituitary adenomas [58, 59].

Medical Therapy

Medical therapy is used to decrease hormone overproduction by functioning pituitary adenomas or block the effects of excess hormone secretion and in some instances may be used to decrease tumor size relieving symptoms of mass effect or to limit further growth.

For patients with prolactinomas, medical treatment with a dopamine agonist is usually the first-line therapy. Cabergoline and bromocriptine are the agents most commonly used, and both are effective in normalizing PRL secretion and decreasing tumor size with cabergoline being more efficacious and more tolerable than bromocriptine [60]. Some patients achieve prolonged remission after 2 or more years of treatment. Cardiac valve disease has been described with cabergoline therapy but is rare in patients treated with the standard doses used for the treatment of hyperprolactinemia. Patients, especially those on doses of cabergoline greater than 2.0 mg/week, should be periodically assessed for valvular heart disease. Impulse control disorders can occur in patients treated with dopamine agonists for Parkinson's disease and restless legs syndrome and has also been reported in patients with prolactinomas [61].

GH-secreting pituitary adenomas are usually initially treated with surgery and/or radiation therapy. Medical therapy is used with persistent disease after surgery, while waiting for the effects of radiation, and occasionally as primary therapy in selected patients unable to tolerate surgery or with clearly unresectable disease [62]. The somatostatin analogues octreotide and lanreotide, given by intramuscular or subcutaneous injection, respectively, act by decreasing GH secretion from the adenoma. Normalization of IGF-1 levels occurs in approximately 60% of patients. Tumor size can decrease in some patients, but the decrease is modest and usually not clinically significant. Common side effects include nausea and diarrhea, but these usually resolve despite continued therapy. Development of gallstones occurs in up to 30% of patients but rarely is symptomatic requiring therapy. In patients with mild GH excess, treatment with the dopamine agonist cabergoline may normalize IGF-1 secretion. Pegvisomant, a GH receptor antagonist, normalizes IGF-1 levels in 90% of patients, is usually well tolerated, but can cause drug-induced hepatitis. Increase in the size of the adenoma has been reported in some patients.

Medical therapy options for patients with ACTH-producing pituitary adenomas and persistent cortisol excess after transsphenoidal surgery or radiation have expanded in recent years. Ketoconazole and metyrapone suppress adrenal cortisol production by inhibiting steroidogenic enzymes [63]. Their efficacy however decreases with time as the continued ACTH stimulation overrides the enzymatic block. Because of this, their role is primarily in correcting severe hypercortisolism in the short term prior to definitive surgical treatment. Hepatotoxicity can occur with ketoconazole requiring monitoring of hepatic enzymes. Pasireotide is a somatostatin analog with high binding affinity for four of the five known somatostatin receptor subtypes (sst_{1-3} and sst_5). ACTH-producing adenomas can express multiple sst receptors, with the predominant receptor being sst_5. Octreotide and lanreotide, which are not effective in treating ACTH-producing adenomas, have high affinity for sst_2 and low affinity for sst_5. Pasireotide, with a 40-fold higher affinity for sst_5 than octreotide, normalized or decreased by $\geq$50% urinary free cortisol in approximately 50% of treated patients after 6 months. Hyperglycemia-related adverse events however occurred in 73% of patients with 46% requiring initiation of or an additional glucose-lowering medication [64]. Mifepristone is a cortisol receptor antagonist shown to improve glycemic parameters, lower diastolic BP, and improve clinical signs and symptoms in patients with Cushing's syndrome from various etiologies [65]. Adverse events however occurred in 88% of the subjects. As cortisol levels rise during treatment, hormonal levels cannot be used to monitor treatment, and overtreatment resulting in adrenal insufficiency may be difficult to detect.

Laparoscopic bilateral adrenalectomy is an established, safe, and effective treatment for patients with persistent Cushing's disease after pituitary surgery. Cortisol excess is immediately and definitively cured, but lifelong hormonal replacement with glucocorticoids and mineralocorticoids is required. There is potential for unrestrained growth of a residual ACTH-producing pituitary adenoma after adrenalectomy (Nelson–Salassa syndrome). The vast majority of patients do not require tumor-directed therapy after adrenalectomy as Nelson–Salassa syndrome typically occurs in the small subset with a clear evidence of invasive pituitary disease at the outset [66]. There are no studies comparing clinical outcomes of bilateral adrenalectomy versus medical therapy for patients with persistent disease after pituitary surgery.

References

1. Molitch ME. Nonfunctioning pituitary tumors and pituitary incidentalomas. Endocrinol Metab Clin N Am. 2008;37:151–71. xi.
2. Bancos I, Natt N, Murad MH, Montori VM. Evidence-based endocrinology—illustrating its principles in the management of patients with pituitary incidentalomas. Best Pract Res Clin Endocrinol Metab. 2012;26(1):9–19.
3. Orija IB, Weil RJ, Hamrahian AH. Pituitary incidentaloma. Best Pract Res Clin Endocrinol Metab. 2012;26(1):47–68.
4. Freda PU, Post KD. Differential diagnosis of sellar masses. Endocrinol Metab Clin N Am. 1999;28:81–117. vi.
5. Al-Sharydah AM, Al-Suhibani SS, Al-Jubran SA, Al-Abdulwahab AH, Al-Bar M, Al-Jehani HM, Al-Issawi WM. Endoscopic management of a typical sellar cavernous hemangioma: a case report and review of the literature. Int J Surg Case Rep. 2018;42:161–4.
6. Goulart CR, Upadhyay S, Ditzel Filho LFS, Beer-Furlan A, Carrau RL, Prevedello LM, Prevedello DM. Newly diagnosed sellar tumors in patients with cancer: a diagnostic challenge and management dilemma. World Neurosurg. 2017;106:254–65.
7. Tajudeen BA, Kuan EC, Adappa ND, Han JK, Chandra RK, Palmer JN, Kennedy DW, Wang MB, Suh JD. Ectopic pituitary adenomas presenting as sphenoid or clival lesions: case series and management recommendations. J Neurol Surg B. 2017;78:120–4.
8. Lee J, Kulubya E, Pressman BD, Mamelak A, Bannykh S, Zada G, Cooper O. Sellar and clival plasmacytomas: case series of 5 patients with systematic review of 65 published cases. Pituitary. 2017;20(3):381–92.
9. Tarabay A, Cossu G, Berhouma M, Levivier M, Daniel RT, Messerer M. Primary pituitary lymphoma: an update of the literature. J Neurooncol. 2016;130(3):383–95.
10. Phillips JJ, Misra A, Feuerstein BG, Kunwar S, Tihan T. Pituicytoma: characterization of a unique neoplasm by histology, immunohistochemistry, ultrastructure, and array-based comparative genomic hybridization. Arch Pathol Lab Med. 2010;34:1063–9.
11. Freda PU, Beckers AM, et al. Pituitary incidentaloma: an endocrine society clinical practice guideline. J Clin Endocrinol Metab. 2011;96(4):894–904.
12. Adam A, Dixon AK. Grainger and Allison's diagnostic radiology: a textbook of medical imaging, vol. 71. 5th ed. Philadelphia: Elsevier Limited; 2008. p. 1705–32.
13. Pisaneschi M, Kapoor G. Imaging the sella and parasellar region. Neuroimaging Clin N Am. 2005;15(1):203–19.
14. Byun WM, Kim OL, Kim D. MR imaging findings of Rathke's cleft cysts: significance of intracystic nodules. Am J Neuroradiol. 2000;21:485–8.
15. Reincke M, Allolio B, Saeger W, Menzel J, Winkelmann W. The 'incidentaloma' of the pituitary gland. Is neurosurgery required? JAMA. 1990;263:2772–6.
16. Feldkamp J, Santen R, Harms E, Aulich A, Mödder U, Scherbaum WA. Incidentally discovered pituitary lesions: high frequency of macroadenomas and hormone secreting adenomas—results of a prospective study. Clin Endocrinol (Oxf). 1999;51:109–13.
17. Yuen KC, Cook DM, Sahasranam P, Patel P, Ghods DE, Shahinian HK, Friedman TC. Prevalence of GH and other anterior pituitary hormone deficiencies in adults with nonsecreting pituitary microadenomas and normal serum IGF-1 levels. Clin Endocrinol (Oxf). 2008;69:292–8.
18. Manojlovic-Gacic E, Engström BE, Casar-Borota O. Histopathological classification of non-functioning pituitary neuroendocrine tumors. Pituitary. 2017; https://doi.org/10.1007/s11102-017-0855-1.
19. Fainstein Day P, Guitelman M, Artese R, Fiszledjer L, Chervin A, Vitale NM, Stalldecker G, De Miguel V, Cornaló D, Alfieri A, Susana M, Gil M. Retrospective multicentric study of pituitary incidentalomas. Pituitary. 2004;7:145–8.
20. Donovan LE, Corenblum B. The natural history of the pituitary incidentaloma. Arch Intern Med. 1995;155:181–3.
21. Petakov MS, Damjanovic SS, Nikolić-Durovic MM, Dragojlović ZL, Obradović S, Gligorović MS, Simić MZ, Popović VP. Pituitary adenomas secreting large amounts of prolactin may give false low values in immunoradiometric assays. The hook effect. J Endocrinol Investig. 1998;21(3):184–8.
22. Buurman H, Saeger W. Subclinical adenomas in postmortem pituitaries: classification and correlations to clinical data. Eur J Endocrinol. 2006;154:753–8.
23. Nieman LK. Difficulty in the diagnosis of Cushing disease. Nat Clin Pract Endocrinol Metab. 2006;2(1):53–7.
24. Snyder PJ. Gonadotroph cell adenomas of the pituitary. Endocr Rev. 1985;6(4):552–63.
25. Garmes HM, Grassiotto OR, et al. A pituitary adenoma secreting follicle-stimulating hormone with ovarian hyperstimulation:

treatment using a gonadotropin-releasing hormone antagonist. Fertil Steril. 2012;97(1):231–4.

26. Beck-Peccoz P, Persani L, Mannavola D, Campi I. Pituitary tumours: TSH-secreting adenomas. Best Pract Res Clin Endocrinol Metab. 2009;23(5):597–606.

27. Stamm AC, Vellutini E, Balsalobre L. Craniopharyngioma. Otolaryngol Clin N Am. 2011;44(4):937–52. viii.

28. Walcott BP, Nahed BV, Mohyeldin A, Coumans JV, Kahle KT, Ferreira MJ. Chordoma: current concepts, management, and future directions. Lancet Oncol. 2012;13(2):e69–76.

29. Wildemberg LE, Vieira Neto L, Taboada GF, Moraes AB, Marcondes J, Conceição FL, Chimelli L, Gadelha MR. Sellar and suprasellar mixed germ cell tumor mimicking a pituitary adenoma. Pituitary. 2011;14(4):345–50.

30. Komninos J, Vlassopoulou V, Protopapa D, Korfias S, Kontogeorgos G, Sakas DE, Thalassinos NC. Tumors metastatic to the pituitary gland: case report and literature review. J Clin Endocrinol Metab. 2004;89(2):574–80.

31. Abele TA, Yetkin ZF, Raisanen JM, Mickey BE, Mendelsohn DB. Non-pituitary origin sellar tumours mimicking pituitary macroadenomas. Clin Radiol. 2012;67(8):821–7.

32. Shapey J, Danesh-Meyer HV, Kaye AH. Diagnosis and management of optic nerve glioma. J Clin Neurosci. 2011;18(12):1585–91.

33. Carpinteri R, Patelli I, Casanueva FF, Giustina A. Pituitary tumours: inflammatory and granulomatous expansive lesions of the pituitary. Best Pract Res Clin Endocrinol Metab. 2009;23(5):639–50.

34. Juszczak A, Gupta A, Karavitaki N, Middleton MR, Grossman AB. Ipilimumab: a novel immunomodulating therapy causing autoimmune hypophysitis: a case report and review. Eur J Endocrinol. 2012;167(1):1–5.

35. Barroso-Sousa R, Barry WT, Garrido-Castro AC, Hodi FS, Min L, Krop IE, Tolaney SM. Incidence of endocrine dysfunction following the use of different immune checkpoint inhibitor regimens a systematic review and meta-analysis. JAMA Oncol. 2017; https://doi.org/10.1001/jamaoncol.2017.3064.

36. Bihan H, Christozova V, Dumas JL, Jomaa R, Valeyre D, Tazi A, Reach G, Krivitzky A, Cohen R. Sarcoidosis: clinical, hormonal, and magnetic resonance imaging (MRI) manifestations of hypothalamic-pituitary disease in 9 patients and review of the literature. Medicine (Baltimore). 2007;86(5):259–68.

37. Hardy J. Atlas of transsphenoidal microsurgery in pituitary tumors. New York: Igaku-Shoin; 1991.

38. Jho HD. Endoscopic transsphenoidal surgery. J Neurooncol. 2001;54:187–95.

39. Atkinson JL, Young WF Jr, Meyer FB, Davis DH, Nippoldt TB, Erickson D, Vella A, Natt N, Abboud CF, Carpenter PC. Sublabial transseptal vs. transnasal combined endoscopic microsurgery in patients with Cushing disease and MRI-depicted microadenomas. Mayo Clin Proc. 2008;83(5):550–3.

40. O'Malley BW Jr, Grady MS, Gabel BC, Cohen MA, Heuer GG, Pisapia J, Bohman LE, Leibowitz JM. Comparison of endoscopic and microscopic removal of pituitary adenomas: single-surgeon experience and the learning curve. Neurosurg Focus. 2008;25(6):E10.

41. Sheehan MT, Atkinson JL, Kasperbauer JL, Erickson BJ, Nippoldt TB. Preliminary comparison of the endoscopic transnasal vs. the sublabial transseptal approach for clinically nonfunctioning pituitary macroadenomas. Mayo Clin Proc. 1999;74(7):661–70.

42. Cappabianca P, Cavallo LM, Colao A, Del Basso De Caro M, Esposito F, Cirillo S, Lombardi G, De Divitiis E. Endoscopic endonasal transsphenoidal approach: outcome analysis of 100 consecutive procedures. Minim Invasive Neurosurg. 2002;45:193–200.

43. D'Haens J, Van Rompaey K, Stadnik T, Haentjens P, Poppe K, Velkeniers B. Fully endoscopic transsphenoidal surgery for functioning pituitary adenomas: a retrospective comparison with tradi-

tional transsphenoidal microsurgery in the same institution. Surg Neurol. 2009;72(4):336–40.

44. Cho DY, Liau WR. Comparison of endonasal endoscopic surgery and sublabial microsurgery for prolactinomas. Surg Neurol. 2002;58:371–5.

45. Frank G, Pasquini E, Farneti G, Mazzatenta D, Sciarretta V, Grasso V, Faustini FM. The endoscopic versus the traditional approach in pituitary surgery. Neuroendocrinology. 2006;83:240–8.

46. Kabil MS, Eby JB, Shahinian HK. Fully endoscopic endonasal vs. transseptal transsphenoidal pituitary surgery. Minim Invasive Neurosurg. 2005;48:348–54.

47. Netea-Maier RT, van Lindert EJ, den Heijer M, van der Eerden A, Pieters GF, Sweep CG, Grotenhuis JA, Hermus AR. Transsphenoidal pituitary surgery via the endoscopic technique: results in 35 consecutive patients with Cushing's disease. Eur J Endocrinol. 2006;154(5):675–84.

48. Dehdashti AR, Ganna A, Karabatsou K, Gentili F. Pure endoscopic endonasal approach for pituitary adenomas: early surgical results in 200 patients and comparison with previous microsurgical series. Neurosurgery. 2008;62(5):1006–15.

49. Ciric I, Ragin A, Baumgartner C, Pierce D. Complications of transsphenoidal surgery: results of a national survey, review of the literature, and personal experience. Neurosurgery. 1997;40:225–37.

50. Wilson PJ, De-Loyde KJ, Williams JR, Smee RI. A single center's experience of stereotactic radiosurgery and radiotherapy for non-functioning pituitary adenomas with the Linear Accelerator (Linac). J Clin Neurosci. 2012;19(3):370–4.

51. Prasad D. Clinical results of conformal radiotherapy and radiosurgery for pituitary adenoma. Neurosurg Clin N Am. 2006;17:129–41.

52. Pollock BE, Jacob JT, Brown PD, Nippoldt TB. Radiosurgery of growth hormone-producing pituitary adenomas: factors associated with biochemical remission. J Neurosurg. 2007;106(5):833–8.

53. Landolt AM, Haller D, Lomax N, Scheib S, Schubiger O, Siegfried J, et al. Stereotactic radiosurgery for recurrent surgically treated acromegaly: comparison with fractionated radiotherapy. J Neurosurg. 1998;88:1002–8.

54. Pouratian N, Sheehan J, Jagannathan J, Laws ER Jr, Steiner L, Vance ML. Gamma knife radiosurgery for medically and surgically refractory prolactinomas. Neurosurgery. 2006;59(2):255–66.

55. Attanasio R, Epaminonda P, Motti E, Giugni E, Ventrella L, Cozzi R, et al. Gamma-knife radiosurgery in acromegaly: a 4-year follow-up study. J Clin Endocrinol Metab. 2003;88:3105–12.

56. Castinetti F, Taieb D, Kuhn JM, Chanson P, Tamura M, Jaquet P, et al. Outcome of gamma knife radiosurgery in 82 patients with acromegaly: correlation with initial hypersecretion. J Clin Endocrinol Metab. 2005;90:4483–8.

57. Leenstra JL, Tanaka S, Kline RW, Brown PD, Link MJ, Nippoldt TB, Young WF Jr, Pollock BE. Factors associated with endocrine deficits after stereotactic radiosurgery of pituitary adenomas. Neurosurgery. 2010;67(1):27–32.

58. Ronson BB, Schulte RW, Han KP, Loredo LN, Slater JM, Slater JD. Fractionated proton beam irradiation of pituitary adenomas. Int J Radiat Oncol Biol Phys. 2006;64(2):425–34.

59. Noel G, Gondi V. Proton therapy for tumors of the base of the skull. Chin Clin Oncol. 2016;5(4):51.

60. Maiter D, Primeau V. 2012 update in the treatment of prolactinomas. Ann Endocrinol (Paris). 2012;73(2):90–8.

61. Bancos I, Nannenga MR, Bostwick JM, Silber MH, Erickson D, Nippoldt TB. Impulse control disorders in patients with dopamine agonist-treated prolactinomas and nonfunctioning pituitary adenomas: a case–control study. Clin Endocrinol. 2014;80:863–8.

62. Katznelson L, Atkinson JL, Cook DM, Ezzat SZ, Hamrahian AH, Miller KK. American Association of Clinical Endocrinologists medical guidelines for clinical practice for the diagnosis and treatment of acromegaly—2011 update. Endocr Pract. 2011;17(Suppl 4):1–44.

63. Feelders RA, Hofland LJ, de Herder WW. Medical treatment of Cushing's syndrome: adrenal-blocking drugs and ketoconazole. Neuroendocrinology. 2010;92(Suppl 1):111–5.

64. Colao A, Petersenn S, Newell-Price J, Findling JW, Gu F, Maldonado M, Schoenherr U, Mills D, Salgado LR, Biller BM, Pasireotide B2305 Study Group. A 12-month phase 3 study of pasireotide in Cushing's disease. N Engl J Med. 2012;366(10):914–24.

65. Fleseriu M, Biller BM, Findling JW, Molitch ME, Schteingart DE, Gross C, SEISMIC Study Investigators. Mifepristone, a glucocor-ticoid receptor antagonist, produces clinical and metabolic benefits in patients with Cushing's syndrome. J Clin Endocrinol Metab. 2012;97(6):2039–49.

66. Porterfield JR, Thompson GB, Young WF Jr, Chow JT, Fryrear RS, van Heerden JA, Farley DR, Atkinson JL, Meyer FB, Abboud CF, Nippoldt TB, Natt N, Erickson D, Vella A, Carpenter PC, Richards M, Carney JA, Larson D, Schleck C, Churchward M, Grant CS. Surgery for Cushing's syndrome: an historical review and recent ten-year experience. World J Surg. 2008;32(5):659–77.

Hyperprolactinemia

Andrea Glezer and Marcello D. Bronstein

Pathophysiology

PRL is secreted by the lactotrophs, present in the anterior pituitary gland, and its secretion is under the inhibitory control of hypothalamic dopamine that reaches the anterior pituitary gland through the portal circulation via the pituitary stalk. Sellar and suprasellar tumors, as well as inflammatory and infectious diseases evolving pituitary stalk, prevent the inflow of the dopamine to lactotrophs, increasing PRL secretion. Moreover, there are several factors releasing PRL secretion, as estrogens, serotonin, thyrotropin-stimulating hormone (TRH), and vasoactive intestinal peptide (VIP) [1].

Hyperprolactinemia, defined by elevated serum PRL levels above the normal range, is the most common hypothalamic-pituitary dysfunction and can result from several causes, as physiological conditions (pregnancy, breastfeeding, stress); pharmacological and pathological status, like kidney and liver failure, hypothyroidism, pituitary adenomas, tumors, or other inflammatory diseases of the hypothalamic-pituitary region; and macroprolactinemia. Prolactinomas, adenomas with autonomous secretion of PRL, are the most common pituitary tumors, with a prevalence of 100 cases per million, more often reaching young women, being ten times more frequent in females aged 20–50 years old than in males. Nevertheless, the prevalence becomes similar between genders in adults over 60 years old [1]. The differential diagnosis of hyperprolactinemia is essential for its proper treatment.

Secretion and pulsatility of gonadotropin-releasing hormone (GnRH) is impaired in hyperprolactinemia, probably via kisspeptin [2], leading to gonadotropin deficiency and consequent hypogonadism. The classic manifestations are sexual dysfunction, infertility, menstrual irregularities, and bone mass loss [1]. Galactorrhea, often found among women with hyperprolactinemia, is not a mandatory or specific sign.

Batrinos et al. evaluated 404 women with galactorrhea, with and without irregular menses, and the prevalence of hyperprolactinemia was 42% and 15%, respectively [3]. Mass effects as headache and visual disturbances are often found [1] in macroprolactinomas and other tumors of the hypothalamic-pituitary region.

Key Points for Diagnosis

Hyperprolactinemia is defined when serum PRL levels are above the normal reference value (usually 20–25 ng/ml in females, 15–20 ng/ml in males) [4]. The stress of venipuncture can increase PRL secretion, frequently at levels slightly above the normal value. When blood collection is performed after rest, about 30% of asymptomatic individuals with mild hyperprolactinemia present with normal hormonal levels [5]. Nevertheless, rest for blood withdrawal is not routinely recommended.

Serum PRL evaluation should be performed only when clinically indicated [1].

Differential Diagnosis

After confirming the diagnosis of hyperprolactinemia, the following etiologies should be evaluated [6]:

- Physiological: pregnancy and lactation and mammary stimulation.
- Pharmacologic: neuroleptic and antipsychotic medications (sulpiride, chlorpromazine, risperidone, haloperidol), antidepressants, opioids, cocaine, antihypertensive medications (verapamil, methyldopa), drugs that act in the gastrointestinal tract (metoclopramide, domperidone), protease inhibitors for AIDS treatment, and the use of estrogens.
- Associated with systemic diseases: kidney and liver failure.

A. Glezer · M. D. Bronstein (✉)
Hospital das Clinicas, University of Sao Paulo, Neuroendocrine Unit, Division of Endocrinology and Metabolism, Sao Paulo, SP, Brazil

- Associated with endocrinological diseases: primary hypothyroidism, polycystic ovarian syndrome (PCOS), and Addison's and Cushing's diseases.
- Other tumors of the hypothalamic-pituitary region or infectious/infiltrative disorders compromising the pituitary stalk [7], as pituitary nonfunctioning macroadenomas, craniopharyngiomas, metastasis, lymphocytic hypophysitis, sarcoidosis, and tuberculosis; in addition post-surgery or radiotherapy status can also lead to hyperprolactinemia.
- Intercostal nerves stimulation.
- Autonomous PRL secretion by pituitary adenomas: prolactinomas, mixed PRL and GH secretion tumors.
- Macroprolactinemia.
- Mutant prolactin receptor.
- Idiopathic.

In pharmacological hyperprolactinemia, a new serum PRL evaluation should be performed after 3 days of withdrawal of the suspected drug, if possible. Otherwise, the patient should undergo magnetic resonance imaging (MRI) of the pituitary to rule out pathological causes [8].

In primary hypothyroidism, increasing PRL secretion is attributed to TRH, and serum PRL levels should decrease and become normal after appropriate levotiroxine replacement [9].

Regarding polycystic ovarian syndrome (PCOS), more recent studies did not confirm any pathophysiological relationship with hyperprolactinemia, and the coexistence of these two conditions could just be a random association [10]. Therefore, in patients who remain with irregular menses after reaching normal serum PRL levels, it is important to exclude other causes for the symptoms, such as PCOS.

Mammary stimulation in nonpregnant women, as chest wall disturbances (herpes zoster, mechanical or chemical trauma), can lead to increased levels of PRL due to neurogenic reflex [11]. Breast clinical examination, mammography, and ultrasound have minimal effect on serum PRL levels [12].

Macroprolactinemia is characterized by the predominance of the PRL isoform big-big-PRL (macroprolactin), which occurs in about 25% of hyperprolactinemic individuals. According to its molecular weight, PRL is classified as monomeric, dimeric, and macroprolactin. Monomeric PRL corresponds to more than 50% of total circulating PRL, and it is considered the biological active isoform, while macroprolactin has low biological activity [13]. In an individual with macroprolactinemia and normal serum concentrations of monomeric PRL, symptoms related to hyperprolactinemia are not expected [14, 15]. Macroprolactinemia is an important cause of dissociation between clinical and laboratory findings, and its screening should be performed in asymptomatic hyperprolactinemic individuals in which the request for the initial PRL evaluation is debatable. However, symptomatic hyperprolactinemia can occur in macroprolactinemic patients when monomeric isoform is also elevated [15].

Dealing with a patient with symptomatic hyperprolactinemia, when pregnancy, use of medications that may cause hyperprolactinemia, kidney failure, liver failure, and hypothyroidism are excluded, sellar MRI should be performed in order to identify a pituitary tumor with autonomous PRL secretion (prolactinoma), or other tumors of the sellar region, as well as infiltrative or infectious diseases, are the cause of hyperprolactinemia by pituitary stalk disconnection. Serum PRL is usually proportional to the tumor size in prolactinomas: in microprolactinomas, serum PRL levels up to 200 ng/ml are expected, while in macroprolactinomas, frequently values above these levels are found [16]. Karavitaki et al. [17] evaluated serum PRL levels in patients with pituitary nonfunctioning tumors with pituitary stalk disconnection, and in 98.7% of the cases, levels were lower than 95 ng/ml. Therefore, in hyperprolactinemia due to disconnection, serum PRL does not exceed 100 ng/ml, with few exceptions. The differentiation between a hyperprolactinemia due to disconnection and prolactinomas is essential, especially in the presence of mass effect, in order to indicate proper therapy.

A heterozygous mutation in prolactin receptor gene was described in three sisters, two of whom presented with oligomenorrhea and one with infertility. The amino acid substitution leads to loss of function and prolactin insensitivity [18]. When all the abovementioned causes were ruled out and sellar MRI is normal, diagnosis of idiopathic hyperprolactinemia is made, albeit the presence of microadenomas not detectable in the image cannot be excluded [6].

Current Therapies and Future Perspectives

Treatment goals include restoration of eugonadism and resolution of galactorrhea. In the presence of macroadenoma, treatment also aims to reduce its size and preserve, or even restore, pituitary function when impaired. The therapeutic modalities available for prolactinomas are medical, surgical, irradiation, and their associations.

Medical Treatment

Dopamine agonists (DA) are the gold standard for the treatment of prolactinomas being most represented by bromocriptine (BRC) and cabergoline (CAB). This class of drugs promotes PRL gene transcription inhibition, PRL secretion decrease, as well as reduction of prolactinoma dimensions [1]. CAB became the drug of choice due to its better tolerance and efficacy, explained by the high affinity and specificity to dopamine receptor subtype 2 [1]. The initial dose of CAB usually is one tablet (0.5 mg) twice per week, after dinner, and the titration is carried out according to the decrease of PRL levels and tumor dimensions [19]. CAB leads to normal serum PRL levels in over 85% of patients and tumor reduction by more than 80% of them, while BRC promotes normal serum PRL levels in 80% and reduction of tumor dimensions in 70% of cases [20].

The most common DA side effects are nausea, vomiting, and postural hypotension and rarely nasal congestion, cramps, and psychiatric disorders [21]. CAB, in higher doses, was related to valvulopathy in patients with Parkinson's disease, usually older patients with other comorbidities that could contribute to increase the risk of heart valve disease. CAB, not BRC, has an agonist activity at serotonin receptor 5HT2B, which can promote fibroblast proliferation and valvular insufficiency, especially in tricuspid and pulmonary valves. However, valvulopathy due to CAB treatment for hyperprolactinemia is still controversial. Among 17 studies published about this issue [22–33], only one showed an association between CAB's use and the presence of moderate tricuspid insufficiency [24]. Moreover, in other four [23, 26, 29, 32] there was a higher prevalence of valvular regurgitation, especially in the tricuspid valve, without clinical repercussion. In two studies, valve structure changes were described, with a greater risk of fibrosis [31] and calcification [32] compared to the control group. Nonetheless, in our opinion individualized monitoring with echocardiography is desirable until more consistent data will be available. Recent data pointed to remission of hyperprolactinemia after withdrawal of the drug in a substantial number of patients. Passos et al. [34] pointed to normoprolactinemia after BRC withdrawal in 20.6% of patients (25.8% in microprolactinomas and 15.9% in macroprolactinomas) after drug use for a median time of 44 months. Even higher remission ratios were observed by Colao et al. [35] using CAB for a median time of 40 months (69% in microprolactinomas and 64% in macroprolactinomas). Notwithstanding, Dekkers et al. [36], in a recent meta-analysis of 19 studies about DA withdraw, showed that the mean number of patients in remission was 21% with a higher nonsignificant tendency toward CAB (35%) compared to BRC (20%). Two other meta-analysis published in 2015 [37] and 2018 [38], including 637 and 1106 patients on DA, showed remission rates of 35% and 36.6%. Lenght of treatment, tumor reduction, normoprolactinemia and low dose of CAB at withdrawal were factors associated with remission. Although the guideline of Endocrine Society [21] suggests that DA suspension should be performed gradually, in patients treated for at least 2 years, we suggest that the removal of DA should be individualized. In the last few years, impulse control disturbance were reported from 8 to 61% in patients harboring prolactinomas on CAB, especially hypersexuality. These symptoms should be actively investigated in the medical interview [39].

In patients with drug-related hyperprolactinemia when drug cannot be discontinued and in patients with idiopathic hyperprolactinemia or microprolactinomas without desire of fertility (particularly with resistance or intolerance to DA), hormonal replacement can be indicated [19].

Surgical Treatment

Considered secondary in the therapeutic algorithm of prolactinomas, the indications for surgery include patient's desire in non-invasive microprolactinomas, DA resistance/persistent intolerance, absence of visual impairment reversal in a short period of DA use, symptomatic apoplexy, cerebrospinal fluid leakage, and/or visual compromise due to tumor shrinkage with chiasma retraction with DA treatment. Surgery is usually performed through microscopic or endoscopic transsphenoidal route, and their results depend on neurosurgeon's experience and skillness, on serum PRL levels, and on tumor's size and the invasiveness. Gillam et al. [40] reviewing 50 surgical series showed remission in 74.7% of microprolactinomas and in 33.9% of macroprolactinomas. Of note, the recurrence rate in this same analysis was 18.2 and 22.8%, for microprolactinomas and macroprolactinomas, respectively.

Radiotherapy

Prolactinomas are among the most radioresistant pituitary adenomas, and therefore radiotherapy is limited to aggressive tumors resistant to usual treatments. Gillam et al. [40] reviewing published data show that the normalization average of PRL levels was similar with radiotherapy by conventional technique (34.1%) or by stereotactic (31.4%) approach. Side effects include optic tract damage, 50% risk of hypopituitarism in 10–20 years, neuropsychological disturbances, development of secondary tumors, and stroke.

Fertility and Pregnancy

Treatment with DA restores fertility in most cases. In the absence of response to drug treatment, and in cases of microprolactinomas or intrasellar macroprolactinomas, ovulation induction with clomiphene citrate or recombinant gonadotropins may be used [41].

The risk of tumor growth with clinical consequences during pregnancy is up to 5% in microprolactinomas, making DA withdrawn upon confirmation of pregnancy a safe procedure. Clinical follow-up should be done in each pregnancy trimester, a systematic assay of PRL not being indicated. In the presence of significant headache or visual complaints confirmed by a neurophthalmologic evaluation, sellar MRI without contrast is indicated, preferably after the first trimester. If a significant tumor growth is detected, DA should be reintroduced. In patients with macroadenomas, however, the risk of clinical significant tumor growth with is higher: 15–35%. Therefore, in patients with expansive macroprolactinomas, tumor reduction within the sellar boundaries preferable for at least 1 year of treatment with DA, before allowing pregnancy, is highly desirable. In cases of no tumor shrinkage, surgical treatment is indicated. The maintenance of DA throughout pregnancy is up to the specialist discretion. Neurophthalmological evaluation should be performed periodically. Reintroduction of the drug is indicated when tumor growth occurs. If this is not effective, surgical treatment should be performed, preferably in the second trimester [42]. A multicentric Brazilian study including 233 pregnancies induced by CAB confirmed previous results of safety in materna and fetal outcomes in CAB-induced pregnancies. Although CAB maintenance after pregnancy comfirmation was associated with higher miscarriage rates [43]. In men, in addition to sexual dysfunction, hypogonadism related to hyperprolactinemia can promote changes in sperm quality, mainly asthenospermia [44]. In men with prolactinoma on DA with persistent hypogonadism, with or without normalization of serum PRL, the use of clomiphene citrate has been proven useful in the recovery of the gonadotropic axis. This approach has advantages over testosterone replacement by restoring fertility [45].

Addressing Prolactinomas Resistant and/or Aggressive

Aggressive pituitary tumors are defined by the presence of extensive expansion or invasiveness of neighboring structures, rapid tumor growth or recurrence, or the presence of giant tumor, with more than 4 cm in diameter. Diagnosis of pituitary carcinoma is performed only in the presence of metastases. They are extremely rare, being PRL secretion tumors the most prevalent. Aggressive prolactinomas are more common in young male patients. The prevalence of prolactinomas resis-

tant to DA is approximately 10% of microprolactinomas and 18% of macroprolactinomas [1]. Reduction of dopaminergic D2 receptors is its principal mechanism [46].

The initial strategy to treat patients partially resistant to DA is the stepwise increase dose. Ono et al. [25] achieved normalization of PRL levels in 96.2% of patients with dose up to 12 mg per week of CAB, an exceeding elevated dose. For agressive/invasive prolactinomas, temozolomide can be used, with or without radiotheraphy, with tumor control in about 60% of cases. Nevertheless, lenght of treatment in responsive cases and failure in second attempt are important questions related to this chemotherapy [47]. Two cases of resistant prolactinomas were sucessfully treated with Pasireotide [48]. Lapatinibe were used in four agressive/invasive prolactinomas, with tumor control in thee [49]. Other therapies as estrogen pathway modulators and mTOR/akt inhibitors may be promising therapies [50].

Surgical treatment, even non-curative, may be effective in obtaining normoprolactinemia in patients partially resistant to DA, who may subsequently respond to cabergoline reintroduction [51, 52].

Summary: Diagnosis and Treatment

Hyperprolactinemia is a major cause of hypogonadism and infertility, especially among young women. Proper diagnostic of its cause is essential for appropriate treatment indication. Figure 5.1 summarizes the steps for diagnosis in

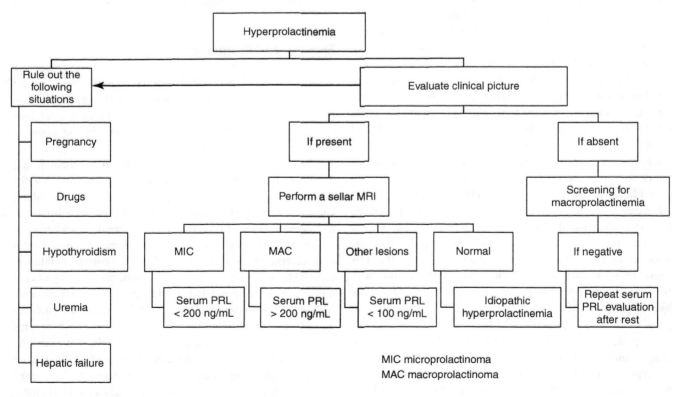

Fig. 5.1 Diagnosis of hyperprolactinemia algorithm

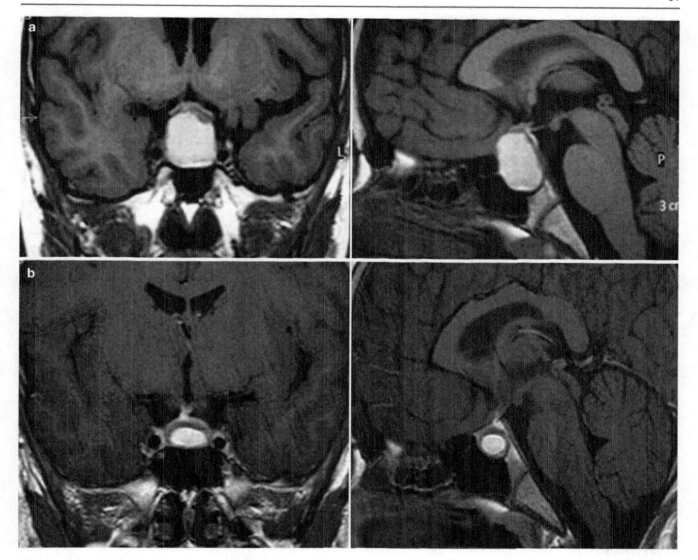

Fig. 5.2 (**a**) Before treatment. Sellar T1-weighted MRI after gadolinium enhancement, coronal (*left*) and sagittal (*right*) depicted a sellar mass impinging optic chiasma. (**b**) After 1 year of treatment with CAB. Sellar T1-weighted MRI after gadolinium enhancement, coronal (*left*) and sagittal (*right*) depicted an important reduction of tumor dimensions, with optic chiasma free of compression

an algorithm. In idiopathic hyperprolactinemia and prolactinomas, the treatment of choice is the use of DA. Surgical treatment and radiation are options for cases of resistance or intolerance to DA. Figure 5.2 depicted sellar MRI of a patient with macroprolactinoma in whom surgery was indicated. The algorithm suggested for the treatment is in Fig. 5.3.

A sellar MRI was performed in a 11-year-old male patient complaining of headache, and a sellar mass was depicted (Fig. 5.2a). Serum PRL level was 1130 ng/ml. The patient also had pubertal impairment development. Neurophthalmologic evaluation was normal. After 4 years of treatment with BRC, there was tumoral reduction without normalization of serum PRL levels. In our department, BRC was substituted for CAB, and dosage was gradually augmented until 3.5 mg a week. After 1 year of treatment with CAB, serum PRL levels were normal, and an additional tumoral reduction occurred (Fig. 5.2b).

Fig. 5.3 Prolactinoma
treatment algorithm

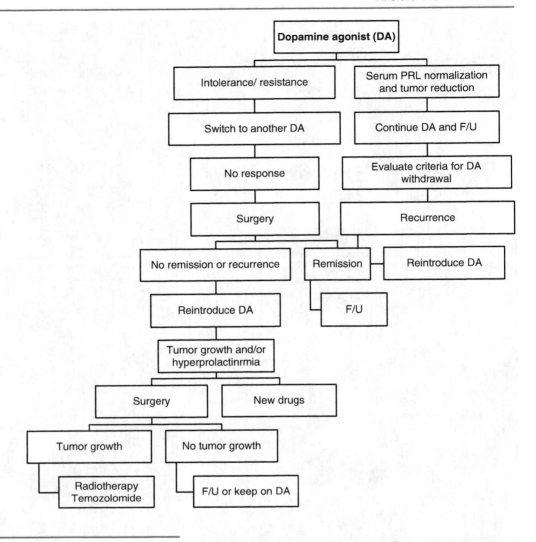

References

1. Bronstein MD. Disorders of prolactin secretion and prolactinomas. In: DeGroot LJ, Jameson JL, editors. Endocrinology. 6th ed. Philadelphia: Saunders; 2010. p. 333–57.
2. Sonigo C, Bouilly J, Carré N, Tolle V, Caraty A, Tello J, Simony-Conesa FJ, Millar R, Young J, Binart N. Hyperprolactinemia-induced ovarian acyclicity is reversed by kisspeptin administration. J Clin Invest. 2012;122(10):3791–5.
3. Batrinos ML, Panitsa-Faflia C, Tsiganou E, Pitoulis G, Liapi C. Contribution to the problem of hyperprolactinaemia: experience with 4,199 prolactin assays and 117 prolactinomas. Int J Fertil Menopausal Stud. 1994;39(2):120–7.
4. Colao A. Pituitary tumours: the prolactinoma. Best Pract Res Clin Endocrinol Metab. 2009;23(5):575–96.
5. Vieira JGHV, Oliveira JH, Tachibana T, Maciel RMB, Hauache OM. Avaliação dos níveis de prolactina sérica: é necessário repouso antes da coleta? Arq Bras Endocrinol Metabol. 2006;50(3):569.
6. Glezer A, Bronstein MD. Approach to the patient with persistent hyperprolactinemia and negative sellar imaging. J Clin Endocrinol Metab. 2012;97(7):2211–6.
7. Glezer A, Bronstein MD. Pituitary autoimmune disease: nuances in clinical presentation. Endocrine. 2012;42(1):74–9.
8. Molitch ME. Drugs and prolactin. Pituitary. 2008;11:209–18.
9. Hekimsoy Z, Kafesçiler S, Güçlü F, Özmen B. The prevalence of hyperprolactinemia in overt and subclinical hypothyroidism. Endocr J. 2010;57(12):1011–5.
10. Robin G, Catteau-Jonard S, Young J, Dewailly D. Physiopathological link between polycystic ovary syndrome and hyperprolactinemia: myth or reality? Gynecol Obstet Fertil. 2011;39(3):141–5.
11. Faubion WA, Nader S. Spinal cord surgery and galactorrhea: a case report. Am J Obstet Gynecol. 1997;177:465–6.
12. Saraç F, Tütüncüoğlu P, Ozgen AG, Saygili F, Yilmaz C, Bilgen I, Memiş A. Prolactin levels and examination with breast ultrasound or mammography. Adv Ther. 2008;25(1):59–66.
13. Glezer A, Soares CR, Vieira JG, Giannella-Neto D, Ribela MT, Goffin V, Bronstein MD. Human macroprolactin displays low biological activity via its homologous receptor in a new sensitive bioassay. J Clin Endocrinol Metab. 2006;91(3):1048–55.
14. Gibney J, Smith TP, McKenna TJ. Clinical relevance of macroprolactin. Clin Endocrinol. 2005;62:633–43.
15. Bronstein MD. Editorial: Is macroprolactinemia just a diagnostic pitfall? Endocrine. 2012;41(2):169–70.
16. Vilar L, Freitas MC, Naves LA, Casulari LA, Azevedo M, Montenegro R Jr, Barros AI, Faria M, Nascimento GC, Lima JG, Nóbrega LH, Cruz TP, Mota A, Ramos A, Violante A, Lamounier Filho A, Gadelha MR, Czepielewski MA, Glezer A, Bronstein MD. Diagnosis and management of hyperprolactinemia: results of a Brazilian multicenter study with 1234 patients. J Endocrinol Investig. 2008;31:436–44.

17. Karavitaki N, Thanabalasingham G, Shore HC, Trifanescu R, Ansorge O, Meston N, Turner HE, Wass JA. Do the limits of serum prolactin in disconnection hyperprolactinaemia need re-definition? A study of 226 patients with histologically verified non-functioning pituitary macroadenoma. Clin Endocrinol (Oxf). 2006;65(4):524–9.

18. Newey PJ, Gorvin CM, Cleland SJ, Willberg CB, Bridge M, Azharuddin M, Drummond RS, van der Merwe PA, Klenerman P, Bountra C, Thakker RV. Mutant prolactin receptor and familial hyperprolactinemia. N Engl J Med. 2013;369(21):2012–20.

19. Webster J, Piscitelli G, Polli A, Ferrari CI, Ismail I, Scanlon MF. A comparison of cabergoline and bromocriptine in the treatment of hyperprolactinemic amenorrhea. Cabergoline Comparative Study Group. N Engl J Med. 1994;331:904–9.

20. Colao A, Savastano S. Medical treatment of prolactinomas. Nat Rev Endocrinol. 2011;7(5):267–78.

21. Melmed S, Casanueva FF, Hoffman AR, Kleinberg DL, Montori VM, Schlechte JA, Wass JA. Endocrine Society. Diagnosis and treatment of hyperprolactinemia: an Endocrine Society clinical practice guideline. J Clin Endocrinol Metab. 2011;96(2):273–88.

22. Valassi E, Klibanski A, Biller BM. Clinical review#: potential cardiac valve effects of dopamine agonists in hyperprolactinemia. J Clin Endocrinol Metab. 2010;95(3):1025–33.

23. Kars M, Pereira AM, Bax JJ, Romijn JA. Cabergoline and cardiac valve disease in prolactinoma patients: additional studies during long-term treatment are required. Eur J Endocrinol. 2008;159(4):363–7.

24. Colao A, Galderisi M, Di Sarno A, Pardo M, Gaccione M, D'Andrea M, Guerra E, Pivonello R, Lerro G, Lombardi G. Increased prevalence of tricuspid regurgitation in patients with prolactinomas chronically treated with cabergoline. J Clin Endocrinol Metab. 2008;93(10):3777–84.

25. Ono M, Miki N, Kawamata T, Makino R, Amano K, Seki T, Kubo O, Hori T, Takano K. Prospective study of high-dose cabergoline treatment of prolactinomas in 150 patients. J Clin Endocrinol Metab. 2008;93(12):4721–7.

26. Nachtigall LB, Valassi E, Lo J, McCarty D, Passeri J, Biller BM, Miller KK, Utz A, Grinspoon S, Lawson EA, Klibanski A. Gender effects on cardiac valvular function in hyperprolactinaemic patients receiving cabergoline: a retrospective study. Clin Endocrinol (Oxf). 2010;72(1):53–8.

27. Lafeber M, Stades AM, Valk GD, Cramer MJ. Teding van Berkhout F, Zelissen PM. Absence of major fibrotic adverse events in hyperprolactinemic patients treated with cabergoline. Eur J Endocrinol. 2010;162(4):667–75.

28. Tan T, Cabrita IZ, Hensman D, Grogono J, Dhillo WS, Baynes KC, Eliahoo J, Meeran K, Robinson S, Nihoyannopoulos P, Martin NM. Assessment of cardiac valve dysfunction in patients receiving cabergoline treatment for hyperprolactinaemia. Clin Endocrinol (Oxf). 2010;73(3):369–74.

29. Boguszewski CL, dos Santos CM, Sakamoto KS, Marini LC, de Souza AM, Azevedo M. A comparison of cabergoline and bromocriptine on the risk of valvular heart disease in patients with prolactinomas. Pituitary. 2012;15(1):44–9.

30. Yarman S, Kurtulmus N, Bilge A. Optimal effective doses of cabergoline and bromocriptine and valvular lesions in men with prolactinomas. Neuro Endocrinol Lett. 2012;33(3):340–6.

31. Elenkova A, Shabani R, Kalinov K, Zacharieva S. Increased prevalence of subclinical cardiac valve fibrosis in patients with prolactinomas on long-term bromocriptine and cabergoline treatment. Eur J Endocrinol. 2012;167(1):17–25.

32. Halperin I, Aller J, Varela C, Mora M, Abad A, Doltra A, Santos AE, Batista E, García-Pavía P, Sitges M, Mirelis JG, Lucas T, Puig-Domingo M. No clinically significant valvular regurgitation in long-term cabergoline treatment for prolactinoma. Clin Endocrinol (Oxf). 2012;77(2):275–80.

33. Drake WM, Stiles CE, Howlett TA, Toogood AA, Bevan JS, Steeds RP, UK Dopamine Agonist Valvulopathy Group. A cross-sectional study of the prevalence of cardiac valvular abnormalities in hyperprolactinemic patients treated with ergot-derived dopamine agonists. J Clin Endocrinol Metab. 2014;99(1):90–6.

34. Passos VQ, Souza JJ, Musolino NR, Bronstein MD. Long-term follow-up of prolactinomas: normoprolactinemia after bromocriptine withdrawal. J Clin Endocrinol Metab. 2002;87(8):3578–82.

35. Colao A, Di Sarno A, Cappabianca P, Di Somma C, Pivonello R, Lombardi G. Withdrawal of long-term cabergoline therapy for tumoral and nontumoral hyperprolactinemia. N Engl J Med. 2003;349(21):2023–33.

36. Dekkers OM, Lagro J, Burman P, Jørgensen JO, Romijn JA, Pereira AM. Recurrence of hyperprolactinemia after withdrawal of dopamine agonists: systematic review and meta-analysis. J Clin Endocrinol Metab. 2010;95(1):43–51.

37. Hu J, Zheng X, Zhang W, Yang H. Current drug withdrawal strategy in prolactinoma patients treated with cabergoline: a systematic review and meta-analysis. Pituitary. 2015;18(5):745–51. https://doi.org/10.1007/s11102-014-0617-2. PMID: 25500765.

38. Xia MY, Lou XH, Lin SJ, Wu ZB. Optimal timing of dopamine agonist withdrawal in patients with hyperprolactinemia: a systematic review and meta-analysis. Endocrine. 2018;59(1):50–61. https://doi.org/10.1007/s12020-017-1444-9. Epub 2017 Oct 17. PMID: 29043560.

39. De Sousa SMC, Baranoff J, Rushworth RL, Butler J, Sorbello J, Vorster J, Thompson T, McCormack AI, Inder WJ, Torpy DJ. Impulse Control Disorders in Dopamine Agonist-Treated Hyperprolactinemia: Prevalence and Risk Factors. J Clin Endocrinol Metab. 2020;105(3):dgz076. https://doi.org/10.1210/clinem/dgz076. PMID: 31580439.

40. Gillam MP, Molitch ME, Lombardi G, et al. Advances in the treatment of prolactinomas. Endocr Rev. 2006;27:485–534.

41. Serafini P, Motta ELA, White JS. Restoration of ovarian cyclicity and ovulation induction in hypopituitary women. In: Bronstein MD, editor. Pituitary tumors in pregnancy. Boston: Kluver Academic Publishers; 2001. p. 173–94.

42. Bronstein MD, Paraiba DB, Jallad RS. Management of pituitary tumors in pregnancy. Nat Rev Endocrinol. 2011;7(5):301–10.

43. Sant' Anna BG, Musolino NRC, Gadelha MR, Marques C, Castro M, Elias PCL, Vilar L, Lyra R, Martins MRA, Quidute ARP, Abucham J, Nazato D, Garmes HM, Fontana MLC, Boguszewski CL, Bueno CB, Czepielewski MA, Portes ES, Nunes-Nogueira VS, Ribeiro-Oliveira A Jr, Francisco RPV, Bronstein MD, Glezer A. A Brazilian multicentre study evaluating pregnancies induced by cabergoline in patients harboring prolactinomas. Pituitary. 2020;23(2):120–8. https://doi.org/10.1007/s11102-019-01008-z. PMID: 31728906.

44. De Rosa M, Ciccarelli A, Zarrilli S, Guerra E, Gaccione M, Di Sarno A, Lombardi G, Colao A. The treatment with cabergoline for 24 month normalizes the quality of seminal fluid in hyperprolactinaemic males. Clin Endocrinol (Oxf). 2006;64(3):307–13.

45. Ribeiro RS, Abucham J. Recovery of persistent hypogonadism by clomiphene in males with prolactinomas under dopamine agonist treatment. Eur J Endocrinol. 2009;161(1):163–9.

46. Passos VQ, Fortes MA, Giannella-Neto D, Bronstein MD. Genes differentially expressed in prolactinomas responsive and resistant to dopamine agonists. Neuroendocrinology. 2009;89(2):163–70.

47. Halevy C, Whitelaw BC. How effective is temozolomide for treating pituitary tumours and when should it be used? Pituitary. 2017 Apr;20(2):261–6.

48. Coopmans EC, van Meyel SWF, Pieterman KJ, van Ipenburg JA, Hofland LJ, Donga E, Daly AF, Beckers A, van der Lely AJ, Neggers SJCMM. Excellent response to pasireotide therapy in an aggressive and dopamine-resistant prolactinoma. Eur J Endocrinol.

2019;181(2):K21-K27. https://doi.org/10.1530/EJE-19-0279. **PMID:** 31167168.

49. Cooper O, Bonert VS, Rudnick J, Pressman BD, Lo J, Salvatori R, Yuen KCJ, Fleseriu M, Melmed S. EGFR/ErbB2-Targeting Lapatinib Therapy for Aggressive Prolactinomas. J Clin Endocrinol Metab. 2021;106(2):e917–e925. https://doi.org/10.1210/clinem/dgaa805. PMID: 33150390; PMCID: PMC7823257.

50. Sari R, Altinoz MA, Ozlu EBK, Sav A, Danyeli AE, Baskan O, Er O, Elmaci I. Treatment Strategies for Dopamine Agonist-Resistant and Aggressive Prolactinomas: A Comprehensive Analysis of the Literature. Horm Metab Res. 2021;53(7):413–24. https://doi.org/10.1055/a-1525-2131. Epub 2021 Jul 19. PMID: 34282593.

51. Vroonen L, Jaffrain-Rea ML, Petrossians P, Tamagno G, Chanson P, Vilar L, Borson-Chazot F, Naves LA, Brue T, Gatta B, Delemer B, Ciccarelli E, Beck-Peccoz P, Caron P, Daly AF, Beckers A. Prolactinomas resistant to standard doses of cabergoline: a multicenter study of 92 patients. Eur J Endocrinol. 2012;167(5):651–62.

52. Primeau V, Raftopoulos C, Maiter D. Outcomes of transsphenoidal surgery in prolactinomas: improvement of hormonal control in dopamine agonist-resistant patients. Eur J Endocrinol. 2012;166(5):779–86.

Acromegaly

6

Francisco Bandeira, Alyne Layane Pereira Lemos,
and Sérgio Ricardo de Lima Andrade

Epidemiology

Acromegaly is a rare, progressive, and chronic disease with high morbidity [1]. It increases all-cause mortality compared with the general population. In Europe, acromegaly has an estimated prevalence of 30 to 70 individuals per million. The disease affects patients between the fourth and fifth decades of life, with a 1:1 ratio between men and women [2, 3]. When it begins before closure of the epiphyses, acromegaly is known as gigantism.

Etiology

Most cases of acromegaly (98%) are the result of hypersecretion of growth hormone by the pituitary gland. Also known as somatotropinomas, GH-producing adenomas are benign tumors, mostly macroadenomas (tumors larger than 1 cm). The disease may occur in the presence of a familial factor or may be associated with other endocrine abnormalities; such as multiple neuroendocrine neoplasia (MEN) types 1 and 4, McCune-Albright syndrome, Carney complex, and familial isolated pituitary adenoma (FIPA). In addition, ectopic tumors producing GH and GNRH may manifest themselves as acromegaly [2, 4–6]. Table 6.1 shows the main characteristics of these syndromes. The genesis of the pituitary tumor is complex and involves several abnormalities in the expression of growth factor and the regulation of cell cycle control. Several mutations have been described. Mutations in the somatic activation of the G alpha (Gs) pro-

Table 6.1 Causes of acromegaly

Family syndrome	Gene	Clinical features
MEN type 1	MEN1 (menin) 11q13 e CDKN1B	Pituitary adenoma associated with parathyroid adenomas and pancreatic neuroendocrine tumors
MEN type 4	Mutation CDKNB1	Similar to MEN1
McCune-Albright syndrome	GNAS 20 q13	Precocious puberty, thyrotoxicosis and Cushing's syndrome. Polyostotic fibrous dysplasia and *café au lait* skin lesions
Carney's complex	PRKAR1A 17q22–24	Associated with thyroid nodules, myxomas, cutaneous pigmentation, and gonadal tumors
FIPA	AIP at 20%, but unknown in most cases	Patients younger than 40 years. They present macroadenomas with extrasellar extension. Less frequently controlled by surgery or somatostatin analogues

tein subunit are found in up to 40% of GH secretory tumors. These cases are more sensitive to treatment with somatostatin analogues. Patients expressing the pituitary tumor transforming gene (PTTG) are more likely to have tumor invasion [2, 4].

Pathophysiology

Approximately 95% of cases of acromegaly are due to a pituitary tumor producing GH. GH is produced by somatotropic cells stimulating the action of hypothalamic GHRH and acts on hepatocytes stimulating the production of IGF-1. This accounts for the typical clinical manifestations of acromegaly. IGF-1, along with steroids and paracrine growth factors, induces a negative feedback on GH release. GH is also suppressed by somatostatin signaling, primarily through the somatostatin receptor (SST) subtype. In rare cases (less than 5%), a hypothalamic or neuroendocrine tumor may release excess GHRH, stimulating the somatotropic cells of the pituitary gland to produce and release GH [2, 5].

F. Bandeira (✉)
Division of Endocrinology, Agamenon Magalhães Hospital,
University of Pernambuco Medical School, Recife, PE, Brazil
e-mail: francisco.bandeira@upe.br

A. L. P. Lemos · S. R. de Lima Andrade
Agamenon Magalhães Hospital, Division of Endocrinology
and Diabetes, University of Pernambuco Medical School,
Recife, Pernambuco, Brazil

© Springer Nature Switzerland AG 2022
F. Bandeira et al. (eds.), *Endocrinology and Diabetes*, https://doi.org/10.1007/978-3-030-90684-9_6

Clinical Features

The clinical presentation of acromegaly is insidious, starting around 4–10 years before the diagnosis of the disease [1]. The systemic complications include cardiovascular disease, sleep apnea, metabolic disorders, and colon neoplasia (Table 6.2). The patient may present with prognathism, frontal protrusion, thickening and increased oiliness of the skin, and cutaneous porosity. Some of these characteristics constitute acromegalic facies as shown in Figs. 6.1 and 6.2. These features occur slowly and progressively and are better identified through the analysis of photographs over time [1, 7].

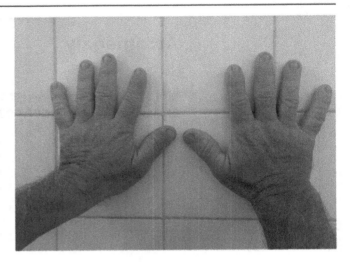

Fig. 6.1 Acromegalic hands

Cardiovascular System

Hypertension occurs in more than 40% of patients and is usually mild and controlled with the usual antihypertensive agents. Cardiac involvement is the major cause of mortality in patients with acromegaly. Cardiomyopathy is present in most patients [8]. Myocardial hypertrophy is biventricular and concentric, compromising mainly the left ventricle. Morphologic changes can lead to arrhythmias, hyperkinesia, increased heart rate, systolic and diastolic dysfunction, and, ultimately, heart failure [2]. In advanced stages, the aortic and mitral valves are also affected. Coronary heart disease occurs mainly due to associated factors such as hypertension and glucose intolerance [1, 2, 5, 7].

Table 6.2 Clinical features of the acromegaly

Cutaneous	Oily skin Hyperhidrosis Acanthosis nigricans
Musculoskeletal	Prognathism, frontal protrusion Arthralgia, osteoarthritis Myopathy, chronic pain Vertebral fractures
Cardiovascular	Arterial hypertension Cardiomyopathy Left ventricular hypertrophy Arrhythmias Cardiac failure
Metabolic	Diabetes mellitus Glucose intolerance
Gastrointestinal	Colonic polyposis Dental changes (malocclusion of the jaw)
Respiratory	Sleep apnea Macroglossia Upper airway obstruction
Visceromegalias	Cardiomegaly Hepatomegaly Splenomegaly
Neurologic	Carpal tunnel syndrome Brain arteries aneurism Headache
Others	Decrease in quality of life

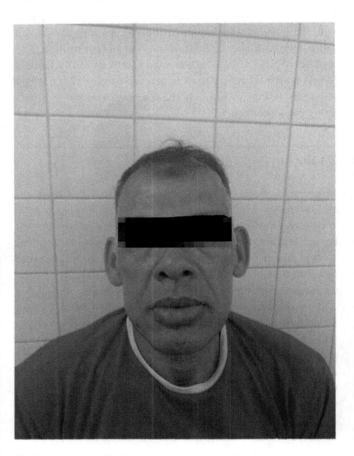

Fig. 6.2 Acromegalic face due to soft tissue thickening

Endocrine and Metabolic Features

Diabetes is more frequent in acromegalic patients than in the general population and is also responsible for the increased mortality. Increased GH levels result in peripheral insulin resistance, hyperinsulinemia, and decreased peripheral glucose uptake. The prevalence of diabetes in patients with acromegaly is reported to be 52% in some studies [9].

Hypogonadism is present in approximately 50% of patients and can occur in cases of hypopituitarism or hyperprolactinemia. Hypopituitarism is found in up to 40% of cases, due to compression of the pituitary gland or destruction of the pituitary tissue. Hyperprolactinemia should be investigated as a cause of hypogonadism [8].

Musculoskeletal Features

Arthropathy affects approximately 75% of patients and is the main cause of morbidity in acromegaly. The condition affects both large and small joints, as well as the vertebrae. Joint changes may be irreversible, depending on the duration of the disease [8]. Carpal tunnel syndrome is also present. Patients present with chronic pain, which impairs their quality of life. Miller et al. evaluated 58 acromegalic patients for musculoskeletal complaints: 90% reported musculoskeletal pain, 84% had hip osteoarthritis, and 34% presented with osteoarthritis of the knees [10]. The bone quality is decreased despite the preserved density. There may be vertebral fractures, usually related to the male sex, hypogonadism, and acromegalic disease activity [11]. There is trabecular bone loss with related preservation of cortical bone. The hands and feet become enlarged due to soft tissue thickening.

Neoplastic Features

Colonic polyps may occur. These are associated with an increased risk of colorectal cancer.

Respiratory System

Sleep apnea is an underestimated condition and may be present in up to 70% of patients. It results from the growth of the soft tissues adjacent to the airways, causing obstruction [2]. This condition is one of the causes of a worsening of hypertension and requires careful evaluation. Apnea may not resolve consistently, even with the proper treatment of the acromegaly, and it requires evaluation by a maxillofacial surgeon and sleep specialists [8]. Macroglossia contributes to upper airway obstruction and may hinder intubation during a surgical procedure [2].

Diagnosis

The serum levels of IGF-1 and GH are persistently high in acromegaly. Serum IGF-1 measurement is the initial test indicated in all patients with suspected clinical features [1, 2, 5].

Table 6.3 Diagnosis of the acromegaly

Test	Comments, interpretations
Serum IGF-1	High values according to age group
Basal GH	GH basal ≥0,4 µg/L GH > 5 µg/L in men and GH > 10 µg/L in women, the presence of characteristic clinical features confirms acromegaly without the need to perform OGTT
Measurement of GH after 75 g oral glucose tolerance test	GH > 0.4 µg/L associated with a high IGF-1, confirms the diagnosis The *Endocrine Society* recommends the cut-off point >1.0 µg/l

Patients with various comorbidities, such as sleep apnea, type 2 diabetes mellitus, debilitating arthritis, carpal tunnel syndrome, hyperhidrosis, and hypertension, even without typical acromegaly characteristics, should undergo IGF-1 measurement. Basal GH measurement should not be done routinely because of its pulsatility. In such cases, the GH level should be evaluated by carrying out an oral glucose tolerance test. This is the gold standard for the diagnosis of acromegaly because it shows the absence of normal suppression of the serum GH concentration during hyperglycemia. During this test, 75 g dextrose is given to the patient, and the GH level is measured at 30, 60, 90, and 120 minutes. Values above 0.4 µg/L (or ng/mL) confirm the diagnosis. A random GH concentration lower than 0.4 µg/L associated with a normal IGF-1 level rules out the diagnosis of acromegaly (Table 6.3) [1, 2, 5].

Plasma testosterone measurement is required for hypogonadism assessment. Patients may have low levels of the sex hormone-binding globulin, making biochemical diagnosis difficult [8].

Pituitary hormone deficiencies may occur because most patients present with large tumors, leading to panhypopituitarism. Gadolinium-enhanced magnetic resonance imaging is used to evaluate tumor extension.

Screening of diseases associated with acromegaly is important and must be done conform to Table 6.4.

Treatment

Transsphenoidal Surgery

Transsphenoidal surgery (TS) is the first-line treatment for control of GH and IGF-1 hypersecretion. The success of this procedure depends on the tumor size, preoperative hormone levels, resection of tumor pseudocapsule, the surgeon's experience, and cavernous sinus invasion [5, 12–14]. Invasive pituitary macroadenomas have a remission rate of less than 50%, whereas the cure rate of patients with noninvasive microadenomas is around 80% [13]. A recent meta-analysis found a remission rate of 74.2% in noninvasive microadenomas, 76.4% in noninvasive macroadenomas, and only 47.6% in invasive macroadenomas [15].

Table 6.4 Screening of diseases associated with acromegaly

Additional tests	Frequency	Comorbidity assessed
Colonoscopy	Should be performed every 5 years in patients with polyps	Intestinal polyposis and colorectal carcinoma
Thyroid USG	Annually	Nodules and/or thyroid neoplasia
Spine radiography	Annually	Evaluation of fractures and morphometric fractures
Echocardiogram and electrocardiogram	Annually	Cardiac abnormalities
Fasting plasma glucose and HbA1c	Every 6 months	Diabetes mellitus
Total serum testosterone	Annually	Hypogonadism
Serum cortisol, FT4, prolactin	Annually	Evaluate pituitary function

Table 6.5 Somatostatin analogs

Somatostatin analogs	Dosing forms	Drug's generation and affinity receptors
Octreotide	100–200 mcg, SQ, 8–12 h	1ª generation SST2 e SST5 receptors
Octreotide LAR	10, 20, or 30 mg, IM, monthly	1ª generation SST2 e SST5 receptors
Sustained-release lanreotide	30 mg, IM, each 10–14 days	1ª generation SST2 e SST5 receptors
Sustained-release lanreotide	60, 90, or 120 mg, SQ, each 28 days	1ª generation SST2 e SST5 receptors
Sustained-release pasireotide	40 or 60 mg, IM, each 28 days	2ª generation SST1, SST2, SST3, SST5 receptors

The AACE recommends carrying out the OGTT and IGF-1 measurement 12 weeks or more after TS to verify the residual disease [12]. The Endocrine Society recommends the measurement of random GH and IGF-1 levels over the same period, with the patient subjected to OGTT if the random GH concentration is >1 ng/mL.

The potential complications of TS are epistaxis, sinusitis, nasal congestion, and gustatory and olfactory changes [5, 12].

Medical Treatment

Somatostatin Analogues

Somatostatin analogues are indicated after surgical failure when there are significant or moderate comorbidities to severe signs and symptoms of excess GH (Table 6.5) [5, 12]. These inhibit GH secretion by binding to somatostatin receptors in various tissues [12, 16] and are able to normalize IGF-1 levels in up to 70% of cases, decreasing the tumor size [12]. They are approved by the FDA as fast- and slow-release octreotide and as slow-release lanreotide and pasireotide [12, 16]. More than 50% of patients do not achieve biochemical control by using somatostatin analogues alone, thus requir-

ing combination therapy [12]. They are also useful in the preoperative management of tumors that are large and not completely resectable, toward decreasing the tumor size [5, 12, 17]. The main side effects of this class of drugs are injection site discomfort, abdominal pain, nausea, vomiting, and diarrhea [5, 12]. First-generation drugs may cause biliary lithiasis, and second-generation ones may cause glucose tolerance and diabetes mellitus [13].

Dopaminergic Agonists

Dopaminergic agonists bind to dopamine-2 receptors on pituitary somatotrophic cells, decreasing the secretion of GH and, consequently, IGF-1 [12]. They can be used before clinical therapy in the case of disease in moderate activity, presenting IGF-1 and GH at modest levels [5, 12, 13]. The most commonly used drug in this group is cabergoline because it offers greater biochemical control and fewer side effects [5, 12]. Despite being an off-label treatment for acromegaly [18], this drug decreases GH levels by 50% and/or IGF-1 concentrations and the tumor size by 33% on average. Bromocriptine, another member of this class of drugs, is rarely used because it achieves poor disease control even when used in high doses and has many side effects. These drugs fail more than somatostatin analogues to achieve biochemical control of the disease [12], and successful treatment with dopaminergic agonists depends on the baseline IGF-1 levels, treatment duration, basal prolactin level, and, less importantly, cabergoline dose [13]. The main side effects of this class of drugs are gastrointestinal intolerance, headaches, and hypotension [5, 12]. The development of cardiac valve disease secondary to high doses of cabergoline in acromegalics is a controversial issue, but this has been proven in patients with Parkinson's disease [12, 13, 18].

GH Receptor Antagonists

Pegvisomant decreases IGF-1 levels by blocking the tissue effects of excess GH. It is indicated for patients who present little response to TS, radiotherapy (RT), and clinical treatment [5, 12], as well as those with moderate to severe signs and symptoms due to hypersecretion of GH [5]. The use of this drug leads to normalization of IGF-1 levels in 76–97% of cases [12], with no significant differences between monotherapy or combined therapy [12, 19]. Better disease control is achieved in those with lower basal GH and IGF-1 levels. Obesity and IGF-1 > 2.7 x upper limit of normality are conditions predictive of resistance to pegvisomant [19]. Successful treatment and dose titration of this drug should be assessed by decreasing the IGF-1 levels [12]. Because pituitary adenoma is not the target of this therapy, the tumor size should be monitored frequently given that such tumors usually grow during pegvisomant monotherapy, even though it is not clinically significant [5, 12]. The main side effect of the drug is the transient elevation of liver function tests in 5% of cases [5, 12].

Combination Therapy

Among the available options, cabergoline in combination with somatostatin analogues decreases IGF-1 levels by 42% compared with monotherapy with such analogues [12]; this treatment decreases IGF-1 concentrations in 40–50% of cases [18]. Cabergoline and pegvisomant at 10 mg/day decrease IGF-1 levels by 68% [12, 13]; such combination allows the use of a low dose of this GH receptor antagonist [18]. Another effective therapeutic combination is the use of somatostatin analogues with a low dose of pegvisomant, which decreases IGF-1 levels by 95% [12]. Pegvisomant monotherapy, when used in patients with a low response to somatostatin analogues or in combination therapy, represents the best option for disease control, especially in long-term treatment [12].

Radiotherapy

Radiotherapy can be done by using the conventional fractional form or by stereotactic radiosurgery (SR) [5, 12]. Fractionated conventional radiotherapy presents a variable time for clinical response, which can occur in up to 10 years [12], requiring combination with other therapeutic modalities until its full effect is achieved [13]. In addition, a second brain tumor can occur as a result of radiotherapy, such as meningioma and glioma. On the other hand, there is also an increased risk of hypopituitarism [12]. Stereotactic radiosurgery can be carried out as Gamma Knife surgery or CyberKnife therapy. Gamma Knife surgery provides biochemical remission with a lower risk of hypopituitarism. CyberKnife therapy, which is no less effective than Gamma Knife surgery, uses a linear accelerator that applies high-energy protons [5, 12]. SR is indicated more than conventional radiotherapy, except when the residual lesion is large after TS or is very close to the optic chiasm, making it impossible to use radiation greater than 8 Gy [5]. Although the remission rate after use of SR is 10–60% in 15 years, this modality of RT still presents shorter remission and treatment periods compared with the conventional one. Annual screening of IGF-1, GH, and hypopituitarism is required after RT [5].

Treatment in Pregnancy

Pregnancy rarely occurs in active acromegaly. In the gestational period, nonuse of drugs is advisable, unless such use is necessary to control the tumor size or headaches, in which case cabergoline, which presents no risk to the fetus, should be used. During pregnancy, the visual field in patients with macroadenomas should be serially monitored because there may be an increased tumor volume. GH and IGF-1 assays during gestation are not necessary because the serum levels are increased due to the increase in placental GH. The assays do not distinguish between placental and pituitary GH [5].

Pasireotide LAR

This drug is more effective than octreotide LAR in virgin treatment, indicating greater biochemical control of the disease (suppression of GH and IGF-1 for up to 25 months). Its main adverse effect is hyperglycemia, which is greater than that caused by octreotide LAR (28.7% vs 8.3%) [12].

Somatoprim

This new somatostatin analogue binds to the SST2, SST4, and SST5 receptors in the pituitary somatotrophic cells, decreasing GH secretion in vitro and in nonresponders to octreotide [12].

Subcutaneous Octreotide

This subcutaneous option requires only small volumes and promotes the prolonged release of octreotide [12]. However, further studies are needed to investigate this treatment alternative.

Oral Octreotide

Despite their convenient route of administration, emulsion-based systems have not yet been proven to be effective in decreasing GH and IGF-1 levels. The conventional options are thus still preferred [12].

Temozolomide

This alkylating chemotherapeutic analogue for aggressive pituitary tumors has no defined role in the treatment of acromegaly but may have some benefit in decreasing GH and IGF-1 levels [12].

References

1. Katznelson L, Atkinson JLD, Cook DM, Ezzat SZ, Hamrahian AH, Miller KK. American Association of Clinical Endocrinologists medical guidelines for clinical practice for the diagnosis and treatment of acromegaly - 2011 update. Endocr Pract. 2011;17:1–44.
2. Capatina C, Wass JAH. Acromegaly. J Endocrinol. 2015;226(2):T141–60.
3. Fernandez-Rodriguez E, Casanueva FF, Bernabeu I. Update on prognostic factors in acromegaly: is a risk score possible? Pituitary. 2015;18(3):431–40.
4. Giustina A, Chanson P, Kleinberg D, Bronstein MD, Clemmons DR, Klibanski A, et al. Expert consensus document: a consensus on the medical treatment of acromegaly. Nat Rev Endocrinol. 2014;10(4):243–8.

5. Katznelson L, Laws ER, Melmed S, Molitch ME, Murad MH, Utz A, et al. Acromegaly: an Endocrine Society clinical practice guideline. J Clin Endocrinol Metab. 2014;99(11):3933–51.

6. Melmed S. Acromegaly pathogenesis and treatment. J Clin Invest. 2009;119(11):3189–202. https://doi.org/10.1172/JCI39375.

7. Zarool-hassan R, Conaglen HM, Conaglen JV, Elston MS. Symptoms and signs of acromegaly: an ongoing need to raise awareness among healthcare practitioners. J Prim Health Care. 2016;8:157–63.

8. Melmed S, Casanueva FF, Klibanski A, Bronstein MD, Chanson P, Lamberts SW, et al. A consensus on the diagnosis and treatment of acromegaly complications. Pituitary. 2013;16(3):294–302.

9. Dreval AV, Trigolosova IV, Misnikova IV, Kovalyova YA, Tishenina RS, Barsukov IA, et al. Prevalence of diabetes mellitus in patients with acromegaly. Endocr Connect. 2014;3(2):93–8.

10. Miller A, Doll H, David J, Wass J. Impact of musculoskeletal disease on quality of life in long-standing acromegaly. Eur J Endocrinol. 2008;158(5):587–93.

11. Mazziotti G, Biagioli E, Maffezzoni F, Spinello M, Serra V, Maroldi R, et al. Bone turnover, bone mineral density, and fracture risk in acromegaly: a meta-analysis. J Clin Endocrinol Metab. 2015;100(2):384–94.

12. Shanik MH. Limitations of current approaches for the treatment of acromegaly. Endocr Pract. 2016;22(2):210–9.

13. Chanson P. Medical treatment of acromegaly with dopamine agonists or somatostatin analogs. Neuroendocrinology. 2016;103(1):50–8.

14. Anik I, Cabuk B, Gokbel A, Selek A, Cetinarslan B, Anik Y, et al. Endoscopic transsphenoidal approach for acromegaly with remission rates in 401 patients: 2010 consensus criteria. World Neurosurg. 2017;108:278–90.

15. Briceno V, Zaidi HA, Doucette JA, Onomichi KB, Alreshidi A, Mekary RA, et al. Efficacy of transsphenoidal surgery in achieving biochemical cure of growth hormone-secreting pituitary adenomas among patients with cavernous sinus invasion: a systematic review and meta-analysis. Neurol Res. 2017;39(5):387–98.

16. Fattah S, Brayden DJ. Progress in the formulation and delivery of somatostatin analogs for acromegaly. Ther Deliv. 2017;8(10):867–78.

17. Losa M, Garbin E, Pedone E, Mortini P. Normal Insulin-like Growth Factor 1 During Somatostatin Receptor Ligand Treatment Predicts Surgical Cure in Acromegaly. J Clin Endocrinol Metab. 2020;105(9):dgaa424. https://doi.org/10.1210/clinem/dgaa424.

18. Kuhn E, Chanson P. Cabergoline in acromegaly. Pituitary. 2017;20(1):121–8.

19. Ragonese M, Grottoli S, Maffei P, Alibrandi A, Ambrosio MR, Arnaldi G, et al. How to improve effectiveness of pegvisomant treatment in acromegalic patients. J Endocrinol Investig. 2017;2017:1–7.

Hypopituitarism

Manuel Faria, Gilvan Cortês Nascimento, André M. Faria, and Manoel R. A. Martins

Hypopituitarism is a complex medical condition with variable clinical manifestations associated with significant morbidity and mortality. The term describes the deficiency of one or more of the hormones of the anterior or posterior pituitary gland. The majority of patients with hypopituitarism have three to five hormone deficits.

Hypopituitarism affects approximately 4 out of every 100,000 individuals each year [1] with a prevalence of approximately 45 cases per 100,000 individuals. The causes, clinical features, diagnosis, management of hypopituitarism (including endocrine replacement therapy), interaction of hormone replacement, and long-term management are considered in this chapter.

Causes

There are numerous causes of hypopituitarism (Tables 7.1 and 7.2). In a Spanish study comprising two cross-sectional surveys, the causes of hypopituitarism included pituitary tumor (61%), non-pituitary tumor (9%), and nontumor cause (30%) [1].

Traumatic brain injury (TBI) has been described to be one of the most common causes of hypopituitarism, with some series reporting a prevalence of chronic dysfunction in more than 25% of patients [2]. However, most clinicians dealing with neuroendocrine diseases and TBI generally do not see such a high incidence of hypopituitarism in this population.

M. Faria (✉) · G. C. Nascimento
Department of Internal Medicine I, Service of Endocrinology and Metabolism, Hospital Universitário Presidente Dutra, Federal University of Maranhão, São Luís, MA, Brazil

A. M. Faria
Hospital das Clínicas da Faculdade de Medicina de São Paulo, Neurofunctional Surgery Division, Neuroendocrine Unit, São Paulo, SP, Brazil

M. R. A. Martins
Department of Clinical Medicine, Hospital Universitário Walter Cantídio, Federal University of Ceará, Fortaleza, Ceará, Brazil

This disproportion is not clearly explained, but recent data indicate that diagnostic testing, which is designed for high-risk populations and not for a cohort of patients with, for example, de novo isolated GH deficiency (the predominant finding in TBI), might have overestimated the true risk and disease burden of hypopituitarism. There is also large variability among studies conducted on hypopituitarism after TBI regarding the use of different hormone assays, test panels, and cut-off limits, which represents obvious sources of variation in the reported prevalence of the condition. In conclusion, causality between TBI and hypopituitarism remains to be demonstrated with more robust, better designed trials that should include confirmatory testing of all test findings of hormone insufficiency. Whether hormonal replacement therapy could result in relevant clinical benefit in cases of mild deficiencies in this specific population also needs to be proven.

The etiologic factors are determinants in the clinical presentation of this condition. For instance, pituitary apoplexy constitutes a medical emergency with the possibility of acute adrenal crisis and sudden loss of vision. On the other hand, functioning pituitary adenomas lead to a clinical picture that predominates the stigmata of the corresponding hormonal hypersecretion. Signs and symptoms related to local mass effect, including associated secondary hypothyroidism and hypocortisolism, may occur as a nonspecific presentation and remain unrecognizable for a long period of time.

Diagnosis

Clinical Presentation

The clinical presentation of hypopituitarism is often vague and nonspecific, leading to a further delay in diagnosis. Nonspecific symptoms include a feeling of general poor health, increased lethargy, feeling cool, chronic tiredness, reduced appetite, weight loss, and abdominal pain [3, 4]. Hypopituitarism can sometimes develop acutely, leading to a rapid onset of symptoms (excruciating headache, menin-

© Springer Nature Switzerland AG 2022
F. Bandeira et al. (eds.), *Endocrinology and Diabetes*, https://doi.org/10.1007/978-3-030-90684-9_7

Table 7.1 Causes of hypopituitarism

Neoplasia	Vascular
Pituitary adenoma	Pituitary tumor apoplexy
Pituitary carcinoma	Sheehan's syndrome
Craniopharyngioma	Intrasellar carotid artery aneurysm
Pituicytoma	
Fibroma	Subarachnoid hemorrhage
Glioma	
Meningioma	Ischemic stroke
Paraganglioma	Genetic
Teratoma	Combined pituitary hormone deficiencies
Chordoma	
Angioma	Isolated pituitary hormone deficiencies
Sarcoma	
Ependymoma	Infectious
Germinoma	Viral
Cysts	Fungal
Rathke's cleft and dermoid	Tuberculosis
Ganglioneuroma	Syphilis
Astrocytoma	Bacterial (others)
Pituitary mestastasis	Primary empty sella functional
Brain damage	
Surgery	Drugs
Radiotherapy	Glucocorticoid excess
Radiosurgery	Megestrol acetate
Traumatic brain injury	Suppressive thyroxine treatment
Infiltrative/inflammatory disease	
Lymphocytic hypophysitis	Dopamine
Granulomatous hypophysitis	Anabolic sex steroids
Xanthomatous hypophysitis	GnRH agonists
Sarcoidosis	Nutritional
Langerhans cell histiocytosis	Obesity
Giant cell granuloma	Malnutrition
Wegener's granulomatosis	Caloric restriction
Hemochromatosis	Chronic/acute critical illness
	Idiopathic

gism, and cardiovascular collapse) necessitating admission and intensive care management, as is often seen in patients with tumor apoplexy.

The signs and symptoms of underlying diseases can sometimes follow hypopituitarism [4]. Symptoms attributed to the local effects of tumoral masses in the sellar region with suprasellar extension, such as headaches, rhinorrhea, and visual disturbances (typically bilateral hemianopsia, but can also occur as unilateral), frequently remain unrecognized by patients, mostly men, for a long period of time.

Deficits of anterior pituitary hormones may be secondary to hormone excess caused by functioning pituitary tumors, which produces a complex picture combining hormone excess and deficiencies, such as suppression of gonadotropins in hyperprolactinemia, growth hormone deficiency (GHD) caused by cortisol excess in Cushing's syndrome [5] or growth hormone (GH)-secreting macroadenoma that causes acromegaly and hypogonadism [6]. In patients with coexisting pituitary hormone abnormalities, the symptoms of hormone deficiencies may be much less obvious than in the isolated conditions themselves. As an example, hot flashes due to hypogonadism may mask the cold intolerance of hypothyroidism. The coexistence of hypothyroidism and hypocortisolism may result in anorexia and weight loss, while acromegalic patients with thyroid hormone deficiency may present with excess sweating.

The presence of central diabetes insipidus (DI) usually indicates a non-pituitary lesion affecting the hypothalamus or pituitary stalk. Preoperatively, pituitary adenomas rarely cause DI, and its occurence should raise the suspicion of other sellar and suprasellar lesions, such as lymphocytic hypophysitis, craniopharyngiomas, germ cell, and metastatic tumors.

Somatotropin Deficiency

Children

GHD in childhood promotes short stature and delayed bone age with slow growth velocity. Idiopathic GHD is the most common etiology. GH does not appear to have a relevant role in fetal growth. Therefore, in general, children are born with normal length, weight, and general appearance. However, microphallus and cryptorchidism may be present, especially with gonadotropin-associated deficiency. Prolonged jaundice, hypoglycemia-associated seizures (when GHD occurs in conjunction with adrenocorticotropic hormone (ACTH) deficiency), and midline abnormalities suggest a congenital etiology.

Recognition of GHD is more common from the first 12–18 months after birth, with slow growth as an early sign and a consequent downward shift in the normal growth curve. Children tend to present with adiposity around the trunk. They have immature body and facial traits, a high-pitched voice, prominent forehead, depressed mid-face development, delayed dentition, and small hands and feet.

Adults

The severity of the clinical manifestations of GHD in adults depends on the timing of onset. In general, patients present nonspecific symptoms, such as fatigue, decreased energy, low mood, and altered body composition with increased fat and decreased lean body mass and muscle strength, as well as reduced bone mineral density, compromised metabolism of glucose and lipids, and poor quality of life [7]. Childhood-onset GHD patients have a lower lean body mass and bone mineral content and better quality of life compared to adult-onset GHD patients.

Table 7.2 Genetic forms of multiple pituitary hormone deficiencies

	HESX1	OTX2	LHX3	LHX4	SOX3	SOX2	PROP1	POU1F1
GH	+	+	+	+	+	+/−	+	+
LH/FSH	+/−	+/−	+	+/−	+/−	+	+	−
PRL	+/−	−	+	−	+/−	−	+	+
TSH	+/−	+/−	+	+/−	+/−	−	+	+/−
ACTH	+/−	+/−	+/−	+/−	+/−	−	+/−	−
ADH	+/−	−	−	−	+/−	−		−
Inheritance	AR/AD	AD	AR	AD	XL	AD	AR	AR/AD
Pituitary involvement	Normal/hypoplastic AP; normal/ectopic PP	Normal/hypoplastic AP; altered stalk; ectopic PP	Hypoplastic, normal or enlarged AP	Normal/hypoplastic AP; normal or ectopic PP	Hypoplastic AP; ectopic PP	Normal/hypoplastic AP; hypothalamic hamartoma	Hypoplastic, normal or enlarged AP and normal PP	Normal/hypoplastic AP
Extra-pituitary phenotype	SOD; normal optic nerves	Anophthalmia or no ocular pathology; chiari malformation	Limited neck rotation or no; SD	Cerebellar anomalies; chiari malformation	Variable learning difficulties; HCC	Anophthalmia; microphthalmia; DD; SD; HCC; esophageal atresia	No involvement	No involvement

AD autosomal dominant, *AP* anterior pituitary, *AR* autosomal recessive, *DD* developmental delay, *PP* posterior pituitary, *HCC* hypoplasia of corpus callosum, *SD* sensorineural deafness, *SOD* septo-optic dysplasia, *XL* X-linked, + deficiency, − no deficiency

Gonadotropin Deficiency

The clinical presentation of male hypogonadism depends on the time of onset of androgen deficiency. In men with recent onset hypogonadism, the physical examination is usually normal, while diminished facial and body hair, gynecomastia, and small soft testes are features of longstanding hypogonadism [3]. The principal signs and symptoms of androgen deficiency in men are loss of libido, decreased sexual potency, loss of body hair (axillary and pubic), infertility, and low bone mineral density. The threshold testosterone level below which symptoms of androgen deficiency and adverse health outcomes occur and testosterone administration improves outcomes in the general population is currently not known [8].

Female adolescents have primary amenorrhea and lack of breast development, whereas in adult women, gonadotropin deficiency leads to reduced secretion of estradiol, resulting in infertility and oligo-/amenorrhea. Low estrogen is also responsible for genital atrophy and decreased breast volume in chronic hypogonadism. There is a reduction of pubic and axillary hair, especially when concomitant dysfunction of the corticotroph axis is present.

At the prepubertal age, no obvious clinical signs or symptoms are present until the normal age of puberty onset (9–14 years in boys and 8–13 years in girls), when a lack of signs of normal pubertal development is then observed. It should be emphasized that micropenis with or without associated cryptorchidism is an important clinical clue that suggests congenital hypogonadotropic hypogonadism (where there is lack of the normal fetal secretion and postnatal surge of gonadotropins) rather than acquired hypogonadotropic hypogonadism [9].

Thyrotropin Deficiency

The clinical picture of central hypothyroidism is very similar to primary hypothyroidism, but is often milder. Symptoms include cold intolerance, dry skin, decreased appetite with mild weight gain, and fatigue [10]. The presence of goiter usually indicates primary thyroid disease. In children, decreased growth velocity with impairment of neurological development is an important sign.

Corticotropin Deficiency

ACTH deficiency leads to decreased glucocorticoid levels. Mineralocorticoid secretion is preserved, since it is primarily modulated by the renin-angiotensin system. Hyperpigmentation is typical of primary adrenal disease and is absent in central disease. Symptoms of ACTH deficiency are largely nonspecific, including weakness, fatigue, anorexia, weight loss, arthralgia, postural hypotension, and tachycardia [11]. Hyponatremia, hypoglycemia, and eosinophilia may also occur. Ultimately, if left untreated, ACTH deficiency may lead to death due to vascular collapse, since cortisol is needed to maintain vascular tone. Mild ACTH deficiency may remain clinically unnoticed when cortisol production is sufficient for preventing symptoms in the absence of clinical stressors (e.g., infections). Hence, laboratorial evaluation is recommended in all patients at risk of ACTH deficiency.

Antidiuretic Hormone (ADH) Deficiency

ADH deficiency results in polyuria (urine volume >3 L/day in adults) and polydipsia. If the thirst mechanism is not present, as is the case in some patients with hypothalamic lesions, then lack of polydipsia leads to a high risk of life-threatening dehydration and hypernatremia [12].

Diagnostic Testing

The diagnosis of hypopituitarism can often be made through simultaneous measurements of basal anterior pituitary and target gland hormone levels. Each axis should be assessed in patients suspected of having partial or complete loss of pituitary function, because the impairment in these patients is often partial rather than complete.

Low or inappropriately normal serum levels of pituitary hormones in conjunction with low peripheral hormones indicate hypopituitarism. FSH, LH, estradiol (women), testosterone (men), prolactin, TSH, free thyroxine (FT4), 9 am cortisol, and insulin-like growth factor-I (IGF-I) tests form the baseline parameters to assess. In addition, dynamic studies are necessary in most cases for documenting hypopituitarism, particularly for assessing GH secretory reserve and the ACTH-adrenal axis (Table 7.3) [6].

Somatotropin Deficiency

Children

GHD in children is based on auxological data, which is considered the gold standard in such diagnosis [13]. An appropriate differential diagnosis must be performed ruling out other causes of growth failure, such as hypothyroidism, Turner syndrome, and systemic diseases.

Evaluation should be considered when patients present with one of the following conditions: (1) short stature of more than 2.5 standard deviations (SD) below the mean; (2) growth failure, which is defined as height velocity less than 2 SD

Table 7.3 Hormone testing for pituitary function

	Criteria for hormone deficiency
Somatotropic axis	
Baseline	
IGF-I	Low/low-normal
GH	No usefulness
Provocative tests (GH measurement)	
Clonidine test (only for children)	<7–10 µg/L
Insulin tolerance test	Children: <7–10 µg/L
	Adults: <5.1 µg/L
	Transition period: <6.1 µg/L
GHRH-Arg test (only for adults)	Adults:
	Lean <11.5 µg/L
	Overweight <8.0 µg/L
	Obese <4.2 µg/L
	Transition period: <19.0 µg/L
Glucagon test	Children: <7–10 µg/L
	Adults: <2.5–3 µg/L
	Overweight/obese: <1.0 µg/L
Macimorelin test	Adults: <2.8 µg/L
Gonadotropic axis	
Baseline	
Male	
Testosterone	Low
FSH/LH	Low or inappropriately normal
Female	
Estradiol	Low
FSH/LH	In younger women: low or inappropriately normal
	In postmenopausal women: inappropriately low
Provocative test	
GnRH	Not useful in adults
Thyrotropic axis	
Baseline	
Free T4	Low, low-normal
TSH	Low, normal, or slightly increased
Provocative test	
TRH	Not useful
Corticotropic axis	
Baseline	
Cortisol (morning)	<3 µg/dL (<80 nmol/L)
	>18 µg/dL (>500 nmol/L): hypocortisolism excluded
ACTH (morning)	Low or normal
Provocative tests	
Insulin tolerance test	Peak cortisol <18 µg/dL (<500 nmol/L)
250 µg ACTH test	Peak cortisol <18 µg/dL (<500 nmol/L)
Overnight metyrapone test	11-deoxicortisol <7 µg/dL (<200 nmol/L), low cortisol
CRH (human or ovine)	ACTH: peak <2–4× baseline
	Cortisol: peak <20 µg/dL (555 nmol/L)

Table 7.3 (continued)

	Criteria for hormone deficiency
Antidiuretic hormone	
Dynamic test	
Water deprivation	Maximal urinary osmolality (MUO)<300 mOsm/kg/H_2O plus >50% increase in MUO after desmopressin (complete DI)

below the mean for age; (3) a combination of less severe short stature (2–2.5 SD below the mean for age) and growth failure (growth velocity less than 1 SD); (4) clinical picture suggesting hypothalamic-pituitary dysfunction, such as hypoglycemia, microphallus, intracranial tumor, or history of cranial irradiation with decelerating growth; and (5) evidence of deficiency in other hypothalamic-pituitary hormones [14].

The pulsatile nature and short half-life of GH preclude the random measurement of serum GH levels as a useful tool for diagnosing GHD. Thus, IGF-I and IGF-binding protein 3 (IGFBP-3) are appropriate initial tests for GHD in children providing that conditions such as poor nutrition, hypothyroidism, and chronic systemic diseases are excluded. These hormones reflect an integrated assessment of GH secretion because of negligible diurnal variation [15].

IGF-I and IGFBP-3 measurements should be interpreted in relation to reference ranges that are standardized for sex and age. An important drawback to using serum IGF-I for GHD diagnosis is that its values are low in very young children and overlap in GHD patients and normal children. In this context, IGFBP-3 levels, which are less related to age, are more discriminatory than IGF-I levels at the lower end of the normal range [16].

These tests present less than adequate sensitivity, although specificity is high. Thus, in patients with severe GHD, IGF-I and IGFBP-3 levels are invariably reduced. On the other hand, patients with milder abnormalities of GH secretion demonstrate normal levels of IGF-I and its binding protein in a significant percentage of cases [17].

Despite these limitations, measurement of IGF-I and IGFBP-3 levels associated with provocative testing in an appropriate clinical context is now commonly performed when investigating GHD in childhood.

GH Stimulation Testing in Children

Provocative GH testing has several caveats. They are not physiological, since the secretagogues used do not reflect normal GH secretion; the cutoff level of normal is arbitrary and the tests are age dependent. Furthermore, the tests rely upon GH assays of variable accuracy and are all uncomfortable, cumbersome, and risky for the patient [13, 18].

Therefore, there is currently no gold standard provocative GH test for GHD in children. As a result, subnormal responses to two secretagogues are necessary for diagnosis, with the exception of patients presenting with a central nervous system disorder, multiple pituitary hormone defects, or a known genetic defect. In these cases, one test is sufficient to establish the diagnosis [19].

These stimulation tests are performed after an overnight fasting. After the pharmacologic stimulus, serum samples are collected at intervals designed to capture the peak GH level. A "normal" response is defined by a serum GH concentration of greater than 7–10 mcg/L, although the ideal threshold may vary with the assay used. Of note, all patients should be euthyroid and should not be under supraphysiological doses of glucocorticoids before any testing is performed (Tables 7.3 and 7.4).

Clonidine, an α-2 adrenergic receptor agonist, promotes GH release, mainly through GHRH secretion. It is a stronger stimulant for growth hormone release, and therefore false-negative results can follow. On the other hand, children presenting with a GH subnormal response to such stimulus rarely secrete normal GH in response to any other stimuli [20]. The test commonly causes hypotension and drowsiness that may last for hours and promote late hypoglycemia.

Insulin-induced hypoglycemia is a potent stimulant of GH release, and, therefore, the insulin tolerance test (ITT) is among the most specific tests for GHD. However, safety concerns have prevented the widespread use of this test. The proposed mechanism by which hypoglycemia promotes GH secretion is through the suppression of somatostatin tone and stimulation of α-adrenergic receptors [21]. This test requires constant supervision by a clinician and is contraindicated in children less than 2 years of age.

Administration of glucagon promotes GH secretion through a poorly understood mechanism, with the activation of central noradrenergic pathways as a plausible hypothesis [22]. Glucagon presents mild and transient side effects, such as nausea, vomiting, and sweating, and therefore is a very good choice for infants and young children who are more susceptible to the risks of insulin-induced hypoglycemia.

Adults

In adults, the clinical picture of GHD is subtle and nonspecific, and therefore the diagnosis relies on biochemical testing. Patients with structural hypothalamic and/or pituitary disease, surgery, or irradiation in these areas as well as TBI,

Table 7.4 Protocols of dynamic tests for investigation of anterior pituitary (GH and ACTH) and posterior pituitary (ADH) deficiencies

Provocative tests	Dosage	Time of hormone collection	Side effects/drawbacks
GH			
Clonidine (only for children)	5 μg/kg, up to 250 μg, PO	GH: 0, 30, 60, 90 min	Drowsiness; false negative results
Insulin tolerance test	Regular insulin 0.05–0.15 IU/kg, IV	GH: 0, 15, 30, 60, 90, 120 min	Severe hypoglycemia and medical surveillance required
Glucagon	0.03 mg/kg (up to 1 mg) IM/SC; if >90 kg, 1.5 mg	GH: 0, 30, 60, 90, 120, 150, 180, 210, 240 min	Late hypoglycemia; very prolonged test; not well validated in adults
GHRH-ARG (only for adults)	GHRH (1 μg/kg, IV bolus) + arginine (0.5 g/kg, up to 30 g, IV, over 30 min)	GH: 0, 30, 60, 90, 120 min	Very influenced by adiposity
Macimorelin	0.5 mg/kg	GH: 0, 30, 45, 60, 75, 90 120, 150 min	Unpleasant taste
ACTH			
ACTH$_{1-24}$	250 μg IV/IM	Cortisol: 0, 30, and 60 min	Adrenal atrophy is required
Insulin tolerance test	Regular insulin 0.05–0.15 IU/kg, IV	Cortisol: 0, 15, 30, 60, 90, 120 min	See above
Overnight metyrapone	30 mg/kg, PO, at midnight (maximum 3 g)	11-deoxycortisol and cortisol: 8 am	Limited availability; adrenal crisis
CRH (human or ovine)	1 μg/kg, up to 100 μg, IV	Cortisol and ACTH: 0, 15, 30, 60, 90, 120 min	Flushing; expensive
Dynamic test	*Procedure*		*Side effects/drawbacks*
ADH			
Water deprivation	Nothing allowed by mouth; patient voids; weight is recorded; serum Na$^+$ and urine Osm are measured at baseline. Weight is checked after each liter of urine is passed. In each voided urine, measure urine Osm and when two consecutive measurements differ <10% and subject has lost 2% of BW, plasma sample for Na$^+$, Osm, and VP should be drawn. DDAVP 2 μg IV/IM is administered and urine Osm and volume are measured every 30 min in the next 2 h. Dehydration is stopped if patient has lost >3% of BW or if serum Na$^+$ becomes elevated		Difficulties in differentiating partial hypothalamic DI from primary polydipsia

PO per oral, *Osm* osmolality, *BW* body weight, *VP* vasopressin

SAH, or evidence of other pituitary hormone deficiencies should be evaluated for acquired GHD. Otherwise, the presence of three or more pituitary hormone deficiencies associated with a low IGF-I is highly predictive of GHD, in which case provocative testing is not necessary [23]. In addition, patients should receive adequate replacement of other deficient hormones before GH stimulation testing is performed.

GH Stimulation Testing in Adults

ITT is considered the most validated test currently available and is the diagnostic test of choice for GHD in adults. However, it is contraindicated in patients with seizure disorders or ischemic heart disease and requires monitoring, even in healthy adults. Adequate hypoglycemia (<2.2 mmol/L) is not always achieved, and therefore, larger doses of insulin up to 0.3 U/kg may be necessary in obese patients and those with fasting blood glucose above 5.5 mmol/L [24]. An assay cutoff of 5.1 µg/L is recommended for diagnosis [23].

A GHRH and arginine test (GHRH-Arg test) is a very potent and reproducible test. Arginine potentiates the response to GHRH presumably through the inhibition of hypothalamic somatostatin secretion [25]. This combined test is not affected by gender or age and shows few side effects with no hypoglycemia. On the other hand, the assay cutoff for GHD diagnosis depends on the body mass index (BMI) [26]. In addition, GHRH directly stimulates the pituitary, and patients with GHD of hypothalamic origin, mainly after radiotherapy, could present a falsely normal GH response [27]. Obesity can decrease the GH response, thereby mimicking, but this effect is reversible with weight loss [28]. BMI-ajusted cutoffs are therefore mandatory for most GH stimulation tests, including the GHRH-Arg [26] and glucagon tests [29] (Table 7.3).

Administration of glucagon allows for the assessment of GH and ACTH-cortisol reserves and has few side effects with minimal contraindications. It is a good choice when other tests are unavailable or contraindicated. It is performed by administering 1 mg of glucagon intramuscularly (or 1.5 mg for those who weigh >90 kg) and measuring GH every 30 minutes for 4 hours. In adults, an assay cutoff between 2.5 and 3.0 µg/L is recommended for GHD diagnosis [23]. However, in overweight/obese patients, a cutoff of 1.0 µg/L gives the best sensitivity and specificity [30]. Side effects, including nausea, vomiting, diaphoresis, and headaches, occur in 10–30%.

Recently, macimorelin, a synthetic oral ghrelin agonist that stimulates GH in a dose-dependent manner [31], has been approved by the FDA for use in the diagnosis of patients with GHD in December 2017. In a study of 50 subjects with adult GHD and 48 healthy controls, a maximally stimulated serum GH level of less than 2.8 ng/mL at 30, 45, 60, and 90 minutes after macimorelin administration confirmed the presence of adult GHD [32]. The accuracy of the macimore-lin test was comparable with the arginine-GHRH test in the 43 patients who underwent both tests. The authors also reported that using separate cut points of less than 6.9 ng/mL for nonobese and 2.8 for obese subjects reduced the misclassification rate.

Transitional Period

In the transitional period (i.e., after the cessation of linear growth and completion of puberty), the majority of GHD patients must be retested. Those patients with conditions causing multiple pituitary hormone deficiencies (MPHD) (i.e., three or more pituitary hormone deficits) can continue on GH therapy but require determination of an adequate dose. Other patients without MPHD but who present with known mutations or irreversible structural hypothalamic-pituitary lesions/damage should be screened for serum IGF-I levels after terminating therapy for at least 1 month. IGF-I levels below −2 SD are sufficient for GH therapy reinstitution. If the IGF-I level is within the normal range, then one provocative testing is mandatory for GH therapy in the case of a subnormal response.

In the remaining patients, mostly with idiopathic causes, a serum IGF-I test and one provocative test must be performed, and in the case of discordant results, a second provocative test is necessary for the diagnosis of persistent GHD [23, 33].

It is unclear whether different assay cutoffs should be adopted during this transitional period, as opposed to GHD assay cutoffs in adults. Some studies suggest that the assay cutoffs in these cases should be higher than for older adults, with levels of 6.1 µg/L and 19.0 µg/L for the ITT and GHRH-arg, respectively [34, 35].

Gonadotropin Deficiency

In men, low or inappropriately normal levels of gonadotropins combined with low levels of serum testosterone are indicative of secondary hypogonadism. Semen analysis is indicated when considering fertility and may demonstrate a reduced sperm count or possibly azoospermia.

In younger women, oligo-/amenorrhoea with low serum estradiol levels and low or inappropriately normal FSH and LH concentrations is consistent with secondary hypogonadism. In postmenopausal women, the absence of the normal rise of FSH and LH levels is sufficient for establishing a diagnosis.

In secondary hypogonadism, serum prolactin should always be measured to exclude hyperprolactinemia, which might occur for several reasons, such as prolactinomas, sellar and parasellar masses causing pituitary stalk compression, and use of drugs with antidopaminergic activity.

In adults, there is no usefulness in performing the gonadotropin-releasing hormone (GnRH) provocative test because it does not provide any additional information [6].

Thyrotropin Deficiency

Evaluation of the thyrotrophic axis is based on the measurement of basal serum TSH and thyroid hormone levels. Central hypothyroidism is diagnosed when serum TSH levels are low or inappropriately normal coupled with low levels of serum free T4. Occasionally, TSH levels may be slightly elevated but usually remain lower than 10 mIU/mL. In these patients, the elevation of serum TSH is associated with decreased bioactivity due to increased sialylation [36]. In patients with concomitant GH and TSH deficiencies, serum-free T4 may be normal (usually at the lower tertile), decreasing only after GH replacement [37, 38]. More recently, it has been proposed that echocardiography can be useful in the evaluation of patients with hypothalamic-pituitary disease and free T4 levels within reference range, as some of these patients present signs of tissue hypothyroidism, a condition that could be named "subclinical central hypothyroidism" [39].

The TRH stimulation test has been performed in the past to diagnose central hypothyroidism [40]. However, this test is not currently recommended due to a lack of accuracy and availability [41].

Corticotropin Deficiency

Cortisol secretion follows a circadian cycle, being highest in the early morning and lowest at midnight. Hence, a basal serum cortisol measurement may not reflect disturbances of the hypothalamus-pituitary-adrenal (HPA) axis. In addition, alterations in the levels of cortisol-binding globulin (CBG), which is frequently seen in clinical practice (e.g., higher levels of CBG, and consequently serum total cortisol, during oral estrogen treatment as a contraceptive), may also mask the diagnosis of central hypoadrenalism. Therefore, early morning serum cortisol (between 07:00 and 09:00) may be measured as a first step in the evaluation [11]. Stimulation tests are frequently required for corticotropic assessment. The most commonly used stimuli in clinical practice are insulin-induced hypoglycemia, metyrapone, synthetic ACTH (ACTH$_{1-24}$), and CRH (Tables 7.3 and 7.4).

Hypoglycemia is a potent activator of the HPA axis, and the ITT is usually regarded as the "gold standard" for diagnosis (see more details in "GH stimulation testing").

ACTH$_{1-24}$ administration is currently the most commonly used test in clinical practice for assessing HPA axis. Adrenal atrophy is required for the test to be positive in cases of ACTH deficiency. Hence, this test should not be performed within 2 weeks of an insult to the hypothalamus or pituitary (e.g., pituitary surgery) [42]. A low-dose (1 μg) ACTH$_{1-24}$ test has been reported to induce improved sensitivity by some studies [43] but not others [44].

Metyrapone decreases serum cortisol by inhibiting the enzyme 11-beta-hydroxylase, and this test is usually not performed due to limited availability of the drug.

CRH has been used to differentiate hypothalamic from pituitary disease in secondary adrenal insufficiency. However, CRH stimulation is not particularly useful in diagnosing secondary adrenal insufficiency because individual responses to exogenous CRH are extremely variable.

ADH Deficiency

DI may be diagnosed with a proper clinical presentation, for example, in a patient with known pituitary/hypothalamic disease if other causes of polyuria (e.g., diabetes mellitus, use of diuretics) are excluded. Serum sodium is usually above the middle of the reference range, but hypernatremia is not seen in patients with an intact thirst mechanism. In situations where diagnosis is not clear-cut, a water deprivation test is warranted. Maximum urine osmolality is less than 300 mOsm/kg H$_2$O in patients with complete DI. In patients with subnormally elevated osmolality after water deprivation (300 mOsm/kg < osmolarity < 800 mOsm/kg H$_2$O), further steps are needed, including magnetic resonance imaging (MRI) of the hypothalamic-pituitary region and/or a therapeutic trial with desmopressin [12].

Imaging

MRI is currently the single best imaging procedure in the investigation for most sellar masses. After hypopituitarism has been confirmed, MRI should be performed to exclude tumors and other lesions of the sellar and parasellar region. When this is not possible, computerized tomography (CT) provides a suitable alternative. Micro- and macroadenomas of the pituitary as well as other sellar masses, such as craniopharyngiomas and meningiomas, usually take up contrast to a lesser degree than the normal pituitary. Craniopharyngiomas and even pituitary adenomas may have a partially cystic content and, therefore, have low-intensity signals. Hemorrhage has a high-intensity signal on both T1- and T2-weighted images. On the other hand, asymptomatic pituitary adenomas are found upon autopsy in approximately 11% of individuals. Such adenomas may also be commonly seen as incidental findings (incidentalomas) on head CT or MRI scans performed for other reasons [45].

Recent MRI studies of the pituitary in patients who had suffered a TBI demonstrated pathological changes consistent with vascular injury. In the acute phase, the pituitary glands of these patients are significantly enlarged and may also present other abnormalities, such as hemorrhage, infarction, and partial stalk transection [46]. In the chronic phase, patients often demonstrate pituitary volume loss or empty sella, perfusion deficits, or lack of a posterior pituitary signal. Such abnormalities were reported to occur in 80% of patients with hypopituitarism compared to 29% of those without hypopituitarism [47].

Neuro-ophthalmic Exam

Patients with a known pituitary tumor must be carefully followed for evidence of growth with early chiasmal-optic nerve compression. The frequency of visual evaluation must be individualized based on the size of the tumor and its relation to critical structures. Goldmann perimetry is useful in plotting the visual field defects and also assists in follow-up.

Management

Understanding the underlying pathophysiology in each patient and recognizing the probability for recovery of function are among the most important issues to be emphasized in the management of patients with hypopituitarism. Treatment is based on the underlying disease that leads to pituitary insufficiency.

Pituitary tumors may be treated with medical therapy, surgery, radiotherapy, or a combination of these modalities depending on the tumor subtype and clinical presentation [6]. Whereas prolactinomas are almost exclusively treated with dopamine agonists, neurosurgical removal is indicated for most other pituitary sellar and parasellar masses. Infections (e.g., meningoencephalitis, tuberculosis, or syphilis) are treated with antibiotics or antivirals, and granulomatous infiltrations (e.g., sarcoidosis) are treated with immunosuppressants.

The goal of hormone replacement therapy is to achieve normal levels of the circulating hormones in order to restore normal physiology as close as possible and to avoid the symptoms of deficiency with minimal side effects. Target peripheral hormones, rather than deficient pituitary hormones, should be replaced, except for GH deficiency, ADH deficiency, and gonadotropins, when fertility is desired [6]. Hormone replacement therapy should be started as soon as the diagnosis of hypopituitarism is made (Box 8.1). It is very important to carefully evaluate whether hypopituitarism is likely to be reversible or whether it is permanent, thereby requiring life-long hormone replacement therapy.

Hormone Replacement Therapy

Hyposomatotropism

Children

Childhood GHD should be treated as soon as possible in order to improve linear growth. The individual response to GH therapy is widely variable and unpredictable. Dosing is mainly based on weight and can range from 0.021 to 0.050 mg/kg/day (0.033 mg/kg/day is the most suitable initial dose) up to 0.1 mg/kg/day in adolescents. It should be given once a day by subcutaneous injection and should be adjusted based on growth response and IGF-I levels [48, 49].

Therapy should be started as early as possible in order to achieve the best results in growth where patients can achieve height within the midparental target height [50].

GH therapy in children is safe and adverse events are uncommon. Idiopathic intracranial hypertension (pseudotumor cerebri) is a rare occurrence that tends to occur early in therapy, and if it occurs, then drug discontinuation and subsequent cautious reintroduction are necessary. Some patients may present increased insulin resistance, which appears not to translate into marked glucose abnormalities [51].

The goals of therapy are to achieve therapeutic levels of IGF-I that are slightly above the mid-normal range (approximately 1 SD above the mean) adjusted for age, pubertal stage, and growth velocity above the 75th percentile curve [52, 53]. An evaluation is performed 4 weeks after beginning treatment, and in the case of an adequate IGF-I response, the length/height should be rechecked every 3–6 months, and IGF-I levels should be rechecked every 6–12 months.

Caution is necessary with unmasking hypothyroidism after GH therapy as previously discussed. Thus, free T4 should be assessed every 3 and 6 months after initiation of this therapy and yearly thereafter.

Adults

In adults, GH dosing regimens are not weight-based as in children, but rather are initialized with a lower dose and then titrated according to clinical parameters and IGF-I levels. The recommended GH starting dose is 0.2–0.3 mg/day for most patients and 0.1–0.2 mg/day for the elderly patients that are more susceptible to adverse events linked to therapy [23]. A target for IGF-I levels is the upper half of normal range.

The most common side effects, which occur in 5–18% of patients, are joint stiffness, peripheral edema, arthralgias, and myalgias. Carpal tunnel syndrome and increased blood pressure are infrequent but, when present, are related to supraphysiological doses in most cases. When this occurs, a reduction in the dose is appropriate [54].

Although there are no conclusive data of a GH role in the development or recurrence of malignant diseases, GH is contraindicated in adult patients with an active malignancy. A slight increase in the risk for DM has been observed with GH therapy, and therefore diabetic patients may require changes in the doses of current medications [23].

Adjustments should be performed every 1–2 months during dose titration. A clinical response, IGF-I levels, and side effects should guide the choice of dose. After titration, evaluation should be performed at 6-month intervals.

Transitional Period

In the transition phase, the recommended dose is 0.4–0.5 mg/day with the goal of achieving IGF-1 levels between 0 and +2 SD with adjustments made at 1–2-month intervals. Reassessment should be made every 6 months thereafter until the patient is in their mid-twenties [23, 33].

Hypogonadism (in the Adult Female)

Estrogen deficiency requires replacement for the relief of symptoms, such as loss of libido and dyspareunia, as well as for the prevention of osteoporosis and premature cardiovascular disease. Epidemiological studies in women with anterior pituitary deficiency have demonstrated excessive cardiovascular mortality in untreated versus treated hypogonadism [55]. Thus, it is strongly recommended to replace sex steroids in younger women until the average age of menopause is reached (approximately 52 years of age in healthy subjects). On the other hand, findings of large studies of sex hormone replacement therapy in non-pituitary postmenopausal patients have shown an increased risk of cardiovascular and neoplastic diseases. Therefore, termination of sex hormone substitution in hypogonadal women after the average menopause age is recommended [56, 57].

The biological potency of 20 μg ethinyl estradiol, 1.25 mg conjugated estrogen, and 100 μg transdermal 17β-estradiol is comparable [58]. In premenopausal women, an oral contraceptive containing 20–35 μg ethinyl estradiol is an effective form of replacement therapy. Alternatively, oral estrogen preparations (conjugated estrogen 0.625–1.25 mg daily or estradiol valerate 1–2 mg) given cyclically or continuously with a progestagen can be administered. Transdermal application of estradiol (50–100 μg/day) is preferred over oral preparations because it avoids hepatic first-pass metabolism. In addition, the transdermal preparation minimizes the synthesis of procoagulatory factors and acute phase proteins, which are potential vascular risk factors [59], and eliminates the growth hormone-resistant effects of estrogen on IGF-I production in the liver [60]. All women who have an intact uterus should receive concomitant progesterone therapy. Breast cancer is clearly an absolute contraindication for sex steroid replacement therapy.

Pubertal Development

The goal for therapy in this case is to approximate normal development, and the appropriate age for intervention is around the chronological age of 11 years. Conjugated estrogens (initial dose 0.15 mg daily or 0.3 mg on alternate days), ethinyl estradiol (2.5–5 μg daily), or 17β-estradiol (initial dose 5 μg/kg daily) may be administered, and the dose should be gradually increased every 6–12 months over the following 2–3 years until the adult replacement dose is reached. After 6 months of therapy or in the case of spotting or menstrual bleeding, cyclic progestagens (usually medroxyprogesterone 5–10 mg daily or norethisterone 0.7–1.0 mg daily) should be added for 12–14 days every month [61].

Estrogen-release patches offer an alternative treatment option. The smallest commercially available patch releases 25 μg 17β-estradiol daily. The patch can be divided into six to eight fragments, and each fragment allows a release of 0.08–0.12 μg/kg daily. Application of the patch may be limited to nighttime in order to mimic the pattern of estrogen secretion that is predominantly nocturnal during the initiation of puberty [62]. The dosage should be increased every 6–12 months until the adult replacement dosage is achieved.

Fertility Treatment

Pulsatile GnRH is mostly used for ovulation induction in patients with hypothalamic hypogonadotropic hypogonadism and normal gonadotropin levels. However, such therapy should only be performed at centers with extensive experience in ovarian stimulation techniques.

Gonadotropin therapy is indicated in patients with gonadotropin deficiency or GnRH resistance but can also be used in patients with GnRH defects [63]. Ovulation induction is initiated with 75 IU daily of a preparation containing only FSH or a mixture of FSH and LH (human menopausal gonadotropins). Careful ultrasound monitoring is recommended to ensure that only one or two follicles develop in order to prevent ovarian superstimulation and prevent multiple pregnancies. Once a follicle has become mature, a single dose of 5000 IU of human chorionic gonadotropin (hCG) is administered to stimulate ovulation, which occurs within 36–48 h of administration. Conception occurs in 5–15% of cycles, and cumulative conception rates average between 30 and 60% [63].

Hypogonadism (in the Adult Male)

The aim of androgen substitution is to restore the serum testosterone concentration to the normal range (in the mid-normal range) in order to maintain secondary sexual characteristics, prevent loss and optimize bone mass, and improve sexual function [8].

The route of delivery depends on availability, patient preference, consideration of pharmacokinetics, treatment burden, and cost. Testosterone therapy is contraindicated in patients with prostate cancer, severe lower urinary tract symptoms, erythrocytosis, untreated severe obstructive sleep apnea, and uncontrolled or poorly controlled heart failure [8].

Oral Testosterone

Oral testosterone undecanoate is commercially available in many countries under various brand names in 40 mg capsules, but is not available in the United States. It is absorbed through the lymphatic system and bypasses the portal vein due to esterification at the 17β position. The daily dose is 80–240 mg given throughout the day with meals. However, this drug has low bioavailability and substantial interindividual and intraindividual variability in absorption [64]. Therefore, it is more suitable for patients who cannot tolerate transdermal or intramuscular administration.

Intramuscular Depot

Testosterone enanthate and testosterone cypionate are 17β esters of testosterone that have been the standard preparations for testosterone treatment for decades and have been proven to be safe with few unwanted side effects. Both esters are more lipophilic than native testosterone and have a long half-life and duration of action.

After intramuscular administration of testosterone enanthate, serum testosterone peaks to maximal supraphysiological levels in approximately 10 h, followed by a gradual decline to low normal or even subnormal levels [65]. Intramuscular doses of testosterone enanthate or cypionate from 100 mg/week or 150–200 mg every 2 weeks are biologically effective. Serum testosterone should be monitored between midway injections aiming at a serum level between 350 ng/dL (12–3 nmol/L) and 750 ng/dL (24–5 nmol/L). Some clinicians prefer to monitor serum testosterone levels immediately prior to the next injection with a goal of achieving a level in the low normal range. Dose adjustment is performed by varying injection intervals or injection dosage.

Testosterone undecanoate (Nebido®) is another ester of testosterone that has a markedly longer half-life (34 days) and duration of effect than testosterone enanthate and cypionate. Intramuscular injection of testosterone undecanoate 1000 mg every 3 months leads to constant physiological serum testosterone levels without the undesired initial peak in drug concentration observed with the other depot formulations. A reduction in the injection interval between the first and second administration is recommended [66], and with this loading dose, sufficient steady state testosterone levels may be achieved more rapidly. Serum testosterone should be monitored at the end of the injection interval with the goal of achieving a serum level of testosterone in the mid-normal range. Dose adjustment is performed by varying the injection intervals.

Transdermal Systems

Transdermal systems are a popular treatment modality for hypogonadal men. Transdermal gel and patches provide a useful delivery system for normalizing serum testosterone in these patients [67]. The transdermal gel has the best pharmacokinetic properties of all the available formulations and can achieve stable serum testosterone concentrations within the normal range using a noninvasive topical application that is applied once a day on non-pressure areas of the body. Potential limitations of transdermal systems include a high rate of skin irritation observed with patches and the possibility that the testosterone gel may be transferred to other individuals through skin contact [68]. Four testosterone gels are currently available in the United States, including AndroGel®, Testim®, Axiron®, and Fortesta®. A multicenter study conducted by Swerdloff et al. [69] (Testosterone Gel Study Group) showed that a daily transdermal application of a hydroalcoholic gel containing 1% testosterone (AndroGel®) at 5.0 and 10.0 g of gel (equivalent to 50 and 100 mg) increased serum testosterone levels in hypogonadal men to within the normal range. Treatment should be started with 5.0 g and adjusted as necessary up to a maximum of 10.0 g. Testim® is another brand of hydroalcoholic gel with the same concentration.

The 2% formulation of testosterone topical solution (Axiron®) is a non-occlusive topical formulation administered to the axilla, instead of the hands. A multicenter study conducted by Wang et al. [70] in hypogonadal men treated with 30–90 mg of this preparation showed that application of the gel restored physiological testosterone levels in 84.8% of treated patients. This finding is similar to results previously reported with testosterone gel and mucoadhesive buccal therapies. The suggested dose of Axiron® is 60 mg (30 mg applied to each axilla once a day), with adjustment of the dose ranging from 30 to 120 mg, as determined by the serum testosterone concentration.

Another 2% testosterone gel for the treatment of hypogonadal male (Fortesta®) is also supplied in a metered dose pump, which is applied to the front and inner thighs. A multicenter study [71] in hypogonadal men followed for 90 days demonstrated that a single daily dose of this preparation restored normal levels of testosterone in more than 75% of hypogonadal patients, with a low risk of supraphysiological testosterone levels. The recommended starting dose is 40 mg once a day (2 g/2 mL of gel) with adjustment of the dose ranging from 10 to 70 mg, as determined by the serum testosterone concentration.

The transdermal system patch (Androderm®) delivers approximately 5 mg of testosterone every 24 h and results in normal serum testosterone concentrations in most hypogonadal men [72]. The application of one or two testosterone patches is recommended to be applied nightly over the skin of the back, thigh, or upper arm, away from pressure areas. Testosterone serum levels can be assessed 3–12 h after the application of the patch. The dose should be adjusted to achieve testosterone levels in the mid-normal range. The scrotal patch is no longer available in the United States.

Testosterone in an adhesive matrix patch is now available in many countries. The recommended regimen consists of 2×60 cm^2 patches that deliver approximately 4.8 mg of testosterone per day and last for approximately 2 days. However, some patients experience skin irritation with this preparation [8].

Buccal Tablet

A controlled release testosterone buccal system (Striant SR®) contains 30 mg of testosterone and mucoadhesive excipients, which rapidly adhere to the buccal mucosa and slowly form a gel. Transbuccal delivery of testosterone substantially circumvents hepatic first-pass metabolism. A study by Wang et al. [73] demonstrated that the administration of this preparation maintained serum testosterone concentrations within the normal range in most hypogonadal men. The recommended dose is 30 mg applied to the buccal region twice a day. Testosterone serum levels can be assessed immediately before or after application of the fresh system. Gum-related adverse events occurred in 16% of treated subjects.

Pellets

Subcutaneous pellets (testospel®) provide stable physiological testosterone levels, but a minor surgical procedure is required for administration [74]. The pellets are implanted into the subdermal fat of the lower abdominal wall, buttock, or thigh. The dose and regimen vary with formulation. The manufacturer recommends implantation of three to six 75 mg pellets every 3–6 months [8]. Extrusion of the pellets and infection are the main risks of this treatment.

Other

Recently, a nasal testosterone gel (Natesto®) was approved in the United States for the treatment of male hypogonadism. The gel is administered into the nostrils with a metered-dose pump applicator. One pump delivers 5.5 mg of testosterone, and the recommended dose is 11 mg (one pump in each nostril), three times a day (total 33 mg/day). One advantage over other formulations is the minimal risk of gel transfer to a partner or child. On the other hand, the three time daily regimen may be inconvenient for many, and its administration can be more troublesome in men with allergies or underlying sinus pathology, since more than 3% of subjects in clinical trials experienced rinorrhea, epistaxis, nasopharyngitis, sinusitis, and nasal scab. A major concern also comes from data in mice studies that showed brain levels twice as high when compared with intravenous testosterone, a finding that is yet unknown in humans. Therefore, until further security data are available with this new formulation, we suggest using the available testosterone gels, patch, or injectable esters.

Monitoring During Androgen Therapy

Men younger than 40 years of age may not need prostate monitoring as they are at low risk for the development of prostate cancer. In men 40 years of age or older with a baseline prostatic specific antigen (PSA) level greater than 0.6 ng/mL, rectal digital examination should be performed before initiating treatment, and PSA levels should be checked 3–6 months after the start of treatment and annually thereafter. A urological consultation is necessary if there is an increase in serum PSA concentration to a level greater than 1.4 ng/mL within any 12-month period of testosterone treatment. Hematocrit should be checked at baseline, at 3–6 months after the start of therapy, and annually thereafter. If the hematocrit is greater than 54%, then the treatment should be stopped until it decreases to a safe level [8].

Infants/Pubertal Development

Infants and children with micropenis (penile length less than 2.5 cm at birth and in infancy) related to congenital hypopituitarism may be treated with three courses of testosterone enanthate 25 mg given IM each month with the goal of increasing penis size. If the desirable increase in penile length (>0.9 cm) has not occurred, then another three-course trial can be repeated [9].

There is no general consensus regarding the best time to induce pubertal development. An acceptable proposal may be to induce pubertal development at 13 years and obtain a slow and progressive increase. A monthly dose of testosterone enanthate or cypionate 25–50 mg IM may be used. The dose should be kept as low as possible in order to preserve maximal growth potential. The dose should be increased every 6–12 months until reaching the adult replacement therapy within 3–5 years [63].

Fertility Treatment

In secondary hypogonadism, spermatogenesis and fertility can be induced. Men with prepubertal onset hypogonadism are more likely to require replacement of FSH as well as LH, whereas men with postpubertal onset are more likely to require replacement of LH only.

The classical gonadotropin regimen combines hCG and human menopausal gonadotropin (hMG) given as IM or subcutaneous (SC) injections, depending on the available preparation [75]. After stopping testosterone treatment, hCG can be used initially at a dose of 2000 IU twice a week to stimulate spermatogenesis. The dose is titrated against testicular volume and serum testosterone, which should be measured every 1–2 months, with the goal of achieving levels between 400 and 900 ng/dL within 3–4 months after initiating treatment. Some patients require as little as 500 IU per dose, while other patients need as much as 10,000 IU per dose. Sperm count is measured every 2–4 weeks, but the value is not used to adjust the hCG dose. Most patients who eventually reach a normal sperm count (over 20 million/mL) do so within 6 months, but some require 12–24 months. The addition of hMG should be considered if the sperm count does not reach one-half of the normal level within 12–24 months. The pharmaceutical preparation of hMG contains FSH and is used to replace FSH for stimulating spermatogenesis in men who are infertile due to secondary hypogonadism. Recombinant human FSH is also available, but has not been as well studied in men and is more expensive. FSH appears to be necessary for the initiation of spermatogenesis, but not for its maintenance or reinitiation. Therefore, for patients with prepubertal onset of secondary hypogonadism, the treatment should be started with both hCG 2000 IU and hMG three times a week while titrating hCG doses based on serum testosterone levels.

Thyrotropin Deficiency

Levothyroxine is the replacement of choice for central hypothyroidism [76]. Most patients use 75–125 mcg/day of L-T$_4$ (for pediatric dosages, see Box 8.1). Laboratory monitoring of serum-free T4 levels should be performed. The FT$_4$ levels should remain in the upper half of the reference range for patients with concomitant untreated GH deficiency in order to ensure adequate replacement [37]. In eusomatotropic patients, the FT$_4$ levels should be in the mid-normal reference range [37, 77] (see "Hormone Replacement Therapy Interactions").

> **Box 8.1 Hormone Replacement Regimens**
> *GH deficiency*
>
> *Adults*: GH therapy 0.1–0.2 mg in elderly; 0.2–0.3 mg in adults; 0.4–0.5 mg, SC, in younger people; adjustment based on clinical response, adverse effects, and IGF-I levels that should be maintained in the middle/upper half of the normal range.
>
> *Children*: GH therapy 0.033 mg/kg/day and up to 0.1 mg/kg/day, SC, during puberty; adjustments based on growth response and IGF-I levels that should be maintained 1 standard deviation (SD) above the mean.
>
> *FSH/LH deficiency*
>
> *Adult male*: 75–100 mg of testosterone enanthate or cypionate IM weekly or 150 mg every 2 weeks; one or two 5 mg nongenital testosterone patches applied nightly over the skin; 5–10 g of a 1% testosterone gel applied daily over skin; 30 mg of bioadhesive buccal testosterone every 12 h. Other options: 2% of testosterone topical solution, 2% testosterone gel, oral testosterone undecanoate, injectable testosterone undecanoate, testosterone-in-adhesive matrix patch, and testosterone pellets.
>
> *Infants/pubertal development* (*boys*): Infants and children with micropenis, three courses of testosterone enanthate 25 mg IM monthly, and another three courses can be repeated if necessary. At 13 years of age, testosterone enanthate or cypionate 25–50 mg IM dosed monthly; increase dose every 6–12 months until the adult replacement level is achieved (3–5 years).
>
> *Adult female*: Oral contraceptive (20–35 μg ethinyl estradiol), conjugated estrogen 0.625–1.25 mg, estradiol valerate 1–2 mg, or transdermal application of estradiol 50–100 μg/day. Add progestagen in case of an intact uterus.
>
> *Pubertal development* (*girls*): At 11 years of age, conjugated estrogen (0.15 mg daily or 0.30 mg on alternate days), ethinyl estradiol 2.5–5 μg, or 17β-estradiol 5 μg/kg daily, or estrogen release patches 25 μg 17β-estradiol (0.08–0.12 μg/kg/day) can be subdivided into six to eight fragments. After 6 months or in the case of spotting or menstrual bleeding, cyclic progestagens should be added.

TSH deficiency

Adults: Levothyroxine, initial dose, 75–125 µg/day in most cases (in elderly, start with 25 µg/day). Adjust the dose based on clinical response and serum free T_4 levels. Serum free T4 levels should be in the upper half of the reference range (see text).

Children: <6 months, 8–10 µg/kg/day; 6–12 months, 6–8 µg/kg/day; 1–5 years, 5–6 µg/kg/day; 6–12 years, 4–5 µg/kg/day

ACTH deficiency

Adults: Hydrocortisone two to three times a day: more commonly 10–15 mg early morning and 5 mg middle of the day; prednisolone 2.5–5.0 mg early morning; prednisone, 2.5–5.0 mg/day. Adjustment based on clinical assessment. Double or triple the oral dose in the case of exercise or mild febrile disease. Use parenteral (IV/IM) dose if vomiting or diarrhea occurs or if surgery is performed (hydrocortisone, 200–300 mg/day in 3–4 divided doses). DHEA 25–50 mg/daily as a trial in symptomatic women.

Children: Oral hydrocortisone 10–24 mg/m²/day or cortisone acetate 13.5–32 mg/m²/day or prednisolone 3–5 mg/m²/day; dexamethasone usually avoided.

ADH deficiency

Adults: Desmopressin, start with 5–10 mcg as a single dose at night before the patient goes to sleep. Increase until there is no nocturia (increments of 5–10 mcg). Add a morning dose if bothersome polyuria is present during the day. Eventually, another dose can be given during the afternoon. Equivalence of nasal solution to pills, 2.5–5.0 mcg (nasal) = 0.1 mg (pill). Dose titration is needed if preparation is changed.

Children (below 12 years of age): Same initial doses of desmopressin, but maximum daily doses are 30 mcg (nasal) and 0.8 mg (oral).

ACTH Deficiency

Glucocorticoid replacement is a priority because its deficiency is potentially life-threatening. Replacement therapy should be initiated before the beginning of thyroxine and/or GH replacement, since these latter treatments may precipitate adrenal crisis. There is no consensus on the best glucocorticoid replacement regimen [11]. Many centers use hydrocortisone (15–20 mg/day) in divided doses in an attempt to mimic circadian variation (e.g., 10–15 mg in the morning and 5 mg in the early afternoon; see Box 8.1). Although dividing the total daily dose into two or even three doses (with the largest dose on arising in the morning) makes sense physiologically and should be initially pursued, many patients cannot remember to take doses in the middle of the day. For them, taking the entire dose in the morning is preferable to missing doses, and many patients may feel well on this regimen. Equivalent doses of prednisone, dexamethasone, or cortisone acetate have also been used. Approximate equivalent doses to 20 mg of hydrocortisone include cortisone acetate, 25 mg; prednisone, 5 mg; and dexamethasone, 0.75 mg. Mineralocorticoid is not required in ACTH-deficient patients, since its secretion is under the control of the renin-angiotensin system. For children, hydrocortisone is usually the glucocorticoid of choice (10–24 mg/m²/day in divided doses). Prednisolone (3–5 mg/m²/day) is also used, albeit less frequently. Due to its higher potency and possible negative effects on growth, dexamethasone is avoided during childhood. Close monitoring and attention should be given to patients being treated for hypopituitarism who also receive enzyme-inducing antiepileptic drugs (e.g., phenytoin, phenobarbital), since these medications can also affect the needed dosages of glucocorticoids and levothyroxine and, thus, patients need to receive education on early signs of adrenal insufficiency.

As a general rule, during acute illness, the usual glucocorticoid replacement dose is increased two to three times over a course of at least 3 days or more, if needed. If patients cannot take oral glucocorticoids or experience severe illness, then IV/IM hydrocortisone is given as 200–300 mg/day in 3–4 doses (e.g., 50 mg every 6 h) [11, 78].

Adult women with hypopituitarism show decreased levels of androgens, including dehydroepiandrosterone (DHEA), dehydroepiandrosterone sulfate (DHEA-S), androstenedione, and testosterone. Some studies on DHEA replacement therapy to these patients have shown beneficial results on quality of life as well as improved mood and sexual function [79–82], whereas other studies have not shown such benefits [83, 84]. A meta-analysis that included randomized studies on the effect of DHEA replacement therapy on the quality of life of primary or secondary adrenal insufficient patients showed a small improvement in quality of life and depression, but no effect on anxiety and sexual well-being [85]. In the same meta-analysis, the most commonly reported side effects were greasy skin, hirsutism, acne, scalp itching, and increased apocrine sweat secretion and odor [85]. However, to date there is insufficient evidence to recommend routine DHEA replacement to these patients [78]. Moreover, in many countries, DHEA is only available as a dietary supplement, and therefore there are often variable and unreliable amounts of the drug in each pill. When DHEA is replaced, the usual dosage ranges from 25 to 50 mg in a single morning dose [86]. Clinical effects are observed only after several weeks of treatment. Monitoring should include measurement of DHEA-S (24 h after the previous dose) as well as free testosterone or total testosterone with sex hormone-binding globulin (SHBG) and estimation of free testosterone. If side effects are observed, then the dosage may be decreased by 50%.

ADH Deficiency

Since polyuria and nocturia impair the quality of life, desmopressin, a vasopressin analogue, should be given to most patients with DI [87]. Desmopressin is usually started as a single dose at night before the patient goes to sleep (e.g., 1 puff), which is increased until nocturia is controlled. A second dose (in the morning) and less commonly a third dose (in the afternoon) may be added as needed. Desmopressin is usually available as nasal spray, with one puff delivering 10 mcg. It is also available as a pill at a concentration of 0.1 mg per dose. In the inpatient setting, Desmopressin may also be given intravenously or subcutaneously at a dosage of 1–4 mcg/day in two divided doses.

Hormone Replacement Therapy Interactions

A critical aspect in the management of patients with hypopituitarism is the interplay between different replacement therapies. Remarkably, GH status impacts thyroid and adrenal replacement, and estrogen influences growth hormone dosages.

GH increases the conversion of T_4 to T_3 [37]. Hence, patients with combined and untreated GH and TSH deficiencies may show normal serum T_4 levels, usually at the lower tertile, which masks the diagnosis of central hypothyroidism. Serum T_4 levels fall below the normal range only after GH replacement in these cases [38]. On the other hand, a decrease in serum T_4 levels after GH replacement should be evaluated carefully, since T_3 levels usually concomitantly rise. If serum T_4 levels fall to the mid-normal range, an increase in the dosage of levothyroxine is usually not necessary. Additionally, during concomitant GH and levothyroxine replacement therapy, serum T_3 measurements may help to detect thyroxine over-replacement [77].

In contrast to the action of GH on thyroid axis, GH enhances the conversion of cortisol to the biologically inactive cortisone through 11β-hydroxysteroid dehydrogenase type 1 [88]. Therefore, GH replacement may induce glucocorticoid insufficiency. This effect has been observed in patients with multiple pituitary deficiencies [89], but not in patients with isolated GH deficiency [90].

Oral estrogen replacement decreases the effect of GH on hepatic tissue, which consequently decreases IGF-I levels. Thus, patients on oral estrogen should have their dosage of GH increased [58, 91]. Since this effect is not observed in patients on transdermal estrogen due to lower concentrations of estrogen in the liver, this mode of administration is usually preferred in GH-deficient patients.

Long-Term Management

While radiotherapy is associated with progressive hypopituitarism, in the case of a pituitary tumor, even if hypofunction is present before surgical treatment, pituitary function should be reassessed postoperatively, as nearly as 50% of pituitary deficiencies will resolve. Lifelong substitution therapy may thus not be necessary.

There is no evidence that GH replacement therapy is associated with the development of cancer, although the association of IGF-I levels and cancer in epidemiological studies has been explored. In addition, the evidence linking GH replacement therapy in GHD patients with the reversal of the highest rates of mortality observed in hypopituitarism is inconclusive.

More studies are needed in order to determine whether testosterone replacement in hypogonadal men increases the risk of developing or converting histological prostate cancer to the clinical form.

Potential Future Therapy

The presence of stem cells in the pituitary gland, which can give rise to all pituitary hormone cells, implies that these cells can be replaced after being lost or damaged. These stem cells could be of great usefulness in the treatment of hypopituitarism and may also have utility in the long-term management of pituitary deficiencies [92].

References

1. Regal M, et al. Prevalence and incidence of hypopituitarism in an adult Caucasian population in northwestern Spain. Clin Endocrinol (Oxf). 2002;55(6):735–40.
2. Klose M, Feldt-Rasmussen U. Chronic endocrine consequences of traumatic brain injury - what is the evidence? Nat Rev Endocrinol. 2018;14(1):57–62.
3. van Aken MO, Lamberts SW. Diagnosis and treatment of hypopituitarism: an update. Pituitary. 2005;8(3–4):183–91.
4. Toogood AA, Stewart PM. Hypopituitarism: clinical features, diagnosis, and management. Endocrinol Metab Clin N Am. 2008;37(1):235–61. x.
5. Hughes NR, Lissett CA, Shalet SM. Growth hormone status following treatment for Cushing's syndrome. Clin Endocrinol (Oxf). 1999;51(1):61–6.
6. Prabhakar VK, Shalet SM. Aetiology, diagnosis, and management of hypopituitarism in adult life. Postgrad Med J. 2006;82(966):259–66.
7. Carroll PV, et al. Growth hormone deficiency in adulthood and the effects of growth hormone replacement: a review. Growth Hormone Research Society Scientific Committee. J Clin Endocrinol Metab. 1998;83(2):382–95.
8. Bhasin S, et al. Testosterone therapy in men with androgen deficiency syndromes: an Endocrine Society clinical practice guideline. J Clin Endocrinol Metab. 2010;95(6):2536–59.

9. Bin-Abbas B, et al. Congenital hypogonadotropic hypogonadism and micropenis: effect of testosterone treatment on adult penile size why sex reversal is not indicated. J Pediatr. 1999;134(5):579–83.

10. Alexopoulou O, et al. Clinical and hormonal characteristics of central hypothyroidism at diagnosis and during follow-up in adult patients. Eur J Endocrinol. 2004;150(1):1–8.

11. Arlt W, Allolio B. Adrenal insufficiency. Lancet. 2003;361(9372):1881–93.

12. Fenske W, Allolio B. Current state and future perspectives in the diagnosis of diabetes insipidus: a clinical review. J Clin Endocrinol Metab. 2012;97:3426–37.

13. Rosenfeld RG, et al. Diagnostic controversy: the diagnosis of childhood growth hormone deficiency revisited. J Clin Endocrinol Metab. 1995;80(5):1532–40.

14. Richmond EJ, Rogol AD. Growth hormone deficiency in children. Pituitary. 2008;11(2):115–20.

15. Martha PM Jr, et al. Alterations in the pulsatile properties of circulating growth hormone concentrations during puberty in boys. J Clin Endocrinol Metab. 1989;69(3):563–70.

16. Bhala A, et al. Insulin-like growth factor axis parameters in sick hospitalized neonates. J Pediatr Endocrinol Metab. 1998;11(3):451–9.

17. Strasburger CJ, Bidlingmaier M. How robust are laboratory measures of growth hormone status? Horm Res. 2005;64(Suppl 2):1–5.

18. Gandrud LM, Wilson DM. Is growth hormone stimulation testing in children still appropriate? Growth Hormon IGF Res. 2004;14(3):185–94.

19. Growth Hormone Research Society. Consensus guidelines for the diagnosis and treatment of growth hormone (GH) deficiency in childhood and adolescence: summary statement of the GH Research Society. GH Research Society. J Clin Endocrinol Metab. 2000;85(11):3990–3.

20. Lanes R, Hurtado E. Oral clonidine-an effective growth hormone-releasing agent in prepubertal subjects. J Pediatr. 1982;100(5):710–4.

21. Sandra P, Popovic V. Diagnosis of growth hormone deficiency in adults. In: Ho K, editor. Growth hormone related diseases and therapy: a molecular and physiological perspective for the clinician. New York: Springer Science + Business Media; 2011.

22. Leong KS, et al. An audit of 500 subcutaneous glucagon stimulation tests to assess growth hormone and ACTH secretion in patients with hypothalamic-pituitary disease. Clin Endocrinol (Oxf). 2001;54(4):463–8.

23. Molitch ME, et al. Evaluation and treatment of adult growth hormone deficiency: an Endocrine Society clinical practice guideline. J Clin Endocrinol Metab. 2011;96(6):1587–609.

24. Lee P, Greenfield JR, Ho KK. Factors determining inadequate hypoglycaemia during insulin tolerance testing (ITT) after pituitary surgery. Clin Endocrinol (Oxf). 2009;71(1):82–5.

25. Ghigo E, et al. Arginine abolishes the inhibitory effect of glucose on the growth hormone response to growth hormone-releasing hormone in man. Metabolism. 1992;41(9):1000–3.

26. Corneli G, Di Somma C, Baldelli R, Rovere S, Gasco V, Croce CG, et al. The cut-off limits of the GH response to GH-releasing hormone-arginine test related to body mass index. Eur J Endocrinol. 2005 Aug;153(2):257–64.

27. Darzy KH, et al. The usefulness of the combined growth hormone (GH)-releasing hormone and arginine stimulation test in the diagnosis of radiation-induced GH deficiency is dependent on the post-irradiation time interval. J Clin Endocrinol Metab. 2003;88(1):95–102.

28. Rasmussen MH, Hvidberg A, Juul A, Main KM, Gotfredsen A, Skakkebaek NE, et al. Massive weight loss restores 24-hour growth hormone release profiles and serum insulin-like growth factor-I levels in obese subjects. J Clin Endocrinol Metab. 1995;80(4):1407–15.

29. Yuen KC, Biller BM, Katznelson L, Rhoads SA, Gurel MH, Chu O, et al. Clinical characteristics, timing of peak responses and safety aspects of two dosing regimens of the glucagon stimulation test in evaluating growth hormone and cortisol secretion in adults. Pituitary. 2013;16(2):220–30.

30. Dichtel LE, Yuen KC, Bredella MA, Gerweck AV, Russell BM, Riccio AD, et al. Overweight/obese adults with pituitary disorders require lower peak growth hormone cutoff values on glucagon stimulation testing to avoid overdiagnosis of growth hormone deficiency. J Clin Endocrinol Metab. 2014;99(12):4712–9.

31. Piccoli F, Degen L, MacLean C, Peter S, Baselgia L, Larsen F, et al. Pharmacokinetics and pharmacodynamic effects of an oral ghrelin agonist in healthy subjects. J Clin Endocrinol Metab. 2007;92(5):1814–20.

32. Garcia JM, Swerdloff R, Wang C, Kyle M, Kipnes M, Biller BM, et al. Macimorelin (AEZS-130)-stimulated growth hormone (GH) test: validation of a novel oral stimulation test for the diagnosis of adult GH deficiency. J Clin Endocrinol Metab. 2013;98(6):2422–9.

33. Clayton PE, et al. Consensus statement on the management of the GH-treated adolescent in the transition to adult care. Eur J Endocrinol. 2005;152(2):165–70.

34. Corneli G, et al. Cut-off limits of the GH response to GHRH plus arginine test and IGF-I levels for the diagnosis of GH deficiency in late adolescents and young adults. Eur J Endocrinol. 2007;157(6):701–8.

35. Maghnie M, et al. Diagnosis of GH deficiency in the transition period: accuracy of insulin tolerance test and insulin-like growth factor-I measurement. Eur J Endocrinol. 2005;152(4):589–96.

36. Oliveira JH, et al. Investigating the paradox of hypothyroidism and increased serum thyrotropin (TSH) levels in Sheehan's syndrome: characterization of TSH carbohydrate content and bioactivity. J Clin Endocrinol Metab. 2001;86(4):1694–9.

37. Behan LA, Monson JP, Agha A. The interaction between growth hormone and the thyroid axis in hypopituitary patients. Clin Endocrinol (Oxf). 2011;74(3):281–8.

38. Portes ES, et al. Changes in serum thyroid hormones levels and their mechanisms during long-term growth hormone (GH) replacement therapy in GH deficient children. Clin Endocrinol (Oxf). 2000;53(2):183–9.

39. Doin FC, et al. Diagnosis of subclinical central hypothyroidism in patients with hypothalamic-pituitary disease by Doppler echocardiography. Eur J Endocrinol. 2012;166(4):631–40.

40. Faglia G. The clinical impact of the thyrotropin-releasing hormone test. Thyroid. 1998;8(10):903–8.

41. Mehta A, et al. Is the thyrotropin-releasing hormone test necessary in the diagnosis of central hypothyroidism in children. J Clin Endocrinol Metab. 2003;88(12):5696–703.

42. Wallace I, Cunningham S, Lindsay J. The diagnosis and investigation of adrenal insufficiency in adults. Ann Clin Biochem. 2009;46(Pt 5):351–67.

43. Thaler LM, Blevins LS Jr. The low dose (1-microg) adrenocorticotropin stimulation test in the evaluation of patients with suspected central adrenal insufficiency. J Clin Endocrinol Metab. 1998;83(8):2726–9.

44. Dorin RI, Qualls CR, Crapo LM. Diagnosis of adrenal insufficiency. Ann Intern Med. 2003;139(3):194–204.

45. Molitch ME. Pituitary tumours: pituitary incidentalomas. Best Pract Res Clin Endocrinol Metab. 2009;23(5):667–75.

46. Maiya B, et al. Magnetic resonance imaging changes in the pituitary gland following acute traumatic brain injury. Intensive Care Med. 2008;34(3):468–75.

47. Schneider HJ, et al. Pituitary imaging abnormalities in patients with and without hypopituitarism after traumatic brain injury. J Endocrinol Investig. 2007;30(4):RC9–12.

48. Wit JM. Growth hormone therapy. Best Pract Res Clin Endocrinol Metab. 2002;16(3):483–503.

49. Mauras N, et al. High dose recombinant human growth hormone (GH) treatment of GH-deficient patients in puberty increases

near-final height: a randomized, multicenter trial. Genentech, Inc., Cooperative Study Group. J Clin Endocrinol Metab. 2000;85(10):3653–60.

50. Reiter EO, et al. Effect of growth hormone (GH) treatment on the near-final height of 1258 patients with idiopathic GH deficiency: analysis of a large international database. J Clin Endocrinol Metab. 2006;91(6):2047–54.

51. Cutfield WS, et al. Incidence of diabetes mellitus and impaired glucose tolerance in children and adolescents receiving growth-hormone treatment. Lancet. 2000;355(9204):610–3.

52. Cohen P, et al. Variable degree of growth hormone (GH) and insulin-like growth factor (IGF) sensitivity in children with idiopathic short stature compared with GH-deficient patients: evidence from an IGF-based dosing study of short children. J Clin Endocrinol Metab. 2010;95(5):2089–98.

53. Ranke MB, Lindberg A. Observed and predicted growth responses in prepubertal children with growth disorders: guidance of growth hormone treatment by empirical variables. J Clin Endocrinol Metab. 2010;95(3):1229–37.

54. Thuesen L, et al. Short and long-term cardiovascular effects of growth hormone therapy in growth hormone deficient adults. Clin Endocrinol (Oxf). 1994;41(5):615–20.

55. Tomlinson JW, et al. Association between premature mortality and hypopituitarism. West Midlands Prospective Hypopituitary Study Group. Lancet. 2001;357(9254):425–31.

56. Rossouw JE, et al. Risks and benefits of estrogen plus progestin in healthy postmenopausal women: principal results from the Women's Health Initiative randomized controlled trial. JAMA. 2002;288(3):321–33.

57. Beral V. Breast cancer and hormone-replacement therapy in the Million Women Study. Lancet. 2003;362(9382):419–27.

58. Mah PM, et al. Estrogen replacement in women of fertile years with hypopituitarism. J Clin Endocrinol Metab. 2005;90(11):5964–9.

59. Menon DV, Vongpatanasin W. Effects of transdermal estrogen replacement therapy on cardiovascular risk factors. Treat Endocrinol. 2006;5(1):37–51.

60. Leung KC, et al. Estrogen regulation of growth hormone action. Endocr Rev. 2004;25(5):693–721.

61. Kiess W, et al. Induction of puberty in the hypogonadal girl—practices and attitudes of pediatric endocrinologists in Europe. Horm Res. 2002;57(1–2):66–71.

62. Ankarberg-Lindgren C, et al. Nocturnal application of transdermal estradiol patches produces levels of estradiol that mimic those seen at the onset of spontaneous puberty in girls. J Clin Endocrinol Metab. 2001;86(7):3039–44.

63. Ascoli P, Cavagnini F. Hypopituitarism. Pituitary. 2006;9(4):335–42.

64. Schurmeyer T, et al. Saliva and serum testosterone following oral testosterone undecanoate administration in normal and hypogonadal men. Acta Endocrinol (Copenh). 1983;102(3):456–62.

65. Schulte-Beerbuhl M, Nieschlag E. Comparison of testosterone, dihydrotestosterone, luteinizing hormone, and follicle-stimulating hormone in serum after injection of testosterone enanthate of testosterone cypionate. Fertil Steril. 1980;33(2):201–3.

66. Schubert M, et al. Intramuscular testosterone undecanoate: pharmacokinetic aspects of a novel testosterone formulation during long-term treatment of men with hypogonadism. J Clin Endocrinol Metab. 2004;89(11):5429–34.

67. Zitzmann M, Nieschlag E. Hormone substitution in male hypogonadism. Mol Cell Endocrinol. 2000;161(1–2):73–88.

68. Jordan WP Jr. Allergy and topical irritation associated with transdermal testosterone administration: a comparison of scrotal and nonscrotal transdermal systems. Am J Contact Dermat. 1997;8(2):108–13.

69. Swerdloff RS, et al. Long-term pharmacokinetics of transdermal testosterone gel in hypogonadal men. J Clin Endocrinol Metab. 2000;85(12):4500–10.

70. Wang C, et al. Efficacy and safety of the 2% formulation of testosterone topical solution applied to the axillae in androgen-deficient men. Clin Endocrinol (Oxf). 2011;75(6):836–43.

71. Dobs AS, et al. A novel testosterone 2% gel for the treatment of hypogonadal males. J Androl. 2012;33(4):601–7.

72. Meikle AW, et al. Pharmacokinetics and metabolism of a permeation-enhanced testosterone transdermal system in hypogonadal men: influence of application site- -a clinical research center study. J Clin Endocrinol Metab. 1996;81(5):1832–40.

73. Wang C, et al. New testosterone buccal system (Striant) delivers physiological testosterone levels: pharmacokinetics study in hypogonadal men. J Clin Endocrinol Metab. 2004;89(8):3821–9.

74. Jockenhovel F, et al. Pharmacokinetics and pharmacodynamics of subcutaneous testosterone implants in hypogonadal men. Clin Endocrinol (Oxf). 1996;45(1):61–71.

75. Vicari E, et al. Therapy with human chorionic gonadotrophin alone induces spermatogenesis in men with isolated hypogonadotrophic hypogonadism—long-term follow-up. Int J Androl. 1992;15(4):320–9.

76. Yamada M, Mori M. Mechanisms related to the pathophysiology and management of central hypothyroidism. Nat Clin Pract Endocrinol Metab. 2008;4(12):683–94.

77. Martins MR, et al. Growth hormone replacement improves thyroxine biological effects: implications for management of central hypothyroidism. J Clin Endocrinol Metab. 2007;92(11):4144–53.

78. Neary N, Nieman L. Adrenal insufficiency: etiology, diagnosis and treatment. Curr Opin Endocrinol Diabetes Obes. 2010;17(3):217–23.

79. Arlt W, et al. Oral dehydroepiandrosterone for adrenal androgen replacement: pharmacokinetics and peripheral conversion to androgens and estrogens in young healthy females after dexamethasone suppression. J Clin Endocrinol Metab. 1998;83(6):1928–34.

80. Bilger M, et al. Androgen replacement in adolescents and young women with hypopituitarism. J Pediatr Endocrinol Metab. 2005;18(4):355–62.

81. Johannsson G, et al. Low dose dehydroepiandrosterone affects behavior in hypopituitary androgen-deficient women: a placebo-controlled trial. J Clin Endocrinol Metab. 2002;87(5):2046–52.

82. van Thiel SW, et al. Effects of dehydroepiandrostenedione, superimposed on growth hormone substitution, on quality of life and insulin-like growth factor I in patients with secondary adrenal insufficiency: a randomized, placebo-controlled, cross-over trial. J Clin Endocrinol Metab. 2005;90(6):3295–303.

83. Libe R, et al. Effects of dehydroepiandrosterone (DHEA) supplementation on hormonal, metabolic and behavioral status in patients with hypoadrenalism. J Endocrinol Investig. 2004;27(8):736–41.

84. Lovas K, et al. Replacement of dehydroepiandrosterone in adrenal failure: no benefit for subjective health status and sexuality in a 9-month, parallel group clinical trial. J Clin Endocrinol Metab. 2003;88(3):1112–8.

85. Alkatib AA, et al. A systematic review and meta-analysis of randomized placebo-controlled trials of DHEA treatment effects on quality of life in women with adrenal insufficiency. J Clin Endocrinol Metab. 2009;94(10):3676–81.

86. Hahner S, Allolio B. Therapeutic management of adrenal insufficiency. Best Pract Res Clin Endocrinol Metab. 2009;23(2):167–79.

87. Schneider HJ, et al. Hypopituitarism. Lancet. 2007;369(9571):1461–70.

88. Filipsson H, Johannsson G. GH replacement in adults: interactions with other pituitary hormone deficiencies and replacement therapies. Eur J Endocrinol. 2009;161(Suppl 1):S85–95.

89. Giavoli C, et al. Effect of recombinant human growth hormone (GH) replacement on the hypothalamic-pituitary-adrenal axis in adult GH-deficient patients. J Clin Endocrinol Metab. 2004;89(11):5397–401.

90. Giavoli C, et al. Effect of growth hormone deficiency and recombinant hGH (rhGH) replacement on the hypothalamic-pituitary-adrenal axis in children with idiopathic isolated GH deficiency. Clin Endocrinol (Oxf). 2008;68(2):247–51.

91. Cook DM, Ludlam WH, Cook MB. Route of estrogen administration helps to determine growth hormone (GH) replace-ment dose in GH-deficient adults. J Clin Endocrinol Metab. 1999;84(11):3956–60.

92. Castinetti F, et al. Pituitary stem cell update and potential implications for treating hypopituitarism. Endocr Rev. 2011;32(4):453–71.

Cushing's Syndrome

8

Krystallenia I. Alexandraki and Ashley B. Grossman

Introduction

Cushing's syndrome (CS) results from long-standing exposure to excessive circulating levels of glucocorticoids [1]. Recently, the prevalence of both exogenous and endogenous CS has shown a marked rise because of the increased use of glucocorticoids in several inflammatory diseases along with an early identification of subclinical forms of endogenous hypercortisolaemia. The early recognition and effective management of CS are of great importance as, when untreated, it is associated with high morbidity due to its metabolic abnormalities and the risk of infection resulting in increased mortality rates.

A florid clinical presentation makes diagnosis straightforward: when the clinical features are less obvious as in subclinical (SCS) or cyclic CS (CyCS), a step-by-step approach may confirm or reject the diagnosis or dictate a longer close follow-up. Later on, specific management targeting to the aetiology or the symptoms of CS may follow.

This chapter will first describe the aetiology of CS and review certain epidemiological data and clinical features, followed by a suggested diagnostic and therapeutic management paradigm.

Aetiology

Exogenous CS includes primarily the administration of glucocorticoids as medical therapy for autoimmune and derma-

K. I. Alexandraki
2nd Department of Surgery, Aretaieion Hospital, Kapodistrian and National University of Athens, Athens, Greece

A. B. Grossman (✉)
Centre for Endocrinology, Barts and the London School of Medicine, Queen Mary University of London, London, UK

Green Templeton College, University of Oxford, Oxford, UK
e-mail: ashley.grossman@ocdem.ox.ac.uk

tological diseases, asthma, atopic reactions, some cancers, and the less common iatrogenic adrenocorticotropin (ACTH) administration and factitious auto-administration. Any topical, inhaled, or injected corticosteroid administration has to be meticulously identified from the drug history [2]. Recently, there has been described a severe hypercortisolaemic state caused by the combination of anti-retroviral drugs used for human immunodeficiency virus (HIV) treatment and synthetic glucocorticoids given for unrelated reason by several routes such as intraocular drops or intra-articular injection. This phenomenon is due to the exaggerated increase of glucocorticoid concentrations after the induction of the hepatic enzyme CYP3A4 and P-glycoprotein export pump by the protease inhibitors used for HIV treatment [3, 4].

Establishing the precise cause of endogenous CS remains challenging since it shares many clinical features with other common conditions. ACTH-dependent CS (80–85%) includes mainly the ACTH-secreting pituitary tumours [Cushing's disease (CD)] (80%) and both ectopic ACTH (20%) and corticotrophin-releasing hormone (CRH) (<1%) syndromes (ECS) [1]. Corticotroph hyperplasia has been also described but seems rare in large surgical series, and we doubt its true existence [5]. CD is mainly caused by microadenomas (<1 cm in diameter) and less by macroadenomas (5–10%), with or without extrasellar extension or invasion; pituitary corticotroph carcinomas defined by extra-pituitary metastases are extremely rare [5, 6]. The molecular pathogenesis of corticotroph adenomas and carcinomas remains unknown but almost always has a monoclonal origin [7, 8], and around one-third show a mutation of USP8 leading to over-expression of the EGF receptor. On the other hand, the tumours that are more frequently associated with ECS are those arising from the lung, small-cell lung carcinoma (SCLC) (3.3–50%) and neuroendocrine tumours (NETs) such as bronchial NETs (5–40%), but can include pancreatic (7.5–25%) or thymic NETs (5–42%), phaeochromocytomas (5%), and medullary thyroid carcinoma (MTC) (2–8%), while in 12–37.5% a source cannot be identified [9]. ECS is mostly associated with tumours sited in the thorax and the

© Springer Nature Switzerland AG 2022
F. Bandeira et al. (eds.), *Endocrinology and Diabetes*, https://doi.org/10.1007/978-3-030-90684-9_8

neck and in only one-third in the abdomen [10]. A further classification regards the identification of the primary site of the source of ECS [11], resulting in *overt* ECS when the tumoural source is present, *covert* ECS when the tumour is identified in a later evaluation or follow-up, and *occult* ECS when the tumoural source cannot be identified [9]. Adrenal rest tissue in the liver, in the adrenal beds, or in association with the gonads may also produce hypercortisolaemia, usually in the context of ACTH-dependent disease after adrenalectomy [5].

ACTH-independent CS (20%) is caused by unilateral adrenocortical tumours or bilateral adrenal hyperplasia or dysplasia. The most common pathology is a cortisol-secreting adrenal adenoma (60%) or carcinoma (40%) and rarely ACTH-independent bilateral macronodular adrenal hyperplasia (BMAH), primary pigmented nodular adrenal disease (PPNAD) or micronodular adrenal disease (<1%) which may be sporadic or associated with Carney complex, the bilateral nodular adrenal disease in McCune-Albright syndrome (<1%), and constitutive activation ACTH receptor by a missense mutation (<1%) [1, 5]. An increased number of eutopic receptors or aberrant receptors such as gastric inhibitory peptide (GIP) receptors has been found to be expressed in adrenal nodules associated with BMAH, resulting in the food-dependent CS where GIP receptors are activated after a meal causing hypercortisolaemia [12]. More lately, other aberrant receptors such as vasopressin, β-adrenergic, luteinising hormone/human chorionic gonadotrophin, serotonin, angiotensin, leptin, glucagon, interleukin-1, and thyroid-stimulating hormone (TSH) have also been described [5]. In McCune-Albright syndrome, adrenal dysplasia is caused by an activating mutation at codon 201 of the α-subunit of the G-protein stimulating cyclic adenosine monophosphate (cAMP) formation resulting in constitutive activation of adenylate cyclase leading to nodule formation and hypercortisolaemia [13]. In PPNAD, the adrenal glands may be of small or normal size with cortical micronodules (2–3 mm) that may be dark or black in colour, mostly in the context of Carney complex where the tumour suppressor gene PRKAR1A (type 1A regulatory subunit of protein kinase A) has been shown to be mutated in approximately half of patients. In isolated cases, mutations in phosphodiesterase 11A (PDE11A) gene have demonstrated as well as a missense mutation of the ACTH receptor resulting in its constitutive activation, all resulting in ACTH-independent CS [5]. However, novel germline mutations can be documented such as of the armadillo repeat-containing-5 (ARMC5) gene, a probable tumour suppressor gene that may be associated with clinically severe forms of CS in the case of macronodular adrenal hyperplasia (BMAH) [14].

Finally, it is of interest to refer to medical conditions mimicking clinically CS features [15] along with mild biochemical evidence of hypercortisolaemia which remains under a physiological feedback hormonal control, so-called pseudo-Cushing states (PC); these entities resolve after the resolution of the pre-disposing condition or require a close follow-up if symptoms and signs increase [1]. These states include the metabolic syndrome, polycystic ovarian syndrome, severe obesity (as opposed to mild obesity where urinary free cortisol may be reduced), poorly controlled diabetes, late pregnancy, psychiatric disorders (depression, anxiety disorder), alcoholism, anorexia nervosa, and generalised resistance to glucocorticoids [16–19]. It is thought that higher brain centres stimulate CRH and/or AVP release in these conditions, with subsequent activation of the entire hypothalamo-pituitary-adrenal (HPA) axis. Thus, distinguishing CS from a PC state is a major clinical challenge for the endocrinologist since no test shows 100% diagnostic accuracy.

Epidemiology

Endogenous CS seems to have an overall incidence of 2.3 per million per year with an incidence of 1.2–1.7 per million per year for CD, 0.6 per million per year for adrenal adenomas, and 0.2 per million per year for adrenal carcinomas, while other CS types are extremely rare [20]. CD is more common in women and between the ages of 25 and 40 years of age, while ECS is more common in men and usually presents one decade older than in CD after the age of 40 years [9]. Adrenal adenomas occur most often around 35 years of age and are significantly more common in women, with an incidence of approximately 0.6 per million per year [5]. Adrenal carcinoma is slightly more common in women and has a bimodal age distribution, with peaks in childhood (then often showing a germline *P53* mutation) and adolescence and then later in life [1, 21]. Regarding BMAH, most cases are sporadic with a few familial cases [5].

Key Points to the Diagnosis and to the Differential Diagnosis (Fig. 8.1)

The most important step for the diagnosis of CS is clinical suspicion along with a detailed past medical and drug history [1]. A vast range of signs, symptoms, and other abnormalities along with a wide range in severity can be seen in CS (Fig. 8.1). When the presentation is florid including central obesity with limb wasting and muscle weakness, a plethoric face with hirsutism and frontal balding, and spontaneous bruising along with metabolic abnormalities (hypertension, prediabetes, or diabetes) and osteoporotic fractures, then the diagnosis is straightforward. Protein wasting, thin skin in the young, easy bruising, and proximal muscle weakness most reliably distinguish CS from PC. In addition, while specific clinical features may suggest one rather than another aetiol-

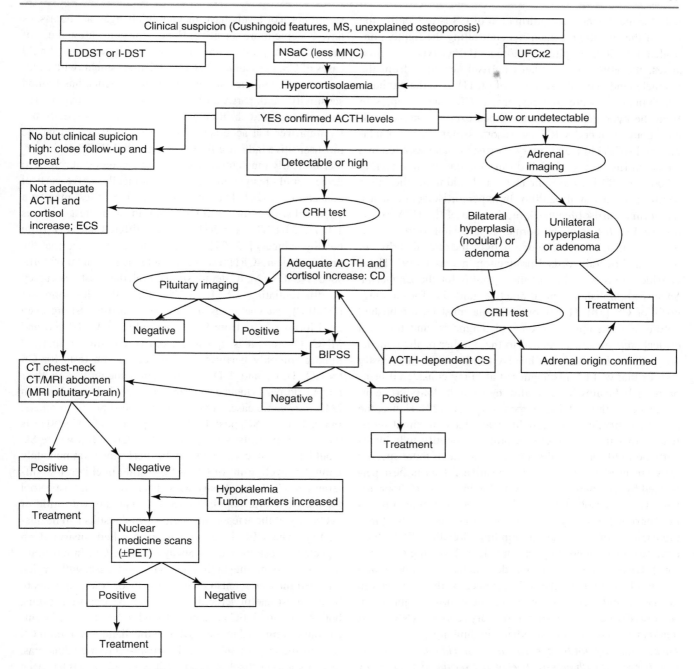

Fig. 8.1 Diagnostic work-up in Cushing's syndrome. (*ACTH* adreno-corticotropin, *BIPSS* bilateral inferior petrosal sinus sampling, *CT* computed tomography, *ECS* ectopic Cushing's syndrome, *LDDST* low-dose dexamethasone test, *NSaC* night salivary cortisol, *MRI* magnetic reso-nance imaging, *MS* metabolic syndrome, *MNC* midnight cortisol, *PET* positron emission tomography, *UFC* 24 hr-urinary free cortisol, *1-DST* 1 mg overnight dexamethasone test)

ogy, the degree of hypercortisolaemia seems to be the major determinant of the clinical features rather than its duration [9, 11]. Severe hirsutism and virilisation strongly suggest an adrenal carcinoma [5]. A gradual onset of signs may be seen with NETs as opposed to SCLCs, which usually have a more rapid onset with symptoms of profound weakness, hyperpigmentation, little or no weight gain, and an absence of overt Cushingoid features, while the severity of the syndrome have

been implicated as the cause of the more frequent presence of skin pigmentation and ankle oedema in SCLCs compared to other causes of ECS [9]. On the other hand, in ECS psychiatric disorders are more prominent in NETs than with SCLCs [9, 22].

It is obvious that the similarity of different types of CS mandates the necessity for a specific step-by-step diagnostic work-up to resolve any diagnostic dilemma [1]. The rationale for the diagnostic confirmation of CS is to identify the loss of the specific mechanisms controlling the tightly controlled hypothalamo-pituitary-adrenal (HPA) axis. In normal states, the HPA axis regulates cortisol secretion from the adrenal gland under the stimulus of ACTH from the pituitary, which in turn is secreted in response to CRH and vasopressin from the hypothalamus. Cortisol then exerts negative feedback control on both CRH and vasopressin in the hypothalamus and ACTH in the pituitary. Cortisol is also secreted in a circadian rhythm; levels fall during the day from a peak at 07.00 h–08.00 h to a nadir at around midnight: they then begin to rise again at 02.00 h. In hypercortisolaemic states, the normal cortisol feedback mechanism of the HPA axis is distorted with loss of the normal suppression to the exogenous administration of glucocorticoids, the circadian rhythm is lost, and overall cortisol production increases [19]. These considerations were in part the stimulus for the *Endocrine Society* to publish a clinical practice guideline for the diagnosis of CS [18]. Hypercortisolaemia must be established before any attempt at differential diagnosis, and this is a critical step since it is related to the number of the patients that will unnecessarily be involved in laborious and costly tests or that will be misdiagnosed as being considered inappropriately healthy but yet suffering from the long-term consequences of the sustained hypercortisolism [23]. Hence, the *initial* biochemical tests should ideally have maximal *sensitivity* rather than specificity in order to identify individuals with the mild forms of this rare disease; later, more specific tests are used to exclude false positives. This is best performed by a combination of the following tests: 24-hour urinary free cortisol (UFC; at least 2–3 measurements) as marker of increased synthesis of cortisol exceeding the binding capacity of corticosteroid binding globulin (CBG), low-dose dexamethasone suppression (LDDST, 0.5 mg every 6 h for 2 days) or 1 mg overnight dexamethasone suppression testing (1-DST) as marker of resistance of the HPA axis to glucocorticoid feedback, and assessment of midnight serum cortisol (MNC) or late-night salivary cortisol (NSaC) as markers of the loss of circadian rhythmicity [18, 24, 25]. *These tests may not be needed when a florid and severe disease is present with massively elevated serum cortisol at any time or in the presence of a urinary free cortisol more than four times the upper limit of normal.* In individuals with normal results in the initial investigation but with strong suspicion or when progression is documented, or when only one of test results is abnormal and clinical suspicion is high, further evaluation at a later stage is crucial to confirm or exclude the diagnosis [25]. It has been suggested that in these particularly difficult cases, a dexamethasone-CRH test is useful, but not all CS experts agree on its superiority over and above the standard LDDST [18]. Diagnostic tests based on a failure of feedback regulation were originally designed for the florid rather than the mild cases we now see, and the thresholds for

serum cortisol levels have inevitably changed as the assays have become more sensitive. Hence, the conventional use of the 1-DST may still be insufficiently sensitive to detect mild cases of CS, particularly in CD; UFC assessment, with accurate assay techniques and in compliant patients, has limited sensitivity, and particularly in cases of mild hypercortisolism, but liquid chromatography tandem-mass spectrometry improves the accuracy [26]. NSaC level should be the most sensitive indicator for CS along with MNC, but the former is clearly much more practical for screening purposes to detect rapid changes in the free biologically active cortisol concentration [24]. The salivary cortisol (SC) test may be a good substitute for serum cortisol in some test such as 1-DST, LDDST, or CRH tests to differentiate CS from healthy subjects [25, 27]. A recent study suggested that the dexamethasone-CRH test and a single measurement of cortisol as NSaC or MNC demonstrated high diagnostic accuracy in differentiating CS from PC. Recently, desmopressin (*DDAVP*) test was suggested as better distinguishing even mild forms of CD from PC compared to UFC, 1-DST, and MNC. Overall, it is apparent from recent studies that the three commonly performed initial diagnostic tests for CS (NSaC, UFC, and 1-DST) are complementary, and their diagnostic performance may increase by their combination [24]. In specific cases some tests may be superior to others. In renal failure SC, post-1-DST is superior to UFC [28] as is the case of patients with cyclic CD (cyCD) [29], where SC would be most convenient to be performed immediately upon the 'cycling-in' of CS or SC testing in children to differentiate CS from obesity as a 'friendlier' diagnostic tool for the paediatric population [30]. In patients with mild or cyCS, any of these tests may yield normal results and be misleading. The UFC in particular, even when measured on repeated occasions, cannot always exclude CS. In our opinion, because of the high sensitivity and ease with which repeated measurements can be performed, NSaC appears to be the most useful screening test [31]. As opposed to this, both NSaC and UFC have been found to be of limited clinical value compared to the 1-DST in the diagnosis of mild CS such as the case of subclinical cortisol-secreting adenomas, 'autonomous cortisol secretion' (SCSA) [32–34]. It has been suggested that one can exclude CS after three normal UFC collections, while values fourfold greater than the upper limit of normal can be considered diagnostic for CS [1]. However, small increases in cortisol production at the circadian nadir may not be detected as an increase in UFC as most of the cortisol secreted during any 24-hour period is generally between 04.00 h and 16.00 h [35, 36], but they might have a small but significant increase in nighttime cortisol secretion. Hence, the recent guidelines for the diagnosis of CS suggest use of the 1-DST or MNC, rather than UFC and NSaC, in patients suspected of having mild CS because of an adrenal incidentaloma [18]. Nevertheless, the diagnosis of

CS should be viewed as probabilistic rather than as algorithmic, and except in the most obvious cases, test procedures have to be assessed with fine judgement.

The second step in the diagnostic cascade is to establish the cause of CS; plasma ACTH measurement will be either very low indicating an adrenal cause causing ACTH suppression or readily detectable. *A plasma ACTH >20 ng/L, and certainly >30 ng/L, will almost immediately establish ACTH dependence, while levels below 10 ng/L will lead to the search for adrenal pathology.* Values in the 'grey zone' are the most challenging since patients with both CD and adrenal pathologies might have intermediate values. In this situation, CRH tests (see below) with measurement of plasma ACTH should help differentiate between ACTH dependence and independence.

With readily detectable ACTH, then the patient either has CD or an ectopic source. Not infrequently, it is difficult to differentiate between them, as both are ACTH-dependent. The rationale for the tests used is that the corticotroph tumour cells in pituitary adenomas retain some responsiveness to the negative feedback effects of glucocorticoids, while tumours ectopically secreting ACTH generally do not [1, 9, 16, 19]. A rise in cortisol and ACTH to corticotrophin-releasing hormone (CRH) test (either alone or in combination with desmopressin) usually suggests CD. An ACTH increase >35% and cortisol >20% above baseline levels are considered to be a specific response for CD when ovine-CRH is used [37] and >105% and >14%, respectively, when human-CRH is used [38]. The CRH test has a sensitivity of 94% for cortisol and ACTH responses, but approximately 5%–17% of patients with ECS respond to CRH administration [9, 19, 37, 38]. Using desmopressin instead of CRH, 40% false-positive responses were observed in patients with ECS, with a reported sensitivity of 77–84% and specificity 73–83% [9, 19, 39, 40]. The high-dose dexamethasone suppression test (HDDST) is no longer in widespread use, but a serum cortisol suppression greater than 50% is considered indicative of CD with sensitivity of 60–100% and a specificity of 65–100% [19, 21, 40]; when the cut-off for serum cortisol suppression was >60%, this occurred in 3% of patients with ECS, and when it was >80%, it did not occur in any patient with EAS [19, 21, 40, 41].

The crucial next step to accurately identify a pituitary source is by direct sampling of the effluent of the pituitary by bilateral inferior petrosal sinus sampling (BIPSS) with CRH stimulation, especially as these tumours are usually microadenomas and may not be visible on magnetic resonance imaging (MRI) [1, 19]. This may be considered as the 'gold standard' test unless there is a clear pituitary abnormality (macroadenoma) or if an ectopic source has been considered highly unlikely or the patient is too ill and requires immediate medical therapy. The criteria used to identify CD is an inferior petrosal sinus-to-peripheral ACTH ratio at baseline >2.0 and a gradient >3.0 following CRH (or desmopressin as a cheaper alternative) stimulation [1]. In patients with ECS, both ratios are expected to be <2.0, but there are reports of false-negative and false-positive responses, particularly when an adequate hypercortisolaemic state is not present [9, 22, 42–46]. This test demands experience and should be performed only in specialised centres since serious complications (stroke, perforation of the arterial wall, hematomas, and transitory arrhythmias) have been described [47]. As previously mentioned, ECS can also have a rapid onset and a paraneoplastic wasting syndrome which may mask hypercortisol features; profound hypokalaemia and less often hyperglycaemia may reveal its presence. Hypokalaemia is related to the degree of hypercortisolaemia since cortisol acts as mineralocorticoid because of the enzyme 11β-hydroxysteroid type 2. With regard to ACTH and potassium levels, no cut-off limit has been defined to distinguish patients with ECS and CD [9] since cortisol-secreting macroadenomas may share a common biochemical profile to the ECS [48]. Measurement of circulating tumour markers also has a role when ECS associated with NETs is suspected. Both calcitonin and gastrin have been found to be the most commonly elevated tumour markers, regardless of tumour type [9] in ECS, while calcitonin and catecholamines need to be measured to exclude an ECS source from MTC or a phaeochromocytoma, respectively. Axial imaging with thin-cut multislice-computed tomography (CT) of the chest and abdomen or with chest and pelvis MRI has the highest detection rate for ECS source identification [9, 11, 22, 49]. MRI of the abdomen is not used routinely because of the bowel movement artefact and because calcification associated with the primary tumour can more easily be identified on a CT scan; CT and MRI failure to localise the source of ECS may fall from 8–50% to 12.5% when an appropriate and meticulous technique is used along with a close prolonged follow-up using additional newer imaging modalities when appropriate [9]. Somatostatin receptor (SSTR) scintigraphy may be proved helpful as ECS may be caused by small NETs expressing SSTRs adding supportive functional data to the conventional imaging techniques [9]. Positron emission tomography (PET) with 18-fluorodeoxyglucose ([18]FDG-PET) is rarely helpful since these tumours have usually low metabolic activity [50]. Whole-body PET with ^{11}C-5-hydroxytryptophan has been proposed as universal imaging technique for NETs, in particular identifying an otherwise occult NET [51]. [131]I- and ^{123}I-meta-iodobenzylguanidine scans have been also used in NET investigation [9, 11]. However, recent data suggest that ^{68}Ga-dotatate-PET/CT may be the most valuable in identifying a source or confirming the nature of an imaging abnormality. All these techniques may also be useful in the investigation of ACTH-secreting pituitary carcinomas [52]. These recent modalities have resulted in only limited use for whole-body venous catheterisation and sampling, while selective abdominal angiography and endoscopic ultrasonography may be useful in suspicion of a pancreatic NET [53] and thyroid ultrasound with fine needle aspiration may be used to exclude or diagnose MTC [54]. More sophisticated imaging techniques with limited experience such as the use of an intraoperative gamma counter in the management of metastatic ACTH-secreting bronchial carcinoids look promising [55]. The appearance of the adrenals on CT scanning may also support a diagnosis, such as the possibility of a phaeochromocytoma as the ECS source; the adrenals may have a normal size in 7–25% of patients with ECS, showing moderate hyperplasia in 56% and marked hyperplasia in 37% compared to 50% either normal or mildly enlarged adrenals in CD; however, macronodular hyperplasia presents similar rates in both clinical settings [9]. *Definitive proof of an ACTH-dependent tumour requires complete resolution of the clinical and biochemical features after tumour resection or partial resolution after tumour debulking and/or the demonstration of ACTH immunohistochemical staining in the tumour tissue or in metastatic deposits* [1, 9].

On the other hand, if ACTH is very low or undetectable, then the next step is imaging of the adrenals. High-resolution CT scanning gives the best resolution of adrenal anatomy, and it is accurate for masses >1 cm. A mass >5 cm in diameter should be considered to be malignant until proven otherwise [1, 9].

Less commonly, genetic testing for mutations of *PRKAR1A* may be needed to confirm Carney complex or *ARMC5* in cases of BMAH.

Summarising international consensus statements for the diagnosis and differential diagnosis of CS, [18] recommend UFC ($\geq$2 values), LDDST, or late night salivary cortisol ($\geq$2 values) to be used as the first-line screening tests. Abnormal results should be confirmed by an additional one of these tests. In patients with discordant results, second-line tests should be used as necessary for confirmation, or they should be repeated a second time if a suspicion of cyclicity/variability has been raised. Once the diagnosis of CS is unequivocal, ACTH levels and CRH testing (combined with the results of the LDDST), together with appropriate imaging, are the most useful non-invasive investigations to determine the aetiology. BIPSS is recommended in cases of ACTH-dependent CS where the clinical, biochemical, or radiological results are discordant or equivocal.

Present and Future Therapies (Fig. 8.2)

Treatment is often complex and may require the use of surgery, radiotherapy, and medical management or their combination. The specific target is to normalise cortisol levels with a reversal of clinical features. Surgical removal of the tumour causing CS is the current first-line approach for all types of CS. Inhibitors of cortisol secretion may be required before surgery after the completion of the biochemical diagnostic work-up to reverse rapidly the metabolic consequences and poor healing, in patients who cannot be submitted to surgical procedures, during the 'waiting follow-up period' until the identification of a covert or occult tumour [53] or as alternative treatment if surgery fails [1, 19, 56]. In cases of SCLCs, appropriate medical therapy is urgently instituted since prompt correction of hypercortisolism is necessary to minimise the side effects of myelo-suppressive cytotoxic chemotherapy [9]. Compounds that target glucocorticoid synthesis (adrenal secretion inhibitors or adrenolytic drugs, such as metyrapone, ketoconazole, etomidate, mitotane, or trilostane) or function (mifepristone) have been broadly used [57]. Metyrapone and ketoconazole (either alone or in combination) are the most frequently used drugs and appear to be more effective and better tolerated than other adrenal inhibitors. *Metyrapone* is rapid in onset and highly effective, but the presence of hirsutism frequently precludes its long-term use. In one study of 195 patients with CS treated with metyrapone, there was a significant improvement when first evaluation and last review were compared [58]. A novel agent having the same therapeutic profile of metyrapone but displaying a threefold more potent and a longer half-life is *osilodrostat* [59]. In one proof-of-concept study of 12 patients with moderate-to-severe CD, all patients achieved UFC levels within the upper limit of normal (ULN) or a >50% decrease from baseline levels, while 92% obtained normalisation of UFC levels in a 10-week treatment [60]. In the extension phase study, UFC levels were normalised in 78.9% of patients at 22 weeks [61]. *Ketoconazole* can be used additionally or in place of metyrapone, although its onset of action is rather slower, occurring over several days, while gynaecomastia or hypogonadism complicates its use in men. *Levoketoconazole* is the single 2S,4R enantiomer of ketoconazole, being 2–7 times more potent than ketoconazole in inhibiting steroidogenesis, possibly displaying a better safety profile being 12 times less potent than ketoconazole to exert hepatoxicity [62]. In a phase I study, when administered to healthy subjects, levoketoconazole (400 mg/day) reduced serum cortisol levels significantly by day 4, compared to placebo and ketoconazole; the drug was well tolerated; headache, back pain, and nausea were the most frequently reported AEs [63]. Intravenous *etomidate* at sub-anaesthetic doses remains an important option when intravenous administration is required for rapid treatment of severely ill patients and is almost always very effective; however, it should usually be used in an intensive care unit in the first instance. The published guidelines suggest a loading dose of 3–5 mg followed by continuous infusion of 0.03–0.10 mg/kg/h (2.5–3.0 mg/hr) with monitoring every 4–6 hrs to prevent

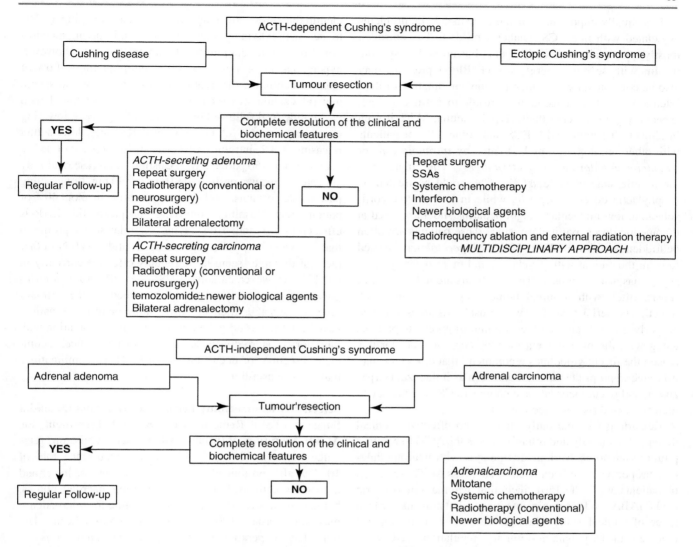

Fig. 8.2 Treatment algorithm in common types of Cushing's syndrome. (*ACTH* adrenocorticotropin, *BIPSS* bilateral inferior petrosal sinus sampling, *CT* computed tomography, *ECS* ectopic Cushing's syndrome, *LDDST* low-dose dexamethasone test, *LNSaC* late night sali-vary cortisol, *MRI* magnetic resonance imaging, *MS* metabolic syndrome, *MSC* midnight serum cortisol, *PET* positron emission tomography, *UFC* 24-hr urinary free cortisol, *SSAs* somatostatin analogues, *1-ODST* 1 mg overnight dexamethasone test)

adrenal insufficiency achieving a stable serum cortisol level between 280–560 nmol/L in physiologically stressed patients and 150–300 nmol/l in an unstressed patient [64]. It should be emphasised that the 11-hydroxylase inhibitors such as metyrapone, osilodrostat, and etomidate all produce elevated levels of 11-deoxycortisol which may cross-react in many conventional cortisol assays. Finally, if all else fails, the glucocorticoid antagonist *mifepristone* can reduce the symptoms and signs of CS with most clinical responders receiving doses ≥600 mg/day, suggesting that higher doses were required to achieve optimal clinical benefit in patients with endogenous CS [65, 66]. Mifepristone is approved in the United States to control carbohydrate metabolism abnormalities (CHA) secondary to hypercortisolism in patients with CD who failed surgery or were not considered to be good surgical candidates, but its drawback is the absence of serum cortisol as a marker of efficacy [66] and the patient risks to become Addisonian unless care is taken; severe hypokalaemia may be induced (treatable with spironolactone), and further evaluation of its safety and follow-up methodologies are needed. **Mitotane** might be an alternative, but the difficulty in monitoring and the adverse effects determine that its use be confined to the minority of patients who are intolerant or not responsive to the previous treatments and who are unsuitable for adrenalectomy [56]. The concomitant administration of mitotane, metyrapone, and ketoconazole was proven to be an effective alternative to avoid adrenalectomy [67], with ketoconazole (200–600 mg/day) and metyrapone (750–1000 mg/ day) and a median duration of treatment of 4 months.

It is equally important to manage the metabolic problems associated with florid CS. Diabetes needs to be controlled mostly with oral antidiabetic agents but possibly requiring insulin with severe hyperglycaemia. Blood pressure may also be controlled by drug therapy; the combination of fluid retention and hypertension may result to cardiac failure, especially in the older patient. Hypokalaemia, which is seen in almost all patients with ECS and some 10% of patients with other aetiologies, may be treated by *spironolactone* or *triamterene/amiloride as alternatives*. The high pro-thrombotic state of patients with CS should be treated by prophylactic doses of *heparin*, while in severe hypercortisolaemia, low molecular weight heparins should be used at therapeutic doses, particularly since these patients are often bedridden or of low mobility [64]. *Haloperidol* may be used to calm the patient with psychosis, and more recently *olanzapine* has also been used. These patients are at high risk of sepsis, often with minimal clinical signs, and any such infection bacterial, fungal, or viral must be vigorously treated properly as is seen in other immunosuppressed patients along with the management of hypercortisolemia. For this reason the recent guidelines recommend that clinicians may offer age-appropriate vaccinations such as influenza, Herpes zoster, and pneumococcal vaccinations to CS patients due to their increased risk of infection [64].

Regarding CD, currently, there is no effective medical therapy that directly and reliably targets the ACTH-secreting pituitary adenoma. Various compounds with neuromodulatory properties have been used to suppress ACTH secretion in patients with CD [56], including gamma-aminobutyric acid (GABA) and serotonin antagonists, but none has proven to be of clinical value. Nuclear hormone receptor ligands involved in hypothalamo-pituitary regulation have been tested; thiazolidinediones were proved to have no effect on pharmaceutical doses used in clinical practice; retinoic acid seems to be of clinical interest since it inhibits ACTH secretion and cell proliferation both in vitro in ACTH-producing tumour cell lines, and cultured human corticotroph adenomas, and in vivo in nude mice [68]; a recent clinical trial showed only minor activity. However, dopamine agonists and somatostatin analogues (SSAs) have shown some promising results. **Pasireotide** targeting mostly both the SSTR5 (not octreotide and lanreotide targeting the SSTR2) and the dopamine agonist cabergoline show therapeutic promise in CD. The 12-month phase 3 published study of pasireotide showed remission of hypercortisolaemia, as measured by UFC, in 15% of patients treated by 600 μg twice daily dose and 26% of patients on the 900 μg twice daily dose; by increasing the daily dose with an additional 300 μg twice daily, they improved to 16% and 29%, respectively [69]. It is of interest that 48% of patients with UFC normalisation at 1 year remained controlled the second year [70]. Mean tumour volume decreased by 44% in 75 patients with an

identifiable lesion on magnetic resonance imaging (MRI) treated with 900 mcg of pasireotide [69], implying an additional role as a neo-adjuvant treatment. Of note, however, hyperglycaemia is a major and frequent problem, and 6% of them discontinued the treatment; more frequent and severe hyperglycaemia was seen in 73% of patients treated with pasireotide [69] followed by the need of a glucose-lowering medication in 46% of patients [69]. Recently, long-acting releasing (LAR) intramuscular once-monthly pasireotide has been given in 150 patients with Cushing's, disease randomly allocated to receive pasireotide 10 mg or 30 mg. Long-acting pasireotide normalised mUFC concentration in about 40% of patients with Cushing's, implying that pasireotide LAR is efficacious at month 7 displaying a similar safety profile to that of twice-daily subcutaneous pasireotide [71]. No other medical therapies seem to be reliably effective currently in CD [72]. However, in some ECS cases, SSTRs as well as dopamine receptors have been identified in the primary tumours, and thus their agonists, alone or in combination, have been tried as drug therapy alone or in combination with inhibitors of steroidogenesis in cases of recurrence, incomplete resection, or occult tumours [9]. These combinations may also be useful in resistant CD [72].

Selective Adenomectomy Performed by Transsphenoidal Surgery (TSS) Remains the Optimal Treatment for ACTH-Secreting Pituitary Adenomas Remission rates range between 60% and 80% with a recurrence rate of 10–25% after prolonged follow-up; these rates are lower and higher, respectively, in patients harbouring macroadenomas, but in experienced hands the remission rate for microadenomas may approach 100%. Persistent disease might mandate immediate reoperation, but this appears to result in remission in only around 50% of cases and with a high risk of hypopituitarism [73]. When the tumour is apparent at transsphenoidal exploration, a selective adenomectomy is performed, but when no tumour is obvious, a hemi-hypophysectomy as guided by the BIPSS or MRI imaged results is often the best course of action [74]. A postoperative concentration of cortisol <50 nmol/L defines cure but is not predictive of permanent cure; this needs glucocorticoid replacement treatment until recovery of the HPA axis, i.e. when the morning cortisol levels or the cortisol response to an ACTH stimulation test is normal. Higher postoperative cortisol levels are more likely to be associated with failed surgery; however, cortisol levels may sometimes gradually decline over 4–6 weeks reflecting either gradual infarction of remnant tumour or some degree of adrenal semiautonomy [75]. It has to be highlighted that patients with CS undergoing surgery should have perioperative prophylaxis for venous thromboembolism, since they bear a thrombotic risk lasting 1 year after hypercortisolaemia remission [64]. It should also be emphasised that a normalised standardised mortality rate is only seen in patients with Cushing's disease cured at their initial surgery.

After surgical failure, patients with cavernous sinus or dural invasion identified at the initial procedure may be considered for radiation therapy. Conventional fractionated external beam radiotherapy achieves control of hypercortisolaemia in 50–60% of patients within 3–5 years but with the risk of long-term hypopituitarism; this treatment seems more effective and is more rapid in onset in children. Stereotactic radiosurgery may also be used if there is a clear target but with higher than initially thought relapse rates [54]. Radiosurgery is not suitable for large lesions near the optic chiasm or optic nerves. Gamma Knife radiosurgery is the most popular technique achieving biochemical remission in about 55% [76] but can be used as salvage therapy in difficult tumours [77]. Radiosurgery using a proton beam has similar efficacy as second-line therapy [78]. Linear accelerator radiotherapy for CD has been reported to be of some success in a small number of patients [79]. As with all the forms of radiotherapy, new hormone deficiencies are the major drawback, and the appropriate replacement regimen has to promptly be initiated. On the other hand, TSS failure should prompt reevaluation of the diagnosis of CD, especially if previous diagnostic test results were indeterminate or conflicting or if no tumour was found on pathological examination. When surgical therapy fails and severe symptoms of CS persist, or when drugs are not effective or tolerated and the rapid control of hypercortisolaemia is crucial, bilateral adrenalectomy should be considered. This option induces a rapid resolution of the clinical features, but patients will need lifelong treatment with glucocorticoids and mineralocorticoids along with careful education and meticulous evaluation in their follow-up visits. A major concern in patients with CD is the development of a locally aggressive pituitary tumour, Nelson's syndrome (NS), seen in 8–29%, which in turn might be treated with further surgery or radiotherapy to reduce tumour size and ameliorate hyperpigmentation [80]. Pituitary radiotherapy at the time of adrenalectomy has been considered to reduce the risk of the syndrome, but this is unproven [9, 17, 53]. Close monitoring with regular MRI scans and plasma ACTH levels should be undertaken 3–6 months after bilateral adrenalectomy and then at regular intervals thereafter. A high plasma ACTH level (>1000 ng/l) in the year after surgery may be a predictive factor for tumour progression [1, 17]. Recently, pasireotide 300–600 μg s.c. twice daily for a month was followed by a 6-month treatment with pasireotide LAR 40–60 mg monthly in seven patients with NS demonstrating a significant reduction of ACTH levels (before the morning dose of glucocorticoids) during the 28 weeks of treatment but without significant change in tumour volumes [81]. Interestingly, an acute response to a test dose predicted the outcome in 80% of patients.

Temozolomide is an oral alkylating precursor of dacarbazine a DNA repair inhibitor showing some results in selected aggressive corticotroph pituitary carcinomas [82]. A temozolomide response in pituitary tumours may be predicted by low expression of the DNA repair enzyme O6-methylguanine-DNA-methyltransferase (MGMT) [83], but in practice the therapeutic response is best determined after three cycles of chemotherapy.

Resection of the causative tumour is the optimum treatment for ectopic CS; curative resection with complete remission was found to be 83% with a single primary lesion, but overall, curative surgery was successful in only 30–47% [11, 22]. Unilateral or complete bilateral adrenalectomy is performed in 30–56% of patients with ECS when hypercortisolaemia cannot be treated by other means; when medical treatment was ineffective, not well tolerated, or rejected by the patient; in young women desiring pregnancy; or when a source of ECS remains occult [9, 11, 22, 47]. A multidisciplinary, individualised approach is needed in metastatic or occult disease, followed by SSAs, systemic chemotherapy, interferon, newer biological agents, chemoembolisation, radiofrequency ablation, and external or peptide radioreceptor radiation therapy used alone or in combination [5] to control tumour growth and symptoms associated with ECS. External radiotherapy directed to the mediastinum has been used for carcinoids directed to the tumour bed or to metastatic deposits [11, 22]. Radiofrequency ablation has been also used to treat hepatic metastases of NETs, and intraoperative 'octreoscanning' with a hand-held gamma detector probe has been proposed to increase the intraoperative detection rate [55]. Chemotherapy with 5-fluorouracil, streptozotocin, cisplatin, etoposide, and/or adriamycin has also been used in metastatic NETs and SCLCs [22]. Hormone analogues and/or radionuclide treatment, chemoembolisation, and ^{131}I-MIBG or ^{177}Lu-octreotate treatment have also been used [11]. No 'gold standard' therapy has been approved when surgical and classical medical therapies have failed. In the context of ectopic CS, despite detailed investigation, the cause of excess and unregulated ACTH production remains occult in 5–15% of patients, and these patients need meticulous follow-up for identification of the primary tumour [9].

Adrenalectomy is either unilateral when associated to adrenal adenoma or carcinoma or bilateral in cases of bilateral hyperplasia or adenomas. In adrenal adenomas cure following surgery in skilled hands approaches 100% and is associated with low morbidity and mortality [84]. Laparoscopic adrenal removal has been shown in experienced hands to be a safe procedure and in many centres has become the approach of choice for non-malignant disease [85]. Prognosis after removal of an adenoma is good. Surgical removal of an adrenal carcinoma can be attempted with limited lesions, but when metastatic these tumours are not very radio- or chemosensitive; aggressive surgical approaches probably account for the increase in life span reported in this disease [86]. Mitotane is thought to be an effective adjuvant therapy [1]. Combination chemotherapy that has been more recently investigated includes etoposide, doxorubicin and cisplatin, or streptozotocin [87]. Newer biological agents are under investigation; recent studies emphasise how the metabolism of many agents can be affected by preceding mitotane [88, 89].

Finally, in BMAH the cortisol secretion may be controlled by blocking the corresponding aberrantly expressed receptor (propranolol for beta-adrenergic receptor, somatostatin analogues for gastric inhibitory peptide receptor, leuprolide for luteinising hormone, etc.) [5], although surgery is usually preferred.

Novel inhibitors of cortisol secretion under investigation include doxazosin, an α1-adrenergic receptor antagonist [90]; gefitinib, a tyrosine kinase inhibitor (TKI) [91]; bevacizumab, a monoclonal antibody that blocks vascular endothelial growth factor receptor 2 (VEGFR2) [92]; R-roscovitine, a CDK2/cyclin E inhibitor [93]; or the selective, peptide melanocortin-2 receptor antagonist, IRC-274 [94].

All patients undergoing treatment should be advised regarding glucocorticoid withdrawal symptoms (skin flaking, fatigue, nausea, joint aches). Hypocortisolism has to be managed with glucocorticoid replacement therapy until the axis recovers, while careful advice and instructions have to be given both orally and written to all patients.

Conclusions

Untreated hypercortisolaemia is associated with excess mortality and increased morbidity, and therefore rapid and lifelong control is vital. The aim of the follow-up is to restore a 24-hour production rate of cortisol within the normal range, even when circadian rhythmicity has not been restored [19]. An individualised follow-up should be tailored to each patient with CS in relation to the cause and the success of the first-line treatment.

References

1. Newell-Price J, Bertagna X, Grossman AB, Nieman LK. Cushing's syndrome. Lancet. 2006;367:1605–17.
2. Matos AC, Srirangalingam U, Barry T, Grossman AB. Cushing's syndrome with low levels of serum cortisol: the role of inhaled steroids. Clin Med. 2011;11:404–5.
3. Alexandraki KI, Grossman AB. Therapeutic strategies for the treatment of severe Cushing's syndrome. Drugs. 2016;76:447–58.
4. Hall JJ, Hughes CA, Foisy MM, Houston S, Shafran S. Iatrogenic Cushing syndrome after intra-articular triamcinolone in a patient receiving ritonavir-boosted darunavir. Int J STD AIDS. 2013;24:748–52.
5. Morris DG, Grossman G. Chapter 7. Cushing's syndrome. In: Neuroendocrinology, hypothalamus, and pituitary a grossman, http://www.endotext.org/neuroendo/.
6. Scheithauer BW, Gaffey TA, Lloyd RV, Sebo TJ, Kovacs KT, Horvath E, et al. Pathobiology of pituitary adenomas and carcinomas. Neurosurgery. 2006;59:341–53.
7. Dworakowska D, Grossman AB. The molecular pathogenesis of pituitary tumors: implications for clinical management. Minerva Endocrinol. 2012;37:157–72.
8. Alexandraki KI, Munayem Khan M, Chahal HS, Dalantaeva NS, Trivellin G, Berney DM, et al. Oncogene-induced senescence in pituitary adenomas and carcinomas. Hormones (Athens). 2012;11:297–307.
9. Alexandraki KI, Grossman AB. The ectopic ACTH syndrome. Rev Endocr Metab Disord. 2010;11:117–26.
10. Isidori AM, Lenzi A. Ectopic ACTH syndrome. Arq Bras Endocrinol Metabol. 2007;51:1217–25.
11. Isidori AM, Kaltsas GA, Pozza C, Frajese V, Newell-Price J, Reznek RH, et al. The ectopic adrenocorticotropin syndrome: clinical features, diagnosis, management and long-term follow-up. J Clin Endocrinol Metab. 2006;91:371–7.
12. Lacroix A, Bolte E, Tremblay J, Dupre J, Poitras P, Fournier H, et al. Gastric inhibitory polypeptide-dependent cortisol hypersecretion--a new cause of Cushing's syndrome. N Engl J Med. 1992;327:974–80.
13. Weinstein LS, Shenker A, Gejman PV, Merino MJ, Friedman E, Spiegel AM. Activating mutations of the stimulatory G protein in the McCune-Albright syndrome. N Engl J Med. 1991;325:1688–95.
14. Faucz FR, Zilbermint M, Lodish MB, Szarek E, Trivellin G, Sinaii N, et al. Macronodular adrenal hyperplasia due to mutations in an armadillo repeat containing 5 (ARMC5) gene: a clinical and genetic investigation. J Clin Endocrinol Metab. 2014;99:E1113–9.
15. Krikorian A, Khan M. Is metabolic syndrome a mild form of Cushing's syndrome? Rev Endocr Metab Disord. 2010;11:141–5.
16. Vilar L, Freitas Mda C, Faria M, Montenegro R, Casulari LA, Naves L, et al. Pitfalls in the diagnosis of Cushing's syndrome. Arq Bras Endocrinol Metabol. 2007;51:1207–16.
17. Arnaldi G, Angeli A, Atkinson AB, Bertagna X, Cavagnini F, Chrousos GP, et al. Diagnosis and complications of Cushing's syndrome: a consensus statement. J Clin Endocrinol Metab. 2003;88:5593–602.
18. Nieman LK, Biller BM, Findling JW, Newell-Price J, Savage MO, Stewart PM, et al. The diagnosis of Cushing's syndrome: an Endocrine Society clinical practice guideline. J Clin Endocrinol Metab. 2008;93:1526–40.
19. Newell-Price J, Trainer P, Besser M, Grossman A. The diagnosis and differential diagnosis of Cushing's syndrome and pseudo-Cushing's states. Endocr Rev. 1998;19:647–72.
20. Steffensen C, Bak AM, Rubeck KZ, Jørgensen JO. Epidemiology of Cushing's syndrome. Neuroendocrinology. 2010;92(Suppl 1):1–5.
21. Invitti C, Giraldi FP, de Martin M, Cavagnini F. Diagnosis and management of Cushing's syndrome: results of an Italian multicentre study. Study Group of the Italian Society of endocrinology on the pathophysiology of the hypothalamic-pituitary-adrenal Axis. J Clin Endocrinol Metab. 1999;84:440–8.
22. Ilias I, Torpy DJ, Pacak K, Mullen N, Wesley RA, Nieman LK. Cushing's syndrome due to ectopic corticotropin secretion: twenty years' experience at the national institutes of health. J Clin Endocrinol Metab. 2005;90:4955–62.
23. Etxabe J, Vazquez JA. Morbidity and mortality in Cushing's disease: an epidemiological approach. Clin Endocrinol. 1994;40:479–84.
24. Alexandraki KI, Grossman AB. Is urinary free cortisol of value in the diagnosis of Cushing's syndrome? Curr Opin Endocrinol Diabetes Obes. 2011;18:259–63.

25. Alexandraki KI, Grossman AB. Novel insights in the diagnosis of Cushing's syndrome. Neuroendocrinology. 2010;92(Suppl 1):35–43.

26. Ceccato F, Barbot M, Zilio M, Frigo AC, Albiger N, Camozzi V, et al. Screening tests for Cushing's syndrome: urinary free cortisol role measured by LC-MS/MS. J Clin Endocrinol Metab. 2015;100:3856–61.

27. Alwani RA, Schmit Jongbloed LW, de Jong FH, van der Lely AJ, de Herder WW, et al. Differentiating between Cushing's disease and pseudo-Cushing's syndrome: comparison of four tests. Eur J Endocrinol. 2014;170:477–86.

28. Issa BG, Page MD, Read G, John R, Douglas-Jones A, Scanlon MF. Undetectable urinary free cortisol concentrations in a case of Cushing's disease. Eur J Endocrinol. 1999;140:148–51.

29. Hermus AR, Pieters GF, Borm GF, Verhofstad AA, Smals AG, Benraad TJ, et al. Unpredictable hypersecretion of cortisol in Cushing's disease: detection by daily salivary cortisol measurements. Acta Endocrinol. 1993;128:428–32.

30. Gafni RI, Papanicolaou DA, Nieman LK. Nighttime salivary cortisol measurement as a simple, noninvasive, outpatient screening test for Cushing's syndrome in children and adolescents. J Pediatr. 2000;137:30–5.

31. Cardoso EM, Arregger AL, Tumilasci OR, Contreras LN. Diagnostic value of salivary cortisol in Cushing's syndrome (CS). Clin Endocrinol. 2009;70:516–21.

32. Masserini B, Morelli V, Bergamaschi S, Ermetici F, Eller-Vainicher C, Barbieri AM, et al. The limited role of midnight salivary cortisol levels in the diagnosis of subclinical hypercortisolism in patients with adrenal incidentaloma. Eur J Endocrinol. 2009;160:87–92.

33. Nunes ML, Vattaut S, Corcuff JB, Rault A, Loiseau H, Gatta B, et al. Late-night salivary cortisol for diagnosis of overt and subclinical Cushing's syndrome in hospitalized and ambulatory patients. J Clin Endocrinol Metab. 2009;94:456–62.

34. Kidambi S, Raff H, Findling JW. Limitations of nocturnal salivary cortisol and urine free cortisol in the diagnosis of mild Cushing's syndrome. Eur J Endocrinol. 2007;157:725–31.

35. Findling JW, Raff H. Cushing's syndrome: important issues in diagnosis and management. J Clin Endocrinol Metab. 2006;91:3746–53.

36. Carroll TB, Findling JW. The diagnosis of Cushing's syndrome. Rev Endocr Metab Disord. 2010;11:147–53.

37. Nieman LK, Oldfield EH, Wesley R, Chrousos GP, Loriaux DL, Cutler GB Jr. A simplified morning ovine corticotropin-releasing hormone stimulation test for the differential diagnosis of adrenocorticotropin-dependent Cushing's syndrome. J Clin Endocrinol Metab. 1993;77:1308–12.

38. Newell-Price J, Morris DG, Drake WM, Korbonits M, Monson JP, Besser GM, et al. Optimal response criteria for the human CRH test in the differential diagnosis of ACTH-dependent Cushing's syndrome. J Clin Endocrinol Metab. 2002;87:1640–5.

39. Terzolo M, Reimondo G, Ali A, Borretta G, Cesario F, Pia A, et al. The limited value of the desmopressin test in the diagnostic approach to Cushing's syndrome. Clin Endocrinol. 2001;54:609–16.

40. Vilar L, Naves LA, Freitas MC, Moura E, Canadas V, Leal E, et al. Endogenous Cushing's syndrome: clinical and laboratorial features in 73 cases. Arq Bras Endocrinol Metab. 2007;51:566–74.

41. Isidori AM, Kaltsas GA, Mohammed S, Morris DG, Jenkins P, Chew SL, et al. Discriminatory value of the low-dose dexamethasone suppression test in establishing the diagnosis and differential diagnosis of Cushing's syndrome. J Clin Endocrinol Metab. 2003;88:5299–306.

42. Castinetti F, Morange I, Dufour H, Jaquet P, Conte-Devolx B, Girard N, et al. Desmopressin test during petrosal sinus sampling: a valuable tool to discriminate pituitary or ectopic ACTH-dependent Cushing's syndrome. Eur J Endocrinol. 2007;157:271–7.

43. Kaltsas GA, Giannulis MG, Newell-Price JD, Dacie JE, Thakkar C, Afshar F, et al. A critical analysis of the value of simultaneous inferior petrosal sinus sampling in Cushing's disease and the occult ectopic adrenocorticotropin syndrome. J Clin Endocrinol Metab. 1999;84:487–92.

44. Swearingen B, Katznelson L, Miller K, Grinspoon S, Waltman A, Dorer DJ, et al. Diagnostic errors after inferior petrosal sinus sampling. J Clin Endocrinol Metab. 2004;89:3752–63.

45. Oldfield EH, Doppman JL, Nieman LK, Chrousos GP, Miller DL, Katz DA, et al. Petrosal sinus sampling with and without corticotropin-releasing hormone for the differential diagnosis of Cushing's syndrome. N Engl J Med. 1991;325:897–905.

46. Yamamoto Y, Davis DH, Nippoldt TB, Young WF Jr, Huston J III, Parisi JE. False-positive inferior petrosal sinus sampling in the diagnosis of Cushing's disease. Rep Two Cases J Neurosurg. 1995;83:1087–91.

47. Salgado LR, Fragoso MC, Knoepfelmacher M, Machado MC, Domenice S, Pereira MA, et al. Ectopic ACTH syndrome: our experience with 25 cases. Eur J Endocrinol. 2006;155:725–33.

48. Howlett TA, Drury PL, Perry L, Doniach I, Rees LH, Besser GM. Diagnosis and management of ACTH-dependent Cushing's syndrome: comparison of the features in ectopic and pituitary ACTH production. Clin Endocrinol. 1986;24:699–713.

49. Grossman AB, Kelly P, Rockall A, Bhattacharya S, McNicol A, Barwick T. Cushing's syndrome caused by an occult source: difficulties in diagnosis and management. Nat Clin Pract Endocrinol Metab. 2006;2:642–7.

50. Pacak K, Ilias I, Chen CC, Carrasquillo JA, Whatley M, Nieman LK. The role of [(18)F]fluorodeoxyglucose positron emission tomography and [(111)in]-diethylenetriaminepentaacetate-D-Phe-pentetreotide scintigraphy in the localization of ectopic adrenocorticotropin-secreting tumors causing Cushing's syndrome. J Clin Endocrinol Metab. 2004;89:2214–21.

51. Nikolaou A, Thomas D, Kampanellou C, Alexandraki K, Andersson LG, Sundin A, et al. The value of 11C-5-hydroxy-tryptophan (5HTP) positron emission tomography (PET) in neuroendocrine tumour diagnosis and management: experience from one center. J Endocrinol Investig. 2010;33:794–9.

52. Kaltsas GA, Nomikos P, Kontogeorgos G, Buchfelder M, Grossman AB. Clinical review: diagnosis and management of pituitary carcinomas. J Clin Endocrinol Metab. 2005;90:3089–99.

53. Biller BM, Grossman AB, Stewart PM, Melmed S, Bertagna X, Bertherat J, et al. Treatment of adrenocorticotropin-dependent Cushing's syndrome: a consensus statement. J Clin Endocrinol Metab. 2008;93:2454–62.

54. Bhansali A, Walia R, Rana SS, Dutta P, Radotra BD, Khandelwal N, et al. Ectopic Cushing's syndrome: experience from a tertiary care Centre. Indian J Med Res. 2009;129:33–41.

55. Grossrubatscher E, Vignati F, Dalino P, Possa M, Belloni PA, Vanzulli A, et al. Use of radioguided surgery with [111In]-pentetreotide in the management of an ACTH-secreting bronchial carcinoid causing ectopic Cushing's syndrome. J Endocrinol Investig. 2005;28:72–8.

56. Alexandraki KI, Grossman AB. Medical therapy of Cushing's disease: where are we now? Front Horm Res. 2010;38:165–73.

57. Alexandraki KI, Grossman AB. Medical therapy for Cushing's disease: past and future modes of treatment. Eur Endocrinol. 2009;4:74–80.

58. Daniel E, Aylwin S, Mustafa O, Ball S, Munir A, Boelaert K, et al. Effectiveness of Metyrapone in treating Cushing's syndrome: a retrospective Multicenter study in 195 patients. J Clin Endocrinol Metab. 2015;100:4146–54.

59. Calhoun DA, White WB, Krum H, Guo W, Bermann G, Trapani A, et al. Effects of a novel aldosterone synthase inhibitor for treatment of primary hypertension: results of a randomized, double-blind, placebo- and active-controlled phase 2 trial. Circulation. 2011;124:1945–55.

60. Bertagna X, Pivonello R, Fleseriu M, Zhang Y, Robinson P, Taylor A, et al. LCI699, a potent 11β-hydroxylase inhibitor, normalizes urinary cortisol in patients with Cushing's disease: results from

a multicenter, proof-of-concept study. J Clin Endocrinol Metab. 2014;99:1375–83.

61. Fleseriu M, Pivonello R, Young J, Hamrahian AH, Molitch ME, Shimizu C, et al. Osilodrostat, a potent oral 11beta-hydroxylase inhibitor: 22week, prospective, phase II study in Cushing's disease. Pituitary. 2016;19:138–48.

62. Castinetti F, Morange I, Jaquet P, Conte-Devolx B, Brue T. Ketoconazole revisited: a preoperative or postoperative treatment in Cushing's disease. Eur J Endocrinol. 2008;158:91–9.

63. Ruth T-E, Philip L, Magid A-G, Nicholas F. Pharmacology of Cor-003 (levoketoconazole), an investigational treatment for endogenous Cushing's syndrome. In: Endocrine Society's 98th Annual Meeting and Expo, April 1–4, 2016, Boston, Pituitary disorders - it's not the anterior pituitary (posters)- SAT-547.

64. Nieman LK, Biller BM, Findling JW, Murad MH, Newell-Price J, Savage MO, et al. Treatment of Cushing's syndrome: an Endocrine Society clinical practice guideline. J Clin Endocrinol Metab. 2015;100:2807–31.

65. Yuen KC, Williams G, Kushner H, Nguyen D. Association between mifepristone dose, efficacy, and tolerability in patients with Cushing syndrome. Endocr Pract. 2015;21:1087–92.

66. Fleseriu M, Biller BM, Findling JW, Molitch ME, Schteingart DE, Gross C, et al. Mifepristone, a glucocorticoid receptor antagonist, produces clinical and metabolic benefits in patients with Cushing's syndrome. J Clin Endocrinol Metab. 2012;97:2039–49.

67. Kamenický P, Droumaguet C, Salenave S, Blanchard A, Jublanc C, Gautier JF, et al. Mitotane, metyrapone, and ketoconazole combination therapy as an alternative to rescue adrenalectomy for severe ACTH-dependent Cushing's syndrome. J Clin Endocrinol Metab. 2011;96:2796–804.

68. Paez-Pereda M, Kovalovsky D, Hopfner U, Theodoropoulou M, Pagotto U, Uhl E, et al. Retinoic acid prevents experimental Cushing syndrome. J Clin Invest. 2001;108:1123–31.

69. Colao A, Petersenn S, Newell-Price J, Findling JW, Gu F, Maldonado M, et al. A 12-month phase 3 study of pasireotide in Cushing's disease. N Engl J Med. 2012;366:914–24.

70. Schopohl J, Gu F, Rubens R, Van Gaal L, Bertherat J, Ligueros-Saylan M, et al. Pasireotide can induce sustained decreases in urinary cortisol and provide clinical benefit in patients with Cushing's disease: results from an open-ended, open-label extension trial. Pituitary. 2015;18:604–12.

71. Lacroix A, Gu F, Gallardo W, Pivonello R, Yu Y, Witek P, et al. Efficacy and safety of once-monthly pasireotide in Cushing's disease: a 12 month clinical trial. Lancet Diabetes Endocrinol. 2018;6:17–26.

72. Alexandraki KI, Grossman AB. Pituitary-targeted medical therapy of Cushing's disease. Expert Opin Investig Drugs. 2008;17:669–77.

73. Locatelli M, Vance ML, Laws ER. Clinical review: the strategy of immediate reoperation for transsphenoidal surgery for Cushing's disease. J Clin Endocrinol Metab. 2005;90:5478–82.

74. Hammer GD, Tyrrell JB, Lamborn KR, Applebury CB, Hannegan ET, Bell S, et al. Transsphenoidal microsurgery for Cushing's disease: initial outcome and long-term results. J Clin Endocrinol Metab. 2004;89:6348–57.

75. Valassi E, Biller BM, Swearingen B, Pecori Giraldi F, Losa M, Mortini P, et al. Delayed remission after transsphenoidal surgery in patients with Cushing's disease. J Clin Endocrinol Metab. 2010;95:601–10.

76. Jagannathan J, Sheehan JP, Pouratian N, Laws ER, Steiner L, Vance ML. Gamma knife surgery for Cushing's disease. J Neurosurg. 2007;106:980–7.

77. Swords FM, Monson JP, Besser GM, Chew SL, Drake WM, Grossman AB, et al. Gamma knife radiosurgery: a safe and effec-

tive salvage treatment for pituitary tumours not controlled despite conventional radiotherapy. Eur J Endocrinol. 2009;161:819–28.

78. Petit JH, Biller BM, Yock TI, Swearingen B, Coen JJ, Chapman P, et al. Proton stereotactic radiotherapy for persistent adrenocorticotropin-producing adenomas. J Clin Endocrinol Metab. 2008;93:393–9.

79. Swords FM, Allan CA, Plowman PN, Sibtain A, Evanson J, Chew SL, et al. Stereotactic radiosurgery XVI: a treatment for previously irradiated pituitary adenomas. J Clin Endocrinol Metab. 2003;88:5334–40.

80. Kelly PA, Samandouras G, Grossman AB, Afshar F, Besser GM, Jenkins PJ. Neurosurgical treatment of Nelson's syndrome. J Clin Endocrinol Metab. 2002;87:5465–9.

81. Daniel E, Debono M, Caunt S, Girio-Fragkoulakis C, Walters SJ, Akker SA, et al. A prospective longitudinal study of Pasireotide in Nelson's syndrome. Pituitary. 2018.

82. Bode H, Seiz M, Lammert A, Brockmann MA, Back W, Hammes HP, et al. SOM230 (pasireotide) and temozolomide achieve sustained control of tumour progression and ACTH secretion in pituitary carcinoma with widespread metastases. Exp Clin Endocrinol Diabetes. 2010;118:760–3.

83. McCormack AI, McDonald KL, Gill AJ, Clark SJ, Burt MG, Campbell KA, et al. Low O6-methylguanine-DNA methyltransferase (MGMT) expression and response to temozolomide in aggressive pituitary tumours. Clin Endocrinol. 2009;71:226–3.

84. Valimaki M, Pelkonen R, Porkka L, Sivula A, Kahri A. Long-term results of adrenal surgery in patients with Cushing's syndrome due to adrenocortical adenoma. Clin Endocrinol. 1984;20:229–36.

85. McCallum RW, Connell JM. Laparoscopic adrenalectomy. Clin Endocrinol. 2001;55:435–6.

86. Bellantone R, Ferrante A, Boscherini M, Lombardi CP, Crucitti P, Crucitti F, et al. Role of reoperation in recurrence of adrenal cortical carcinoma: results from 188 cases collected in the Italian National Registry for adrenal cortical carcinoma. Surgery. 1997;122:1212–8.

87. Fassnacht M, Terzolo M, Allolio B, Baudin E, Haak H, Berruti A, et al. Combination chemotherapy in advanced adrenocortical carcinoma. N Engl J Med. 2012;366:2189–97.

88. Mariniello B, Rosato A, Zuccolotto G, Rubin B, Cicala MV, Finco I, et al. Combination of sorafenib and everolimus impacts therapeutically on adrenocortical tumor models. Endocr Relat Cancer. 2012;19:527–39.

89. Kroiss M, Quinkler M, Johanssen S, van Erp NP, Lankheet N, Pöllinger A, et al. Sunitinib in refractory adrenocortical carcinoma: a phase II, single-arm. Open-Label Trial J Clin Endocrinol Metab. 2012;97:3495–503.

90. Fernando MA, Heaney AP. Alpha1-adrenergic receptor antagonists: novel therapy for pituitary adenomas. Mol Endocrinol. 2005;19:3085–96.

91. Fukuoka H, Cooper O, Ben-Shlomo A, Mamelak A, Ren SG, Bruyette D, et al. EGFR as a therapeutic target for human, canine, and mouse ACTH-secreting pituitary adenomas. J Clin Invest. 2011;121:4712–21.

92. Ortiz LD, Syro LV, Scheithauer BW, Ersen A, Uribe H, Fadul CE, et al. Anti-VEGF therapy in pituitary carcinoma. Pituitary. 2012;15:445–9.

93. Liu NA, Jiang H, Ben-Shlomo A, Wawrowsky K, Fan XM, Lin S, et al. Targeting zebrafish and murine pituitary corticotroph tumors with a cyclin-dependent kinase (CDK) inhibitor. Proc Natl Acad Sci U S A. 2011;108:8414–9.

94. Halem HA, Ufret M, Jewett I, Mattei A, Bastille A, Beech J, et al. In Vivo Suppression of Corticosterone in Rodent Models of Cushing's Disease with a Selective, Peptide MC2 Receptor Antagonist. Pituitary Development and Neoplasia. In: Endocrine Society's 98th Annual Meeting and Expo, April 1–4, 2016, Boston Pituitary Development and Neoplasia, OR29–6.

Adrenal Failure

Kavinga Gunawardane and Ashley B. Grossman

Introduction

Adrenal insufficiency results from the failure of production of corticosteroid hormone and/or mineralocorticoids and adrenal androgens. It could be due to several reasons: either adrenocortical disease (primary) or secondary to the lack of ACTH secretion from the pituitary (secondary) and/or lack of CRH/AVP secretion form the hypothalamus (tertiary).

Although primary adrenal insufficiency can present at any age, it commonly presents between 30 and 50 years of age and more frequently in women. The estimated incidence of primary adrenal insufficiency is between 4.4 and 6 new cases per million population per year [1, 2]. However, secondary adrenal insufficiency is more frequent (estimated prevalence of 150–280 per million), while tertiary adrenal insufficiency is commonly due to chronic hypothalamic suppression due to prolonged exogenous glucocorticoid use.

The presentation of adrenal insufficiency can be acute or insidious depending on the underlying aetiology. Life-threatening adrenal crisis is more commonly seen in primary disease rather than in secondary or tertiary adrenal insufficiency [3]. However, regardless of the aetiology, adrenal insufficiency is a life-threatening condition which poses frequent challenges in diagnosis and management.

Presentation of Adrenal Insufficiency

1. Severe acute adrenal insufficiency or adrenal crisis.
   - Hypotension and shock (>90%).
   - Abdominal, flank, back or lower chest pain (86%).
   - Fever (66%).
   - Anorexia, nausea or vomiting (47%).
   - Neuropsychiatric symptoms such as confusion or disorientation (42%).
   - Abdominal rigidity or rebound tenderness (22%).
   - Hypoglycaemia (rare in adults, common in children).
   - Sudden severe headache, loss of vision or visual field defect (pituitary apoplexy).
2. Non-acute or insidious presentation.
   - Chronic malaise.
   - Lassitude.
   - Fatigue.
   - Generalised weakness.
   - Anorexia.
   - Weight loss.
   - Nausea and vomiting, abdominal pain, diarrhoea.
   - Hyperpigmentation (only in primary adrenal insufficiency, noted in sun-exposed or pressure areas, scars after adrenal insufficiency, buccal mucosa, palmar creases).
   - Dizziness and postural hypotension.
   - Improved blood pressure control in hypertensive patient.
   - Salt craving (22%).
   - Psychiatric manifestations.
   - Vitiligo (as a marker of autoimmune disease).
   - Reduced axillary and pubic hair and reduced libido in females (DHEA deficiency).
   - Amenorrhoea (in 25% due to chronic illness, weight loss or associated premature ovarian failure).
   - Features of other associated endocrinopathies (autoimmune polyglandular syndrome).
   - Headache, visual field defects and other features of pituitary hormone deficiency (secondary or tertiary adrenal insufficiency).

K. Gunawardane
Provincial General Hospital – Ratnapura, Diabetes and Endocrinology Unit, Ratnapura, Sri Lanka

A. B. Grossman (✉)
Oxford Centre for Diabetes, Endocrinology and Metabolism, University of Oxford, Oxford, UK

Barts and the London School of Medicine, London, UK
e-mail: Ashley.grossman@ocdem.ox.ac.uk

© Springer Nature Switzerland AG 2022
F. Bandeira et al. (eds.), *Endocrinology and Diabetes*, https://doi.org/10.1007/978-3-030-90684-9_9

Biochemical Findings in Adrenal Insufficiency

- Hyponatraemia, 85–90% (due to cortisol deficiency).
- Hyperkalaemia, 60–65% (due to mineralocorticoid deficiency).
- Elevated blood urea.
- Low blood bicarbonate (metabolic acidosis in primary adrenal insufficiency).
- Elevated TSH with normal or low normal T4.
- Elevated ESR.
- Mild anaemia (normocytic normochromic).
- Eosinophilia.
- Mild hypercalcaemia (uncommon).

Pathophysiology

In primary adrenal insufficiency, all three zones of the adrenal cortex are affected by the disease process resulting in inadequate glucocorticoid, mineralocorticoid and adrenal androgen production; this initially leads to partial adrenal insufficiency, manifest by inadequate cortisol responses during stress, followed by a complete insufficiency [4]. However, acute insufficiency may occur due to adrenal haemorrhage or infarction. The clinical features appear following 90% destruction of the adrenal glands.

Combined glucocorticoid and mineralocorticoid deficiency leads to increased urinary sodium loss and hypovolaemia resulting in hypotension and electrolyte imbalance (hyponatraemia and hyperkalaemia). In addition, appropriate anti-diuretic hormone release (in this context, *not* inappropriate and thus not SIADH) and action on the renal tubule due to glucocorticoid deficiency contribute to the hyponatraemia. The lack of glucocorticoid negative feedback increases the release of ACTH and other POMC peptides; it is the β-MSH sequence within ACTH which is responsible for the hyperpigmentation by acting on the MSH (MCR1) receptors in the skin [5].

Mineralocorticoid deficiency is not seen in secondary adrenal insufficiency, as mineralocorticoids are principally regulated by the plasma renin-angiotensin system. Hypotension in secondary adrenal insufficiency occurs due to decreased vascular tone as a result of reduced vascular responsiveness to angiotensin II and noradrenaline. ACTH and POMC secretion is reduced, and, unlike primary adrenal insufficiency, hyperpigmentation is not a feature of secondary adrenal insufficiency [6] (Table 9.1) [7–11].

Table 9.1 Aetiology

Causes of primary adrenal insufficiency
Acute or insidious presentation
Autoimmune adrenalitis or Addison's disease (80%, in developed countries)
Autoimmune polyglandular syndrome (APS1, APS2)
Metastatic deposits from the lung, breast, kidney, etc.
Bilateral adrenal infiltration (lymphoma, amyloidosis, haemochromatosis)
Infectious adrenalitis (tuberculosis, histoplasmosis, cryptococcosis, CMV, HIV (up to 5% patients with AIDS))
Infarction due to adrenal venous thrombosis (anti-phospholipid syndrome, heparin-induced thrombocytopenia syndrome)
Genetic disorders
Congenital adrenal hyperplasia (21-hydroxylase deficiency, 11β-hydroxylase deficiency, 3β-hydroxysteroid dehydrogenase II deficiency, etc.)
Adrenoleukodystrophy (X-linked disorder of very long chain fatty acid metabolism (VLCFAs), presents in childhood, may progress to severe neurological problems due to white matter demyelination)
Congenital adrenal hypoplasia (X-linked, SF 1 gene linked)
Familial glucocorticoid deficiency (types 1, 2, 3; mineralocorticoids usually spared).
Congenital lipoid adrenal hyperplasia (StAR mutations)
P450 oxidoreductase deficiency
Genetic disorders associated with sphingolipid metabolism [7] (SGPL1, sphingosine-1-phosphate lyase) [8, 9]
Bilateral adrenalectomy
Drugs (ketoconazole, fluconazole, phenytoin, rifampicin, etomidate, aminoglutethimide, some novel tyrosine kinase-targeting drugs (e.g. sunitinib)
Acute presentation [10, 11]
Haemorrhage (trauma, anticoagulants)
Waterhouse-Friderichsen syndrome (meningococcal septicaemia)
Causes of secondary and tertiary adrenal insufficiency
Withdrawal of exogenous glucocorticoid: Very common (suppression of the hypothalamo-pituitary-adrenal axis, abrupt withdrawal can cause adrenal crisis)
Pituitary tumours
Pituitary apoplexy (acute presentation)
Pituitary surgery
Pituitary radiotherapy
Infiltration: Tuberculosis, sarcoidosis, Langerhans cell histocytosis, haemochromatosis, lymphocytic hypophysitis
Isolated ACTH deficiency (rare)
Trauma to the pituitary

Diagnostic Tests (Tables 9.2 and 9.3) [12]

In the first instance, adrenal insufficiency needs to be confirmed with dynamic tests unless there is an Addisonian crisis. The next step is differentiation of primary from secondary adrenal insufficiency by measuring the level of ACTH. Once the primary or secondary diagnosis has been established, fur-

Table 9.2 Investigations to confirm adrenal insufficiency

Tests	Procedure	Interpretation of the result	Comments
Short Synacthen test (SST) (considered as "gold standard" for the diagnosis of primary adrenal insufficiency)	Take blood sample for 9 a.m. cortisol and 9 a.m. ACTH level Administer 250 µg Synacthen/tetracosactrin (ACTH) i.m. or i.v. 30 mins or 60 mins later, collect blood sample for serum cortisol level	Peak cortisol levels below 450 nmol/L (18 µg/dL) (assay dependent) at 30 minutes indicate adrenal insufficiency (*but note, highly dependent on cortisol assay*)	Different criteria may apply according to cortisol assay Recent onset secondary adrenal failure may produce a normal response SST can be done at any time of the day Oestrogens can give falsely high cortisol levels by elevating cortisol-binding globulin; discontinue oestrogen at least for 4–6 weeks prior to the SST If already on glucocorticoid replacement, omit steroid dose before the test
9 a.m. cortisol level	Collect serum cortisol level at 9 a.m.	9 a.m. cortisol <140 nmol/L (5 µg/dL) suggests adrenal insufficiency	Can be useful in recent onset secondary adrenal insufficiency (2 weeks) or if a corticotropin stimulation test is not feasible In severe stress such as sepsis, a "normal" level may still indicate adrenal insufficiency
Random cortisol	Collect random serum cortisol level if adrenal insufficiency is suspected, prior to steroid replacement	Undetectable level suggests adrenal insufficiency	Not very reliable, unless very low

Table 9.3 Investigations to differentiate primary from secondary adrenal insufficiency [12]

Tests	Procedure	Interpretation of the results	Comments
9 a.m. serum ACTH level	Take venous blood sample at 9 a.m.	In patients with confirmed cortisol deficiency, a plasma ACTH >two-fold the upper limit of the reference range is consistent with primary adrenal insufficiency Low ACTH level (<10 ng/L) confirms secondary or tertiary adrenal insufficiency	ACTH 10–20 ng/L can be equivocal, consider long Synacthen test
Long Synacthen test	Take blood sample for 9 a.m. cortisol and ACTH level Administer 1 mg depot Synacthen i.m. Collect blood sample for serum cortisol level at 30, 60, 120 min, 4, 8, 12 and 24 h	Progressive rise in cortisol response in secondary adrenal insufficiency Little or no response in primary adrenal insufficiency	Useful in differentiating primary from secondary adrenal insufficiency when ACTH level is equivocal

blood sample taken at this time for cortisol and if possible ACTH is extremely helpful. Furthermore, simultaneous measurement of plasma renin and aldosterone in primary adrenal insufficiency to determine the presence of mineralocorticoid deficiency is recommended [12].

Investigations to Establish the Underlying Cause of Adrenal Insufficiency

- Adrenal autoantibodies: Although measurement of autoantibodies against CYP21A2 can be of value, one must keep in mind that these tests are not standardised and are subjected to wide variations.
- Screening in autoimmune polyglandular syndrome (APS): In children with primary adrenal insufficiency, other autoimmune polyglandular pathologies should be considered. Other autoimmune markers and hormonal assays to assess autoimmune polyglandular syndrome are:
  - Thyroid function (autoimmune hypothyroidism).
  - Plasma glucose (diabetes mellitus type 1).
  - Serum calcium and PTH (autoimmune hypoparathyroidism).

ther investigations, e.g. imaging and auto-antibodies or microbiological screening, should be arranged to identify the underlying cause of the adrenal insufficiency. There is no need to wait for the biochemical confirmation in a clear or suspected adrenal crisis; treatment should be initiated without any delay as soon as suspected clinically. However, a

- Anti-parietal cell antibody, intrinsic factor antibody (pernicious anaemia).
- Endomyseal antibody or tissue transglutaminase (coeliac disease).
- Liver function tests (autoimmune hepatitis).

Antibodies to interferon-ω or interferon-α have a high diagnostic sensitivity and specificity in APS-1 [13].

- Adrenoleukodystrophy: Males who are negative to auto-antibody screening should be screened for adrenoleukodystrophy by the measurement of very long fatty acids [14].
- Microbial and serological tests—tuberculosis, other infective causes.
- CT adrenals and MRI adrenals.
  - Large adrenals with or without calcification seen in tuberculosis and metastatic deposits.
  - Small atrophic glands in autoimmune primary adrenal insufficiency, but can also be seen in chronic secondary adrenal insufficiency.
  - Adrenal haemorrhage and adrenal vein thrombosis (MRI better than CT).
- MRI pituitary and hypothalamus—secondary or tertiary adrenal insufficiency.
- 17-OH progesterone and 24-hour urine steroid profile (classic CAH, in neonates).

Other Investigations

- Plasma renin activity, high in primary adrenal insufficiency due to mineralocorticoid deficiency.
- DHEAS (> 60 μg/dL indicate normal adrenal function).

Differential Diagnosis

Many of the changes seen in adrenal insufficiency are non-specific, and it overlaps with mild depression, chronic fatigue syndrome and generalised malignancy or sepsis, especially slow-onset infections such as TB. One of the most useful discriminants for Addison's disease is the presence of hyperpigmentation [15], which should always be sought. For secondary and tertiary adrenal failure, critical features such as features of hypopituitarism, headache and visual failure must be looked for. However, it should be noted that ACTH deficiency is generally a feature of advanced pituitary failure other than in lymphocytic hypophysitis, when it may occur early or as an isolated endocrine feature.

Treatment

Management of Adrenal Crisis

This is a life-threatening medical emergency which requires prompt treatment with hydrocortisone and fluid replacement. Once clinically suspected, there should be no delay in initiating treatment pending biochemical confirmation. The management approach should be similar to the resuscitation of any critically ill patient.

- Maintain airway and breathing and blood pressure.
- Establish venous access with two large bore cannulae.
- Check capillary blood glucose and correct and hypoglycaemia.
- Collect venous blood sample for:
  - Urea and electrolytes.
  - Serum creatinine.
  - Full blood count.
  - Bicarbonate.
  - Infection screen.
  - Random cortisol, ACTH and plasma renin.
- *Steroid replacements.*
  - iv hydrocortisone 100 mg immediately followed by 200 mg/d, ideally as a continuous infusion for 24 hours [12].
  - Hydrocortisone can be reduced to 100 mg/d, the following day.
  - Switch to oral hydrocortisone with a tapering dose (usually 20–10–10 mg) after 48 h if oral intake is resumed and if there is no other major illness.
  - If hydrocortisone is unavailable, prednisolone can be used as an alternative. Dexamethasone is the least preferred alternative and should only be given if no other glucocorticoid is available.
- *Intravenous fluids.*
  - Rapid infusion of 1000 mL isotonic saline within the first hour or 5% glucose in isotonic saline, followed by continuous iv isotonic saline guided by individual patient needs [12].
  - But caution should be taken in correcting chronic hyponatraemia (not more than 8 mmol/L in 24 h) to prevent central pontine myelinolysis.
  - Treatment of hyperkalaemia is advisable if potassium fails to fall following hydrocortisone injection.
- There is no need for fludrocortisone replacement in an acute crisis. The mineralocorticoid activity of high-dose hydrocortisone and 0.9% saline infusion are sufficient to correct electrolyte imbalances.

Management of Chronic or Insidious Onset of Adrenal Insufficiency

Glucocorticoid Replacements

There are various types of cortisol replacement regimens, and no head-to-head comparison data are available to advocate one over the other. Clinicians can make their decision based on the form of glucocorticoid available locally and the clinical need.

- Hydrocortisone.
  - Short-acting, 15–25 mg given in two to three divided doses.
  - The first and largest dose is given upon waking, the second dose after lunch, and, in case of a three-dose regimen, the last and smallest dose not later than 4–6 hours before bedtime (avoid high doses in the evening, which may compromise sleep and insulin sensitivity) [16].
  - This approximately mimics the endogenous glucocorticoid diurnal rhythm.
  - Adequacy of replacement can be monitored with biochemical testing of hydrocortisone replacement day curves, but most importantly seeking patient subjective feedback.
- Cortisone acetate.
  - Short-acting (but longer than hydrocortisone).
  - 25–35 mg in three divided doses: highest dose given in the morning on waking.
  - Metabolised in liver to active form, hydrocortisone.
  - No iv preparation.
- Prednisolone.
  - 3–5 mg on waking
  - Long-acting, once-daily dose is sufficient.
  - Some may need additional 2.5 mg in the evening.
  - Does not mimic diurnal rhythm of endogenous cortisol.
  - Better choice in non-compliant patients due to multiple daily dose problems.
  - Cross-reacts in most cortisol assays.
- Dexamethasone.
  - Not currently recommended for replacement due to risk of over-replacement.

Mineralocorticoid Replacement

- Required only in primary adrenal insufficiency.
- 50–100 mcg in adults and no restriction in their salt intake.

- May need to increase dose in hot weather with increased perspiration.
- Available in oral preparation only.
- Monitoring is based on clinical assessment (salt craving, postural hypotension or oedema), plasma renin and serum electrolytes.

DHEA Replacement [17]

- Can be offered to women with low energy, low mood and lack of libido.
- Some variable evidence of benefit.
- Initially 25–50 mg daily for 3 to 6 months and continued if clinical response is positive.

Modified Release Hydrocortisone

Slow-release hydrocortisone, which has a pharmacokinetic profile similar to the physiological levels of cortisol, is now available in many countries. It is taken once daily and is thus clearly more convenient for patients and may aid compliance. The usual daily dose ranges from 20 to 30 mg, early in the morning. However, it is considerably more expensive than immediate-release hydrocortisone, and its specific advantages remain unclear.

Follow-Up

The aim in follow-up is to ensure adequate physiological glucocorticoid and mineralocorticoid (in primary adrenal insufficiency) replacement and to reduce the risk of adrenal crisis by providing necessary education to patients.

The dose of steroids should be adjusted according to clinical symptoms as well as biochemical parameters.

Assess Glucocorticoid Replacement

- Inadequate replacement.
  - Lethargy, tiredness, especially in the morning.
  - Low serum cortisol level on cortisol day curve (useful for hydrocortisone or cortisone replacement only).
- Over-replacement.
  - Cushingoid appearance.
  - High 24-h urinary free cortisol.
  - High serum cortisol on hydrocortisone day curve (useful for hydrocortisone or cortisone replacement only).
  - Low bone mineral density.

Assess Mineralocorticoid Replacement

- Inadequate replacement.
  - Postural hypotension.
  - High plasma renin activity (should be at the upper level of normal).
- Over-replacement.
  - Hypertension.
  - Oedema.
  - Hypokalaemia.

Patient Education

This is crucial in the management of adrenal insufficiency. All patients with adrenal insufficiency should be educated about their condition and the emergency measures they should take at home to prevent adrenal crisis. This information should be reinforced during the annual follow-up visits by the clinicians and, if possible, through a structured patient education programme.

- Steroid "sick day" rules [18].
  - Need to double the routine oral glucocorticoid dose when the patient experiences fever or illness requiring bed rest; when requiring antibiotics for an infection; or before a small outpatient procedure (e.g. dental work).
  - If the patient remains unwell after 24–72 h, they should contact the physician.
  - There should always be a supply of additional oral glucocorticoids on prescription for "sick days".
  - There is no need to increase the mineralocorticoid dose.
- Steroid emergency pack.
  - Every patient should be provided with this pack to keep at home.
  - The pack contains a vial of 100 mg hydrocortisone, a syringe and a needle (alternatively, also hydrocortisone or prednisolone suppositories). Ideally, this should be in the form of a premixed injection for simplified use.
  - The patient and/or any responsible family member should be educated to administer this medication intramuscularly *or subcutaneously* during an emergency situation, i.e. a severe accident, significant haemorrhage, fracture, unconsciousness, diarrhoea and vomiting, and they should call the emergency medical personnel immediately.
  - The expiry date on the pack should be checked regularly and replaced with a new pack if expired.
  - The patient should be advised to take the pack when travelling.
- Medical Alert bracelet or pendant and emergency steroid card.
  - Every patient should wear or carry these in which the diagnosis and daily medication should be clearly documented.
  - Reinforce education and confirm understanding during each follow-up visit.

References

1. Løvås K, Husebye ES. High prevalence and increasing incidence of Addison's disease in western Norway. Clin Endocrinol. 2002;56(6):787–91.
2. Kong MF, Jeffocoate W. Eighty-six cases of Addison's disease. Clin Endocrinol. 1994;41(6):757–61.
3. Tanaka M, Suganuma K, Funase Y, et al. Hypoglycaemic coma due to adrenal failure in a chronic haemodialysis patient. NDT Plus. 2011;4:36–8.
4. Scheys JO, Heaton JH, Hammer GD. Evidence of adrenal failure in aging Dax1-deficient mice. Endocrinol. 2011;152:3430–9.
5. Bakalov VK, Vanderhoof VH, Bondy CA, Nelson LM. Adrenal antibodies detect asymptomatic auto-immune adrenal insufficiency in young women with spontaneous premature ovarian failure. Hum Reprod. 2002;17:2096–100.
6. Lin L, Gu WX, Ozisik G, To WS, Owen CJ, et al. Analysis of DAX1 (*NR0B1*) and steroidogenic factor-1 (*NR5A1*) in children and adults with primary adrenal failure: ten years' experience. J Clin Endocrinol Metab. 2006;91:3048–54.
7. Lucki NC, Sewer MB. The interplay between bioactive sphingolipids and steroid hormones. Steroids. 2010 Jun;75(6):390–9.
8. Prasad R, et al. Sphingosine-1-phosphate lyase mutations cause primary adrenal insufficiency and steroid-resistant nephrotic syndrome. J Clin Invest. 2017;127(3):942–53.
9. Lovric S, et al. Mutations in sphingosine-1-phosphate lyase cause nephrosis with ichthyosis and adrenal insufficiency. J Clin Invest. 2017;127(3):912–28.
10. Presotto F, Fornasini F, Betterle C, Federspil G, Rossato M. Acute adrenal failure as the heralding symptom of primary antiphospholipid syndrome: report of a case and review of the literature. Eur J Endocrinol. 2005;153:507–14.
11. Rao RH, Vagnucci AH, Amico JA. Bilateral massive adrenal hemorrhage: early recognition and treatment. Ann Intern Med. 1989;110(3):227.
12. Bornstein SR, Allolio B, Arlt W, Barthel A, Don-Wauchope A, Hammer GD, Husebye ES, Merke DP, Murad MH, Stratakis CA, Torpy DJ. Diagnosis and treatment of primary adrenal insufficiency: an endocrine society clinical practice guideline. J Clin Endocrinol Metabol. 2016;101(2):364–89.
13. Meager A, Visvalingam K, Peterson P, et al. Anti-interferon autoantibodies in autoimmune polyendocrinopathy syndrome type 1. PLoS Med. 2006;3:e289.
14. Horn MA, Erichsen MM, Wolff AS, et al. Screening for X-linked adrenoleukodystrophy among adult men with Addison's disease. Clin Endocrinol (Oxf). 2013;79:316–20.
15. Nerup J. Addisons disease—clinical studies. A report of 108 cases. Acta Endocrinol (Copenh). 1974;76(1):127.

16. Simon N, Castinetti F, Ouliac F, Lesavre N, Brue T, Oliver C. Pharmacokinetic evidence for suboptimal treatment of adrenal in- sufficiency with currently available hydrocortisone tablets. Clin Pharmacokinet. 2010;49:455–63.

17. Alkatib AA, Cosma M, Elamin MB, Erickson D, et al. A systematic review and meta-analysis of randomized placebo-controlled trials of DHEA treatment effects on quality of life in women with adrenal insufficiency. J Clin Endocrinol Metab. 2009;94:3676.

18. Bancos I, Hahner S, Tomlinson J, Arlt W. Diagnosis and man- age ment of adrenal insufficiency. Lancet Diabetes Endocrinol. 2015;3:216–26.

Adrenal Incidentalomas

Francisco Bandeira, Manoel Aderson Soares Filho, and Sérgio Ricardo de Lima Andrade

Epidemiology

Most cases of AI are due to cortical adenomas, whose prevalence in large series ranges from 70 to 90%. Although inactive adenoma is considered the most common adrenal lesion, other adrenal lesions may be functionally active, requiring hormonal investigation, along with subsequent medical and surgical treatment [1, 2] (Table 10.1).

Prevalence increases with age, especially in the fifth and seventh decades of life, but is regarded as uncommon in individuals with less than 40 years of age and is rare in children and adolescents. Hypertension, obesity, and diabetes have been frequently reported, particularly in bilateral lesions, and this may be due to the presence of subclinical hypercortisolism [3, 4].

Imaging Procedures

CT scan is the primary and preferred method used for evaluation of adrenal glands because it is a procedure that is readily available while offering the highest spatial resolution. Contrast enhancement and deenhancement (washout) in late phases (15 min) are helpful to characterize the lesions; however, noncontrast CT is often sufficient for the diagnosis of AI (Fig. 10.1).

Among the characteristics for identification of potentially malignant lesions, the first to be observed is the size of the mass. Various cut points have been proposed ranging between 3 and 6 cm (more often 4 cm) of diameter based on the fact that primary carcinomas of the adrenal with measurements lower than these are quite rare. However, adrenal carcinomas of 2.5 cm have been documented, and the use of these cutoff

Table 10.1 Etiology, prevalence, and laboratory evaluation of adrenal incidentalomas

Etiology	Prevalence (%)	Laboratory screening
Nonfunctional adenoma	85	Normal
Subclinical Cushing's syndrome	7	1 mg DST(serum cortisol >3 µ/dl) Plasma ACTH (<5 pg/ml)
Phaeochromocytoma	3.5	24-h urine metanephrines>2 mg/g Cr
Hyperaldosteronism	0.7	Plasma aldosterone ≥15 ng/dl with a APRR ≥20
Nonfunctional adrenocortical carcinoma	2	Normal

limits can exclude patients harboring carcinomas that are still small and, therefore, offer the greatest likelihood of being able to be treated and cured if operated upon in early stages [5, 6].

The next, and probably the most important, aspect to be seen is related to the noncontrast attenuation of the lesion when evaluated by CT. The rationale is that adrenal adenomas, due to their high content of intracellular lipids, usually exhibit low attenuation. In this regard, using a cutoff level of 10 HU (Hounsfield units) or less, a sensitivity of 96–100%, and a specificity of 50–100% have been reported for diagnosing a benign lesion [4, 7–9]. However, 40% of the benign lesions have a pre-contrast attenuation above 10 HU [4, 9]. Several authors reported high sensitivity and specificity in CT after using contrast. Percentage deenhancement, the so-called washout, of at least 60% in 15 min has been shown to be 98% sensitive and 92% specific for benign lesion [8] (Fig. 10.1).

Other features of benign lesions that can be evaluated by CT, such as regular margins and homogeneous attenuation, have low accuracy and are less useful in diagnosis. Calcifications, necrosis, and hemorrhages are atypical events but occur more specifically in larger lesions.

In adrenal hemorrhage, a clinical condition associated with sepsis, coagulation disorders, adrenal tumors (such as pheochromocytomas), and abdominal trauma, CT scan initially shows high density that gradually decreases as the hematoma subsides which may in turn become a pseudocyst.

F. Bandeira (✉) · M. A. S. Filho
Division of Endocrinology, Agamenon Magalhães Hospital, University of Pernambuco Medical School, Recife, PE, Brazil
e-mail: francisco.bandeira@upe.br

S. R. de Lima Andrade
Agamenon Magalhães Hospital, Division of Endocrinology and Diabetes, University of Pernambuco Medical School, Recife, Pernambuco, Brazil

© Springer Nature Switzerland AG 2022
F. Bandeira et al. (eds.), *Endocrinology and Diabetes*, https://doi.org/10.1007/978-3-030-90684-9_10

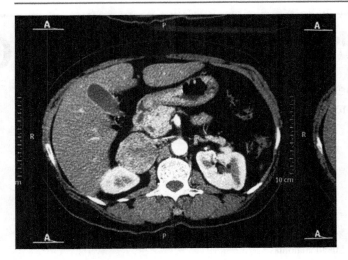

Fig. 10.1 A 52-year-old woman with primary hyperparathyroidism and hypertension had a CT scan to evaluate for renal calculi. A lesion (5.5 cm) in right adrenal gland was discovered. Noncontrast attenuation: 39 HU. Contrast washout: 42% in 15 min

Other lesions with characteristic features include cysts and myelolipomas. Endothelial cysts and pseudocysts are the most common, accounting for more than 80% of the cases. CT is useful in demonstrating the presence of liquid (hypodense) and generally thick capsules, whereas MRI shows hypointensity on T1 and hyperintensity on T2. Patients with adrenal cysts can, in some cases, benefit from fine needle aspiration (FNA) biopsy guided by ultrasound or CT for decompression and/or cytologic evaluation of the aspirated fluid. Since pseudocysts can originate from pheochromocytomas, measurements of serum or urinary catecholamines or metanephrines are always recommended [2, 5, 6].

Myelolipomas, in turn, are benign tumors composed of mature adipose tissue and normal hematopoietic tissue, corresponding to around 7–15% of AI cases. They are almost always asymptomatic lesions. Seen by CT, they appear as hypo-dense lesions (−40 HU), due to the presence of fat. Calcifications and hemorrhages may also be present [4]. Bilateral lesions occur in about 20% of AI cases and are usually due to metastases, granulomatous diseases, adrenal hemorrhage, or congenital adrenal hyperplasia. In this regard, positron emission tomography (PET) using 2-^{18}F-fluoro-2-deoxy-d-glucose has been used in cancer patients to evaluate the possibility of adrenal metastasis by demonstrating increased uptake, as well as being able to differentiate these cases from adenomas, which may not demonstrate the same uptake [8, 10].

Fine Needle Aspiration (FNA)

This procedure is useful in cases where there is known malignant disease (prior or concurrent) and suspicion that the adrenal nodule is metastatic [4, 6, 8, 10]. Diagnosis of metastasis in this situation has corresponded on average to about half the

cases. The incidental finding of metastatic adrenal lesions in a patient with no clinical symptoms is considered to be rare. FNA should always be preceded by hormonal evaluation to rule out pheochromocytoma as catecholamines may be released with subsequent increase in blood pressure during the procedure. FNA should not be performed in the suspicion of adrenocortical carcinoma due to the risk of tumor seeding. FNA is now rarely necessary due to the improved accuracy of the emerging procedures [6, 8–10].

Hormonal Evaluation

The prevalence of autonomous adenomas that produce cortisol among cases of incidentalomas is from 5 to 20%. This condition has been classified as possible autonomous cortisol secretion (PACS), formerly named anteriormente denominada subclinical Cushing's syndrome (SCCS). Diagnosis can be made by a combination of 1 mg dexamethasone suppression test and plasma ACTH concentrations. Various cutoff values for cortisol have been proposed ranging from 2 to 5 μg/dl [4, 8, 11].

The natural history of SCCS is not completely understood. In many patients the condition does not progress, but in some it may evolve to clinical Cushing's syndrome. Patients must be evaluated for the presence of arterial hypertension, obesity, and glucose intolerance. Patients who demonstrate clinical consequences attributable to cortisol excess are likely to benefit from surgery. In asymptomatic patients, conservative management is appropriate, along with clinical and laboratory monitoring [4].

The prevalence of primary hyperaldosteronism, as a cause of arterial hypertension in the general population, has been growing due to its increasing recognition and diagnosis, especially in normokalaemic patients, through routine measurements of aldosterone and plasma renin activity (PARA). Hypertensive patients, hypokalemic or not, demonstrating AI should be evaluated, initially with the aldosterone-plasma renin activity ratio (APRR), providing a diet with normal amount of sodium and, if possible, stopping medications such as spironolactone, diuretics, and beta-blockers that may interfere with measurements [8, 10]. Plasma aldosterone values of more than 15 ng/dl in the presence of an APRR of 20 or more should be considered a positive screening, and dynamic tests are necessary. Additional test should include aldosterone suppression test with 2 L of normal saline infusion over 4 h followed by measurement of plasma aldosterone. Oral captopril 50 mg may be given after 2 h of infusion. At the end of 4-h infusion, plasma aldosterone level above 10 ng/dl confirms the diagnosis of hyperaldosteronism [4].

Pheochromocytomas comprise about 10% of AI cases. Many of these patients are asymptomatic, and half of them have arterial hypertension and adrenergic symptoms which may be paroxysmal. Metaiodobenzylguanidine scintigraphy (MIBG) has almost 100% specificity (albeit with much lower sensitivity than MRI and CT) and can be used to confirm cases with positive hormonal screening. This should be done with measurements of plasma-free metanephrines or urinary fractioned metanephrines [4, 10]. Plasma catecholamines above 2000 pg/ml or urine norepinephrine above 100 μg/g urine creatinine/24 h or urine epinephrine above 10 μg/g urine creatinine/24 h or urine metanephrine above 2 mg/g urine creatinine is suggestive of the presence of phaeochromocytoma. Highest specificity may be obtained with a plasma free metanephrine value above 1.4 pmol/ml [1, 4, 7, 10]. If this initial endocrine evaluation is normal, a follow-up workup would be necessary only in the setting of clinical symptoms [4].

Patient Follow-Up

The clinical evolution of AI patients who exhibit radiological characteristics suggesting a benign and normal hormonal profile is usually favorable. Some patients (about 20%) progress to hormonal hyperfunction, notably clinically evident hypercortisolism, or PACS and more rarely pheochromocytomas. In those patients with nonfunction lesion with noncontrast attenuation less than 10 HU, a one-time follow-up CT scan in 12 months is recommended [7, 10]. Those with lesion less than 4 cm but more than 10HU should have a CT scan done in 3–6 months and then yearly for 2 years (Fig. 10.2a, b).

Figs. 10.2 (**a** and **b**) Approach to the patient with incidentally discovered adrenal mass, with low (**a**) and high (**b**) attenuation

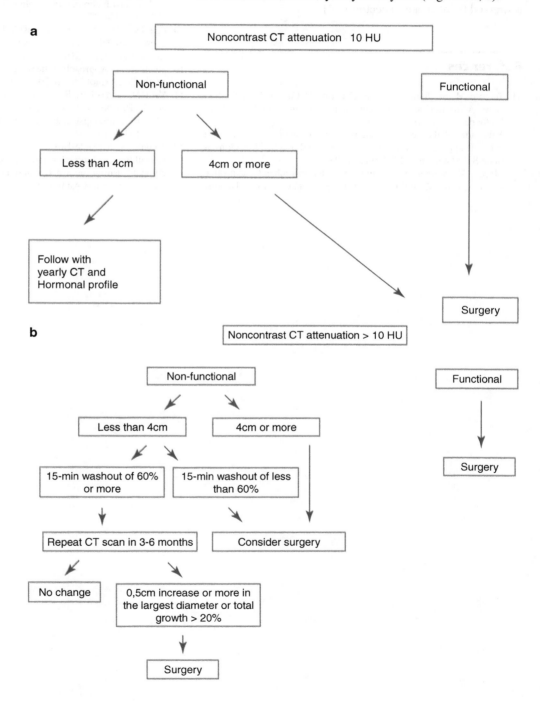

Treatment

Most lesions can be removed by laparoscopic surgery, including pheochromocytomas, cortisol-producing adenomas (Cushing's syndrome), aldosteronomas, nonfunctional adenomas, lesions suspected of malignancy without signs of local invasion, and, more rarely, cysts or myelolipomas. Tumors larger than 10 cm in diameter should preferably be operated with conventional techniques due to the increased risk of malignancy and the greater difficulty involved in the laparoscopic procedure [4, 12]. Suspected malignancy lesions with evidence of local invasion at imaging should be addressed by open adrenalectomy [4].

References

1. Terzolo M, Stigliano A, Chiodini I, Loli P, Furlani L, Arnaldi G, et al. AME position statement on adrenal incidentaloma. Eur J Endocrinol. 2011;164:851–70.
2. NIH State-of-the-Science Statement on management of the clinically in apparent adrenal mass ("incidentaloma"). NIH Consens State Sci Statements. 2002;19(2):1–23.
3. Morelli V, Palmieri S, Salcuni AS, Eller-Vainicher C, Cairoli E, Zhoukouskaya V, Scillitani A, Beck-Peccoz P, Chiodini I. Bilateral and unilateral adrenal incidentalomas: biochemical and clinical characteristics. Eur J Endocrinol. 2013;168:235–41.
4. Fassnacht M, Arlt W, Bancos I, Dralle H, Newell-Price J, Sahdev A, et al. Management of adrenal incidentalomas: European society of endocrinology clinical practice guideline in collaboration with the European network for the study of adrenal tumors. Eur J Endocrinol. 2016;175(2):G1–G34.
5. Sohaib SA, Reznek RH. Adrenal imaging. Br J Urol Int. 2000;86(Suppl 1):95–110.
6. Zeiger MA, Thompson GB, Duh QY, Hamrahian AH, Angelos P, Elaraj D et al. AACE/AAES adrenal incidentaloma guidelines. EndocrPract. 2009;15(Suppl 1).
7. Arnaldi G, Boscaro M. Adrenal incidentaloma. Best Pract Res Clin Endocrinol Metab. 2012;26(4):405–19.
8. Zeiger M, Siegelmen SS, Hamrahian AH. Medical and surgical evaluation of adrenal incidentalomas. J Clin Endocrinol Metab. 2011;96:2004–15.
9. Lee JM, Kim MK, Ko SH, Koh JM, Kim BY, Kim SW, et al. Clinical guidelines for the management of adrenal incidentaloma. Endocrinol Metab. 2017;32(2):200–18.
10. Nieman LK. Approach to the patient with an adrenal incidentaloma. J Clin Endocrinol Metab. 2010;95(9):4106–13.
11. Valli N, Catargi B, Ronci N, Vergnot V, Leccia F, Ferriere JM, et al. Biochemical screening for subclinical cortisol-secreting adenomas amongst adrenal incidentalomas. Eur J Endocrinol. 2001;144:401–8.
12. Toniato A, Merante-Boschin I, Opocher G, Pelizzo MR, Schiavi F, Ballotta E. Surgical versus conservative management for subclinical Cushing syndrome in adrenal incidentalomas: a prospective randomized study. Ann Surg. 2009;249(3):388–91.

Endocrine Hypertension

Francisco Bandeira, Morgana Barbosa Duarte, and Ana Maíra Quental da Nóbrega

Introduction

Endocrine hypertension is responsible for 5–10% of secondary hypertension cases and is characterized by elevated blood pressure levels resulting from an endocrine disorder [1]. Although some features may be suggestive, various patterns of hypertension exist in a patient with an endocrine disorder, including recent-onset hypertension in a previously normotensive individual, loss of control of blood pressure, or labile blood pressure in the setting of either of these two standards. Most cases result from primary aldosteronism (PA) and other existing conditions such as pheochromocytoma (PCC) [2].

Primary Aldosteronism

Primary aldosteronism (PA) is characterized by excessive production of aldosterone independent of the renin-angiotensin system and results in excessive activation of mineralocorticoid receptors [3–5]. This inappropriate production of aldosterone leads to cardiovascular damage, plasma renin suppression, hypertension, sodium retention, and potassium excretion, which, if prolonged and severe, can lead to hypokalemia [5, 6]. It is estimated that 4–19% of patients with systemic arterial hypertension (SAH) and 3–14% of normotensive patients may be considered as PA patients [6].

Conn et al. (1955) estimated PA prevalence at approximately 10% among the hypertensive population; however, such estimation was never confirmed, and for decades, PA prevalence was found to be almost always below 1% [7].

F. Bandeira (✉)
Division of Endocrinology, Agamenon Magalhães Hospital, University of Pernambuco Medical School, Recife, PE, Brazil
e-mail: francisco.bandeira@upe.br

M. B. Duarte · A. M. Q. da Nóbrega
Division of Endocrinology, Diabetes and Metabolic Bone Diseases, Agamenon Magalhães Hospital, University of Pernambuco Medical School, Recife, PE, Brazil

However, with improved screening methodologies, PA is now considered as a common cause of secondary hypertension, as it accounts for more than 10% of all forms of high blood pressure [3]. Today, it is recognized that normocalcemic hypertension is the most common presentation of PA; hypokalemia is present in only a minority of PA patients (9–37%), and only 17% of patients with idiopathic hyperaldosteronism (IHA) present with serum potassium concentrations <3.5 mmol/l. Thus, the presence of hypokalemia has low sensitivity for diagnosis of PA. On the other hand, the absence of hypokalemia has a low negative predictive value for diagnosis of PA [8].

Etiology

Aldosterone-producing adenoma (APA) and bilateral IHA are the most common PA subtypes, accounting for about 35% and 60% of PA cases, respectively. The much less common form, unilateral hyperplasia or primary adrenal hyperplasia (PAH), which accounts for 2% of cases, is caused by micronodular or macronodular hyperplasia of the zona glomerulosa of the adrenal gland. Ectopic tumors with aldosterone secretion, such as ovarian or renal neoplasms, are extremely rare [3]. Familial hyperaldosteronism (FH) is rare as well, and three types of FH have been described: FH types I, II, and II [9].

FH type I, or glucocorticoid remediable aldosteronism (GRA), has autosomal dominant inheritance and is responsible for 1% of PA cases [10]. The gene mutation usually found in patients with GRA is the fusion of the CYP11B1 gene promoter region and the CYP11B2 gene coding sequences, which results in a chimeric CYP11B1/CYP11B2 gene. Such gene mutation leads to form of hyperaldosteronism wherein aldosterone hypersecretion is dependent on the endogenous secretion of ACTH, which subsequently activates aldosterone synthesis. GRA presentation is highly variable, with some patients having normal BP and some with elevated aldosterone levels, suppressed plasma renin activity

(PRA), and early-onset hypertension, which is generally severe and refractory to conventional antihypertensive therapies [8].

FH type II is an autosomal dominant and a possibly genetically heterogeneous disorder, and, unlike FH type I, it is not suppressed by dexamethasone, and the GRA mutation test is negative [8]. Its molecular basis is unclear, although several binding analyses have associated FH type II with chromosome 7p22 [8].

FH type III was first described in a population that presented with severe hypertension in early childhood, associated with hyperaldosteronism and hypokalemia, and is refractory to antihypertensive therapy, thus requiring bilateral adrenalectomy. Its etiology is a mutation in the KCNJ5 gene, which encodes the potassium channel [8].

Clinical Presentation

PA is characterized by excessive production of aldosterone, suppression of PRA, hypertension, hypokalemia, and alkalosis. Only a few symptoms are pathognomonic for PA. Furthermore, its clinical manifestations gradually progress and are dependent on the degree of blood pressure elevation and in the reduction of plasma potassium concentration [3, 7]. Blood pressure levels are variable and tend to be higher in IHA than in APA. Patients with hypokalemia may present with muscle weakness, cramps, paresthesia, intermittent paralysis, tetany, polydipsia, polyuria, nocturia, cardiac and electrocardiographic abnormalities, and nephrogenic diabetes insipidus [3, 7].

A 3-year case-control study of 124 patients with PA and 465 patients with essential hypertension (EHT) randomly matched for age, gender, and systolic and diastolic blood pressure reported that patients with PA had more cardiovascular events (stroke, atrial fibrillation, and myocardial infarction) as compared to patients with EHT, regardless of blood pressure (BP) [11]. In addition, excess aldosterone is known to be associated with increased left ventricular (LV) wall thickness and reduced diastolic function, even in the absence of EHT, as observed in the study by Stowasser et al., who analyzed eight normotensive individuals with PA type 1 and 24 normotensive controls [12].

Diagnosis

The diagnosis of PA comprises of three steps: screening, confirmation or exclusion test, and subtype diagnosis (Fig. 11.1).

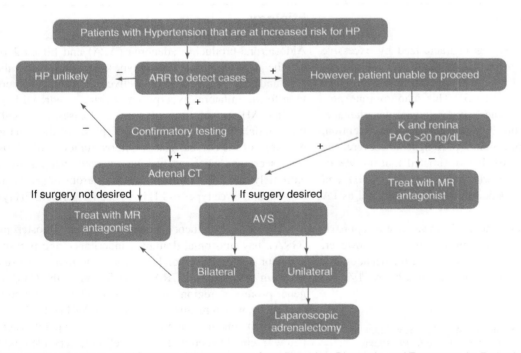

Reference: The Management of Primaery Aldosteronism: Case Detection, Diagnosis, and Treatment: An Endocrine Society Clinical Practice Guideline, 2016 HP: Primary Hiperaldosteronism / ARR: plasma aldosterone/renin ratio / PAC: plasma aldosterone concentration / CT: computed tomography / AVS: adrenal venous sampling / MR: mineralocorticoid receptor

Fig. 11.1 Evaluation of primary hyperaldosteronism

Screening

PA screening should be done in patients with BP >150/100 mmHg in each three measurements obtained on different days; BP >140/90 mmHg even when using three conventional antihypertensive drugs, including a diuretic; controlled hypertension (BP <140/90 mmHg) using four or more antihypertensive drugs; SAH and diuretic-induced or spontaneous hypokalemia; SAH and adrenal incidentaloma; SAH and sleep apnea; and SAH and family history of hypertension, with early-onset hypertension or stroke in <40 years of age and in all first-degree hypertensive relatives of patients with PA [8].

The plasma aldosterone-to-renin ratio (ARR) is currently the most reliable means of PA screening, being superior to either potassium or aldosterone measurement (both of which have lower sensitivity) or isolated renin (which is less specific). Certain substances, such as spironolactone, eplerenone, amiloride, triamterene, potassium-losing diuretics, and licorice root products, affect ARR measurement and should be discontinued for at least 4 weeks prior to collection. Salt intake should not be restricted, and antihypertensive drugs with minimal effect on aldosterone levels, such as slow-release verapamil, hydralazine, prazosin, doxazosin, and terazosin, are usually preferred [8].

Therefore, ARR can be considered as a screening test and should be repeated if the initial results are inconclusive, under suboptimal conditions, or if there is a strong PA suspicion but initial results are negative. Table 11.1 presents the cutoff values. As ARR is mathematically and highly dependent on renin, renin assays should be sufficiently sensitive to measure levels as low as 0.2–0.3 ng/ml/h [8].

Confirmatory Tests

Patients with positive ARR must undergo one or more confirmatory tests to definitively confirm or exclude the diagnosis of PA. Four assays, namely, oral sodium overload, saline infusion, fludrocortisone suppression, and captopril tests, are commonly used; there is no sufficient direct evidence as to which of the tests is superior. Although these tests may differ in terms of sensitivity, specificity, and reliability, preference of a test is commonly determined by considering costs and local experience (Table 11.2) [8].

Table 11.1 Plasma aldosterone/renin ratio (ARR) cutoff values

	PRA(ng/ml/h)	PRA(pmol/L/min)
CAP (ng/ml)	30	1.6
		2.5
CAP (pmol/L)	750	60
		80

Table 11.2 Confirmatory tests for diagnosis of primary aldosteronism (PA)

Test	Procedure	Interpretation
Oral sodium overload	Increase sodium intake to >200 mmol (~ 6 g)/d for 3 days. Receive adequate supplementation of potassium chloride. Measure urinary aldosterone in the urine for 24 hours from the morning of day 3 to the morning of day 4	PA is unlikely for urinary aldosterone <10 μg/24 h (28 nmol/d) in the absence of renal disease Elevated urinary excretion of aldosterone >12 μg/24 h or >14 μg/24 h makes PH highly likely
Fludrocortisone Suppression test	Administer 0.1 mg of oral fludrocortisone every 6 h for 4 days, along with supplements of KCl and NaCl. On day 4, PAC and PRA are measured at 10 o'clock with the patient seated, and plasma cortisol is measured at 7 and 10 o'clock in the morning	CAP >6 ng/dl (170 nmol/L) on day 4 at 10 o'clock confirms PH, provided that PRA is <1 ng/ml/h and plasma cortisol concentration is lower than the value obtained at 7 o'clock in the morning.
Saline infusion test	Remain in the reclined position for at least 1 h before and during the infusion of 2 L of 0.9% EV saline over 4 h (start at 8 o'clock). Collect blood samples for PRA, PAC, cortisol, and plasma potassium at time 0 and after 4 h, with BP and heart rate monitored throughout the test	Post-infusion CAP <5 ng/dl (140 pmol/L) makes the diagnosis of PH unlikely Levels >10 ng/dl (280 nmol/L) are a very likely PA signal Values between 5 and 10 ng/dl are indeterminate
Captopril test	Administer 25–50 mg captopril orally after sitting for at least 1 hour. Dosing PRA, CAP, and cortisol at time 0 and at 1 or 2 h after	CAP is usually suppressed by captopril (>30%) but remains high in patients with PA and suppressed PRA

In the setting of spontaneous hypokalemia, with suppressed plasma renin and plasma aldosterone concentration (PAC) >20 ng/dl (550 pmol/L), confirmatory test is not necessary [8].

Imaging Tests

After confirmation of PA, the patient should undergo computed tomography (CT) to exclude large masses that may represent adrenocortical carcinoma. APA may appear as small hypodense nodules, usually <2 cm in diameter. In contrast, IHA may be normal or present as nodular changes. Aldosterone-producing adrenal carcinomas are usually greater than 4 cm in diameter. Large unilateral benign masses may represent a secretory adenoma of aldosterone and cortisol [8].

Nevertheless, adrenal CT has several limitations. Radiologists may incorrectly interpret small APAs as IHA based on findings of bilateral nodularity or normal-appearing adrenals. In addition, apparent adrenal microadenomas may actually represent areas of nonfunctional hyperplasia or nodularity; hence, unilateral adrenalectomy would be inadequate. In addition, nonfunctional unilateral adrenal macroadenomas are common, especially in patients older than 35 years, and are indistinguishable from APAs in CT [8].

In the study by Young et al., 203 patients with PA were analyzed and evaluated through CT and adrenal vein sampling (AVS), wherein it was demonstrated that CT was accurate in only 53% of patients. Therefore, with low CT accuracy, 42 patients (22%) may be incorrectly excluded as candidates for adrenalectomy, and 48 (25%) may have undergone unnecessary or inadequate surgery [13].

Magnetic resonance imaging has no advantage over CT in PA subtype evaluation [8].

Adrenal Vein Sampling

Lateralization of the source of excessive aldosterone secretion is fundamental in the management of HP. AVS is the "gold standard" in distinguishing unilateral disease (APA or unilateral adrenal hyperplasia (UAH)) from bilateral disease (IHA) in patients with PA. In detecting excessive unilateral aldosterone levels, it has a sensitivity and specificity of around 95% and 100%, respectively, which are relatively higher as compared to that of adrenal CT (78% and 75%, respectively) [8].

Some centers perform catheterization in all patients with PA. However, in patients under 35 years of age with spontaneous hypokalemia, CAP>30 ng/dl (831 pmol/L), and solitary unilateral adenoma found in CT, unilateral adrenalectomy can be performed without previous AVS [8].

AVS should be performed only in patients with confirmed PA and after CT; patients with FH types I and III should be excluded, and subclinical hypercortisolism should be excluded in aldosterone-producing adenomas greater than 10 mm [8, 14]. Moreover, cortisol and aldosterone should be measured in each sample, and the patient should remain in a decubitus position for at least 1 hour before the procedure [14]. Medications that may interfere with renin-angiotensin system and stimulate the secretion of renin are contraindicated. Therefore, α1-adrenergic receptor blockers and calcium channel blockers are the preferred drugs for BP control [8].

The procedure involves the catheterization of the adrenal veins through percutaneous approach on the femoral vein. The adrenal veins are sequentially catheterized under fluoroscopy. The correct position of the catheter is checked by injecting a small volume (3 ml) of contrast and by collecting blood sample through slow aspiration. Cannulation of the left adrenal vein is relatively easy; however, the right adrenal vein is shorter and smaller, and it usually drains directly into the inferior vena cava (IVC), thus making cannulation difficult [8, 14]. As per review of 47 reports, the success rate of right adrenal vein cannulation in 384 patients was estimated to be 74%. With experience, the success rate increases to 90–96% [8].

To determine the success of catheterization, calculation of the selectivity index must be carried out through the ratio between cortisol level measured in the adrenal vein and in the peripheral vein [8]. The ratio of adrenal cortisol to peripheral cortisol concentrations typically should be greater than 5:1 with continuous cortrosyn infusion protocol (infusion 50 µg/30 minutes prior to adrenal catheterization and continue throughout the procedure or infusion of 250 µg bolus) or greater than 3:1 under basal conditions [8]. However, there is no consensus on the ideal selectivity index, with slices between 1 and 1 at baseline, with most authors using a selectivity index between two and three and between two and ten after cortrosyn stimulation and, more commonly, between three and five [14]. Sampling of the adrenal vein with selectivity <2 (basal) or <3 (after cortrosyn stimulation) should be ruled out as nondiagnostic [8].

After confirming a correct catheterization, the lateralization index should be calculated through the aldosterone/cortisol ratio. With continued administration of cortrosyn, the aldosterone/cortisol ratio cutoff point greater than 4:1 indicates unilateral aldosterone excess, whereas a ratio of less than 3:1 is suggestive of bilateral aldosterone hypersecretion [8]. With these cutoff values, AVS has a 95% sensitivity and 100% specificity in detecting unilateral aldosterone hypersecretion (APA or UAH) [8].

Patients with 3:1 and 4:1 lateralization rates may have unilateral or bilateral disease. Thus, AVS results should be interpreted cautiously in conjunction with the clinical setting, CT, and, if possible, repeat AVS. Contralateral suppression of aldosterone secretion has recently been reported as beneficial in the diagnosis of unilateral PA. In the absence of cortrosyn administration, an aldosterone/cortisol ratio greater than 2:1 is consistent with unilateral disease [8].

If both adrenal veins are not successfully catheterized, AVS may be repeated, treat the patient clinically, or consider surgery. A posture stimulation test can guide in this context [8].

Postural Test

In patients with unsuccessful AVS and with CT results indicative of a unilateral adrenal mass, some experts employ the posture stimulation test. This test, developed in the 1970s, was based on the discovery that CAP in patients with APA presented diurnal variation and was relatively unaffected by changes in angiotensin II levels, in contrast to IHA, which is characterized by exaggerated sensitivity to fluctuations in angiotensin II levels [8]. Postural test should be performed by collecting basal blood sample after lying down for 40 minutes and 2 hours after in the upright position. In cases of APA, CAP increases by three to four times; however, in patients with IHA, CAP either remains unchanged or decreases [15].

The lack of precision of this test can be attributed to the fact that some APAs are sensitive to angiotensin II and that some patients with IHA have diurnal variation in aldosterone secretion [8].

Genetic Tests

Genetic testing by Southern blot polymerase chain reaction or determination of the CYP11B1/CYP11B2 hybrid mutation is sensitive and specific for GRA and should replace indirect tests such as urinary 18-oxocortisol and 18-hydroxycortisol levels and dexamethasone suppression test, which may be misleading. It should be considered for patients with early-onset hypertension and family history of PA or stroke [8].

Treatment

The aim of the treatment is to avoid the morbidity and mortality associated with PA. Excess aldosterone has deleterious effects on the cardiovascular system, regardless of blood pressure levels. Studies have demonstrated PA complications, such as increased LV dimensions and myocardial fibrosis, increased carotid intima-media thickness and femoral pulse wave velocity, and reduced endothelial function [8, 12], and provide evidence that patients with PA are at risk of cardiovascular and renal complications, as compared to EHT patients [8, 11].

In patients with unilateral PA (APA or PAH), unilateral laparoscopic adrenalectomy is recommended. Serum potassium levels decrease by about 100% postoperatively [16], and SAH is treated (BP <140/90 mmHg) without the aid of antihypertensive drugs in about 50% of APA patients [17]. In the postoperative period, aldosterone and PRA levels should be measured, and the antihypertensive therapy should be reduced if appropriate. There should be no sodium restriction in the diet. In 5% of patients operated on, persistent hypoaldosteronism may develop, which would require

fludrocortisone replacement therapy. Blood pressure levels usually decrease in 1–6 months after unilateral adrenalectomy for unilateral APA, but it may continue to drop for up to 1 year in some patients.

If the patient does not undergo surgery, a mineralocorticoid receptor antagonist (MRA) should be used [8]. In the retrospective study by Ghose et al., 24 APA patients treated for 5 years with spironolactone or amiloride were analyzed; and it was noted that their systolic and diastolic BP decreased from 175/106 to 129/79 mmHg, with 83% of these patients requiring additional antihypertensive medication to achieve this result [18]. Therefore, in the long term, adrenalectomy is more profitable and is the therapy of choice [8].

In patients with bilateral adrenal disease (IHA, bilateral APA, and GRA), clinical treatment with MRAs is recommended [8]. Currently, only two classes of MRAs are used: spironolactone (12.5 to 25 mg/day, maximum dose of 100 mg/day) and eplerenone (25 mg twice/day). Spironolactone has been the agent of choice, with eplerenone being an alternative, as it has only 50% of the potency of spironolactone and is more expensive. In patients with stage III chronic kidney disease, these drugs should be administered with caution due to risk of hyperkalemia; both drugs are contraindicated in patients with stage IV chronic kidney disease [8].

In patients with GRA, it is necessary to administer the lowest dose of glucocorticoid as the first-line treatment to lower ACTH levels and thus normalize BP and potassium levels. If BP does not normalize with the glucocorticoid alone, an MRA may be used as an adjunct. Administration of dexamethasone (0.125–0.25 mg daily) or prednisone (2.5–5 mg daily) is recommended before bedtime.

Pheochromocytoma and Paraganglioma

Pheochromocytoma (PCC) and paraganglioma (PG) are rare neuroendocrine tumors originating from cells derived from the neural crest of the sympathetic and parasympathetic nervous system and confer high morbidity and mortality. PCC arises from the adrenal medulla, whereas PG is derived from extra-adrenal chromaffin cells of sympathetic and parasympathetic ganglia, which are found in the abdomen, pelvis, thorax, head, and neck. PCCs and most of the thoracoabdominopelvic PGs distributed along the paraaortic and paravertebral axes are of sympathetic origin, while most of the parasympathetic PGs are found in the head or neck along the branches of the glossopharyngeal and vagus nerves and generally do not produce catecholamines [19].

Epidemiology and Pathophysiology

PCC is a rare tumor with an annual incidence of 1–4/10 [6] individuals and is commonly seen with SAH, in which it is an uncommon cause, and is estimated in approximately 0.1–1% of hypertensive patients. It also corresponds to 4% of adrenal incidentalomas [20]. Such tumors occur in any age group, with a mean age of diagnosis at 40 years of age, manifesting earlier in patients with an established mutation or hereditary syndrome than in patients with sporadic disease [21].

Most of the catecholamines secreted are epinephrine, norepinephrine, and dopamine (Fig. 11.2). Normal adrenals mainly secrete epinephrine, and most PCCs predominantly secrete epinephrine and can produce up to 27 times more the normal adrenal capacity. This high rate of production causes accumulation of catecholamines and their metabolites, leading to the diffusion of metanephrines in the cytoplasm of chromaffin cells into the bloodstream. Dopamine beta-hydroxylase, a dopamine-converting enzyme of norepinephrine, may be absent in immature tumors. Therefore, the dominant production of dopamine indicates a greater probability of malignancy [20, 22]. Flowchart 2 demonstrates the synthesis cascade of catecholamines. Norepinephrine acts on alpha-1 adrenergic receptors, causing vasoconstriction in peripheral arteries and veins; on alpha-2 adrenergic receptors leading to coronary vasoconstriction; and on beta-1 adrenergic receptors causing a positive inotropic effect and stimulating renin release, resulting in increased blood pressure. Epinephrine acts on beta-1 adrenergic receptors as well as on beta-2 adrenergic receptors, promoting arterial vasodilation and increased secretion of norepinephrine by the sympathetic ganglia [20, 22].

Recent studies suggest that up to 32% of patients with PCC present a mutation in the germ line in one of the known genes of common susceptibility (NF1, VHL, RET, SDHB, SDHD, and SDHC genes). A retrospective review by Fishbein et al. on 139 PCC/PG patients followed at the University of Pennsylvania Hospital reported a global detection rate of 41% of hereditary mutation, with SDHB as the most commonly mutated gene, which presents a higher risk of malignancy [23].

FLUXOGRAMA 2: CATECHOLAMINE SYNTHESIS

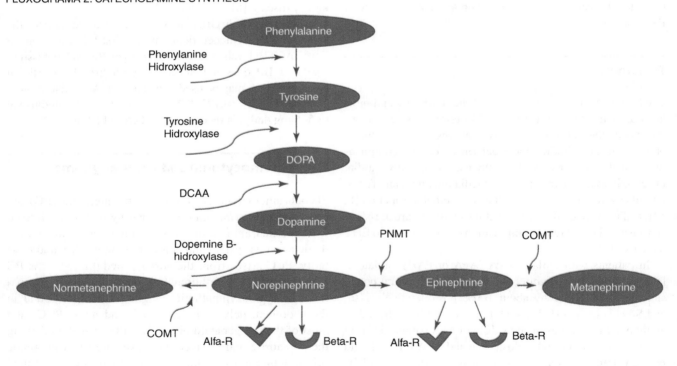

Reference: Perioperative Management of Pheochromocytoma. Journal of Cardiothoracic and Vascular Anesthesia. 2017.

DCCA: Aromatic Acid Decarboxilase; PNMT: Phenylethanolamine N-methyltransferase; COMT: Catechol-O-methyltransferase; DOPA: Dihydroxyphenyllalanine; Alfa-R: receptoralfa; Beta-R: Receptor beta.

Fig. 11.2 Catecholamine synthesis pathway

Clinical Presentation

The clinical presentation of the PCC/PG is mainly attributable to the exaggerated production of catecholamines, which can either be continuous or paroxysmal, presenting in a nonspecific way, and may be confused with several clinical entities [22].

The paroxysmal release of catecholamines leads to the classic triad: headache, sweating, and palpitation. Anesthesia and tumor manipulation are the most well-known triggers of catecholaminergic attacks, which may occur after exercise, change in position, and use of medications such as opioids, metoclopramide, and iodinated contrast [20]. Patients may present with dyspnea, anxiety, hyperthermia, nausea, vomiting, abdominal pain, tremor, flushing, dizziness, visual changes, and paresthesias. The state of hypermetabolism due to elevated catecholamines can result in asthenia, fatigue, weight loss, and intestinal changes [20, 24].

The cardiovascular system is especially affected, with hypertension being the most common cardiovascular manifestation. It can present in two ways: sustained hypertension, in which the tumor preferentially produces norepinephrine, or paroxysmal hypertension, wherein the mainly produced hormone is epinephrine. Arrhythmias, myocardial or peripheral ischemia, aortic dissection, hypotension due to reduced venous return secondary to prolonged vasoconstriction and shock, and irreversible myocardial fibrosis may occur if chronic exposure to the adrenergic stimulus occurs [20, 22]. In more extreme situations, the multisystemic crisis characterized by hemodynamic instability with eventual hemodynamic collapse, encephalopathy, hyperthermia, and multiple organ failure may occur [22].

Table 11.3 demonstrates the frequency of signs and symptoms of patients with PCC/PG.

Laboratory Tests

Plasma free metanephrine measurement is the initial screening approach for the diagnosis of PCC, with a sensitivity of 96–100% and specificity of 89–98%. The upper limit of normality can be elevated in 80% of the patients with PCC/PG by three to four times, leading to the diagnosis of this disease. Moreover, a value within the normal range excludes the diagnosis. Measurement of 24-hour urinary free metanephrine confirms serum elevations of plasma metabolites, but it has slightly lower sensitivity and specificity (86–97% and 86–95%, respectively); it is indicated in cases of discrete elevations in the plasma test [25].

False-positive results may occur secondary to the use of medications such as tricyclic antidepressants, beta blockers, monoamine oxidase inhibitors, calcium channel inhibitors, phenoxybenzamine, etc. In these situations, the suppression test can be performed with clonidine (300 ug/70 kg) and serum normetanephrine dosage 3 hours later. Persistently high metanephrine levels after administration of the medication suggests the diagnosis of PCC, while the 50% reduction in metanephrine levels after the test is defined as false-positive, with sensitivity of 97% and specificity of 100% [25, 26]. It is recommended to measure metanephrines through liquid chromatography with electrochemical or fluorometric detection, liquid chromatography with tandem mass spectrometry, or immunoassay methods [26].

Chromogranin A is a polypeptide secreted by chromaffin cells and is found in 91% of PCC/PG carriers. Although it is a nonspecific marker of neuroendocrine tumors, in some patients, it may be a valuable marker for disease monitoring. When combined with the measurement of serum catecholamine levels, the diagnostic sensitivity of PCC may be as close to 100% [27]. Studies suggest that metoxiquimine, a

Table 11.3 Frequency of signs and symptoms in patients with PCC/PG

Signs	Frequency	Symptoms	Frequency
Hypertension	++++	Headache	++++
Sustained	++		
Paroxysmal	++		
Postural hypotension	+	Palpitation	++++
Tachycardia or reflex bradycardia	+++	Anxiety/nervousness	+++
Excessive sweating	++++	Tremors	++
Pallidness	++	Fatigue	++
Flushing	+	Nausea/vomiting	+
Weight loss	+	Chest/abdominal pain	+
Fasting hyperglycemia	++	Dizziness	+
Decreased bowel motility	+	Constipation (rarely diarrhea)	+
Tachypnea	+	Paresthesia	+

dopamine metabolite, may be useful in the detection of tumors that exclusively produce dopamine and may serve as a marker of malignancy [27].

Imaging Tests

Contrast CT and abdominal MRI confer similar sensitivities for the diagnosis of PCC/PG, with abdominal and pelvic CT being the first option. However, MRI may be more capable of detecting extra-adrenal tumors [26, 27]. In CT, the tumors may appear as homogeneous or heterogeneous, with necrotic, calcified, solid areas, aside from cystic areas. It presents an average attenuation of more than 10 units of Hounsfield in 87–100% of cases and, occasionally, a washout greater than 60% in the contrast phase [26, 27].

In MRI, tumors usually appear with T2-weighted hyper-signal lesions, although cystic and necrotic components may affect the classic appearance. In T1-weighted images, the PCC is isointense to the muscle and is relatively less intense than the liver [25, 27].

MIBG (metaiodobenzylguanidine) scintigraphy assists in the detection of primary or metastatic tumors that may not be identified in CT/MRI. False-negative results occur in extra-adrenal tumors or are associated with SDHB mutation. Medications, such as antihypertensives, tricyclic antidepressants, and opioids, can affect MIBG absorption and lead to false-negative results. Scintigraphy with pentetreotide (Octreoscan) explores the somatostatin receptors present in the PCC/PG cell membrane, which is important in the evaluation of metastases or in carriers of SDHB mutation [27].

Positron emission tomography (PET) has recently become widely used in the PCC/PG field because of its sensitivity, as well as its ability to quantify tracer's absorption and some aspect of tumor metabolism. The most widely used marker is fluorodeoxyglucose (FDG), which is a glucose analogue. This technique is particularly valuable for patients with DHBG mutation or other metastatic diseases. However, FDG is not specific for PCC and may present with positive results for other tumors [27].

Other more specific tracers for neuroendocrine tumors have been developed but are not yet fully disseminated. Fluorodopa is an amino acid analogue and catecholamine precursor that is specific for neuroendocrine tumors. FDOPA-PET is extremely sensitive to PGs of the head and neck. It is still particularly effective for patients with biochemically silent SDHB and/or PCC/PG mutation. Fluorodopamine (FDA) is a marker similar to dopamine and is absorbed by norepinephrine transporters. FDA-PET is particularly useful in the identification of abdominal tumors, with a greater sensitivity than MIBG or Octreoscan. It also proves to be a valuable modality for patients with metastatic tumors [27, 28].

Genetic Tests

Genetic tests should be considered in all patients and are strongly indicated for specific patients, such as those with a positive family history of PCC/PG or genetic mutations that increase tumor susceptibility, as well as in those patients with genetic syndromes or metastatic tumors. It is advisable to perform these tests in individuals with risk factors for underlying mutation: young, with multifocal or bilateral adrenal tumors, and paraganglioma carriers. Genetic mutation screening in these patients can result in early detection of the tumor and allow a more personalized approach, therefore reducing morbidity and improving the survival of affected patients [23, 28, 29]. Depending on the characteristics associated with each mutation, one can establish the order of the genes to be tested, as shown in Fig. 11.3.

Treatment

Preoperative Clinical Management

The clinical treatment of the PCC/PG aims at controlling the blood pressure and alleviating the symptoms and reducing risk of hypertensive crises and other cardiovascular complications that may occur during the perioperative period [28]. Alpha-adrenergic receptor blockers are indicated as first-line medications. However, there is no consensus yet on the use of selective or nonselective alpha blockers, with phenoxybenzamine as the most commonly used long-acting nonselective blocker. Doxazosin and prazosin, which are selective blockers with comparable efficacies, are also used [22, 26, 28]. The calcium channel blocker has been used as additional drug for BP optimization. Some studies suggested the use of this class as monotherapy, but this practice is not indicated unless the patient has a mild hypertensive condition or presents with severe orthotropic hypotension with the use of alpha blockers [26, 28].

Administration of beta blockers is indicated for heart rate control but only after the initiation of alpha blockers to avoid hypertensive crisis due to unopposed stimulation of alpha adrenergic receptors. There is no consensus on the use of beta-selective or nonselective beta blockers. However, it is advised to avoid labetalol as initial therapy, because, despite having both alpha and beta inhibition capabilities, the beta blocker effect is predominant and may result in paradoxical hypertension [26].

Alpha-methylparatyrosine (metyrosine) inhibits the synthesis of catecholamines and may be used in combination with alpha blockers for a short time in the preoperative period for a more optimal hemodynamic stabilization and reduction of intraoperative volume depletion. It is recom-

FLUXOGRAMA 3: DECISIONAL FLOW-CHART FOR GENETIC TESTING IN PATIENTS WITH A PROVEN FCC/PGG

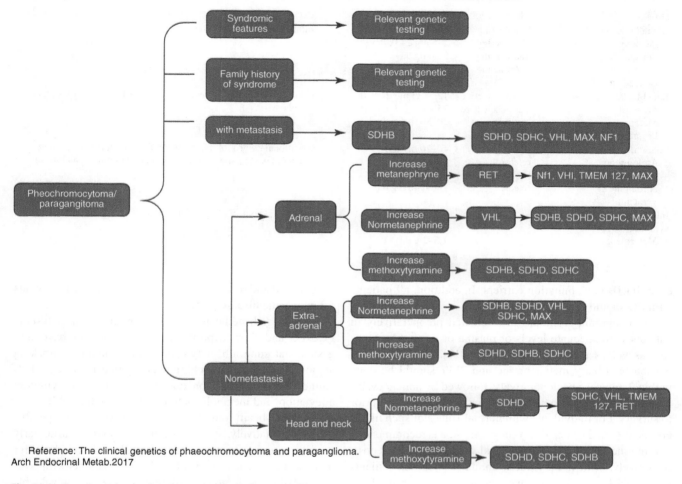

Reference: The clinical genetics of phaeochromocytoma and paraganglioma.
Arch Endocrinal Metab.2017

Fig. 11.3 Genetic testing in pheochromocytoma and paragangliomas

mended to start clinical treatment 7–14 days before the surgical procedure [26, 28].

The main medications used and their dosages are presented in Table 11.4.

Perioperative Management

Surgical resection is the definitive treatment for PCC. Laparoscopic adrenalectomy is the technique of choice when feasible. It can be performed by two different approaches: transperitoneal approach, which is considered for larger masses and obese patients, and retroperitoneal route, which is a more recent approach in which the patient is in the inclined or lateral position and is preferable for bilateral tumors. Both modalities are considered safe, and the decision depends on the experience and preference of the surgeon [30]. For tumors greater than 6 cm, this modality can still be used, although there is a possibility of conversion to open surgery intraoperatively [22].

For multiple, metastatic, or recurrent tumors, open surgery confers a greater likelihood of complete tumor removal and is thus preferable [30]. Robotic assistance can also be used, with a similar success rate [27]. In some patients wherein surgery cannot be performed, tumors in accessible locations can be managed through radiofrequency [27].

Follow-Up

There are currently no validated reliable histopathological criteria that can predict malignancy or risk of primary tumor metastasis; hence, long-term follow-up with laboratory and imaging tests is necessary [27]. In this way, a tumor is considered malignant when at follow-up, lymph node metastasis or metastasis to distant sites is detected [19].

Screening for metastatic tumors with CT or PET is recommended for patients with PG, PCC patients with elevated levels of serum or urinary 3-methoxytyramine (3MT), or

Table 11.4 Medications used to control symptoms and preoperative treatment

Drug	Classification	Dose	Recommendation
Alpha blockers	Long acting	10 mg 1–3x day	First choice of treatment
Phenoxybenzamine	Short acting	2–5 mg 2–3x day	
Prazosin	Short acting	2–5 mg day	
Terazosin	Short acting	2–8 mg day	
Doxazosin			
Beta blockers	Cardioselective	12.5–25 mg 2–3x day	Control of tachycardia secondary to catecholamines or alpha blockade
Atenolol	Cardioselective	25–50 mg 3–4x day	
Metoprolol	Not selective	20–80 mg 1–3x day	
Propranolol			
Calcium channel blockers	Prolonged release	10–20 mg day	Additional control of hypertension for patients already using alpha blockers; patients with contraindication to alpha blockade
Amlodipine		60–90 mg day	
Nicardipine	Prolonged release	30–90 mg day	
Nifedipine		180–540 mg day	
Verapamil			
Inhibitors of catecholamine synthesis	–	250 mg 2–3x day (maximum dose 1.5–2 g day)	Additional control of hypertension
Metyrosine			

even SDHB gene mutation carriers. In addition, all patients with PG should undergo genetic testing.

Chromogranin A should be evaluated preoperatively in patients with adequate levels of plasma or urine metanephrine, as well as adequate levels of 3MT [19]. Measurement of plasma or urinary metanephrine and 3MT should be done within 2–6 weeks postoperatively, followed by annual evaluations for patients who had alterations in these markers prior to surgery. For individuals with normal values of such markers and elevated levels of chromogranin A, it is recommended that the measurement be performed within 2–6 weeks postoperatively, with a subsequent annual evaluation. Patients with SDHB mutation may have normal metanephrine level and elevated plasma chromogranin A level [19].

Imaging tests should be performed 3 months after complete surgery in patients who had postoperatively altered metanephrines or 3MT or in patients without preoperative exams [19]. It is suggested to follow these patients for at least 10 years, with consultations every 1–2 years for relapse surveillance or detection of new tumors. For high-risk patients (young, with genetic disease, large tumor, and diagnosed with PG), lifetime annual follow-up should be offered [19].

Treatment of Malignant Pheochromocytoma

For patients with metastatic disease, chemotherapy (QT) may be helpful in relieving symptoms and in disrupting or even reducing the rate of tumor growth. Although no QT regimen showed long-term efficacy, some can maintain the disease state for an extended period, improving the survival and quality of life of patients [27]. Traditional QT with cyclophosphamide, vincristine, and dacarbazine has been widely used and remains one of the most effective treatments for metastatic disease [27].

New drugs have been studied for treatment of metastatic PCC/PG and showed promising effects. Studies have suggested that sunitinib, a tyrosine kinase inhibitor blocking angiogenesis, directly inhibits the synthesis of catecholamines; however, data on tumor size reduction, symptom alleviation, and metabolic activity are conflicting [27].

External beam radiation can be used for inoperable tumors, palliatively, symptom reduction and is particularly useful for bone metastases. They may also be considered for nonresectable head and neck PG [27]. For patients with positive MIBG scintigraphy, radiotherapy may be a valuable treatment option, requiring a recent scan of MIBG tumors to determine the degree of absorption. The therapy is based on the emission of beta particles, as the radioactive compound is absorbed by the tumor cells, leading to their destruction [27].

A better understanding of the pathogenesis of PCC/PG has led to significant progress in this field. However, successful long-term treatments for patients with metastatic disease are still yet to be determined [27].

References

1. Thomas RM, Ruel E, Shantavasinkul PC, Corsino L. Endocrine hypertension: an overview on the current etiopathogenesis and management options. World J Hypertens. 2015;5(2):14–27.
2. Sica DA. Endocrine causes of secondary hypertension. J Clin Hypertension. 2008;10(7):534–40.
3. Young WF. Primary aldosteronism: renaissance of a syndrome. Clin Endocrinol. 2007;66(5):607–18.
4. Brown JM, Cohen CR, Fernandez MAL, Allison MA, Baudrand R, Ix JH, et al. The spectrum of subclinical primary Aldosteronism and incident hypertension: a cohort study. Ann Intern Med. 2017;167(9):630–41.

5. Capeletti JT, Barbosa RR, Cestari PF, Peres GMTLSR, Ibañez TLP, Gonzaga CC, et al. Primary aldosteronism: diagnosis and clinical outcomes. Rev Bras Hipertens. 2009;16(1):65–8.

6. Hundemer GL, Curhan GC, Yozamp N, Wang M, Vaidya A. Cardiometabolic outcomes and mortality in medically treated primary aldosteronism: a retrospective cohort study. Lancet Diabetes Endocrinol. 2017; https://doi.org/10.1016/S2213-8587(17)30367-4.

7. Kater CE. Primary hyperaldosteronism. Arq Bras Endocrinol Metabvol. 2002;46(1):106–15.

8. Funder JW, Carey RM, Mantero F, Murad MH, Reincke M, Shibata H, et al. The Management of Primary Aldosteronism: case detection, diagnosis, and treatment: an Endocrine Society clinical practice guideline. J Clin Endocrinol Metab. 2016;101(5):1889–916.

9. So A, Duffy DL, Gordon RD, Jeske YW, Lin-Su K, New MI, et al. Familial hyperaldosteronism type II is linked to the chromosome 7p22 region but also shows predicted heterogeneity. J Hypertens. 2005;23(8):1477–84.

10. Mulatero P, Tizzani D, Viola A, et al. Prevalence and characteristics of familial hyperaldosteronism: the PATOGEN study (primary Aldosteronism in torino-genetic forms). Hypertension. 2011;58:797–803.

11. Milliez P, Girerd X, Plouin PF, Blacher J, Safar ME, Mourad JJ. Evidence for an increased rate of cardiovascular events in patients with primary aldosteronism. J Am Coll Cardiol. 2005;45:1243–8.

12. Stowasser M, Sharman J, Leano R, et al. Evidence for abnormal left ventricular structure and function in normotensive individuals with familial hyperaldosteronism type I. J Clin Endocrinol Metab. 2005;90:5070–6.

13. Young WF, Stanson AW, Thompson GB, Grant CS, Farley DR, et al. Role for adrenal venous sampling in primary aldosteronism. Surgery. 2004;136:1227–35.

14. Monticone S, Viola A, Rossato D, Veglio F, Reincke M, Gomez-Sanchez C, et al. Adrenal vein sampling in primary aldosteronism: towards a standardised protocol. Lancet Diabetes Endocrinol. 2015;3(4):296–303.

15. Kater CE. Rastremento, comprovação e diferenciação laboratorial do hiperaldosteronismo primário. Arq Bras Endocrinol Metabol. 2002;46:106–15.

16. Sawka AM, Young WF, Thompson GB, et al. Primary aldosteronism: factors associated with normalization of blood pressure after surgery. Ann Intern Med. 2001;135:258–61.

17. Rossi GP, Cesari M, Cuspidi C, et al. Long-term control of arterial hypertension and regression of left ventricular hypertrophy with treatment of primary aldosteronism. Hypertension. 2013;62:62–9.

18. Ghose RP, Hall PM, Bravo EL. Medical management of aldosterone-producing adenomas. Ann Intern Med. 1999;131:105–8.

19. Plouin PF, Amar L, Dekkers OM, Fassnacht M, Gimenez-Roqueplo AP, Lenders JWM, et al. European Society of Endocrinology Clinical Practice Guideline for long-term follow-up of patients operated on for a phaeochromocytoma or a paraganglioma. Euro J Endocrinol. 2016;174:5. Available from https://doi.org/10.1530/EJE-16-0033.

20. Pourian M, Mostafazadeh DB, Soltani A. Does this patient have pheochromocytoma? A systematic review of clinical signs and symptoms. J Diabetes Metabolic Disorders. 2016;15:11. Available from https://doi.org/10.1186/s40200-016-0230-1.

21. Bausch B, Wellner U, Bausch D, Schiavi F, Barontini M, Sanso G, et al. Long-term prognosis of patients with pediatric pheochromocytoma. Endocr Relat Cancer. 2014;21(1):17–25.

22. Castelino T, Mitmaker E. Pheochromocytoma Crisis. Crisis, Clinical Management of Adrenal Tumors, Dr. John Lew (Ed.). 2017. https://doi.org/10.5772/intechopen.69338. Available from: https://www.intechopen.com/books/clinical-management-of-adrenal-umors/pheochromocytoma-crisis.

23. Fishbein L, Merrill S, Fraker DL, Cohen DL, Nathanson KL. Inherited mutations in pheochromocytoma and paraganglioma: why all patients should be offered genetic testing. Ann Surg Oncol. 2013;20(5):1444–50.

24. Wei GY, Jennifer P, Mehta K, Monica S, Irene W. Cardiovascular Manifestations of Pheochromocytoma. Cardiol Rev. 2017;25(5):215–22.

25. Galati SJ, Said M, Gospin R, Babic N, Brown K, Geer EB, et al. The Mount Sinai clinical pathway for the management of pheochromocytoma. Endocr Pract. 2015;21(4):368–82.

26. Lenders JW, Duh QY, Eisenhofer G, Gimenez-Roqueplo AP, Grebe SK, Murad MH, et al. Pheochromocytoma and paraganglioma: an endocrine society clinical practice guideline. J Clin Endocrinol Metab. 2014;99(6):1915–42.

27. Martucci VL, Pacak K. Pheochromocytoma and paraganglioma: diagnosis, genetics, management, and treatment. Curr Probl Cancer. 2014;38(7):41.

28. Lenders JWM, Eisenhofer G. Update on modern Management of Pheochromocytoma and Paraganglioma. Endocrinol Metab. 2017;32:152–61.

29. Gunawardane PTK, Grossman A. The clinical genetics of phaeochromocytoma and paraganglioma. Arch Endocrinol Metab. 2017. Available from https://doi.org/10.1590/2359-3997000000299.

30. Naranjo J, Dodd S, Martin YN. Perioperative Management of Pheochromocytoma. J Cardiothorac Vasc Anesth. 2017;31:1427–39.

Hirsutism and Virilization

12

Alessandra Gambineri, Antonio Balsamo, and Renato Pasquali

Epidemiology of Hirsutism and Virilization

Hirsutism is one of the commonest medical complaints among women of reproductive age [1]. The actual prevalence of hirsutism in adults ranges from 3 to 15% in Blacks and Whites [2–5] but is somewhat lower in Asians (1–3%) [6].

Recent epidemiological surveys have added data concerning hirsutism restricted to adolescence and youth and demonstrated that this condition is still very frequent from the post-menarchal years, with a prevalence ranging from 8 to 13% [7–9].

At variance, virilization is a rare condition, but it may present from prenatal to adult life, involving also the neonatal, prepubertal, and adolescent periods with a prevalence varying with the cause and the date of appearance of the disorder. In particular, the most frequent causes of virilization in the prenatal/neonatal periods of life are some monogenic enzymatic adrenal deficiencies, CCAH, due to 21-hydroxylase, 11-hydroxylase, 3β-hydroxysteroid-dehydrogenase, P450-oxidoreductase, or aromatase defects [10, 11] that have an overall prevalence of about 1:20,000 female newborns per year. The prevalence of virilization decreases switching to prepubertal, pubertal, and adolescent periods, where the principal cause is represented by rare adrenocortical tumors, whose worldwide annual incidence ranges from 0.3 to 0.38 per million children below the age of 15 years [12–15]. In adults, the prevalence of virilization is even more rare, being mainly caused by rare forms of ovarian androgen-secreting tumors, the sex cord-stromal tumors, that account for less than 0.5% of all ovarian neoplasms [16].

A. Gambineri (✉)
Division of Endocrinology, Department of Medical and Surgical Sciences, St. Orsola-Malpighi Hospital, University of Bologna, Bologna, Italy
e-mail: alessandra.gambiner3@unibo.it

A. Balsamo
Pediatric Unit, Department of Medical and Surgical Sciences, St. Orsola-Malpighi Hospital, University of Bologna, Bologna, Italy
e-mail: antonio.balsamo@unibo.it

R. Pasquali
Department of Medicine, University of Bologna, Bologna, Italy
e-mail: renato.pasquali@unibo.it

Etiology of Hirsutism and Virilization

Functional causes account for most of cases of hirsutism. They include polycystic ovary syndrome (PCOS), idiopathic hyperandrogenism, and idiopathic hirsutism. PCOS, the most common cause of hirsutism, is characterized by the combination of hirsutism and/or biochemical hyperandrogenism with anovulatory cycles and/or polycystic ovarian morphology [17]. Idiopathic hyperandrogenism is characterized by the combination of hirsutism with biochemical hyperandrogenism but normal ovulatory cycles and normal ovarian morphology [18]; idiopathic hirsutism is characterized by hirsutism in the presence of normal androgens, ovulatory cycles, and normal ovaries [19].

Less common but an important cause of hirsutism are different forms of non-classic congenital adrenal hyperplasia (NCCAH), mainly represented by 21-hydroxylase deficiency, while adrenal or ovarian androgen-secreting tumors, gestational hyperandrogenism, drug-induced hirsutism, ovarian hyperthecosis, Cushing's syndrome, acromegaly, hypothyroidism, and hyperprolactinemia are very uncommon but should always be considered in the diagnostic approach to hirsutism [2].

The latter causes become much more consistent when virilism is present. The more frequent causes of virilization according to age of onset are shown in Table 12.1.

Pathophysiology of Hirsutism and Virilization

There are three structural types of hair on the human body: lanugo is a soft hair that covers the skin of the fetus but disappears soon after the birth; vellus is a soft hair, usually non-pigmented and with a diameter less than 0.03 mm covering much of the body in men and women; and terminal hair is longer, pigmented, and coarser in texture and with different extents of expression in men and women. In particular, females have terminal hairs only in the eyebrows, eyelashes,

Table 12.1 Causes of female virilization according to age

Age	Adrenals	Ovaries	Others
Prenatal/neonatal	46,XX CCAH:	Maternal androgenizing tumors	Maternal drugs
Prepubertal	46,XX NCCAH Adrenal adenomas Adrenal carcinomas Adrenal hyperplasia 11β-HSD1 deficiency	Androgen-producing tumors (sex cord stromal; gonadoblastoma)	
Pubertal/adolescence	Adrenal adenomas Adrenal carcinomas Adrenal hyperplasia Cushing's syndrome	Androgen-producing tumors (sex cord stromal; gonadoblastoma)	Hyperprolactinemia
Adult	Adrenal adenomas Adrenal carcinomas Adrenal hyperplasia Cushing's syndrome	Androgen-producing tumors (sex cord stromal) Hyperthecosis	Hyperprolactinemia Exogenous DHEA intake
Pregnancy	Maternal adenomas/carcinomas	Luteoma	Placental aromatase deficiency Fetal PORD
Post-menopausal	Adrenal adenomas Adrenal carcinomas	Androgen-producing tumors (sex cord stromal) Hyperthecosis	

CCAH classic congenital adrenal hyperplasia, *NCCAH* non-classic congenital adrenal hyperplasia, *11β-HSD1* 11β-hydroxysteroid dehydrogenase type 1, *PORD* cytochrome P450 oxidoreductase deficiency

scalp, pubis, and axillae [20]. Hair arises from a complex and highly dynamic structure—the hair follicle, which consists of several components and has a rhythmic growth cycle [21]. The hair follicle growth cycle is made up of three major phases: anagen (a stage of rapid growth), telogen (a stage of relative quiescence), and catagen (apoptosis-mediated regression) [22]. Hirsutism follows an alteration of the hair follicle cycle, in particular a prolongation of the anagen phase with a consequent transformation of vellus into terminal hairs. This alteration appears under the effect of androgens that are triggered and involved in the regulation of growth of sexual hair. Androgens active on hair follicle are testosterone (T) and dihydrotestosterone (DHT), which may be generated via a de novo synthetic pathway from cholesterol and/or via a shortcut pathway from circulating dehydroepiandrosterone sulfate (DHEA-S) [23]. Cutaneous testosterone may arrive from the circulation, principally synthesized in the adrenals and ovaries, and/or may be locally generated, since hair follicles are equipped with all the necessary enzymes for biosynthesis and metabolism of androgens [23]. DHT is almost entirely synthesized locally in a step catalyzed by the enzyme 5α-reductase [24]. Therefore, circulating androgen levels do not quantify the real exposure of hair follicle to androgens, since a quota is locally generated. Furthermore, cutaneous androgen effects also depend on the local expression and activity of the androgen receptor [22]. This justifies why the severity of hirsutism is always not correlated with circulating androgen concentrations.

Similarly, virilization results from the interaction between androgen concentration and local sensitivity to androgens. However, virilization also results from an excessive widespread exposure to androgens (mainly T and DHT), involving not only hair follicles but also sebaceous glands, muscle mass, adipose tissue, and external genitalia. Similar to hirsutism, also for virilization the source of androgens is mainly represented by the adrenals (from prenatal to prepubertal periods) and ovaries (after puberty until menopause), but a quota is peripherally or locally synthesized [25, 26]. The most deleterious effect of hyperandrogenism in females is certainly when it appears in the prenatal period, because it may cause ambiguous external genitalia [27].

At the start of life, in fact, the external genitalia are identical, regardless of the genetic or gonadal sex, and consist of the genital tubercle, the urogenital folds, and the genital swellings (Fig. 12.1a). In a normal female fetus, when androgenic effects are lacking, the genital tubercle forms a clitoris, and the urethral folds and the genital swellings develop into the labia minora and majora, respectively (Fig. 12.1a, left side) [28]. On the contrary, when hyperandrogenism takes place in utero, such as in a 46,XX fetus affected by CCAH, male genital differentiation occurs due to the elevated amounts of adrenal testosterone, which is produced from the seventh to eighth week of gestation. In this case the genital tubercle grows into a penis, the urethral folds fuse to create a tubular penile urethra with the tendency of the meatus to locate at the tip of the penis, and the genital swellings join to form a scrotum (Fig. 12.1a; right side). In cases of milder androgen exposure (before the 14th week of gestational age), the posterior labial fusion results in an increased anal-genital distance (Fig. 12.1b). Since internal genitalia are not sensitive to androgens, the uterus, fallopian tubes, and the upper part of the vagina develop normally.

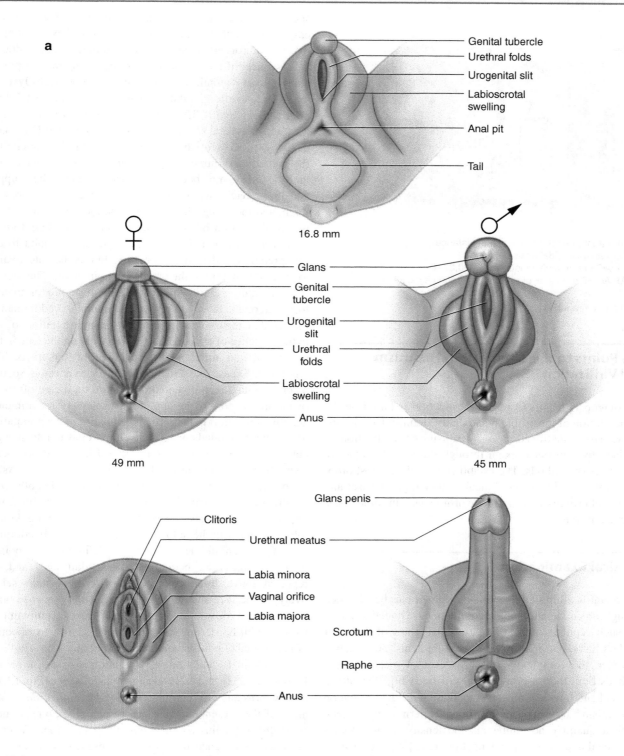

Fig. 12.1 (**a**) External genitalia development in females and males; (**b**) anal-genital distance

b

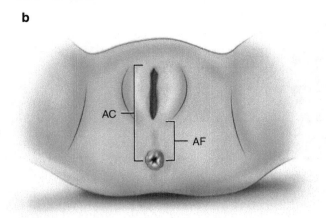

- AF= anal-posterior forket fusion distance
- AC= anal-clitoridal basis distance
- AF/AC= anal-genital distance (v.n. 0.37±0.07)
- AF/AC >0.5 = index of prenatal androgen exposition.

Fig. 12.1 (continued)

Key Points to the Diagnosis of Hirsutism and Virilization

The diagnosis of hirsutism and virilization is based on the quantification of the problem and on the definition of the etiology. The quantification of hirsutism or virilization is obtained by a physical exam through the use of subjective and objective methods. The establishment of the most probable etiology is based on clinical history (age of onset and rapidity of progression), hormone profile, and, in some cases, genetic analysis.

Physical Examination

The quantification of hirsutism in women can be obtained through objective and subjective methods. Objective methods, such as photographic evaluations, weighing of shaved or plucked hairs, and microscopic measurements, are reliable. However, the complexity and high cost of most of these methods limit their use in clinical practice [29]. Recently, a practical and low-cost objective technique for the evaluation of hirsutism has been proposed, the videodermoscopy, which is able to quantify the number and the density of hair follicles in selected androgen-dependent skin areas [30]. More studies are needed to validate this interesting and objective method and to justify the substitution of the widespread used subjective methods for the evaluation of hirsutism. Subjective methods mainly refer to visually scoring terminal hairs in specified areas. These methods have the advantage of being easy, convenient, cheap, and fast; however, they are subject to some interobserver variation. This limitation can be drastically reduced if the visual score is applied by trained physicians at least 3 months after the use of laser or electrolysis, at least 4 weeks after depilation or waxing, and at least 5 days after shaving and if the number of examiners is minimized [29]. Of the visual scores available, the modified Ferriman-Gallwey (mFG) score has now become the gold standard for the evaluation of hirsutism [31]. This method applies a similar 0–4 scale to nine body areas (upper lip, chin, chest, upper and lower back, upper and lower abdomen, arm, forearm, thigh, and lower leg) that appear to be the best areas indicative of the action of androgens on the female hair follicle [29]. There are actually two open questions related to the interpretation of the mFG score. The first is the cutoff value to be used to diagnose the presence of hirsutism. The second is what interpretation to give to hirsutism predominantly localized on the face with respect to hirsutism predominantly localized on the trunk or arms and what interpretation to give to the presence of terminal hairs selectively on the face in the absence of an mFG score indicative of hirsutism. The Androgen Excess and Polycystic Ovary Syndrome Society recently issued recommendations regarding the cutoff value of the mFG score to be applied. The Society recommends adapting the cutoff to the race and ethnicity of the population to which it is applied and, if this value is unavailable, using a cutoff value of 8 or above for White, Black, and Southeast Asian women and a cutoff of 3 or above for Far-East Asian women [21]. Given the importance of the topic in both clinical practice and scientific research, how to define hirsutism requires more intensive research, possibly involving dermatologists and with the help of new technologies. In addition, other factors should be considered in defining cutoff points, including age (i.e., pediatric versus adult age) and, as reported above, how the presence of terminal hairs selectively on the face should be evaluated with respect to body hair. In fact, this often represents a major complaint in women with borderline hirsutism mFG scores, irrespective of age, social condition, and health problems.

The clinical evaluation of virilization is based on genital Prader staging (Fig. 12.2) and anogenital distance (Fig. 12.1b) in newborns and on a complete physical examination (evaluation of the presence or absence of palpable gonads, measurement of phallus length, urethral opening identification, presence or absence of a vagina, presence or absence of clitoral hypertrophy) thereafter. When virilization is clinically suspected, the diagnosis usually needs to be confirmed by imaging such as abdominal/pelvic ultrasound, genitourethrogram, and, if necessary, MRI.

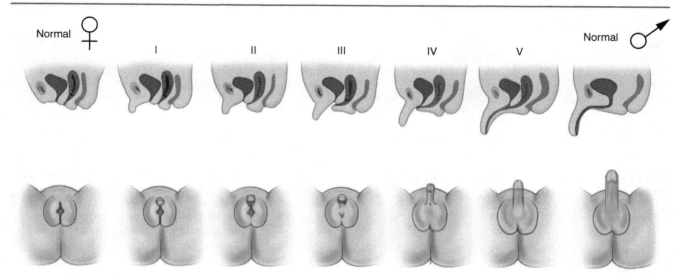

Fig. 12.2 Prader stages of genital androgenization

Hormone Profile

As previously mentioned, hirsutism and virilization are markers of excessive tissue exposure to androgen action, which results from the interaction between local androgen concentration and tissue sensitivity to androgens. Therefore, the diagnosis of hirsutism and virilization does not necessarily reflect high circulating androgen levels. This means that serum androgen measurements are often not sufficient to diagnose the presence of hirsutism or virilization, or to establish their severity, although they are extremely useful to define the etiology. However, the assay performance of the analytical methods used to measure androgens in the circulation has to be seriously taken into account for the correct interpretation of the results. The performance of modern immunoassay methods in terms of specificity and accuracy is poor, particularly for some androgens (17OH-progesterone, androstenedione, DHEA) and for low circulating concentrations, such as those enriched by testosterone in prepuberty and in the normal adult female range (<1 ng/mL) [32]. In addition, immunoassay methods routinely used are unable to measure some androgens that could impact the clinical expression of hyperandrogenism in terms of hirsutism or virilization. Liquid chromatography combined with tandem mass spectrometry (LC-MS/MS) is an innovative technique displaying good precision, sensitivity, and high accuracy for measuring female androgen levels throughout all stages of life, with the advantages of the high throughput and the low cost required for the analysis [33, 34]. Therefore, it represents a convenient and reliable assay when androgen mea-

surement in females is required, provided that a reference normal range is determined in house, by using a carefully selected healthy non-hyperandrogenic control female population [21]. In addition, LC-MS/MS makes it possible to measure important steroids such as 11-deoxycortisol and deoxycorticosterone (DOC) that cannot be measured with immunoassay methods and that are triggers for the diagnosis of uncommon forms of CCAH and NCCAH. Due to the numerous advantages of this technique, LC-MS/MS has recently been introduced in laboratories in critical fields that strongly rely on the reliability and rapidity of the measurement, such as newborn screening for congenital diseases including CCAH [35].

For example, the use of LC-MS/MS to diagnose hyperandrogemia in PCOS women gave importance to androstenedione and introduced the concept that a subset of women with PCOS has an isolated increase in androstenedione levels, thus reducing the number of subjects affected by isolated hirsutism [36]. In addition, a significant link between high androstenedione levels and an adverse metabolic phenotype has been found in PCOS patients [36, 37].

Genetic Analysis

Genetic analyses are warranted when NCCAH or CCAH is strongly suspected as cause of hirsutism or virilization, because they are genetic disorders with autosomal recessive inheritance. The genes involved in all defects have been isolated and characterized, and specific mutations have been

Table 12.2 Genes involved in congenital adrenal hyperplasia (CAH)

Gene/protein type	Chromosome location	Inheritance	Gonads	Müllerian structures	External genitalia	Other associated features
HSD3B2/ enzyme	1p13.1	AR	Ovary	Yes	Female or ambiguous	CAH, adrenal insufficiency
CYP21A2/ enzyme	6p21.23	AR	Ovary	Yes	Female, ambiguous or male	CAH, +/− adrenal insufficiency
CYP11B1/ enzyme	8q21.22	AR	Ovary	Yes	Female, ambiguous or male	CAH, +/− hypertension
POR/CYP electron donor	7q11.2	AR	Ovary	Yes	Female or ambiguous	Mixed features of 21-OHDef, 17-OHDef/17–20-lyaseDef, aromatase Def; +/− Antley–Bixler syndrome
CYP19/enzyme	15q21	AR	Ovary	Yes	Ambiguous	Maternal virilization during pregnancy, absent breast development at puberty, except partial cases

identified (Table 12.2). Genetic analysis for identification of mutations of the genes involved is informative for the index case (type and severity of the disorder) and for future prenatal diagnosis.

21-Hydroxylase deficiency, the most frequent cause of NCCAH and CCAH, is caused by cytochrome P450c21 enzyme impairment. The *CYP21A2* gene, encoding for 21-hydroxylase, is homologous at 98% in exons and at 96% in introns to the nonfunctional *CYP21A1P* pseudogene. The high degree of sequence homology and tandem repeating order of RCCX module sequences is the cause of sequence misalignments during meiosis, which result in frequent unequal meiotic crossovers, as these modules are located in the HLA region of the genome (where recombination events occur at a particularly high level to ensure high immunological diversity) [38]. This mechanism generates gene deletions as well as the commonly called "large gene conversions," both consisting in chromosomes with a chimeric gene (with a 5′ part of pseudogenic origin fused with a 3′ CYP21A2 region), but without a *CYP21A2* gene [39]. The majority of disease-causing mutations are small mutations that arise from micro-conversions (transfer of small DNA sequences) from *CYP21A1P* to *CYP21A2*: P30L, IVS2-13A/C > G (I2 splice), Del 8 bp E3, I172N, Cluster E6, V281L, 1762_1763insT (L307 Frameshift), Q318X, R356W; the P453S mutation, which is not pseudogene-derived, is usually added to this list. The remaining 10% of alleles have new/rare mutations due to random events [40]; over 90 rare pseudogene-independent mutations are actually listed in the Human Cytochrome P450 (*CYP*) Allele Nomenclature Committee at http://www.imm.ki.se/CYPalleles/cyp21.htm. The phenotype derives from the type(s) of genetic mutations with a final influence on the total residual enzymatic activity [41] (Fig. 12.3). The CCAH forms result from deletions/conversions or point mutations associated with <10% residual enzymatic activity (Null, A, B, mutation groups of Fig. 12.3); the NCCAH forms result from point mutations with residual

enzymatic activity comprised between 15 and 60% (C mutation groups of Fig. 12.3). As for genital appearance, while the presence of "group C" mutations is highly predictive of forms without external genital virilization, a clear predicting capacity does not exist for stages of virilization within the Null, A, and B mutation groups. In fact, although more severe virilization tends somehow to be present in patients with the most severe genotypes [42], Prader stages from II to V have, however, been reported in each of the previous mutation groups [43] (Fig. 12.3). When patients are compound heterozygotes, with two or more different mutations on the two alleles, the severity of the phenotype depends principally on the mutation with the less impaired residual activity [41].

Differential Diagnosis

Hirsutism is a marker of excessive tissue exposure to androgens and, therefore, always deserves to be investigated. Various disorders enter into the differential diagnosis, some more frequent (PCOS, idiopathic hirsutism, idiopathic hyperandrogenism), others more rare (NCCAH due to 21-hydroxylase deficiency, hyperprolactinemia, hypothyroidism, drugs, gestation), and others very occasional (androgen-secreting tumors, Cushing's syndrome, acromegaly, NCCAH not due to 21-hydroxylase deficiency, CCAH). However, all these causes must be taken into account in the correct approach to a patient who complains of hirsutism. In addition, a correct medical approach to hirsutism assumes the need to exclude whether it accompanies signs of virilization or, alternatively, it is isolated. A diagnostic algorithm is suggested in Fig. 12.4. All patients presenting with hirsutism should be firstly subjected to a careful evaluation of the clinical history and a thorough physical examination. Age of onset and rapidity of progression are key factors that should often be investigated. Functional causes or NCCAH, in fact, almost always show a peripubertal onset and a slow progres-

Fig. 12.3 CYP21A2P derived mutations: phenotypic spectrum. (Modified from Ref. [38, 43])

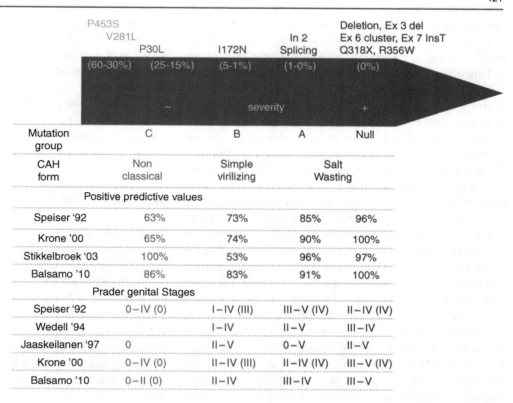

Mutation group	C	B	A	Null
CAH form	Non classical	Simple virilizing	Salt Wasting	
Positive predictive values				
Speiser '92	63%	73%	85%	96%
Krone '00	65%	74%	90%	100%
Stikkelbroek '03	100%	53%	96%	97%
Balsamo '10	86%	83%	91%	100%
Prader genital Stages				
Speiser '92	0–IV (0)	I–IV (III)	III–V (IV)	II–IV (IV)
Wedell '94		I–IV	II–V	III–IV
Jaaskeilanen '97	0	II–V	0–V	II–V
Krone '00	0–IV (0)	II–IV (III)	II–IV (IV)	III–V (IV)
Balsamo '10	0–II (0)	II–IV	III–IV	III–V

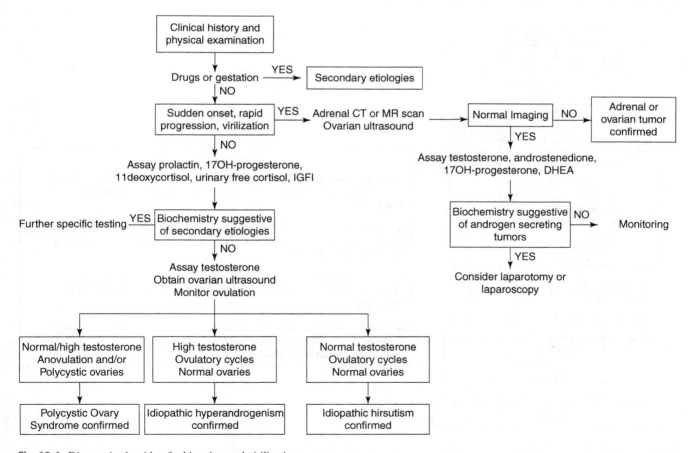

Fig. 12.4 Diagnostic algorithm for hirsutism and virilization

sion over years and are generally not associated with signs of virilization. In contrast, androgen-secreting tumors usually manifest at any age with sudden onset and rapid progression and are usually associated with signs of virilization. Clinical screening is also essential to rule out secondary forms of hirsutism or virilization that, however, usually need serum or urine measurements of the relevant hormones and, if necessary, specific testing in order to be confirmed. Functional forms of hirsutism (PCOS, idiopathic hirsutism, idiopathic hyperandrogenism) must be considered and dealt with only after androgen-secreting tumors and the other forms have been excluded. At this point, measurement of testosterone and *androstenedione* in serum, assessment of ovulatory function, and ovarian ultrasound evaluation are essential for the differential diagnosis between the three forms. CCAH is generally diagnosed in neonatal age because of external ambiguous genitalia, salt-losing crisis, or, rarely, hypertension (Fig. 12.5). CCAH due to 21-hydroxylase deficiency is the commonest cause of ambiguous genitalia of the newborn. Ambiguous genitalia at neonatal age may depend more rarely on 11-hydroxylase, 3β-hydroxysteroid dehydrogenase, and P450-oxidoreductase deficiencies [10, 44]. All these forms of CCAH are generally characterized by varying degrees of genital virilization (Prader staging, Fig. 12.2) possibly accompanied by genital pigmentation (expression of

excessive ACTH production). Salt-losing crisis may be associated with 21-hydroxylase and 3β-hydroxysteroid dehydrogenase deficiencies [10, 45]. Hypertension due to DOC excess is extremely rare in newborns affected by 11-hydroxylase deficiency. Measurement of 17OH-progesterone, 17OH-pregnenolone, androstenedione, DHEA, testosterone, 11-deoxycortisol, and DOC in the circulation is essential for a differential diagnosis of the various causes of virilizing 46,XX CCAH (Fig. 12.5).

Management of Hirsutism and of Virilization

Hirsutism is a clinical sign and not a disease by itself. Therefore, its presence does not necessarily require treatment. However, physicians should decide whether hirsutism is to be treated or not by evaluating not only the severity of the phenomenon but also the subjective perception of the patient that does not necessarily correspond to the true extent of hair growth. Interestingly, a recent population-based study performed on adolescent and young adult Italian students confirmed that, among the hyperandrogenic disorders (i.e., isolated menstrual irregularity, isolated biochemical hyperandrogenism, isolated hirsutism, or polycystic ovary syndrome (PCOS)), hirsutism is the worse in terms of

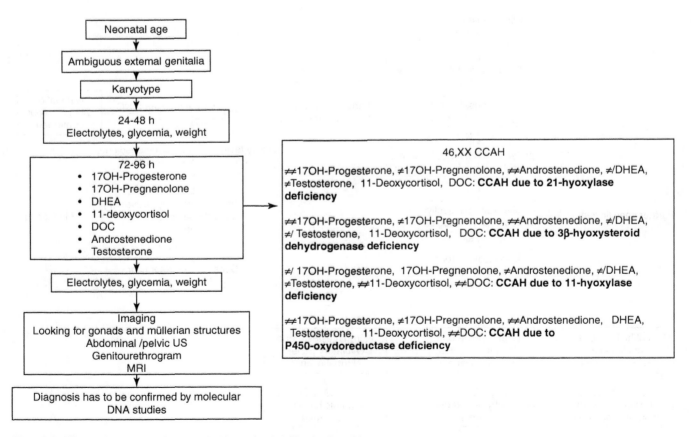

Fig. 12.5 Diagnostic algorithm for an early diagnosis of virilization in newborns

psychological distress and quality of life, because it is associated with reduced quality of life, anxiety, and depression [46]. The correct management of hirsutism is, obviously, the treatment of the underlying cause, if possible. Usually, however, treatment targeted at ameliorating hirsutism directly is also necessary.

Cosmetic measures are effective as individual therapy in controlling mild and localized hirsutism. In addition, they are recommended as an adjuvant to pharmacological therapy in cases of clinically moderate to severe hirsutism. Among the cosmetic measures available, only electrolysis and the newer methods, such as laser therapy and intense pulse light, may result in permanent amelioration of hirsutism in the treated area [47, 48]. Data of comparisons between different laser methods are few and give contradictory results. However, from the studies available, diode and alexandrite offer the highest success rate, whereas Nd:Yag gives the lowest success rate [49]. There are very few and low-quality studies comparing laser and intense pulsed light devices.

In cases of mild hirsutism localized on the face, an alternative to the cosmetic approach is the topical application of a 13.9% eflornithine HCl cream [50]. Eflornithine is an irreversible inhibitor of l-ornithine decarboxylase, an enzyme that catalyzes the conversion of ornithine to putrescine, a polyamine that is critical to the regulation of cell growth and differentiation within the hair follicle [50]. Some evidence exists for the efficacy of topical eflornithine applied twice daily in reducing facial hirsutism [51, 52]. Drawbacks included nonresponse in 30% of users and regrowth to pretreatment levels within 8 weeks of discontinuation. The safety profile was good and percutaneous absorption was minimal. Other evidences demonstrate the ability of topical eflornithine added to photoepilation to promote more rapid and complete laser removal of facial hirsutism and to reduce hair regrowth between laser sessions and after cessation of IPL therapy [52, 53]. Limited and contradictory results are available on the effect of topical finasteride on hirsutism.

A systemic pharmacological approach is usually required when hirsutism is moderate to severe and/or widespread. Drugs that are safer and more cost-effective are oral contraceptive pills (OCPs). Their efficacy is mainly justified by the ability of progestin to suppress luteinizing hormone levels and thus ovarian androgen production and by the ability of estrogen (ethinyl estradiol (EE)) to increase sex hormone-binding globulin (SHBG), thus reducing bioavailable free androgens [54]. Moreover, OCPs induce a moderate reduction of adrenal androgens, probably through a direct interaction with adrenal steroid synthesis [55]. In addition to these effects, which are common to all OCPs, some progestins have anti-androgenic properties, due to their antagonizing effects on the androgen receptor (cyproterone acetate, drospirenone, dienogest) and to the inhibition of 5α-reductase activity [cyproterone acetate, chlormadinone acetate, "third-generation" progestins (desogestrel, gestodene, norgestimate), drospirenone, and dienogest] [54]. Although all OCPs are efficacious in reducing hirsutism, OCPs containing a progestin with antiandrogen properties are preferable for the treatment of hirsutism [56, 57].

In cases of moderate to severe forms of hirsutism not responsive to OCPs or, alternatively, when OCPs are contraindicated, the use of antiandrogens alone or combined with OCPs is indicated. Antiandrogens (androgen receptor blockers (flutamide, spironolactone) and 5α reductase inhibitors (finasteride, spironolactone)) are, in fact, the most effective drugs for hirsutism currently available [58]. At present there is not enough information to establish a scale of efficacy for these drugs. Some comparative studies did not find significant differences in efficacy between antiandrogens, whereas in other studies flutamide appeared to have the greatest efficacy and finasteride the lowest [22]. Furthermore, these drugs do not appear to extend dose-dependent effects against hirsutism [22]. Therefore, the minimum effective dose is recommended, in order to reduce the side effects. A recent randomized controlled study tested bicalutamide, an androgen receptor antagonist that interferes with the DHT-induced events required for activation of androgen receptor gene expression by androgens, with interesting results on hirsutism, but further studies are needed [30]. It must be stressed that antiandrogens cannot be given to pregnant women for the risk of feminization of male fetuses and should only be prescribed to women using secure contraception. An algorithm for the management of hirsutism is suggested in Fig. 12.6.

Conversely, virilization always deserves treatment, with an approach that may be medical and/or surgical depending upon the underlying disorder. Surgery is the treatment of choice for all patients with hormone-secreting adrenal or ovarian tumors [59, 60] and for those patients with virilization due to pituitary adenomas secreting ACTH, GH, or prolactin, if indicated.

CCAH always needs glucocorticoid treatment (associated with mineralocorticoid supplementation in the salt-wasting forms) and surgical correction of virilization. Standard treatment at diagnosis until growth is complete is hydrocortisone at 10–20 mg/m²/day, possibly divided into three doses, orally. Sometimes, in sick infants, 2 mg/kg of hydrocortisone hemisuccinate by i.v. bolus, followed by 20–30 mg/m²/day by constant i.v. infusion, may be a more appropriate initial treatment. After growth is complete, other more potent synthetic glucocorticoids may be used in a double (prednisone, prednisolone: hydrocortisone equivalent dose = 5) or a single (dexamethasone: hydrocortisone equivalent dose = 70) administration. Blood electrolytes need monitoring daily from day 3 of life, and if K⁺ rises or Na⁺ falls (salt loss occurs most frequently between day 6 and 21 of life), 9α-fludrocortisone should be started at 0.05–0.2 mg/day in

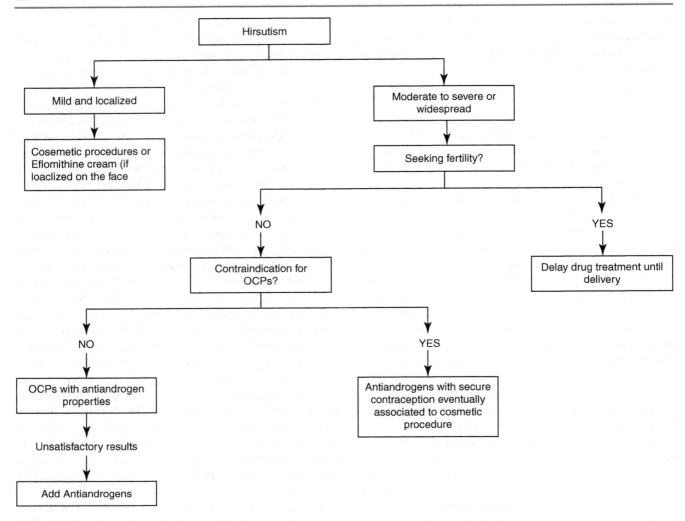

Fig. 12.6 Algorithm for the management of hirsutism

two divided doses. Salt supplementation (5 mEq/kg/day; NaCl = 1 g = 17 mEq) is a fundamental complement to mineralocorticoid treatment, at least in the first 6 months of life. Significant controversy exists on the timing of feminizing genitoplasty in girls with virilizing CCAH. When possible, feminizing genitoplasty should be a one-stage repair using the newest techniques. Clitoroplasty should only be considered in cases of severe virilization (Prader III–V) with prominence for functional outcome rather than cosmetic appearance. Vaginoplasty should be performed in infancy only if the persistence of a urogenital sinus causes complications. Surgical improvement generally needs to be done at puberty. Vaginal dilation is not recommended in childhood, while during young adulthood it may be useful to avoid the need for bowel vaginoplasty [27].

In families at risk for a virilized female newborn (index case affected by classic 21-hydroxylase or 11-hydroxylase deficien-

cies), prenatal diagnosis and treatment may be undertaken. Early administration (before 8 weeks of gestational age) of dexamethasone to the mother (20 μg/kg/pre-pregnancy), in fact, is able to prevent genital virilization in most affected females. Treatment should be started in all pregnancies at risk for virilized female newborn until chorionic villous sampling for sex and genetic analyses can be performed (10–11 weeks of gestational age). Thereafter, only affected female fetuses need to continue the treatment throughout pregnancy. To reduce the number of fetuses exposed to dexamethasone unnecessarily, polymerase chain reaction (PCR) for cell-free Y DNA in maternal blood at 5–6 weeks of gestation for prenatal sexing screening is now available as an experimental technique [61, 62]. In any case, due to possible maternal side effects (Cushing's syndrome) and the lack of long-term trials for its safety, antenatal dexamethasone treatment should only be carried out in specialized centers with the use of approved protocols [63].

References

1. Escobar-Morreale HF. Diagnosis and management of hirsutism. Ann N Y Acad Sci. 2010;1205:166–74.

2. Asuncion M, Calvo RM, San Millan JL, Sancho J, Avila S, Escobar-Morreale HF. A prospective study of the prevalence of the polycystic ovary syndrome in unselected Caucasian women from Spain. J Clin Endocrinol Metab. 2000;85:2434–8.

3. Sagsoz N, Kamaci M, Orbak Z. Body hair scores and total hair diameters in healthy women in the Kirikkale region of Turkey. Yonsei Med J. 2004;45:483–91.

4. DeUgarte CM, Woods KS, Bartolucci AA, Azziz R. Degree of facial and body terminal hair growth in unselected black and white women: toward a populational definition of hirsutism. J Clin Endocrinol Metab. 2006;91:1345–50.

5. Sanchón R, Gambineri A, Alpañés M, Martínez-García MÁ, Pasquali R, Escobar-Morreale HF. Prevalence of functional disorders of androgen excess in unselected premenopausal women: a study in blood donors. Hum Reprod. 2012;27:1209–16.

6. Cheewadhanaraks S, Peeyananjarassri K, Choksuchat C. Clinical diagnosis of hirsutism in Thai women. J Med Assoc Thail. 2004;87:459–63.

7. Noorbala MT, Kefaie P. The prevalence of hirsutism in adolescent girls in Yazd, Central Iran. Iran Red Crescent Med J. 2010;12:111–7.

8. Hickey M, Doherty DA, Atkinson H, Sloboda DM, Franks S, Norman RJ, et al. Clinical, ultrasound and biochemical features of polycystic ovary syndrome in adolescents: implications for diagnosis. Hum Reprod. 2011;26:1469–77.

9. Gambineri A, Prontera O, Fanelli F, Repaci A, Di Dalmazi G, Pagotto U, et al. Epidemiological survey on the prevalence of hyperandrogenic states in adolescent and young women. In: 15th International & 14th European congress of endocrinology, 5–9 2012, Florence, Italy.

10. New MI. Inborn errors of adrenal steroidogenesis. Mol Cell Endocrinol. 2003;211:75–83.

11. Balsamo A, Cacciari E, Piazzi S, Cassio A, Bozza D, Pirazzoli P, et al. Congenital adrenal hyperplasia: neonatal mass screening compared with clinical diagnosis only in the Emilia-Romagna region of Italy, 1980–1995. Pediatrics. 1996;98:362–7.

12. Stiller CA. International variations in the incidence of childhood carcinomas. Cancer Epidemiol Biom Prev. 1994;3:305–10.

13. Cagle PT, Hough AJ, Pysher TJ, Page DL, Johnson EH, Kirkland RT, et al. Comparison of adrenal cortical tumors in children and adults. Cancer. 1986;57:2235–7.

14. Federici S, Galli G, Ceccarelli PL, Ferrari M, Cicognani A, Cacciari E, et al. Adrenocortical tumors in children: a report of 12 cases. Eur J Pediatr Surg. 1994;4:21–5.

15. Balsamo A, Cacciari E. Le malattie del cortico-surrene. Edited by Prof. G. Saggese, Pacini Editore SPA, Via della Gherardesca 1, Ospedaletto, Pisa; in Monography n. 4. Endocrinologia Pediatrica; 2000, p. 31–56.

16. Young RH, Scully RE. Ovarian Sertoli-Leydig cell tumors. A clinicopathologic analysis of 207 cases. J Surg Pathol. 1985;9:543–69.

17. Azziz R, Carmina E, Dewailly D, Diamanti-Kandarakis E, Escobar-Morreale HF, Futterweit W, et al. The androgen excess and PCOS society criteria for the polycystic ovary syndrome: the complete task force report. Fertil Steril. 2009;91:456–88.

18. Carmina E. The spectrum of androgen excess disorders. Fertil Steril. 2006;85:1582–5.

19. Azziz R, Carmina E, Sawaya ME. Idiopathic hirsutism. Endocr Rev. 2000;21:347–62.

20. Uno H. Biology of hair growth. Semin Reprod Endocrinol. 1986;4:131–41.

21. Escobar-Morreale HF, Carmina E, Dewailly D, Gambineri A, Kelestimur F, Moghetti P, et al. Epidemiology, diagnosis and management of hirsutism: a consensus statement by the androgen excess and polycystic ovary syndrome. Hum Reprod Update. 2012;18:146–70.

22. Chen WC, Zouboulis CC. Hormones and the pilosebaceous unit. Dermatoendocrinol. 2009;1:81–6.

23. Thiboutot D, Jabara S, McAllister JM, Sivarajah A, Gilliland K, Cong Z, et al. Human skin is a steroidogenic tissue: steroidogenic enzymes and cofactors are expressed in epidermis, normal sebocytes, and an immortalized sebocyte cell line (SEB-1). J Invest Dermatol. 2003;120:905–14.

24. Longcope C. Adrenal and gonadal androgen secretion in normal females. Clin Endocrinol Metab. 1986;15:213–28.

25. Chrousos GP. Adrenal hyperandrogenism. http://www.UpToDate.com. 2012.

26. Orentreich N, Brind JL, Rizer RL, Vogelman JH. Age changes and sex differences in serum dehydroepiandrosterone sulfate concentrations throughout adulthood. J Clin Endocrinol Metab. 1984;59:551–5.

27. Balsamo A, Cicognani A, Ghirri P, Scaramuzzo RT, D'Alberton F, Bertelloni S, et al. Disorders of sexual development. In: Bonocore G, Bracci R, Weidlings M, editors. Neonatology: a practical approach to neonatal management. Milan, Italy: Springer-Verlag; 2011. Chapter 123, p. 1004–17.

28. Yamada G, Satoh Y, Baskin LS, Cunha GR. Cellular and molecular mechanisms of development of external genitalia. Differentiation. 2003;71:445–70.

29. Yildiz BO, Bolour S, Woods K, Moore A, Azziz R. Visually scoring hirsutism. Hum Reprod Update. 2010;16:51–64.

30. Moretti C, Guccione L, Di Giacinto P, Simonelli I, Exacoustos C, Toscano V, Motta C, De Leo V, Petraglia F, Lenzi A. Combined Oral contraception and Bicalutamide in polycystic ovary syndrome and severe hirsutism - a double-blind RTC. J Clin Endocrinol Metab. 2017; [Epub ahead of print]

31. Hatch R, Rosenfield RL, Kim MH, Tredway D. Hirsutism: implications, etiology, and management. Am J Obstet Gynecol. 1981;140:815–30.

32. Legro RS, Schlaff WD, Diamond MP, Coutifaris C, Casson PR, Brzyski RG, et al. For the reproductive medicine network. Total testosterone assays in women with polycystic ovary syndrome: precision and correlation with hirsutism. J Clin Endocrinol Metab. 2010;95:5305–13.

33. Fanelli F, Belluomo I, Di Lallo VD, Cuomo G, De Iasio R, Baccini M, et al. Serum steroid profiling by isotopic dilution-liquid chromatography-mass spectrometry: comparison with current immunoassays and reference intervals in healthy adults. Steroids. 2011;76:244–53.

34. Janse F, Eijkemans MJC, Goverde AJ, Lentjes EGWM, Hoek A, Lambalk CB, et al. Assessment of androgen concentration in women: liquid chromatography-tandem mass spectrometry and extraction RIA show comparable results. Eur J Endocrinol. 2011;165:925–33.

35. Balsamo A, Rinaldini D, Marsigli A, Monti S, Bettocchi I, Baronio F, et al. Screening e diagnosi dell'iperplasia surrenale congenita: dalle vecchie alle nuove tecnologie. Ligand Assay. 2012;17:1–10.

36. Pasquali R, Zanotti L, Fanelli F, Mezzullo M, Fazzini A, Morselli Labate AM, Repaci A, Ribichini D, Gambineri A. Defining hyperandrogenism in women with polycystic ovary syndrome: a challenging perspective. J Clin Endocrinol Metab. 2016;101:2013–22.

37. O'Reilly MW, Taylor AE, Crabtree NJ, Hughes BA, Capper F, Crowley RK, Stewart PM, Tomlinson JW, Arlt W. Hyperandrogenemia predicts metabolic phenotype in polycystic ovary syndrome: the utility of serum androstenedione. J Clin Endocrinol Metab. 2014;99:1027–36.

38. Balsamo A, Baldazzi L, Menabò S, Cicognani A. Impact of molecular genetics on congenital adrenal hyperplasia management. Sex Dev. 2010;4:233–48.

39. Koppens PF, Hoogenboezem T, Degenhart HJ. Duplication of the CYP21A2 gene complicates mutation analysis of steroid 21-hydroxylase deficiency: characteristics of three unusual haplotypes. Hum Genet. 2002;111:405–10.

40. White PC, Speiser PW. Congenital adrenal hyperplasia due to 21-hydroxylase deficiency. Endocr Rev. 2000;21:245–91.

41. Speiser PW, Dupont J, Zhu D, Serrat J, Buegeleisen M, Tusie-Luna MT, et al. Disease expression and molecular genotype in congenital adrenal hyperplasia due to 21-hydroxylase deficiency. J Clin Invest. 1992;90:584–95.

42. Welzel M, Schwarz HP, Hedderich J, Dörr HG, Binder G, Brämswig JH, et al. No correlation between androgen receptor CAG and GGN repeat length and the degree of genital virilization in females with 21-hydroxylase deficiency. J Clin Endocrinol Metab. 2010;95:2443–50.

43. Krone N, Arlt W. Genetics of congenital adrenal hyperplasia. Best Prac Res Clin Endocrinol Metab. 2009;23:181–92.

44. Arlt W, Walker EA, Draper N, Ivison HE, Ride JP, Hammer F, et al. Congenital adrenal hyperplasia caused by mutant P450 oxidoreductase and human androgen synthesis: analytical study. Lancet. 2004;363:2128.

45. Bongiovanni AM, Root AW. The adrenogenital syndrome. N Engl J Med. 1963;268:1283.

46. Guidi J, Gambineri A, Zanotti L, Fanelli F, Fava GA, Pasquali R. Psychological aspects of hyperandrogenic states in late adolescent and young women. Clin Endocrinol. 2015;83:872–8.

47. Richards RN, Meharg GE. Electrolysis: observations from 13 years and 140,000 hours of experience. J Am Acad Dermatol. 1995;33:662–6.

48. Haedersdal M, Wulf HC. Evidence-based review of hair removal using lasers and light sources. J Eur Acad Dermatol Venereol. 2006;20:9–20.

49. Sadighha A, Mohaghegh ZG. Meta-analysis of hair removal laser trials. Lasers Med Sci. 2009;24:21–5.

50. Barman Balfour JA, McClellan K. Topical Eflornithine. Am J Clin Dermatol. 2001;2:197–201.

51. Wolf JE Jr, Shander D, Huber F, Jackson J, Lin CS, Mathes BM, et al. Randomized, double-blind clinical evaluation of the efficacy and safety of topical eflornithine HCl 13.9% cream in the treatment of women with facial hair. Int J Dermatol. 2007;46:94–8.

52. Somani N, Turvy D. Hirsutism: an evidence-based treatment update. Am J Clin Dermatol. 2014;15:247–66.

53. Vissing AC, Taudorf EH, Haak CS, Philipsen PA, Hædersdal M. Adjuvant eflornithine to maintain IPL-induced hair reduction in women with facial hirsutism: a randomized controlled trial. J Eur Acad Dermatol Venereol. 2016;30:314–9.

54. Vrbíková J, Cibula D. Combined oral contraceptives in the treatment of polycystic ovary syndrome. Hum Reprod Update. 2005;11:277–91.

55. De Leo V, Morgante G, Piomboni P, Musacchio MC, Petraglia F, Cianci A. Evaluation of effects of an oral contraceptive containing ethinylestradiol combined with drospirenone on adrenal steroidogenesis in hyperandrogenic women with polycystic ovary syndrome. Fertil Steril. 2007;88:113–7.

56. Lello S, Primavera G, Colonna L, Vittori G, Guardianelli F, Sorge R, et al. Effects of two estroprogestins containing ethynilestradiol 30 microg and drospirenone 3 mg and ethynilestradiol 30 microg and chlormadinone 2 mg on skin and hormonal hyperandrogenic manifestations. Gynecol Endocrinol. 2008;24:718–23.

57. Batukan C, Muderris II, Ozcelik B, Ozturk A. Comparison of two oral contraceptives containing either drospirenone or cyproterone acetate in the treatment of hirsutism. Gynecol Endocrinol. 2007;23:38–44.

58. Swiglo BA, Cosma M, Flynn DN, Kurtz DM, Labella ML, Mullan RJ, et al. Clinical review: antiandrogens for the treatment of hirsutism: a systematic review and metaanalyses of randomized controlled trials. J Clin Endocrinol Metab. 2008;93:1153–60.

59. Chrousos GP. Is laparoscopic adrenalectomy suitable for all adrenal masses? Nat Clin Pract Endocrinol Metab. 2007;3:210.

60. Burges A, Schmalfeldt B. Ovarian cancer: diagnosis and treatment. Dtsch Arztebl Int. 2011;108:635–41.

61. Shearer BM, Thorland EC, Gonzales PR, Ketterling RP. Evaluation of a commercially available focused aCGH platform for the detection of constitutional chromosome anomalies. Am J Med Genet. 2007;143:2357–70.

62. Zimmermann B, Zhong XY, Holzgreve W, Hahn S. Real-time quantitative polymerase chain reaction measurement of male fetal DNA in maternal plasma. Methods Mol Med. 2007;132:43–9.

63. Lajic S, Nordenström A, Hirvikoski T. Long-term outcome of prenatal treatment of congenital adrenal hyperplasia. Endocr Dev. 2008;13:82–98.

Menopause

Thyciara Fontenelle, Alyne Layane Pereira Lemos, and Luiz Griz

Epidemiology

The Stages of Reproductive Aging Workshop (STRAW), in 2001, proposed a staging system, including menstrual and hormonal criteria, to define each stage of the process of reproductive senescence, constituting the gold standard to characterize all steps of the period [1].

Although the average age at menopause is 51 years, in 5% of women it occurs after 55 years of age, which is considered late menopause and in 5% between 40 and 45 years, which defines premature menopause. The cessation of cycles that occurs before the age of 40 is considered premature ovarian failure [2].

Various factors are considered as determinants of age at menopause. Thirteen common genetic variants located on chromosomes 5, 6, 19, and 20 related to age at menopause were identified [3]. Genetic variation in the estrogen receptor gene may be another determining factor, as well as permutations in the FMR1 gene that defines fragile X syndrome and causes premature ovarian failure [4].

Women with a family history of early menopause are at increased risk of developing amenorrhea earlier on. Women whose mothers started the phase of menopause at a young age have a sixfold greater likelihood of early menopause [5]. Race and ethnicity may also affect age at menopause. In two prospective, multiethnic studies, natural menopause occurred earlier among Hispanic women and later on in Americans and Japanese, when compared with a Caucasian population [6].

Smoking reduces age at menopause by about 2 years [7]. A study of 10,606 middle-aged women showed that 31% of female smokers developed natural menopause earlier than nonsmokers [8]. Other factors also seem to be involved, such as the consumption of galactose, a history of type 1 diabetes, intrauterine exposure to diethylstilbestrol, and nulliparity [3, 9].

Hormonal changes begin years before the menopause. In the final years of reproductive life, menstrual cycles are ovulatory, but gradually, the duration of the follicular phase begins to decrease. In the initial transition to menopause, women experience some menstrual irregularity, and in this phase inhibin B concentrations begin to fall due to a decline in the number of ovarian follicles, whereas FSH levels begin to rise with a relative maintenance of estradiol levels, but with low concentrations of progesterone [10].

In late transition there is an increase in the variability of the cycle, with fluctuations in serum levels of FSH and estradiol. Following menopause, when there is a total loss of ovarian follicles, the ovary can no longer synthesize estradiol but keep producing and secreting the androgenic hormones under the stimulus of luteinizing hormone (LH) [11].

Other endocrine changes present in the menopausal transition include the reduction of the anti-Müllerian hormone (AMH), a product of the granulosa cell, and the reduction in antral follicle count (AFC) of the ovary, defined as follicles of 2–10 mm in diameter on the transvaginal ultrasound [1].

After 12 months of amenorrhea in a woman aged over 45 years and in the absence of other physiological or pathological causes, we identify the presence of menopause.[4, 6]

Clinical Manifestations

Clinically women experience drastic changes in the body (Table 13.1). Chronic anovulation and progesterone deficiency can lead to long periods of uterine exposure to estrogen, thereby generating anovulatory bleeding and endometrial hyperplasia. Hot flashes, which are manifested in 75% of women, are the most common acute change during menopause. They are self-limited, with an average duration of 5 years, begin suddenly, and are characterized by a feeling of warmth in the face and chest that spreads rapidly. The heat sensation lasts about 2–4 min and is associated with intense

T. Fontenelle · A. L. P. Lemos (✉)
Endocrinology and Metabology, Hospital Agamenom Magalhães, Recife, PE, Brazil

L. Griz
Division of Endocrinology and Diabetes, University of Pernambuco Medical School, Hospital Agamenom Magalhães, Recife, PE, Brazil

© Springer Nature Switzerland AG 2022
F. Bandeira et al. (eds.), *Endocrinology and Diabetes*, https://doi.org/10.1007/978-3-030-90684-9_13

Table 13.1 Prevalence of menopausal symptoms

Symptoms	Prevalence
Hot flashes	41–79%
Sleep disturbance	38–43%
Depression	33%
Dementia	Uncertain
Vaginal dryness	20–47%
Sexual function	Uncertain
Cognitive changes	Uncertain
Joint pain	Uncertain
Fat mass gain	Uncertain
Skin changes	Uncertain
Breast pain	Uncertain

sweating, palpitations, and anxiety. It occurs predominantly at night, causing severe sleep disturbances [6].

Sleep disorders may be present in postmenopausal women, even in the absence of hot flashes at night. Anxiety and depression also influence, reducing patients' quality of life. Sexual dysfunction may be associated with impaired sleep [12].

As the epithelia of the vagina and urethra are sensitive to the action of estrogen, its thinning occurs during menopause, resulting in vaginal atrophy and related symptoms, a genitourinary syndrome of menopause (GSM) such as vaginal dryness, vaginitis, itching and pain during intercourse, and urethral atrophy, causing greater susceptibility to infections, overactive bladder, and urinary incontinence [13].

Sexual dysfunctions are highly prevalent in this period. Estradiol deficiency significantly reduces blood flow to the vagina and vulva, resulting in decreased vaginal lubrication and pudendal nerve neuropathy [14]. Vaginal dryness and dyspareunia, as previously mentioned, may contribute to decreased sexual function in this period [15].

Studies investigating the relationship between menopause and depression present conflicting findings. Some longitudinal studies have found no association. However, several others have shown a significant association between the menopausal transition and depression [16]. The largest prospective study to date, the Study of Women's Health Across the Nation (SWAN) trial, reported that perimenopausal women showed a higher rate of depressive symptoms (14.9–18.4%) than premenopausal women (8–12%), the most common symptoms being irritability, nervousness, and emotional lability [17].

Other, less common, symptoms are breast tenderness, headache, skin aging, and joint pain [18].

Diagnosis

Menopause is clinically defined as a period of 12 months of amenorrhea in a woman over 45 years of age in the absence of other biological or physiological causes. The best approach to the diagnosis of perimenopause is a longitudinal evaluation of the history of the menstrual cycle and menopausal symptoms (vasomotor waves, mood swings, sleep disturbances). There is no need for measurement of serum FSH, estradiol, or inhibin levels for diagnostic purposes.

Some medical conditions can mimic conditions of menopause, such as hyperthyroidism, which should always be considered in the differential diagnosis, and occur together with irregular menstruation, sweats (although different from typical hot flushes), and mood changes. Other causes for menstrual cycle changes should be considered, including pregnancy, hyperprolactinemia, and other thyroid diseases. Atypical hot flashes and night sweats may be present in other disorders, such as drug use, pheochromocytoma, carcinoid tumors, or other malignancies [19].

Hormone Therapy

Hormone therapy (HT) in postmenopausal women is currently recommended for use in short-term treatment of moderate to severe vasomotor symptoms. Long-term use for primary or secondary prevention of cardiovascular disease and osteoporosis is no longer recommended [20].

According to the recommendations of the American Association of Clinical Endocrinologists (AACE) 2017, the use of hormone therapy in postmenopausal symptomatic women should take into account all risk factors for cardiovascular disease, age, and time of menopause [21].

Vasomotor Symptoms

Hormone therapy, estrogen with or without progesterone, remains the gold standard treatment for the relief of menopausal vasomotor symptoms and their consequences. In a systematic review involving 24 trials and 3329 women, estrogen therapy was able to reduce 75% of frequency and 87% of the intensity of vasomotor symptoms when used at a standard dose. However, lower doses are also capable of minimizing 65% of the heat waves [22, 23]. It is therefore a reasonable option for most postmenopausal women, except those with a history of breast cancer and coronary heart disease, previous thromboembolic event or stroke, or at high risk for these complications. In healthy women, the absolute risk of an adverse event is extremely low [20]. The exclusive use of progesterone also reduces vasomotor symptoms, but less efficiently than estrogen therapy [24].

Genitourinary Tract

Both vaginal and urethral epithelia are sensitive to estrogen, and estrogen deficiency leads to their thinning, resulting in vaginal atrophy, which may generate symptoms of vaginal dryness, itching, and often dyspareunia. Both systemic and local estrogen therapy are effective for symptoms of genito-urinary atrophy. Vaginal administration (available as creams, tablets, or rings) is an extremely effective therapy, making it an excellent choice for nearly all postmenopausal women (with the exception of patients with breast cancer) and can be administered in the long term, since systemic absorption is minimal [20].

Local estrogen therapy may benefit some women with an overactive bladder. A clinical study demonstrated that using an estradiol ring showed clinical efficacy similar to the use of oxybutynin in women suffering from an overactive bladder [25]. The use of low-dose transdermal estradiol, however, did not affect the development of urinary incontinence [26]. A recent clinical trial reported an increased risk of nephroli-thiasis in healthy women on hormone therapy, but the mechanisms involved have not been elucidated [27]. Two studies have shown a reduced risk of recurrent urinary tract infection in women using vaginal estrogen therapy [28, 29].

Sexual Function

Hormone therapy is not recommended for the treatment of sexual dysfunction, including decreased libido [20]. There is no evidence that estrogen therapy acts independently in sexual interest, arousal, and orgasmic response. Low doses of local estrogen can improve sexual function merely by increasing local blood flow and vaginal lubrication [30].

Quality of Life

Although there is no approval for the use of hormone therapy for the sole purpose of improving the quality of life of women, data shows that symptomatic women show an improvement in some areas of quality of life through relief of vasomotor symptoms. There is no evidence to support this improvement in asymptomatic women [20].

Osteoporosis

Some randomized controlled trials and those controlled with placebo support the use of estrogen therapy for the prevention of osteoporosis and fractures, including hip fractures and treatment of proven osteoporosis [20]. However, to date, there has been no approval for their use in the treatment of osteoporosis in postmenopausal women without vasomotor symptoms. When prescribed for the prevention of postmenopausal osteoporosis, hormone therapy should only be considered for women with a significant risk of osteoporosis and fractures and for whom non-estrogenic drugs are considered inappropriate.

The results of the WHI trials indicated some benefits with hormone therapy. Women randomly assigned to estrogen and progesterone had a 34% reduction in the risk of vertebral and hip fractures (hip, 6 fewer per 10,000 woman-years; vertebral, 6 fewer per 10,000 woman-years; and total, 46 fewer per 10,000 woman years) [31].

Women randomly assigned to estrogen alone had fewer fractures (hip, 7 fewer per 10,000 woman-years; vertebral, 6 fewer per 10,000 woman-years; and total, 56 fewer per 10,000 woman-years). However, fractures were a major pre-defined secondary outcome and were determined by clinical criteria [31].

In a cross-sectional study, Papadakis and colleagues evaluated data from the OsteoLaus cohort involving 1279 menopausal women in 2016, investigating the positive impact of hormone therapy on the preservation of bone mineral density (BMD) and, for the first time, on the trabecular index (TBS), persistent effects for up to 2 years after withdrawal of hormone therapy [32].

When there are failures or adverse effects of standard therapy for osteoporosis, prolonged use of hormone therapy is an option for women at high risk of osteoporotic fractures. However, its beneficial effects on bone mass and fracture reduction are minimized quickly after its administration has been discontinued [33].

In women who experience premature menopause, unless there are contraindications, hormone therapy should be used for the purpose of bone loss prevention, rather than the standard therapy for osteoporosis, until they reach the age of menopause, when the treatment should be reevaluated [20].

Cardiovascular Effect

Based on extensive observational data, it was believed that estrogen exerted a cardioprotective effect, and as a result, estrogen therapy was routinely prescribed for primary and secondary prevention of cardiovascular disease (CVD).

In 1995, the PEPI Trial evaluated cardiovascular risk in healthy postmenopausal women. A total of 875 women between the ages of 45 and 64 years were evaluated. Participants were randomized into five groups: the placebo group; those who used conjugated equine estrogen at a dose of 0.625 mg/day alone; associated with cyclic medroxyprogesterone acetate, 10 mg daily for 12 days per month; conjugated equine estrogen associated with medroxyprogesterone of continuous use at the dose of 2.5 mg/day; and estrogen at the dose of 0.625 mg/day associated with cyclic micronized progesterone 200 mg/day for 12 days in the month. It was concluded that the use of estrogen alone or in combination with progesterone improved lipoproteins and reduced levels of fibrinogen, without significant effects on insulin or blood pressure. When estrogen alone was evaluated, it was ideal for the elevation of HDL, but restricted for hysterectomized women. In women with uterus, estrogen with the cyclic micronized progesterone had a more favorable effect on HDL [34].

Data from the Heart and Estrogen/Progestin Replacement Study (HERS I and II), other small controlled trials and two meta-analyses have not confirmed this protective effect on the heart [35–37]. The HERS I study demonstrated a twofold to threefold increase in the risk of venous thrombosis and pulmonary embolism with hormone therapy. However, the absolute risk was low, ranging from one case to two or three cases per 100,000 women. The data is related to the oral use of the hormone. The HERS II study found a 2.89 times risk of thromboembolism in users of combined hormone therapy, estrogen/progesterone, compared with the placebo and a trend toward an increased risk of pulmonary embolism.

In 2002, the subgroup of women in the WHI who used the estrogen-progestin combination showed an increased risk of coronary heart disease and breast cancer, and the study was discontinued prematurely. The results of the subgroup that used only estrogen therapy, published in 2004, showed a tendency to a decreased risk of breast cancer, but an increased risk of stroke and thromboembolic disease, and no benefits on coronary heart disease [20, 31].

Some, but not all, observational studies suggest that long-term hormonal therapy is associated with a smaller accumulation of calcium in the coronary arteries, data which is strongly correlated with the presence of atheromatous plaques and the risk of future coronary events [38].

The WHI trial found a risk twice higher of pulmonary embolism in users of combined hormone therapy, representing eight more cases of pulmonary embolism in 10,000 women/year. This risk was attributed to the combination of estrogen and progestin [20, 31]. There is no data for other, non-oral forms of administration of hormonal therapy.

The WHI showed an increase in the risk of stroke, but no effect on hemorrhaging. When all women in that trial were analyzed, there were 8 additional cases of stroke per 10,000 women/year in combined therapy and 11 cases per 10,000 women/year in estrogen-alone therapy, and in both, the risk was eliminated after discontinuation of treatment [31]. In a recent data analysis from the WHI trial involving only women aged 50–59 years, there was no significant effect on the risk of stroke [39]. The risk of stroke did not significantly increase in the HERS I and II studies [40, 41]. The data from observational studies on the association between hormone therapy and stroke have been inconsistent. Various studies have indicated a positive association, but others showed no effect on the risk of stroke [20].

One difference between observational studies and the WHI study is the fact that the women enrolled in the latter presented an average age of 63 years at the start of the use of hormone therapy, about 12 years after menopause had begun [20, 31]. Participants in the observational studies began therapy immediately after the beginning of menopause, with a mean age of 51 years, that is, women from the WHI were older and began using the hormone later, which is unusual in clinical practice. As the atherosclerotic lesions develop early, it is likely that the WHI participants already presented subclinical coronary disease and therefore would not be candidates for hormonal regime, since hormonal therapy appears to be more effective in primary prevention than in secondary prevention. The idea that differences in age or time since menopause at the start of hormone therapy are responsible for differences in cardiovascular outcomes has become known as the "window of opportunity" [42].

In the observational studies and in animal models that suggested beneficial cardiovascular effects of hormone therapy, the subjects generally initiated therapy at the time of menopause (often for management of vasomotor symptoms), or in animal studies, treatment began immediately after ovariectomy. This contrast with the WHI, which treatment was initiated more than a decade after menopause in most study participants, led to the development of the "window of opportunity." This theory proposed that initiation of HT at or shortly after menopause is cardioprotective, whereas starting treatment at a time remote from menopause may be harmful. Indeed, in the WHI, the trend toward lower rates of CVD events was noted in women who were within 10 years of menopause or who were aged 50–59 years at the time of entry into the trial. In the estrogen and progestin arm, women within 10 years of the menopausal transition had a hazard ratio (HR) of coronary heart disease (CHD) events of 0.89, compared with 1.71 in those more than 20 years from menopausal transition. In the conjugated equine estrogen (CEE) alone arm, those aged 50–59 years had an HR of 0.56, compared with older women, whose HR was almost 1.0 [42].

In addition, women enrolled in the CEE arm and aged 50–59 at baseline had coronary calcium measured by computed tomography; women who received CEE had significantly lower scores at trial completion than those who received placebo [38]. In this young population, the incidence of coronary events was low, and the absolute risk of clinical CHD events was small. In a more recent analysis, the results were examined after pooling the data from the WHI estrogen-alone and estrogen and progestin trials [42]. Women enrolled within 10 years of the onset of menopause had a HR for CHD of 0.76 (CI, 0.50–1.16). The HR continued to rise years after the menopause. Initiating therapy from 10 to 19 years after menopause gave a HR of 1.10 (CI, 0.84–1.45), and when initiated after 20 or more years, the HR was 1.28 (CI, 1.03–1.58). The P value for the trend was 0.02, supporting the timing hypothesis, which predicts that protection from atherosclerosis is evident only when hormone therapy is initiated shortly prior to the onset of menopause and before the development of advanced atherosclerotic plaques.

The timing hypothesis is further supported by several recent studies. A Bayesian meta-analysis of hormone therapy mortality in younger postmenopausal women (mean age, 55 years) presented the combined results of 19 randomized clinical trials that enrolled 16,000 women at a mean age of 55 years, totaling 83,000 patient-years. This study showed a relative risk of mortality of 0.73 [20]. The analysis also demonstrated a cardiovascular benefit when HT was initiated early, supporting the timing hypothesis. Current ongoing prospective randomized trials will formally test this hypothesis.

Despite this reassuring data, HT in postmenopausal women is still indicated only for the management of vasomotor symptoms, since there is no data to support its use in primary or secondary prevention of coronary disease.

The Kronos Early Estrogen Prevention Study (KEEPS) evaluated cardiovascular risk in 728 women aged 42 to 58 years who started hormone therapy in the first months of menopause (6–36 months postmenopausal). HT consisted of oral conjugated estrogens (Premarin®, 0.45 mg), transdermal estradiol (Climara®, 50 μg), or placebo with micronized progesterone (Prometrium®, 200 mg) for 12 days per month or placebo for women with an intact uterus. The endpoints were the coronary artery calcification score measured by computed tomography and the intima carotid thickness (IMT). Preliminary results showed no difference in the rate of progression of intima carotid thickness in the three groups. No estrogenic formulation raised blood pressure. Conjugated oral estrogens increased HDL and reduced LDL and increased triglycerides and C-reactive protein. Transdermal estradiol improved glucose levels and insulin sensitivity. In this study there were no significant differences in rates of clinical events including breast and endometrial cancer and cardiovascular disease among the three groups. It should be noted that the population studied consisted of a small group of healthy and relatively young women. In the group treated with hormones, symptoms such as heat waves were reduced; BMD and sexual function improved when compared to controls [21, 43].

The Early versus Late Intervention Trial with Estradiol (ELITE) [44] evaluated a total of 643 healthy postmenopausal women using estradiol 1 mg daily and progesterone 45 mg during 10 days of each 30-day cycle with women with preserved uterus for 5 years, comparing them with distinct times of the beginning of HT (<6 years, early onset, or >10 years, late onset). Women treated with estradiol in both age groups/timing had lower LDL and higher levels of HDL and triglycerides compared to untreated women in both groups. The rate of progression of coronary artery calcification measured by CT was lower in the postmenopausal group treated with estrogen than in its placebo group or the group treated with estrogen later on in the menopause. The group treated later in menopause did not differ from the cohort

taken with placebo. The study concluded that oral estradiol therapy was associated with a lower progression of subclinical atherosclerosis (measured as IMT) than placebo when therapy was initiated within 6 years after menopause but not when 10 or more [21, 44].

A subgroup analysis of the Danish Osteoporosis Prevention Study, involving 1006 women aged 45 to 58 years, randomized to the use of three-phase estradiol and norethisterone acetate in those with uterus and estradiol 2 mg day in those hysterectomized versus placebo demonstrated, after 10-year and 16-year follow-up, that 16 women in the treatment group had the primary composite outcome (death, hospital admission for heart failure, and myocardial infarction) compared to 33 in the control group (hazard ratio 0.48, confidence interval 95%, 0.26 to 0.87, $P = 0.015$), and 15 died compared to 26 (0.57, 0.30 to 1.08, $P = 0.084$). Reduction in cardiovascular events was not associated with increased cancer (36 in the treated group, 39 in the control group, 0.92, 0.58 to 1.45, $P = 0.71$) or with breast cancer (10 in the treated group, 17 in the control group, 0.58, 0.27 to 1.27, $P = 0.17$). The risk ratio for deep vein thrombosis (2 in treated group, 1 in the control group) was 2.01 (0.18 to 22.16) and for stroke (11 in treated group, 14 in the control group) was 0.77 (0.35 to 1.70). After 16 years, the reduction in the primary outcome result was still present and not associated with an increase in cancer. After 10 years of treatment, women who received HT early after menopause had a significantly reduced risk of mortality, heart failure, or myocardial infarction without any apparent increase in the risk of cancer, venous thromboembolism, or stroke [21].

Another topic of constant debate is the role of the mode of administration of the hormone in relation to the adverse effects observed in large studies. The oral route is associated with an increase in thrombotic effects and decreased synthesis of thrombolytic factors in the liver, induced by the hepatic first pass of estradiol, which could justify a two- to threefold increase in the risk of thromboembolism observed with the use of oral, but not transdermal, estrogen [20, 45]. Low-dose, cyclic, and transdermal formulations have been suggested as potentially favorable alternatives. Unfortunately, no large, prospective, randomized trials exist that carefully compare these alternative regimens.

Diabetes Mellitus

Large clinical trials have shown that hormone therapy reduces the appearance of type 2 diabetes mellitus (T2DM), despite not having been approved as a prevention measure in this disease. Women in the WHI and HERS studies who received estrogen/progesterone showed an average reduction of 21% in the incidence of T2DM [46].

Endometrial Cancer

Women constantly exposed to endogenous or exogenous estrogens not neutralized by progesterone are at increased risk of developing hyperplasia and endometrial cancer. The risk of endometrial cancer is six to eight times higher in women using estrogen compared with women who do not use it [47].

Breast Cancer

The relationship between breast cancer and hormone therapy is complex. There are dozens of observational, case-control, and cohort studies, with results which are not very consistent. A meta-analysis of observational studies, carried out in 1997, summed up 90% of the literature (53,705 women with breast cancer, compared with 108,411 controls) and showed that each year of hormone therapy confers a relative risk for breast cancer of 2.3%, attributable to the use of progesterone [48].

Despite demonstrating an increased incidence, the present study, like others, showed no increase in mortality from the disease. The use of estrogen/progestin for the group of women in the WHI study was discontinued because of the 26% increase in the risk of breast cancer, that is, for every 10,000 women, 38 developed breast cancer, while among nonusers of hormone therapy, 30 cases of breast cancer in 10,000 women were found [31].

Studies have not clarified whether the risk of breast cancer differs between continuous and intermittent use of progesterone, with observational studies suggesting that the risk may be greater with the continuous use of this drug. It is also unclear whether there is a class effect of progesterone or if a specific agent influences a higher risk of breast cancer. Data from a large observational study suggests that hormone therapy with micronized progesterone carries a low risk of breast cancer with short-term use but generates an increased risk if used for long periods [49].

It is known that combination therapy and, to a lesser extent, estrogen-alone therapy promote increased proliferation of breast cells, breast tenderness, and increased mammographic density, complicating the interpretation of mammography and delaying the diagnosis of breast cancer [20].

In The Million Women Study (MWS), researchers reported an increased risk of breast cancer in women who start hormone therapy soon after menopause [50]. Women in the WHI study who used estrogen alone had no increased risk of developing breast cancer after an average of 7.1 years of use, and there was even a decrease in the risk in this arm of the study, despite having shown an increase in risk early in treatment. It is claimed that the hypothesis that justifies this reduction in risk is the probable apoptotic effect exerted by estrogen on neoplastic mammary cells in an environment with low levels of estrogen [20]. This finding was not demonstrated in the MWS [50].

Ovarian Cancer

The association between hormone therapy and ovarian cancer is unclear. A cohort study of 44,241 postmenopausal women concluded that women who used estrogen alone as hormone therapy for more than 10 years had a significant risk of developing ovarian cancer, while those who used combined therapy for a short period showed no increased risk [51]. According to data from the MWS, women using hormone therapy are at increased risk for ovarian cancer [52]. Another observational study found a strong association between estrogen and death due to ovarian cancer. Moreover, the risk is increased in women who used estrogen for 10 years or more [20].

In a post hoc analysis of the arm of WHI using combination therapy for an average of 7.1 years, the incidence of non-small cell lung cancer did not increase significantly; there was, however, a significant increase in the number of deaths from this cancer, as well as the presence of metastatic and poorly differentiated tumors. This association was found exclusively in women over 60 years who were smokers or who had a history of smoking. The arm that used only estrogen therapy exhibited no increase in incidence or mortality from lung cancer [53].

Cognition and Dementia

Randomized controlled studies of short duration, comparing estrogen with placebo, show inconsistent results. The methodology, the type of estrogen, age, the type of menopause (natural or surgical), and, in particular, the tests performed are different. Some studies show benefits in some tests, focused mainly on memory and verbal fluency in patients using estrogen [20]. A meta-analysis concluded that the evidence is still scanty and inconsistent and does not explain the improvement in symptoms and relief from depression, indicating the need to evaluate the various types of hormone therapy used [54].

WHIMS reported hormone therapy (HT), conjugated equine estrogen (CEE) with or without medroxyprogesterone acetate (MPA), increased the risk for dementia [HR 1.76 (95% CI, 1.19–2.60); $P = 0.005$] and global cognitive decline, with a mean decrement relative to placebo of 0.21 points on the Modified Mini-Mental State Examination in women aged 65 and older. A subset of WHIMS participants joined the ancillary WHI Study of Cognitive Aging

(WHISCA) trials, in which domain-specific cognitive tests and mood were measured annually. Compared with placebo, CEE + MPA had a negative impact on verbal memory over time and CEE-alone was associated with lower spatial rotational ability at the initial assessment, but the difference diminished over time. The ancillary WHIMS-MRI study measured subclinical cerebrovascular disease to possibly explain the negative cognitive findings reported by WHIMS and the increased clinical stroke in older women reported by the WHI. WHIMS-MRI reported that while CEE + MPA and CEE-alone were not associated with increased ischemic brain lesion volume relative to placebo, both CEE + MPA and CEE-alone were associated with lower mean brain volumes in the hippocampus, frontal lobe, and total brain [55].

The evidence linking estrogen use with the prevention of Alzheimer's disease is still inconsistent. Some observational, case-control, and cohort studies have shown reduced incidence of Alzheimer's disease in women using estrogen compared with nonusers. Not all studies have shown favorable results [20].

Principles of Treatment

Patient Selection

In view of the results of the new clinical trials and the legacy brought by WHI, a risk stratification for the use of hormone therapy was developed, suggesting that a certain group of women would have a lower risk of adverse cardiovascular outcome. An age less than 60 years, onset of HT in the first 10 years postmenopausal, LDL less than 130 mg/dl or LDL/HDL ratio <2.5, absence of metabolic syndrome, and absence of genotype for Leiden factor V confer less risk. When analyzing the clinical impact of the KEEPS, WHI, and ELITE studies, we found that the results are reassuring for patients who require HT to treat menopausal symptoms at a young age [21, 44].

Although there are alternative therapies for the treatment of vasomotor symptoms, none appear to be as effective in the short term as hormone therapy, which is the gold standard treatment for most women with postmenopausal symptoms, except for those with a history of breast cancer and coronary heart disease, with a previous thromboembolic event or CHD, or at high risk for these complications. In the past, short-term therapy was defined as less than 5 years. This definition is somewhat arbitrary, since there is no consensus on the duration of treatment.

To date, postmenopausal HT, either using estrogen alone or in combination, should not be initiated for the prevention of cardiovascular diseases. Furthermore, postmenopausal HT is no longer considered a first-line option for the prevention and treatment of osteoporosis [20].

Preparations

Both estrogen and progesterone present common features typical of the class of drug, but also with potentially different properties (Table 13.2). In the absence of clinical trials designed to compare different hormonal formulations, it is necessary to generalize the results to all drugs belonging to this class. It is possible, however, to find differences within each family, such as potency, androgenicity, glucocorticoid effect, bioavailability, and route of administration.

Progesterone is recommended for all postmenopausal women with an indication for hormone therapy to prevent the risk of endometrial cancer in those women with an intact uterus [20].

Dose and Route of Administration

Although it is not known whether lower doses of estrogen and progesterone have less effect on the cardiovascular system and the risk of breast cancer, it is recommended to use low hormone doses, when possible (e.g., 0.3–0.45 mg of oral conjugated estrogens, 0.5 mg of oral estradiol, or 0.014–0.0375 mg of transdermal estradiol). In some studies, these doses have proved to be suitable for the treatment of symptoms. Many studies on the efficacy and safety of use of estrogen have used conjugated estrogen at a dose of 0.625 mg, considered to be the standard dose. Low-dosage preparations generally contain half this dose [56].

Low-dose estrogen formulations are also available in the form of gel, cream, ova pill, and spray. The use of low hormonal doses sometimes requires a longer period of treatment to achieve maximum effectiveness in reducing vasomotor symptoms. Individualization of doses according to the woman's needs presents a good therapeutic strategy. Lower doses are associated with a lower incidence of side effects such as uterine bleeding and breast tenderness and may have a more favorable risk-benefit ratio [20].

In a case-control study, the risk of CHD was not increased with the use of low-dose transdermal estrogen (0.05 mg) but showed an increase with the use of oral and transdermal formulation with a higher dosage [57]. All routes of administration can effectively treat vasomotor symptoms. Non-oral routes of administration, including vaginal and intrauterine ones, and transdermal patches, may offer both advantages and disadvantages compared to the oral route, but the long-term risk-benefit ratio has still not been demonstrated in clinical trials [20].

There are differences regarding the role of the hepatic first-pass effect, the hormone concentrations in the blood, and the biological activity of preparations. With transdermal therapy there is no significant increase in triglyceride levels, C-reactive protein, hormone-binding globulin, and the effect

Table 13.2 Types of hormonal therapy for vasomotor symptoms

Drug	Route	Dose
17β-Estradiol	Oral	1–2 mg/day
Ethinyl estradiol	Oral	0.02–0.05 mg 1–3 times daily
Conjugated equine estrogens	Oral	0.3–1.25 mg/day
17β-Estradiol patch	Transdermal	0.014 mg/d–0.0375 mg/day 1 patch twice/week
17β-Estradiol gel	Transdermal	0.25 mg/d or 0.75 mg/d 0.25 g gel daily 1.25 g gel daily
Estradiol 1 mg + norethindrone acetate 0,5 mg	Oral	1 tab daily
Ethinyl estradiol 5mcg + norethindrone acetate 1 mg	Oral	1 tab daily
17β-Estradiol 1 mg + norgestimate 0.09 mg	Oral	First 3 tablets contain estrogen, next 3 contain both hormones, alternate pills every 3 days
CEE 0.625 mg + medroxyprogesterone acetate 5 mg	Oral	First 14 tablets contain estrogen only and remaining 14 tablets contain both hormones
CEE 0.625 mg + medroxyprogesterone acetate 2.5 mg or 5 mg	Oral	1 tab daily
17β-Estradiol + norethindrone acetate	Transdermal	0.05 mg/0.14 mg daily; 1 patch twice/week
17β-Estradiol + levonorgestrel	Transdermal	0.45 mg/0,015 mg daily; 1 patch weekly
CEE 0.45 mg + Bazedoxifene 20 mg	Oral	1 tablet daily
Medroxyprogesterone acetate	Oral	1.5–2.5 mg daily
Norethindrone acetate	Oral	0.1 mg daily in combination preparations or 14 days/month
Drospirenone	Oral	0.25 mg daily
Micronized progesterone	Oral	100 mg/d continuously or 200 mg/d for 12 days/month
Norethindrone acetate	Transdermal	0.14 mg/d 1 patch twice/week
Levonorgestrel	Transdermal	0.015 mg/d 1 patch/week

on arterial pressure. It is suggested by the AACE 2017 recommendations that the transdermal route may be advantageous for diabetic women and other cardiovascular risk factors as well as for women in old age [21]. There is a growing observational evidence that the transdermal route may be associated with a lower risk of deep vein thrombosis, CHD, and myocardial infarction [20].

There are various dosage options of progesterone with no harm to the endometrium. The dose varies according to the progestin chosen and the estrogen system used, starting with the lowest effective doses, such as 1.5 mg of medroxyprogesterone acetate, 0.1 mg of norethindrone acetate, 0.5 mg of drospirenone, or 100 mg micronized progesterone. Oral progestogens, oral estrogen combinations, and combinations in the form of a patch have demonstrated endometrial protection and have been approved for use in postmenopausal hormone therapy.

Duration of Treatment

For postmenopausal women with moderate to severe vasomotor symptoms, and no contraindication for the use of estrogen, hormonal therapy is suggested as the treatment of choice. The lowest effective dose of estrogen should be used, with the shortest possible duration. Short-term therapy is considered for 2–3 years and generally not more than 5 years. Only a minority of women unable to successfully discontinue treatment without the persistence of symptoms may be considered for a longer period of use, under close medical supervision [20]. Hormone therapy does not need to be routinely discontinued in women over 60 or 65 years old, and maintenance of its use may be considered beyond 65 years for persistent vasomotor symptoms, severe impairment of quality of life, or prevention of osteoporosis after adequate evaluation and advice on benefits and risks. Annual reassessment including review of comorbidities and periodic HT reduction or discontinuation testing or change to low-dose transdermal patch routes should be considered [58].

Discontinuation of Treatment

Many women do not have problems at the time of discontinuation of treatment. Observational studies suggest that 40–50% of women discontinue hormone therapy 1 year after starting treatment, and 65–75% stop in the second year, most often without medical follow-up. For other women the abrupt discontinuation of medication provokes the return of vasomotor symptoms and requires the resumption of treatment [20].

The North American Menopause Society suggests that after a failed attempt to stop the therapy, prolonged use of postmenopausal hormone therapy may be reasonable for women who find that the benefits of symptom relief outweigh the risks. In this context, additional attempts are required at a later date for the discontinuation of postmenopausal hormone therapy [58].

Complementary and Alternative Therapies

Nonhormonal Therapy for Vasomotor Symptoms

α-Adrenergic agonists such as clonidine have been used with variable success, although scientific data is contradictory [59]. A randomized clinical trial using oral clonidine showed no reduction in vasomotor symptoms. Normally, doses of 0.1 mg a day are required. Sometimes it can cause postural hypotension and have side effects in 50% of users, including insomnia. Beta-blockers have been used for the control of anxiety and palpitation but are not useful for hot flashes [60].

Serotonin selective reuptake inhibitors such as fluoxetine, paroxetine, and citalopram have been used in some studies. The most favorable finding indicates paroxetine at a dose of 10 mg per day, as higher doses were not associated with better symptom control. It may have adverse effects on the libido and should not be prescribed in patients with breast cancer using tamoxifen because it may modify the action of that drug [61].

Selective noradrenaline reuptake inhibitors, such as venlafaxine, have been reported as effective in some small studies, especially in women with breast cancer unable to use hormone therapy. Usually venlafaxine is initiated at a dose of 37.5 mg and adjusted to a dose of 75 mg a day if necessary [61].

Gabapentin has also been used to relieve vasomotor symptoms in women with breast cancer. The dose used is usually 300 mg three times a day, but in order to reduce side effects, the dose may be gradually titrated, in other words, 300 mg per day for 2 weeks, 300 mg twice a day for 2 weeks, and finally, 300 mg three times a day after the first month (Table 13.3) [61].

Table 13.3 Nonhormonal pharmacological therapy for vasomotor symptoms

Class	Drug	Dose
α-Adrenergic agonists	Clonidine	0.1 mg a day
Serotonin selective reuptake inhibitors	Fluoxetine	20 mg a day
Anticholinergic	Oxybutynin	5–10 mg a day
Serotonin selective reuptake inhibitors	Paroxetine	7.5–10 mg a day
Serotonin selective reuptake inhibitors	Citalopram	20 mg a day
Selective noradrenaline reuptake inhibitors	Venlafaxine	75 mg a day
Selective noradrenaline reuptake inhibitors	Desvenlafaxine	100 mg a day
Structural analogue gamma aminobutyric acid	Gabapentin	900 mg a day

Other Hormone Therapies

In the USA dehydroepiandrosterone (DHEA) has been used to relieve vasomotor symptoms but has not been widely used in other countries such as the UK. Some studies have shown beneficial effects on libido, bone metabolism, cognition, well-being, and vaginal lubrication. An uncontrolled pilot study showed a slight decrease in hot flashes using DHEA. The treatment of GSM in estrogen-sensitive cancer survivors is challenging, since vaginal estrogen may be contraindicated. In a randomized study comparing two doses of vaginal DHEA with a nonhormonal vaginal moisturizer in postmenopausal cancer survivors, especially breast cancer, all three groups reported similar improvement in dyspareunia and vaginal dryness symptoms after 12 weeks of treatment, but only the group that used DHEA at the highest dose reported significant improvement in sexual function. Although it is a promising treatment for this specific subgroup of women, safety data are required [62]. Evidence on the use of natural progesterone cream is limited, with studies showing no symptom relief compared with placebo [63].

Phytohormones

Phytoestrogens, nonsteroidal compounds that are naturally present in many plants, fruits, and vegetables, present both estrogenic and antiestrogen activities. They are usually found in soybeans, lentils, flaxseed, grains, fruits, and vegetables. Data suggests that the lower risk of heart disease among Asian women compared with Western populations is due to the high consumption of soy products. This observation has led to an increasing interest in the potential use of phytoestrogens as an alternative to hormone therapy in postmenopausal women. In fact, an increasing percentage of women (including women with a history of breast cancer) use soy products in their diet to help control the symptoms of menopause. Moreover, many women believe that phytoestrogens, because they are "natural," are safer than hormone therapy, although this has never been proven [64].

A review of the Cochrane Database of 30 randomized trials evaluated the efficacy, safety, and acceptability of foods and supplements, including all phytoestrogens. The reviewers concluded that there was no evidence that phytoestrogens help relieve menopausal symptoms [64].

Botanicals

There is a wide range of natural products that have been used as a complementary therapy in menopause, without scientific evidence, such as St. John's wort, *Cimicifuga racemosa*, ginseng, dong quai, agnus castus, and *Gingko biloba* [65].

Tibolone

Tibolone, a drug that has been widely used in Europe and other countries for almost 20 years, is a synthetic steroid whose metabolites have estrogenic, androgenic, and progestogenic properties. It reduces vasomotor symptoms when compared to placebo and has a beneficial effect on bone mineral density. Limited data suggests that it may also have a modest effect on symptoms of sexual dysfunction. However, tibolone has been associated with an increased risk of stroke recurrence and possibly breast cancer, based on data from the LIFT and LIBERATE studies, respectively, and is therefore not recommended for routine use in the management of menopausal symptoms [66]. The LIFT trial, designed to examine the effect of tibolone on vertebral fractures in postmenopausal women, reported a reduction in the absolute risk of vertebral and non-vertebral fractures (8.6 and 6.9 per 1000 person-years, respectively, relative hazards of 0.55, 95% CI 0.41–0.74 and 0.74, 95% CI 0.58–0.93, respectively). However, this trial was discontinued early, owing to an increased risk of stroke [67].

Ospemifene

Ospemifene is a SERM with agonist action of estrogen in the vaginal epithelium and without estrogenic effect clinically significant in the endometrium or in the breast. Ospemifene was approved by the US Food and Drug Administration (FDA) in 2013 for the treatment of moderate to severe dyspareunia caused by vulvovaginal atrophy in menopausal women. Its use is indicated for women with symptomatic vulvovaginal atrophy refractory to non-pharmacological therapy, with contraindication to the use of vaginal estrogen or in those with difficulty of application, as in patients with severe obesity. Its disadvantages in relation to the use of vaginal estrogen are the need for daily use, the appearance of heat waves, and the potential risk of thromboembolism [68].

Bazedoxifene, a selective estrogen receptor modulator (SERM) with breast and endometrial safety, combined with conjugated estrogens, is available in the USA and Europe for the treatment of vasomotor symptoms and prevention of osteoporosis. The combination of conjugated estrogen at the dose of 0.45 mg and bazedoxifene 20 mg in women with moderate to severe heat waves decreases their frequency by approximately 75% versus 50% for placebo. To date no serious adverse events have been reported [69, 70].

Others

A neurokinin 3 receptor antagonist (NK3R) is a potential non-hormonal therapy for the control of heat waves. In a randomized, placebo-controlled clinical trial of an oral NK3R antagonist administered for 4 weeks in symptomatic postmenopausal women, the average weekly number of heat waves decreased from approximately 85 at the baseline to 20 and 50 in the treatment and placebo, respectively. The residual heat waves in the treatment group were also less severe. While the results of this assay are encouraging, long-term trials are required to determine the efficacy and safety of this drug [71].

Vitamin E has been associated with decreased vasomotor symptoms in an isolated clinical trial [72]. Herbs of traditional Chinese medicine, reflexology, and magnetic devices have been studied but have no beneficial effects [73]. Acupuncture has been studied as a potential therapy for hot flashes, but results so far are not promising [74].

The Future

Although there is a real need to treat vasomotor symptoms and sleep disturbance in the menopausal transition, the long-term risks of hormone therapy preclude extended duration of use for the prevention of chronic disease. Although studies are currently under way to determine whether CHD risk will be impacted by the timing of initiation, the cancer risks are present at all ages, and some seem to persist after cessation of hormone therapy. The reduction in hip and vertebral fracture dissipates after stopping hormone therapy, whereas the long-term risk of breast cancer and possibly lung and ovarian cancers continues. Alternative therapies for menopausal symptoms that would not increase the risk of cancer are sorely needed. Because breast cancer seems significantly impacted by the use of progestin, ways to oppose estrogen's effect on the uterus without the use of a progestin are currently being developed.

References

1. Soules MR, Sherman S, Parrott E, et al. Executive summary: stages of reproductive aging workshop (STRAW). Climacteric. 2001;4:267–72.
2. Cramer DW, Barbieri RL, Xu H, Reichardt JK. Determinants of basal follicle-stimulating hormone levels in premenopausal women. J Clin Endocrinol Metab. 1994;79(4):1105.
3. Stolk L, Zhai G, van Meurs JBJ, et al. Loci at chromosomes 13, 19 and 20 influence age at natural menopause. Nat Genet. 2009;41:645.
4. De Vries BB, Halley DJ, Oostra BA, Niermeijer MF. The fragile X syndrome. J Med Genet. 1998;35(7):579.
5. Cramer DW, Xu H, Harlow BL. Family history as a predictor of early menopause. Fertil Steril. 1995;64:740–5.
6. Soules MR, Sherman S, Parrott E, Rebar R, Santoro N, Utian W, Woods N. Executive summary: stages of reproductive aging workshop (STRAW). Fertil Steril. 2001;76(5):874.
7. McKinlay SM, Bifano NL, McKinlay JB. Smoking and age at menopause in women. Ann Intern Med. 1985;103(3):350.
8. Cramer DW, Harlow BL, Xu H, Fraer C, Barbieri R. Cross-sectional and case-controlled analyses of the association between smoking and early menopause. Maturitas. 1995;22(2):79–87.

9. Cooper GS, Hulka BS, Baird DD, Savitz DA, Hughes CL Jr, Weinberg CR, Coleman RA, Shields JM. Galactose consumption, metabolism, and follicle-stimulating hormone concentrations in women of late reproductive age. Fertil Steril. 1994;62(6):1168.

10. Hall JE. Neuroendocrine physiology of the early and late menopause. Endocrinol Metab Clin N Am. 2004;33(4):637.

11. Nagamani M, Stuart CA, Doherty MG. Increased steroid production by the ovarian stromal tissue of postmenopausal women with endometrial cancer. J Clin Endocrinol Metab. 1992;74(1):172.

12. Kling JM, Manson JE, Naughton MJ, Temkit M, Sullivan SD, Gower EW, et al. Association of sleep disturbance and sexual function in postmenopausal women. Menopause. 2017;24(6):604–12.

13. Woods NF, Mitchell ES. Symptoms during the perimenopause: prevalence, severity, trajectory, and significance in women's lives. Am J Med. 2005;118(12B):14S–24S.

14. Berman JR, Berman L, Goldstein I. Female sexual dysfunction: incidence, pathophysiology, evaluation, and treatment options. Urology. 1999;54(3):385.

15. Dennerstein L, Dudley EC, Hopper JL, Burger H. Sexuality, hormones and the menopausal transition. Maturitas. 1997;26(2):83.

16. Freeman EW, Sammel MD, Liu L, Gracia CR, Nelson DB, Hollander L. Hormones and menopausal status as predictors of depression in women in transition to menopause. Arch Gen Psychiatry. 2004;61(1):62.

17. Bromberger JT, Meyer PM, Kravitz HM, Sommer B, Cordal A, Powell L, Ganz PA, Sutton-Tyrrell K. Psychologic distress and natural menopause: a multiethnic community study. Am J Public Health. 2001;91(9):1435.

18. Matthews KA, Wing RR, Kuller LH, Meilahn EN, Plantinga P. Influence of the perimenopause on cardiovascular risk factors and symptoms of middle-aged healthy women. Arch Intern Med. 1994;154(20):2349.

19. Mohyi D, Tabassi K, Simon J. Differential diagnosis of hot flashes. Maturitas. 1997;27(3):203.

20. North American Menopause Society. The 2012 hormone therapy position statement of the North American Menopause Society. Menopause. 2012;19(3):257–71.

21. Cobin RH, Goodman NF. Position Statement American Association of Clinical Endocrinologists and American College of Endocrinology Position Statement on Menopause – 2017 Update. 2017;23(7):869–80.

22. Maclennan AH, Broadbent JL, Lester S, Moore V. Oral oestrogen and combined oestrogen/progestogen therapy versus placebo for hot flushes. Cochrane Database Syst Rev. 2004;4:CD002978.

23. Ettinger B. Rationale for use of lower estrogen doses for postmenopausal hormone therapy. Maturitas. 2007;57(1):81–4. Epub 2007 Mar 23.

24. Schiff I, Tulchinsky D, Cramer D, Ryan KJ. Oral medroxyprogesterone in the treatment of postmenopausal symptoms. JAMA. 1980;244:1443–5.

25. Nelken RS, Ozel BZ, Leegant AR, Felix JC, Mishell DR. Randomized trial of estradiol vaginal ring versus oral oxybutynin for the treatment of overactive bladder. Menopause. 2011;18:962–6.

26. Waetjen LE, Brown JS, Vittinghoff E, et al. For the ULTRA low dose transdermal Estrogen assessment (ULTRA) study. The effect of ultralow-dose transdermal estradiol on urinary incontinence in postmenopausal women. Obstet Gynecol. 2005;106:946–52.

27. Maalouf NM, Sato AH, Welch BJ, et al. Postmenopausal hormone use and the risk of nephrolithiasis: results from the Women's health initiative hormone therapy trials. Arch Intern Med. 2010;170:1678–85.

28. Raz R, Stamm WE. A controlled trial of intravaginal estriol in postmenopausal women with recurrent urinary tract infections. N Engl J Med. 1993;329:753–6.

29. Eriksen BC. A randomized, open, parallel-group study on the preventive effect of an estradiol-releasing vaginal ring (Estring) on recurrent urinary tract infections in postmenopausal women. Am J Obstet Gynecol. 1999;80:1072–9.

30. Gass M, Cochrane BB, Larson JC, et al. Patterns and predictors of sexual activity among women in the hormone therapy trials of the Women's health initiative. Menopause. 2011;18:1160–71.

31. Rossouw JE, Anderson GL, Prentice RL, et al. Risks and benefits of estrogen plus progestin in healthy postmenopausal women: principal results from the Women's health initiative randomized controlled trial. JAMA. 2002;288(3):321.

32. Papadakis G, Hans D, Gonzalez-Rodriguez E, Vollenweider P, Waeber G, Marques-Vidal PM, Lamy O. The benefit of menopausal hormone therapy on bone density and microarchitecture persists after its withdrawal. J Clin Endocrinol Metab. 2016;101(12):5004–11. Epub 2016 Nov 17.

33. LaCroix AZ, Chlebowski RT, Manson JE, et al. for the WHI Investigators. Health outcomes after stopping conjugated equine estrogens among postmenopausal women with prior hysterectomy: a randomized controlled trial. JAMA. 2011;305:1305–14.

34. Valery TM, John L, Vanessa B, et al. Effects of estrogen or estrogen/progestin regimens on heart disease risk factors in postmenopausal women. The Postmenopausal Estrogen/Progestin Interventions (PEPI) Trial. JAMA 1995;274(21):1676.

35. Hulley S, Grady D, Bush T, et al. Randomized trial of estrogen plus progestin for secondary prevention of coronary heart disease in postmenopausal women. Heart and Estrogen/progestin Replacement Study (HERS) Research Group. JAMA. 1998;280(7):605.

36. Grady D, Herrington D, Bittner V, et al. Cardiovascular disease outcomes during 6.8 years of hormone therapy: Heart and Estrogen/progestin Replacement Study follow-up (HERS II). JAMA. 2002;288(1):49.

37. Hulley S, Furberg C, Barrett-Connor E, et al. Noncardiovascular disease outcomes during 6.8 years of hormone therapy: heart and Estrogen/progestin Replacement Study follow-up (HERS II). JAMA. 2002;288(1):58.

38. Manson JE, Allison MA, Rossouw JE, et al. For the WHI and WHICACS investigators. Estrogen therapy and coronary-artery calcification. N Engl J Med. 2007;356:2591–602.

39. Prentice RL, Manson JE, Langer RD, et al. Benefits and risks of postmenopausal hormone therapy when it is initiated soon after menopause. Am J Epidemiol. 2009;170:12–23.

40. Simon JA, Hsia J, Cauley JA, et al. Postmenopausal hormone therapy and risk of stroke: the heart and Estrogen-progestin replacement study (HERS). Circulation. 2001;103:638–42.

41. Viscoli CM, Brass LM, Kernan WN, Sarrel PM, Suissa S, Horwitz RI. A clinical trial of estrogen-replacement therapy after ischemic stroke. N Engl J Med. 2001;345:1243–9.

42. Taylor HS, Manson JE. Update in hormone therapy use in menopause. J Clin Endocrinol Metab. 2011;96(2):255–64.

43. Miller VM, Black DM, Brinton EA, et al. Using basic science to design a clinical trial: baseline characteristics of women enrolled in the Kronos early Estrogen prevention study (KEEPS). J Cardiovasc Transl Res. 2009;2:228–39.

44. Hodis HN, Mack WJ, Henderson VW, Shoupe D, Budoff MJ, Hwang-Levine J, et al. Vascular effects of early versus late postmenopausal treatment with Estradiol. N Engl J Med [Internet]. 2016;374(13):1221–31.

45. Canonico M, Oger E, Plu-Bureau G, et al. Hormone therapy and venous thromboembolism among postmenopausal women: impact of the route of estrogen administration and progestogens. The ESTHER Study Circulation. 2007;115:840–5.

46. Margolis KL, Bonds DE, Rodabough RJ, et al. Effect of estrogen plus progestin on the incidence of diabetes in postmenopausal women: results from the Women's health initiative hormone trial. Diabetologia. 2004;47:1175–87.

47. Grady D, Gebretsadik T, Kerlikowske K, Ernster V, Petitti D. Hormone replacement therapy and endometrial cancer risk: a meta-analysis. Obstet Gynecol. 1995;85:304–13.

48. Collaborative Group on Hormonal Factors in Breast Cancer. Breast cancer and hormone replacement therapy: collaborative reanalysis of data from 51 epidemiological studies of 52,705 women with breast cancer and 108,411 women without breast cancer. Collaborative Group on Hormonal Factors in Breast Cancer. Lancet. 1997;350:1047–59.

49. Chlebowski RT, Hendrix SL, Langer RD, et al. for the WHI Investigators. Influence of estrogen plus progestin on breast cancer and mammography in healthy postmenopausal women: the Women's Health Initiative Randomized Trial. JAMA. 2003;289:3243–53.

50. Beral V, Reeves G, Bull D, Green J. For the million women study collaborators. Breast cancer risk in relation to the interval between menopause and starting hormone therapy. J Natl Cancer Inst. 2011;103:296–305.

51. Lacey JV Jr, Mink PJ, Lubin JH, et al. Menopausal hormone replacement therapy and risk of ovarian cancer. JAMA. 2002;288: 334–41.

52. Beral V, Bull D, Green J, Reeves G. Million women study collaborators. Ovarian cancer and hormone replacement therapy in million women study. Lancet. 2007;369:1703–10.

53. Chlebowski RT, Schwartz AG, Wakelee H, et al. for the Women's Health Initiative Investigators. O estrogen plus progestin and lung cancer in postmenopausal women (Women's Health Initiative trial): a post-hoc analysis of a randomised trial. Lancet. 2009;374:1243–51.

54. Hogervorst E, Williams J, Budge M, Riedel W, Jolles J. The nature of the effect of female gonadal hormone replacement therapy on cognitive function in postmenopausal women: a meta-analysis. Neuroscience. 2000;101:485–512.

55. Maki PM, Henderson VW. Hormone therapy, dementia, and cognition: the Women's health initiative 10 years on. Climacteric. 2012;15(3):256–62.

56. Bachmann GA, Schaefers M, Uddin A, Utian WH. Lowest effective transdermal 17A-estradiol dose for relief of hot flushes in postmenopausal women: a randomized controlled trial. Obstet Gynecol. 2007;110:771–9.

57. Renoux C, Dell'aniello S, Garbe E, Suissa S. Transdermal and oral hormone replacement therapy and the risk of stroke: a nested case control study. BMJ. 2010;340:c2519.

58. The NAMS. 2017 hormone therapy position statement advisory panel. The 2017 hormone therapy position statement of the North American Menopause Society. Menopause. 2017;24(7):728–53.

59. Pitkin J. Alternative and complementary therapies for the menopause. Menopause Int. 2012;18(1):20–7.

60. Wren BG, Brown LB. A double blind trial with clonidine and a placebo to treat hot flushes. Med J Aust. 1986;144:369–70.

61. Nelson H, Vesco K, Haney E, et al. Non-hormonal therapies for menopausal hot flushes : systematic review and meta-analysis. JAMA. 2006;295:2057–71.

62. Barton DL, Sloan JA, Shuster LT, Gill P, Griffin P, Flynn K, Terstriep SA, Rana FN, Dockter T, Atherton PJ, Tsai M, Sturtz K, Lafky JM, Riepl M, Thielen J, Loprinzi CL. Evaluating the efficacy of vaginal dehydroepiandosterone for vaginal symptoms in postmenopausal cancer survivors: NCCTG N10C1 (Alliance). Support Care Cancer. 2017;

63. Panjari M, Davis SR. DHEA for postmenopausal women: a review of the evidence. Maturitas. 2010;66:172–9.

64. Lissin LW, Cooke JP. Phytoestrogens and cardiovascular health. J Am Coll Cardiol. 2000;35(6):1403.

65. Elsabagh S, Hartley S, File S. Limited cognitive benefits in stage þ2 postmenopausal women after 6 weeks of treatment with Ginkgo biloba. J Psychopharmacol. 2005;19:173–81.

66. Koebnick C, Reimann M, Carlsohn A, et al. The acceptability of isoflavones as a treatment of menopausal symptoms: a European survey among postmenopausal women. Climacteric. 2005;8:230–42.

67. Cummings SR, Ettinger B, Delmas PD, et al. The effects of tibolone in older postmenopausal women. N Engl J Med. 2008;359(7):697.

68. Portman DJ, Bachmann GA, Simon JA, Ospemifene Study Group. Ospemifene, a novel selective estrogen receptor modulator for treating dyspareunia associated with postmenopausal vulvar and vaginal atrophy. Menopause. 2013;20(6):623.

69. Lobo RA, Pinkerton JV, Gass ML, Dorin MH, Ronkin S, Pickar JH, Constantine G. Evaluation of bazedoxifene/conjugated estrogens for the treatment of menopausal symptoms and effects on metabolic parameters and overall safety profile. Fertil Steril. 2009;92(3):1025; Epub 2009 Jul 26.

70. Pinkerton JV, Utian WH, Constantine GD, Olivier S, Pickar JH. Relief of vasomotor symptoms with the tissue selective estrogen complex containing bazedoxifene/conjugated estrogens: a randomized, controlled trial. Menopause. 2009;16(6):1116–24.

71. Prague JK, Roberts RE, Comninos AN, Clarke S, Jayasena CN, Nash Z, Doyle C, Papadopoulou DA, Bloom SR, Mohideen P, Panay N, Hunter MS, Veldhuis JD, Webber LC, Huson L, Dhillo WS. Neurokinin 3 receptor antagonism as a novel treatment for menopausal hot flushes: a phase 2, randomised, double-blind, placebo-controlled trial. Lancet. 2017;389(10081):1809–20.

72. Barton DL, Loprinzi CL, Quella SK, et al. Prospective evaluation of vitamin E for hot flashes in breast cancer survivors. J Clin Oncol. 1998;16(2):495.

73. Nedrow A, Miller J, Walker M, et al. Complementary and alternative therapies for the management of menopause-related symptoms: a systematic evidence review. Arch Intern Med. 2006;166(14):1453.

74. Deng G, Vickers A, Yeung S, et al. Randomized, controlled trial of acupuncture for the treatment of hot flashes in breast cancer patients. J Clin Oncol. 2007;25(35):5584.

Male Hypogonadism

14

Alexandre Hohl and Marcelo Fernando Ronsoni

Pathophysiology

The male reproductive tract is in constant interaction with the hypothalamic–pituitary–testes, to produce and secrete androgenic hormones (HAs) and produce, maintain, and transport sperm and seminal fluid, thus enabling male fecundity. The HAs are critical for embryonic differentiation of internal and external male genitalia, development and maintenance of secondary sexual characteristics, and androgenic extra-gonadal effects [1].

During embryonic development, primordial gonads during the first weeks of pregnancy suffer a cascade of events that culminate in sexual differentiation. The undifferentiated germ cells of the gonads subsequently differentiate into Sertoli cells and interstitial cells differentiate into Leydig cells constituting the endocrine testicular tissue. In the presence of sex chromosomes XY, from the seventh week of pregnancy, the activity of the gene SRY (sex-determining region on the Y chromosome) starts, located on the short arm of the Y chromosome, which encodes a protein that, together with other factors encoded by other chromosomes (autosomal or X chromosome), act in embryonic differentiation from the primordial gonad. Sertoli cells secrete the anti-Mullerian hormone that promotes regression of Mullerian ducts. After about 8 weeks of gestation, the Leydig cells already have the capacity to produce steroids and, together with the stimulation of human chorionic gonadotropin (hCG) produced by the placenta, secrete testosterone, beginning the process of stabilizing Wolff ducts and with that the differentiation of the internal sexual organs. The differentiation of testosterone into dihydrotestosterone (DHT) by the enzyme 5α-reductase causes DHT to stimulates the differentiation of the external genitalia [2, 3].

The synthesis of testosterone occurs in Leydig cells (interstitial compartment) in response to the stimulation of luteinizing hormone (LH). The spermatogenesis in the somniferous tubules is dependent on the action of follicle-stimulating hormone (FSH) in Sertoli cells (germ cells) and by the action of testosterone. Approximately 95% of the testes match compartment germ cells, which explains the enormous daily production of sperm. The gonadotropins (LH and FSH) are produced in the pituitary in its anterior portion (gonadotrophs) through stimulation of GnRH produced in the hypothalamus, which is transported through the pituitary portal system [4]. Testosterone is the principal androgen plasma in men, is synthesized predominantly in the testes, and small quantities in the adrenal glands. The circulating testosterone (total testosterone) represents the set of existing forms, being the absolute value of testosterone, 2% in its free form, coupled with 44% of androgen binding protein (steroid hormone binding globulin [SHBG]) and 54% bound to albumin [3].

Testosterone is the most important testicular androgen in men. Low serum testosterone levels are associated with cardiovascular morbidity, metabolic syndrome, type 2 diabetes mellitus, atherosclerosis, osteoporosis, sarcopenia, and mortality. There is increasing evidence that serum testosterone is a major biomarker status of men's health in general. Studies in twins indicate that in an individual there is a strong heritability of serum testosterone. Research based on genomes has sought to evaluate the effects of genetic variants on serum concentrations of testosterone. Analysis of 14,429 men showed that genetic variants in SHBG and on their locus on the X chromosome are associated with a wide variation in serum testosterone concentrations and an increased risk of low levels. A genetic variant that affects the affinity of testosterone to SHBG, interfering directly in its free fraction, could influence the mathematical calculations that estimate their serum. Thus, in the future it may be necessary to evaluate the affinity of testosterone to SHBG and this is taken into account in the measurement of serum levels, as well as analysis of genetic polymorphisms closely related to these variables [5].

A. Hohl (✉) · M. F. Ronsoni
University Hospital (Federal University of Santa Catarina), Endocrinology and Metabolism Department, Florianópolis, Santa Catarina, Brazil
e-mail: alexandrehohl@endocrino.org.br

© Springer Nature Switzerland AG 2022
F. Bandeira et al. (eds.), *Endocrinology and Diabetes*, https://doi.org/10.1007/978-3-030-90684-9_14

The testicular disorders can be classified into disorders of production and/or action of sex steroids, disorders of spermatogenesis, and testicular neoplasms. Male hypogonadism and gynecomastia are the most prevalent disorders in the production of sex steroids in men. Defects in androgen action include mutations in different receptors (androgen, estrogen-alpha) and enzymes (5-α reductase, aromatase). The defects of spermatogenesis characterize infertility or sub-fertility [1].

Male hypogonadism is a syndrome associated with disturbances of the production or action of testosterone and/or disorders in spermatogenesis. Testosterone deficiency can result from abnormalities in testicular function, such as disorders in testosterone production and/or spermatogenesis disorders (primary hypogonadism), the regulation of the hypothalamic pituitary or testicular function (secondary hypogonadism), or disorder of hormone action due to a reduced or absent function of the androgen receptor (androgen insensitivity). Testosterone deficiency may occur as a result of Leydig cell dysfunction in primary hypogonadism by insufficient secretion of GnRH and/or LH at secondary hypogonadism (pituitary and hypothalamic) [6].

Primary gonadal failure may be due to congenital and acquired disorders. Already, a secondary gonadal failure may be due to functional or organic abnormalities (congenital and acquired; Table 14.1). Primary testicular failure is

Table 14.1 Causes of hypogonadism

Primary hypogonadism
Congenital
1. Chromosomal disorders
   (a) *Klinefelter syndrome and related syndromes (such as Male 46 XX)*
   (b) *Enzyme defects in the biosynthesis of testosterone*
   (c) *Myotonic dystrophy*
2. Developmental disorders
   (a) *Exposure to prenatal endocrine disruptors*
   (b) *Cryptorchidism*
   (c) *Anorchia due to bilateral torsion testes syndrome*
   (d) *Noonan syndrome*
Acquired
1. Orchitis
2. Mumps and other viruses
3. Infiltrative diseases (such as amyloidosis, hemochromatosis)
4. Acquired immunodeficiency syndrome (AIDS)
5. Granulomatous diseases (such as leprosy and tuberculosis)
6. Irradiation
7. Surgical lesions
8. Trauma and testicular torsion of the testicle
9. Varicocele
10. Autoimmune testicular failure
    (a) *Isolated*

Table 14.1 (continued)

   (b) *Associated (as Hashimoto's thyroiditis, type 1 diabetes mellitus)*
11. Drugs
    (a) *Anti-androgenic steroids (as flutamide, cimetidine, cyproterone, spironolactone, ketoconazole)*
    (b) *Cytotoxic*
12. Endocrine disruptors (such as insecticides, heavy metals, gossypol, environmental estrogens)
Androgen resistance syndrome
1. Testicular feminization syndrome (Morris syndrome)
2. Reifenstein syndrome
Secondary hypogonadism
Congenital
1. Multiple pituitary hormone deficiency
2. Pituitary aplasia or hypoplasia
3. Defects in the secretion or action of GnRH
   (a) *Mutation Kalig-1*
   (b) *Mutation in GnRH receptor*
4. Defects in the action or secretion of gonadotropins
   (a) *Inactivating mutations of the LH-β gene*
   (b) *Inactivating mutations of the LH receptor gene*
   (c) *Inactivating mutations of the FSH-β gene*
   (d) *Mutation in DAX-1 and SF*
5. GnRH deficiency
   (a) *Isolated (idiopathic hypogonadotropic or isolated hypogonadism)*
   (b) *With anosmia (Kallmann syndrome)*
   (c) *Associated with other abnormalities (Prader–Willi syndrome, Laurence–Moon, and Bardet–Biedl syndrome, CHARGE syndrome, Rud syndrome, multiple lentigines, basal encephalocele, cerebellar ataxia)*
   (d) *Partial deficiency of GnRH (fertile eunuch syndrome)*
Acquired
1. Traumatic brain injury
2. Post-radiation central nervous system, post-surgery, pituitary infarction, carotid aneurysm
3. Neoplasms
   (a) *Pituitary adenomas: prolactinomas, nonfunctioning adenomas, other adenomas*
   (b) *Craniopharyngiomas, germinomas, gliomas, lymphomas*
4. Autoimmune hypophysitis
5. Functional disorders: anorexia nervosa, dysfunction secondary to stress or other systemic diseases
6. Infiltrative disease: sarcoidosis, Langerhans cell histiocytosis, hemochromatosis
7. Infectious diseases: tuberculosis, histoplasmosis, abscesses
8. Drugs
9. Endocrine disruptors
Combined hypogonadism
1. Aging
2. Alcoholism
3. Hemochromatosis
4. Sickle cell anemia
5. Congenital adrenal hypoplasia (mutation of DAX-1)
6. Endocrine disruptors

characterized by low levels of testosterone and/or disorders of spermatogenesis associated with high concentrations of LH and FSH (hypergonadotropic hypogonadism). Secondary testicular failure is associated with low testosterone levels and inappropriately normal or low concentrations of LH and FSH (hypogonadotropic hypogonadism).

Secondary hypogonadism is usually associated with similar decreases in sperm and testosterone production. This occurs because the reduction in LH secretion promotes a reduction of testosterone production in the testes and, consequently, of intratesticular testosterone (primary hormonal stimulus for the production of sperm). In primary hypogonadism there may be a decrease in spermatogenesis in major damage in the cells of the seminiferous tubules (Sertoli cells) compared with Leydig cells. When this occurs, the subjects may present normal LH and testosterone levels, even with a number of ejaculated sperm very low or near zero. In these cases, FSH levels will be high.

In cases of secondary hypogonadism there is also less susceptibility to the occurrence of gynecomastia, probably due to normal or low levels of FSH and LH, which do not stimulate testicular aromatase, not increasing the conversion of testosterone to estradiol.

Causes of Hypogonadism

Primary Hypogonadism (Hypergonadotropic)

Congenital Causes

Klinefelter Syndrome

The Klinefelter syndrome (KS) is the most common sex chromosomal disorder in men, affecting one in every 660 children born alive [7]. It was first described in 1942. KS has a genetic background, with characteristics involving various specialties as embryology, pediatrics, endocrinology, cardiology, psychology, psychiatry, urology, and epidemiology.

Genetic inheritance is the extra X chromosome, which can be inherited from either parent. Most genes undergo additional X inactivation, but some may escape and serve as a genetic cause of the syndrome. Of these genes, the one that has been clearly shown to influence the phenotype of KS was short-stature home box-containing gene on chromosome X (SHOX) located pseudoautosomal region 1 in Xp. The haploinsufficiency of SHOX gene has been implicated in growth retardation and bone abnormalities in Turner syndrome and Leri–Weill dyschondrosteosis, and is also implicated in the slightly accelerated growth in KS [8]. The more frequent karyotype in men with KS is 47, XXY (93%) but karyotypes 46, XY/47, XXY; 48, XXXY; 48, XXYY; and 49, XXXXY have been reported [7].

Klinefelter syndrome is commonly under-diagnosed or is diagnosed late. Most men with KS live without a diagnosis. Boys with KS are likely to receive a diagnosis during evaluation for developmental delay and behavioral issues. Men with KS usually come to attention during evaluation for infertility or hypogonadism. Only 25% of cases are diagnosed and the average age of diagnosis is 30 years. A recent Australian study found a prevalence of 223 cases per 100,000 live births in boys [9], proposing an increase in the prevalence observed in several previous studies [10] and suggesting that it might differ between populations.

Klinefelter syndrome is associated with increased morbidity resulting in loss of life, and an increase in mortality owing to various diseases. Large epidemiological studies in KS were performed in two main cohorts: a British [11] and a Danish [12]. Together these studies show that the expected lifetime was reduced by 1.5–2 years, with increased mortality from various diseases, including diabetes, pulmonary disease, epilepsy, cerebrovascular disease, and vascular insufficiency of the intestine. In both studies, mortality among men with KS was significantly greater (hazard ratio: 1.9) and remained so after adjustment for social cohesion and education level (hazard ratio: 1.5), indicating that socioeconomic parameters can explain some but not all excess mortality in KS.

The main findings of KS are small testes, hypergonadotropic hypogonadism, and cognitive impairment. Other abnormalities are associated with KS and its frequency is varied (Table 14.2) [7].

Azoospermia is found in the vast majority of men with KS who have the karyotype 47, XXY. The mechanism by which an extra X chromosome causes infertile patients is not well known. Men with germ cell mosaics can present in their testicles, especially at a younger age. The testicular histology in men with KS shows hyalinization of seminiferous tubules and an absence of spermatogenesis. Patients with mosaics may show normal-sized testes and spermatogenesis in puberty. However, the progressive degeneration and hyalinization of seminiferous tubules occur soon after puberty. Therapeutic advances with the use of intracytoplasmic sperm injection allow 47, XXY men with azoospermia to achieve biological fatherhood [13].

The behavioral phenotype of KS is characterized by language, executive, and socioemotional dysfunction and psychomotor impairment. Boys with KS often need speech therapy, and many suffer from learning difficulties and may benefit from special education. The prevalence of schizophrenia, attention deficit hyperactivity disorder, autism spectrum disorders, and problems with mood regulation is increased. Neuroimaging studies of children and adults with KS show increases in the volume of gray matter sensorimotor and parieto-occipital regions, as well as significant reductions in the amygdala, hippocampus, insular, temporal, and inferior frontal volumes of gray matter [14].

Table 14.2 Abnormalities associated with Klinefelter syndrome

Feature	Frequency (%)
Infertility (adults)	91–99
Small testes (both testes <6 ml)	>95
Increased gonadotropin	>95
Azoospermia (adults)	>95
Commitment to learning (children)	>75
Decreased testosterone	63–85
Decreased facial hair (adults)	60–80
Decreased pubic hair (adults)	30–60
Gynecomastia (teens/adults)	38–75
Delayed speech development (children)	40
Increased height (prepubertal/adults)	30
Adiposity (adults)	50
Metabolic syndrome (adults)	46
Osteopenia (adults)	5–40
Type 2 diabetes mellitus	10–39
Cryptorchidism	27–37
Reduced penis size (children)	10–25
Psychiatric disorders (children)	25
Congenital malformations, ogival palate, inguinal hernia	18
Osteoporosis (adults)	10
Mitral valve prolapse (adults)	0–55
Breast cancer (adults)	Increased risk (50 times)
Mediastinum cancer (children)	Increased risk (500 times)
Fractures	Increased risk (2–40 times)

Hypogonadism in KS may lead to changes in body composition and a risk of developing metabolic syndrome and diabetes type 2. Medical treatment is mainly testosterone replacement therapy to relieve acute and long-term hypogonadism, as well as treatment or prevention of comorbidities.

Other Chromosomal Abnormalities

Other chromosomal abnormalities that result in testicular hypo function were reported, including rare diseases 46, XY/XO and 47, XYY. The karyotype 46, XY/XO leads to a syndrome characterized by short stature and other typical features of Turner syndrome. The gonad digenesis varies from the normal testes. The risk for gonadoblastoma is about 20% of digenesis. Gonadectomy should therefore be conducted in these patients [15, 16]. The karyotype 47, XXY was initially associated with hypogonadism, but other reports have not confirmed this relationship further. Micro deletion-specific regions of the long arm of chromosome Y can be detected in approximately 20% of men with severe oligospermia or azoospermia. Some of these men have no other testicular lesions, but others have cryptorchidism [17].

Myotonic dystrophy, an autosomal-dominant disease, leads to muscle atrophy and is accompanied by hypogonadism that is usually not recognized until adulthood. Small tes-

tes and decreased production of sperm are more common than reduction of serum testosterone levels [18, 19].

Disorders of Androgen Synthesis

Mutations in genes encoding the enzymes necessary for the biosynthesis of testosterone may result in a decrease in their serum. The rare mutations found are enzyme cleavage of the side chain of cholesterol, 3β-hydroxysteroid dehydrogenase, 17α-hydroxylase (present in the adrenals and testes), and 17β-hydroxysteroid dehydrogenase (present only in the testes). Depending on the degree of mutation differing degrees of fetal virilization are met [20].

Mutation in FSH and LH Genes

Changes in LH and FSH receptors are rare causes of primary hypogonadism. The mutation in the FSH receptor induces a variable sperm count, which tends to be generally low and concentrations of inhibin B and FSH levels. Mutations in LH receptor results in hypoplasia and Leydig cell testosterone deficiency in the first trimester in utero, resulting in different degrees of disorder of sexual development DDS [21–23].

Cryptorchidism

Cryptorchidism is a condition in which one or both of the testes fail to descend from the abdomen into the scrotum. The main sites are the inguinal canal and abdominal cavity. It is necessary to differentiate between the possible cryptorchid testes and shrunken testicles, that on manipulation, return to the scrotum normally. Cryptorchidism can affect one or both testes. If only one testes is affected, the sperm count is subnormal in 30% of cases (and the concentration of FSH is slightly raised), suggesting that even in the presence of one normolocated testicle, this may present different degrees of testicular dysfunction. If both testes are cryptorchid, the sperm count is usually severely impaired and serum testosterone may also be reduced. The risk of gonadoblastoma also increases if the testicle is not in its normal position [24, 25].

Congenital Anorchia

Congenital anorchia occurs in disorders (after 20 weeks of gestation) that lead to testes regression. The male sex differentiation at birth is normal, but the testes are absent and hypogonadism in general is important [26]. The diagnosis is confirmed after anorchia with a full search of imaging studies (both in the scrotum and in the abdominal cavity) and, if necessary, laparotomy. There are case reports that testosterone treatment in adult men with congenital anorchia and micropenis can lead to penis enlargement.

Acquired Causes

Varicocele

Damage to the seminiferous tubules due to varicosity of the venous plexus within the scrotum has been considered a possible cause of male infertility. Current data are conflicting about the real benefit of varicocele correction in relation to fertility [27].

Orchitis

Several infections may be associated with testicular damage. The most common cause is mumps and orchitis is a frequent manifestation when occurring in adulthood. The incidence has decreased owing to the vaccination of the population. The involvement of testicular mumps causes increased painful testicles, followed by atrophy. The seminiferous tubules are often severely affected, often resulting in infertility, especially when both testicles are involved. The Leydig cells can also be damaged, resulting in decreased production of testosterone.

Chronic Diseases

Gonadal dysfunction is a common finding in men with chronic kidney disease (CKD) and end-stage kidney disease. Testosterone deficiency, generally accompanied by elevated serum gonadotropin, is present in 26–66% of men with varying degrees of renal impairment. Uremia-associated hypogonadism is multifactorial in origin, and rarely improves with the onset of dialysis, although usually it normalizes after renal transplantation. Although there are encouraging data suggesting benefits of testosterone replacement therapy for CKD patients, more studies are needed regarding the safety and efficacy [28].

The gonadal function requires a normal liver function. It is well known that the clinical symptoms of hypogonadism are common in patients with liver cirrhosis. The pathogenesis of hypogonadism in cirrhotic patients is complex and not well explained. It involves both a gonadal dysfunction and a central disturbance [29]. Hypogonadism is a potential complication of hemochromatosis, usually seen in patients with severe iron overload and liver cirrhosis [30].

Other infiltrative or granulomatous disease may promote primary gonadal failure, varying clinical demonstrations, and testicular dysfunction according to the degree of involvement of the underlying disease. Examples are tuberculosis and leprosy.

HIV Infection

Men who have HIV may have hypogonadism to varying degrees. The premature decline of serum testosterone is common (16%) among young and middle-aged HIV-infected men and is associated with inappropriately low or normal LH and accumulation of visceral adipose tissue. Testosterone deficiency may be regarded as a process of accelerated or premature aging. The role of HIV and/or treatment of HIV infection have yet to be elucidated [31]. The frequency of hypogonadism and its severity appear to have decreased since the introduction of antiretroviral therapy.

Irradiation

Direct radiation to the testes, as the treatment for leukemia, can damage them. Even when radiation is indirect, damage may occur in the seminiferous tubules. The degree of damage is proportional to the amount of radiation exposure. Radioactive iodine may cause a decrease in sperm count when the doses administered are high for the treatment of differentiated thyroid carcinoma.

Gonadal Toxicity of Cancer Chemotherapy

The number of surviving young men with cancer has increased dramatically over the past 20 years as a result of early detection and better treatment protocols for cancer. Over 75% of cancer patients diagnosed in youth are long-term survivors.

The gonadal dysfunction has emerged as an important long-term complication of cancer chemotherapy, especially in young patients with hematological and testicular malignancies. Infertility can be a significant issue for many cancer survivors. The male hypogonadism after chemotherapy may contribute to fatigue, sexual dysfunction, irritability, loss of lean mass, and osteopenia. Quality of life and recovery from cancer treatment is worsened by this clinical symptom.

Cytotoxic chemotherapy may cause gonadal injury, and the nature and extent of the damage depends on the drug, the dose received, and the age of the patient. Many drugs are toxic (Table 14.3), including procarbazine, cisplatin, and alkylating drugs such as cyclophosphamide, melphalan, and chlorambucil. However, all chemotherapeutic drugs can cause damage to gonadal function [32]. The relative contribution of each individual drug can be difficult to determine because most treatments are conducted with multiple drug regimens [33].

Trauma and Torsion of Testes

Any trauma in the testes may be sufficient to damage both the seminiferous tubules and the Leydig cells. Testicular torsion is one of the most common reasons for the loss of a testicle before puberty. The torsion of a testes is a twist in the spermatic cord, which results in severe loss of blood to the

Table 14.3 Estimated risk of gonadal dysfunction with cytotoxic agents

High risk	Medium risk	Low risk
Cyclophosphamide	Cisplatin	Vincristine
Ifosfamide	Carboplatin	Methotrexate
Chlormethine	Doxorubicin	Dactinomycin
Busulfan	BEP	Bleomycin
Melphalan	ABVD	Mercaptopurine
Procarbazine		Vinblastine
Chlorambucil		
MOPP		

ABVD adriamycin, bleomycin, vinblastine, and dacarbazine, *BEP* bleomycin, etoposide, and cisplatin, *MOPP* nitrogen mustard, oncovin (vincristine), procarbazine, and prednisone testes. The loss of the testes can occur owing to a lack of blood if the twist is not reverted spontaneously or surgically corrected within a few hours. The degree of damage depends on the length of the twist. A twist that lasts more than 8 h can promote enough damage to decrease the sperm count. Even when the twist involves only one testicle, both testicles may be damaged; however, it is not clear how this can occur [34–36].

Medications

Ketoconazole directly inhibits the biosynthesis of testosterone, thereby causing a deficiency in production [37]. Chronic use of glucocorticoids can also decrease testosterone levels in about one third of individuals. The mechanism is not clear, but the inhibition can occur in both testes and in the pituitary gland [38, 39].

Autoimmune Testicular Failure

It may occur in isolation or as a manifestation of polyglandular autoimmune syndrome and should be considered in all patients with other concomitant autoimmune diseases [40].

Secondary Hypogonadism (Hypogonadotropic)

Congenital Causes

The etiology of congenital gonadotropin dysfunction is rare. Clinical findings vary among individuals mainly because of the time of onset of dysfunction of gonadotropins. Sexual differentiation is normal because testosterone secretion by Leydig cells in the fetal first trimester of pregnancy is dependent on the stimulation of placental hCG. Penile development occurs primarily during the third trimester of pregnancy, and is often subnormal because testicular testosterone secretion at this stage is dependent on fetal LH secretion, which is also subnormal. This results in many cases in micropenis. The linear growth in childhood is normal, deficits occurring only when associated with deficiency in the production of growth hormone or thyroid hormone. Most diagnoses are made during puberty. Pubertal development can start and progress slowly, becoming it incomplete in many cases. In some patients, depending on the degree of gonadotropin deficiency, delayed puberty may present or absent [41].

Isolated Hypogonadotropic Hypogonadism

It is characterized by isolated deficiency of gonadotropins, without changes in smell and due to deficient secretion of GnRH, GnRH receptor mutation, or mutations of β fractions of LH or FSH. Several genetic mutations may be involved in the production process, hormonal secretion, or action (Table 14.4). Many cases remain of unknown etiology [42, 45].

Kallmann Syndrome

Kallmann syndrome is characterized by hypogonadotropic hypogonadism and another congenital abnormality that is not gonadal, including anosmia or hyposmia, red–green daltonism, midline facial defects, abnormalities of the urogeni-

Table 14.4 Genes involved in the etiology of hypogonadotropic hypogonadism [22, 23, 42–44]

Gene	Product	Function	Clinical
CHD7	Protein linker of chromodomain-type DNA helicase-7	Development of the neural crest, protein bound to DNA	CHARGE syndrome — semicircular canal aplasia, hypoplasia of the olfactory bulb, GH deficiency, hypothyroidism, congenital malformations that include hypogonadotropic hypogonadism (with micropenis and/or cryptorchidism)
DAX1/NR0B1A	Gene 1 of sex reversal	Development of adrenal secretion of gonadotropin control	Adrenal hypoplasia congenital X-linked (primary adrenal insufficiency that is expressed in the early stages of life)
FGF8	Fibroblast growth factor type 8	FGFR1 Binder/migration of GnRH neurons	Kallmann syndrome
FGFR1	Receptor type 1 fibroblast growth factor (FGF receptor 1)	Migration of GnRH neurons	Kallmann syndrome
FSHβ	B subunit of FSH	Binder receptor FSH	Isolated FSH deficiency (azoospermia, small testes in soft and undetectable serum FSH)
GnRH1	Pre-hormone GnRH	GnRH synthesis and cell signaling	Isolated hypogonadotropic hypogonadism
GnRHR	GnRH receptor	Synthesis of LH and FSH	Isolated hypogonadotropic hypogonadism, LH-isolated deficiency (partial mutations)
GPR54/Kiss1R	Receptor 1 of Kisspeptin	Stimulation of secretion of GnRH	Isolated hypogonadotropic hypogonadism with attenuated LH response to exogenous GnRH stimulation
HESX-1	Homeobox protein ANS	Marking the previous visceral endoderm embryo	Syndrome of septo-optic dysplasia (optic nerve hypoplasia, radiological changes of online medical and hypoplastic anterior pituitary (hypopituitarism with neuro-ectopic posterior pituitary) and Pickhardt–Fahlbusch syndrome
HS6ST1	6-O-sulfotransferase heparin sulfate	Catalyzes transfer of the sulfate at position-6 in the biogenesis of heparin sulfate	Hypogonadotropic hypogonadism

Table 14.4 (continued)

Gene	Product	Function	Clinical
KAL1	Anosmin-1	Cell adhesion glycoprotein (expressed in embryonic development in olfactory bulb, cerebellum, spinal cord, kidney, and retina), migration of GnRH neurons	Kallmann syndrome
LEP	Leptin	Hormone regulating food intake, energy expenditure, and hypothalamic reproductive function	Homozygous mutation in the leptin exhibits morbid obesity and hypogonadism (apparently of hypothalamic origin)
LEPR	Leptin receptor	Membrane receptor	Morbid obesity and hypogonadism (apparently of hypothalamic origin)
LHX3		Transcription factor required for the development of pituitary	Hypopituitarism (corticotropic-preserving function) associated with limitation of neck rotation (rigid cervical spine), elevated and anteverted shoulders
LHβ	B subunit of LH	Binder receptor LH	Isolated FSH deficiency (fertile eunuch syndrome — deficient production of testosterone associated with varying degrees of spermatogenesis)
NELF	Factor nasal embryonic LHRH	Neuronal migration	Hypogonadotropic hypogonadism
PROK2	Type 2 prokineticin	Migration of GnRH neurons	Kallmann syndrome
PROKR2	Receptor type 2 prokineticin	Migration of GnRH neurons	Kallmann syndrome
TAC3	Neurokinin B	Binder TACR3, stimulates GnRH secretion	Hypogonadotropic hypogonadism
TAC3R	Neurokinin B receptor	Stimulates the secretion of GnRH	Hypogonadotropic hypogonadism
WDR11	Protein WD	Interaction with transcription factor EMX1/GnRH neuronal migration	Hypogonadotropic hypogonadism

tal tract, synkinesis (mirror movements), and sensorineural hearing loss. Hypogonadism is due to deficient secretion of GnRH owing to defects in the migration of GnRH-secreting neurons that have the same embryological origin as those olfactory neurons. Most cases are sporadic, but there may be a familial transmission (X-linked inheritance is autosomal dominant or recessive). Studies have shown mutations in genes encoding several adhesion molecules on the cell surface, receptors or necessary for the migration of neurons, such as fibroblast growth factor receptor 1 (also called KAL1) procineticina-2 (PROK2) and its receptor (PROKR-2). These mutations together represent less than half of the cases described [22, 23, 43, 45].

Laurence–Moon and Bardet–Biedl Syndrome

These are etiologies of hypogonadism associated with retinitis pigmentosa and developmental delay. Laurence–Moon syndrome is associated with spastic paraplegia and Bardet–Biedl is associated with post-axial polydactyly, renal dysplasia, and early-onset obesity [46, 47].

Deficiencies of Transcription Factors

Some individuals have involvement of other hormonal axes in association with gonadotropin deficiency. Mutations in PROP-1 mutations represent the most common known genetic cause of hypopituitarism both in sporadic and familial cases [22, 23].

Acquired Causes

Hypogonadotropic hypogonadism can be caused by any disease that interferes with the hypothalamic–pituitary axis. The mechanisms that may be involved (one or more) are hypothalamic disorders (that impair the GnRH secretion), disorders of the pituitary stalk (that interfere with the passage of GnRH into the pituitary gland), and pituitary disorders (that directly decrease the secretion of LH and FSH).

Disorders of Gonadotropin Secretion

Hyperprolactinemia

Hyperprolactinemia of any cause can suppress gonadotropin secretion and thus testicular function [48]. Hypogonadism is reversible with normalization of prolactin.

Drugs

– *Sexual steroids*:

The use of androgen, estrogen, or progesterone may alter the secretion of gonadotropins. The recreational use of male sex hormones can interfere with the aim of anabolism in the secretion of gonadotropins during the period they are being used and, after several months of drug withdrawal when high doses are used. Recent data show that abuse of androgens can lead, in addition, to hypogonadism, increased cardiovascular morbidity, and mortality [49]. Estrogens and progestins used as appetite stimulants can promote secondary hypogonadism in some individuals.

– *Glucocorticoids*:

Chronic treatment with glucocorticoids can lead to hypogonadism. Prolonged use in various diseases in current medical settings, and the indiscriminate use of steroids, showed the effect of medication on the pulsatility of gonadotropins and consequently on gonadal function [38].

– *Opiates*:

When administered chronically, especially when continuing to control chronic pain, opiates often cause pronounced hypogonadism [50, 51]. Opioids, endogenous and exogenous, modulate gonadal function, acting mainly on opioid receptors in the hypothalamus, decreasing the secretion or causing loss of pulsatility of normal gonadotropin-releasing hormone (GnRH). Opioids may also have direct effects on the pituitary gland and testes [52].

– *GnRH Analogs*:

The prolonged administration of GnRH analogs leads to a decrease in the secretion of LH and hence in the secretion of testosterone. Currently, drugs as triptorelin and histrelin are much used in the adjuvant treatment of prostate cancer [53].

Chronic Diseases
Several systemic and chronic diseases, including cirrhosis, chronic kidney failure, chronic lung disease, and AIDS, cause hypogonadism by a combination of primary and secondary effects [54].

Critical Conditions
Any serious illness, surgery, myocardial infarction can cause hypogonadism. Decreased levels of LH are found in critically ill patients, suggesting an involvement in the pituitary gonadal function [55, 56].

Anorexia Nervosa
Although less common in adolescent males, anorexia may also be associated with secondary hypogonadism, characterized by functional hypothalamic changes, and interfering with the proper secretion of GnRH [57].

Diabetes Mellitus
Male patients with type 2 diabetes mellitus (T2DM) have a higher prevalence of low serum concentrations of testoster-

one than men without diabetes. The pathogenesis of this disorder is still uncertain, but it is known that there is a decrease in both total testosterones as its free fraction. Patients with T2DM have other signs and symptoms of metabolic syndrome, which may contribute to further enhancing the hormonal deficit [58–62].

Obesity
The European Male Aging Study demonstrated that men who are overweight (BMI 25–29 kg/m^2) and those who are obese (BMI $\geq$ 30 kg/m^2) tend to have lower serum concentrations of the hormone binding globulin (SHBG) and, therefore, lower serum total testosterone, inasmuch as the concentration of total serum testosterone to SHBG is due to a low concentration of free testosterone is normal. However, men who are obese may also have low levels of free testosterone. At all ages, total testosterone and SHBG concentrations were lower in overweight men than in men of normal weight and even lower in obese men. Free testosterone was similar in men with normal weight and overweight, but lower in obese men. Serum concentrations of LH did not increase in patients with BMI above the normal range, demonstrating a disorder in the central gonadal axis [61–63].

Disorders of Direct Gonadotroph

Benign Tumors and Cysts
Pituitary adenomas and sellar cysts can cause decreased cell function by a gonadotropic local mass effect, decreasing the release of LH and FSH.

Neoplasms
Malignant tumors of the central nervous system (CNS), metastases, or other malignancies can affect the functioning of the gonadal axis by interfering with the production of gonadotropins. Meningiomas are among the most common primary tumors and metastatic lesions of lung cancer and prostate cancer.

Infiltrative Diseases
Sarcoidosis and Langerhans cell histiocytosis (eosinophilic granuloma) can cause hypothalamic hypogonadism. The iron deposition in patients with hemochromatosis directly on the pituitary can induce secondary hypogonadism.

Infections
Tuberculosis meningitis and other causes of CNS infections may promote central hypogonadism. In most cases there is a concomitant impairment of another hypothalamic-pituitary axis (somatotropic or adrenocorticotropic axis).

Traumatic Brain Injury

The external carotid artery has been described in recent years as an important cause of hypopituitarism, including GH deficiency and male hypogonadism. Whiplash injury leading to concussions, brain trauma and the skull base can pull the pituitary stalk and sectional portal circulation. However, most of the dysfunctions of the hypothalamic–pituitary axis are still poorly understood, demonstrating a high rate of hypogonadism during acute trauma with subsequent recovery of gonadal function in a group of patients remaining in permanent hypogonadism (10–15% of individuals 1 year after the event). The time of recovery of gonadal function and the reason for the fall in gonadotropins at an acute moment are still matters of discussion and research [64].

Endocrine Disruptors and the Gonadotropic Axis

Endocrine disruptor compounds (EDCs) are exogenous compounds that have the potential to interfere in regulating the endocrine system and therefore may predispose to disease in man and animals [65]. The EDCs can be naturally derived from plants (phytoestrogens) in animals and man. Currently, artificial chemical compounds are of major concern worldwide. EDCs can interfere with the production, secretion, metabolism, transport, or in the peripheral action of endogenous hormones through its binding to hormone receptors.

Evidence for changes in the human male reproductive tract associated with EDCs is still limited. Humans are exposed to hundreds or thousands of environmental chemicals and a major limitation of epidemiological studies is that they generally measure human exposure to a single EDC [65, 66].

The male sex differentiation is androgen dependent. Thus, various diseases can be observed in males owing to exposure to EDCs. Postnatal exposures also have an impact on the development and maintenance of gonadal males (Table 14.5).

Quality of Semen

The decline in semen lifelong quality has been followed in several countries. Some studies suggest that semen quality decreases before 50 years of age, whereas others do not observe this decline [66].

Table 14.5 Association of endocrine disruptor compounds and possible diseases of the human male reproductive system

Stage of development	Disease/associated amendment
Fetal	Cryptorchidism, hypospadias, testes dysgenesis syndrome
Prepubertal	Precocious pubarche
Pubertal	Testes atrophy, precocious puberty, delayed puberty
Adult	Infertility, testes cancer, and enlarged prostate

Despite the importance and relevance of exposure to EDCs, especially polychlorinated biphenyls (PCBs), pesticides, and phthalates, the epidemiological evidence for the relationship with semen quality in adults is still limited, mainly because many of the data were obtained transversely.

Testes Dysgenesis Syndrome

Testes dysgenesis syndrome (TDS) is the association between cryptorchidism, hypospadias, and testicular cancer oligozoospermia resulting from altered testicular development. This association may mean that several elements acted at different times throughout the life of an individual, and may be due to exposure to a particular EDC or mixture. However, epidemiological data concerning EDCs with this syndrome in humans are still indirect [67].

The decreased anogenital distance, a marker of prenatal androgen activity, was observed in rats exposed to phthalates in the prenatal period and later identified in an epidemiological study with newborn human males [68].

Male Urogenital Tract Malformation

The association of the exposure of father and/or mother or a community to pesticides with the presence of hypospadias or cryptorchidism in newborns is suggestive of the involvement of EDCs. Epidemiological data supporting this link are those from individuals living in agricultural areas and/or that directly assessed the exposure of parents to organochlorine pesticides [69].

Testicular Germ Cell Cancer

The frequency of testicular germ cell tumors (TGCTs), which comprise more than 95% of all testicular cancers, has increased significantly during the past four decades, well beyond the expected population growth. To date, the evidence for the relationship between EDCs and risk of TGCTs has been limited. Interestingly, in a case–control study, no association was observed between serum concentrations of organochlorine compounds in patients with controls and TGCT, but an association was observed with serum levels of organochlorines in their mothers during antenatal care being a predictive factor for increased risk for TGCT in adulthood [70].

Gynecomastia

Di-(2-ethylhexyl) phthalate (DEHP) is one of the most commonly used phthalates in plastics manufacture. DEHP has been reported as an androgen receptor antagonist. Mono-(2-ethylhexyl) phthalate (MEHP) is known as the first and primary metabolite of DEHP. It was observed that plasma levels of DEHP and MEHP were significantly higher in patients with gynecomastia compared with pubertal controls [71].

Diagnosis

The diagnosis of androgen deficiency occurs in three stages. Initially, it should include a general health assessment to look for signs and symptoms of androgen deficiency and exclude systemic disease, eating disorders, and lifestyle problems, such as excessive exercise or drug abuse. The signs and symptoms of androgen deficiency are nonspecific and are modified by age of onset, severity, and duration of disability, comorbidities, use of androgen sensitivity, and prior therapies. If an androgen deficiency is initiated before the patient has completed pubertal development, it often appears as delayed or incomplete sexual development and eunuchoid proportions (arm span greater than height by more than 5 cm). In men in whom androgen deficiency develops after complete pubertal maturation, symptoms include reduced sexual desire and activity, reduced spontaneous erections, loss of body hair and reduced frequency of shaving, infertility, decreased muscle mass and strength, small or shrinking testicles, and breast enlargement. In older men, there may be a background of nonspecific symptoms associated with aging.

After the initial clinical investigation, serum total testosterone (TT) should be measured, preferably in the morning, using a reliable biochemical assay. An examination with a low value should be repeated at least once for confirmation. Measurement of testosterone should be avoided during the period of acute disease as there is suppression of the hypothalamic–pituitary–gonadal axis resulting in decreased serum levels of TT. Also, conditions that elevate the serum androgen-binding protein (SHBG) decrease the dosage of TT (Table 14.6). The TT measured represents the set of presentation forms of serum testosterone. The absolute value of TT is equal to 2% free testosterone, 44% bound to SHBG, and 54% bound to albumin. Therefore, it is recommended that free testosterone (FT) is determined in some individuals, particularly those that have altered levels of SHBG, as in the

case of obese patients. The method of measuring TT considered more accurate is liquid chromatography–tandem mass spectrometry, but it is not available in the vast majority of laboratories. Thus, the measurement of total testosterone by direct and automated methods (such as electrochemiluminescent assay - ECLIA) fulfills its role in most diagnoses [72]. As most laboratories do not have this methodology and use radioimmunoassay for their evaluation, it is recommended to obtain the FT values from the construction proposed by Vermeulen, based on the values of TT, SHBG, and albumin (Table 14.7). Other causes of low testosterone levels should be discarded, such as hyperprolactinemia, thyroid disorders, chronic diseases, or other disorders. Estradiol should be measured in all adult patients with gynecomastia. DHT is measured in cases of abnormal differentiation of the genitalia and when this is suspected. Semen analysis is of great importance in assessing the fertility and gonadal function of the individual [73].

The cutoff points of normal TT for the diagnosis of hypogonadism in adult males is a subject of discussion between different researchers and medical companies. The Endocrine Society (ES) requires TT values below 280–300 ng/dL to be monitored and repeated measurement of SHBH for the calculation of FT [74]. The ES recognizes that there is variation in the normal values between laboratories and according to the dosage methodology used. As the cutoff for FT, Endocrine Society suggests 5–9 ng/dL. But the consensus established by various international medical societies (International Society of Andrology, International Society for the Study of the Aging Male, European Association of Urology, European Academy of Andrology, American Society of Andrology) presents a different proposition [75]. Symptomatic patients with a TT above 350 ng/dl do not require androgen replacement. If the TT value is below 230 ng/dl, the diagnosis of male hypogonadism is made. However, if the TT result is in the so-called "gray area" (between 230 and 350 ng/dl) dosage of SHBG and calculation of FT are indicated. Hypogonadal patients are considered to be those with a calculated FT below 6.5 ng/dL. Very low values of TT (below 150 ng/dL) should be investigated to rule out secondary hypogonadism or hyperprolactinemia associated with hyperprolactinemia. Recently, Anawalt and coworkers suggested a new "gray area" for TT between 150 and 400 ng/dl [76].

Table 14.6 Conditions associated with changes in serum steroid hormone binding globulin

Decreased concentrations	Obesity
	Nephrotic syndrome
	Hypothyroidism
	Glucocorticoids
	Progestins
	Androgenic steroids
	Acromegaly
	Diabetes mellitus
Increased concentrations	Aging
	Hepatitis and liver cirrhosis
	Hyperthyroidism
	Use of anticonvulsants
	Use of estrogen
	HIV/AIDS

Table 14.7 Vermeulen formula: Calculation of free testosterone

Vermeulen formula: FT = TT (nM/l)/SHBG (nM/l) × 100[a, b]

FT free testosterone, *TT* total testosterone, *SHBG* sex hormone binding globulin

[a]Assuming that the albumin concentration is normal

[b]The calculation of free testosterone, conducted by the formula of Vermeulen, can be obtained at the website: http://www.issam.ch/freetesto.htm

The third step is to measure the level of LH of those who allegedly have an androgen deficiency to determine whether the fault lies at or in the region of the hypothalamic–pituitary–testicular axis. Other laboratory tests and imaging should be evaluated according to each case. On suspicion of testicular diseases, testicular ultrasound can be requested for evaluation of characteristics, location, and associated abnormalities. MRI is performed in suspected cases of CNS diseases and for pituitary evaluation in selected cases. An olfactory test must be performed in order to detect the presence of anosmia, hyposmia, and as part of the evaluation for Kallmann syndrome. Karyotype is indicated in cases of suspected chromosomal abnormalities as part of hypogonadism. Genotyping for known monogenic causes monogenic is currently a research procedure and is not performed in routine clinical practice. It may be performed when there is a specific positive family history or when the patient has phenotypic signs suggestive of a specific mutation. When performed, genetic testing should always be accompanied by genetic counseling.

Treatment

The main goal of treatment of patients with hypogonadism is the re-establishment of sexual function and its subsequent maintenance, along with the secondary sexual characteristics and sexual extra effect of androgens (bone mineral density, muscle hypertrophy, wellness, among others) [77–79]. According to the etiology of hypogonadism, after assessment of the fertility of an individual, one can suggest the induction of spermatogenesis, if there is a desire for fertility.

If primary hypogonadism is diagnosed early, replacement with testosterone is the best option. For congenital secondary hypogonadism, some medical centers recommend starting with gonadotropins to allow the testicles to reach the size at puberty. After testicular growth, the testosterone replacement therapy may be administered until the moment that fertility is desired. Right now, the gonadotropins should be employed in order to To stimulate sperm production, the use of gonadotropins can be helpful [80]. Anti-estrogens may be an alternative therapy; however, their effectiveness has not been adequately tested. In the presence of symptoms of increased estrogen production (gynecomastia and breast tenderness), a short course with the non-aromatizable androgens (dihydrotestosterone, mesterolone, or oxandrolone) may be advisable. However, after a few months of therapy, switching to other aromatizable preparations is recommended to prevent bone loss. When there is concern about the safety of the prostate, the use of steroids or modulators of the nonselective androgen receptor (less susceptible 5α-reductase) may be advisable. One interesting possibility is combined use with inhibitors of testosterone 5α-reductase. Theoretically, Estrogen receptor-beta ligands could be used

and studies are underway. however, the development of these compounds, although promising, is still at the preliminary research stage [80].

The major routes of androgen administration [78] are described in the following sections.

Oral Androgens

The use of prepared 17α-alkylated anabolic steroids (fluoxymesterone and methyltestosterone) should not be prescribed because of the high rate of hepatotoxicity. The ester testosterone undecanoate (40–80 mg, 2–3 times daily) is only effective via oral administration owing to its absorption via the lymphatic system, thus minimizing the side effects of its use. The disadvantages are multiple daily doses and variability in serum hormone. It has not been approved for use in the US.

Transdermal Androgens

Marketed since the 1990s, this form is widespread throughout the world and provides ease of use and a close to physiological replacement. Present in the form of gels and adhesives [81].

Testosterone Gel (1%)

Hydroalcoholic formulation, applied in doses of 50–100 mg per day, is applicable in body regions with little hair. It is practical and has good tolerability, allowing flexibility in dosage with few side effects, mostly limited to local irritation. The disadvantages are the potential transfer of the gel to the partner through direct contact with skin [81].

Testosterone Topical Solution (2%) Applied to the Axillae

The 2% formulation of testosterone topical solution, approved by the US Food and Drug Administration (FDA) in November 2010, is a non-occlusive topical formulation administered to the axillae with an applicator instead of the hands. About 5–10% of the testosterone applied to the axilla is absorbed and appears in serum [82].

Transdermal Patches

Both scrotal and nonscrotal, they can be applied once a day, at night. They are easy to apply and can be ready to interrupt if necessary. The gel is less well tolerated owing to the high rate of local irritation. An area is needed that is clear for adhesion. The application can provide scrotal testicular atrophy light.

Injectable Androgens

The existing drugs on the market are oily formulations that allow an increased dosing interval and the prolongation of the action of the testosterone derivative [83, 84].

– *Testosterone cypionate (200 mg ampoules)*:

An oil formulation that can be safely administered intramuscularly. It elevates serum testosterone levels, reaching a peak serum rapidly around the first 2–5 days with a mean nadir around 15–20 days. Doses are administered at intervals ranging from 2 to 4 weeks, depending on the clinical response of the patient. The advantages are that fewer applications are needed, the low cost, and easy access. The disadvantage is that it does not mimic the physiological hormonal cycle, with supraphysiological levels achieved in the first days after application.

– *Testosterone esters (ampoules containing 250 mg of four esters: propionate, phenylpropionate, testosterone decanoate, and isocaproate)*:

Also an oily formulation that is administered intramuscularly. The mixture of four kinds of testosterone esters with different proportions and peaks of activity confers hormone peaks at different times. Try to avoid the peak supraphysiological initial cycle and get closer to normal hormonal levels. The advantages and disadvantages are similar to those of testosterone cypionate.

– *Undecylate (or undecanoate) testosterone (ampoules 1000 mg)*:

Oil formulation and administration intramuscularly, using the castor oil vehicle. It shows no peak action and its action is longer, keeping close to physiological levels for a period of 10–14 weeks. At the time of the first application the range for the second dose should be 6 weeks and it settles down after a mean interval between doses of 12 weeks, individually adjusted according to the clinical response and the laboratory. The advantages are mimicry of the normal hormonal cycle, longer duration of action of application, and convenience in dosing. The disadvantage is the high cost.

Subcutaneous Implants

Subcutaneous implants come in the form of pellets. The dose and regimen vary with the formulation used, but generally have a duration of action of about 3–6 months and the dose varies between 150 and 450 mg. The disadvantages are local complications, discomfort, infection at the site of application, and the possibility of extrusion of the pellet. The advantage is dosage for long-term use.

Other forms of treatment

Adhesive oral 30 mg applicable gum twice a day [85]. Another option is the hCG. Although not an androgen, it stimulates the testes to produce testosterone and is especially useful when one wishes to stimulate the production of sperm and hence male fertility.

Male Hypogonadism Associated with T2DM and Obesity: To Treat or Not to Treat?

Only in the last decade, the main consensus on male hypogonadism started adding conditions between T2DM risk for decreased testosterone, drawing attention to the need for the treatment of these patients [74, 75]. The TIMES2 Study is an important work that evaluated hypogonadal patients with T2DM and metabolic syndrome. Their results show a significant decrease in homeostatic model assessment-insulin resistance among hypogonadal diabetic patients after 6 months of treatment with testosterone replacement gel and a better control of HbA1c after 9 months of treatment [86]. Heufelder et al. evaluated hypogonadal men with a newly diagnosed T2DM treated with testosterone and a change in lifestyle (CL) compared with placebo and CL. After 52 weeks, testosterone replacement resulted in better control of HbA1c and a significant reduction in waist measurement (14.6 cm versus a loss of 6.7 cm respectively) [87].

A number of studies demonstrated that treatment of hypogonadism improves weight loss in hypogonadal obesity. Svartberg et al. found in a case–control study an improvement in body shape of elderly hypogonadal men treated with testosterone for 1 year [88]. The study evaluated 184 hypogonadal men with metabolic syndrome from Moscow [89]. After 30 weeks of administration of parenteral testosterone undecanoate, a significant drop in weight, BMI, and waist circumference, as well as improvement of some components of metabolic syndrome and inflammatory markers [89].

Thus, treatment of hypogonadism in obese men can be effective in helping weight loss because it improves energy and mood, reduces fatigue, and may motivate men to adhere to diet and exercise, which is fundamental in combating obesity [90].

Testosterone and Cardiovascular Disease

Longitudinal cohort studies examining the association of sex hormones measured using immunoassays at baseline with the incidence of cardiovascular disease (CVD) events during follow-up and the results have been controversial [91–93]. In a large population-based cohort of older men, TT or FT in the lowest quartile of values predicted an increased incidence of stroke or transient ischemic attacks [94] whereas higher LH was associated with the incidence of ischemic heart disease events [95]. Most of the studies evaluated older patients and other inclusion criteria were variable and questionable. A small study (also in older men) reported testosterone in the lowest and highest quintiles to be associated with CVD events, suggesting a U-shaped association [96].

In a recent large cohort sex steroids were evaluated using mass spectrometry. In the Osteoporotic Fractures in Men (MrOS) Study, the risk of experiencing a cardiovascular event was 30% lower in men with higher total testosterone [97]. In the Cardiovascular Study, testosterone was not associated with cardiovascular death, or nonfatal myocardial infarction or stroke [98]. In an updated analysis from the Western Australian Health In Men Study (HIMS), testosterone was not associated with incident myocardial infarction and, by contrast, higher testosterone was associated with a lower incidence of stroke [99]. The Atherosclerosis Risk in Communities Study showed that lower testosterone was associated with adverse cardiovascular risk factors, but not with incidence of coronary heart disease events [100]. The recent studies have demonstrated that low testosterone as an independent predictor for higher incidence of stroke in older men has been confirmed by the Copenhagen Study [101].

Cohort studies based on the use of immunoassays for sex steroids provide limited evidence but demonstrate an association of low TT or FT with incidence of stroke and transient ischemic attack [94, 101]. The two largest cohort studies, which measured testosterone using mass spectrometry, reported associations of low testosterone with CVD events in MrOS [97], and stroke in HIMS [99].

Based on current evidence, lower circulating testosterone seems to be a biomarker for CVD risk, particularly an increased incidence of stroke. An age differential should be highlighted. In younger and middle-aged men, lower testosterone levels are associated with adverse cardiovascular risk factors rather than incidence of CVD, whereas in older men, lower testosterone is associated with an increased incidence of CVD manifesting as stroke more prominently than myocardial infarction.

In the last few years, some randomized controlled trials (RCTs) have been published that have shown the effects of testosterone supplementation on protecting against myocardial ischemia. The Testosterone in Older Men with Mobility Limitations (TOM) trial promoted several discussions on the subject due to discontinuous of the trial by the excess of cardiovascular adverse events in the testosterone arm [102]. Others RCTs demonstrated different results than the TOM study [103–109]. In the absence of definitive RCT data, meta-analyses of testosterone RCTs have been undertaken to explore the association between testosterone supplementation and cardiovascular adverse events and, in general, have not found testosterone supplementation to be associated with excess cardiovascular adverse effects [110–115].

Monitoring and Follow-Up

In adolescent or young adult patients, the prostate is not a concern. However, in older men, especially after the age of 40, the prostate should be monitored. Currently, it is known that testosterone replacement does not cause the appearance of prostate cancer in patients who do not have a background for it. However, testosterone and mainly dihydrotestosterone can stimulate prostate tissue [116]. In the last decade, some case series described the use of testosterone therapy in hypogonadal men after treatment for prostate cancer and no clinical or biochemical progression of the tumor. This is not yet an established practice, but it can be a safe treatment in these cases [117–123]. Similarly, with increasing recognition that men with low-grade prostate cancer are at a low risk for morbidity and mortality, there is a growing practice of deferring treatment until there is evidence for more aggressive pathology (active surveillance) Some of these men have symptomatic testosterone deficiency and desire treatment, but the use of testosterone replacement therapy in these men is highly controversial, although small studies have shown some that it is somewhat safe to use [124–126].

Initiation of testosterone therapy is not recommended in men with breast cancer or prostate cancer, with a palpable nodule or indurations, with prostate-specific antigen (PSA) greater than 4 ng/ml or undiagnosed urological treatment, hematocrit above 50%, obstructive sleep apnea, severe, untreated urinary tract symptoms with an International Prostate Symptom Score over 19, heart failure, uncontrolled or poorly controlled (Table 14.8) [74].

Table 14.8 Conditions in which testosterone replacement is associated with a high risk for adverse events and should be contraindicated

High risk for adverse events (absolute contraindication)	Metastatic prostate cancer or activity
	Breast cancer
Moderate risk for adverse events (relative contraindication)	Palpable nodule or induration prostate
	Prostate-specific antigen greater than 4 ng/ml or undiagnosed urological treatment (or greater than 3 ng/ml in subjects at a high risk for prostate cancer, such as African Americans or men with first-degree relatives with a history of prostate cancer)
	Hematocrit above 50%
	Obstructive sleep apnea, severe, untreated
	Severe urinary tract symptoms (International Prostate Symptom Score above 19)
	Heart failure, uncontrolled or poorly controlled

Table 14.9 Monitoring testosterone therapy

1. Evaluate the patient 3–6 months after treatment initiation and then annually to assess whether symptoms have responded to treatment and whether the patient is suffering from any adverse effects
2. Monitor testosterone level 3–6 months after initiation of testosterone therapy

   Therapy should be aimed at raising serum testosterone level to the mid-normal range

   Injectable testosterone enanthate or cypionate: measure serum testosterone level midway between injections. If testosterone is >700 ng/dl (24.5 nmol/l) or <400 ng/dl (14.1 nmol/l), adjust dose or frequency

   Transdermal patches: assess testosterone level 3–12 h after application of the patch; adjust dose to achieve testosterone level in the mid-normal range

   Buccal testosterone bioadhesive tablet: assess level immediately before or after application of fresh system

   Transdermal gels: assess testosterone level any time after the patient has been on treatment for at least 1 week; adjust dose to achieve serum testosterone level in the mid-normal range

   Testosterone pellets: measure testosterone levels at the end of the dosing interval. Adjust the number of pellets and/or the dosing interval to achieve serum testosterone levels within the normal range

   Oral testosterone undecanoate[a]: monitor serum testosterone level 3–5 h after ingestion

   Injectable testosterone undecanoate: measure serum testosterone level just prior to each subsequent injection and adjust the dosing interval to maintain serum testosterone within the mid-normal range
3. Check hematocrit at baseline, at 3–6 months, and then annually. If hematocrit is >54%, stop therapy until hematocrit decreases to a safe level; evaluate the patient for hypoxia and sleep apnea; reinitiate therapy with a reduced dose
4. Measure bone mineral density of lumbar spine and/or femoral neck after 1–2 years of testosterone therapy in hypogonadal men with osteoporosis or low trauma fracture, consistent with regional standard of care
5. In men 40 years of age or older with baseline PSA greater than 0.6 ng/ml, perform digital rectal examination and check PSA level before initiating treatment, at 3–6 months, and then in accordance with guidelines for prostate cancer screening depending on the age and race of the patient
7. Obtain urological consultation if there is:

   An increase in serum PSA concentration >1.4 ng/ml within any 12-month period of testosterone treatment

   A PSA velocity of >0.4 ng/ml year using the PSA level after 6 months of testosterone administration as the reference (only applicable if PSA data are available for a period exceeding 2 years)

   Detection of a prostatic abnormality on digital rectal examination

   An AUA/IPSS of >19
8. Evaluate formulation-specific adverse effects at each visit

   Buccal testosterone tablets: inquire about alterations in taste and examine the gums and oral mucosa for irritation

   Injectable testosterone esters (enanthate, cypionate, and undecanoate): ask about fluctuations in mood or libido, and rarely coughing after injections

   Testosterone patches: look for skin reaction at the application site

   Testosterone gels: advise patients to cover the application sites with a shirt and to wash the skin with soap and water before having skin-to-skin contact, because testosterone gels leave a testosterone residue on the skin that can be transferred to a woman or child who might come in close contact. Serum testosterone levels are maintained when the application site is washed 4–6 h after application of the testosterone gel

   Testosterone pellets: look for signs of infection, fibrosis, or pellet extrusion

[a]Not approved for clinical use in the USA
PSA prostate-specific antigen, *AUA/IPSS* American Urological Association/International Prostate Symptom Score

When testosterone therapy is instituted, one should achieve the average normal levels of testosterone during treatment with any of the formulations adopted. The choice of formulation of testosterone must take into account the patient's preference, the pharmacokinetics, and the cost. Men receiving testosterone therapy should be monitored continuously through a standardized plan that includes medical consultation with a physical examination and laboratory tests (PSA and hematocrit; Table 14.9) [74].

References

1. Krausz C. Male infertility: pathogenesis and clinical diagnosis. Best Pract Res Clin Endocrinol Metab. 2011;25(2):271–85.
2. Grinspon RP, Loreti N, Braslavsky D, Bedecarrás P, Ambao V, et al. Sertoli cell markers in the diagnosis of paediatric male hypogonadism. J Pediatr Endocrinol Metab. 2012;25(1–2):3–11.
3. Grinspon RP, Rey RA. New perspectives in the diagnosis of pediatric male hypogonadism: the importance of AMH as a Sertoli cell marker. Arq Bras Endocrinol Metabol. 2011;55(8):512–9.
4. Tsutsumi R, Webster NJ. GnRH pulsatility, the pituitary response and reproductive dysfunction. Endocr J. 2009;56(6):729–37.
5. Ohlsson C, Wallaschofski H, Lunetta KL, Stolk L, Perry JRB, et al. Genetic determinants of serum testosterone concentrations in men. PLoS Genet. 2011;7(10):1–11.
6. Salenave S, Trabado S, Maione L, Brailly-Tabard S, Young J. Male acquired hypogonadotropic hypogonadism: diagnosis and treatment. Ann Endocrinol (Paris). 2012;73(2):141–6.
7. Groth KA, Skakkebaek A, Host C, Gravholt CH, Bojesen A. Klinefelter syndrome-a clinical update. J Clin Endocrinol Metab. 2012;98(1):20–30.
8. Ottesen AM, Aksglaede L, Garn I, Tartaglia N, Tassone F, Gravholt CH, et al. Increased number of sex chromosomes affects height in a nonlinear fashion: a study of 305 patients with sex chromosome aneuploidy. Am J Med Genet A. 2010;152A(5):1206–12.
9. Herlihy AS, Halliday JL, Cock ML, RI M. The prevalence and diagnosis rates of Klinefelter syndrome: an Australian comparison. Med J Aust. 2011;194(1):24–8.

10. Morris JKAE, Scott C, Jacobs P. Is the prevalence of Klinefelter syndrome increasing? Eur J Hum Genet. 2008;16(2):163–70.

11. Swerdlow AJ, Higgins CD, Schoemaker MJ, Wright AF, Jacobs PA. Mortality in patients with Klinefelter syndrome in Britain: a cohort study. J Clin Endocrinol Metab. 2005;90(12):6516–22.

12. Bojesen A, Juul S, Birkebaek NH, Gravholt CH. Morbidity in Klinefelter syndrome: a Danish register study based on hospital discharge diagnoses. J Clin Endocrinol Metab. 2006;91(4):1254–60.

13. Oates RD. The natural history of endocrine function and spermatogenesis in Klinefelter syndrome: what the data show. Fertil Steril. 2012;98(2):266–73.

14. Savic I. Advances in research on the neurological and neuropsychiatric phenotype of Klinefelter syndrome. Curr Opin Neurol. 2012;25(2):138–43.

15. Mendeluk GR, Pardes EM, López-Costa S. 45,X/46,XY qh- karyotype and aspermia. A case report. Tsitol Genet 2012;46(4):27–30.

16. Lindhardt Johansen M, Hagen CP, Rajpert-De Meyts E, Kjærgaard S, Petersen BL. 45, X/46, XY mosaicism: phenotypic characteristics, growth, and reproductive function–a retrospective longitudinal study. J Clin Endocrinol Metab. 2012;97(8):1540–9.

17. Templado C, Vidal F, Estop A. Aneuploidy in human spermatozoa. Cytogenet Genome Res. 2011;133(2–4):91–9.

18. Cruz Guzmán Odel R, Chávez García AL, Rodríguez-Cruz M. Muscular dystrophies at different ages: metabolic and endocrine alterations. Int J Endocrinol. 2012;2012:1–12.

19. Al-Harbi TM, Bainbridge LJ, McQueen MJ, Tarnopolsky MA. Hypogonadism is common in men with myopathies. J Clin Neuromuscul Dis. 2008;9(4):397–401.

20. Belchetz PE, Barth JH, Kaufman JM. Biochemical endocrinology of the hypogonadal male. Ann Clin Biochem. 2010;47(6):503–15.

21. Menon KM, Menon B. Structure, function and regulation of gonadotropin receptors—a perspective. Mol Cell Endocrinol. 2012;356(1–2):88–97.

22. Brioude F, Bouvattier CE, Lombès M. Hypogonadotropic hypogonadism: new aspects in the regulation of hypothalamic-pituitary-gonadal axis. Ann Endocrinol (Paris). 2010;71 suppl 1:s33–41.

23. Pitteloud N, Durrani S, Raivio T, Sykiotis GP. Complex genetics in idiopathic hypogonadotropic hypogonadism. Front Horm Res. 2010;39:142–53.

24. Robin G, Boitrelle F, Marcelli F, Colin P, Leroy-Martin B, et al. Cryptorchidism: from physiopathology to infertility. Gynecol Obstet Fertil. 2010;38(10):588–99.

25. Hutson JM, Balic A, Nation T, Southwell B. Cryptorchidism. Semin Pediatr Surg. 2010;10(3):215–24.

26. Brauner R, Neve M, Allali S, Trivin C, Lottmann H, et al. Clinical, biological and genetic analysis of anorchia in 26 boys. PLoS One. 2011;6(8):23292.

27. Shiraishi K, Matsuyama H, Takihara H. Pathophysiology of varicocele in male infertility in the era of assisted reproductive technology. Int J Urol. 2012;19(6):538–50.

28. Iglesias P, Carrero JJ, Díez JJ. Gonadal dysfunction in men with chronic kidney disease: clinical features, prognostic implications and therapeutic options. J Nephrol. 2012;25(1):31–42.

29. Foresta C, Schipilliti M, Ciarleglio FA, Lenzi A, D'Amico D. Male hypogonadism in cirrhosis and after liver transplantation. J Endocrinol Investig. 2008;31(5):470–8.

30. Young J. Endocrine consequences of hemochromatosis. Presse Med. 2007;36(9):1319–25.

31. Rochira V, Zirilli L, Orlando G, Santi D, Brigante G, et al. Premature decline of serum total testosterone in HIV-infected men in the HAART-Era. PLoS One. 2011;6(12):e28512.

32. Wallace WH, Anderson RA, Irvine DS. Fertility preservation for young patients with cancer: who is at risk and what can be offered? Lancet Oncol. 2005;6(4):209–18.

33. Dohle GR. Male infertility in cancer patients: review of the literature. Int J Urol. 2010;17(4):327–31.

34. Davis JE, Silverman M. Scrotal emergencies. Emerg Med Clin North Am. 2011;29(3):469–84.

35. Dajusta DG, Granberg CF, Villanueva C, Baker LA. Contemporary review of testicular torsion: new concepts, emerging technologies and potential therapeutics. J Pediatr Urol. 2012;S1477–5131(12):00221–5.

36. Woodruff DY, Horwitz G, Weigel J, Nangia AK. Fertility preservation following torsion and severe ischemic injury of a solitary testes. Fertil Steril. 2010;94(1):352.

37. Ankley GT, Cavallin JE, Durhan EJ, Jensen KM, Kahl MD, et al. A time-course analysis of effects of the steroidogenesis inhibitor ketoconazole on components of the hypothalamic-pituitary-gonadal axis of fathead minnows. Aquat Toxicol. 2012;114–115:88–95.

38. Salehian B, Kejriwal K. Glucocorticoid-induced muscle atrophy: mechanisms and therapeutic strategies. Endocr Pract. 1999;5(5):277–81.

39. Hu GX, Lian QQ, Lin H, Latif SA, Morris DJ, et al. Rapid mechanisms of glucocorticoid signaling in the Leydig cell. Steroids. 2008;73(9–10):1018–24.

40. Viswanathan V, Eugster EA. Etiology and treatment of hypogonadism in adolescents. Pediatr Clin N Am. 2011;58(5):1181–200.

41. Young J. Approach to the male patient with congenital hypogonadotropic hypogonadism. J Clin Endocrinol Metab. 2012;97(3):707–18.

42. Bonomi M, Libri DV, Guizzardi F, Guarducci E, Maiolo E, et al. New understandings of the genetic basis of isolated idiopathic central hypogonadism. Asian J Androl. 2012;14(1):49–56.

43. Hardelin JP, Dodé C. The complex genetics of Kallmann syndrome: KAL1, FGFR1, FGF8, PROKR2, PROK2, et al. Sex Dev. 2008;2(4–5):181–93.

44. Semple RK, Topaloglu AK. The recent genetics of hypogonadotrophic hypogonadism — novel insights and new questions. Clin Endocrinol. 2010;72(4):427–35.

45. Raivio T, Falardeau J, Dwyer A, Quinton R, Hayes FJ, et al. Reversal of idiopathic hypogonadotropic hypogonadism. N Engl J Med. 2007;357(9):863–73.

46. Bahceci M, Dolek D, Tutuncuoglu P, Gorgel A, Oruk G, et al. A case series of Bardet-Biedl syndrome in a large Turkish family and review of the literature. Eat Weight Disord. 2012;17(1):e66–9.

47. Iannello S, Bosco P, Cavaleri A, Camuto M, Milazzo P, et al. A review of the literature of Bardet-Biedl disease and report of three cases associated with metabolic syndrome and diagnosed after the age of fifty. Obes Rev. 2002;3(2):123–35.

48. Bolyakov A, Paduch DA. Prolactin in men's health and disease. Curr Opin Urol. 2011;21(6):527–34.

49. Kanayama G, Pope HG Jr. Illicit use of androgens and other hormones: recent advances. Curr Opin Endocrinol Diabetes Obes. 2012;19(3):211–9.

50. Smith HS, Elliott JA. Opioid-induced androgen deficiency (OPIAD). Pain Physician. 2012;15(3 Suppl):145–56.

51. Elliott JA, Opper SE, Agarwal S, Fibuch EE. Non-analgesic effects of opioids: opioids and the endocrine system. Curr Pharm Des. 2012;18(37):6070–8.

52. De Maddalena C, Bellini M, Berra M, Meriggiola MC, Aloisi AM. Opioid-induced hypogonadism: why and how to treat it. Pain Physician. 2012;15:ES111–8.

53. Chauhan S, Diamond MP. Effect of gonadotropin-releasing-hormone-induced hypogonadism on insulin action as assessed by euglycemic clamp studies in men. Fertil Steril. 2005;84(1):186–90.

54. Jóźków P, Mędraś M. Psychological stress and the function of male gonads. Endokrynol Pol. 2012;63(1):44–9.

55. Nierman DM, Mechanick JI. Hypotestosteronemia in chronically critically ill men. Crit Care Med. 1999;27(11):2418–21.

56. Mechanick JI, Brett EM. Endocrine and metabolic issues in the management of the chronically critically ill patient. Crit Care Med. 2002;18(3):619–41.

57. Miller KK. Endocrine dysregulation in anorexia nervosa update. J Clin Endocrinol Metab. 2011;96(10):2939–49.

58. Isidro ML. Sexual dysfunction in men with type 2 diabetes. Postgrad Med J. 2012;88(1037):152–9.

59. Phé V, Rouprêt M. Erectile dysfunction and diabetes: a review of the current evidence-based medicine and a synthesis of the main available therapies. Diabetes Metab. 2012;38(1):1–13.

60. Dandona P, Dhindsa S. Update: hypogonadotropic hypogonadism in type 2 diabetes and obesity. J Clin Endocrinol Metab. 2011;96(9):2643–51.

61. Traish AM, Miner MM, Morgentaler A, Zitzmann M. Testosterone deficiency. Am J Med. 2011;124(7):578–87.

62. Aftab SS, Kumar S, Barber T. The role of obesity and type 2 diabetes mellitus in the development of male obesity-associated secondary hypogonadism. Clin Endocrinol. 2013;78(3):330–7.

63. Du Plessis SS, Cabler S, McAlister DA, Sabanegh E, Agarwal A. The effect of obesity on sperm disorders and male infertility. Nat Rev Urol. 2010;7(3):153–61.

64. Hohl A, Mazzuco TL, Coral MHC, Schwarzbold M, Walz R. Hypogonadism after traumatic brain injury. Arq Bras Endocrinol Metabol. 2009;53(8):908.

65. Diamanti-Kandarakis E, Bourguignon JP, Giudice LC, Hauser R, Prins GS, Soto AM, et al. Endocrine-disrupting chemicals: an Endocrine Society scientific statement. Endocr Rev. 2009;30(4):293–342.

66. Carlsen EGA, Keiding N, Skakkebaek NE. Evidence for decreasing quality of semen during past 50 years. Evidence for decreasing quality of semen during past 50 years. BMJ. 1992;305(6854):609–13.

67. Skakkebaek NE, Toppari J, Soder O, Gordon CM, Divall S, Draznin M. The exposure of fetuses and children to endocrine disrupting chemicals: a European Society for Paediatric Endocrinology (ESPE) and Pediatric Endocrine Society (PES) call to action statement. J Clin Endocrinol Metab. 2011;96(10):3056–8.

68. Swan SH, Main KM, Liu F, Stewart SL, Kruse RL, Calafat AM, et al. Decrease in anogenital distance among male infants with prenatal phthalate exposure. Environ Health Perspect. 2005;113(8):1056–61.

69. Pierik FH, Burdorf A, Deddens JA, Juttmann RE, Weber RF. Maternal and paternal risk factors for cryptorchidism and hypospadias: a case-control study in newborn boys. Environ Health Perspect. 2004;112(15):1570–6.

70. Hardell L, Van Bavel B, Lindstrom G, Carlberg M, Dreifaldt AC, Wijkstrom H, et al. Increased concentrations of polychlorinated biphenyls, hexachlorobenzene, and chlordanes in mothers of men with testicular cancer. Environ Health Perspect. 2003;111(7):930–4.

71. Durmaz E, Ozmert EN, Erkekoglu P, Giray B, Derman O, Hincal F, et al. Plasma phthalate levels in pubertal gynecomastia. Pediatrics. 2010;125(1):e122–9.

72. Vieira JGH, Nakamura OH, Ferrer CM, Tachibana TT, Endo MHK, et al. Importância da Metodologia na Dosagem de Testosterona Sérica: Comparação entre um Imunoensaio Direto e um Método Fundamentado em Cromatografia. Líquida de Alta Performance e Espectrometria de Massa em Tandem (HPLC/MS-MS). Arq Bras Endocrinol Metabol. 2008;52(6):1050–5.

73. Appelbaum H, Malhotra S. A comprehensive approach to the spectrum of abnormal pubertal development. Adolesc Med State Art Rev. 2012;23(1):1–14.

74. Bhasin S, Cunningham GR, Hayes FJ, Matsumoto AM, Snyder PJ, et al. Testosterone therapy in men with androgen deficiency syndromes: an endocrine society clinical practice guideline. J Clin Endocrinol Metab. 2010;95:2536–59.

75. Wang C, Nieschlag E, Swerdloff R, Behre HM, Hellstrom WJ, et al. Investigation, treatment and monitoring of late-onset hypogonadism in males. Eur J Endocrinol. 2008;159:507–14.

76. Anawalt BD, Hotaling JM, Walsh TJ, Matsumoto AM. Performance of total testosterone measurement to predict free testosterone for the biochemical evaluation of male hypogonadism. J Urol. 2012;187:1369–73.

77. Corona G, Rastrelli G, Forti G, Maggi M. Update in testosterone therapy for men. J Sex Med. 2011;8(3):639–54.

78. Giagulli VA, Triggiani V, Corona G, Carbone D, Licchelli B, et al. Evidence-based medicine update on testosterone replacement therapy (TRT) in male hypogonadism: focus on new formulations. Curr Pharm Des. 2011;17(15):1500–11.

79. Meirelles RM, Hohl A. Saúde masculina: tão negligenciada, principalmente pelos homens. Arq Bras Endocrinol Metabol. 2009;53(8):899.

80. Corona G, Rastrelli G, Vignozzi L, Maggi M. Emerging medication for the treatment of male hypogonadism. Expert Opin Emerg Drugs. 2012;17(2):239–59.

81. Wang C, Swedloff RS, Iranmanesh A, Dobs A, Snyder PJ, Cunningham G, et al. Transdermal testosterone gel improves sexual function, mood, muscle strength and body composition parameters in hypogonadal men: Testosterone Gel Study. J Clin Endocrinol Metab. 2000;85:2839.

82. Wang C, Ilani N, Arvert S, McLachlan RI, Soulis T, Watkinson A. Efficacy and safety of the 2% formulation of testosterone topical solution applied to the axillae in androgen-deficient men. Clin Endocrinol. 2011;75:836–43.

83. Fennell C, Sartorius G, Ly LP, Turner L, Liu PY, Conway AJ, et al. Randomized cross-over clinical trial of injectable vs. implantable depot testosterone for maintenance of testosterone replacement therapy in androgen deficient men. Clin Endocrinol. 2010;73(1):102–9.

84. Hohl A, Marques MOT, Coral MHC, Walz R. Evaluation of late-onset hypogonadism (andropause) treatment using three different formulations of injectable testosterone. Arq Bras Endocrinol Metabol. 2009;53(8):989–95.

85. Dinsmore WW, Wyllie MG. The long-term efficacy and safety of a testosterone mucoadhesive buccal tablet in testosterone-deficient men. BJU Int. 2012;110(2):162–9.

86. Jones TH, Arver S, Behre HM, Buvat J, Meuleman E, et al. Testosterone replacement in hypogonadal men with type 2 diabetes and/or metabolic syndrome (the TIMES2 Study). Diabetes Care. 2011;34(4):828–37.

87. Heufelder AE, Saad F, Bunck MC, Gooren L. Fifty-two-week treatment with diet and exercise plus transdermal testosterone reverses the metabolic syndrome and improves glycemic control in men with newly diagnosed type 2 diabetes and subnormal plasma testosterone. J Androl. 2009;30:726–33.

88. Svartberg J, Agledahl I, Figenschau Y, Sildnes T, Waterloo K, et al. Testosterone treatment in elderly men with subnormal testosterone levels improves body composition and BMD in the hip. Int J Impot Res. 2008;20:378–87.

89. Kalinchenko SY, Tishova YA, Mskhalaya GJ, Gooren LJ, Giltay EJ, et al. Effects of testosterone supplementation on markers of the metabolic syndrome and inflammation in hypogonadal men with the metabolic syndrome: the double-blinded placebo controlled Moscow study. Clin Endocrinol. 2010;73:602–12.

90. Saad F, Aversa A, Isidori AM, Gooren LJ. Testosterone as potential effective therapy in treatment of obesity in men with testosterone deficiency: a review. Curr Diabetes Rev. 2012;8(2):131–43.

91. Smith GD, Ben-Shlomo Y, Beswick A, et al. Cortisol, testosterone, and coronary heart disease. Prospective evidence from the Caerphilly Study. Circulation. 2005;112:332–40.

92. Arnlov J, Pencina MJ, Amin S, et al. Endogenous sex hormones and cardiovascular disease incidence in men. Ann Intern Med. 2006;145:176–84.

93. Vikan T, Schirmer H, Njolstad I, Svartberg J. Endogenous sex hormones and the prospective association with cardiovascular disease and mortality in men: the Tromso study. Eur J Endocrinol. 2009;161:435–42.

94. Yeap BB, Hyde Z, Almeida OP, et al. Lower testosterone levels predict incident stroke and transient ischemic attack in older men. J Clin Endocrinol Metab. 2009;94:2353–9.

95. Hyde Z, Norman PE, Flicker L, et al. Elevated luteinizing hormone predicts ischaemic heart disease events in older men. The Health In Men Study. Eur J Endocrinol. 2011;164:569–77.

96. Soisson V, Brailly-Tabard S, Helmer C, et al. A J-shaped association between plasma testosterone and risk of ischemic arterial event in elderly men: the French 3C Cohort Study. Maturitas. 2013;75:282–8.

97. Ohlsson C, Barrett-Connor E, Bhasin S, et al. High serum testosterone is associated with reduced risk of cardiovascular events in elderly men. J Am Coll Cardiol. 2011;58:1674–81.

98. Shores MM, Biggs ML, Arnold AM, et al. Testosterone, dihydrotestosterone, and incident cardiovascular disease and mortality in the cardiovascular health study. J Clin Endocrinol Metab. 2014;99:2061–8.

99. Yeap BB, Alfonso H, Chubb SAP, et al. In older men, higher plasma testosterone or dihydrotestosterone are independent predictors for reduced incidence of stroke but not myocardial infarction. J Clin Endocrinol Metab. 2014;99:4565–73.

100. Srinath R, Golden SH, Carson KA, Dobs A. Endogenous testosterone and its relationship to preclinical and clinical measures of cardiovascular disease in the Atherosclerosis Risk in Communities Study. J Clin Endocrinol Metab. 2015;100:1602–8.

101. Holmegard HN, Nordestgaard BG, Jensen GB, et al. Sex hormones and ischemic stroke: a prospective cohort study and meta-analyses. J Clin Endocrinol Metab. 2016;101:69–78.

102. Basaria S, Coviello AD, Travison TG, et al. Adverse events associated with testosterone administration. N Engl J Med. 2010;363:109–22.

103. Shores MM, Smith NL, Forsberg CW, et al. Testosterone treatment and mortality in men with low testosterone levels. J Clin Endocrinol Metab. 2012;97:2050–8.

104. Muraleedharan V, Marsh H, Kapoor D, et al. Testosterone deficiency is associated with increased risk of mortality and testosterone replacement improves survival in men with type 2 diabetes. Eur J Endocrinol. 2013;169:725–33.

105. Vigen R, O'Donnell CI, Baron AE, et al. Association of testosterone therapy with mortality, myocardial infarction, and stroke in men with low testosterone levels. JAMA. 2013;310:1829–36.

106. Finkle WD, Greenland S, Ridgeway GK, et al. Increased risk of non-fatal myocardial infarction following testosterone therapy prescription in men. PLoS One. 2014;9:e85805.

107. Baillargeon J, Urban RJ, Kuo Y-F, et al. Risk of myocardial infarction in older men receiving testosterone therapy. Ann Pharmacother. 2014;48:1138–44.

108. Sharma R, Oni OA, Gupta K, et al. Normalization of testosterone level is associated with reduced incidence of myocardial infarction and mortality in men. Eur Heart J. 2015;36:2706–15.

109. Anderson JL, May HT, Lappe DL, et al. Impact of testosterone replacement therapy on myocardial infarction, stroke and death in men with low testosterone concentrations in an integrated health care system. Am J Cardiol. 2016;117:794–9.

110. Haddad RM, Kennedy CC, Caples SM, et al. Testosterone and cardiovascular risk in men: a systematic review and meta-analysis of randomized placebo-controlled trials. Mayo Clin Proc. 2007;82:29–39.

111. Fernandez-Balsells MM, Murad MH, Lane M, et al. Adverse effects of testosterone therapy in adult men: a systematic review and meta-analysis. J Clin Endocrinol Metab. 2010;95:2560–75.

112. Xu L, Freeman G, Cowling BJ, Schooling CM. Testosterone therapy and cardiovascular events among men: a systematic review and meta-analysis of placebo-controlled randomized trials. BMC Med. 2013;11:108.

113. Ruige JB, Ouwens DM, Kaufman J-M. Beneficial and adverse effects of testosterone on the cardiovascular system in men. J Clin Endocrinol Metab. 2013;98:4300–10.

114. Corona G, Maseroli E, Rastrelli G, et al. Cardiovascular risk associated with testosterone-boosting medications: a systematic review and meta-analysis. Expert Opin Drug Saf. 2014;13:1327–51.

115. Borst SE, Shuster JJ, Zou B, et al. Cardiovascular risks and elevation of serum DHT vary by route of testosterone administration: a systematic review and meta-analysis. BMC Med. 2014;12:21.

116. Rhoden EL, Averbeck MA. Câncer de próstata e testosterona: riscos e controvérsias. Arq Bras Endocrinol Metabol. 2009;53(8):956–62.

117. Kaufman JM, Graydon RJ. Androgen replacement after curative radical prostatectomy for prostate carcinoma in hypogonadal men. J Urol. 2004;172:920; Agarwal PK, Oefelein MG. Testosterone replacement therapy after primary treatment for prostate carcinoma. J Urol. 2005;173:533.

118. Khera M, Grober ED, Najari B, Colen JS, Mohamed O, Lamb DJ, Lipshultz LI. Testosterone replacement therapy following radical prostatectomy. J Sex Med. 2009;6(4):1165–70.

119. Sarosdy MF. Testosterone replacement for hypogonadism after treatment of early prostate carcinoma with brachytherapy. Cancer. 2007;109:536.

120. Pastuszak AW, Khanna A, Badhiwala N, et al. Testosterone therapy after radiation therapy for low, intermediate and high risk prostate cancer. J Urol. 2015;194(5):1271–6.

121. Balbontin FG, Moreno SA, Bley E, Chacon R, Silva A, Morgentaler A. Long-acting testosterone injection for treatment of testosterone deficiency after brachytherapy of prostate cancer. BJU Int. 2014;114(1):125–30.

122. Morales A, Black AM, Emerson LE. Testosterone administration to men with testosterone deficiency syndrome after external beam radiotherapy for localized prostate carcinoma: preliminary observations. BJU Int. 2009;103:62.

123. Pastuszak AW, Pearlman AM, Lai WS, et al. Testosterone replacement therapy in patients with prostate cancer after radical prostatectomy. J Urol. 2013;190:639.

124. Morgentaler A. Two years of testosterone therapy associated with decline in prostate-specific antigen in a man with untreated prostate cancer. J Sex Med. 2009;6(2):574–7.

125. Morgentaler A, Lipshultz LI, Bennett R, Sweeney M, Avila D Jr, Khera M. Testosterone therapy in men with untreated prostate cancer. J Urol. 2011;185(4):1256–60.

126. Kacker R, Hult M, San Francisco IF, Conners WP, Rojas PA, Dewolf WC, Morgentaler A. Can testosterone therapy be offered to men on active surveillance for prostate cancer? Preliminary results. Asian J Androl. 2016;18:16.

Hormone Therapy in the Transgender Patient

Mary O. Stevenson and Vin Tangpricha

Introduction and Terminology

People who have a gender identity that differs from the gender assigned at birth have existed for centuries. The term used to describe the discomfort with having a gender identity that differs from the gender assigned at birth is gender dysphoria [1]. Transgender has been used as the term to describe people who do not express a gender identity that fits their assigned gender and/or societal norms for accepted gender expression [2]. Most but not all transgender people will have gender dysphoria. Transgender people may differ in their approach in handling their gender dysphoria, which may range from a social transition (living in the gender role of the affirmed gender), hormone therapy, and gender-affirming surgery [2].

The previous terms, transsexual or transsexualism, are no longer preferred since they imply a more negative connotation and that transgender people only had a "binary" gender identity, meaning only male or female. Terminologies such as gender nonconforming or gender incongruence have been proposed as terms that recognize the broad spectrum of gender identity and expression.

There are other entities that share some overlap with transgender and gender-nonconforming people. Persons with differences of sexual differentiation or disorders of sex development (DSD) or intersex often represent a separate entity of people from transgender persons. Some people with DSD may have gender dysphoria and seek therapies to align their external appearance to match their gender identity. However, some people with DSD reject the notion that they have a gender dysphoria and/or that surgery is required to align with their gender expression [3]. People that cross-dress (dress in the clothes of a different gender than their birth-assigned gender) represent an understudied population of people who may or may not fall under the terminology of transgender. Some people that initially cross-dress may be exploring different gender expressions, while others have a solidified gender expression but cross-dress for enjoyment. Other entities that may overlap with transgender and gender nonconforming include eunuchs and people with body dysmorphic syndrome. Sexual orientation is often confused with gender identity. There are a number of sexual orientations, and these occur independently from a person's gender identity. One cannot assume a person's sexual orientation based on their gender identity or sex assigned at birth.

The purpose of this chapter is to focus on the hormonal and surgical treatment of people who identity as transgender and gender nonconforming. The criteria for diagnosis, available guidelines on the initiation and monitoring of hormone therapy, and the criteria for referral for gender-affirming surgery will be discussed.

Diagnosis and Guidelines

Specific criteria for the diagnosis for gender dysphoria are available in the Diagnostic and Statistical Manual of Mental Disorders, Fifth Edition (DSM-V) [1]. In brief, the criteria establish that there exists a marked incongruence of greater than 6-month duration between the affirmed gender and the sex assigned at birth that causes significant psychosocial stress which impairs functioning. There is controversy over the classification of gender dysphoria under the category of sexual dysfunctions. Professionals and transgender stakeholders are proposing to move gender dysphoria under the category of sexual health in the next revision of the International Classification of Diseases (ICD) [4]. The qualifications of professionals making the diagnosis of gender dysphoria and the timing and eligibility of hormone therapy for children and adults are proposed by the World Professional Association for Transgender Health's Standards of Care, version 7 (SOC7) [2]. In brief, gender-nonconforming adults can start on hormone therapy if they

M. O. Stevenson · V. Tangpricha (✉)
Division of Endocrinology, Metabolism and Lipids, Emory University Department of Medicine, Atlanta, GA, USA
e-mail: MOSTEVE@emory.edu; vin.tangpricha@emory.edu

have a "persistent, well-documented gender dysphoria," have the "capacity to make a fully informed decision and can consent for treatment," "are of age [an adult] in a given country," and have "significant medical concerns" well-controlled prior to the initiation of hormone therapy [2]. For gender-nonconforming children, hormone therapy can be initiated once the child has reached the age of consent (typically 16 years old in most countries) but ideally also with parental consent, has documented a long period of gender dysphoria during childhood, or emerges or is exacerbated by the initiation of puberty, and has had all psychological, medical, and social issues addressed prior to hormone therapy. The hormone regimens used in children and adults differ according to the stage of puberty which will be addressed in the following sections.

Once the diagnosis of gender dysphoria has been established and the person is deemed eligible and ready to initiate hormone therapy, the 2017 Endocrine Society provides specific evidence-based and consensus recommendations on the initiation, monitoring, and long-term follow-up of hormone therapy and criteria for referral for gender-affirming surgery [5, 6]. The guidelines reaffirm that special expertise in children and adolescent psychology and psychopathology is required to make the diagnosis of gender dysphoria in children and that a multispecialty of medical and mental health providers participates in the management of children prior and during the treatment with hormone therapy. The guidelines reaffirm that the DSM-V should be used when diagnosing gender dysphoria.

Gender-Affirming Hormone Therapy in Children

Once the multispecialty team of medical and mental health providers endorses that a child is eligible for hormone therapy, the regimens used in children depend on the stage of puberty. For pre-pubertal children, no hormone therapy is recommended. During this stage, the child should work with a mental health care professional and/or mental health team regarding issues on social role change (e.g., name and pronoun change, gender role change at school, etc.). For children who are in the earliest stages of puberty, gonadotropin-releasing hormone (GnRH) agonists are recommended initially to halt puberty until the time that the expert multispecialty team deems that sex hormone therapy should be started. Earlier studies have suggested that children have not yet affirmed their adult gender identity prior to the age of 16 [7, 8]. However, more recent studies have suggested that selected children who have intense gender dysphoria prior to the age of 16 may be good candidates for earlier hormone therapy [9]. For children presenting in later stages of puberty, GnRH agonists can be started along with

sex hormone therapy for the desired gender once deemed appropriate by the expert multispecialty team.

Long-term data for pubertal suppression along with hormone therapy in children do not currently exist. The longest published follow-up time was 22 years in a transboy started on hormone therapy at age 13 [10]. In this reported case, there were no reported long-term medical or mental health consequences from the hormone therapy. Recent studies have indicated that trans-children ($n = 55$) cared by a multidisciplinary team had improvements of psychosocial functioning after pubertal suppression, hormone therapy, and gender-affirming surgery [11]. Important to consider are the impacts of therapies on fertility especially if puberty is blocked making future retrieval of gametes difficult for fertility preservation therapies [12]. Other considerations include the lower doses of hormones used in children compared to adults as children have not yet reached full adult size. Finally, the continuation of GnRH agonists in transgender children into adulthood should be reassessed. The GnRH agonist therapy may be stopped particularly in transboys on testosterone. However, in transgirls, GnRH agonists still act as very effective testosterone-lowering agents [13].

Transfeminine Hormone Therapy and Long-Term Monitoring

Endocrinologists should discuss individual expectations and the time course of physical and emotional changes with each individual to ensure that these two align (Fig. 15.1). Transfeminine hormone therapy refers to hormone regimens provided to a person who is sex assigned at birth as male who is wishing to transition into the affirmed gender of a female. Some individuals may not wish to develop all of the primary and secondary sex characteristics of a female; therefore, it is important to discuss these expectations with each individual. For transfeminine hormone therapy, the Endocrine Society guidelines recommend that physicians target blood sex steroid levels in the reference normal range for females, estradiol levels 100–200 pg/mL and testosterone levels <50 ng/dL [5]. Two major classes of medications are required for transgender women: estrogen and testosterone-lowering drugs.

Estrogens can be given as an oral pill, transcutaneous gel, skin patch, or intramuscular injection. The choice of estrogen depends on the local pharmacy coverage, the individual's comorbidities, and patient preference. Estradiol is considered the safest form of estrogen to be given orally as opposed to other formulations of estrogen including ethinyl estradiol and conjugated estrogens, which have been associated with increased thromboembolism [14]. Oral estradiol preparations have the advantage that estradiol can be measured in blood to ensure adequate therapeutic concentrations and to avoid supraphysiologic levels, providing an advantage

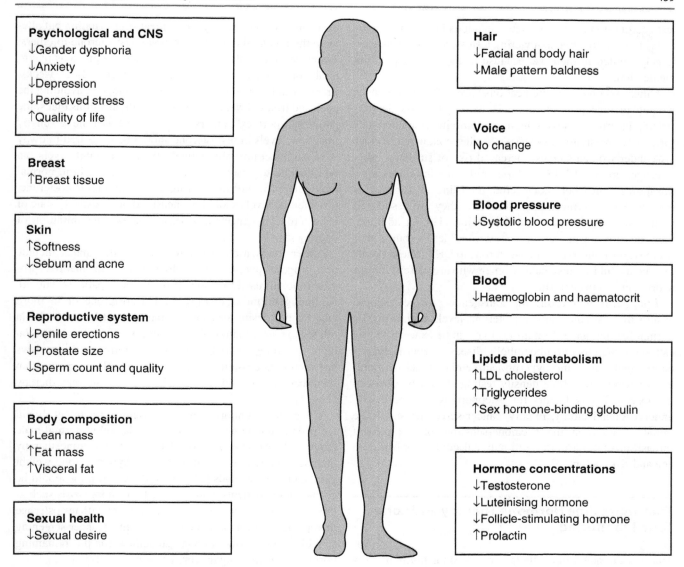

Psychological and CNS
↓Gender dysphoria
↓Anxiety
↓Depression
↓Perceived stress
↑Quality of life

Breast
↑Breast tissue

Skin
↑Softness
↓Sebum and acne

Reproductive system
↓Penile erections
↓Prostate size
↓Sperm count and quality

Body composition
↓Lean mass
↑Fat mass
↑Visceral fat

Sexual health
↓Sexual desire

Hair
↓Facial and body hair
↓Male pattern baldness

Voice
No change

Blood pressure
↓Systolic blood pressure

Blood
↓Haemoglobin and haematocrit

Lipids and metabolism
↑LDL cholesterol
↑Triglycerides
↑Sex hormone-binding globulin

Hormone concentrations
↓Testosterone
↓Luteinising hormone
↓Follicle-stimulating hormone
↑Prolactin

Fig. 15.1 Expected changes in response to transfeminine hormone therapy. (From Tangpricha and Den Heijer [16] Reprinted with permission from Elsevier)

over other oral formulations of estrogen. Estradiol patches have the advantage of avoiding the first-pass liver effect and thus have less stimulation on blood-clotting proteins. Estradiol patches and gels appear to have a better safety profile in terms of thromboembolism [15]. Intramuscular estrogen can be given as estradiol ester, typically estradiol valerate or cypionate [5]. Intramuscular estrogen can be given every 1–2 weeks and also has the advantage of avoiding the first-pass liver effect; however, supraphysiologic levels of estradiol can occur if levels are not carefully monitored and the dose of estrogen is not adjusted accordingly. In general, all forms of estrogen should be initiated at a low dose and titrated up over a few months until the target estradiol level is reached.

In general, a testosterone-lowering agent is also required to lower serum testosterone levels into the female range, at least initially. In the USA, the most commonly prescribed testosterone-lowering medication is spironolactone, which antagonizes androgen activity at the androgen receptor and has additional testosterone-lowering action by an unclear mechanism [5]. Given spironolactone's properties as a potassium-sparing diuretic, potassium levels and kidney function should also be monitored. In Europe, cyproterone is used as a testosterone antagonist which also has progestin-like properties. However, recent reports suggest that cyproterone is associated with increased risk of hyperprolactinemia and meningiomas which has limited its use, especially in the UK [16]. In the UK, GnRH agonists are preferred as the testosterone-lowering medication in adults [14]. GnRH ago-nists are very effective in lowering testosterone levels but are largely limited in their use because of the high cost of the medication.

Other second-line medications used for transgender women include progesterones. However, the data demonstrating its effectiveness in inducing feminine characteristics (primarily breast) are very sparse. Studies conducted in older cis-gender women suggest increased risk of stroke in users of progesterones [17, 18]. 5-Alpha-reductase inhibitors, e.g., finasteride, are not considered first-line agents as a testosterone-lowering medication since they are associated with sexual dysfunction and depression [19]. In addition, they do not lower serum testosterone levels but rather decrease the conversion of testosterone to DHT. These agents may be useful in transgender women who are suffering from androgenic alopecia [20].

Long-term monitoring in transgender women should ensure that estradiol and testosterone levels remain in the normal female range. Conditions that can be exacerbated by estrogens such as thromboembolic disease, hypertriglyceridemia, gallstones, and hyperprolactinemia should be monitored periodically. Bone density testing should be obtained in those with risk factors for osteoporosis and those who undergo gonadectomy. Finally, cancer screening should be initiated based on the hormone-sensitive organs present (breast, prostate) according to national guidelines based on age and risk factors [5].

Transmasculine Hormone Therapy and Long-Term Monitoring

Transmasculine hormone therapy refers to the hormone therapy provided to a person who is sex-assigned female at birth and wishes to transition into the affirmed gender of male. As compared to transfeminine hormone therapy, transmasculine therapy is more straightforward as it requires the administration of only one medication, testosterone, to achieve secondary sex characters of male. The expected time course of changes should be discussed with each individual (Fig. 15.2). The concept of transmasculine therapy, including the preparations and hormone laboratory goals, follows the general approach of treating male hypogonadism [21]. The Endocrine Society guidelines recommend a goal to achieve testosterone values in the normal male range, typically 400–700 ng/dL [5].

Testosterone can be given transdermally, as a patch or gel, or as an injection, either subcutaneously or intramuscularly. Again, the choice of regimen depends on patient preference and insurance factors. Transdermal gel preparations require daily application, and androgen can be inadvertently transferred to close contacts if patients are not mindful of application site and do not wash their hands after application.

Testosterone patches may cause local skin irritation but alleviate the potential risk of transferring testosterone to others. Testosterone enanthate or cypionate may be given as parenteral or subcutaneous injections every 1–2 weeks. Transdermal preparations have the advantage of avoiding the peak and trough levels that are seen with injections that some patients report as bothersome. For testosterone given by injection, levels of testosterone should be measured midway between injections; alternatively, peak and trough levels can be obtained to ensure levels are maintained within normal male range [5]. For monitoring of transdermal testosterone, testosterone levels should be measured once a steady state of testosterone is expected, at least a week after initiation of therapy [5].

Other medications used for transgender males include oral progesterone, GnRH analogs, and depot medroxyprogesterone, all used to stop menses in those patients who are beginning hormone therapy with testosterone or in those who do not desire testosterone therapy but have dysphoria related to menstruation. The time course of menses cessation on testosterone is variable, and several retrospective reviews have reported cessation as early as 1 month but more often seen between 6 and 12 months on testosterone therapy [22–24].

Long-term monitoring of transmasculine treatment should focus on maintaining testosterone levels within normal male range. Adverse events associated with testosterone therapy include erythrocytosis, sleep apnea, hypertension, weight gain, and lipid changes [25]. Bone density testing should be considered in patients who are at risk of osteoporosis such as those patients who stop or are noncompliant with testosterone therapy and have undergone gonadectomy. Cancer screening should again follow national guidelines for the remaining hormone-sensitive organs (breast tissue, cervix) [5].

Surgical Considerations

There are many surgical options for both transgender women and men to align their primary and secondary sex characteristics with their affirmed gender. The Endocrine Society guidelines identify two main types of surgeries, those that affect fertility and those that do not [5]. Surgeries that do not affect fertility have less stringent criteria for approval. For transwomen, these would include surgeries such as breast augmentation, facial feminization surgeries, as well as removal of facial or body hair by electrolysis or laser treatments. For transmen, a mastectomy is an example of fertility sparing surgery that may be desired.

Gender-affirming surgery, formerly known as sex reassignment surgery, affects fertility and is irreversible. Because of this, the Endocrine Society guidelines propose several criteria for gender-affirming surgery: "(1) persistent, well-

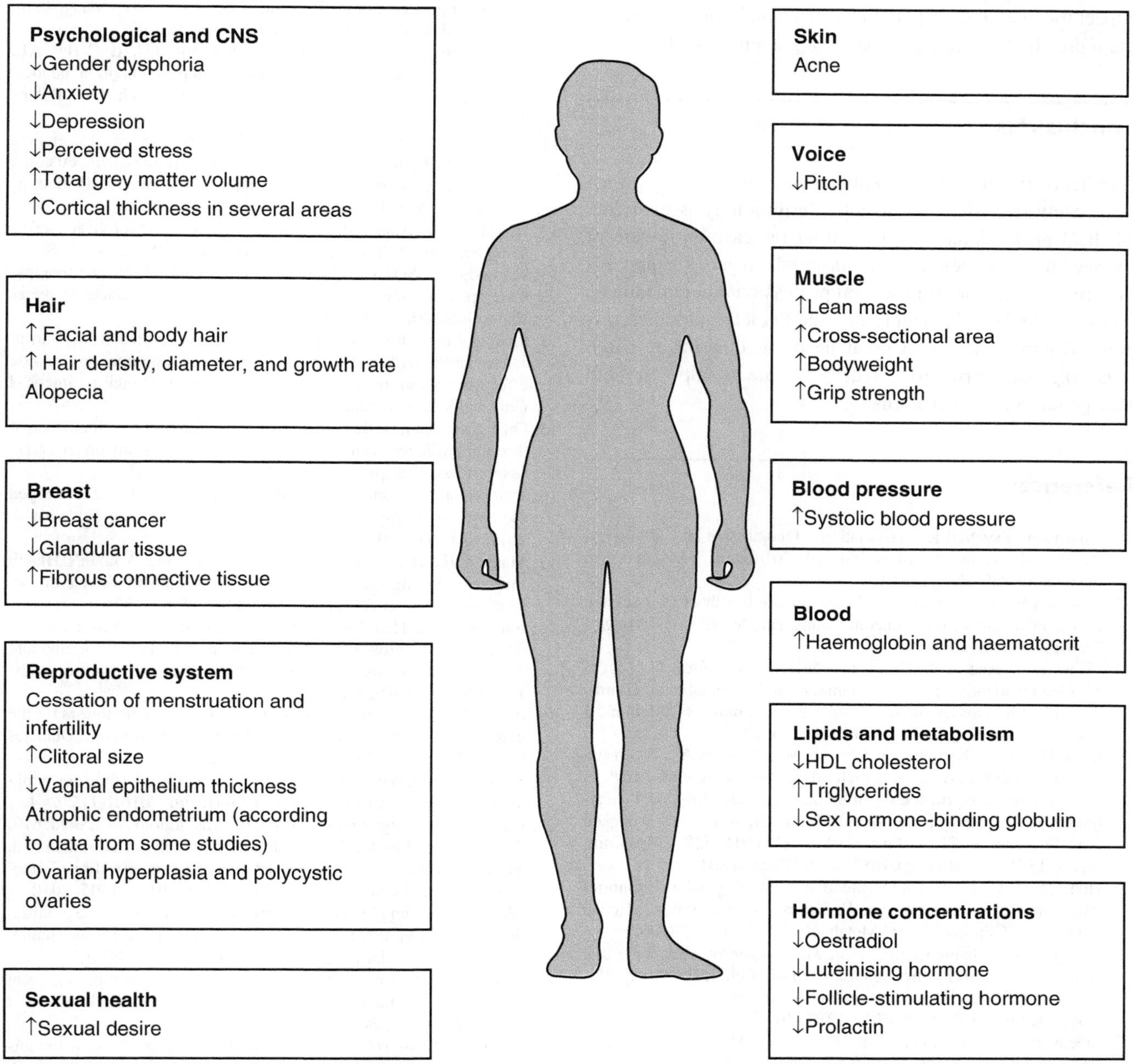

Psychological and CNS
↓Gender dysphoria
↓Anxiety
↓Depression
↓Perceived stress
↑Total grey matter volume
↑Cortical thickness in several areas

Hair
↑ Facial and body hair
↑ Hair density, diameter, and growth rate
Alopecia

Breast
↓Breast cancer
↓Glandular tissue
↑Fibrous connective tissue

Reproductive system
Cessation of menstruation and infertility
↑Clitoral size
↓Vaginal epithelium thickness
Atrophic endometrium (according to data from some studies)
Ovarian hyperplasia and polycystic ovaries

Sexual health
↑Sexual desire

Skin
Acne

Voice
↓Pitch

Muscle
↑Lean mass
↑Cross-sectional area
↑Bodyweight
↑Grip strength

Blood pressure
↑Systolic blood pressure

Blood
↑Haemoglobin and haematocrit

Lipids and metabolism
↓HDL cholesterol
↑Triglycerides
↓Sex hormone-binding globulin

Hormone concentrations
↓Oestradiol
↓Luteinising hormone
↓Follicle-stimulating hormone
↓Prolactin

Fig. 15.2 Expected changes in response to transmasculine hormone therapy. (From Irwig MS. Testosterone therapy for transgender men. Lancet Diabetes Endocrinol. 2017;5(4):301–11. Reprinted with permission from Elsevier)

documented gender dysphoria, (2) legal age of majority in a given country, (3) having continuously and responsibly used gender-affirming hormones for 12 months, and (4) successful continuous full-time living in the new gender role for 12 months" in addition to good control of any existing medical or mental health conditions and proficiency in the practical aspects of surgery [5].

These surgeries are typically under the regulation of the state or country in which they are performed, and most surgeons require at least one letter of recommendations from a mental health provider. Examples of gender-affirming surgeries for transgender women include penectomy, gonadectomy, and creation of a neovagina. For transgender men, hysterectomy, oophorectomy, vaginectomy, and creation of a neopenis and scrotum are all considerations.

For all transgender patients considering gender-affirming surgery, fertility preservation should be offered and discussed prior to referral for surgical procedures. Fertility preservation should be offered for all patients initiating hormone therapy as well as those patients already on medical therapy. The duration and dosages of hormone therapy that will affect fertility are not known though it is reasonable to expect that the longer a patient has been on hormone therapy, the more challenging the retrieval of gametes may be.

Conclusions

The fields of transgender medicine and surgery have grown immensely over the past decade. Terminology is evolving. Medical professionals are becoming increasingly aware of the need for competent care of transgender persons. Standards of care are available from several professional organizations, including the WPATH and Endocrine Society guidelines referenced here. There is a great need for ongoing research regarding long-term effects of hormone therapy in both transgender youth and adults.

References

1. American Psychiatric Association. Diagnostic and statistical manual of mental disorders. 5th ed. Arlington, VA: American Psychiatric Publishing; 2013.
2. Coleman E, et al. Standards of care for the health of transsexual, transgender and gender-nonconforming people, version 7. Inter J Transgenderism. 2012;13(4).
3. Fisher AD, Ristori J, Fanni E, Castellini G, Forti G, Maggi M. Gender identity, gender assignment and reassignment in individuals with disorders of sex development: a major of dilemma. J Endocrinol Investig. 2016;39(11):1207–24.
4. Beek TF, Cohen-Kettenis PT, Bouman WP, de Vries AL, Steensma TD, Witcomb GL, Arcelus J, Richards C, De Cuypere G, Kreukels BP. Gender incongruence of childhood: clinical utility and stakeholder agreement with the World Health Organization's proposed ICD-11 criteria. PLoS One. 2017;12(1):e0168522. https://doi.org/10.1371/journal.pone.0168522. eCollection 2017.
5. Hembree WC, et al. Endocrine treatment of gender-dysphoric/gender-incongruent persons: an Endocrine Society clinical practice guideline. J Clin Endocrinol Metab. 2017;102(11):3869–903.
6. Tangpricha V, Hannema SE, Irwig MS, Meyer WJ 3rd, Safer JD, Hembree WC. 2017 American association of clinical endocrinologists/endocrine society update on transgender medicine: CASE discussions. Endocr Pract. 2017;23(12):1430–6.
7. Steensma TD, Kreukels BP, de Vries AL, Cohen-Kettenis PT. Gender identity development in adolescence. Horm Behav. 2013;64(2):288–97.
8. Wallien MS, Cohen-Kettenis PT. Psychosexual outcome of gender-dysphoric children. J Am Acad Child Adolesc Psychiatry. 2008;47(12):1413–23.
9. Steensma TD, McGuire JK, Kreukels BP, Beekman AJ, Cohen-Kettenis PT. Factors associated with desistence and persistence of childhood gender dysphoria: a quantitative follow-up study. J Am Acad Child Adolesc Psychiatry. 2013;52(6):582–90.
10. Cohen-Kettenis PT, Schagen SE, Steensma TD, de Vries AL, Delemarre-van de Waal HA. Puberty suppression in a gender-dysphoric adolescent: a 22-year follow-up. Arch Sex Behav. 2011;40(4):843–7.
11. de Vries AL, McGuire JK, Steensma TD, Wagenaar EC, Doreleijers TA, Cohen-Kettenis PT. Young adult psychological outcome after puberty suppression and gender reassignment. Pediatrics. 2014;134(4):696–704.
12. Rosenthal SM. Approach to the patient: transgender youth: endocrine considerations. J Clin Endocrinol Metab. 2014;99(12):4379–89.
13. Mamoojee Y, Seal LJ, Quinton R. Transgender hormone therapy: understanding international variation in practice. Lancet Diabetes Endocrinol. 2017;5(4):243–6.
14. Seal LJ, Franklin S, Richards C, Shishkareva A, Sinclaire C, Barrett J. Predictive markers for mammoplasty and a comparison of side effect profiles in transwomen taking various hormonal regimens. J Clin Endocrinol Metab. 2012;97(12):4422–8.
15. Ott J, Kaufmann U, Bentz EK, Huber JC, Tempfer CB. Incidence of thrombophilia and venous thrombosis in transsexuals under cross-sex hormone therapy. Fertil Steril. 2010;93(4):1267–72.
16. Tangpricha V, den Heijer M. Oestrogen and anti-androgen therapy for transgender women. Lancet Diabetes Endocrinol. 2017;5(4):291–300.
17. Manson JE, Hsia J, Johnson KC, et al, for the Women's Health Initiative Investigators. Estrogen plus progestin and the risk of coronary heart disease. N Engl J Med. 2003;349:523–534.
18. Barsoum MK, Heit JA, Ashrani AA, Leibson CL, Petterson TM, Bailey KR. Is progestin an independent risk factor for incident venous thromboembolism? A population-based case-control study. Thromb Res. 2010;126:373–8.
19. Irwig MS. Safety concerns regarding 5α reductase inhibitors for the treatment of androgenetic alopecia. Curr Opin Endocrinol Diabetes Obes. 2015;22(3):248–53.
20. Stevenson MO, Wixon N, Safer JD. Scalp hair regrowth in hormone-treated transgender woman. Transgend Health. 2016;1(1):202–4.
21. Bhasin S, Cunningham GR, Hayes FJ, Matsumoto AM, Snyder PJ, Swerdloff RS, Montori VM. Testosterone therapy in adult men with androgen deficiency syndromes: an endocrine society clinical practice guideline. J Clin Endocrinol Metab. 2006;91(6):1995–2010.
22. Ahmad S, Leinung M. The response of the menstrual cycle to initiation of hormonal therapy in transgender men. Transgender Health. 2017;2(1):176–9. https://doi.org/10.1089/trgh.2017.0023.
23. Pelusi C, Costantino A, Martelli V, et al. Effects of three different testosterone formulations in female-to-male transsexual persons. J Sex Med. 2014;11:3002–11.
24. Deutsch MB, Bhakri V, Kubicek K, et al. Effects of cross-sex hormone treatment on transgender women and men. Obstet Gynecol. 2015;125:605–10.
25. Bhasin S, Cunningham GR, Hayes FJ, Matsumoto AM, Snyder PJ, Swerdloff RS, Montori VM. Testosterone therapy in adult men with androgen deficiency syndromes: an endocrine society clinical practice guideline. J Clin Endocrinol Metab. 2006;91(6):1995–2010.

Idiopathic Short Stature: Diagnostic and Therapeutic Approach

Ana P. M. Canton and Alexander A. L. Jorge

Case Report

Our clinical case for discussion is about a short statured boy who was 14.6 years old at his first evaluation. He was born after a 39-week gestation as the third child of a non-consanguineous marriage. His birth weight was 3.250 g (−0.3 SDS), and his birth length was not available. His neuropsychomotor development was normal, his school performance was good, and there were no remarkable findings in his medical history. His father's height was 174 cm (−0.1 SDS) and his mother's height was 154 cm (−1.3 SDS), resulting in a target height of 170.6 cm (−0.6 SDS). His father and mother apparently had normal pubertal development, and his mother's age of menarche was 13 years old. His older brother's height was not available, but he had a previous history of pubertal spurt after 16 years of age. Likewise, his older sister's height was also not available, but she had a previous history of menarche at 14.

At the presentation, the height of the patient was 142.5 cm (−2.6 SDS), his weight was 29.4 kg (−3.9 SDS), his body mass index was 14.5 kg/m^2 (−3.1 SDS), and his sitting height was 73 cm (−0.3 SDS). Physical examination was unremarkable, without dysmorphic features. His pubertal staging was G2P1, as determined by Marshall and Tanner criteria. His bone age was 11 years old, as determined by Greulich and Pyle criteria. At this moment, his adult height prediction was 173.1 cm (−0.2 SDS), as determined by the Bayley–Pinneau method.

A. P. M. Canton · A. A. L. Jorge (✉)
Unidade de Endocrinologia Genetica, Laboratorio de Endocrinologia Celular e Molecular LIM/25, Disciplina de Endocrinologia, Hospital das Clinicas da Faculdade de Medicina da Universidade de São Paulo, São Paulo, SP, Brazil
e-mail: alexj@usp.br

Introduction

Growth is an essential process for the development of a healthy adult, and it is a sensitive marker of child health status. It comprises a dynamic, nonhomogeneous, and complex process of replication and differentiation of cells from several tissues. It is generally assumed that growth is regulated by a multitude of genetic and epigenetic mechanisms, which interact with influences from internal and external environments. With respect to genes, it is assumed that both adult height and growth pattern are largely genetically programmed [1].

Growth intensity differs depending on the stage of life, from intrauterine to adult life. During the prenatal period, growth velocity varies greatly according to gestational age, with a median growth of 1.2–1.5 cm per week. In late gestation, growth velocity takes on a process of deceleration that persists until pubertal onset. In the first and second years of life, children's growth velocity is, in average, 25 and 12 cm/year, respectively. After that, it decelerates gradually to an average of 4–6 cm/year until the pubertal spurt starts. During puberty, there is an acceleration of growth, and children can reach an average height velocity (HV) of 12 cm/year. Pubertal spurt onset time is dependent on the age children start puberty. Girls start a rhythm of growth acceleration in the early pubertal development, while boys start this same process in the late pubertal development [2, 3].

Growth disorders are associated with different diseases, which encompass different systems and mechanisms. Therefore, short stature is one of the most common concerns presented to pediatric endocrinologists and other child-caring physicians. Despite the complexity of the matter, some diagnoses can be obtained by a careful analysis of medical history and a comprehensive physical examination [3, 4].

In this chapter, we present referral criteria for children with short stature, diagnostic procedures to detect the causes of this condition, involved differential diagnosis, and possible therapeutic approaches. Idiopathic short stature diagnosis and approach will be specifically emphasized.

Short Stature Diagnosis

Criteria for Investigation of Short Stature

Height has an almost perfect Gaussian distribution in large-scale growth studies. Therefore, the first key point in the diagnostic approach of children with short stature is the application of referral criteria for diagnostic workup. With this application we can distinguish if they are simply within the shortest part of the "normal" distribution or if they effectively are with a disorder restricting growth [1, 3].

In the initial evaluation of growth, there are basically three parameters that can be assessed. First, height can be compared with age and sex references and expressed as standard deviation score (SDS) or centile position. Height SDS is a measure of the deviation of the individual height from the mean and is expressed as the number of standard deviation below or above the mean height of the population for the same age and sex [5]. Therefore, by definition, individuals are defined as short statured when they present a height SDS < −2.0 or a height below the 2.3% percentile for a given age, sex, and population.

Second, height SDS can be compared with the sex-corrected parental height (target height) SDS [5]. The target height is a mathematical calculation, which expresses the genetic potential of height of an individual. It can be calculated by the arithmetic mean of parental height with the addition or subtraction of 6.5 cm for boys and girls, respectively [3]. Children should be referred for a diagnostic workup when he/she is "short for the target height," i.e., when the height SDS minus target height SDS is below −2.0.

Third, a longitudinal analysis of growth can be used, either expressed as height velocity (cm/year or SDS) in comparison to age and sex references or as a height SDS change (deflection or deviation) from the original SDS position (height SDS change is the difference in height SDS between two measurements, preferably 1 year apart from each other) [5]. A growth deflection (or a "crossing" of height percentiles) is defined as a height SDS decrease >1 SD and should also be considered abnormal requiring further evaluation.

Diagnostic Approach

Short stature can be the presenting symptom or the suggestive symptom of numerous conditions and diseases. There are different classifications for its differential diagnosis, but most of them include three main groups: primary short stature (skeletal abnormalities), secondary short stature, and short stature without recognizable cause (Tables 16.1 and 16.2). The latter group includes the diagnosis known as idiopathic short stature (ISS).

Clinical evaluation starts with a detailed medical and family history and a thorough physical examination (Table 16.3). A key point is a detailed description of the child's growth pattern, including the time when the growth deficit was first observed. Birth characteristics must be evaluated (gestation and delivery conditions or complications; gestational age, birth weight, length and head circumference). This information is important to distinguish short children in two groups by the onset of the growth impairment: short stature with prenatal or postnatal onset. Medical history must be investigated, with a focus in neuropsychomotor development, nutritional status, medication use, and cardiac, renal, pulmonary, and gastrointestinal diseases. Evaluation of a child's height must take into account the familial patterns of growth and puberty [3–5].

Physical examination should be complete, including the description of anthropometric measurements, facial and body dysmorphic features, and any other clues for one of the many causes of short stature. In children younger than 2 years of age, supine length, weight, weight-for-length, and head circumference will be measured, and fontanelles as well as dentition should be evaluated. In older children, erect height, weight, body mass index (BMI), head circumference, arm

Table 16.1 Differential diagnosis in short stature

Primary short stature—Skeletal abnormalities
With recognizable skeletal dysplasia (achondroplasia, hypochondroplasia)
Without recognizable skeletal dysplasia (turner syndrome, heterozygous *NPR2* and *SHOX* defects)
Secondary short stature
Malnutrition
Psychosocial deprivation
Chronic diseases
Renal (renal failure, tubular acidosis, nephrotic syndrome)
Intestinal (celiac disease, intestinal inflammatory disease)
Hematological (chronic anemia)
Cardiac
Pulmonary (cystic fibrosis)
Endocrine
Hypothyroidism
Disorders of the GH/IGF-1 axis
Cushing's syndrome
Pseudohypoparathyroidism
Rickets
Short stature without recognizable cause
Intrauterine growth retardation without recognizable cause (small for gestational age with failure of catch-up growth)
Idiopathic short stature
Familial short stature
Constitutional delay of growth and puberty

NPR2 natriuretic peptide receptor 2, *SHOX* short stature homeobox, *GH* growth hormone, *IGF-1* insulin-like growth factor type 1

Table 16.2 Disorders of the GH/IGF-1 axis

GH deficiency
Idiopathic
Acquired (craniopharyngioma, pituitary tumors, autoimmune diseases, granulomatous diseases, central nervous system infections, post-radiotherapy, head trauma)
Genetic
    GH secretion (*GH1* and *GHRHR* genes).
    Pituitary cell differentiation (*POU1F1* and *PROP1* genes).
    Pituitary development (*HESX1, GLI2, LHX3, LHX4,* and *SOX3* genes).
Bioinactive GH
    GH1 gene mutation.
GH insensitivity
Primary
    Laron syndrome (*GHR* gene defect).
    Associated with immunodysfunction (abnormalities of GH signal transduction, e.g., *STAT5B* gene defect).
Secondary or acquired (anti-GH antibodies, malnutrition, liver disorders, diabetes mellitus poorly controlled, uremia)
Ternary complex defects (IGF-1/IGFBP-3/ALS)
    Acid-labile subunit deficiency (*IGFALS* gene).
    Defects on proteolytic cleavage of IGFBPs (*PAPPA2* gene).
IGF deficiency
    IGF1 gene mutation.
    IGF2 gene mutation (paternal allele).
Bioinactive IGF-1
    IGF1 gene mutation.
IGF-1 insensitivity
    IGF1R defects and post-receptor defects.

GH growth hormone, *IGF-1* insulin-like growth factor type 1, *IGFBP-3* insulin-like growth factor binding protein 3, *ALS* acid-label subunit, *IGFs* insulin-like growth factors

Table 16.3 Specific diagnostic findings and key points in medical history and physical examination of children with short stature

Findings and key points	Interpretation and application
Medical history	
Birth length, weight, head circumference, gestational age	Classification as SGA or AGA
Previous growth data	Height velocity and growth pattern analysis
Age at start of pubertal signs	Early, normal, or delayed puberty
Previous diseases, surgeries, and medication use	Organic or iatrogenic causes
Medical history of the various systems	Search for chronic and systemic diseases
Feeding and nutrition history	As example, silver–Russell and Prader–Willi syndromes can lead to feeding difficulties
Neuropsychomotor development delay and/or intellectual disability	Syndromes, chromosomal disorders, metabolic disorders
Consanguinity	To assess disorders with autosomal dominant or recessive inheritance
If short stature is diagnosed in other family members, it is indicated to draw the family pedigree	
Parental height (measured)	To estimate the target height
Parents' age at the start of puberty	To assess likelihood of a familiar pattern of delayed puberty
Physical examination	
Length or height SDS	Severity of growth deficit
Body proportions (sitting height-total height ratio SDS; arm spam)	Altered sitting height-height ratio is suggestive of skeletal dysplasia
Weight-for-height or BMI showing underweight	Weight more affected than height, low weight-for-height and low BMI are suggestive of malnutrition
Weight-for-height or BMI showing overweight or obesity	Hypothyroidism, Cushing's syndrome, GH deficiency, pseudohypoparathyroidism
Head circumference SDS	Microcephaly and macrocephaly are important findings, indicating potential diagnosis
Dysmorphic features	Syndromes
Pubertal stage	Early, normal, or delayed puberty
General physical exam	Search for chronic and systemic diseases

SGA small for gestational age, *AGA* adequate for gestational age, *BMI* body mass index, *GH* growth hormone

span, and sitting height (SH) should be measured [3, 5]. In the latter, the pubertal staging has to be evaluated, as determined by Marshall and Tanner criteria [6, 7]. Evaluation of a child's height must be done in the context of normal standards for sex and age with the international data at hand. Such standards can be either cross-sectional (by calculation of height SDS) or longitudinal (by plotting in growth charts). Serial measurements with a minimum interval of 6 months are necessary to determine the height velocity. Because genetic factors are important determinants of growth and height, all children should be assessed considering siblings and parents. For that purpose, the parental target height is calculated and expressed as mentioned above. When a child's growth pattern clearly deviates from that of parents and siblings, the possibility of an underlying pathology should be considered [2].

Many abnormal growth states are characterized by disproportionate growth, which is strongly suggestive of skeletal dysplasia. Therefore, body proportion measurements should be part of the evaluation of short stature. We recommend the use of sitting height-height ratio (SH-H) for age and sex, which can also be expressed in SDS, according to published standards [8]. This ratio allows for the observation of body proportion changes throughout development.

Children with short stature and an increased SH-H ratio for age and sex have a disproportional short stature caused by limb abnormalities, while children with short stature and a decreased SH-H ratio for age and sex have a disproportional short stature caused by axial segment abnormalities [8] (Fig. 16.1).

It is assumed by most groups that a radiograph of the left hand and wrist is a useful adjunct. On this radiograph, bone age can be determined by comparison with the normal age and sex-related standards published by Greulich and Pyle [9]. Skeletal maturation can be used to predict adult height.

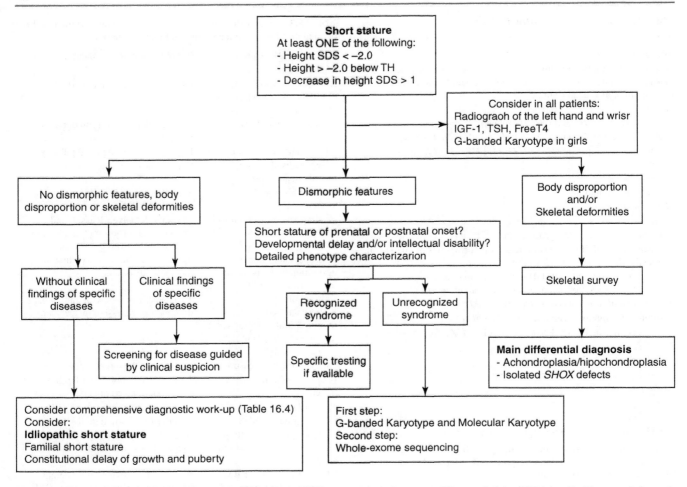

Fig. 16.1 Diagnostic approach in children with short stature. (*SDS* standard deviation score, *TH* target height, *IGF-1* insulin-like growth factor 1, *TSH* thyroid-stimulating hormone, *SHOX* short stature homeobox)

The most commonly used method for height prediction is the Bayley and Pinneau method [10]. We also consider the measurement of serum concentrations of IGF-1 and TSH/free T4 as initial screening tests for most patients, due to the importance of these hormonal axes to normal growth. Besides the aforementioned, it is generally advised to request initially a karyotype in short girls, even in the absence of typical signs of Turner syndrome [4, 5] (Fig. 16.1 and Table 16.4).

Depending on specific clinical clues at medical history and physical examination, special investigations are required. When skeletal dysplasia is suspected, skeletal survey analysis is indicated for a more precise diagnosis, including the following parts: skull, spine, pelvis, upper limb, and lower limb (Fig. 16.1) [11]. Likewise, when dysmorphic features are suggestive of syndromic causes, diagnostic investigations have to prioritize them. When a specific syndrome is recognized by clinical evaluation, the patient should be specifically tested. On the other hand, if no syndrome is clinically recognizable, patients with short stature associated with dysmorphic features should undergo genetic testing,

including molecular karyotyping (single nucleotide polymorphism array or array-comparative genomic hybridization) and whole-genome sequencing [12, 13].

When initial clinical evaluation does not point to a specific diagnosis, including absence of dysmorphisms, body disproportion, or skeletal deformities in physical exam, the diagnostic workup may include tests for a wide group of diseases that can be associated with short stature [5, 14] (Fig. 16.1 and Table 16.4).

One of the most important parameters to be evaluated is the growth hormone/insulin-like growth factor-1 (GH/IGF-1) axis. There are several defects that affect this axis (Table 16.2); among them, growth hormone deficiency (GHD) is the most prevalent. However, the latter is responsible for only 5% of short stature cases.

Laboratorial investigation of GHD is made by direct and/or indirect analysis of the GH secretion. The direct analysis is made by provocative tests (also called stimulation tests), and pharmacological ones are the most appropriate [15]. The most important tests are insulin, clonidine, arginine, and glucagon, which are comparable in terms of sensitivity and

Table 16.4 Most common laboratorial, radiographic, and genetic tests in diagnostic workup of patients with short stature

Exam	Objective (to detect or exclude)
Initial screening tests to be considered in all patients	
Radiograph of the left hand and wrist	Bone age
IGF-1	GH/IGF-1 axis disorders, poor nutritional status
TSH and free T4	Thyroid disorders
Karyotype in female patients	Turner syndrome
Diagnostic workup tests to be considered in patients depending on their clinical evaluation	
Blood cell count, erythrocyte sedimentation rate	Anemia, infections, chronic inflammatory diseases
Albumin, ferritin	Poor nutritional status
AST, ALT, γGT	Chronic liver diseases
Creatinine, sodium, potassium, venous blood gas analysis, urinalysis	Renal disorders, renal tubular acidosis[a]
Calcium, phosphate, alkaline phosphatases	Calcium/phosphate disorders
IgA-anti-endomysium antibodies, IgA-anti-tissue transglutaminase antibodies and total IgA	Celiac disease
GH and IGFBP-3	GH/IGF-1 axis disorders
Skeletal survey analysis (skull, spine, pelvis, upper limb, and lower limb, in two views)	Skeletal dysplasias
Molecular karyotyping (aCGH or SNParray)	Chromosomal copy number variants
Whole-exome sequencing	Pathogenic mutations (monogenic disorders)

IGF-1 insulin-like growth factor type 1, GH growth hormone, TSH thyroid-stimulating hormone, Free T4 free tetraiodothyronine, IGFBP-3 insulin-like growth factor binding protein 3, aCGH array-comparative genomic hybridization, SNParray single nucleotide polymorphism array

[a]Renal tubular acidosis should be excluded in children younger than 4 years old with short stature and difficulty in gaining weight

specificity. The choice of a test to provoke GH secretion is dependent on the center experience and on the test availability. A substantial number of healthy short statured children without GHD may have an inadequate response to one test. Because of this, two provocative tests must be made for GHD diagnosis [15] (Fig. 16.2). A technical topic related to provocative tests is the use, or not, of sexual steroid priming. It is well known that the peak of GH level after a stimulation test is higher if the patient has been recently exposed to sex steroids. Clinical practice guidelines suggest that priming should be used mainly in children with pubertal delay, in order to prevent unnecessary GH treatment of children with constitutional delay of growth and puberty [15].

The indirect analysis of the GH secretion is made by serum concentrations of IGF-1 and insulin-like growth factor binding protein 3 (IGFBP-3). Both of them are directly related to GH action and are used as screening tests to select short statured children for GHD diagnostic tests. The IGF-1

and IGFBP-3 serum levels vary with age, sex, and pubertal staging [16, 17]. When the hormonal diagnostic is established, a hypothalamic–pituitary magnetic resonance imaging (MRI) is requested for anatomical evaluation (Fig. 16.2).

It is noteworthy to highlight that recently several genomic approaches have been transforming the diagnostic investigation of growth disorders in an attempt to identify monogenic etiologies of short stature phenotype [18, 19]. These approaches include mutational analysis of candidate genes, large-scale genome-wide association studies, molecular karyotyping, and whole-exome sequencing. This technological development is revealing novel causes of short stature, involving hormone signaling, paracrine factors, matrix molecules, and intracellular pathways [20]. Consequently, some authors are now proposing a new conceptual framework for understanding growth disorders, with a diagnostic classification centered on epiphyseal growth plate [21].

In this "genomic approach" context, the selection of patients for genetic testing should take into account several factors and key points that increase the likelihood of a monogenic etiology for short stature: the severity of growth failure, the presence of associated clinical features, the familial segregation (family members with similar phenotype), and consanguinity [18, 20]. Besides the etiology definition of growth retardation, the genetic testing approaches may be valuable tools for genetic counseling and future therapies [20].

Case Report Evolution and the Diagnosis of Idiopathic Short Stature (ISS)

Continuing our clinical case discussion, we can conclude that the boy met the referral criteria to initiate diagnostic workup: height SDS −2.6 (<2.5) and height below target height (difference of 2.0 SD). Skeletal maturation analysis showed a significant bone age delay (chronological age of 14.6 years with a bone age of 11 years). Serum concentrations of IGF-1 and IGFBP3 were both < −2.0 SDS. As the patient presented a proportional short stature (SH-H SDS of −0.3), skeletal survey analysis was not performed. Likewise, as he did not present dysmorphic features, karyotype or other diagnostic investigations for specific syndromic causes were not necessary. Additional laboratory analyses, including TSH, free T4, blood cell count, erythrocyte sedimentation rate, creatinine, sodium, potassium, calcium, phosphate, alkaline phosphatase, venous blood gas analysis, ferritin, albumin, AST, ALT, γGT, IgA-anti-endomysium antibody, and urinalysis analysis, were all normal. As such, a clonidine test was performed, but the GH peak after the pharmacological stimulus was 17 μ/L, ruling out GHD.

At this moment, we had excluded the most recognizable diseases associated with short stature, and we formulated a hypothesis of idiopathic short stature (ISS). The term ISS does

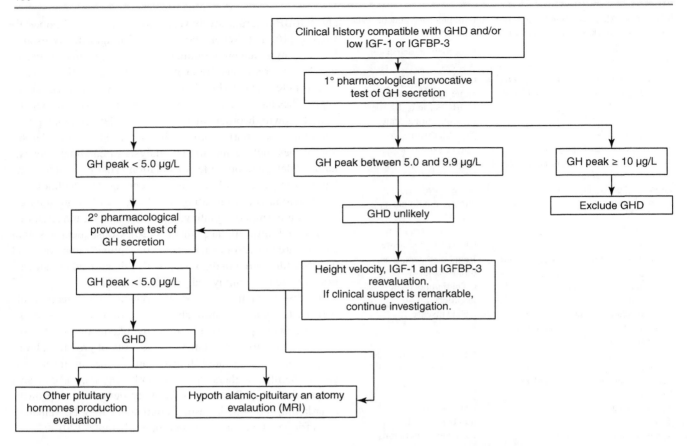

Fig. 16.2 Investigation protocol of children with suspected GHD. (*GH* growth hormone, *GHD* growth hormone deficiency, *IGF*-1 insulin-like growth factor type 1; *IGFBP*-3 insulin-like growth factor binding protein 3, *MRI* magnetic resonance imaging)

not reflect an exactly defined diagnosis. It is usually used for children whose shortness compared to age-matched normal population cannot be attributed to specific diseases [22]. According to the Consensus Statement on the diagnosis of ISS, "it is defined as a condition in which the height of an individual is more than 2 SDS below the corresponding mean for height for a given age, sex and population group, without evidence of systemic, endocrine, nutritional or chromosomal abnormalities; it describes a heterogeneous group of children consisting of many presently unidentified causes of short stature" [4]. It is estimated that 60–80% of all short children presented to pediatric or endocrinological evaluation can be labeled according to this definition. ISS can be subcategorized. The main distinction is between children with a familial history of short stature (familial short stature, FSS) and those children who are short for their parents (nonfamilial short stature, non-FSS) [4]. In FSS, children are short compared with the relevant population but remain within the expected target range for the family. In non-FSS, children are short for the population as well as for the target range. In addition, ISS children can also be subcategorized according to the age of puberty onset, presenting a constitutional delay of growth and puberty (CDGP). The diagnosis of CDGP is based on lack of breast development by the age of

13 in girls and testicular volume <4.0 ml by the age of 14 in boys (Tanner stage 2), absence of other identifiable causes of delayed puberty, delayed bone age, as well as spontaneous and complete achievement of pubertal development during follow-up [1].

In the presenting case, we could classify the patient with a nonfamilial proportional short stature of postnatal onset. And, because he presented a remarkable bone age delay and a delayed puberty, the most appropriate hypothesis was CDGP. The patient was evaluated every 6 months, when the auxological data were repeatedly measured (Fig. 16.3). He started puberty at the age of 15. His bone age was 12 years and at that time height velocity increased from 3.7 to 5.1 cm/year. The peak height velocity was 8.8 cm/year, observed at 16.5 years old and pubertal staging G4P3 (Fig. 16.4). At 17.5 years old, his height was 165.3 cm (−1.4 SDS), his bone age was 14.5 years, his pubertal staging was G5P5, and his adult height prediction was 174.3 cm (0.0 SDS). At 20 years old, he reached his final height (or adult height) in 170 cm (−0.7 SDS) (Figs. 16.3 and 16.4).

The abovementioned case report is a common example in clinical practice. It brings out two important points in the management of patients with ISS. First, ISS is not a diagnos-

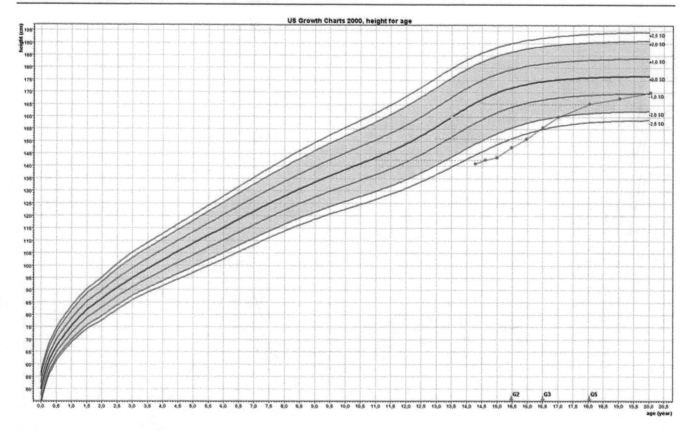

Fig. 16.3 Height for age growth chart of the patient presented. (*Red marks* = height measures in follow-up visits; *yellow marks* = bone age as determined by Greulich and Pyle criteria; G2, G3, and G5 = pubertal stages 2, 3, and 5, respectively, as determined by Marshall and Tanner)

tic entity in terms of etiology or pathogenesis. It is a term used to describe such forms of growth failure that cannot be attributed to any known cause of short stature and are usually considered normal variants of growth [22]. Secondly, the choice whether using growth-promoting therapies or not has to take into account the natural history and the growth pattern of children with ISS.

Several studies have been published about the natural history of ISS. In most of them, it is assumed that FSS and CDGP are different. Children with FSS tend to be younger at presentation of short stature, reach an adult height SDS similar to the initial height SDS, and reach the target height more precisely than the predicted adult height. Conversely, children with CDGP tend to be older at presentation and reach an adult height SDS higher than initial height SDS and more compatible with predicted adult height based on bone age [1, 22].

In an important study evaluating the spontaneous adult height in ISS, Ranke et al. found that 67% of children with FSS reached adult height within the normal range, whereas 81% of children with CDGP reached it as well. As a group, only 5% of children with ISS did not reach an adult height above −2.0 SDS, thus becoming short adults. Moreover, 10% of children with ISS did not reach an adult height within

the range of their target height. In clinical observation of the natural history of ISS, there are three main indicators of a poor adult height outcome: younger age at presentation, lower target height, and lower predicted adult height at presentation (as measured by BP method) [22]. Once aware of the spontaneous growth pattern of children with ISS, growth-promoting therapies to improve final height are no longer widely justified.

Present Therapies for Short Stature

When a specific disease is known to be the cause of growth retardation, the treatment of this condition is considered the best therapy for short stature. Current available treatments, used for different causes of short stature, are recombinant human GH (rhGH), recombinant human IGF-1 (rhIGF-1), gonadotropin-releasing hormone analogs (GnRHa), and aromatase inhibitors.

The rhGH is the main hormonal treatment of short stature and is accepted as a safe and effective therapy up to now. Presently, according to the US Food and Drug Administration (FDA), the indications for its use are GHD, small for gestational age (SGA), Turner syndrome, Prader–Willi syn-

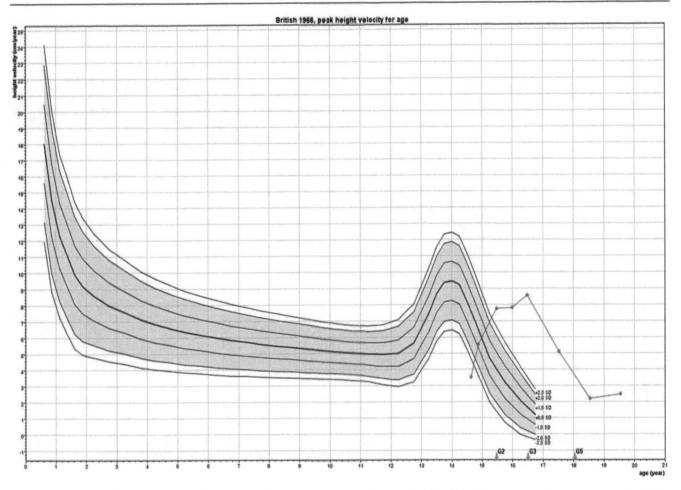

Fig. 16.4 Height velocity for age growth chart of the patient presented. (*Red marks* = height velocity measures in follow-up visits; G2, G3, and G5 = pubertal stages 2, 3, and 5, respectively, as determined by Marshall and Tanner)

drome, chronic kidney disease, *SHOX* gene haploinsufficiency, Noonan syndrome, and ISS. According to the European Medicines Agency (EMA), indications are the same, except for Noonan syndrome and ISS, which are not included. Several studies assessed different variables which can influence final height after rhGH therapy in children with different conditions. Duration of treatment, height at the start of treatment, bone age delay, height at puberty onset, midparental height, and first year of treatment growth velocity were positively correlated, whereas age at the beginning of treatment had a negative correlation [2, 15].

GHD is the most accepted indication for rhGH treatment. In these cases, the reposition of physiological doses of GH (33 μg/kg/day) allows for growth normalization and should be initiated as soon as the diagnosis is established [15]. Children with severe GHD have higher height velocity in initial treatment and greater height gain in overall treatment than other causes of short stature. When initiated early, GH reposition results in adult height close to target height [23].

The use of rhGH to increase adult height in ISS is controversial. Most studies indicate that height velocity increases in short term and that final height gain is modest, with a mean increase of 4 cm [24]. Studies about the natural history of ISS show that most children become normal adults with adequate stature outcome, even without treatment [22]. In addition, in children with ISS, there is a great interindividual variability in the response to GH therapy, and there are no effective tools to predict the individual response. The treatment has a high cost and is not completely free of adverse effects. Most studies do not show sufficient evidence with respect to safety and psychosocial benefits in this condition [25]. For these reasons, in recent clinical practice guidelines, Grimberg et al. suggest that GH treatment for ISS patients should be made on a case-by-case basis after assessment of physical and psychological burdens and discussion of risks and benefits [15] with the family and the patient, if possible [25].

Besides rhGH, alternative growth-promoting therapies have been assessed in ISS as well as in other causes of short stature. Some studies evaluated the use of GnRHa, with or without concomitant GH in short stature. Those that kept the agonists for 3 or more years showed a modest final height gain in children with GHD, ISS, and SGA [26–28]. However, the consequences of its use in long terms are still unclear.

The use of aromatase inhibitors has also been evaluated in boys with short stature. They are capable of inhibiting the conversion of testosterone in estradiol and thus enhancing height potential by delaying epiphyseal fusion while promoting linear growth [29]. Initial questions about bone health are still not completely elucidated. Despite that, trials in CDGP boys and ISS pubertal boys show promising results with a well-tolerated and safe use [29–31].

Recombinant human IGF-1 is the treatment of choice in children with primary or secondary forms of GH insensitivity, and its use is recommended to increase height in these conditions [15].

Last but not least, we should take into account the importance of ethical aspects on growth promotion and the challenge to resist cosmetic endocrinology. The advent of recombinant human GH brought the narrative of "GH for height," meaning "increasing height gain and attainment in children who are short for reasons other than GHD," mostly in ISS children [25]. This narrative considers a psychosocial belief that "distress in short children is due to their shortness," which is biased, uncertain, and not proved by quality of life studies. In agreement with Allen [25], we believe that our responsibility is putting on the scale the most appropriate choice for these children: indicating them necessary treatments or protecting them from unnecessary ones.

Acknowledgments This work was supported by grants from the Conselho Nacional de Desenvolvimento Científico e Tecnológico (The National Council for Scientific and Technological Development—CNPq) (301477/2009-4 to A.A.L.J).

References

1. Wit JM, Clayton PE, Rogol AD, Savage MO, Saenger PH, Cohen P. Idiopathic short stature: definition, epidemiology and diagnostic evaluation. Growth Hormon IGF Res. 2008;18:89–110.
2. Cooke DW, DiVall SA, Radovick S. Normal and aberrant growth in children. In: Melmed S, Polonsky KS, Larsen PR, Kronenberg MH, editors. Williams textbook of endocrinology. 13th ed. Philadelphia: Saunders Elsevier; 2016. p. 964–1073.
3. Rogol AD, Hayden GF. Etiologies and early diagnosis of short stature and growth failure in children and adolescents. J Pediatr. 2014;164:S1–S14.
4. Cohen P, Rogol AD, Deal CL, Saenger P, Reiter EO, Ross JL, Chernausek SD, Savage MO, Wit JM. Consensus statement on the diagnosis and treatment of children with idiopathic short stature: a summary of the growth hormone research society, the Lawson Wilkins Pediatric Endocrine Society, and the European Society for Paediatric Endocrinology Workshop. J Clin Endocrinol Metab. 2008;93(11):4210–7.
5. Oostdijk W, Grote FK, Muinck Keizer-Schrama SMPF, Wit JM. Diagnostic approach in children with short stature. Horm Res. 2009;72:206–17.
6. Marshall WA, Tanner JM. Variations in pattern of pubertal changes in girls. Arch Dis Child. 1969;44(235):291–303.
7. Marshall WA, Tanner JM. Variations in pattern of pubertal changes in boys. Arch Dis Child. 1970;45(239):13–23.
8. Malaquias AC, Scalco RC, Fontenele EGP, Costalonga EF, et al. The sitting height/height ratio for age in healthy and short individuals and its potential role in selecting short children for SHOX analysis. Horm Res Paediatr. 2013;80:449–56.
9. Greulich WW, Pyle SI. Radiographic atlas of skeletal development of the hand and wrist. 2nd ed. Stanford, CA: Stanford University Press; 1959.
10. Bayley N, Pinneau SR. Tables for predicting adult height from skeletal age: revised for use with the Greulich-Pyle hand standards. J Pediatr. 1952;40:423.
11. Kant SG, Grote F, de Ru MH, Oostdijk W, Zonderland HM, Breuning MH, Wit JM. Radiographic evaluation of children with growth disorders. Horm Res. 2007;68:310–5.
12. Canton APM, Costa SS, Rodrigues TC, Bertola DR, et al. Genome-wide screening of copy number variants in children born small for gestational age reveals several candidate genes involved in growth pathways. Eur J Endocrinol. 2014;171(2):253–62.
13. De Bruin C, Dauber A. Insights from exome sequencing for endocrine disorders. Nat Rev Endocrinol. 2015;11(8):455–64.
14. Sisley S, Trujillo MV, Khoury J, Backeljauw P. Low incidence of pathology detection and high cost of screening in the evaluation of asymptomatic short children. J Pediatr. 2013;163:1045–51.
15. Grimberg A, DiVall SA, Polychronakos C, Allen DB, et al. Guidelines for growth hormone and insulin-like growth factor-1 treatment in children and adolescents: growth hormone deficiency, idiopathic short stature, and primary insulin-like growth factor-1 deficiency. Horm Res Paediatr. 2016;86:361–97.
16. Lee PD, Wilson DM, Rountree L, Hintz RL, Rosenfeld RG. Efficacy of insulin-like growth factor I levels in predicting the response to provocative growth hormone testing. Pediatr Res. 1990;27(1):45–51.
17. Elmlinger MW, Kuhnel W, Weber MM, Ranke MB. Reference ranges for two automated chemiluminescent assays for serum insulin-like growth factor I (IGF-I) and IGF-binding protein 3 (IGFBP-3). Clin Chem Lab Med. 2004;42(6):654–64.
18. Dauber A, Rosenfeld RG, Hirschhorn JN. Genetic evaluation of short stature. J Clin Endocrinol Metab. 2014;99(9):3080–92.
19. Jorge AAL. Whole exome sequencing in the investigation of growth disorders, including patients with primary IGF-1 deficiency. Horm Res Paediatr. 2017; https://doi.org/10.1159/000481792
20. Wit JM, Oostdijk W, Losekoot M, van Duyvenvoorde HA, et al. Novel genetic causes of short stature. Eur J Endocrinol. 2016;174:R145–73.
21. Baron J, Savendahl L, De Luca F, Dauber A, Philip M, Wit JM, Nilsson O. Short and tall stature: a new paradigm emerges. Nat Rev Endocrinol. 2015;11(12):735–46.
22. Ranke MB, Grauer MI, Kistner K, Blum WF, Wollmann HA. Spontaneous adult height in idiopathic short stature. Horm Res. 1995;44:152–7.
23. Guyda HJ. Four decades of growth hormone therapy for short children: what have we achieved? J Clin Endocrinol Metab. 1999;84:4307–16.
24. Deodati A, Peschiaroli E, Cianfarani S. Review of growth hormone randomized controlled trials in children with idiopathic short stature. Horm Res Paediatr. 2011;76(3):40–2.
25. Allen DB. Growth promotion ethics and the challenge to resist cosmetic endocrinology. Horm Res Paediatr. 2017;87:145–52.
26. Saggese G, Federico G, Barsanti S, Fiore L. The effect of administering gonadotropin-releasing hormone agonist with

recombinant-human growth hormone (GH) on the final height of girls with isolated GH deficiency: results from a controlled study. J Clin Endocrinol Metab. 2011;86:1900–4.

27. Yanovski JA, Rose SR, Municchi G, Pescovitz OH, Cassorla FG, Cutler GB Jr. Treatment with a luteinizing hormone-releasing hormone agonist in adolescents with short stature. N Engl J Med. 2003;348:908–17.

28. Kamp GA, Mul D, Waelkens JJ, Jansen M, et al. A randomized controlled trial of three years growth hormone and gonadotropin-releasing hormone agonist treatment in children with idiopathic short stature and intrauterine growth retardation. J Clin Endocrinol Metab. 2001;86:2969–75.

29. Mauras N, Ross JL, Gagliardi P, Miles Yu Y, et al. Randomized trial of aromatase inhibitors, growth hormone, or combination in pubertal boys with idiopathic short stature. J Clin Endocrinol Metab. 2016;101:4984–93.

30. Wickman S, Sipil I, Ankarberg-Lindgren C, Norjavaara E, Dunkel L. A specific aromatase inhibitor and potential increase in adult height in boys with delayed puberty. Lancet. 2001;357(9270):1743–8.

31. Hero M, Norjavaara E, Dunkel L. Inhibition of estrogen biosynthesis with a potent aromatase inhibitor increases predicted adult height in boys with idiopathic short stature: a randomized controlled trial. J Clin Endocrinol Metab. 2005;90(12):6396–402.

Delayed Puberty

Caroline Colvin, Gayathri Devineni, Bhuvana Sunil, and Ambika P. Ashraf

Introduction

Puberty is an indelible period of metamorphosis of the human lifecycle, which culminates in sexual maturation and reproductive capability. The failure to develop in a normal and timely fashion can, therefore, cause profound anxiety in individuals and families. Furthermore, awareness that pubertal delay can indicate significant underlying pathology compels physicians to investigate any perceived deviation from a rigidly defined acceptable pattern of development. The ability to distinguish between various causes of delay and to differentiate significant underlying pathology from common benign delay can be daunting often requiring prudent investigation. Depending on the ultimate diagnosis, treatment options vary, but most patients can ultimately expect to achieve pubertal maturation and fertility.

Puberty is initiated when the hypothalamic gonadotropin-releasing hormone (GnRH) pulse generator begins secreting brief nocturnal pulses of GnRH from the hypothalamic arcuate nucleus which subsequently stimulate the pituitary to release luteinizing hormone (LH) and follicle-stimulating hormone (FSH) [1]. Kisspeptin acts on the hypothalamic GnRH neurons, stimulating GnRH secretion [2]. The gonadotropins (LH and FSH) promote gonadal maturation, and gonads synthesize sex steroids, including testosterone and estrogen, and other proteins. LH acts on theca cells and interstitial cells to produce progestins and androgens which diffuse into adjacent granulosa cells. FSH acts on granulosa cells to stimulate aromatization of these androgens to estrogen. Estrogen and testosterone then promote pubertal changes throughout the body and provide negative feedback effect on the GnRH and gonadotropins (Fig. 17.1).

The first physical signs of puberty are typically breast development in girls and testicular enlargement in boys (testicular volume > 3 ml/ ≥ 2.5 cm in length). Some children, especially girls, have the appearance of pubic hair prior to the initiation of breast development, but in the absence of other puberty signs this usually represents adrenarche [adrenal source of androgens, independent of hypothalamic-pituitary-gonadal (HPG) axis maturation] and not true puberty. The trigger(s) for re-activation of the HPG axis is not completely understood, but modifying factors include general health, nutrition, genetic determinants, pubertal timing among primary relatives, endocrine-disrupting chemicals, and body mass index. Elevated body mass index (BMI) is often associated with delayed puberty in boys [3, 4]. Many of the genes involved in the HPG axis maturation are still unknown. Kisspeptin-1 and its cognate receptor (GPR54, a G protein-coupled receptor) are integral to the normal function of HPG axis and play critical role in the physiologic regulation of puberty [2, 5]. Kisspeptin is co-expressed with neurokinin B and dynorphin, and these signaling pathways are also important in physiologic regulation of puberty [6]. There is evidence that leptin, a 16 kDa hormone product of the Ob gene, synthesized by adipocytes, plays a permissive role [7, 8].

In delayed puberty, 16–40% of the population has loss of function mutation in the GnRH receptor. HS6ST1, FGFR1, KLB, and variants in several HH genes including GNRHR, TAC3, TACR3, IL17RD, and SEMA3A have been identified by whole exome sequencing; however, the exact pathogenicity of all these mutations is unknown [9–12]. Recently, in a Finnish family with delayed puberty, a gene of the immunoglobulin superfamily, IGSF10, has been described to cause

C. Colvin · B. Sunil
Department of Pediatrics/Division of Pediatric Endocrinology and Metabolism, Children's of Alabama, University of Alabama at Birmingham, Birmingham, AL, USA
e-mail: bsunil@uabmc.edu

G. Devineni
EndoHealth Atlanta, Department of Endocrinology, Kennesaw, GA, USA
e-mail: GKD@endohealthatlanta.com

A. P. Ashraf (✉)
Department of Pediatrics/Division of Pediatric Endocrinology and Metabolism, Children's of Alabama, University of Alabama at Birmingham, Birmingham, AL, USA

Children's Hospital, UAB, Birmingham, AL, USA
e-mail: AAshraf@peds.uab.edu

Fig. 17.1 Schematic illustration of pubertal regulation

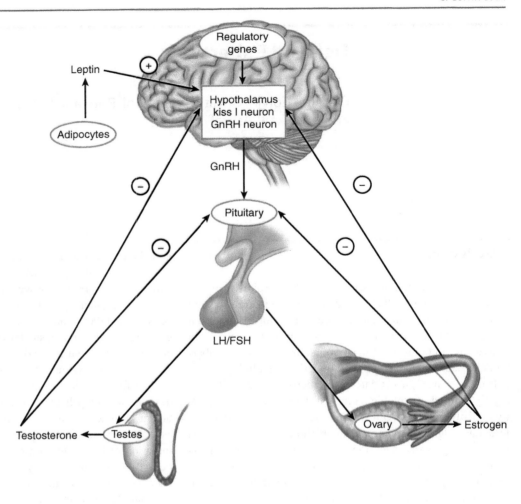

delay by a defective neuroendocrine network of the GnRH pulse regulator [13].

Although the lower limit of normal for the onset of puberty is contestable, the average age for this process is generally accepted to be 9–10 years for girls and 10–11 years for boys [1, 14]. Delayed puberty can be defined as failure to demonstrate signs of pubertal maturation by an age that is ≥2 standard deviations above the population mean [1]. Delayed puberty is considered when there is lack of testicular enlargement by age 14 in males, lack of breast development by age 13 in females, absence of menarche by age 16 years in girls, or absence of menarche within 5 years of pubertal onset [15, 16]. Parenthetically, males present far more often for evaluation of delayed puberty, but it has been suggested that this is in part due to a referral bias [17, 18].

Key Points to the Diagnosis

There is a wide range of conditions that can present with a delay in puberty [17], which requires a systematic tapered approach fundamental to the diagnostic process. In consider-

ing a patient with delayed puberty, the most important initial assessment is the gonadotropin status. Disorders of pubertal delay can be broadly categorized into hypogonadotropic, hypergonadotropic, and eugonadotropic hypogonadism (Table 17.1).

Hypogonadotropic Hypogonadism (HH)

Hypogonadotropic hypogonadism (HH) is the commonest of the groups in both sexes and includes many pathologic disorders that can be further subdivided into constitutional delay of growth and puberty (CDGP), functional hypogonadotropic hypogonadism (FHH), and permanent hypogonadotropic hypogonadism (PHH). This classification can facilitate the diagnostic process by appropriately directing early evaluation efforts. HH is defined as lack of normal gonadal function secondary to low or absent gonadotropin secretion. In this case, the defect can be in the pituitary gland itself, or it can be related to hypothalamic dysfunction (delayed activation of the GnRH pulse generator). The delay in puberty can be either temporary or permanent. Isolated hypogonado-

Table 17.1 Etiology of delayed puberty

Hypogonadotropic hypogonadism (low LH and FSH)

1. Constitutional delay of growth and puberty (CDGP)

2. Functional hypogonadotropic hypogonadism: Delayed, but spontaneous, pubertal development

3. Permanent hypogonadotropic hypogonadism:

   Hypothalamic and pituitary dysfunction: Isolated gonadotropin deficiency, panhypopituitarism

   Acquired causes: Hypophysitis, Langerhans histiocytosis, radiation therapy, head trauma, anorchia, testicular torsion, mumps, chronic disease states including malnutrition, anorexia nervosa, untreated autoimmune diseases, inflammatory bowel disease, cystic fibrosis

   CNS tumors: Germinoma, optic glioma, oligodendroglioma, Rathke's pouch/cleft cyst astrocytoma, pituitary tumor, craniopharyngioma

   Congenital malformation with midline central defect (septo-optic dysplasia)

   Mutations in the *PROP1, LHX3, LHX4, SOX2,* and *HESX1* genes

   Mutations in the *NROB1, GPR54* genes, GnRH receptor gene mutations, inactivating mutations of *KISS1 and KISS1 R genes,* loss of function mutations in genes encoding neurokinin B and its receptor, *FGF8, FGFR1, KAL1, PROK2, PROKR2, NELF* mutations

   Syndromes: Prader-Willi syndrome, coffin-Lowry syndrome, CHARGE syndrome, Laurence-moon-Biedl syndrome, Gordon syndrome, Holmes syndrome, and others

Hypergonadotropic hypogonadism (increased LH and FSH)

1. Gonadotropin receptor mutations.

2. FSH-β subunit gene mutation.

3. LH/FSH receptor mutation.

4. Gonadal dysgenesis: Turner syndrome, mixed gonadal dysgenesis, Klinefelter syndrome.

5. Premature ovarian failure.

6. Resistant ovary syndromes.

7. Gonadal injury/loss: Irradiation, cytotoxic therapy, trauma, infections, galactosemia, AIS with gonadectomy.

8. Glycoprotein syndrome type 1.

9. Androgen resistance.

Eugonadotropic hypogonadism (normal LH and FSH)

1. Steroidogenic enzyme defects

   (a) Cholesterol desmolase complex deficiency (lipoid adrenal hyperplasia)

   (b) 3-β OH-steroid dehydrogenase deficiency

   (c) 17 α-hydroxylase deficiency

   (d) C17,20-Desmolase deficiency

   (e) 17-β OH-steroid oxidoreductase deficiency

   (f) 21-hydroxylase deficiency in girls

2. Anatomic abnormalities: Imperforate hymen, vaginal atresia, vaginal and uterine agenesis (Mayer-Rokitansky-Küster-Hauser syndrome)

3. Polycystic ovary syndrome

4. Prolactinoma

tropic hypogonadism is diagnosed if there is no evidence of puberty by the age of 18 years [1].

Evaluation: In addition to low or absent LH/FSH, sex steroid concentrations will be in the pre-pubertal range, and bone age is typically delayed. Serum concentrations of adrenal androgens may be normal.

Constitutional Delay of Growth and Puberty (CDGP)

Constitutional delay of growth and puberty is the most common cause of delayed puberty, especially in males (65% of boys and 30% of girls with delayed puberty) [17]. It is a benign variant of normal growth and development and is, notably, a diagnosis of exclusion. Typically, a child will be normal size at birth and in infancy. At some point in early childhood, a decrease in growth velocity (GV) begets a decline in height centile for age. Normal growth then resumes with the child growing at an age-appropriate GV and at a consistent but low height percentile for age. This represents a global delay in biologic maturity affecting puberty and bone maturation. Height is usually appropriate for genetic potential when plotted for bone age. Often, there is a family history of "late bloomers" in the family history of delayed puberty in the patient's parents or siblings (77%) [19]. Pedigree studies show that children with CDGP are mainly autosomal dominant with variable penetrance [20]. They exhibit a relatively normal pre-pubertal growth velocity and protracted pre-pubertal growth nadir. The discordance in height vs. peers is exacerbated by a relatively lower growth velocity compared to peers who are undergoing a pubertal growth spurt. The growth velocity and height, however, should remain normal for bone age and pubertal stage. After HPG axis maturation, secondary sexual characteristics appear in their natural sequence with normal secondary sexual characteristics development. In 93% of cases, spontaneous pubertal maturation occurs by 18 years and has an excellent height phenotype. In some cases, the constitutional delay of puberty superimposed on constitutional short stature and final height may be shorter than genetic potential [21].

Diagnosis of this common condition is ultimately a matter of watchful waiting with close monitoring of growth and development. However, judicious evaluation to rule out other conditions and support the likelihood of CDGP is important. Clustering of CDGP has been clearly established [17, 19], and the pericentromeric region of chromosome 2 harbors a gene predisposing to pubertal delay [19]. Growth charts, if available, should be reviewed to demonstrate typical CDGP pattern. In CDGP, both adrenarche and gonadal enlargement occur later than average. In isolated hypogonadotropic hypogonadism (IHH), there is dissociation of adrenarche and gonadarche, with adrenarche occurring at normal age [17, 22]. GV and serum somatomedin-c (IGF1) should be monitored and remain normal for pubertal status.

Evaluation: Patients can have low/normal serum gonadotropins and a delayed bone age. Even though gonadotropin-releasing hormone (GnRH) agonist stimulation testing is often ambiguous in differentiating CDGP and permanent HH [23], a positive response to GnRH agonist is suggestive of CDGP. To date, no single lab test or hormone stimulation protocol has the sensitivity and specificity to confirm this diagnosis. Response to sex steroid replacement therapy, which will often trigger activation of the HPG axis in CDGP but not permanent HH, may aid in the diagnosis. Baseline, morning testosterone concentration of ≥ 20 ng/dl suggests the appearance of pubertal signs within 12–15 months [24]. A very low basal serum FSH (<0.2 IU/L by ICMA and < 1.0 U/L by IFMA) infers permanent HH [25, 26]. Serum inhibin B (INHB) measurement will help to discriminate permanent HH from CDGP. INHB is produced by Sertoli cells upon FSH stimulation and is a reflection of Sertoli cell integrity [27]. A baseline INHB concentration of >35 pg/ml is highly suggestive of CDGP [27].

Functional Hypogonadotropic Hypogonadism (FHH)

Functional hypogonadotropic hypogonadism represents another form of temporary, reversible HH. It accounts for about 20% of children with delayed puberty [17]. Within this category is a broad range of pathology that highlights the complexity of the HPG axis and the diverse factors that must coordinate to initiate puberty. The most common diagnoses are related to chronic or underlying illnesses, such as hypothyroidism, cystic fibrosis, Crohn's disease, inflammatory disorders that produce cytokines, immunosuppression seen in perinatally HIV-infected children, and chronic renal failure [17, 28, 29]. The mechanism of pubertal delay in the case of underlying illness is thought to be manifold, involving a combination of factors that include, but not limited to, undernutrition, stress, and medications such as corticosteroids resulting in abnormal gonadotropin secretion [28]. The implicated genetic variations are in genes that have been associated with idiopathic hypogonadotropic hypogonadism [30]. As aforementioned, a common cause of FHH is malnutrition, as seen in anorexia nervosa or intense exercise resulting in HPG dysfunction. The connection between weight, especially body fat mass and puberty, has been extensively studied [7, 31, 32]. On the other extreme, bulk training exercises, especially in sports like boxing and wrestling, may also lead to transient interruption in puberty.

Evaluation: A thorough and detailed history may disclose systemic complaints, eccentric eating habits, or an obsession with exercise and weight loss. Physical exam may be revealing at times: weight and BMI will typically be low for age, and erosion of dental enamel, lanugo hair, and callused knuckles may suggest eating disorders. Elevated sedimentation rate and/or other inflammatory markers may be detected. Further evaluation depends on general clinical picture.

Isolated Gonadotropin Deficiency

Isolated GnRH deficiency resulting in low or inappropriately normal gonadotropins and absent or incomplete puberty could be associated with abnormalities in craniofacial, skeletal, neurologic, renal, and olfactory systems. This could be due to molecular defects that alter the regulation of GnRH release, GnRH neurons, the action of GnRH or gonadotropins, or both GnRH and gonadotropins. Rare sequence variants (RSVs) in genes involved in GnRH neuronal migration (*FGF8*, *FGFR1*, *KAL1*, *PROK2*, *PROKR2*, and *NELF*), secretion (*GNRH1*, *GPR54*, *TAC3*, and *TACR3*), and receptivity (*GNRHR*) have been reported to contribute to GnRH deficiency in both men and women [33–35].

Kallmann syndrome (KS) is a well-known cause of gonadotropin deficiency due to abnormalities in the *KAL1* gene and is inherited as X-linked dominant or autosomal recessive disorder [33, 36]. This condition is caused by abnormal migration of embryonic GnRH and olfactory neuronal cells to the hypothalamus, resulting in HH and anosmia or hyposmia.

FGFR1 mutations are autosomal dominant and are often associated with cleft lip/cleft palate, syndactyly, or skeletal abnormalities. Other cases of permanent isolated HH have historically been referred to as idiopathic HH (IHH). More recently, several genetic mutations have been reported in some of these cases.

Multiple GnRH receptor mutations causing GnRH insensitivity and G protein-coupled receptor 54 mutations causing impaired gonadotropin secretion have been identified [36]. At the time of puberty, the affected patients may have adrenarche – some pubic hair may be there, but little or no breast development or axillary hair and present with primary amenorrhea.

HH is reported in leptin deficiency and puberty can be induced by recombinant leptin [8]. HH has also been reported in DAX1 mutations. DAX1 is a nuclear receptor protein encoded by the *NR0B1* and associated with X-linked congenital adrenal hypoplasia and HH, secondary to attenuated production of gonadotropins by the pituitary [37].

A reversible form of congenital GnRH deficiency also has been identified where the activation of the GnRH-gonadotropins axis is markedly delayed, yet the affected subject undergoes a sustained reversal of hypogonadotropism by the age of 18 [38].

A few neurological conditions are also known to be associated with delayed puberty. The 4H syndrome is caused by mutations in POLR3A/B and causes myelination defects (hypomyelination), hypodontia, and hypogonadotropic hypogonadism [39]. Gordon Holmes syndrome is associated with RNF216, OTUD4, and PNPLA6 mutations and presents as HH and ataxia [40]. A syndrome complex of polyneuropathy, endocrinopathies, and HH has been studied in children with DMXL2 mutation. Warburg Micro syndrome may be associated with ocular and neurodevelopmental issues and HH due to mutations in the RAB2GAP1 dysregulation of the RAB cycle.

Evaluation: In all cases of isolated HH, other pituitary hormones should be assessed to confirm that the defect is truly isolated to gonadotropin secretion. In KS there is often associated decreased olfaction, synkinesia (mirror movements), sensorineural deafness, unilateral renal agenesis, and pes cavus. Brain MRI with contrast imaging in cases of KS may show aplasia/hypoplasia of olfactory bulb and sulci. Some patients with isolated HH will have a positive family history, but most cases are sporadic. Genetic testing for associated mutations is possible, but frequently not diagnostic insofar as the majority of isolated HH is idiopathic, that is, not associated with identified genetic abnormalities [2]. It can be particularly challenging to differentiate between CD and isolated HH. Definitive diagnosis of GnRH deficiency cannot be established before 18 years.

Multiple Pituitary Hormone Deficiencies

Hypogonadotropic hypogonadism as part of a constellation of multiple pituitary hormone deficiencies (MPHDs) can occur in the setting of central nervous system (CNS) tumors (i.e., craniopharyngioma, germinoma, hypothalamic glioma, prolactinoma), non-tumoral lesions (i.e., histiocytosis, granuloma, hydrocephalus, vascular lesions, dermoid and epidermoid cysts), cerebral dysgenesis, CNS trauma or infection, and destructive medical therapies such as radiation therapy. Genetic mutations, including defects in transcription factors involved in pituitary formation such as PROP1, HESX1, LHX3 and LHX4, and SOX2, have also been incriminated [36].

In children, craniopharyngiomas are the predominant cause of permanent HH [17]. They are benign tumors that arise in the suprasellar region of the brain and may cause symptoms related to increased intracranial pressure and/or pituitary gland and optic nerve dysfunction [41]. Growth hormone deficiency is the most common endocrinologic disorder, but all pituitary hormones can be affected, and most adolescents presenting with these tumors will have delay in puberty [42]. Surgery and radiation therapy may further damage pituitary and hypothalamic function leading to permanent hormone deficiencies. Depending on dose and anatomical location, intracranial radiation therapy, in particular, causes irreversible damage to the hypothalamic-pituitary axis. It usually affects the hypothalamus to a greater extent than the pituitary gland; precocious puberty is more common than delayed puberty [43].

Septo-optic dysplasia (SOD) with midline cerebral dysgenesis can cause pubertal delay. It is characterized by congenital absence of the septum pellucidum, bilateral optic nerve hypoplasia, and hypopituitarism. There is significant variability in the severity of affected children but typically involves visual impairment and pituitary hormone deficiency with radiologic abnormalities of the septum pellucidum or corpus callosum. It is occasionally associated with HESX1 gene mutations [44]. The *FGF8* mutation has been associated with Moebius syndrome and septo-optic dysplasia as well.

Histiocytosis X is a condition that usually presents with diabetes insipidus but may also present with multiple pituitary hormone abnormalities leading to pubertal delay.

Evaluation: In any case of MPHD, laboratory assessment of thyroid function, adrenal function, growth, and electrolyte balance is indicated. Physical exam should include a thorough neurologic examination. A careful history should include review of past or recent head trauma, CNS infection, or intracranial radiation therapy. A review of systems should be performed with particular attention to visual change, headache, vomiting, fever, polyuria, polydipsia, poor growth, and salt craving. In most cases of MPHD, brain and pituitary imaging is a requisite, and, if SOD is considered, an ophthalmologic exam is a requisite to evaluate optic nerves and vision. Genetic testing is not indicated in all patients, but for those with a family history of MPHD and specific radiographic findings, targeted testing for specific mutations may be indicated [45].

Genetic Syndromes

There are several congenital syndromes that have HH as one of the primary findings. The most well-known syndrome is Prader-Willi syndrome (PWS). It is caused by loss of imprinted genetic material from the paternally derived chromosome 15. In addition to HH, it is marked by neonatal hypotonia, feeding problems in infancy, obesity, hyperphagia, developmental delay, small hands/feet, and short stature. It is usually sporadic.

CHARGE syndrome is another common syndromic cause of HH [17]. This acronym stands for coloboma, heart defects, choanal atresia, impaired growth and development, genital hypoplasia, and ear abnormalities and/ or hearing loss. Mutations in the CHD7 gene have recently been identified in approximately 2/3 of affected patients [46], and it has been suggested that the developmental abnormality causing HH in this condition may be similar to that seen in KS [47]. It can be an autosomal dominant mutation, but most cases are sporadic. Bardet-Biedl syndrome also includes HH as a primary feature. Other manifestations of this rare, autosomal recessive condition include rod-cone dystrophy, obesity, renal dysfunction, developmental delay, and postaxial polydactyly. Rud syndrome is also characterized by ichthyosis, HH, and epilepsy. Alstrom syndrome, associated with cardiomyopathy and cone rod abnormalities, and Bloom syndrome are other syndromes associated with HH.

The presence of other dysmorphic characteristics associated with a syndrome in addition to HH warrants further evaluation. For PWS, genetic testing, preferably with DNA-based methylation testing [48]. CHARGE and Bardet-Biedl syndromes are both diagnosed clinically. CHARGE syndrome diagnosis is based on major and minor criteria, but genetic testing for CHD7 mutation is available. Similarly, there is genetic testing for 14 associated genetic mutations for Bardet-Biedl, but the diagnosis is based on the presence of primary and secondary phenotypic features [49].

Hypergonadotropic Hypogonadism (HHG)

Hypergonadotropic hypogonadism (HHG) causes delayed puberty due to primary gonadal failure. By definition, these disorders have elevated levels of gonadotropins without concomitant increase in sex steroid concentrations and without signs of pubertal maturation. Within this category lie primarily disorders of gonadal dysgenesis and gonadal injury.

Gonadal Dysgenesis

Gonadal dysgenesis is the most common cause of hypergonadotropic hypogonadism in children [17]. It is usually related to chromosomal abnormalities, and hence chromosomal analysis is fundamental in the evaluation of children with HHG. In females, Turner's syndrome (TS) is a condition of X-monosomy (45, X) or structural abnormalities of an X chromosome. Mosaicism is common (50% may have 45X/mosaic karyotype). Girls have short stature and lack of normal pubertal development secondary to streak ovaries and premature ovarian failure. The degree of pubertal maturation is variable with occasional spontaneous menarche and rare fertility [50]. Other characteristics include heart and renal abnormalities, webbed neck, and broad chest. Mixed gonadal dysgenesis (MGD) can also occur similarly with X-monosomy/XY mosaicism. This protean genetic disorder can range in phenotypic presentation depending on degree of mosaicism, from phenotypic female to phenotypic male.

Klinefelter syndrome is a chromosomal abnormality found in males presenting with delayed puberty. In this case the underlying karyotype is 47-XXY. Along with HHG, this condition is characterized by tall stature; gynecomastia; small, firm, fibrotic testes; decreased upper to lower segment body ratio; and learning disabilities. Klinefelter is typically characterized by declining inhibin B and AMH levels due to Sertoli cell dysfunction. Other less prevalent disorders of gonadal

dysgenesis in 46XY karyotype are Swyer syndrome (46XY, streak gonads), Drash syndrome, Frasier syndrome, mutations of SOX-9, DAX1 with duplication of Xp21, and mutations in the SF1 [16]. 46,XX males, who may be SRY positive or negative, can present with hypergonadotropic hypogonadism, small testes, and normal-appearing external genitalia at birth.

Disorders of Sex Development

Certain disorders of sex development can present as hypergonadotropic hypogonadism. For example, children with AIS or 5-alpha reductase deficiency (5-ARD) are genetically XY but are often raised female because of ambiguous or female external genitalia. They may present with pubertal delay or primary amenorrhea when there is a failure to progress through normal female puberty.

Rare cases of gonadotropin receptor mutations (LH/FSH receptor mutation in XX females) with normal breast development, primary or secondary amenorrhea, elevated serum LH/ FSH [depending on mutation of LH/FSH receptor], low estradiol level, and infertility have been reported. LH receptor mutation (homozygous or compound heterozygous inactivating mutations of the LH receptor) in XY males presents with male pseudohermaphroditism – female external genitalia/micropenis, absence of Müllerian structures, Leydig cell hypoplasia, lack of breast development, or hypergonadotropic hypogonadism [15, 51, 52].

FSH-β subunit gene mutation presents with delayed puberty, primary amenorrhea, elevated LH, and low or undetectable FSH [53, 54]. FSH receptor mutation presents with primary gonadal failure and HHG in females [53]. FSH is required for follicular development and ovarian androgen and estrogen synthesis in females. Males present with oligospermia but are fertile as FSH is not necessary for spermatogenesis [54].

Recently, mutations in the HAX1 gene have been implicated as important in gonadal development and may present as premature ovarian failure in girls.

Gonadal Injury or Loss

Hypergonadotropic hypogonadism also occurs in children who have suffered gonadal damage. Some causes are iatrogenic (i.e., surgery, radiation, chemotherapy), environmental factors, viral infections, metabolic and autoimmune diseases, and genetic alterations. Gonadal tissue is particularly sensitive to radiation damage but can also be affected by many chemotherapeutic agents [17]. Testicular tissue is more sensitive to damage by these cytotoxic therapies compared to ovarian tissue, and in all cases the risk is agent and dose dependent [55].

Gonadal tissue can also be injured by a wide spectrum of other processes, including trauma, infarction, and infection. In addition, certain disease processes can affect gonadal tissue and lead to pubertal dysfunction and infertility. Autoimmune polyendocrine syndrome type 1 (APS 1), for example, is associated with autoimmune-induced damage to gonadal tissue. Gonadal failure is much more common in females with this disorder, and there is correlation between SCC autoantibodies and ovarian failure in women with APS1 [56]. Galactosemia is also associated with HHG in female patients, especially those for whom treatment was delayed. It is thought that this is caused by cellular galactose toxicity occurring very early in life [57].

Complete loss of gonadal tissue can also present with delayed puberty. There are several indications for gonadectomy in the prevention and treatment of malignancy, including mixed gonadal dysgenesis and selective cases of androgen insensitivity syndrome (AIS) [58]. Additionally, anorchia is a male condition in which testes form normally in utero, as evidenced by normal male genitalia, but are absent at the time of birth, indicating loss sometime after the 14th week gestational age. The cause is unknown. "Resistant ovary syndrome" is a condition due to abnormalities in gonadotropin receptors or antibodies to these receptors seen in 46,XX karyotypes, typically presenting with sexual immaturity and primary amenorrhea and small ovaries with primordial follicles despite elevated gonadotropin concentrations [59, 60].

Evaluation of Hypergonadotropic Hypogonadism: A careful history should disclose past surgeries, exposure to chemotherapy (especially of alkylating agents) or radiation, gonadal trauma or testicular torsion, prior episodes of orchitis, and the presence of other medical problems, including sickle cell disease, galactosemia, and autoimmune illnesses (especially hypoparathyroidism and Addison's disease). If autoimmunity is suspected, certain autoantibodies associated with APS1 can be measured with those against 21-hydroxylase being the most common. If an undiagnosed underlying process is suspected based on history or physical examination, further evaluation should be tailored specifically as needed. Ultrasound examination of abdominal gonads and/or chromosomal analysis is often warranted.

Eugonadotropic Hypogonadism (EH)

There are several conditions that can present with normal, pubertal gonadotropin levels with delayed or abnormal pubertal progression. Hormonal imbalances, for example, can cause failure to mature appropriately despite normal gonadotropin levels. Females with polycystic ovarian syndrome (PCOS) can undergo puberty appropriately but fail to proceed to menarche. These girls, usually obese, have normal reproductive anatomy and secondary sex characteristics but may have signs of insulin resistance and hyperandrogenism including severe acne or hirsutism. Hyperprolactinemia can also present with hypogonadism. Males will often have gynecomastia and females can have galactorrhea. The most common cause of elevated prolactin levels is prolactinoma.

Anatomic abnormalities are another cause of delayed puberty. Vaginal outflow obstruction such as imperforate hymen can prevent menstrual outflow, a so-called pseudo-primary amenorrhea. Müllerian duct anomalies (MDAs) are another type of anatomic abnormality that can present with primary amenorrhea. MDAs are classified according to level and degree of malformation. Class 1 represents segmental or complete agenesis or hypoplasia that can involve any combination of the vagina, cervix, fundus, and fallopian tubes (American Fertility Society, 1988) and is referred to as Müllerian aplasia [61]. Mayer-Rokitansky-Küster-Hauser syndrome is associated with uterine and vaginal hypoplasia/aplasia, where ovaries and fallopian tubes are preserved [16].

Evaluation: A careful physical examination including assessment of weight, acanthosis, hirsutism, acne, gynecomastia or galactorrhea, neurologic or visual abnormalities, secondary sex characteristics, and external genitalia is warranted. Laboratory tests should include a serum prolactin. If PCOS is suspected, an elevated free testosterone level can strengthen the diagnosis, and a 17-OHP level should be obtained to rule out nonclassical congenital adrenal hyperplasia. Chromosomal analysis is warranted if a disorder of sex development is entertained. If serum prolactin level is elevated, an MRI of the brain/pituitary to detect prolactinoma is indicated. Abdominal and pelvic ultrasound is often helpful in EH cases and can identify polycystic ovaries, vaginal obstruction, and the presence of gonads and other internal reproductive organs.

Diagnostic Tests

Table 17.2 summarizes the diagnostic evaluation. A detailed history (especially of parental consanguinity, age of puberty and history of infertility in family members, anosmia, nutritional history, systemic illness), thorough physical examination (special attention to stature, BMI, accurate sexual maturity staging/Tanner staging, stigmata of known conditions and systemic illnesses, galactorrhea, etc.), bone age evaluation, and appropriate laboratory evaluations as indicated (i.e., karyotype, LH, FSH, estradiol/testosterone, other pituitary hormones, thyroid function and prolactin) will be a reasonable starting point. The aim of initial evaluation is to rule out underlying disorders causing delayed puberty. The assay methodology of serum LH and FSH determination is

Table 17.2 Diagnostic evaluation of delayed puberty

History
Physical exam (height, BMI, Tanner staging, known stigmata)
Bone age
Baseline LH, FSH, testosterone (boys), estradiol (girls)
TSH, free T4

Hypogonadotropic hypogonadism	Hypergonadotropic hypogonadism	Eugonadotropic hypogonadism
Serum inhibin B	Karyotype/CGH	Pelvic ultrasound
Pituitary hormones	Pelvic ultrasound	Serum prolactin
Prolactin	Serum inhibin B	17-OH progesterone
LHRH agonist test		Free testosterone
HCG stimulation test		
MRI		
Genetic test		

important as values obtained by immunochemiluminometric assays (ICMA) are less than half of those obtained by immunofluorometric assays (IFMA) [62]. Serum LH is a more specific marker of pubertal onset than FSH; the latter is a more specific marker of primary gonadal failure [62]. Basal levels of LH and FSH may discriminate between hypo−/eugonadotropic and hypergonadotropic causes.

A delay in bone age is commonly seen in delayed puberty. If the bone age is >2 years delayed, the height prediction by Bayley-Pinneau tables overestimate predicted target height in CDGP [1, 62]. Karyotype and/or comparative genomic hybridization is indicated in hypergonadotropic hypogonadism. Pelvic ultrasound (US) in girls will help to delineate the presence of absence of uterus and ovaries as well as any evidence of stimulation. Brain imaging is also indicated, especially in cases of hypogonadotropic hypogonadism. Serum INHB corroborates the functional integrity of the Sertoli cells. Depending on the clinical and laboratory assessment, imaging of brain and pelvic ultrasound is indicated. If basal gonadotropin levels are inconclusive, stimulation tests may assist in differentiating CDGP vs. HH. However, no single test has 100% specificity/sensitivity.

Role of stimulation tests If basal gonadotropin levels are inconclusive, stimulation tests may be helpful in differentiating CDGP vs. hypogonadotropic hypogonadism (HH). However, no single test has 100% specificity/sensitivity.

1. *GnRH or a GnRH agonist stimulation test*: This is the gold standard for biochemical evaluation of HPG axis activation determined by the LH response to a classical GnRH stimulation test. LHRH agonist stimulation test is more popular due to its wide availability and is also considered to be more discriminative than provocative LHRH test [63]. There is a significant overlap in LH and FSH responses between CDGP and HH patients. Persistence of low basal or GnRH agonist stimulated LH and FSH in a late teen with a bone age > 12 years may be suggestive

of defective gonadotropin secretion. A positive response (i.e., predominant LH response over FSH response or peak LH >5 IU/L by ICMA and > 8 by IFMA) is more consistent with CDGP. In primary ovarian failure in which the gonadotropin levels are only mildly elevated, a GnRH agonist stimulation will reveal partial gonadal failure.

A variety of hormone stimulation protocols exist, but an often used one is leuprolide acetate injection 20mcg/kg (maximum 500mcg) administered subcutaneously. Draw blood levels for FSH, LH, and estradiol/testosterone. Some institutions use blood draws at 0 hour, 30 minutes, and 60 minutes. At our institution, blood is sampled at 0 hour, 4 hours, and 24 hours. If the HPG axis is activated, a two- to threefold rise in FSH and LH is observed with maximal pituitary response of LH >5 IU/L at 4 hours and maximal gonadal response of estradiol (E2) of >150 pmol/L (>40.86 pg/ml) and testosterone >3.15 nmol/L (>90 ng/dl) [64–66].

2. *Human chorionic gonadotropin (hCG) stimulation test*: Likewise, there are disparate protocols for this test [67–71]. The protocol commonly used in our institution is hCG administered intra-muscularly at a dose of 3000 IU/m^2 once a day for 3 days. Baseline LH, FSH, testosterone, as well as blood sampling for testosterone need to be drawn 24 hours after the third injection. An absolute serum testosterone concentration on day 4 of ≥150 ng/dl is normal and ≤ 50 ng/dl in HH.

3. *Growth hormone stimulation testing*: In subjects with short stature, delayed puberty, poor growth velocity, and delayed bone age, evaluation of serum IGF1 and provocative growth hormone testing will be helpful to assess growth hormone deficiency. If there is significant short stature to warrant provocative growth hormone testing, sex steroid priming with estrogen/testosterone is recommended necessarily as this may restore the physiologic depressed growth hormone secretion associated with low estrogen levels [1].

Present and Future Therapies

Inadequate gonadal steroid secretion is the fundamental basis of delayed puberty.

Therapeutic goals are to develop secondary sex characteristics, to amass and sustain normal bone development, to maximize final height, and to restore fertility. Treatment of delayed puberty is variable and depends on diagnosis.

Observation Most cases of temporary hypogonadism and EH do not require hormonal treatment to induce puberty. With GDGP, observation and "watchful waiting" are generally adequate, but short-term hormone therapy to "jump start" puberty is sometimes justified to prevent significant psychological distress, initiate a growth spurt, and/ or activate the HPG axis.

In functional HH related to exercise, eating disorder, or chronic illness, the treatment is to improve overall health and nutrition. In regard to disorders of sex development, there is significant controversy surrounding the appropriate time for cosmetic surgery, gonadectomy, and HRT – current recommendations are complex and beyond the scope of this review [58].

Hormone replacement therapy (HRT) Permanent HH and HHG generally require sex steroid HRT to induce puberty and maintain physiologic hormone levels. Replacement of other pituitary hormones is also frequently required, especially in the case of *MPHD*. When using HRT to induce puberty, there are several important considerations. Initiation of therapy must be timed appropriately to balance the benefits of developing according to population and physiologic norms with risk of premature epiphyseal closure and attenuated final adult height. Studies on boys with CDGP and girls with TS have shown that initiation of hormone therapy at very low doses after around 14 years of age in boys or 12 years in girls has no significant negative impact on final adult height while simultaneously promoting a natural emergence in the development of secondary sex characteristics [72–75]. In girls with any type of hypogonadism, HRT is the best treatment option as this will result in adequate development of secondary sex characteristics as well as that of the uterus.

Estrogen therapy to induce female puberty is typically initiated with transdermal preparations of 17β-estradiol given the very low doses of hormone replacement that is required. Typically treatment starts with using half of the lowest dose patch with 3.1–6.2 μg daily (1/8–1/4 of the 25 μg patch) and increased gradually by 3.1–6.2 μg daily every 6 months [1] over the next 2 years to an adult dose of 100–200ug daily to mimic physiologic levels seen in puberty. Estradiol (E2) levels can be monitored to ensure appropriate dosing. On the other hand, HRT that is provided too rapidly tends to promote unnatural development, including breast growth that occurs disproportionately in the nipple and areola [76]. Once full E2 dosing is reached and breast maturation is almost complete, cyclic oral progesterone at normal adult dose is added every 1–3 months to induce menstruation, a necessity to decrease the risk of uterine cancer. Once menstruation has been established, contraception preparations can be used for HRT depending on patient preference [77]. In cases of HH in which permanent hypogonadism has not been confirmed, brief trials off HRT can be attempted once regular cycles occur in order to assess for activation of the HPG axis. If transdermal preparations are unavailable, HRT may be initiated with conjugated estrogens (Premarin®) 0.1625 mg daily, increase every 3–6 months to 0.325 mg daily or ethinylestradiol 2 μg daily and increase every 3–6 months up to 10 μg daily.

Initial therapy is with estrogen alone to maximize breast growth and to induce uterine and endometrial proliferation. Adding a progestin prematurely or administering combinations of estrogens and progestins early on may reduce ultimate breast size. Progestin is added to mimic the normal menstrual cycle after breast growth ceases (when full contour breast growth plateaus) or menses occur. Once menstruation established with cyclic hormone treatment, discontinue intermittently for 1–3-month periods to determine if spontaneous menstruation occurs (in girls with CD and FHH). In permanent hypogonadism, OCP should be continued till the average age of menopause, ~50 years.

Testosterone therapy to initiate male puberty is generally started at 50 mg of depot testosterone as intramuscular injection once monthly for 3–6 months [1]. This will result in pubertal activation in CDG P [38]. If testes do not grow and reach a volume of 4 ml within 1 year of treatment, it is highly likely that the patient will not develop puberty spontaneously (most likely, not CGDP). In that scenario, treatment may be discontinued for 3 months, and HPG axis activation may be re-evaluated. Subsequently, testosterone is increased to 100 mg per month with 25–50 mg increment in dose for approximately 18 months to complete the growth spurt (dosing should increase gradually to mimic physiologic puberty and prevent accelerated bone maturation). After growth is complete, further increase in dose can be made to 100 mg twice monthly. Testosterone levels and, in the case of hypergonadotropic hypogonadism, LH levels should be monitored and used to adjust dose up to a maximum adult dose of 200 mg twice monthly as needed to achieve serum concentrations in the normal range. Thereafter, the increment of testosterone is 250 mg, every 3–4 weeks. It has to be kept in mind that HRT in males only result in virilization without testicular development. Oral testosterone preparations provide less consistent serum testosterone levels, and there is a risk for hepatic damage or carcinogenesis. Testosterone topical products, nasal spray, and gels, frequently used in adults, are not well studied in children.

Pulsatile GnRH or gonadotropin therapy Patients with permanent hypogonadism can occasionally achieve fertility through treatment with gonadotropin or GnRH-based therapies and should be referred to reproductive endocrinology as needed. When fertility is desired, treat with either exogenous gonadotropins or pulsatile GnRH. Pulsatile administration of exogenous GnRH is effective therapy for stimulation of endogenous gonadotropin secretion, follicular development, and ovulation in women with GnRH deficiency. Mutations in the GPR54 (encoding the kisspeptin receptor, also known as KISS1R) reportedly can be corrected by the administration of GnRH [5, 36]. In male hypogonadotropic hypogonadism, GnRH treatment will promote a physiologic puberty with testicular development, virilization, and spermatogenesis. When spermatogenesis is achieved, maintenance therapy consists of subcutaneous hCG injections once or twice a week [15].

Human chorionic gonadotropin (hCG) HCG has been used to treat subjects with permanent HH. A typical starting dose of 500 IU is administered subcutaneously on Mondays, Wednesdays, and Fridays. Dilute the 10,000-unit vial of powder with 5 mL of diluent for a 2000 unit/mL concentration. Obtain serum testosterone measurement in 1 month on a Monday prior to an injection. If the testosterone is <200 ng/dL, increase the dose to 1000 units subcutaneously, up to a maximum dose of 1500 IU (on M-W-F) and repeat a "trough" testosterone in another month. The hCG treatment will result in testicular enlargement, testosterone production, Sertoli cell maturation, and spermatogenesis and thus offers better chances of future fertility.

Leptin has been used in the management of amenorrhea in adults, but there is no pediatric data available. Other treatment options such as combination of hMG/hCG or recombinant FSH/hCG [15] that are used in the management of hypogonadotropic males for fertility are beyond the scope of this chapter.

Future Therapies

Although current treatment of delayed puberty centers revolves around replacement of sex steroid hormones, advances in the identification of genetic mutations that underlie HH promise to increase our understanding of the physiology behind pubertal initiation [78]. This information could result in the development of improved targeted therapies and allow for normal pubertal progression. A potential future therapeutic agent for treatment of delayed puberty is agonists of kisspeptin peptides and neurokinin B agonists. In boys with CDGP and short stature, a potential therapeutic approach is aromatase inhibition, which may increase the final adult height [1, 79]. The treatments targeted to preserve future fertility such as cryopreservation of ovarian fragments prior to anticipated ovarian failure secondary to gonadotoxic treatment [10] and pulsatile hCG treatment for HH are not discussed in this chapter.

References

1. Palmert MR, Dunkel L. Clinical practice. Delayed puberty. N Engl J Med. 2012;366(5):443–53.
2. Seminara SB, Crowley WF Jr. Kisspeptin and GPR54: discovery of a novel pathway in reproduction. J Neuroendocrinol. 2008;20(6):727–31.
3. Lee JM, Kaciroti N, Appugliese D, Corwyn RF, Bradley RH, Lumeng JC. Body mass index and timing of pubertal initiation in boys. Arch Pediatr Adolesc Med. 2010;164(2):139–44.
4. Nathan BM, Sedlmeyer IL, Palmert MR. Impact of body mass index on growth in boys with delayed puberty. J Pediatr Endocrinol Metab. 2006;19(8):971–7.
5. Messager S, Chatzidaki EE, Ma D, Hendrick AG, Zahn D, Dixon J, et al. Kisspeptin directly stimulates gonadotropin-releasing hormone release via G protein-coupled receptor 54. Proc Natl Acad Sci U S A. 2005;102(5):1761–6.
6. Silveira LG, Noel SD, Silveira-Neto AP, Abreu AP, Brito VN, Santos MG, et al. Mutations of the KISS1 gene in disorders of puberty. J Clin Endocrinol Metab. 2010;95(5):2276–80.
7. Gueorguiev M, Goth ML, Korbonits M. Leptin and puberty: a review. Pituitary. 2001;4(1–2):79–86.
8. Farooqi IS, Jebb SA, Langmack G, Lawrence E, Cheetham CH, Prentice AM, et al. Effects of recombinant leptin therapy in a child with congenital leptin deficiency. N Engl J Med. 1999;341(12):879–84.
9. Tornberg J, Sykiotis GP, Keefe K, Plummer L, Hoang X, Hall JE, et al. Heparan sulfate 6-O-sulfotransferase 1, a gene involved in extracellular sugar modifications, is mutated in patients with idiopathic hypogonadotrophic hypogonadism. Proc Natl Acad Sci U S A. 2011;108(28):11524–9.
10. Poirot C, Vacher-Lavenu MC, Helardot P, Guibert J, Brugieres L, Jouannet P. Human ovarian tissue cryopreservation: indications and feasibility. Hum Reprod. 2002;17(6):1447–52.
11. Xu C, Messina A, Somm E, Miraoui H, Kinnunen T, Acierno J Jr, et al. KLB, encoding beta-klotho, is mutated in patients with congenital hypogonadotropic hypogonadism. EMBO Mol Med. 2017;9(10):1379–97.
12. Zhu J, Choa RE, Guo MH, Plummer L, Buck C, Palmert MR, et al. A shared genetic basis for self-limited delayed puberty and idiopathic hypogonadotropic hypogonadism. J Clin Endocrinol Metab. 2015;100(4):E646–54.
13. Howard SR, Guasti L, Ruiz-Babot G, Mancini A, David A, Storr HL, et al. IGSF10 mutations dysregulate gonadotropin-releasing hormone neuronal migration resulting in delayed puberty. EMBO Mol Med. 2016;8(6):626–42.
14. Parent AS, Teilmann G, Juul A, Skakkebaek NE, Toppari J, Bourguignon JP. The timing of normal puberty and the age limits of sexual precocity: variations around the world, secular trends, and changes after migration. Endocr Rev. 2003;24(5):668–93.
15. Delemarre EM, Felius B, Delemarre-van de Waal HA. Inducing puberty. Eur J Endocrinol. 2008;159(Suppl 1):S9–15.

16. Fenichel P. Delayed puberty. Endocr Dev. 2012;22:138–59.

17. Sedlmeyer IL, Palmert MR. Delayed puberty: analysis of a large case series from an academic center. J Clin Endocrinol Metab. 2002;87(4):1613–20.

18. Rosenfield RL. Clinical review 6: diagnosis and management of delayed puberty. J Clin Endocrinol Metab. 1990;70(3):559–62.

19. Wehkalampi K, Widen E, Laine T, Palotie A, Dunkel L. Association of the timing of puberty with a chromosome 2 locus. J Clin Endocrinol Metab. 2008;93(12):4833–9.

20. Sedlmeyer IL, Hirschhorn JN, Palmert MR. Pedigree analysis of constitutional delay of growth and maturation: determination of familial aggregation and inheritance patterns. J Clin Endocrinol Metab. 2002;87(12):5581–6.

21. Albanese A, Stanhope R. Predictive factors in the determination of final height in boys with constitutional delay of growth and puberty. J Pediatr. 1995;126(4):545–50.

22. Counts DR, Pescovitz OH, Barnes KM, Hench KD, Chrousos GP, Sherins RJ, et al. Dissociation of adrenarche and gonadarche in precocious puberty and in isolated hypogonadotropic hypogonadism. J Clin Endocrinol Metab. 1987;64(6):1174–8.

23. Kelch RP, Hopwood NJ, Marshall JC. Diagnosis of gonadotropin deficiency in adolescents: limited usefulness of a standard gonadotropin-releasing hormone test in obese boys. J Pediatr. 1980;97(5):820–4.

24. Wu FC, Brown DC, Butler GE, Stirling HF, Kelnar CJ. Early morning plasma testosterone is an accurate predictor of imminent pubertal development in prepubertal boys. J Clin Endocrinol Metab. 1993;76(1):26–31.

25. Grinspon RP, Ropelato MG, Gottlieb S, Keselman A, Martinez A, Ballerini MG, et al. Basal follicle-stimulating hormone and peak gonadotropin levels after gonadotropin-releasing hormone infusion show high diagnostic accuracy in boys with suspicion of hypogonadotropic hypogonadism. J Clin Endocrinol Metab. 2010;95(6):2811–8.

26. Resende EA, Lara BH, Reis JD, Ferreira BP, Pereira GA, Borges MF. Assessment of basal and gonadotropin-releasing hormone-stimulated gonadotropins by immunochemiluminometric and immunofluorometric assays in normal children. J Clin Endocrinol Metab. 2007;92(4):1424–9.

27. Coutant R, Biette-Demeneix E, Bouvattier C, Bouhours-Nouet N, Gatelais F, Dufresne S, et al. Baseline inhibin B and anti-Mullerian hormone measurements for diagnosis of hypogonadotropic hypogonadism (HH) in boys with delayed puberty. J Clin Endocrinol Metab. 2010;95(12):5225–32.

28. Simon D. Puberty in chronically diseased patients. Horm Res. 2002;57(Suppl 2):53–6.

29. Buchacz K, Rogol AD, Lindsey JC, Wilson CM, Hughes MD, Seage GR 3rd, et al. Delayed onset of pubertal development in children and adolescents with perinatally acquired HIV infection. J Acquir Immune Defic Syndr. 2003;33(1):56–65.

30. Caronia LM, Martin C, Welt CK, Sykiotis GP, Quinton R, Thambundit A, et al. A genetic basis for functional hypothalamic amenorrhea. N Engl J Med. 2011;364(3):215–25.

31. Kaplowitz P. Clinical characteristics of 104 children referred for evaluation of precocious puberty. J Clin Endocrinol Metab. 2004;89(8):3644–50.

32. Wyshak G, Frisch RE. Evidence for a secular trend in age of menarche. N Engl J Med. 1982;306(17):1033–5.

33. Semple RK, Topaloglu AK. The recent genetics of hypogonadotrophic hypogonadism – novel insights and new questions. Clin Endocrinol. 2010;72(4):427–35.

34. Shaw ND, Seminara SB, Welt CK, Au MG, Plummer L, Hughes VA, et al. Expanding the phenotype and genotype of female GnRH deficiency. J Clin Endocrinol Metab. 2011;96(3):E566–76.

35. Wang Y, Gong C, Qin M, Liu Y, Tian Y. Clinical and genetic features of 64 young male paediatric patients with congenital hypogonadotropic hypogonadism. Clin Endocrinol. 2017;87(6):757–66.

36. de Roux N, Genin E, Carel JC, Matsuda F, Chaussain JL, Milgrom E. Hypogonadotropic hypogonadism due to loss of function of the KiSS1-derived peptide receptor GPR54. Proc Natl Acad Sci U S A. 2003;100(19):10972–6.

37. Achermann JC, Gu WX, Kotlar TJ, Meeks JJ, Sabacan LP, Seminara SB, et al. Mutational analysis of DAX1 in patients with hypogonadotropic hypogonadism or pubertal delay. J Clin Endocrinol Metab. 1999;84(12):4497–500.

38. Raivio T, Falardeau J, Dwyer A, Quinton R, Hayes FJ, Hughes VA, et al. Reversal of idiopathic hypogonadotropic hypogonadism. N Engl J Med. 2007;357(9):863–73.

39. Wolf NI, Vanderver A, van Spaendonk RM, Schiffmann R, Brais B, Bugiani M, et al. Clinical spectrum of 4H leukodystrophy caused by POLR3A and POLR3B mutations. Neurology. 2014;83(21):1898–905.

40. Topaloglu AK, Lomniczi A, Kretzschmar D, Dissen GA, Kotan LD, McArdle CA, et al. Loss-of-function mutations in PNPLA6 encoding neuropathy target esterase underlie pubertal failure and neurological deficits in Gordon Holmes syndrome. J Clin Endocrinol Metab. 2014;99(10):E2067–75.

41. de Vries L, Weintrob N, Phillip M. Craniopharyngioma presenting as precocious puberty and accelerated growth. Clin Pediatr (Phila). 2003;42(2):181–4.

42. Halac I, Zimmerman D. Endocrine manifestations of craniopharyngioma. Childs Nerv Syst. 2005;21(8–9):640–8.

43. Darzy KH, Shalet SM. Pathophysiology of radiation-induced growth hormone deficiency: efficacy and safety of GH replacement. Growth Hormon IGF Res 2006;16 Suppl A:S30–40.

44. Dattani MT, Martinez-Barbera JP, Thomas PQ, Brickman JM, Gupta R, Martensson IL, et al. Mutations in the homeobox gene HESX1/Hesx1 associated with septo-optic dysplasia in human and mouse. Nat Genet. 1998;19(2):125–33.

45. Reynaud R, Gueydan M, Saveanu A, Vallette-Kasic S, Enjalbert A, Brue T, et al. Genetic screening of combined pituitary hormone deficiency: experience in 195 patients. J Clin Endocrinol Metab. 2006;91(9):3329–36.

46. Zentner GE, Layman WS, Martin DM, Scacheri PC. Molecular and phenotypic aspects of CHD7 mutation in CHARGE syndrome. Am J Med Genet A. 152A(3):674–86.

47. Pinto G, Abadie V, Mesnage R, Blustajn J, Cabrol S, Amiel J, et al. CHARGE syndrome includes hypogonadotropic hypogonadism and abnormal olfactory bulb development. J Clin Endocrinol Metab. 2005;90(10):5621–6.

48. Goldstone AP, Holland AJ, Hauffa BP, Hokken-Koelega AC, Tauber M. Recommendations for the diagnosis and management of Prader-Willi syndrome. J Clin Endocrinol Metab. 2008;93(11):4183–97.

49. Beales PL, Elcioglu N, Woolf AS, Parker D, Flinter FA. New criteria for improved diagnosis of Bardet-Biedl syndrome: results of a population survey. J Med Genet. 1999;36(6):437–46.

50. Pasquino AM, Passeri F, Pucarelli I, Segni M, Municchi G. Spontaneous pubertal development in Turner's syndrome. Italian study Group for Turner's syndrome. J Clin Endocrinol Metab. 1997;82(6):1810–3.

51. Latronico AC, Arnhold IJ. Inactivating mutations of LH and FSH receptors–from genotype to phenotype. Pediatr Endocrinol Rev. 2006;4(1):28–31.

52. Beranova M, Oliveira LM, Bedecarrats GY, Schipani E, Vallejo M, Ammini AC, et al. Prevalence, phenotypic spectrum, and modes of inheritance of gonadotropin-releasing hormone receptor mutations in idiopathic hypogonadotropic hypogonadism. J Clin Endocrinol Metab. 2001;86(4):1580–8.

53. Layman LC. Mutations in the follicle-stimulating hormone-beta (FSH beta) and FSH receptor genes in mice and humans. Semin Reprod Med. 2000;18(1):5–10.

54. Layman LC, Lee EJ, Peak DB, Namnoum AB, Vu KV, van Lingen BL, et al. Delayed puberty and hypogonadism caused by mutations in the follicle-stimulating hormone beta-subunit gene. N Engl J Med. 1997;337(9):607–11.

55. Howell SJ, Shalet SM. Spermatogenesis after cancer treatment: damage and recovery. J Natl Cancer Inst Monogr. 2005;34:12–7.

56. Myhre AG, Halonen M, Eskelin P, Ekwall O, Hedstrand H, Rorsman F, et al. Autoimmune polyendocrine syndrome type 1 (APS I) in Norway. Clin Endocrinol. 2001;54(2):211–7.

57. Kaufman FR, Kogut MD, Donnell GN, Goebelsmann U, March C, Koch R. Hypergonadotropic hypogonadism in female patients with galactosemia. N Engl J Med. 1981;304(17):994–8.

58. Lee PA, Houk CP, Ahmed SF, Hughes IA. Consensus statement on management of intersex disorders. International consensus conference on intersex. Pediatrics. 2006;118(2):e488–500.

59. Arici A, Matalliotakis IM, Koumantakis GE, Goumenou AG, Neonaki MA, Koumantakis EE. Diagnostic role of inhibin B in resistant ovary syndrome associated with secondary amenorrhea. Fertil Steril. 2002;78(6):1324–6.

60. Mueller A, Berkholz A, Dittrich R, Wildt L. Spontaneous normalization of ovarian function and pregnancy in a patient with resistant ovary syndrome. Eur J Obstet Gynecol Reprod Biol. 2003;111(2):210–3.

61. ACOG Committee Opinion No. 355: vaginal agenesis: diagnosis, management, and routine care. Obstet Gynecol. 2006;108(6):1605–9.

62. Wit JM, Rekers-Mombarg LT. Final height gain by GH therapy in children with idiopathic short stature is dose dependent. J Clin Endocrinol Metab. 2002;87(2):604–11.

63. Ibanez L, Potau N, Zampolli M, Virdis R, Gussinye M, Carrascosa A, et al. Use of leuprolide acetate response patterns in the early diagnosis of pubertal disorders: comparison with the gonadotropin-releasing hormone test. J Clin Endocrinol Metab. 1994;78(1):30–5.

64. Lanes R. A GnRH analog test in diagnosing gonadotropin deficiency in males with delayed puberty. J Pediatr. 2006;149(5):731; author reply –2

65. Wilson DA, Hofman PL, Miles HL, Unwin KE, McGrail CE, Cutfield WS. Evaluation of the buserelin stimulation test in diagnosing gonadotropin deficiency in males with delayed puberty. J Pediatr. 2006;148(1):89–94.

66. Zamboni G, Antoniazzi F, Tato L. Use of the gonadotropin-releasing hormone agonist triptorelin in the diagnosis of delayed puberty in boys. J Pediatr. 1995;126(5 Pt 1):756–8.

67. Segal TY, Mehta A, Anazodo A, Hindmarsh PC, Dattani MT. Role of gonadotropin-releasing hormone and human chorionic gonadotropin stimulation tests in differentiating patients with hypogonadotropic hypogonadism from those with constitutional delay of growth and puberty. J Clin Endocrinol Metab. 2009;94(3):780–5.

68. Dunkel L, Perheentupa J, Virtanen M, Maenpaa J. Gonadotropin-releasing hormone test and human chorionic gonadotropin test in the diagnosis of gonadotropin deficiency in prepubertal boys. J Pediatr. 1985;107(3):388–92.

69. Dunkel L, Perheentupa J, Virtanen M, Maenpaa J. GnRH and HCG tests are both necessary in differential diagnosis of male delayed puberty. Am J Dis Child. 1985;139(5):494–8.

70. Degros V, Cortet-Rudelli C, Soudan B, Dewailly D. The human chorionic gonadotropin test is more powerful than the gonadotropin-releasing hormone agonist test to discriminate male isolated hypogonadotropic hypogonadism from constitutional delayed puberty. Eur J Endocrinol. 2003;149(1):23–9.

71. Kauschansky A, Dickerman Z, Phillip M, Weintrob N, Strich D. Use of GnRH agonist and human chorionic gonadotrophin tests for differentiating constitutional delayed puberty from gonadotrophin deficiency in boys. Clin Endocrinol. 2002;56(5):603–7.

72. Arrigo T, Cisternino M, Luca De F, Saggese G, Messina MF, Pasquino AM, et al. Final height outcome in both untreated and testosterone-treated boys with constitutional delay of growth and puberty. J Pediatr Endocrinol Metab. 1996;9(5):511–7.

73. Buyukgebiz A. Treatment of constitutional delayed puberty with a combination of testosterone esters. Horm Res. 1995;44(Suppl 3):32–4.

74. Soliman AT, Khadir MM, Asfour M. Testosterone treatment in adolescent boys with constitutional delay of growth and development. Metabolism. 1995;44(8):1013–5.

75. Ankarberg-Lindgren C, Elfving M, Wikland KA, Norjavaara E. Nocturnal application of transdermal estradiol patches produces levels of estradiol that mimic those seen at the onset of spontaneous puberty in girls. J Clin Endocrinol Metab. 2001;86(7):3039–44.

76. Brook CG. Management of delayed puberty. Br Med J (Clin Res Ed). 1985;290(6469):657–8.

77. Bondy CA. Care of girls and women with turner syndrome: a guideline of the turner syndrome study group. J Clin Endocrinol Metab. 2007;92(1):10–25.

78. Achermann JC, Jameson JL. Advances in the molecular genetics of hypogonadotropic hypogonadism. J Pediatr Endocrinol Metab. 2001;14(1):3–15.

79. Wickman S, Sipila I, Ankarberg-Lindgren C, Norjavaara E, Dunkel L. A specific aromatase inhibitor and potential increase in adult height in boys with delayed puberty: a randomised controlled trial. Lancet. 2001;357(9270):1743–8.

Precocious Puberty

Elizabeth Fudge

Introduction

Puberty is the stage of development leading to sexual maturation and reproductive potential. Normal puberty is regulated by the hypothalamic–pituitary–gonadal (HPG) axis which is activated at the onset of puberty from the quiescent prepubertal state. Precocious puberty is the onset of pubertal changes at an earlier age than is expected for the population. Precocious pubertal development may occur by either premature activation of the HPG axis (central precocious puberty) or exposure to endogenous or exogenous sex steroids independent of HPG axis activation (peripheral precocious puberty). Although some children evaluated for precocious puberty will have variants of normal development such as premature thelarche (breast development), pathologic causes will need to be ruled out in others [1].

Hypothalamic–Pituitary–Gonadal Axis

At the onset of puberty, the hypothalamus increases gonadotropin-releasing hormone (GnRH) secretion which stimulates the anterior pituitary to produce luteinizing hormone (LH) and follicle-stimulating hormone (FSH). LH and FSH enter the systemic circulation and increase sex steroid production by the ovaries and testes. The primary sex steroid produced by the ovary is estradiol which promotes breast and reproductive system maturation in females. Estradiol, along with the inhibin and follistatin molecules produced by the ovary (follistatin is produced in other tissues as well), has a negative feedback effect on hypothalamic GnRH and pituitary gonadotropin release. In the testis, LH stimulates production of testosterone (and estradiol to a lesser extent) from Leydig cells, while FSH stimulates Sertoli cells to produce

E. Fudge (✉)
Pediatric Endocrinology, University of Florida,
Gainsville, FL, USA
e-mail: efudge@peds.ufl.edu

the inhibin peptides and to mature into cells capable of supporting spermatozoa through the stages of spermatogenesis. Testosterone is responsible for growth of sexual hair, apocrine gland maturation, and increase in somatic (especially muscle) growth during puberty. Testosterone also stimulates longitudinal bone growth and promotes osseous maturation by aromatization to estradiol. Both testosterone and inhibins exert feedback inhibition on the hypothalamic–pituitary–gonadal (HPG) axis in males [2, 3] (Fig. 18.1).

The HPG axis matures during fetal life, with gonadotropin release persisting into infancy. Peaks in gonadotropin and sex steroid levels occur between 6 and 8 weeks of life with levels comparable to those in early to mid-puberty. Generally, peripheral effects of these sex steroids do not occur during this "mini-puberty," possibly due to the transient nature of the sex steroid increase. Gonadotropin levels reach a nadir at 6 months of life, although females may retain variable degrees of GnRH release during the first few years of life. The activation of HPG axis early in life is followed by a long period of quiescence through the prepubertal years when hypothalamic activity is suppressed. During the childhood years, GnRH is released in low amplitude pulses at a low frequency. During this time, the pituitary gland remains responsive to GnRH stimulation, with a characteristic response of greater FSH release than that of LH.

At the onset of puberty, the hypothalamus is reactivated, with enhanced, pulsatile GnRH secretion. The mechanisms that control pubertal onset and increase in GnRH secretion involve a balance between inhibitory and stimulatory neurotransmitters of the central nervous system. The earliest identified neuroendocrine change of puberty is the production of kisspeptin from hypothalamic neurons in the arcuate nucleus and anteroventral periventricular area. Kisspeptin is known to promote GnRH secretion. Neurokinin B and dynorphin are coproduced from kisspeptin-producing hypothalamic neurons and appear to have local stimulatory and inhibitory effects respectively on kisspeptin release. In addition, the onset of puberty is influenced by energy status of an individual: leptin and ghrelin which reflect energy stores

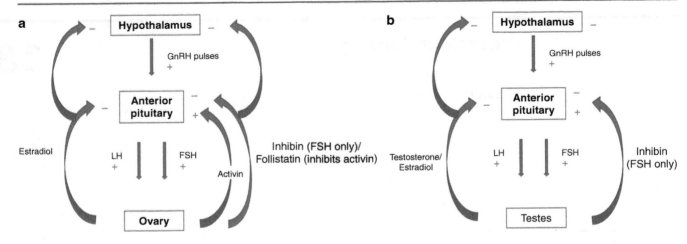

Fig. 18.1 (**a**) Hypothalamic–pituitary–ovarian axis. (**b**) Hypothalamic–pituitary–testicular axis

modulate kisspeptin secretion. Hypothalamic astrocytes and other neuroglial cells are postulated to regulate puberty by the secretion of growth factors which act on GnRH neurons as well as by direct apposition to GnRH neurons modulating GnRH release.

In early puberty, GnRH pulse frequency and amplitude increase primarily at night and extend into daytime hours as puberty progresses. LH and FSH production increases in response to GnRH, initially rising during the night and then during the day with pubertal advancement [4–9].

Normal Puberty

Girls

The increase in sex steroids from the gonad, as well as adrenal androgens, is responsible for the physical changes of puberty. In girls, estradiol stimulates the onset and progression of breast maturity, genital growth (elongation of the vulva and growth of the labia minora), maturation of vaginal mucosa, uterine growth, and changes in body composition, mainly accumulation and localization of fat. Breast budding, or thelarche, is often the first sign of puberty in females. However, one-third of girls may experience pubic hair development, pubarche, before thelarche. Progression of breast development and pubic hair growth may be classified into Tanner stages (Table 18.1). A substantial number of girls may not progress to Tanner stage 5 breast development and have persistent Tanner stage 4 breast development throughout adulthood [10].

The adolescent growth spurt is seen early in puberty in girls, driven by the increase in estrogen and the augmentation of growth hormone release by sex steroids. Menarche occurs approximately 2 years after the onset of puberty. Age at menarche correlates positively with skeletal maturity and

Table 18.1 Pubertal stages in females

Tanner stage	Pubic hair	Breast	Growth rate
1	No pubic hair	Papilla elevation; prepubertal	5–6 cm/year
2	Sparse, pigmented hair primarily on labia	Palpable breast buds; enlargement of areola	7–8 cm/year
3	Coarser, darker hair spread over Mons pubis	Areola and breast enlargement; no projection of areola	Peak growth rate at 8 cm/year
4	Adult hair type but smaller area, not spreading to thighs	Projection of areola and papilla to form secondary mound	7 cm/year
5	Adult hair type and distribution	Mature breast development with projection of papilla only	Linear growth complete after epiphyseal closure

inversely with the remaining height potential. The average girl will gain an additional 4–6 cm after menarche. The duration of puberty is on average 3–4 years, although the tempo of puberty can vary as widely as 2–7 years between individuals.

The historical ranges of normal pubertal timing were based on the data of Tanner and Marshall from the 1960s. In these observational studies of primarily middle-class Caucasian children, 95% of girls experienced breast development between ages 8.5 and 13 years, with an average age of 11.2 years. Black girls have been found to enter puberty earlier than girls of other ethnic groups, followed by Mexican-American girls, and then white girls [11, 12].

Other data on pubertal timing further support racial differences in the age of onset. These studies show that the early age limit and mean of Tanner stage 2 breast development for white girls is 8.0 and 10.4 years, for black girls is 6.6 and 9.5 years, and for Mexican-American girls is 6.8 and

9.8 years. The duration between pubertal onset and menarche was found to be approximately 2.3 years in these studies, with median age of menarche of 12.06 years in black girls, 12.25 years in Mexican-American girls, and 12.55 years in white girls [11–18].

Boys

Testicular enlargement is the first sign of normal puberty in boys, with pubic hair growth often occurring around this time. A testicular volume ≥ 3 ml, or a longitudinal axis of ≥2.2 cm, is indicative of puberty. Axillary hair growth begins at mid-puberty, and hair growth in androgen-sensitive areas progresses. Male puberty can be classified according to Tanner stages of genital development and pubic hair (Table 18.2).

Peak growth velocity in boys occurs in mid-puberty with increasing testosterone production. Males experience an increase in lean body mass and a relative decline in body fat during this time. Estradiol levels increase during mid-puberty as the result of conversion of increasing levels of testosterone, potentiating growth and skeletal maturation. Spermarche, which is the onset of sperm production, occurs at an average age of 14 years [19].

The median age of development of Tanner stage 2 pubic hair is 11.2 years in black boys, 12.0 years in white boys, and 12.3 years in Mexican-American boys based on NHANES III data. In the earlier reports from Marshall and Tanner, 95% of boys entered puberty between 9.5 and 13.5 years with an

Table 18.2 Pubertal stages in males

Tanner stage	Genital changes; pubic hair	Growth rate	Other changes
1	No pigmented hair; penis size prepubertal; testes <4 ml	5–6 cm/year	
2	Sparse pubic hair at base of penis; early penile and scrotal growth; testes 4–8 ml	5–6 cm/year	Early voice changes; scrotal thinning
3	Coarse, dark hair over pubis; increasing penile length and width; testes 10–15 ml	Increase growth rate to 7–8 cm/year	Voice breaks; light hair on upper lip; muscle mass increasing
4	Increasing pubic hair but less than adult distribution; increasing pigmentation of scrotum; increase in penile size; testes 15–20 ml	Peak growth velocity 10 cm/year	Voice changes; axillary hair
5	Adult distribution of pubic hair; adult size and shape of penis; testes >20 ml	Linear growth complete after epiphyseal closure	Beard growth; mature male physique

average of 11.6 years. The average duration of puberty in boys is 3 years [20–22].

Precocious Puberty

Definition

Pubertal development at a younger age than expected for gender and population is considered precocious. The features include progression of pubertal signs, linear growth acceleration, and advancement of skeletal maturity. Classically, pubertal onset before the age of 8 in girls and age of 9 in boys has been defined as precocious. However, racial differences in the timing of pubertal onset must be taken into consideration.

The lower age limit for defining precocious pubertal onset in girls has been controversial. Some experts suggest that the lower age cutoff should be 6 years for black girls and 7 years for white girls, with individuals older than these limits evaluated only if they meet certain criteria: significant skeletal advancement, predicted adult height < 2SD below genetic target, features suspicious of a central nervous system (CNS) lesion, rapid tempo of puberty, or psychosocial concerns. These recommendations have not been universally endorsed due to concerns that the lower age cutoff would fail to identify pathology in some individuals. For example, a retrospective review of patients referred for precocious puberty to a tertiary care center found that application of these lower age limits would have resulted in failure to identify treatable etiologies (such as congenital adrenal hyperplasia, pituitary adenoma, and neurofibromatosis) in 12% of patients [23].

Until more data are available, careful evaluation of children with signs of secondary sexual development is warranted for girls younger than 8 years and boys younger than 9 years. A comprehensive history and physical exam with clinical follow-up may be sufficient in those individuals between the lower and upper suggested age cutoffs whose evaluations indicate slow progression that do not raise concerns for underlying pathology [24].

Normal Variants

Premature Thelarche: When evaluating children referred for precocious puberty, normal variants must be considered. For instance, premature thelarche is isolated breast development in girls without other signs suggestive of true puberty. Premature thelarche often occurs within the first 2 years of life, with a second peak between the ages of 6 and 8 years. Breast development in these patients is minimal or nonprogressive and is not associated with linear growth acceleration, skeletal age advancement, or other signs of puberty. In most cases, there is no underlying pathology, although some instances have been associated with the use of cosmetic or hair products containing lavender oil, tea tree oil, or placental extracts. Clinical follow-up is warranted in these individuals to monitor for pubertal progression as some may progress to true central precocious puberty [25–28].

Premature Adrenarche: Adrenarche is the component of puberty that is not dependent on the HPG axis and may, therefore, vary in time of onset in relation to HPG activation. Adrenarche results when the adrenal cortex matures and increases production of androgens, including dehydroepiandrosterone (DHEA), dehydroepiandrosterone-sulfate (DHEA-S), and androstenedione. These androgens are responsible for some of the physical changes of puberty such as acne, growth of sexual hair, and body odor from the development of apocrine glands. The appearance of these physical signs is referred to as pubarche. Adrenarche usually occurs just before or around the onset of puberty.

Adrenarche before the age of 8 years in females and 9 years in males is referred to as premature. The factors initiating premature adrenarche are not clearly understood. Children with benign premature adrenarche have features that are non- or slowly progressive. In addition, these children do not have growth acceleration, substantial bone age advancement, or other signs of true puberty such as breast development or testicular enlargement. Levels of DHEA, DHEA-S, and androstenedione are often mild to moderately elevated and consistent with Tanner stage of pubic hair. A small percentage of individuals with premature adrenarche may have a pathological cause such as central precocious puberty, nonclassical congenital adrenal hyperplasia, or androgen-producing tumor. Therefore, thorough clinical evaluation and follow-up are warranted in this group of patients. In addition, premature adrenarche has been associated with insulin resistance and polycystic ovarian syndrome later in life [29–33].

Differential Diagnosis

Precocious puberty may occur either by premature activation of the HPG axis which is termed central, or GnRH-dependent precocious puberty (GDPP), or by sex steroid exposure that is independent of hypothalamic–pituitary control, termed peripheral, or GnRH-independent precocious puberty (GIPP). The differential diagnosis is outlined in Table 18.3.

Gonadotropin-Dependent Precocious Puberty

In GDPP, there is premature maturation of the HPG axis, with pubertal changes resulting from centrally mediated sex steroid production. The cause of the early onset of HPG activation may be congenital or acquired CNS abnormalities (e.g., hypothalamic hamartoma, astrocytoma, granulomatous disease, trauma). GDPP may also be idiopathic, which is estimated to occur 10–20 times more commonly in females compared to males. In addition, chronic exposure to sex steroids such as with untreated congenital adrenal hyperplasia may accelerate hypothalamic maturation and HPG activation resulting in GDPP.

In GDPP, the timing and sequence of pubertal events evolve in a normal pattern. The clinical signs are those of normal puberty including development of secondary sexual characteristics, linear growth acceleration, skeletal age advancement, and pubertal levels of sex steroids and gonadotropins.

Gonadotropin-Independent Precocious Puberty

In GIPP, pubertal changes are induced by sex steroids from exogenous sources or from endogenous production that is not directed by hypothalamic GnRH secretion. Endogenous production of steroids may be derived from either gonadal or non-gonadal tissue. For example, precocious puberty may develop in individuals with elevated levels of adrenal androgens such as with congenital adrenal hyperplasia or adrenal tumors. Ovarian and testicular tumors secreting sex steroids may cause early pubertal development. In addition, tumors such as choriocarcinomas or hepatoblastomas can produce gonadotropins and cause GIPP. Gonadotropin receptors may be activated independently of gonadotropin activity, as in LH receptor-activating mutations. For instance, McCune–Albright syndrome (MAS) involves constitutive activation of G protein-coupled receptor signaling through G_s protein; the receptors for LH, FSH, TSH, GHRH, PTH, ACTH, and MSH function by this mechanism, and activation of these receptors can result in a variable number of endocrinopathies including precocious pubertal development. A more specific form of GIPP is seen in boys with dominantly transmitted sex-limited activation of the LH receptor at a young age. Rarely, long-standing untreated primary hypothyroidism may result in GIPP, thought to be due to chronically elevated TSH levels stimulating structurally similar LH receptors, known as the Van Wyk–Grumbach syndrome [34–37].

Key Points to the Diagnosis

Which Children with Early Pubertal Development Should Be Evaluated?

In general, females younger than 8 years and males younger than 9 years with pubertal signs should be evaluated. Younger age heightens the concern for a pathological

Table 18.3 Differential diagnosis of precocious puberty

Category	Presentation	Diagnosis	Treatment
GnRH dependent (central)			
Idiopathic	Pubertal changes in normal sequence, although may be more rapidly progressive Female-male >10:1	Pubertal gonadotropins and sex steroids, either basal or stimulated Skeletal age advanced	GnRH agonist

CNS abnormalities
  Tumors
    Hypothalamic hamartomas
    Craniopharyngeomas
    Optic gliomas (may be associated with neurofibromatosis)
  Structural abnormalities
    Septo-optic dysplasia
    Hydrocephalus
    Arachnoid cysts
    Intracranial abscesses
  Other causes
    Granulomatous disease
    Infiltrative disease
    Trauma
    Surgery
    Radiation
	Features of pubertal development similar to idiopathic Clinical symptoms or signs of underlying CNS abnormality	Similar to idiopathic Imaging (MRI or CT) showing CNS lesion in cases of tumor or structural abnormality	Therapy aimed at underlying lesion GnRH agonist in cases of hypothalamic hamartoma and some CNS lesions

Chronic exposure to sex steroids with advanced maturation	Initial development out of sequence and/or progresses rapidly due to peripheral cause HPG activation results in onset of true puberty with features similar to idiopathic	Similar to idiopathic Laboratory findings consistent with underlying peripheral etiology (e.g., CAH)	Treatment of underlying disorder GnRH agonist required in most cases
GnRH independent (peripheral)			
General features	Isosexual or contrasexual pubertal changes which may progress rapidly and/or out of normal sequence		

Adrenal tumors
  Adenoma
  Carcinoma
	Virilization in girls, and precocious sexual development in boys Gonads prepubertal	Elevated adrenal androgens such as DHEA, DHEA-S, androstenedione Other adrenocortical hormones such as cortisol may be elevated Imaging revealing adrenal tumor	Therapy directed at tumor including surgery and possibly chemotherapy

Ovarian tumors
  Carcinoma
  Gonadoblastoma
  Granulosa cell
  Theca cell
	Rapid pubertal progression in girls; feminization in boys	Elevated estradiol Prepubertal gonadotropins CT or ultrasound showing ovarian tumor	Tumor resection

Testicular tumors Leydig cell	Virilization in girls, and precocious sexual development in boys Asymmetrical testes in boys	Elevated testosterone Prepubertal gonadotropins CT or ultrasound showing testicular tumor	Tumor resection

Gonadotropin or hCG producing
  Choriocarcinoma
  Dysgerminoma
  Hepatoblastoma
  Teratoma
	Pubertal development with testicular enlargement in males Rare in females; associated with isosexual pubertal development	Elevated LH, FSH, or β-hCG Elevated sex steroids Evidence of tumor on imaging	Tumor resection Chemotherapy and radiation in some cases

Congenital adrenal hyperplasia
  Classical
  Nonclassical
	Premature pubarche and rapid growth Virilization in females Gonads prepubertal May lead to central precocious puberty	Elevated 17-OH progesterone and other adrenal precursors either basally or in response to ACTH stimulation	Glucocorticoid and mineralocorticoid replacement

(continued)

Table 18.3 (continued)

Category	Presentation	Diagnosis	Treatment
Male-limited familial precocious puberty (testotoxicosis)	Occurs in males Virilization and rapid growth early in life Testicular enlargement	Pubertal testosterone levels Prepubertal gonadotropins	Ketoconazole Aromatase inhibitors Antiandrogens
McCune–Albright syndrome	Isosexual development that occurs in unusual sequence Affects girls more commonly than boys Polyostotic fibrous dysplasia Café au lait lesions Other endocrinopathies	Pubertal sex steroid levels Pelvic ultrasound in females may show ovarian cysts GNAS1 mutation in samples from affected tissue	Tamoxifen Aromatase inhibitors GnRHa if central precocious puberty develops
Primary hypothyroidism	Isosexual pubertal changes associated with lack of expected growth acceleration Gonadal enlargement	Elevated TSH and low thyroxine level Gonadotropins prepubertal	Thyroid hormone replacement
Exogenous exposure to sex steroids	Various presentations depending upon substance	Variable; some compounds measurable in serum Gonadotropins prepubertal	Identify and remove exposure to compound

etiology and warrants a more extensive evaluation. In those children who are approaching the lower age limit, a careful history, physical examination, and bone age determination may be sufficient if no other concerns arise during the initial evaluation.

Are the Pubertal Changes Progressive? If so, What Are the Sequence and Tempo of Changes?

Precocious puberty is associated with progressive pubertal changes which can be differentiated from normal variants such as benign premature thelarche in which pubertal signs are non- or minimally progressive. Precocious puberty is associated with advancement of skeletal maturity and linear growth acceleration, features which are not seen in normal variants of development.

In GDPP, pubertal changes occur in a normal sequence with a tempo similar to normal puberty. On the other hand, children who have GIPP are more likely to have features of puberty outside of the normal sequence and with aberrant timing. For example, a young boy with development of sexual hair and virilizing features without testicular enlargement is likely to have a peripheral source of androgen production such as an adrenal tumor. Furthermore, children who have a normal sequence of pubertal changes, but have rapid tempo of changes, are more likely to have GIPP. For instance, a young girl with breast development who progresses to menarche within 12 months is likely to have a peripheral source of estrogen production such as an ovarian tumor.

Are the Pubertal Signs Suggestive of the Source of Sex Steroids?

Elevated estradiol levels will result in signs of puberty in girls but will lead to feminization in males, with gynecomastia. Conversely, elevated androgen levels in females will lead to signs of virilization including hirsutism, acne, and clitoromegaly, but signs of puberty in males. Therefore, isolated virilization in females suggests a peripheral etiology and excludes GDPP. Feminization in males also excludes a central etiology and most testicular etiologies with the exception of rare testicular tumors such as a feminizing Sertoli cell tumor.

Does the Patient Have Features of an Underlying Disorder?

- Neurological signs such as changes in gait or vision, or symptoms of pituitary hormone deficiencies such as diabetes insipidus or growth hormone deficiency, raise suspicion for CNS abnormalities.
- MAS should be considered if there are café au lait spots, bone deformities on the face or long bones, or accelerated growth. In addition, patients with MAS often develop pubertal signs that are outside of the normal sequence. For example, menstrual bleeding often precedes breast development in girls with this disorder and may occur as early as 4–6 months of age.
- Neurofibromatosis type 1 (NF1) may be associated with GDPP, usually but not exclusively in those with optic pathway gliomas. Primary features of NF1 are café au lait macules, axillary freckling, neurofibromas, optic nerve gliomas, and hamartomas of the iris (Lisch nodules).
- Signs of precocious puberty with absent linear growth are suggestive of primary hypothyroidism, although this is extremely rare with only approximately 12 reported cases in the literature [38].
- In patients with primary adrenal failure with precocious puberty, a DAX-1 (dosage-sensitive sex reversal, adrenal hypoplasia critical region, on chromosome X, gene 1) mutation should be considered. Rarely, patients with adrenal hypoplasia congenital (AHC) due to DAX-1 mutation may develop GDPP; these individuals may have primary adrenal failure during infancy. DAX-1 mutations

may also be associated with Duchenne muscular dystrophy and glycerol kinase deficiency due to a contiguous gene deletion syndrome.

Evaluation

Medical History

Pertinent history includes the age of onset of pubertal signs and their rate of progression, as well as timing of puberty in family members. Growth data are helpful to determine if there is growth acceleration. Symptoms of a CNS lesion such as headaches or seizures should be sought. Exposure to exogenous hormones should be explored; this may be from the cosmetic products noted above or contact with a parent's topical testosterone [39, 40].

Physical Examination

Important anthropometric data include height, weight, and height velocity (if possible). A thorough neurological examination including visual fields and fundoscopic examination should be performed to evaluate for a CNS lesion. Careful examination of the skin may provide clues to the diagnosis, for example, café au lait macules suggest MAS or NF1.

Pubertal signs should be assessed to determine Tanner stage. In girls, the diameter of glandular breast tissue and areola should be measured. Examination of the genitalia for signs of maturation may be helpful. In addition to the labial and vulvar changes noted above, an increase in clear mucous secretions and changes in vaginal mucosa from a thin, red mucosa to a thickened, pink-appearing mucosa are seen in girls with puberty.

In boys, testicular size and pubertal staging should be determined. Testicular volume $\geq$ 3 cc or longitudinal axis $\geq$ 2.2 cm suggests gonadotropin stimulation and likely GDPP. In a male with pubertal signs, but without testicular enlargement, a peripheral source of sex steroids should be sought. For instance, boys with constitutive activation of the LH receptor in the testis have relatively small testes for their degree of sexual maturation. If significant asymmetry of the testes is present, a testicular tumor such as a Leydig cell tumor should be considered; some asymmetry, however, is common.

Imaging Studies

A bone age film to determine skeletal maturity should be obtained in children with early pubertal development, recognizing the subjectivity and normal variation of this test. Significant skeletal advancement is present in GDPP, along with other signs such as growth acceleration and pubertal findings on physical examination. In individuals with signs of puberty which are progressive without bone age advancement, a peripheral source should be sought; more rapid increases in sex steroid levels can occur with GIPP compared to GDPP, and ossification of the growth centers lags behind sex hormone stimulation by some 6 months. In addition, those with normal variants of puberty such as premature adrenarche have skeletal age that is normal or slightly advanced and pubertal signs that are nonprogressive.

Pelvic ultrasonography in girls to assess ovarian and uterine volumes can be useful in establishing whether an individual is pubertal and for monitoring the progress of puberty. In cases of GIPP, abdominal-pelvic ultrasound should be performed to evaluate for an ovarian tumor or cyst. In addition, a testicular ultrasound study may be indicated in boys with GIPP to evaluate for a testicular mass [41].

Imaging of the CNS with magnetic resonance imaging (MRI) is indicated in most children with GDPP to evaluate for an intracranial lesion. There has been conflicting data about whether MRI should be performed in low-risk categories such as girls over the age of 6 years with GDPP. For example, one series reported no CNS abnormalities found in a group of females with the onset of GDPP after 6 years of age with estradiol levels <12 pg/ml. However, another report found that 15% of girls in this age group had CNS lesions. A careful neurological examination, consideration of ethnicity, and estradiol levels can be used to determine whether an MRI of the brain is indicated in girls older than 6 years with GDPP. The vast majority of the brain lesions found in these girls are nonprogressive hamartomas that do not require surgical intervention. As idiopathic GDPP is less common in boys, an MRI of the brain is warranted in all males due to the higher likelihood of identifying intracranial pathology [42–44].

Biochemical Studies

Initial laboratory assessment includes measurement of basal hormone levels including LH, FSH, and estradiol in girls and testosterone in boys. Basal LH above 0.3 IU/L, estradiol level > 20 pg/ml, and testosterone level > 50 ng/dl have been used to define GDPP, although these cutoffs depend upon the sensitivity of the individual assay. If basal hormone levels are consistent with puberty, then dynamic testing is not necessary [45].

As LH is pulsatile and initially elevated nocturnally in early puberty, a GnRH stimulation test may be needed to diagnose GDPP. To perform this test, a GnRH analog (GnRHa) is given with measurement of LH and FSH levels at baseline and 30–60 min after GnRHa is administered. LH response to GnRHa stimulation becomes more pronounced than that of FSH with pubertal maturation. A peak LH of >5 µIU/ml is suggestive of GDPP, while lack of response is indicative of either prepuberty or GIPP. FSH response does not increase as dramatically as that of LH during pubertal development, and LH/FSH ratios may be helpful in determining pubertal status. A peak LH/peak FSH ratio of >0.66 has also been used as criterion for diagnosis of GDPP [46].

In patients suspected of having GIPP, biochemical evaluation for peripheral sources of sex steroids should be performed. Serum cortisol, DHEA, DHEA-S, and 17-hydroxyprogesterone should be measured in addition to the aforementioned tests. In boys, serum B-hCG can be measured for the possibility of a tumor-secreting hCG [47–49].

Present and Future Therapies

Treatment of precocious puberty depends upon whether or not the process is gonadotropin mediated. In GDPP, therapy is aimed at decreasing pulsatile GnRH release from the hypothalamus and, therefore, pituitary production of gonadotropins. In GIPP, treatment is directed at the underlying etiology of sex steroid production which may involve the gonads, adrenal glands, or exogenous sources.

Treatment of Gonadotropin-Dependent Precocious Puberty

As noted previously, GDPP may be idiopathic in nature or be associated with a CNS lesion. Children who have CNS lesions should undergo appropriate surgery, radiation, or chemotherapy as indicated. Hypothalamic hamartomas are generally not resected because there is significant morbidity from damage to the hypothalamus and pituitary function associated with surgical intervention. Hypothalamic hamartomas are typically monitored radiologically and rarely cause neurological manifestations. Individuals with hypothalamic hamartomas may be treated with GnRHa therapy (discussed below) [50].

Precocious sexual development results in accelerated skeletal maturation and linear growth rate which may compromise adult height due to premature fusion of epiphyses. The extent of adult height potential that is lost depends upon the age of onset and rate of progression of pubertal changes. Younger age and more rapid progression of puberty result in greater loss of adult height. In addition, precocious puberty may be associated with psychosocial stress due to earlier development compared to peers; anxiety, withdrawal, and depression may occur in those with early puberty. The decision to treat a child with early pubertal development depends upon both the degree of compromise of adult height and psychosocial factors [51].

GnRHa therapy is the primary treatment for GDPP. GnRH agonists act by providing a tonic elevation of GnRH which occupies GnRH receptors on the pituitary gland, decreasing pituitary responsiveness to GnRH, thereby blunting pulsatile gonadotropin release. This continuous GnRH exposure restores the prepubertal state of the HPG axis. GnRHa is the only effective treatment for GDPP [52].

Patients being considered for GnRHa therapy should have pubertal basal or stimulated gonadotropin concentrations, progressive pubertal changes, linear growth acceleration, and advanced skeletal maturation. Treatment should be considered for those with compromised adult height prediction (relative to genetic height target) and those with significant psychosocial concerns from the parents or the child about further pubertal development.

Children with the onset of GDPP at a younger age will have early epiphyseal fusion and loss of adult height potential if not treated and will have greatest benefit from therapy. Those children who are nearing the age of normal puberty at the time of diagnosis or who have slow progression of puberty are likely to have less benefit from GnRHa therapy and may not require intervention. For instance, girls with GDPP who are started on GnRHa therapy before 6 years old have an average adult height gain of 9–10 cm, and those started on therapy between 6 and 8 years old have average height gains of 4–7 cm. Although fewer data are available for boys, those starting on GnRHa therapy at an average age of 7.6 years had a mean height gain of 6.2 cm. Height gains are likely to be less in those with more advanced bone ages. Because some children with precocious puberty may have slow progression of puberty, they may not require medical intervention with GnRHa to preserve height potential, especially in those nearing the age of normal puberty. Monitoring patients to assess the tempo of puberty before treatment is indicated in those who are not rapidly progressing or who are older [53–59].

GnRHa Dosing and Monitoring

GnRHa are available as depot injections, short-acting injections, subcutaneous implants, and nasal spray, with the depot formulations and subcutaneous implants being the most commonly prescribed therapies. The depot formulation, leuprolide acetate, is available in either monthly or 3-monthly dosing which appear to be comparably effective in suppressing the HPG axis. The implantable form of GnRHa, histrelin, is also an effective therapy and may provide HPG suppression for up to 1 year [60–62].

The recommended dose of GnRHa therapy is sufficient to achieve pubertal suppression in most patients. Patients should be examined every 3–6 months, and skeletal maturity is determined every 6–12 months. During the first 6 months of therapy, skeletal maturation may continue to accelerate at the pretreatment rate as a result of ossification of preexisting cartilaginous maturation. Adequacy of dosing may be determined by clinical and biochemical parameters. If HPG axis suppression is achieved, there will be lack of progression of pubertal signs such as breast development and testicular enlargement. Height velocity and rate of bone age advancement should decline.

In addition, levels of LH and estradiol (in girls) and testosterone (in boys) may provide evidence of HPG axis suppression. Two to three months after initiating therapy, LH and sex steroid levels may be obtained either just before the next dose or at 30–60 min after therapeutic GnRHa dose is given. Prepubertal LH and sex steroid levels obtained before the next dose generally reflect HPG axis suppression. Normative data for LH levels post-therapeutic dose may guide whether further investigation is necessary. For instance, one study found that an LH level of <2.5 µIU/ml measured 90 min after GnRHa administration correlated with adequate pubertal suppression compared to GnRH stimulation testing. Biochemical parameters should be interpreted along with other clinical data, as LH and sex steroid levels are not well correlated with clinical response to GnRHa therapy. When pubertal suppression is not achieved, GnRHa dose should be increased with appropriate clinical follow-up to determine dose adequacy [63, 64].

The decision to discontinue GnRHa therapy must be individualized. In general, therapy is discontinued at an age when normal puberty would be occurring. Psychosocial factors including the child's preparedness for pubertal progression and menarche must be considered. Prolonged suppression of adolescent development can have a deleterious effect on accrual of peak bone mass. In some cases, therapy may be continued for a longer time if there are concerns about adult height potential, although height gains decrease with advancing age.

Safety

Treatment with GnRHa appears to be safe and without significant long-term effects on the HPG axis. The HPG axis is reactivated within weeks to months after discontinuation of GnRHa therapy, with pubertal gonadotropin levels occurring within 6 months after cessation. Most girls experience menarche within 18 months of discontinuing GnRHa, and small studies show normal testicular function in males after treatment. In addition, gonadal function in adulthood does not appear to be affected by GnRHa therapy [65].

Bone mineral density (BMD) may decrease for age during treatment with GnRHa due to suppression of sex steroids during a critical time of bone mineral accrual. Individuals with precocious puberty have greater than average BMD for age before therapy and have little change in BMD during therapy, yielding a lower than average BMD at the end of the treatment. However, as puberty resumes after therapy is discontinued, the resulting increase in sex steroids normalizes BMD by mid-puberty. Due to these concerns, adequate intake of calcium and vitamin D is encouraged in patients receiving GnRHa therapy [66, 67].

Data on adult height gain from GnRHa therapy are variable due to the wide spectrum of ages and degrees of advanced bone age when therapy is initiated. Factors associated with greater gains in adult height are earlier onset of puberty, younger age, less advanced skeletal age, longer duration of therapy, and initiation of therapy close to the onset of puberty. Growth rates and adult height after cessation of GnRHa therapy are often less than predicted based on skeletal maturity and height at the time treatment is discontinued [68–71].

Treatment of Gonadotropin-Independent Precocious Puberty

GIPP treatment is directed at the underlying etiology and does not respond to GnRHa therapy. For example, individuals with congenital adrenal hyperplasia (CAH) should be placed on corticosteroid replacement to decrease production of adrenal androgens leading to precocity and bone age advancement. Many children with CAH develop GDPP due to delayed diagnosis with long-term exposure to sex steroids and require GnRHa therapy.

Children with tumors secreting sex steroids or gonadotropins should undergo appropriate surgical or medical treatment for those conditions. Tumors of the gonads and adrenal gland are treated by surgery. Adjuvant chemotherapy may be necessary with some adrenal tumors depending upon surgical results, histology, and presence of metastases. Individuals with hCG-secreting tumors possibly require surgery, chemotherapy, and radiation depending upon the location and histological type of tumor.

In children who have premature development due to exogenous exposure to sex steroids, the exposure must be identified and removed. A careful history is critical in determining the exposure. Removal of the offending agent often results in regression of pubertal changes.

Precocious sexual development is the most common endocrine manifestation in MAS, which is far more common in girls than boys. Estrogen and testosterone are produced autonomously by the gonads, in girls and boys, respectively.

Other endocrinopathies may include overproduction of thyroid hormone, growth hormone, and cortisol.

Treatment of GIPP in girls with MAS is targeted at inhibiting the aromatization of testosterone to estradiol and at the blockade of estrogen receptors. Aromatase inhibitors (such as testolactone, letrozole, and anastrozole) reduce ovarian estrogen production, decrease menses, and slow the rate of skeletal maturation in MAS. Tamoxifen, an antiestrogen, may slow pubertal progression and skeletal maturation, as well as reduce the frequency of menses. Some patients with MAS develop GDPP and may respond to GnRHa therapy. MAS in males is manifested as overproduction of testosterone, although males are rarely affected. The treatment of males with MAS is similar to that for male-limited precocious puberty (MLPP) outlined below [72–74].

MLPP, or familial testotoxicosis, is an autosomal dominant disorder characterized by GIPP in males due to autonomously functioning LH receptors. An activating mutation of the LH receptor in Leydig cells results in unregulated testosterone production and precocious puberty most commonly between the ages of 1 and 4 years. As in MAS, treatment for MLPP is directed at inhibiting the production and blocking the action of sex steroids. Inhibitors of androgen biosynthesis such as ketoconazole are effective in reducing testosterone levels and decreasing the growth velocity and the rate of skeletal age advancement. Ketoconazole therapy may also improve adult height, especially if started at an early age. Alternatively, combination therapy with antiandrogens and aromatase inhibitors such as spironolactone and anastrozole may be beneficial in reducing pubertal progression and slowing linear growth and skeletal maturation. These therapies appear to improve predicted adult height based on skeletal maturity, although data on adult height are lacking. Secondary GDPP may develop in individuals with MLPP necessitating treatment with GnRHa [75–82].

Conclusions

In summary, the child presenting with precocious puberty may be classified into three categories: GDPP, GIPP, or a normal variant. A thorough evaluation is warranted for girls younger than 8 years of age and boys younger than 9 years of age or in those whose evaluation is concerning for underlying pathology. The goals of therapy in children with precocious puberty are to preserve adult height potential and alleviate psychosocial stress that may accompany early puberty. Treatment with GnRHa is safe and effective in individuals with GDPP, with greater height preservation in those of younger age who have less advanced skeletal ages and on longer duration of therapy. Treatment should be aimed at the underlying etiology or the mechanism of the sex steroids in those with GIPP.

References

1. Kaplowitz P. Clinical characteristics of 104 children referred for evaluation of precocious puberty. J Clin Endocrinol Metab. 2004;89(8):3644–50.
2. Kaplan SL, Grumbach MM. Clinical review 14: pathophysiology and treatment of sexual precocity. J Clin Endocrinol Metab. 1990;71(4):785–9.
3. de Kretser DM, Hedger MP, Loveland KL, Phillips DJ. Inhibins, activins and follistatin in reproduction. Hum Reprod Update. 2002;8(6):529–41.
4. Apter D, Butzow TL, Laughlin GA, Yen SS. Gonadotropin-releasing hormone pulse generator activity during pubertal transition in girls: pulsatile and diurnal patterns of circulating gonadotropins. J Clin Endocrinol Metab. 1993;76(4):940–9.
5. Fuqua J. Treatment and outcomes of precocious puberty: an update. JCEM. 2013;98(6):2198–207.
6. Sisk CL, Foster DL. The neural basis of puberty and adolescence. Nat Neurosci. 2004;7(10):1040–7.
7. Penny R, Olambiwonnu NO, Frasier SD. Serum gonadotropin concentrations during the first four years of life. J Clin Endocrinol Metab. 1974;38(2):320–1.
8. Schmidt H, Schwarz HP. Serum concentrations of LH and FSH in the healthy newborn. Eur J Endocrinol. 2000;143(2):213–5.
9. Parent AS, Matagne V, Bourguignon JP. Control of puberty by excitatory amino acid neurotransmitters and its clinical implications. Endocrine. 2005;28(3):281–6.
10. Rosenbloom A, Rohrs H, Haller M, Malasanos T. Tanner stage 4 breast development in adults: forensic implications. Pediatrics. 2012;130(4):978–81.
11. Marshall WA, Tanner JM. Variations in pattern of pubertal changes in girls. Arch Dis Child. 1969;44(235):291–303.
12. Marshall WA, Tanner JM. Variations in the pattern of pubertal changes in boys. Arch Dis Child. 1970;45(239):13–23.
13. Sun SS, Schubert CM, Chumlea WC, et al. National estimates of the timing of sexual maturation and racial differences among US children. Pediatrics. 2002;110(5):911–9.
14. Sun SS, Schubert CM, Liang R, et al. Is sexual maturity occurring earlier among U.S. children? J Adolesc Health. 2005;37(5):345–55.
15. Chumlea WC, Schubert CM, Roche AF, et al. Age at menarche and racial comparisons in US girls. Pediatrics. 2003;111(1):110–3.
16. Freedman DS, Khan LK, Serdula MK, Dietz WH, Srinivasan SR, Berenson GS. Relation of age at menarche to race, time period, and anthropometric dimensions: the Bogalusa Heart Study. Pediatrics. 2002;110(4):e43.
17. Kaplowitz PB, Slora EJ, Wasserman RC, Pedlow SE, Herman-Giddens ME. Earlier onset of puberty in girls: relation to increased body mass index and race. Pediatrics. 2001;108(2):347–53.
18. Lee PA, Kulin HE, Guo SS. Age of puberty among girls and the diagnosis of precocious puberty. Pediatrics. 2001;107(6):1493.
19. Weise M, De-Levi S, Barnes KM, Gafni RI, Abad V, Baron J. Effects of estrogen on growth plate senescence and epiphyseal fusion. Proc Natl Acad Sci U S A. 2001;98(12):6871–6.
20. Herman-Giddens ME, Wang L, Koch G. Secondary sexual characteristics in boys: estimates from the national health and nutrition examination survey III, 1988–1994. Arch Pediatr Adolesc Med. 2001;155(9):1022–8.
21. Tinggaard J, Mieritz MG, Sorensen K, et al. The physiology and timing of male puberty. Curr Opin Endocrinol Diabetes Obes. 2012;19(3):197–203.
22. Blizzard RM, Martha PM, Kerrigan JR, Mauras N, Rogol AD. Changes in growth hormone (GH) secretion and in growth during puberty. J Endocrinol Investig. 1989;12(8 Suppl 3):65–8.
23. Midyett LK, Moore WV, Jacobson JD. Are pubertal changes in girls before age 8 benign? Pediatrics. 2003;111(1):47–51.

24. Kaplowitz PB, Oberfield SE. Reexamination of the age limit for defining when puberty is precocious in girls in the United States: implications for evaluation and treatment. Drug and Therapeutics and Executive Committees of the Lawson Wilkins Pediatric Endocrine Society. Pediatrics. 1999;104(4 Pt 1):936–41.

25. Palmert MR, Malin HV, Boepple PA. Unsustained or slowly progressive puberty in young girls: initial presentation and long-term follow-up of 20 untreated patients. J Clin Endocrinol Metab. 1999;84(2):415–23.

26. Pasquino AM, Pucarelli I, Passeri F, Segni M, Mancini MA, Municchi G. Progression of premature thelarche to central precocious puberty. J Pediatr. 1995;126(1):11–4.

27. Pescovitz OH, Hench KD, Barnes KM, Loriaux DL, Cutler GB Jr. Premature thelarche and central precocious puberty: the relationship between clinical presentation and the gonadotropin response to luteinizing hormone-releasing hormone. J Clin Endocrinol Metab. 1988;67(3):474–9.

28. Salardi S, Cacciari E, Mainetti B, Mazzanti L, Pirazzoli P. Outcome of premature thelarche: relation to puberty and final height. Arch Dis Child. 1998;79(2):173–4.

29. Ghizzoni L, Milani S. The natural history of premature adrenarche. J Pediatr Endocrinol Metab. 2000;13(Suppl 5):1247–51.

30. Ibanez L, Dimartino-Nardi J, Potau N, Saenger P. Premature adrenarche—normal variant or forerunner of adult disease? Endocr Rev. 2000;21(6):671–96.

31. Ibanez L, Virdis R, Potau N, et al. Natural history of premature pubarche: an auxological study. J Clin Endocrinol Metab. 1992;74(2):254–7.

32. Ibanez L, Potau N, Virdis R, et al. Postpubertal outcome in girls diagnosed of premature pubarche during childhood: increased frequency of functional ovarian hyperandrogenism. J Clin Endocrinol Metab. 1993;76(6):1599–603.

33. Rosenfield RL. Normal and almost normal precocious variations in pubertal development premature pubarche and premature thelarche revisited. Horm Res. 1994;41(Suppl 2):7–13.

34. Baranowski E, Hogler W. An unusual presentation of acquired hypothyroidism: the Van Wyk-Grumbach syndrome. Eur J Endocrinol. 2012;166(3):537–42.

35. Jaruratanasirikul S, Patarapinyokul S, Mitranun W. Androgen-producing adrenocortical carcinoma: report of 3 cases with different clinical presentations. J Med Assoc Thail. 2012;95(6):816–20.

36. Kunz GJ, Klein KO, Clemons RD, Gottschalk ME, Jones KL. Virilization of young children after topical androgen use by their parents. Pediatrics. 2004;114(1):282–4.

37. Durbin KL, Diaz-Montes T, Loveless MB. Van wyk and grumbach syndrome: an unusual case and review of the literature. J Pediatr Adolesc Gynecol. 2011;24(4):e93–6.

38. Barnes ND, Hayles AB, Ryan RJ. Sexual maturation in juvenile hypothyroidism. Mayo Clin Proc. 1973;48(12):849–56.

39. Li ST, Lozano P, Grossman DC, Graham E. Hormone-containing hair product use in prepubertal children. Arch Pediatr Adolesc Med. 2002;156(1):85–6.

40. Yu YM, Punyasavatsu N, Elder D, D'Ercole AJ. Sexual development in a two-year-old boy induced by topical exposure to testosterone. Pediatrics. 1999;104(2):e23.

41. Buzi F, Pilotta A, Dordoni D, Lombardi A, Zaglio S, Adlard P. Pelvic ultrasonography in normal girls and in girls with pubertal precocity. Acta Paediatr. 1998;87(11):1138–45.

42. De Sanctis V, Corrias A, Rizzo V, et al. Etiology of central precocious puberty in males: the results of the Italian Study Group for Physiopathology of Puberty. J Pediatr Endocrinol Metab. 2000;13(Suppl 1):687–93.

43. Faizah M, Zuhanis A, Rahmah R, et al. Precocious puberty in children: a review of imaging findings. Biomed Imaging Interv J. 2012;8(1):e6.

44. Mogensen SS, Aksglaede L, Mouritsen A, et al. Pathological and incidental findings on brain MRI in a single-center study of 229 consecutive girls with early or precocious puberty. PLoS One. 2012;7(1):e29829.

45. Neely EK, Wilson DM, Lee PA, Stene M, Hintz RL. Spontaneous serum gonadotropin concentrations in the evaluation of precocious puberty. J Pediatr. 1995;127(1):47–52.

46. Brito VN, Batista MC, Borges MF, et al. Diagnostic value of fluorometric assays in the evaluation of precocious puberty. J Clin Endocrinol Metab. 1999;84(10):3539–44.

47. Carel JC, Leger J. Clinical practice. Precocious puberty. N Engl J Med. 2008;358(22):2366–77.

48. Chemaitilly W, Trivin C, Adan L, Gall V, Sainte-Rose C, Brauner R. Central precocious puberty: clinical and laboratory features. Clin Endocrinol. 2001;54(3):289–94.

49. Iughetti L, Predieri B, Ferrari M, et al. Diagnosis of central precocious puberty: endocrine assessment. J Pediatr Endocrinol Metab. 2000;13(Suppl 1):709–15.

50. de Brito VN, Latronico AC, Arnhold IJ, et al. Treatment of gonadotropin dependent precocious puberty due to hypothalamic hamartoma with gonadotropin releasing hormone agonist depot. Arch Dis Child. 1999;80(3):231–4.

51. Kim EY, Lee MI. Psychosocial aspects in girls with idiopathic precocious puberty. Psychiatry Investig. 2012;9(1):25–8.

52. Crowley WF Jr, Comite F, Vale W, Rivier J, Loriaux DL, Cutler GB Jr. Therapeutic use of pituitary desensitization with a long-acting lhrh agonist: a potential new treatment for idiopathic precocious puberty. J Clin Endocrinol Metab. 1981;52(2):370–2.

53. Rosenfield RL. Selection of children with precocious puberty for treatment with gonadotropin releasing hormone analogs. J Pediatr. 1994;124(6):989–91.

54. Mul D, Bertelloni S, Carel JC, Saggese G, Chaussain JL, Oostdijk W. Effect of gonadotropin-releasing hormone agonist treatment in boys with central precocious puberty: final height results. Horm Res. 2002;58(1):1–7.

55. Klein KO, Barnes KM, Jones JV, Feuillan PP, Cutler GB Jr. Increased final height in precocious puberty after long-term treatment with LHRH agonists: the National Institutes of Health experience. J Clin Endocrinol Metab. 2001;86(10):4711–6.

56. Bar A, Linder B, Sobel EH, Saenger P, DiMartino-Nardi J. Bayley-Pinneau method of height prediction in girls with central precocious puberty: correlation with adult height. J Pediatr. 1995;126(6):955–8.

57. Comite F, Cassorla F, Barnes KM, et al. Luteinizing hormone releasing hormone analogue therapy for central precocious puberty. Long-term effect on somatic growth, bone maturation, and predicted height. JAMA. 1986;255(19):2613–6.

58. Kletter GB, Kelch RP. Clinical review 60: effects of gonadotropin-releasing hormone analog therapy on adult stature in precocious puberty. J Clin Endocrinol Metab. 1994;79(2):331–4.

59. Weise M, Flor A, Barnes KM, Cutler GB Jr, Baron J. Determinants of growth during gonadotropin-releasing hormone analog therapy for precocious puberty. J Clin Endocrinol Metab. 2004;89(1):103–7.

60. Badaru A, Wilson DM, Bachrach LK, et al. Sequential comparisons of one-month and three-month depot leuprolide regimens in central precocious puberty. J Clin Endocrinol Metab. 2006;91(5):1862–7.

61. Eugster EA, Clarke W, Kletter GB, et al. Efficacy and safety of histrelin subdermal implant in children with central precocious puberty: a multicenter trial. J Clin Endocrinol Metab. 2007;92(5):1697–704.

62. Fuld K, Chi C, Neely EK. A randomized trial of 1-and 3-month depot leuprolide doses in the treatment of central precocious puberty. J Pediatr. 2011;159(6):982–987 e981.

63. Bhatia S, Neely EK, Wilson DM. Serum luteinizing hormone rises within minutes after depot leuprolide injection: implications for monitoring therapy. Pediatrics. 2002;109(2):E30.

64. Kunz GJ, Sherman TI, Klein KO. Luteinizing hormone (LH) and estradiol suppression and growth in girls with central precocious

puberty: is more suppression better? Are pre-injection LH levels useful in monitoring treatment? J Pediatr Endocrinol Metab. 2007;20(11):1189–98.

65. Cassio A, Bal MO, Orsini LF, et al. Reproductive outcome in patients treated and not treated for idiopathic early puberty: long-term results of a randomized trial in adults. J Pediatr. 2006;149(4):532–6.

66. Antoniazzi F, Zamboni G, Bertoldo F, et al. Bone mass at final height in precocious puberty after gonadotropin-releasing hormone agonist with and without calcium supplementation. J Clin Endocrinol Metab. 2003;88(3):1096–101.

67. Unal O, Berberoglu M, Evliyaoglu O, Adiyaman P, Aycan Z, Ocal G. Effects on bone mineral density of gonadotropin releasing hormone analogs used in the treatment of central precocious puberty. J Pediatr Endocrinol Metab. 2003;16(3):407–11.

68. Carel JC, Eugster EA, Rogol A, et al. Consensus statement on the use of gonadotropin-releasing hormone analogs in children. Pediatrics. 2009;123(4):e752–62.

69. Arrigo T, Cisternino M, Galluzzi F, et al. Analysis of the factors affecting auxological response to GnRH agonist treatment and final height outcome in girls with idiopathic central precocious puberty. Eur J Endocrinol. 1999;141(2):140–4.

70. Lee PA. Central precocious puberty. An overview of diagnosis, treatment, and outcome. Endocrinol Metab Clin N Am. 1999;28(4):901–18.

71. Tanaka T, Niimi H, Matsuo N, et al. Results of long-term follow-up after treatment of central precocious puberty with leuprorelin acetate: evaluation of effectiveness of treatment and recovery of gonadal function. The TAP-144-SR Japanese Study Group on Central Precocious Puberty. J Clin Endocrinol Metab. 2005;90(3):1371–6.

72. Eugster EA, Rubin SD, Reiter EO, Plourde P, Jou HC, Pescovitz OH. Tamoxifen treatment for precocious puberty in McCune-Albright syndrome: a multicenter trial. J Pediatr. 2003;143(1):60–6.

73. Feuillan P, Calis K, Hill S, Shawker T, Robey PG, Collins MT. Letrozole treatment of precocious puberty in girls with the McCune-Albright syndrome: a pilot study. J Clin Endocrinol Metab. 2007;92(6):2100–6.

74. Mieszczak J, Lowe ES, Plourde P, Eugster EA. The aromatase inhibitor anastrozole is ineffective in the treatment of precocious puberty in girls with McCune-Albright syndrome. J Clin Endocrinol Metab. 2008;93(7):2751–4.

75. Reiter EO, Norjavaara E. Testotoxicosis: current viewpoint. Pediatr Endocrinol Rev. 2005;3(2):77–86.

76. Haddad N, Eugster E. An update on the treatment of precocious puberty in McCune-Albright syndrome and testotoxicosis. J Pediatr Endocrinol Metab. 2007;20(6):653–61.

77. Bertelloni S, Baroncelli GI, Lala R, et al. Long-term outcome of male-limited gonadotropin-independent precocious puberty. Horm Res. 1997;48(5):235–9.

78. Kreher NC, Pescovitz OH, Delameter P, Tiulpakov A, Hochberg Z. Treatment of familial male-limited precocious puberty with bicalutamide and anastrozole. J Pediatr. 2006;149(3):416–20.

79. Leschek EW, Jones J, Barnes KM, Hill SC, Cutler GB Jr. Six-year results of spironolactone and testolactone treatment of familial male-limited precocious puberty with addition of deslorelin after central puberty onset. J Clin Endocrinol Metab. 1999;84(1):175–8.

80. Reiter EO, Mauras N, McCormick K, et al. Bicalutamide plus anastrozole for the treatment of gonadotropin-independent precocious puberty in boys with testotoxicosis: a phase II, open-label pilot study (BATT). J Pediatr Endocrinol Metab. 2010;23(10):999–1009.

81. Soriano-Guillen L, Lahlou N, Chauvet G, Roger M, Chaussain JL, Carel JC. Adult height after ketoconazole treatment in patients with familial male-limited precocious puberty. J Clin Endocrinol Metab. 2005;90(1):147–51.

82. Almeida MQ, Brito VN, Lins TS, et al. Long-term treatment of familial male-limited precocious puberty (testotoxicosis) with cyproterone acetate or ketoconazole. Clin Endocrinol. 2008;69(1):93–8.

Ambiguous Genitalia

19

Bruno Cesar Caldas, Aline Alves Lopes,
and Maria Paula Costa Bandeira E. Farias

Epidemiology and Classification

Disorders of sex *development* (DSD) are congenital conditions in which the development of chromosomal, gonadal, and anatomical sex is atypical. This can affect from 1:1000 to 1:1500 individuals, being the most severe ambiguities seen in up to 1:5000 born [1, 2]. The DSD nomenclature and its distinction were originally established at the Chicago conference in 2005, according to the consensus of the largest pediatric endocrinology societies [3], and distributed the patients in three subgroups:

- DSD sex chromosome.
- 46,XX DSD (formerly called female pseudohermaphroditism): they have ovarian gonadal tissue at their origin, but their external genitalia is ambiguous or even masculine
- 46,XY DSD (formerly called male pseudohermaphroditism): they have testes, but their genital ducts and/or external genitalia undergoes incomplete virilization (Fig. 19.1).

Differentiation of Genitalia and Hormonal Control

Within the genital bud, the gonads of males and females are undifferentiated until the sixth week. Under the action of the Sry/Sox9 set and other genes, the gonad begins the differentiation in the testis. Support cells give rise to Sertoli cells, and steroidogenic cells give rise to Leydig cells (around 60 days). The gonad predestined to an ovary remains undifferentiated until about 77 to 84 days, when the first oocytes

arise. The supporting cells form the granulosa and the steroidogenic cells form the theca.

The expression of the SRY gene on the Y chromosome initiates the cascade leading to the formation of a testis, which secretes testosterone (Leydig cells) and anti-Müllerian hormone (AMH) (Sertoli cells), responsible for the differentiation of the Wolffian ducts in the seminal vesicles, ductus deferens, and epididymis, as well as regression of the Müllerian ducts. Leydig cells also produce insulin-like factor 3 (INSL3), which acts on the testicular descent [4]. In the absence of the Y chromosome, the testicle does not form, the Wolff ducts regress, and the Müllerian ducts develop the tubas, uterus, and upper third of the vagina [1]. The external genitalia remains undifferentiated until about the eighth week of life. An important concept is that the female genitalia occurs when there is an ovary or in the absence of any gonad. The hormonal regulation of the differentiation process of the genitalia is dynamic and involves steroidogenic production in the gonads and adrenals.

The ovaries do not secrete steroids in the prenatal period, and the female genitalia is not influenced by adrenal androgens at the beginning of gestation, as they are converted into estrogens by placental aromatase. Critical transient period (around 12-week gestation) occurs, in which the adrenals begin to express 3β-HSD2 and produce more cortisol instead of DHEA-S. This transition is marked by the decreased androgenic receptors in the labioscrotal folds, and these will not undergo fusion even under high posterior exposures of T/DHT. When the adrenal starts producing greater amounts of androgens again, the aromatase activity will also be increased, resulting in an even greater production of estrogens, ensuring that female genitalia is formed.

If during this window (where aromatase is low) testicular Leydig cells appear, there will be a large fetal exposure to testosterone, under the influence of human chorionic gonadotropin (hCG), and late fetal luteinizing hormone (LH), which determines the masculinization of the internal genitalia. Testosterone, under the action of 5α-reductase, is converted into dihydrotestosterone (DHT), responsible for

B. C. Caldas (✉) · A. A. Lopes
Fellowship of Endocrinology of Agamenon Magalhães Hospital – Division of Endocrinology and Diabetes, Recife, PE, Brazil

M. P. C. B. E. Farias
Faculdade Pernambucana de Saúde, Recife, PE, Brazil

© Springer Nature Switzerland AG 2022
F. Bandeira et al. (eds.), *Endocrinology and Diabetes*, https://doi.org/10.1007/978-3-030-90684-9_19

Sex chromossome DSDs / Gonadal disorders

Mixed and partial gonadal dysgenesis (mosaicisms, 45X/46XY)

Ovotesticular DSD (most 45XX)

Urogenital abnormalities

Testicular Regression syndrome (46XY)

SF1, WT1, Denys Drash

Virilization in 46XX

Excess androgen production

    congenital Adrenal Hyperplasia (CAH):

    21 hydroxylase deficiency

    11-β hydroxilase deficiency

    3-β hydroxysteroid dehydorgenase deficiency

P450 oxidoreductase deficiency

Maternal androgen source

    luteoma

    maternal CAH

    hyperreaction luteinalis

Causes of genital ambiguity in the newborn

Undervirilization of 46XY

Defects in testosterone synhtesis

    Smith-Lemli-Optiz syndrome

    5α reductase deficiency

    Leydig Cell Hypoplasia

congenital adrenal hyperplasia

    3-β hydroxysteroid dehydorgenase deficiency

    17 alfa hydroxylase / 17.20 lyase defiiency

    17-β hydroxysteroid dehydrogeneaese 3 deficiency

    Steroid Acute regulatory protein deficiency (StAR)

Defects in testosterone action

    Partial Androgen insenitivity syndrome (PAIS)

Others

    Denys-Drash Syndrome

    SRY, SF1, DAX1, Wnt4, SOX9

Fig. 19.1 Causes of genital ambiguity in the newborn

masculinization of the external genitalia and urogenital sinus [5]. Genitalia virilization may occur without the presence of testis in cases of congenital adrenal hyperplasia, in which the enzymatic blockage deviates steroidogenic production to DHEA-S during the critical period (when aromatase is low). In addition the high production of 17-hydroxyprogesterone can be used by the alternative routes for the production of dihydrotestosterone, which causes clitoromegaly even after the downregulation of the androgenic receptors.

In humans, as well as in other primates, androgens appear to have a considerable effect on gender behavior [6]. However, the association between prenatal exposure to androgens and behavior is not uniform.

Genetics

- For the development of the bipotential gonad, the action of WT1 (Wilms' Tumor 1), which acts on urogenital development, is essential. Aside from being fundamental in the formation of all steroid-producing glands, SF-1 (steroidogenic factor-1) nuclear receptor is required for the synthesis of testosterone in Leydig cells and regulation of AMH in Sertoli cells.
- The interaction of the SRYry gene with other genes is the determining step for sexual differentiation. It also potentiates the SOXox9 gene (main for the lower SRYry), inhibiting the Rspo1 (R-spondin-1)-Wnt4-β-catenin-FOXL2 pathway, which promotes the formation of Sertoli cells and inhibits ovarian development.

- In the case of a gonad predestined to become an ovary, the action of the WNT4 gene, which inhibits testicular formation by upregulation of DAX1, is important in stabilizing β-catenin-FOXL2 (a complex pathway, which, as stated above, will be inhibited by Sry/Sox9).
- Some mutations of the above genes are responsible for many cases of AG in DSD. For example, the expression of a single copy of SOXox9, SF1, and WT1 or duplication of DAX1 and WNT4 in individuals 46,XY may lead to gonadal dysgenesis. On the other hand, duplications of Sox9 or Sox3 may lead to 46,XX testicular DSD [1].

Figure 19.2. Dashed arrows show the alternative routes of androgen production. These pathways produce DHT without DHEA, androstenedione or T as intermediates. In the cases of 17OH, 21OH, and POR, there is an increase of 17OH as a substrate. Another synthetic route involves the generation of 11-oxygenated C19 steroids via CYP11β1, including 11-ketotestosterone and 11-ketodihydrotestosterone. CYP11A1 (cholesterol side-chain cleavage enzyme, P450scc), StAR (steroidogenic acute regulatory protein), CYP17A1 (17 α-hydroxylase/17,20-lyase, P450c17), CYP21A2 (21 α-hydroxylase), CYP11b1 and CYP11b2 (11β-hydroxylase type 1 and 2) 3βHSD2 (3β-hydroxysteroid dehydrogenase, type 2), 17βHSD3 (17b-hydroxysteroid dehydrogenase, type 3), 5α-reductase 2 (5α-reductase, type 2), 5α-reductase 1 (5α-reductase, type 1), AKR1C1/3 (3a-reductase, type 1/3), and 17βHSD6 (3-hydroxyepimerase, encoded by *Flück CE*) [7]

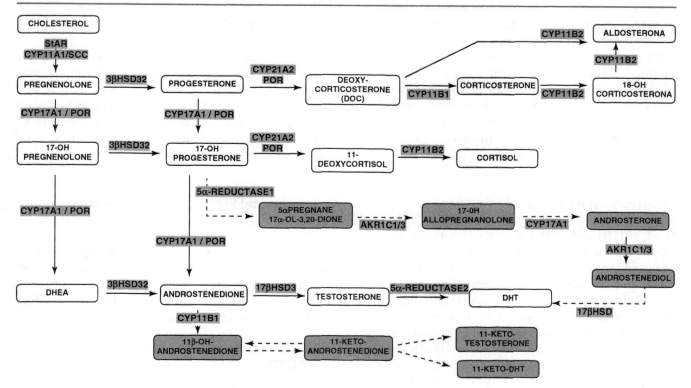

Fig. 19.2 Classic and alternative adrenal steroid synthesis pathways

Causes of Ambiguous Genitalia

Sex Chromosome DSD

This group contained the variants of Turner (45,X0) and Klinefelter (47,XXY), as well as the mosaicisms. The latter have the most common 45,X/46,XY karyotype, corresponding to mixed gonadal dysgenesis. The external genitalia commonly shows asymmetries and inguinal hernias. There may even be occurrence of virilization only on the side where the dysgenetic testis is present and Müllerian structures on the other side. Gender affirmation is a challenge due to the broad phenotypic spectrum.

Ovotesticular DSD

This rare disease was called true hermaphroditism, because there is a presence of viable testicular and ovarian tissue in the same patient, in the same gonad, or vice versa. They commonly present asymmetric AG, and inguinal hernias are frequent. The most common karyotype is 46,XX (60% of cases), followed by mosaicism [8]. This diagnosis should be made in all cases of ambiguous genitalia, especially if a bilobed gonad of non-scrotal location is evidenced. The gender affirmation is variable and can follow both sides, and the degree of virilization and response to stimulation with Hcg (testis viability) should be taken into account.

46,XX DSD

46,XX are the most prevalent forms of DSD, and about 90% of them are due to congenital adrenal hyperplasia (CAH). The latter is a group of seven autosomal recessive and monogenetic diseases, caused by mutations in the genes involved in the cortisol synthesis pathways, with consequent elevation of ACTH, hyperplasia of the adrenal glands, and elevation of androgens in the stages prior to enzymatic blockade during steroidogenesis. Most cases are heterozygous, and the allele with the highest enzymatic activity determines the phenotype. Both sexes can be affected, but suspecting in boys becomes more difficult when there are no exuberant clinical manifestations.

21-Hydroxylase (21-OH) Deficiency

It is the main cause of CAH, corresponding to more than 95% of the cases [9]. Such an enzyme is encoded by the CYP21A2 gene, and the mutations are due to recombinant events of meiosis. The classic forms are divided into salt losers, which manifest itself in the first 2 weeks of life, with adrenal crisis, and simple virilizations, which maintain about 1–2% of the enzymatic activity, preventing the crises. Those with the nonclassical forms retain more than 50% of the enzymatic activity, preventing virilization, but may present low reserve of cortisol [10]. It is suspected in all cases of AG with karyotype 46,XX and ovaries/uterus in the USG, especially if there are signs of adrenal insufficiency (shock, hypoglycemia, electrolyte disturbance).

11β-Hydroxylase (11-OH) Deficiency

The CYP11B1 and CYP11B2 genes encode two enzymes: p450c11B1 (ACTH dependent), which is responsible for the 11-hydroxylation of 11-deoxycortisol in cortisol and deoxycorticosterone (DOC) in corticosterone in the fasciculate zone, and isoenzyme p450c11B2 (angiotensin-dependent), with the same action of the first isoform (but much more potent) in addition to converting corticosterone into 18-OH-corticosterone and the latter into aldosterone. Most of the affected patients have minimal or absent enzymatic activity (nonclassical forms are very rare). Although the conversion attributed to 11bOH is minimal, elevated levels of DOC, a weak mineralocorticoid, may suppress the renin-angiotensin-aldosterone axis. Clinically, they present virilization, volumetric expansion, and consequent hypertension but low renin activity (as compared to those with 21-OH deficiency that have more hypertension than salt loss).

P450 Oxidoreductase (POR) Deficiency

This type of CAH, of fetal-placental origin, arises from the flavoprotein defect that transfers electrons to all the microsomal P450 (21-OH, 17-OH, P450 aromatase). Most patients retain some enzymatic action, since their total blockage would be impracticable, which determines highly variable phenotypes. The mineralocorticoid pathway is not compromised, and the intermediates may rise causing hypertension. Virilization may be due to the DHT production by the retrograde pathway, as well as poor placental aromatization, including cases of maternal virilization. POR deficiency is also involved in other non-steroidogenic enzymes, which may explain other findings such as bone dysplasia. Craniosynostosis, radioulnar or radiohumeral synostosis, facial hypoplasia, and other aspects of Antley-Bixler syndrome can be seen.

P450 Aromatase Deficiency

With the fetal-placental origin, it results from mutations in the CYP19 gene and determines a defective placental conversion of androgens (C19) to estrogens (C18). Virilization of the female external genitalia, and often of the mother, occurs. The diagnosis is made by elevated levels of T and androstenedione, low estrogens, and elevated gonadotrophins.

Androgens and Progestogens of Maternal Origin

In addition to the use of testosterone, certain progestogens may be involved in the masculinization of the female fetus: norethindrone, ethisterone, and medroxyprogesterone acetate. It is a diagnosis of exclusion and only surgical correction of the external genitalia is conducted.

46,XY DSD

The prevalence of 46,XY DSD is much lower than those of 46,XX DSD as it covers a broader etiologic spectrum and does not necessarily present itself with ambiguity. The assumed gender is commonly discordant (female) of the karyotype in this type of DSD (more than 33%) [11]. They are patients whose gonads are testes, but genital ducts and/or external genitalia are not completely masculinized. The causes of CAH that undergo subvirilization in 46,XY DSD are rarer: 3βHSD2, 17αOH, SCC, and CAH lipoid. In these cases, the ambiguity is exacerbated at puberty. Other rare disorders are deficiencies of 5α-reductase and 17βHSD3, which often present more severe subvirilization, or even female genitalia, and more difficult clinical suspicion at birth.

Androgen Insensitivity Syndrome (CAIS and PAIS)

In its complete form (CAIS), it does not present with AG. Partial forms, however, range from isolated hypospadias to perineoscrotal hypospadias, micropenis, and bifid scrotum (similar to 5α-reductase deficiency). Most 46,XY DSD with no defined cause are determined to have partial androgen insensitivity.

46,XY Partial or Total Gonadal Dysgenesis

Pure gonadal dysgenesis (*Swyer syndrome*) does not cause ambiguous genitalia as it will be female. Partial forms, however, determine gonadal subvirilization and Müllerian duct persistence, due to the capacity of the dysgenetic testis to produce AMH and testosterone (although at lower levels than expected). Dax1, Sox9, and Gata4 are examples of genes involved in gonadal dysgenesis; but most patients do not yet have a specific genetic cause. There is an increased risk of Wilms tumor related to the WT1 gene in these patients [12].

17-OH Deficiency

The CYP17A1 gene encodes both the 17 hydroxylase and 17,20 lyase enzymes in the fasciculate and reticulate zones. There is a deficiency in adrenal and gonadal production, with accumulation of DOC (sodium retention, hypertension, hypokalemia, suppression of aldosterone), and corticosterone, preventing adrenal crises (glucocorticoid effect). Isolated 17,20 lyase deficiency is extremely rare [13].

3βHSD2 Deficiency

This enzyme exists in two isoforms: type 1, expressed in the placenta and peripheral tissues, and type 2, highly expressed in adrenals. The deficiency results in the decrease in aldosterone, cortisol, and androstenedione. In this case, a little production of 17-OH-progesterone by peripheral 3β-HSD may occur, allowing production of DHT by the retrograde pathway, or even excess S-DHEA can be converted by the placenta. Clinically, the patient has salt loss and subvirilized genitalia.

StAR Deficiency (Lipoid CAH)

Deficiency of all steroid hormones is due to the mutations in the StAR gene, which regulates the transfer of cholesterol from the outer membrane to the internal mitochondria and is a key step for steroidogenesis. It is one of the rarest forms of CAH. There are nonclassical forms, which retain 20–30% of StAR gene's activity [14], and may be confused with Addison's disease or isolated familial glucocorticoid deficiency, and 46,XY may be born with normal or ambiguous genitalia. Laboratory diagnosis is by the low or absent levels of all steroids, with an unresponsiveness in ACTH or hCG tests.

SCC Deficiency

This is coded by the CYP11A1 gene, presenting clinical and laboratory findings identical to lipoid CAH, with few cases reported in the literature, being differentiated only by the DNA genetic test.

Smith-Lemli-Opitz Syndrome

This syndrome caused by a failure in the synthesis of cholesterol leads to micrognathia, mental retardation, microcephaly, complete hypospadia, micropenis, growth retardation, and, rarely, suprarenal insufficiency. In the laboratory findings, we have low cholesterol levels and high levels of 7-dehydrocholesterol.

5α-Reductase Deficiency

This enzyme is responsible for the transformation of T into DHT. It has two forms: type I, which is present in the skin, and type II, which is present in the genital epithelium, accessory glands, and prostate. During uterine development, the external genitalia and the urogenital sinus suffer a little differentiation, whereas the T-dependent Wolffian structures develop normally. The phenotype ranges from micropenis to hypospadias with pseudovagina. The 46,XY develop virilization during puberty, with descent of testis and penile enlargement, without gynecomastia (probably by the peripheral conversion of type 1 enzyme, with increased activity during puberty). Commonly, gender change occurs from female to male. In the laboratory findings, until the onset of puberty, the T/DHT ratio is very high (> 10.5 basal, or > 8.5 after stimulation with hCG).

17β-Hydroxysteroid-Dehydrogenase Type 3 Deficiency

This enzyme is expressed exclusively in the testis and converts androstenedione to T and estrone into estradiol. Affected 46,XY individuals are born with female or ambiguous external genitalia, with male ducts present, absence of Müllerian structures, short vagina, and undescended testicles. During puberty, clitoromegaly may occur due to some peripheral conversion, and the breasts grow by the influence of estrone. In the laboratory findings, gonadotrophins, androstenedione, estrone are elevated, while estradiol and T are low. Likewise, there is an increase in the proportions of androstenedione/T and estrone/estradiol after hCG stimulation test.

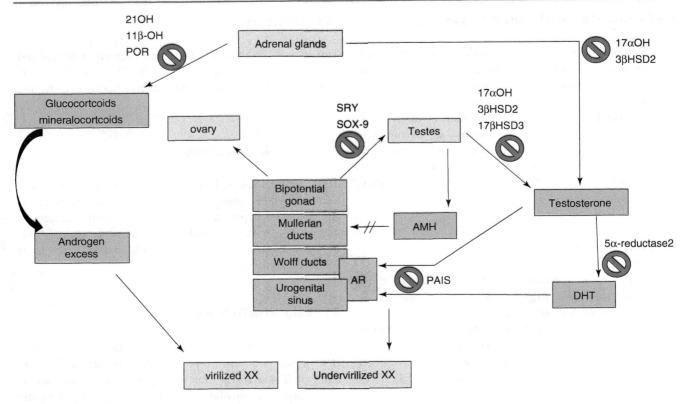

Fig. 19.3 Development of internal and external genitalia and conditions that may affect the final phenotype

Figure 19.3 Once SRY gene triggers testes, testosterone should stabilize the Wolffian ducts, and anti-Müllerian hormone leads to regression of Müllerian ducts. The main hormone responsible for the male differentiation of the urogenital sinus and external genitalia is dihydrotestosterone that needs proper production and action at androgenic receptors (AR). The red symbols indicate blockages that may impair the final route of differentiation Fig. 19.4.

Initial Approach of Newborns with Ambiguous Genitalia

The first step is to differentiate genuinely ambiguous genitalia from minor genital abnormalities, such as discrete clitoral augmentation and isolated distal hypospadias. Those who fit the criteria should be followed by a multidisciplinary team using the best level of evidence available. Family acquaintance and clarification should be clear and detailed, knowing that diagnostic research and conduct can take days to months to be taken. One should investigate consanguinity, family history of DSD, maternal use of steroids or progestogens, and use of assisted reproductive technology. A history of maternal virilization during pregnancy (a rare condition) may point to maternal androgen-secreting tumors (such as luteomas of the ovary) or hyperreactio luteinalis, which is a result of increased serum concentrations of human chorion gonadotropin (β-hCG) and increased receptor's sensibility to β-hCG. Aromatase deficiency is a possible diagnosis in these cases, but the onset of ovarian pathology is more common.

Physical Exam

It begins with the inspection of the phallic structure (length, erectile tissue, thickness), number of perineal orifices and their topographies, labioscrotal folds (pigmentation, roughness, degree of fusion), as well as position and anal patency. Asymmetries may be an important clinical sign as ovotesticular DSD and mixed gonadal dysgenesis may virilize only one side of the genitalia. Palpation may reveal gonads in the scrotum or labioscrotal folds and inguinal canal or be impalpable. In the case of females, the degree of virilization can be evaluated by the Prader scale [15], ranging from 1, discrete clitoromegaly with distinct openings to the vagina and urethra, up to 5, elongated phallus and long urogenital sinus (common canal) that resembles a male urethra. Regarding the anterior structures, it is still important to evaluate the exact location of the convergence of the urethra with the vagina (not evaluated by the Prader scale) for surgical planning. Likewise, subvirilized males will present varying degrees of hypospadias, which may also be associated with

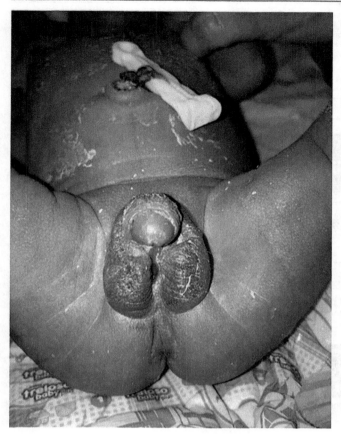

Fig. 19.4 Virilized female genitalia due to androgen excess

bifid scrotum, ventral penile curvature, and penoscrotal transposition. Even those with apparent normal male genitalia should be assessed more extensively if the penile compartment is smaller than 2.0–2.5 cm.

Diagnostic Tests

The first to be ordered are the karyotype (always mandatory), pelvic ultrasonography, and sodium, potassium, and 17OHP levels after 48 hours of life. Following the known pathophysiology, other tests to determine the diagnosis are pregnenolone, 17-OH-pregnenolone, testosterone, DHEA, dihydrotestosterone, androstenedione, cortisol, gonadotrophins, and AMH tests. Children aged 3–6 years, or those suspected of having defective androgen production, may require a human chorionic gonadotrophin (HCG) stimulation test:

- Abdominopelvic ultrasonography: aimed primarily to detect Müllerian structures. The vagina and uterus are well visualized in the newborn; but intra-abdominal gonads hardly are. This test may also show adrenal hyperplasia.

- Magnetic resonance: may be useful for determining renal abnormalities and more detailed pelvic structure (more useful for surgical programming than diagnosis).

- The dosage of 17-OHP (17-hydroxyprogesterone) is intended to identify the main cause of CAH (21-OH deficiency). It may be high within the first 48 hours, dropping to <100–200 ng/dL. Premature and those under acute stress may have falsely elevated levels of 17-OHP. Some cases of 21-OH may require the cortrosyn test to close diagnosis. It should be remembered that deficiencies of 11βOH and POR also occur with high 17-OHP [10].

- At more advanced ages (denoting a nonclassical form), screening for 21-OH is based on the measurement of 17-OHP before 8:00 AM. However, the cortrosyn test is usually required for an accurate diagnosis and to differentiate it from the classical form.

- The anti-Müllerian and inhibin B hormone dosage in patients with 46,XY DSD is useful to differentiate between gonadal dysgenesis and defects in the synthesis or action of testosterone.

- High concentrations of 11-DOC and DOC (baseline or after ACTH stimulation) associated with low levels of renin and aldosterone help in cases of suspected diagnostic doubt between 21-OH deficiency and 11-βOH.

- Pregnenolone and 17-OH-pregnenolone aid in the evaluation of deficiencies of 3βHSD2 and 17-OH.

- Preferably, serum steroid determinations in neonates and infants should be performed with liquid chromatography-mass spectrometry/mass spectrometry (LC-MS/MS), as antibody-based assays cannot accurately discriminate the different deviations from steroidogenesis.

- Testing of hCG tests can be done with hCG 1000–1500 U intramuscularly for 3 consecutive days, with the physiological response being twice as large as the testosterone baseline [16]. HCG will elicit an increased T response in patients with partial androgen resistance and 5α-reductase deficiency. 5α-Reductase deficiency can generally be ruled out by a T/DHT ratio of less than 8.5 after hCG.

Figure 19.5 The first and faster steps regard to clinical history, examination looking for palpable gonads, and imaging of pelvic/labioscrotal content. Determination of karyotype is always mandatory. The presence of Müllerian structures leads to a clinical diagnosis and further analysis of biochemical profile. In 46,XX DSD patients whose congenital adrenal hyperplasia is the main cause of ambiguous genitalia, cortrosyn test is usually necessary to access 17OHP, androgen, and cortisol response. In case of 46,XY DSD patients, the hCG stimulation test permits exploring androgen secretion by Leydig cells from the first months of life to early adolescence (when testes produce low levels of androgens). Despite assays for anti-Müllerian hormone (AMH),

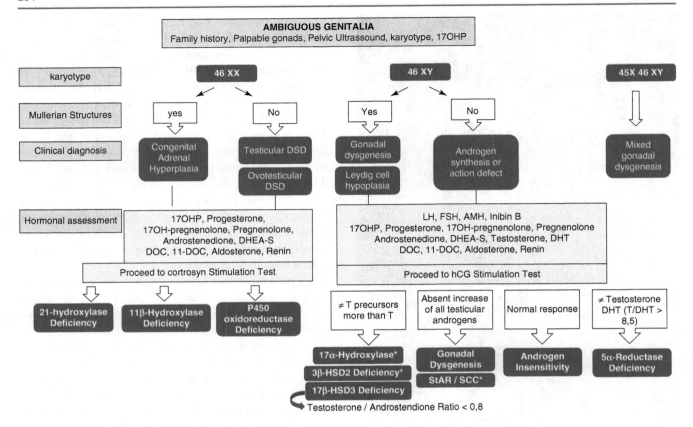

Fig. 19.5 Diagnostic Algorithm of ambiguous genitalia

inhibin B, and Insl3 may be excellent tools to demonstrate presence of functional testicular tissue, they are not always available and do not determine testicular androgen production. 17OHP, 17-hydroxyprogesterone; T, testosterone; DHT, dihydrotestosterone; 3β-HSD2, 3 β-hydroxysteroid dehydrogenase type 2; 17β-HSD3, 17-β-hydroxysteroid dehydrogenase type 3* may require cortrosyn test for final diagnosis (rare forms of CAH)

Hormonal Treatment

Hormonal treatment is basically reserved for those with CAH, as well as its main cause: 21-OH deficiency.

- Glucocorticoids: Due to their effects on growth suppression, chronic glucocorticoid therapy is avoided in children. In classical forms, it aims to replace deficient cortisol and reduce excess (androgens in 21-OH and 11beta-OH, or DOC in 17-OH) – in children, hydrocortisone 8–15 mg/m² divided into three doses, and in adolescents and adults, hydrocortisone 2–3 times/day, or prednisone 5–7.5 mg/day, once or twice, or dexamethasone 0.25–0.5 mg/day [10]. Lower doses are required in nonclassical forms in which children are treated only if

there are signs of virilization with advanced bone age; women with excess androgens can be treated only with oral contraceptives (and in some cases in conjunction with spironolactone). In this group, the cortrosyn test may reveal suboptimal cortisol response (<18 µg/dL), but patients generally only need to replace glucocorticoids if they are symptomatic or under stress conditions.

- Glucocorticoid dose in stress: For all types, there must be education regarding the adrenal crisis and increased dose in case of intercurrences. Patients with classic 21-OH also have epinephrine deficiency, due to impaired adrenal medulla formation, predisposing the patient to bouts of hypoglycemia, especially when they become ill or when fed. A dosage of 50 mg/m² hydrocortisone is recommended for children and 100 mg IV for adults, followed by 200 mg in the next 24 hours [10].
- *Mineralocorticoids*: The goal of using fludrocortisone is to achieve a physiological renin activity in salt-losing forms. Higher doses are required in the first 6 months of life due to neonatal resistance to mineralocorticoids [17]. Despite some production of aldosterone in the simple virilizing forms, there is a relative deficiency of the hormone. The association also allows the glucocorticoid dose to be reduced. The dose is 50–200 µg daily.

- *Sexual steroids*: In cases of 17-OH, 3βHD2, CAH lipoid, POR, and SCC, replacement occurs at the time of physiological puberty. For women, estradiol 0.5–2.0 mg/day is required for 2–3 years; progestogen is added after 2 years of estrogen (or when menarche occurs) with micronized progesterone 100–200 mg/day, or medroxyprogesterone 5–10 mg/day or norethindrone 2.5–5.0 mg, for 5–10 days, in those with uterus, is necessary. For men, 50–200 mg of testosterone ester per month, or transdermal testosterone 25–100 g per day, is required. The replacement of DHT in cases of 5α-reductase deficiency and 17βHSD3, if diagnosed early, becomes important for phallic growth and surgical management.

Monitoring

The child's linear growth, weight/height, signs of puberty, and symptoms of salt loss should be taken into account. An X-ray for determination of bone age should be performed every 2 years. Although 17-OHP levels tend to normalize with appropriate treatment, this should not be a primary goal because it denotes a high dose of glucocorticoid. Instead, it is better to evaluate the signs of virilization, in girls, and levels of androgens.

Surgical Treatment

Genital surgery is a complex task and full of controversy. In the last two decades, some groups have advocated that surgery should be delayed until the patient is able to participate in the decision. The family should always be educated about the benefits and risks of the procedure, involving a multidisciplinary team. Surgical treatment should, ideally, reconstitute the cosmetic appearance and functionality of the genitalia, preserving fertility in the best possible way. Sexual intercourse may or may not be possible after surgical repair, and this should be discussed with those who present themselves to the surgeon in adolescence or adulthood.

Intervention should be considered for 46,XX patients with CAH by 21-OH, when there is considerable virilization, ideally between the third and ninth months of life [11]. The feminizing surgery consents in clitoroplasty, labiaplasty, and vaginoplasty, which can be performed at the same time or not, with the intention of exteriorizing the vagina and creating separate openings for the vagina and urethra. This procedure becomes more difficult with the greater degree of virilization, because in these cases, the vagina is implanted higher in the urogenital sinus (common canal). Cosmetic results and long-term functionality are scarce. In cases of 21-OH, gender dysphoria is extremely rare, despite behavioral changes reported due to intrauterine androgens exposure, and it is prudent to proceed with feminizing surgery [18].

Reconstruction in 46,XY cases is complex. The corrections of distal hypospadias have high success rates, as opposed to proximal ones, which denote greater complications. In the case of those with 5α-reductase deficiency, an old approach in those highly subvirilized was to offer surgery for feminization. However, these partially virilized patients show the highest rate of gender dysphoria among all patients with DSD, with great dissatisfaction with surgical modifications [19]. Thus, it is reasonable to assume the male gender for 46,XY DSD patients with at least one functioning testis and reasonable penile tissue. Most boys will need repair of hypospadias with or without orchiopexy, and the approach is performed in the first year of life [20]. Patients with complete insensitivity to androgens usually have their gonads preserved until at least puberty, avoiding future hormone replacement needs, although the chances of malignancy are not fully known [21]. For pure gonadal dysgenesis, early gonadectomy is advisable because of the high risk of malignancy and female gender identity in this group [22].

Affirmation of Gender

Although the treatment includes hormonal and surgical options, many patients have been treated according to a traditional binary concept of the sexes. It is important to know that dealing with DSD requires acceptance of the deviations from traditional definitions of gender, and the karyotype is not necessarily determinative of it.

Generally, children with 46,XX karyotype and 21-OH deficiency are raised as females, even if strong virilization has occurred. On the other hand, those with 46,XY karyotype and androgen deficiency (17βHSD3 or 5α-reductase 2 deficiency) are usually raised as men, even if severe underandrogenization occurs. These decisions are justified by the current knowledge of the high potential of alternative routes of androgen synthesis, as well as in the cases of gender dysphoria in patients with DSD and in the possibility of preservation of fertility.

In 46,XX patients with CAH, studies show that patients live and identify themselves as women, despite the more masculine behavior. In a study by Dessens [23], 46,XX patients with CAH raised as boys had a change from male to female of 12.1%, while the opposite (female to male) was 5.2%.

In the case of 46,XY patients raised as women, another study showed a change from female to male in 64% of those with 17βHSD3 deficiency (no cases of male to female) and up to 66% in 46,XY patients with 5α-reductase 2 deficiency [24]. In the latter case, despite the blockage of external virilization by lack of DHT, testosterone still maintains strong masculinizing effects on the brain and behavior. 46,XY patients with incomplete insensitivity to androgens, with partial subvirilization enough to be raised as girls, tend to masculinize behavior [25].

It is possible that many patients who present themselves in the transition period for adolescence have not received much information about their diagnosis during pediatric care, complicating the clinical history for management in adult life. This fact reinforces the need for a multidisciplinary team to manage these patients, with support groups, psychologists, endocrinologists, gynecologists, and urologists.

References

1. Ostrer H. Disorders of sex development (DSDs): an update. J Clin Endocrinol Metab. 2014;99:1503.
2. Thyen UK, Lanz PM, Holterhus, et al. Epidemiology and initial management of ambiguous genitalia at birth in Germany. Horm Res. 2006;66:195–203.
3. Hughes IA, Houk C, Ahmed SF, Lee PA, LWPES Consensus Group; ESPE Consensus Group. Consensus statement on management of intersex disorders. Arch Dis Child. 2006;91(7):554–63.
4. Ferlin A, Foresta C. Insulin-like factor 3: a novel circulating hormone of testicular origin in humans. Ann N Y Acad Sci. 2005;1041:494–505.
5. Hanley NA, Arlt W. The human fetal adrenal cortex and the window of sexual differentiation. Trends Endocrinol Metab. 2006;17:391.
6. Jurgensen M, Hiort O, Holterhus T, U. Gender role behavior in children with XY karyotype and disorders of sex development. Horm Behav. 2007;51:443–53.
7. Flück CE, Meyer-Böni M, Pandey AV, Kempná P, Miller WL, Schoenle EJ, Biason-Lauber A. Why boys will be boys: two pathways of fetal testicular androgen biosynthesis are needed for male sexual differentiation. Am J Hum Genet. 2011;89(2):201–18.
8. Matsui F, Shimada K, Matsumoto F, et al. Long-term outcome of ovotesticular disorder of sex development: a single center experience. Int J Urol. 2011;18(3):231–6.
9. Speiser PW, Azziz R, Baskin LS, et al. Congenital adrenal hyperplasia due to steroid 21-hydroxylase deficiency: an endocrine society clinical practice guideline. J Clin Endocrinol Metab. 2010;95:4133.
10. El-Maouche D, Arlt W, Merke DP. Congenital adrenal hyperplasia. Lancet. 2017;390(10108):2194–210.
11. Romao RL, Salle JL, Wherrett DK. Update on th management of disorders of sex development. Pediatr Clin N Am. 2012;59:853–69.
12. Kohler B, Biebermann H, Friedsam V, et al. Analysis of the Wilm's tumor suppressor gene (WT1) in patients 46, XY disorders of sex development. J Clin Endocrinol Metab. 2011;96(7):E1131–6.
13. Geller DH, Archus RJ, Mendonça BB, Miller WL. The genetic and functional basis of isolated 17,20-lyase deficiency. Nat Genet. 1997;17:201–5.
14. Baker BY, Lin L, Kim CJ, et al. Nonclassic congenital lipoid adrenal hyperplasia: a new disorder of the steroidogenic acute regulatory protein with very late presentation and normal male genitalia. J Clin Endocrinol Metab. 2006;91:4781–5.
15. Prader A. Genital findings in the female pseudo-hermaphroditism of the congenital adrenogenital syndrome: morphology, frequency, development and heredity of the different genital forms. Helv Paediatr Acta. 1954;9:231–48.
16. Ahmed SF, Rodie M. Investigation and clinical management of ambiguous genitalia. Best Pract Res Clin Endocinol Metab. 2010;24:197–218.
17. Martinerie L, Pussard E, Foix-L'Hélias L, et al. Physiological partial aldosterone resistance in human newborns. Pediatr Res. 2009;66:323–8.
18. Fisher AD, Ristori J, Fanni E, Castellini G, Forti G, Maggi M. Gender identity, gender assignment and reassignment in individuals with disorders of sex development: a major dilemma. J Endocrinol Investig. 2016;39:1207–24.
19. Kohler B, Kleinemeier E, Lux A, et al. Satisfaction with genital surgery and sexual life of adults with XY disorders os sex development: results from the German clinical evaluation study. J Clin Endocrinol Metab. 2012;97(2):577–88.
20. Hutson JM, Clarke MC. Current management of the undescendend testicle. Semin Pediatr Surg. 2007;16(1):64–70.
21. Papadimitriou DT, Linglart A, Morel Y, et al. Puberty in subjects with complete androgen insensitivity syndrome. Horm Res. 2006;65:126–31.
22. Capito C, Leclair M-D, Arnaud A, et al. 46, XY pure gonadal dysgenesis: clinical presentations and management of the tumor risk. J Pediatr Urol. 2011;7(1):72–5.
23. Dessens AB, Slipjer FM, Drop SL. Gender dysphoria and gender change in chromosomal females with congenital adrenal hyperplasia. Arch Sex Behav. 2005;34:389–97.
24. Cohen-Kettenis PT. Gender change in 46, XY persons with 5α-reductase-2-deficiency and 17β-hydroxysteroid dehydrogenase-3 deficiency. Arch Sex Behav. 2005;34(4):399–410.
25. Hines M, Ahmed SF, Hughes IA. Psychological outcomes and gender-related development in complete androgen insensitivity syndrome. Arch Sex Behav. 2003;32(2):93–101.

Non-parathyroid Hypercalcemia

Daniele Fontan and Luiz Griz

Non-parathyroid Hypercalcemia

Hypercalcemia is a clinical condition defined as total serum calcium >10.3 mg/dl (>2.6 nmol/L) or ionized calcium >5.6 mg/dl (>1.4 nmol/L). It affects about 0.5–1% of the general population. It is well tolerated if serum calcium levels are <12 mg/dl, but when severe it can be a life-threatening condition [1]. It is known that hypercalcemia is one of the most common metabolic disorders in clinical practice. The participation of calcium in numerous organic processes, such as coagulation cascade, enzymatic reactions, and neuromuscular transmission, determine the importance of maintaining its homeostasis.

Calcium in the body corresponds to 2% of an individual's body, and approximately 99% is found within the crystal structure of hydroxyapatite in the mineralized bone matrix and 1% is in the soluble form in the intra- and extracellular fluid compartments. Of this solution, 50% are linked to proteins, 45% in the form of ionized calcium, and 5% linked to organic and inorganic anions such as sulfate, phosphate, lactate, and citrate [2, 3].

Factors such as venous stasis (e.g., tourniquet use), liver cirrhosis, and malnutrition may affect the measurement of total calcium, so in such situations, we must calculate the corrected calcium or, preferably, dose the ionizable calcium that is not influenced by albumin levels.

The formula to calculate corrected calcium is as follows: corrected calcium = total calcium + (4-albumin) × 0.8. The ionizable fraction of calcium is regulated by parathyroid hormone (PTH) and vitamin D. It can also vary with blood PH, where acidosis increases the concentration of ionizable calcium and alkalosis reduces it. Alteration of 0.1 unit in serum pH modifies the protein-calcium binding by 0.12 mg/dl.

Hypercalcemia may be classified as mild (10.4–11.9 mg/dl), moderate (12–13.9 mg/dl), or severe (≥14 mg/dl) [4].

Etiology

There are several causes of hypercalcemia, but about 90% of cases are caused by primary hyperparathyroidism (most frequent cause in outpatients) and malignant neoplasms (in inpatients) [5]. Other causes of hypercalcemia are less frequent. Hypercalcemia occurs by combining excess bone resorption, increased intestinal calcium absorption, and decreased renal excretion. In some disorders, more than one mechanism may be involved; however, the common finding in almost all hypercalcemic disorders is increased bone resorption (Table 20.1).

Table 20.1 Etiology of hypercalcemia

Bone resorption	Calcium absorption	Decrease in the excretion of calcium
pHPTH	Hypervitaminosis D	Chronic renal disease
Malignancy	Granulomatous disease	Rhabdomyolysis and acute renal failure
Thyrotoxicosis	Parenteral nutrition	Thiazide diuretics
Immobilization	Milk alkali syndrome	
Downregulation of the calcium receptor sensor	**Medication**	**Endocrinal disorders**
FHH	Lithium	Pheochromocytoma
	Hypervitaminosis A	Adrenal insufficiency

pHPTH primary hyperparathyroidism, *FHH* familial hypocalciuric hypercalcemia

D. Fontan (✉)
Endocrinology and Metabology, Hospital Agamenon Magalhães, Recife, PE, Brazil

Agamenon Magalhães Hospital, Department of Endocrinology and Diabetes, Recife, PE, Brazil

L. Griz
School of Medicine, University of Pernambuco School of Medicine, Recife, Brazil

© Springer Nature Switzerland AG 2022
F. Bandeira et al. (eds.), *Endocrinology and Diabetes*, https://doi.org/10.1007/978-3-030-90684-9_20

Bone Resorption

Primary Hyperparathyroidism

Primary hyperparathyroidism (PHPT) is a disorder resulting from hypersecretion of the parathyroid hormone. Most cases are sporadic, but 5–10% correspond to familial forms that may be isolated or associated with autosomal dominant inherited endocrine diseases, such as multiple endocrine neoplasia type 1 (MEN 1) and type 2A (MEN 2A). Its incidence has increased significantly in some countries since the mid-1970s, when systematic dosing of serum calcium began. Hypercalcemia in this disorder occurs due to the activation of osteoclasts mediated by the parathyroid hormone, culminating with the increase of bone resorption. PHPT occurs more frequently because of the presence of parathyroid adenoma (~85%), less frequently due to parathyroid hyperplasia (~15%), and rarely results from parathyroid carcinoma (<1%) [6]. Patients can evolve with small increases in serum calcium (elevations below 11 mg/dL or 2.75 nmol/L) or with intermittent hypercalcemia [7–9].

Secondary and Tertiary Hyperparathyroidism

Patients with chronic renal disease and secondary hyperparathyroidism usually have normal or low serum calcium levels, but with the progression of the disease, they may develop hypercalcemia. Increased serum calcium occurs more frequently in patients with adynamic bone disease and marked reduction in bone turnover. Hypercalcemia in these patients is observed due to a marked reduction in bone calcium uptake, as occurs after ingestion of calcium carbonate to treat hyperphosphatemia [10].

In other patients with advanced renal disease, hypercalcemia is due to the autonomic production of PTH, a disorder known as tertiary hyperparathyroidism.

Malignant Neoplasms

Malignant neoplasms are the most frequent cause of hypercalcemia in hospitalized patients [11, 12]. Its frequency ranges from 20% to 30% of cancer patients and could reach up to 40% in some casuistic, depending on the duration of the disease, the primary site, the presence of metastases, and the type of malignancy. Hypercalcemia usually occurs in patients with advanced disease, and survival beyond 6 months is uncommon.

The humoral hypercalcemia of malignancy (HHM) is the main cause of hypercalcemia associated with neoplasias, being responsible for approximately 80% of cases [13].

Hypercalcemia is due to tumor secretion of the parathormone-related peptide (PTH-rp). Among the solid tumors, lung carcinoma, particularly squamous cell carcinoma, is the most frequent. Other tumors associated with HHM are squamous cell carcinomas of the head and neck and adenocarcinoma of the kidneys, breast, bladder, pancreas, and ovaries [14]. Therefore, humoral hypercalcemia of malignancy should be suspected in any patient with a solid tumor, in the absence of bone metastases, and with low PTH concentration. The diagnosis can be confirmed when a high concentration of PTH-rp is demonstrated.

In tumors such as breast cancer with skeletal metastasis, multiple myeloma and lymphomas are common to tumor cell production of osteoclast stimulating factors in bone such as PTHrp, DKKI, lymphotoxins, interleukins, TGF, and prostaglandins [13].

In some lymphomas, hypercalcemia is due to the extrarenal production of calcitriol from calcidiol (independent of PTH) through the activation of mononuclear cells (macrophages) [15]. Finally, ectopic PTH secretion is a rare cause of hypercalcemia, documented only in a few patients.

In general, consumptive malignancy syndrome precedes the picture of hypercalcemia which tends to be more severe than that observed in PHPT. Generally, values higher than 13 mg/dl (3.25 nmol/L) are observed. Hypercalcemia is associated with poor life expectancy in the patient with neoplasia, independent of the response of calcemia to the treatment.

Thyrotoxicosis

Mild hypercalcemia is seen in about 15–20% of patients with thyrotoxicosis [16, 17]. The thyroid hormone has bone resorption properties, causing a state of high bone turnover, which can culminate in osteoporosis. Hypercalcemia typically disappears after the correction of hyperthyroidism. If hypercalcemia persists after the restoration of euthyroidism, serum PTH should be measured in order to evaluate concomitant hyperparathyroidism.

Another less frequent cause of hypercalcemia due to increased bone resorption includes immobilization with high turnover bone disease, as in PAGET disease.

Increase in Intestinal Calcium Absorption

High calcium intake is, in isolation, a rare cause of hypercalcemia, since the initial elevation of serum calcium concentration inhibits both PTH release and calcitriol synthesis, but when combined with reduced urinary excretion, it can lead to hypercalcemia.

Alkaline Milk Syndrome

In the absence of renal insufficiency, hypercalcemia may occur following the ingestion of large amounts of calcium with absorbable substances (sodium bicarbonate and calcium carbonate), leading to hypercalcemia, metabolic alkalosis, renal dysfunction, and, usually, nephrocalcinosis, a situation known as alkaline milk syndrome [18, 19]. Alkaline milk syndrome typically occurs in the scenario of excess calcium carbonate supplementation in the treatment of osteoporosis or dyspepsia. One study found that this syndrome accounted for 8.8% of cases of hypercalcemia in the period 1998 and 2003 [20]. It represents one of the few examples of purely absorptive hypercalcemia.

Hypervitaminosis D

Vitamin D poisoning is a rare cause of hypercalcemia. The dose of vitamin D required to induce toxicity varies among patients, reflecting differences in absorption, storage, and metabolism, but serum levels of 25(OH)D, the main metabolite of vitamin D, >150 ng/ml, generally indicate intoxication. Elevated serum concentrations of $1,25(OH)_2D_3$ may be observed after ingestion of calcitriol for treatment of hypoparathyroidism. Due to its short half-life, calcitriol-induced hypercalcemia usually lasts for 1–2 days. Suspension of calcitriol and venous hydration with saline may be the only treatment needed in these cases. On the other hand, hypercalcemia caused by high intake of calcidiol may take several weeks, since excess vitamin D is slowly cleared by the body (weeks to months). More aggressive therapy with glucocorticoids, which antagonize the action of calcitriol, and intravenous bisphosphonates may be necessary [21–23].

Granulomatous Diseases

Hypercalcemia can be observed in around 10% of the patients with sarcoidosis, and an even greater percentage of these individuals evolve with hypercalciuria. The primary disturbance of hypercalcemia in these cases is the extrarenal activation of 25-dihydroxyvitamin D by 1α-hydroxylase in activated macrophage tissue, which is resistant to normal feedback control. Other granulomatous diseases that may cause hypercalcemia by the same mechanisms include tuberculosis, berylliosis, disseminated coccidioidomycosis, histoplasmosis, leprosy, and pulmonary eosinophilic granulomatosis [24]. Although most patients are normocalcemic at presentation, they may be hypercalciuric, with urinary calcium excretion analysis as part of the diagnostic investigation. In addition, hypercalcemia and hypercalciuria may not be apparent until calcium and vitamin D intake occurs.

Decrease of Calcium Excretion

Chronic Renal Insufficiency

It is known that in chronic renal failure alone, although associated with decreased calcium excretion, hypercalcemia does not occur due to hyperphosphatemia and decreased synthesis of calcitriol. On the contrary, these patients usually present hypocalcemia with hyperphosphatemia. Hypercalcemia, however, may be seen in patients receiving carbonate or calcium acetate in conjunction with dietary phosphate, particularly if they are being treated with calcitriol, in an attempt to reverse a hypocalcemia or secondary hyperparathyroidism.

Rhabdomyolysis and Acute Renal Failure

Hypercalcemia has been described during the diuretic phase of acute renal failure, often seen in patients with rhabdomyolysis. Hypercalcemia is due to the mobilization of calcium from the injured muscle [25].

Thiazide Diuretics

The administration of thiazide diuretics may increase serum calcium, and this fact cannot be fully explained by hemoconcentration. Thiazide diuretics have the ability to reduce urinary calcium excretion and are used in the treatment of patients with recurrent hypercalciuria and nephrolithiasis. Rarely, they cause hypercalcemia in healthy individuals but may cause hypercalcemia in patients with underlying increase in bone resorption, such as in those with hyperparathyroidism.

Downregulation of Calcium-Sensing Receptor

Familial Hypocalciuric Hypercalcemia (FHH)

Familial hypocalciuric hypercalcemia is a rare autosomal dominant disorder characterized by a genetic defect in calcium receptors in the parathyroid and kidney. It presents with mild hypercalcemia, the most marked laboratory finding being hypocalciuria, suggesting an increased tubular reabsorption of calcium. The urinary calcium level is generally <50 mg/24 h and the calcium/creatinine clearance <0.01

[26]. The diagnosis should be considered in any asymptomatic patient with mild to moderate hypercalcemia, hypocalciuria, and a family history of hypercalcemia. Its diagnostic importance is with the differential diagnosis with primary hyperparathyroidism in order to avoid unnecessary parathyroidectomy.

Medicines

Lithium

Patients who use chronic lithium may develop mild to moderate hypercalcemia, probably due to increased secretion of PTH, by an increase in levels at which calcium inhibits the release of PTH. Hypercalcemia usually, but not always, regresses when therapy is discontinued. Lithium therapy may also unmask a PHPT framework; on the other hand, lithium may raise serum PTH concentration, but it does not alter serum calcium [27].

Hypervitaminosis A

Excessive intake of vitamin A (>50,000 IU/d) leads to increased bone resorption, culminating with osteoporosis, fractures, hypercalcemia, and hyperostosis. The mechanism by which vitamin A stimulates bone resorption has not yet been fully elucidated [28].

Other medications that may rarely evolve with hypercalcemia are omeprazole, theophylline, and foscarnet.

Other Endocrinopathies

Pheochromocytoma

Hypercalcemia is a rare complication of pheochromocytoma. It may occur in NEM-2A due to hyperparathyroidism or to pheochromocytoma itself. In this case, hypercalcemia appears to be due to the tumor production of PTHrp. Its serum concentration may be reduced with the use of β-adrenergic blockers, suggesting a role of β-adrenergic stimulation in the pathogenesis [29].

Adrenal Insufficiency

Hypercalcemia may be a finding in adrenal crisis. Multiple factors appear to contribute to hypercalcemia, including increased bone resorption, increased tubular calcium reabsorption, increased hemoconcentration, and increased calcium-protein binding. The use of glucocorticoids reverses hypercalcemia [30, 31].

Uncommon Causes of Hypercalcemia

In certain situations, the differential diagnosis of hypercalcemia can become a real challenge in the clinical practice of the endocrinologist and general practitioner. Some etiologies so unusual that are not listed in many reviews of hypercalcemia and even rarely seen in patients with hypercalcemia of obscure etiology are summarized below (Table 20.2).

Hypercalcemia Mediated by Elevated Levels of Calcitriol

Similar to sarcoidosis, tuberculosis, and some fungal infections, other less frequent diseases characterized by granuloma formation have been associated with hypercalcemia secondary to elevated 1,25-dihydroxyvitamin D levels, such as Wegener's granulomatosis, Crohn's disease, cat-scratch disease, acute granulomatous pneumonitis (rare complication of methotrexate therapy), and hepatic granulomatosis [32].

Hypercalcemia Caused by PTHrp

Although recognition of humoral hypercalcemia in malignant neoplasms is well established, hypercalcemia due to

Table 20.2 Rare causes of hypercalcemia

Rare causes of hypercalcemia
Wegener's granulomatosis
Cat scratch fever
Crohn's disease
Acute granulomatous pneumonia
BCG therapy
HIV-associated lymphadenopathy
Massive mammary hyperplasia during pregnancy
Omeprazole in acute interstitial nephritis
Theophylline toxicity
Parenteral nutrition
Foscarnet
Eosinophilic granuloma
Leprosy in rheumatoid arthritis
Mycobacterium avium complicating AIDS
Cytomegalic virus infection in AIDS
Chronic berylliosis
Nocardia asteroides pericarditis
Diffuse octeoclastosis
Lymphedema of chest and pleural cavities
Brucellosis

high PTHrp levels in the benign disease setting is very unusual. This has already been described in a patient with systemic lupus erythematosus (SLE) with multiple organ involvement, in HIV-associated lymphadenopathy, diffuse mammary hyperplasia of pregnancy, and benign ovarian and renal tumors [32].

Hypercalcemia of Unknown Mechanism

Hypercalcemia has been reported in several clinical settings where the mechanisms of hypercalcemia have not been fully elucidated.

Clinical Manifestations

Increased serum calcium causes changes in all organ systems, as their extracellular levels interfere with the tissue functions of the brain, peripheral nerves, visceral smooth muscle, and cardiac and renal musculature. The severity of the clinical presentation does not depend exclusively on the serum calcium level but on the speed of installation, age, clinical conditions, presence of metastases, liver and renal dysfunctions, and evolution of the underlying disease (Table 20.3).

Gastrointestinal

Intestinal constipation is the most frequent complaint. Other symptoms include anorexia, nausea, vomiting, and vague abdominal complaints. Rarely, severe hypercalcemia can cause acute pancreatitis [33–35].

Renal

The most important renal manifestations are nephrolithiasis, renal tubular dysfunction, and renal failure, which may be acute or chronic. Chronic hypercalcemia leads to a defect in the ability to concentrate urine, which can lead to polyuria in up to 20% of patients, and the mechanism by which this occurs is not well understood. Chronic hypercalcemic nephropathy has the clinical features of interstitial nephritis with polyuria, natriuresis, and hypertension. Hypertension, nephrolithiasis, obstruction, and possible infections may contribute to the additional loss of renal function [36].

Cardiovascular

In chronic hypercalcemia, calcium deposits can be seen in cardiac valves, coronary arteries, and myocardial fibers.

A short QT interval is also observed, which does not appear to be clinically important in cardiac conduction or in the prevalence of supraventricular or ventricular arrhythmias [37–39].

Neuropsychiatric

The most common neuropsychiatric symptoms were anxiety, depression, and cognitive deficiency. More severe symptoms are observed in elderly patients with severe hypercalcemia. Personality changes and affective disorders may occur when calcium concentrations exceed 12 mg/dl (3 nmol/L), while confusion, psychosis, hallucinations, somnolence, and coma are rare [40, 41].

Physical Findings

There is no specific physical finding of hypercalcemia, in addition to those that could be related to an underlying disease, such as in the malignancy syndrome. Band keratopathy reflects the deposition of calcium phosphate in the subepithelial layer of the cornea, a very rare finding, usually discovered through an ophthalmological examination with a slit lamp [42].

Table 20.3 Clinical manifestations of hypercalcemia

Gastrointestinal	Renal	Cardiovascular	Neuropsychiatric	Musculoskeletal
Constipation	Nephrolithiasis	Shortened QT interval	Anxiety	Muscle weakness
Anorexia	DI nephrogenic	Deposition of calcium in heart valves,	Depression	Bone pain[b]
Nausea	Renal tubular acidosis (type 1)	Coronary arteries, and myocardial fibers	Cognitive dysfunction	
Peptic ulcer disease[a]	Tubular renal dysfunction	Hypertension	Lethargy	
Acute pancreatitis[a]	Renal insufficiency	Cardiomyopathy	Confusion[a]	
	Chronic hypercalcemic nephropathy		Stupor[a]	
	Nephrocalcinosis		Coma[a]	

DI diabetes insipidus
[a]Rare
[b]Primary hyperparathyroidism or malignancy

Diagnostic Evaluation/Laboratory Diagnosis

Hypercalcemia is a relatively common clinical problem. As the great majority of causes of hypercalcemia are due to primary hyperparathyroidism and malignant diseases, laboratory diagnosis typically involves the distinction between these two clinical entities. In general, there is no difficulty in distinguishing them. Symptoms of malignancy are often present at the time of diagnosis of hypercalcemia, and serum calcium levels are usually higher than in patients with PHPT (Fig. 20.1).

A single elevated serum calcium value does not diagnose hypercalcemia, and this dosage should be repeated to confirm the diagnosis, preferably without the use of the tourniquet. If available, previous serum calcium values should be reviewed. The presence of long-term asymptomatic hypercalcemia is more suggestive of primary hyperparathyroidism and also increases the possibility of familial hypocalciuria hypercalcemia. The degree of hypercalcemia may also be useful in the diagnostic distinction. Primary hyperparathyroidism is usually associated with mild hypercalcemia (values <11 mg/

dl). Values >13 mg/dl are more consistent with hypercalcemia of malignancy.

In patients with hypoalbuminemia, chronic disease, or malnutrition, total serum calcium may be normal, but ionizable calcium will be elevated. In this situation, serum calcium should be corrected for the value of albumin or, as some authorities prefer, to dose the ionizable calcium.

Since hypercalcemia has been confirmed, the next step is to measure serum PTH in order to distinguish parathyroid-mediated hypercalcemia (PHPT and HHF) from those not mediated by PTH (malignant diseases, vitamin D intoxication, granulomatous diseases).

In the presence of non-suppressed PTH, the next step is to assess the relationship of calcium clearance to creatinine clearance. If the ratio is >0.02, then the diagnosis will be PHPT, and < 0.01 will be indicative of HHF. On the other hand, if PTH is suppressed PTH-rp and vitamin D metabolites (1,25OH2D and 25OHD) should be requested.

If PTHrp is >12 mg/dl (or > 4.0 nmol/L), the diagnosis will be humoral hypercalcemia of malignancy. Levels of 25OHD

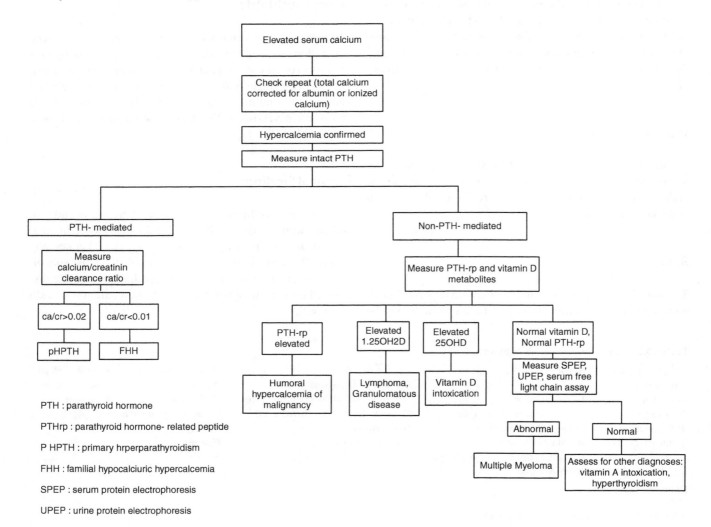

PTH : parathyroid hormone

PTHrp : parathyroid hormone- related peptide

P HPTH : primary hrperparathyroidism

FHH : familial hypocalciuric hypercalcemia

SPEP : serum protein electrophoresis

UPEP : urine protein electrophoresis

Fig. 20.1 Diagnostic approach to hypercalcemia. PTH parathyroid hormone, PTHrp parathyroid hormone-related peptide, PHPTH primary hyperparathyroidism, FHH familial hypocalciuric hypercalcemia, SPEP serum protein electrophoresis, UPEP urine protein electrophoresis

>100 ng/ml probably indicate intoxication. If 1,25OH2D is elevated, we must think of lymphoproliferative disorders and/or chronic granulomatous diseases. In the presence of normal levels of PTHrp and vitamin D metabolites, other causes of hypercalcemia should be considered. Additional laboratory data include serum protein electrophoresis to screen for multiple myeloma, TSH, and vitamin A. In most cases, this laboratory assessment will lead to the correct diagnosis.

Serum phosphate concentration and urinary calcium excretion are also useful in the differential diagnosis. PHPT and humoral neoplastic hypercalcemia (mediated by PTHrp) frequently present hypophosphatemia, a result of the inhibition of renal phosphate reabsorption [43]. In contrast, phosphate concentration is normal or elevated in granulomatous diseases, vitamin D intoxication, immobilization, thyrotoxicosis, alkaline milk syndrome, and bone metastatic diseases. In hypercalcemia of the family hypocalciuria, the dosage of phosphate is variable [43]. Dosage of alkaline phosphatase (AP) may also be useful in differentiating the causes of hypercalcemia. AP is elevated in osteoblastic bone metastasis, as in prostate cancer, but not in osteoclast disorders, such as multiple myeloma [24].

Urinary calcium excretion is usually increased in hyperparathyroidism and hypercalcemia of malignancy. In contrast, there are three disorders in which the increase of renal calcium reabsorption leads to relative hypocalciuria (<100 mg/day or 2.5 nmol/day); they are alkaline milk syndrome, thiazide diuretics, and familial hypocalciuria hypercalcemia, where fraction of calcium excretion is less than 1% [44, 45].

Finally, the review of the therapeutic regimen (prescribed drugs or not, use of calcium and vitamin D supplements) and dietary plan is useful to evaluate alkaline milk syndrome and drug-induced hypercalcemia.

Treatment

Treatment of hypercalcemia is aimed at reducing serum calcium concentrations and, when possible, treating the causative condition. Calcium levels may be reduced by measures that act on intestinal absorption, increasing renal excretion or inhibiting bone resorption. The choice of treatment will depend on the cause and severity of hypercalcemia (Table 20.4).

Table 20.4 Treatment of hypercalcemic crisis

Intervention	Mode of action	Dose	Beginning of action	Duration of action	Comments
Hydration	Restore intravascular volume Increase calcium excretion	SF 0.9% 500–1000 ml/hour Followed 150–250 ml/hour **Cardiac monitoring**	Hours	During infusion	Caution in patients with cardiac and/or renal dysfunction
Loop diuretics*	Increase urinary calcium excretion	Furosemide 40 mg EV 12/12 H Begin only after adequate hydration	Hours	During therapy	They should not be used routinely. In patients with cardiac and/or renal dysfunction, judicious use may be necessary in order to avoid volume overload during intravenous hydration
Glucocorticosteroids	Reduces absorption of intestinal calcium. Decreases 1,25OH2D by activated mononuclear cells in patients with lymphomas or granulomatous diseases	Hydrocortisone 200–300 mg IV/day	3–5 days	2 weeks	Effective in the treatment of hematological malignancies with increase of 1,25OH2D, vitamin D intoxication, and granulomatous diseases
Bisphosphonates	Inhibits bone resorption via interference in osteoclast function and recruitment	**Pamidronate** Dose: 60–90 mg IV diluted in SF 0.9% infused in 4–6 hours (+ − 2 h) interval between doses, at least 7 days **Zoledronic acid** Dose: 4 mg IV diluted SF 0.9% for 15–20 minutes	24–72 hours	2–4 weeks	Effective in hypercalcemia of malignancy
Denosumab	Inhibits bone resorption via inhibition of RANKL	120 mg, SC Can be repeated within 1 week if needed	24 hours	4 weeks	Effective in hypercalcemia of malignancy. It should be considered in patients refractory to bisphosphonates, in those with GFR <35 ml/minute, or even as a first option

*Use with caution

Asymptomatic or symptomatic patients with mild hypercalcemia (<12 mg/dl or 3 nmol/L) do not require immediate therapeutic intervention, but increased oral hydration is recommended, and they should avoid prolonged immobilization and medications which elevate calcemia such as thiazide diuretics and vitamin D supplements. Similarly, patients with calcium levels between 12 and 14 mg/dL may not require immediate treatment if hypercalcemia is chronic. However, a sudden increase in the concentration of serum calcium levels may lead to altered consciousness, demanding more vigorous measures. In addition, patients with serum calcium concentration > 14 mg/dl require treatment, regardless of symptoms.

Increase in Calcium Urinary Excretion

The filtered calcium is reabsorbed, mainly, in the proximal tubules and in the ascending limbs of the loop of Henle. This process is passive and results from favorable electrochemical gradients created by sodium and chloride reabsorption. The active resorption of calcium occurs mainly in the distal tubule due to the influence of PTH. Urinary calcium excretion may be increased in patients with hypercalcemia, inhibiting sodium reabsorption in the proximal tubules and the loop of Henle, thereby reducing passive calcium reabsorption. Proximal resorption is inhibited by volume expansion with intravenous saline infusion, as it increases the concentration of sodium, calcium, and water in the loop of Henle.

A reasonable scheme is to initiate the administration of saline solution to 500–1000 ml in the first hour, followed by an infusion rate of 150–250 ml/hour until intravascular volume restoration. Diuretics of the loop should not be used routinely. However, in patients with cardiac or renal dysfunction, judicious use of the diuretic may be necessary in order to avoid volume overload during hydration. The patient should be monitored to avoid hypovolemia and electrolyte disturbances, especially potassium and magnesium.

Decrease in Intestinal Calcium Absorption

Increased intestinal calcium absorption in the diet is the main mechanism by which excessive vitamin D administration or endogenous overproduction of calcitriol leads to hypercalcemia.

Corticosteroids may be effective in patients with hematologic malignancies with an increase of 1,25OH2D, vitamin D intoxication, and chronic granulomatous diseases [46]. In such patients, prednisone at a dose of 20–40 mg/day reduces the serum calcium concentration within 2–5 days, decreasing the production of calcitriol by the activated mononuclear cells of the lung and lymph nodes.

Inhibition of Bone Resorption

Bisphosphonates have become one of the main instruments for the treatment of hypercalcemia, especially severe and malignant hypercalcemia. These drugs are effective inhibitors of osteoclasts and thus influence one of the most important pathophysiological mechanisms of hypercalcemia. The maximum effect occurs in 2–4 days, so they are usually given along with saline or calcitonin when quick serum calcium normalization is desired.

Among the currently available agents for the treatment of hypercalcemia of malignancy are pamidronate, zoledronate, and ibandronate, with pamidronate and zoledronate being the ones of choice.

Pamidronate can be used at a dose of 60–90 mg, depending on the initial calcium levels, and is effective in normalizing serum calcium in 70–100% [47]. Its therapeutic response is dose dependent, and the maximum effect on the normalization of calcium is seen with a dose of 90 mg intravenously [48]. It is usually given as a single intravenous infusion diluted in isotonic saline solution in 4–6 hours. A therapeutic scheme of infusion of 24 hours has also been proposed. It is well tolerated, with a low incidence of side effects such as transient fever, myalgia, and leukopenia (easily bypassed with the use of simple analgesics). Frequently, the response is continuous for up to 2–4 weeks, with maintenance of normocalcemia for up to 15 days [49–51].

In three clinical studies, two in breast cancer and one in multiple myeloma, pamidronate improved all skeletal-related events (bone pain, fracture, and hypercalcemia). The drug also extended the time for the onset of skeletal events and reduced the need for analgesics [52].

Zoledronate has been shown to be the most potent bisphosphonate in the treatment of hypercalcemia, especially when associated with malignancy. In a study of 275 patients with moderate to severe hypercalcemia of malignancy, the efficacy and maintenance of zoledronate response at doses of 4 and 8 mg were compared to those of pamidronate at a dose of 90 mg. Zoledronic acid was given at doses of 4 and 8 mg in intravenous infusions of 5 min, while pamidronate was infused at a dose of 90 mg in 2 h. This study concluded that both doses of zoledronate were superior to pamidronate. The normalization rate of calcemia on the tenth day was 88.4% with 4 mg and 86.7% with 8 mg of zoledronate and 69.7% with 90 mg of pamidronate. Calcium normalization occurred on the fourth day in approximately 50% of zoledronate-treated patients versus 33.3% of those using pamidronate. The mean duration of control was longer with zoledronate (32 and 43 days) compared to pamidronate (18 days). Finally, the authors conclude that zoledronate is superior to pamidronate, and the recommended dose is 4 mg, reserving the dose of 8 mg for refractory or recurrent cases [53].

Although renal toxicity was reported more frequently with zoledronate than pamidronate, in trials evaluating the chronic use of these drugs in the treatment of metastatic bone disease, no difference was observed between drugs with regard to renal dysfunction. The efficacy of 4 and 8 mg of zoledronic acid was similar, but at the dose of 4 mg a lower incidence of renal toxicity was observed ($5.2 \times 2.3\%$ with 4 mg) [54].

Ibandronate has also been shown to be effective in the treatment of hypercalcemia of malignancy. In a study involving more than 320 patients, the dose of 2 mg intravenously normalized serum calcium in 67% of patients and doses of up to 6 mg intravenously were shown to be safe and well tolerated [55, 56]. The response frequency was significantly higher with 4 or 6 mg than with 2 mg; however, the duration of response was not dose dependent.

In a trial involving 72 patients with hypercalcemia of malignancy, ibandronate (2–4 mg) was compared with pamidronate (15–90 mg IV). The number of patients responding to both agents was similar ($77 \times 76\%$ for ibandronate and pamidronate, respectively), but ibandronate was more effective in maintaining normocalcemia (14×4 days) [57].

Bisphosphonates are known to be nephrotoxic drugs, but in clinical trials involving zoledronate in the treatment of hypercalcemia of malignancy, patients with creatinine levels above 4.5 mg/dl were eligible to enter the study [53]. In addition, there were three reports of successful use of both ibandronate and pamidronate for patients with renal insufficiency and multiple myeloma [58], patients with renal insufficiency (creatinine >1.5 mg/dl) [59], and patients on hemodialysis with severe hypercalcemia [60, 61]. However, caution is suggested in the use of intravenous bisphosphonates to treat hypercalcemia in the setting of renal failure. We should reduce the dose of bisphosphonates (4 mg of zoledronate, 30–45 mg of pamidronate, and 2 mg of ibandronate) and prolong the infusion time in order to minimize the risk of deterioration of renal function.

Salmon calcitonin is another therapeutic agent available in the treatment of acute hypercalcemia. Like bisphosphonates, it inhibits bone resorption via osteoclasts. It can be administered IM or SC [62]. Intranasal calcitonin has not been shown to be effective in the treatment of hypercalcemia [63]. The recommended dose is 4 U/kg every 12 hours, and the dose may be increased to 6–8 U/kg every 6 hours [64]. The great advantage of calcitonin is its quick action, with reduction of serum calcium in a few hours. Maximum calcium reduction is seen in 12–24 hours. It is not a potent agent, and calcium levels fall to a maximum of 1–2 mg/dl; another disadvantage is the development of tachyphylaxis, probably by downregulation of the receptor. Thus, we must associate it with bisphosphonates to lead to a more pronounced and lasting decline in serum calcium.

Denosumab

Denosumab is a human monoclonal antibody that binds to the receptor activator of nuclear factor kappa-B ligand (RANKL) and inhibits the differentiation, function, and survival of osteoclasts. Like bisphosphonates, it represents an important therapeutic option in the modulation of hypercalcemia of malignancy, especially in patients with hypercalcemia refractory to bisphosphonates or with a glomerular filtration rate < 35 ml/minute since, as they are metabolized by peptidases and cleared by the reticuloendothelial system, it has minimal nephrotoxic effects.

In a phase III trial of patients with prostate cancer resistant to castration and bone metastasis, denosumab at the dose of 120 mg SC every 4 weeks was shown to be superior to zoledronic acid 4 mg IV in the reduction of skeletal-related events (bone pain, pathological fracture, bone radiation, bone marrow compression, and hypercalcemia) [65].

In a single-arm and open-label study, patients with corrected serum calcium (CSC) >12.5 mg/dL despite recent treatment with venous bisphosphonate received denosumab, SC, on days 1, 8, 15, and 29 and then every 4 weeks. The primary endpoint of this study was to assess the proportion of patients with CSC levels ≤11.5 mg/dl within 10 days of starting treatment. The mean calcemia in this study was 13.6 mg/dl. The secondary endpoint included the duration of response and the proportion of patients who achieved a response considered complete with CSC levels ≤10.8 mg/dl on the tenth day. Eighty percent of the patients responded to denosumab treatment, reaching CSC levels ≤11.5 mg/dl. All responses occurred on the tenth day. The mean duration of response was 26 days, and 67% of the patients had a response considered complete with CSC ≤10.8 mg/dl in the tenth day of the treatment [66].

Another recent phase III study investigated the use of denosumab for the treatment of hypercalcemia refractory to bisphosphonates. In this trial, as in the previous one, patients had CSC >12.5 mg/dl at least 7 days after treatment with bisphosphonates. The study also showed that denosumab was able to reduce CSC to ≤ 11.5 mg/dl, within the tenth day of the treatment, in 64% of patients [67]. In December 2014, the FDA approved the use of denosumab for the treatment of hypercalcemia of malignancy refractory to bisphosphonate therapy.

Other Therapies

Calcimimetics

Calcimimetics (cinacalcet, the only one currently available) reduces serum calcium concentration in patients with severe hypercalcemia due to parathyroid carcinoma, hemodialysis patients with increased calcium-phosphorus product, and patients with secondary hyperparathyroidism. Calcimimetics has been evaluated in the treatment of primary hyperparathyroidism, but it is not standard therapy [68].

Dialysis

Dialysis therapy, whether in the form of hemodialysis or by peritoneal dialysis, is an effective way of treating hypercalcemia. Dialysis is particularly useful in patients with renal and cardiac insufficiency, in whom salt solutions cannot be infused safely [69].

References

1. Carrol R, Matfin G. Endocrine and metabolic emergencies: hypercalcaemia. Ther Adv Endocrinol Metab. 2010;1(5):225–34.
2. Bourke E, Yanagawa N. Assessment of hyperphosphatemia and hypophosphatemia. Clin Lab Med. 1993;13(1):183–207.
3. Chan FKW, Koberle LC, Thys-jacobs S, et al. Differential diagnosis, causes and management of hypercalcemia. Curr Probl Surg. 1997;34:450–523.
4. Bilezikian JP. Management of acute hypercalcemia. N Engl J Med. 1992;326:1196–203.
5. Minisola S, Pepe J, Piemonte S, Cipriani C. The diagnosis and management of hypercalcaemia. Clinical review. BMJ. 2015;350:h2723.
6. Wermers RA, Khosla S, Atkinson EJ, Hodgson SF, O'Fallon WM, Melton LJ III. The rise and fall of hyperparathyroidism: a population-based study in Rochester, Minnesota,1965–1992. Ann Intern Med. 1997;126:443–0.
7. Silverberg E, Lewiecki M, Mosekilde L, Peacock M, Rubin MR. Presentation of asymptomatic primary hyperparathyroidism: proceedings of the third international workshop. J Clin Endocrinol Metab. 2009;94:351–65.
8. Bilezikian JP, Khan AA, Potts JT Jr. Guidelines for the management of asymptomatic primary hyperparathyroidism: summary statement from the third international workshop. J Clin Endocrinol Metab. 2009;94:335–9.
9. Eastell R, Arnold A, Brandi ML, Brown EM, D'Amour P, Hanley DA, et al. Diagnosis of asymptomatic primary hyperparathyroidism Proceedings of the Third international Workshop. J Clin Endocrinol Metab. 2009;94:340–50.
10. Meric F, Yap P, Bia MJ. Etiology of hypercalcemia in hemodialysis patients on calcium carbonate therapy. Am J Kidney Dis. 1990;16:459.
11. Frolick A. Prevalence of hypercalcemia in normal and in hospital populations. Dan Med Bull. 1998;45:436–9.
12. Lee C-T, Yang C-C, Lam K-K, Kung C-T, Tsai C-J, Chen H-C. Hypercalcemia in the emergency department. Am J Med Sci. 2006;331:119–23.
13. Stewart AF. Hypercalcemia associated with cancer. N Engl J Med. 2005;352:373–9.
14. Pi J, Kang Y, Smith M, et al. A review in the treatment of oncologic emergencies. J Oncol Pharm Pract. 2016;22(4):625–38.
15. Tebben P, Singh R, Kumar R. Vitamin D-mediated hypercalcemia: mechanisms, diagnosis, and treatment. Endocr Rev. 2016;37:521–47.
16. Burman KD, Monchik JM, Earll JM, Wartofsky L. Ionized and total serum calcium and parathyroid hormone in hyperthyroidism. Ann Intern Med. 1976;84:668.
17. Alikhan Z, Singh A. Hyperthyroidism manifested as hypercalcemia. South Med J. 1996;89:997.
18. Beall DP, Scofield RH. Milk-alkali syndrome associated with calcium carbonate consumption. Report of 7 patients with parathyroid hormone levels and an estimate of prevalence among patients hospitalized with hypercalcemia. Medicine (Baltimore). 1995;74:89.
19. Abreo K, Adlakha A, Kilpatrick S, et al. The milk-alkali syndrome. A reversible form of acute renal failure. Arch Intern Med. 1993;153:1005.
20. Picolos MK, Lavis VR, Orlander PR. Milk-alkali syndrome is a major cause of hypercalcemia among non-end-stage renal disease(non-ESRD) inpatients. Clin Endocrinol (Oxf). 2005;63:566.
21. Tebben P, Singh R, Kumar R. Vitamin D- mediated hypercalcemia: mechanisms, diagnosis, and treatment. Endocr Rev. 2016;37:521–47.
22. Hoeck HC, Laurberg G, Laurberg P. Hypercalcaemic crisis after excessive topical use of a vitamin D derivative. J Intern Med. 1994;235:281.
23. Selby PL, Davies M, Marks JS, Mawer EB. Vitamin D intoxication causes hypercalcaemia by increased bone resorption which responds to pamidronate. Clin Endocrinol (Oxf). 1995;43:531.
24. David B. Endres. Investigation of hypercalcemia. Clin Biochem. 2012;45:954–63.
25. Llach F, Felsenfeld AJ, Haussler MR. The pathophysiology of altered calcium metabolism in rhabdomyolysis-induced acute renal failure. Interactions of parathyroid hormone, 25Ohydroxycholecalciferol, and 1,25-diydrocholecalciferol. N Engl J Med. 1981;305:117.
26. Schwartz SR, Futran ND. Hypercalcemic hypocalciuria: a critical differential diagnosis for hyperparathyroidism. Otolaryngol Clin N Am. 2004;37:887.
27. Mark TW, et al. Effects of lithium therapy on bone mineral metabolism: a two-year prospective longitudinal study. J Clin Endocrinol Metab. 1998;83:3857.
28. Bhalla K, Ennis DM, Ennis ED. Hypercalcemia caused by iatrogenic hypervitaminosis a. J Am Diet Assoc. 2005;105:119.
29. Stewart AF, Hoecker J, Segre JV, et al. Hypercalcemia in pheochromocytoma: evidence for a novel mechanism. Ann Intern Med. 1985;102:776.
30. Vasikaran SD, Tallis GA, Braund WJ. Secondary hypoadrenalism presenting with hypercalcaemia. Clin Endocrinol (Oxf). 1994;41:261.
31. Fujikawa M, Kamihira K, Sato K, et al. Elevated bone resorption markers in a patient with hypercalcemia associated with postpartum thyrotoxicosis and hypoadrenocorticism due to pituitary failure. J Endocrinol Invest. 2004;27:782.
32. Jacobs TP, Bilezikian JP. Clinical review: rare causes of hypercalcemia. J Clin Endocrinol Metab. 2005;90:6316–22.
33. Bourgain A, Acker O, Lambaudie E, et al. Small cell carcinoma of the ovary of the hypercalcemic type revealed by a severe acute pancreatitis: about one case. Gynecol Obstet Ferttil. 2005;33:35.
34. Mithofer K, Fernández-del Castillo C, Frick TW, et al. Acute hypercalcemia causes acute pancreatitis and ectopic trypsinogen activation in the rat. Gastroenterology. 1995;109:239.
35. Ward JB, Petersen OH, Jenkins SA, Sutton R. Is an elevated concentration of acinar cytosolic free ionized calcium the trigger for acute pancreatitis? Lancet. 1995;346:1016.
36. Peacock M. Primary hyperparathyroidism and the kidney: biochemical and clinical spectrum. J Bone Miner Res. 2002;17(sppl 2):87.

37. Kiewiet RM, Ponssen HH, Janssens EN, Fels PW. Ventricular fibrillation in hypercalcaemic crisis due to primary hyperparathyroidism. Neth J Med. 2004;62:94.

38. Diercks DB, Shumaik GM, Harrigan RA, et al. Electrocardiographic manifestations: electrolyte abnormalities. J Emerg Med. 2004;27:153.

39. Nishi SP, Barbagelata NA, Atar S, et al. Hypercalcemia-induced ST-segment elevation mimicking acute myocardial infarction. J Electrocardiol. 2006;39:298.

40. Shane E, Dinaz I. Hypercalcemia: pathogenesis, clinical manifestations, differential diagnosis and management. In: Favus MJ, editor. Primer on the metabolic bone diseases and disorders of mineral metabolism, vol. 26. 6th ed. Philadelphia: Lippincott, Williams and wilkins; 2006. p. 176.

41. Inzucchi SE. Understanding hypercalcemia. Its metabolic basis, signs and symptoms. Postgrad Med. 2004;115:69.

42. Wilson KS, Alexander S, Chisholm IA. Band keratopathy in hypercalcemia of myeloma. Can Med Assoc J. 1982;126:1314.

43. Elizabeth S, Clifford J, Jean E. Diagnostic approach to hypercalcemia. http://www.uptodate.com. Accessed 20 Nov 2017.

44. Patel AM, Goldfarb S. Got calcium? Welcome to the calcium-alkali syndrome. J Am Soc Nephrol. 2010;21:1440–3.

45. Medarov BI. Milk-alkali syndrome. Mayo Clin Proc. 2009;84:261–7.

46. Bilezikian JP. Management of hypercalcemia. J Clin Endocrinol Metab. 1993;77:1445.

47. Coleman RE. Bisphosphonates: clinical experience. Oncologist. 2002;9:14.

48. Nussbaum SR, Younger J, Vandepol CJ, et al. Single-dose intravenous therapy with pamidronate for the treatment of hypercalcemia of malignancy: comparison of 30, 60-, and 90-mg dosages. Am J Med. 1993;95:297.

49. Gurney H, Grill V, Martin TJ. Parathyroid hormone-related protein and response to pamidronate in tumor-induced hypercalcemia. Lancet. 1993;341:1611.

50. Walls J, Ratcliffe WA, Howell A, Bundred NJ. Response to intravenous bisphosphonate therapy in hypercalcaemic patients with and without bone metastases: the role of parathyroid hormone-related protein. Br J Cancer. 1994;70:169.

51. Wimalawansa SJ. Significance of plasma PTH-rp in patients with hypercalcemia of malignancy treated with bisphosphonates. Cancer. 1994;73:2223.

52. Conte PF, Latreille J, Mauriac L, et al. Delay in progression of bone metastases in breast cancer patients treated with intravenous pamidronate: results from a multinational randomized controlled trial. The Aredia Multinational Cooperative Group. J Clin Oncol. 1996;14(9):2552–9.

53. Major P, Lortholary A, Hon J, Abdi E, Mills G, Menssen HD, et al. Zoledronic acid is superior to pamidronate in the treatment of hypercalcemia of malignancy: a pooled analysis of two randomized, controlled clinical trials. J Clin Oncol. 2001;19:558–67.

54. Schwaetz LM, Woloshin S. Lost in transmission- FDA drug information that never reaches clinicians. N Engl J Med. 2009;361:1717.

55. Ralston SH, Thiébaud D, Herrmann Z, et al. Dose-response study of ibandronate in the treatment of cancer-associated hypercalcemia. Br J Cancer. 1997;75:295.

56. Pecherstorfer M, Herrmann Z, Body JJ, et al. Randomized phase II trial comparing different doses of the bisphosphonate ibandronate in the treatment of hypercalcemia of malignancy. J Clin Oncol. 1996;14:268.

57. Pecherstorfer M, Steinhauer EU, Rizzoli R, et al. Efficacy and safety of ibandronate in the treatment of hypercalcemia of malignancy: a randomized multicentric comparison to pamidronate. Support Care Cancer. 2003;11:539.

58. Henrich D, Hoffman M, Uppenkamp M, Bergner R. Ibandronate for the treatment of hypercalcemia or nephrocalcinosis in patients with multiple myeloma and acute renal failure: case reports. Acta Haematol. 2006;116:165.

59. Machado CE, Flombaum CD. Safety of pamidronate in patients with renal failure and hypercalcemia. Clin Nephrol. 1996;45:175.

60. Trimarchi H, Lombi F, Forrester M, et al. Disodium pamidronate for treating severe hypercalcemia in a hemodialysis patient. Nat Clin Pract Nephrol. 2006;2:459.

61. Davenport A, Goel S, Mackenzie JC. Treatment of hypercalcemia with pamidronate in patients with end stage renal failure. Scand J Urol Nephrol. 1993;27:447.

62. Austin LA, Heath H 3rd. Calcitonin: physiology and pathophysiology. N Engl J Med. 1981;304:269.

63. Dumon JC, Magritte A, Body JJ. Nasal human calcitonin for tumor-induced hypercalcemia. Calcif Tissue Int. 1992;51:18.

64. Wisneski LA. Salmon calcitonin in the acute management of hypercalcemia. Calcif Tissue Int. 1990;46(Suppl):26.

65. Smith MR, Coleman RE, Klotz L, et al. Denosumab for the prevention of skeletal complications in metastatic castration-resistant prostate cancer: comparison of skeletal- related events and symptomatic skeletal events. Ann Oncol. 2015;26:368–74.

66. Hu MI, Glezerman I, Leboulleux S, et al. Denosumab for patients with persistent or relapsed hypercalcemia of malignancy despite recent bisphosphonate treatment. J Natl Cancer Inst. 2013;105:1417–20.

67. Hu MI, Glezerman IG, Leboulleux S, et al. Denosumab for treatment of hypercalcemia of malignancy. J Clin Endocrinol Metab. 2014;99:3144–52.

68. Silverberg SJ, Rubin MR, Faiman C, Peacock M, Shoback DM, Smallridge RC, et al. Cinacalcet hydrochloride reduces the serum calcium concentration in inoperable parathyroid carcinoma. J Clin Endocrinol Metab. 2007;92(10):3803.

69. Leehey DJ, Ing TS. Correction of hypercalcemia and hypophosphatemia by hemodialysis using a conventional, calcium-containing dialysis solution enriched with phosphorus. Am J Kidney Dis. 1997;29:288.

Hypocalcemia

Vivien Lim and Bart L. Clarke

Key Points to the Diagnosis

Serum calcium concentration is determined by the balance between calcium influx into extracellular fluid from intestinal absorption, skeletal resorption, and renal reabsorption and calcium efflux from extracellular fluid through intestinal secretion, skeletal uptake, and renal excretion [1]. Hypocalcemia usually results from decreased skeletal resorption or intestinal absorption, in conjunction with normal or increased renal excretion, but it may result from normal calcium influx in association with increased renal excretion or skeletal mineralization [2]. Decreased skeletal resorption is typically due to decreased osteoclast recruitment and activation, most often due to decreased parathyroid hormone (PTH), parathyroid hormone-related protein (PTHrP), or 1,25-dihydroxyvitamin D levels [3]. Deficiencies of other cytokines that normally stimulate osteoclast recruitment or function, including interleukin (IL)-1α, IL-1β, IL-6, tumor necrosis factor-α, lymphotoxin, or transforming growth factor-β, might also lead to decreased skeletal resorption, but by themselves do not cause hypocalcemia. Decreased intestinal absorption of calcium is fairly common, typically occurring due to decreased 1,25-dihydroxyvitamin D or malabsorption. Regardless of the cause of decreased calcium influx into extracellular fluid, serum calcium levels do not typically decrease unless the kidneys fail to compensate with appropriately increased urinary calcium reabsorption.

Other factors may indirectly affect serum calcium. Decreased PTH and PTHrP lead to decreased renal tubular reabsorption of filtered calcium, which results in increased urinary calcium excretion. Increased fluid intake may result in hemodilution, and volume overload may result in polyuria resulting in increased renal calcium clearance. Physical activity may directly decrease bone resorption and thereby reduce serum calcium.

The seven-transmembrane segment G protein-coupled extracellular calcium-sensing receptor (CaSR) plays a major role in regulation of extracellular calcium [4]. This receptor is found on parathyroid, renal tubular, osteoblast, intestinal mucosal, and adipocyte cells, as well as other cells in other tissues. The CaSR regulates secretion of PTH by parathyroid cells and renal tubular reabsorption of calcium, as it regulates bone turnover and intestinal absorption of calcium. The CaSR has a large extracellular portion that binds ionized calcium and a shorter intracellular portion that interacts with a variety of G proteins and signal transduction pathways. It may be part of a larger family of calcium- or cation-binding receptors.

Signs and Symptoms

Patients with mild hypocalcemia may be completely asymptomatic, whereas those with severe hypocalcemia are often incapacitated due to profound metabolic derangements. The magnitude of symptoms and signs present depends largely on the severity and chronicity of the hypocalcemia (Table 21.1). Patients with chronically low levels of ionized calcium may be asymptomatic except for a positive Chvostek's sign. Chvostek's sign may be present in up to 15% of healthy subjects without hypocalcemia, however, so it is not pathognomic of hypocalcemia. Neuromuscular irritability is the most common cause of symptoms, ranging from tingling paresthesias around the fingertips, toes, or lips to tetany, carpopedal spasm, extremity muscle twitching or cramping, or abdominal cramps. Neuromuscular irritability is often most clearly demonstrated by eliciting facial muscle twitching after tapping over the facial nerve just anterior to the ear (Chvostek's sign) [5] or by carpal spasm with inflation

V. Lim
Gleneagles Hospital, Singapore, Singapore

B. L. Clarke (✉)
Department of Medicine, Division of Endocrinology, Diabetes, Metabolism, and Nutrition, Mayo Clinic College of Medicine, Rochester, MN, USA
e-mail: clarke.bart@mayo.edu

© Springer Nature Switzerland AG 2022
F. Bandeira et al. (eds.), *Endocrinology and Diabetes*, https://doi.org/10.1007/978-3-030-90684-9_21

Table 21.1 Symptoms and signs of hypocalcemia

Symptoms
Circumoral and acral tingling paresthesias
Increased neuromuscular irritability
  Tetany
  Muscle cramps and twitching
  Abdominal cramps
Laryngospasm
Bronchospasm
Altered CNS function
  Seizures of all types
  Papilledema or pseudotumor cerebri
  Choreoathetoid movements
  Depression
  Coma
Congestive heart failure
Generalized fatigue
Signs
Chvostek's sign
Trousseau's sign
Prolongation of QTc interval
Cataracts
Basal ganglia and other intracerebral calcifications

Table 21.2 Causes of hypocalcemia

PTH-related
Acquired hypoparathyroidism
  Postsurgical
  Infiltration with iron
    Hemochromatosis
    Thalassemia with repeated transfusions
  Infiltration with copper: Wilson's disease
  Parathyroid metastases
  Neck radiation therapy
  Hypomagnesemia or hypermagnesemia
  Autoimmunity: Parathyroid gland antibodies
Congenital or inherited hypoparathyroidism
  APECED syndrome
  Autosomal dominant hypocalcemia
  Isolated hypoparathyroidism: Familial or X-linked
  Parathyroid agenesis
  Mutations in PTH gene
  Syndromes associated with hypoparathyroidism: DiGeorge syndrome, mitochondrial disorders with hypoparathyroidism
PTH resistance
  Pseudohypoparathyroidism types 1a, 1b, 1c, and 2
  Hypomagnesemia
Vitamin D-related
Vitamin D deficiency:
  Nutritional deficiency
  Malabsorption
  Lack of adequate sunlight exposure
  Hyperpigmentation
  Anticonvulsant therapy
  Pseudovitamin D deficiency rickets (vitamin D-dependent rickets type 1)
  Chronic renal disease
  Severe liver disease
Vitamin D resistance
  Hereditary vitamin D-resistant rickets (vitamin D-dependent rickets type 2)
Others
Hyperphosphatemia
Chronic renal failure
Tumor lysis syndrome
Rhabdomyolysis
Acute pancreatitis
Burns
Hungry bone syndrome
Osteoblastic bone metastasis
Transfusion with citrated blood products
Critical illness
Pseudohypocalcemia: Gadolinium-based contrast agents: gadodiamide and gadoversetamide B
Medications
  Hypocalcemia with decreased PTH levels
    Drug-induced hypomagnesemia: Cisplatin, diuretics, aminoglycosides, amphotericin
    Drug-induced hypermagnesemia: Magnesium-containing antacids or laxatives, tocolytic therapy
    Cinacalcet
    Alcohol abuse
  Hypocalcemia with increased PTH levels

of an upper arm blood pressure cuff to 20 mmHg above systolic blood pressure for 3 minutes (Trousseau's sign) [6]. Trousseau's sign may be present in up to 1–2% of healthy subjects without hypocalcemia, so it is also not pathognomonic of hypocalcemia.

More severe hypocalcemia may cause bronchospasm, laryngospasm, seizures, cardiac dysrhythmias associated with QT interval prolongation, coma, or sudden death. Head CT, MRI, or X-ray imaging may demonstrate calcification of the basal ganglia and other intracerebral structures. Patients may develop posterior subcapsular cataracts related to long-standing treatment-related increases in the calcium x phosphate product, or pseudotumor cerebri. Prolonged hypocalcemia may cause congestive heart failure due to cardiomyopathy, which may reverse with appropriate management of hypocalcemia. Patients often report feeling weak, fatigued, or depressed until hypocalcemia is corrected.

Differential Diagnosis

Causes of hypocalcemia may be broadly divided into PTH-related and non-PTH-related causes (Table 21.2). PTH-related hypocalcemia is most often due to PTH deficiency or resistance. A large portion of non-PTH-related causes are due to vitamin D deficiency or resistance, with a wide variety of other less common causes. This section briefly reviews the multiple causes of hypocalcemia and gives several case illustrations of different causes.

Table 21.2 (continued)

Calcium-chelating agents: EDTA, citrate, foscarnet, hydrofluoric acid

Vitamin D deficiency or resistance: Phenytoin, phenobarbital, carbamazepine, valproate, isoniazid, theophylline, glutethimide, rifampicin

Skeletal antiresorptive agents: Bisphosphonates, denosumab, estrogens, raloxifene, calcitonin, plicamycin, colchicine overdose

Loop diuretics

PPIs and H2-blockers

Glucocorticoid therapy

Others:

Propylthiouracil (PTU)

Dobutamine

Calcium channel blockers

Strontium-89

Deferasirox

Bicarbonate therapy

Electroconvulsive therapy

PTH-Mediated Hypocalcemia

Hypoparathyroidism

By far the most common cause of hypoparathyroidism in adults is postsurgical hypoparathyroidism [7]. Postsurgical hypoparathyroidism occurs after anterior neck surgery, not just due to surgery targeting the parathyroid glands. The parathyroid glands may be adversely affected by compromised blood supply after manipulation during surgery on other neck structures, or by inadvertent removal. Postsurgical hypoparathyroidism usually results in hypocalcemia within 24–48 h after surgery and is usually temporary. Different centers have reported different rates of symptomatic hypoparathyroidism after thyroid cancer surgery, ranging from 1 to 46% of cases [8], whereas long-term postsurgical hypoparathyroidism is usually limited to less than 1–2% of cases, depending on surgical expertise. The rate of postthyroidectomy hypoparathyroidism increases with the stage of thyroid cancer and is dependent on the extent of surgery, with about half of stage IV patients suffering from postsurgical hypoparathyroidism. Thyroidectomy for Graves' disease was an independent predictor of both transient and permanent hypoparathyroidism [9].

Illustration: Case 1

A 29-year-old female was referred for post-thyroidectomy tetany. She had undergone surgery for a benign multinodular goiter, without evidence of malignancy at pathology review. The morning after surgery, her serum total calcium was decreased at 5.8 mg/dL (normal, 8.9–10.1), serum phospho-

rus mildly increased at 4.8 mg/dL (normal, 2.5–4.5), and serum creatinine normal at 0.9 mg/dL (normal, 0.8–1.3). Her serum 25-hydroxyvitamin D was normal at 38 ng/mL (optimal, 20–50 ng/mL). Her serum parathyroid hormone was undetectable at <6 pg/mL (normal, 15–65). Her serum magnesium was normal at 1.9 mg/dL (normal, 1.7–2.3 mg/dL). These findings indicate that postsurgical hypoparathyroidism was the cause of her hypocalcemia and hyperphosphatemia. Unfortunately about 75% of adults diagnosed with acquired hypoparathyroidism are postsurgical, with surgery sometimes being done for benign causes such as goiter or primary hyperparathyroidism, but more often for thyroid or other head or neck cancers.

Most patients with postsurgical hypoparathyroidism have transient hypoparathyroidism. Experience of the surgeon performing surgery generally predicts the incidence of postsurgical hypoparathyroidism. Immediate postoperative PTH levels may be useful in predicting which patients will develop permanent hypocalcemia due to postsurgical hypoparathyroidism [10].

Nonsurgical hypoparathyroidism may be due to deficiency or excess of serum magnesium [11, 12]. Hypomagnesemia usually causes hypoparathyroidism when serum magnesium is less than 1.0 mg/dL. Up to 11% of hospitalized patients may have hypomagnesemia, while up to 9% may have hypermagnesemia [13]. Hypomagnesemia may be due to gastrointestinal losses associated with vomiting related to excessive alcohol intake, chronic diarrhea, steatorrhea, malabsorption, or intestinal resection; renal tubular losses due to medications such as furosemide, aminoglycosides, cisplatin, cyclosporin, amphotericin B, pentamidine, tacrolimus, or proton pump inhibitors [14]; or rare genetic disorders such as Gitelman syndrome. Hypomagnesemia occurs frequently in critically ill patients, which contributes to the hypocalcemia frequently seen in intensive care unit patients. Hypermagnesemia may occur in the setting of late-stage chronic kidney disease in patients treated with magnesium antacids, enemas, or infusions, tocolytic therapy during labor, or acute renal failure associated with rhabdomyolysis or tumor lysis syndrome [15].

Illustration: Case 2

A 48-year-old male was referred for possible hypoparathyroidism. His serum calcium was decreased at 6.7 mg/dL (normal, 8.9–10.1 mg/dL), with serum phosphorus increased at 5.5 mg/dL (normal, 2.5–4.5 mg/dL), and serum creatinine normal at 1.3 mg/dL (normal, 0.8–1.3 mg/dL). His serum 25-hydroxyvitamin D was normal at 45 ng/mL (optimal, 20–50 ng/mL). His serum PTH was decreased at 8 pg/mL (normal, 15–65 pg/mL). His serum magnesium was very low at 0.8 mg/dL (normal, 1.7–2.3 mg/dL). These findings indicate that significant magnesium deficiency was the primary cause of his hypoparathyroidism leading to hypocalcemia and hyperphosphatemia. Further evaluation demonstrated renal tubular magnesium wasting due to previous use of outdated aminoglycoside antibiotics.

Primary intestinal hypomagnesemia results from a rare inherited disorder causing magnesium malabsorption leading to hypomagnesemia in early infancy. This condition is thought to primarily occur due to deficient intestinal magnesium absorption, but there may also be defects in renal magnesium reabsorption. Patients usually present with neurological symptoms, including tetany, muscle spasms, and seizures due to both hypomagnesemia and hypocalcemia associated with hypoparathyroidism. Lifelong high oral intake of magnesium supplements decreases symptoms and restores serum calcium levels to normal. Mutations in the TRMP6 gene on chromosome 9 have been identified to cause this disorder [16, 17]. The TRMP6 protein is a member of the transient receptor membrane potential channel family that complexes to TRPM7, a calcium- and magnesium-permeable cation channel.

Other acquired causes of hypoparathyroidism are much rarer. Infiltration and destruction of the parathyroid glands by iron overload may occur in hemochromatosis, or thalassemia requiring multiple blood transfusions [18]. Copper overload occurring due to Wilson's disease may also result in hypoparathyroidism [19].

Hypoparathyroidism may result from metastases to the parathyroid glands in extremely rare circumstances [20]. External beam radiation therapy to the neck for treatment of malignant disease in this region, or radioactive iodine therapy for Graves' disease, may also rarely result in destruction of the parathyroid glands [21].

Inherited causes of hypoparathyroidism include autosomal dominant hypocalcemia (ADH), a condition in which there is a gain-of-function mutation in the CaSR [22]. This type of mutation changes the threshold of PTH secretion by parathyroid cells in response to circulating ionized calcium, leading to low or inappropriately normal PTH secretion despite hypocalcemia. Most of the mutations reported to date affect the extracellular amino-terminal or transmembrane domains of the receptor. The mutant receptors may show both increased receptor sensitivity to calcium and increased maximal signal transduction capacity.

Since this activating mutation is also expressed in the CaSR on proximal renal tubular cells in the thick ascending limb of Henle, absolute or relatively increased 24-h urinary calcium excretion is a hallmark of the disorder. Most patients with ADH are asymptomatic and have mild hypocalcemia with significant hypercalciuria, but occasional patients may present with moderate or severe hypocalcemia. This form of

CaSR-mediated hypoparathyroidism may cause increased risk of nephrocalcinosis compared to other forms of hypoparathyroidism. In one series, almost half of the patients evaluated had nephrocalcinosis associated with hypercalciuria [23]. Calcium supplementation must therefore be monitored carefully in this condition.

Occasional reports have described patients with CaSR gain-of-function mutations associated with a Bartter-like syndrome, suggesting that the CaSR may also play a role in sodium chloride regulation [24]. These patients present with hypocalcemia, hypercalciuria, and nephrocalcinosis, associated with hypokalemic alkalosis, renal salt wasting that may cause hypotension, hyperreninemic hyperaldosteronism, and increased urinary prostaglandin excretion. Extensive burns may lead to upregulation of the CaSR, with lower than normal serum calcium suppressing PTH secretion, resulting in hypocalcemia and hypoparathyroidism.

Autoimmune hypoparathyroidism is thought to be the second most common form of acquired hypoparathyroidism, after postsurgical hypoparathyroidism. Isolated autoimmune destruction of the parathyroid glands may occur, resulting in idiopathic hypoparathyroidism, or autoimmune destruction may occur in association with other autoimmune conditions as part of autosomal recessive autoimmune polyglandular endocrinopathy candidiasis ectodermal dystrophy (APECED) syndrome [25]. This syndrome is caused by mutations in the autoimmune regulator gene AIRE, which results in abnormal thymic expression of tissue antigens, generation of autoreactive T cells, ultimate loss of central tolerance to specific self-antigens, and the development of multiple autoimmune disorders [26]. Antibodies against the CaSR have been identified in some individuals with both idiopathic hypoparathyroidism or APECED syndrome [27, 28], but it is not yet clear if these antibodies are causative or simply markers of disease [29]. Idiopathic autoimmune hypoparathyroidism most often occurs in the teens or the young adulthood but may occur at any age. APECED usually presents in childhood and is characterized by chronic mucocutaneous candidiasis and Addison's disease, in addition to the variable expression of endocrine and other autoimmune diseases. Variation in the clinical phenotype of individuals with identical mutations in the AIRE gene is incompletely understood, but this suggests that other genetic loci or environmental factors are important in the development of the phenotype.

Hypoparathyroidism may be diagnosed at birth or during childhood due to a variety of genetic mutations causing congenital syndromes, the most widely known being the DiGeorge (velocardiofacial) syndrome [30]. This disorder is caused by abnormal development of neural crest cells in the third and fourth branchial pouches. In 90% of cases, the syndrome is caused by heterozygous chromosomal deletion of the *TBX1* gene in the region of chromosome 22q11. Thirty-five genes have been identified in this region, so deletion of other genes, alone or in combination, could also cause this syndrome, but the *TBX1* gene is a major determinant of cardiac, thymus, and parathyroid cell phenotypes. A region on chromosome 10p (DiGeorge critical region II) has also been linked to the syndrome. DiGeorge syndrome is associated with distinctive facial abnormalities, cleft lip and/or palate, conotruncal cardiac anomalies, and mild-to-moderate immune deficiency. Hypocalcemia due to hypoparathyroidism has been reported in 17–60% of affected children [31]. DiGeorge syndrome is estimated to occur in as many as 1:2000–1:3000 births, with the incidence rate of new mutations estimated at 1:4000–1:6000. Because the clinical phenotype varies, findings may be subtle and therefore overlooked, and mild hypocalcemia may be easily missed. In one study of adults with chromosome 22q11.2 deletion, about half were hypocalcemic, with a median age of presentation of 25 years and a maximum age of diagnosis of up to 48 years [32]. This disorder may rarely be diagnosed for the first time as late as the mid-60s, with late onset of mild hypocalcemia, and is not infrequently diagnosed in an affected parent in the 20s or 30s after birth of an affected child.

Finally, a variety of other rare genetic or inherited disorders may cause hypocalcemia that is recognized in infancy or childhood. Familial isolated hypoparathyroidism due to autosomal recessive or dominant mutations in the *pre–proPTH* gene on chromosome 11p15 [33, 34], or parathyroid gland dysgenesis due to mutations in various transcription factors regulating parathyroid gland development such as *GCMB* (glial cells missing B) [35] or *GCM2* (glial cells missing 2) [36], *GATA3* [37, 38], or Sry-box 3 (*SOX3*) [39], is thought to be very rare. Autosomal dominant hypoparathyroidism associated with deafness and renal anomalies has been linked to mutations in the *GATA3* gene on chromosome 10p14-10-pter [37, 38]. Hypoparathyroidism has been very rarely associated with X-linked recessive mutations on Xq26-27, leading to disruption of SOX3 transcription [39]. The syndrome of autosomal recessive hypoparathyroidism, growth and mental retardation, and dysmorphism due to mutations in the *TBCE* gene on chromosome 1q42-q43 is another very rare

cause of hypoparathyroidism [40]. Hypoparathyroidism with metabolic disturbances and congenital anomalies has been associated with rare maternal mitochondrial gene defects [41, 42].

PTH Resistance

Pseudohypoparathyroidism (PHP) is a complex disorder with several recognized subtypes, characterized biochemically by hypocalcemia, hyperphosphatemia, and hyperparathyroidism due to tissue unresponsiveness to PTH [43] (Table 21.3). Most often hypocalcemia is not present at birth and typically develops during childhood. The previous gold standard for diagnosis of PHP was the Ellsworth–Howard test, in which bovine PTH was infused to determine if urinary cyclic AMP increased normally. In most forms of PHP, urinary cyclic AMP does not increase as expected. This test is rarely performed today due to lack of bovine PTH, and the diagnosis is often based on the constellation of biochemical findings, family history when present, and genetic analysis.

PHP is further classified as types 1a, pseudo-PHP, 1b, 1c, or 2. In PHP type 1a, the most common subtype, loss-of-function mutations in the coding region of the maternally inherited *GNAS* gene encoding the Gsα subunit of G proteins causes the disorder, with resultant 50% loss of Gsα protein expression [44]. PHP type 1a patients have PTH resistance at the renal tubule, resulting in a blunted phosphaturic and cAMP response to PTH. This blunted response is due to lack of normal signaling by the PTH receptor due to reduced stimulatory G protein expression.

PHP type 1a is characterized by Albright's hereditary osteodystrophy (AHO), which includes obesity, round facies, mild mental retardation, and a skeletal phenotype involving short stature, brachydactyly of hands and/or feet, and heterotopic ossifications in subcutaneous tissues. This disorder is frequently associated with multiple hormone resistance involving thyroid-stimulating hormone (TSH), luteinizing hormone (LH), follicle-stimulating hormone (FSH), calcitonin, and/or growth hormone-releasing hormone (GHRH).

Patients with PHP type 1a have renal tubule PTH resistance because they inherit a mutated maternally imprinted *GNAS* allele. *GNAS* alleles undergo differential imprinting in

Table 21.3 Characteristics of pseudohypoparathyroidism subtypes

Type	Gsα activity	AHO	PTH resistance	Urinary cAMP response	Multiple hormone resistance	Molecular defect
1a	Reduced	Yes	Yes	Reduced	Yes	Heterozygous mutations in *GNAS*
Pseudo-PHP	Reduced	Yes	No	Normal	No	Heterozygous mutation in *GNAS*
1b	Normal	No	Kidney	Reduced	No	Imprinting defect in *GNAS*
1c	Normal	No	Yes	Reduced	Yes	Unknown
2	Normal	No	Kidney	Normal	No	Unknown

AHO indicates Albright's hereditary osteodystrophy, *cAMP* cyclic adenosine monophosphate, *PTH* parathyroid hormone mothers and fathers, with tissue-specific expression of alleles in offspring. Only the maternal allele is expressed in the kidney and in the relevant endocrine organs associated with hormone resistance in this form of the disorder, but the rest of the body expresses both maternal and paternal alleles. An affected allele in other body tissues leads to haploinsufficiency and AHO expression, but PTH resistance occurs only in the tissues expressing the maternal allele.

Patients with paternally inherited *GNAS* mutations who have AHO without renal or endocrine gland resistance are designated as having pseudo-PHP. Patients with pseudo-PHP have a normal urinary cAMP response to PTH, unlike PHP type 1a patients. Patients with both PHP type 1a or pseudo-PHP may occur in the same kindred. In some cases both forms are found in the same generation, but more often the two forms are found in different generations.

PHP type 1b patients lack typical features of AHO but may have mild brachydactyly [45]. Levels of Gsα in accessible tissues are normal, but patients have renal tubular PTH resistance without resistance to other hormones, although some may have mildly increased TSH levels. Skeletal manifestations are similar to those seen in patients with hyperparathyroidism, with bone loss or changes of osteitis fibrosa cystica. Most cases are due to switching of the maternal *GNAS* allele to a paternal pattern of methylation, caused by microdeletions in the *STX16* gene located 220 kB centromeric from *GNAS* exon 1A, or deletions removing the differentially methylated region involving exon NESP55 or exons 3 and 4 of the antisense transcript [46]. In both situations, inheritance of a mutation from a female, or spontaneous mutation of a maternally derived allele, removes the maternal *GNAS* epigenotype, leading to transcriptional silencing of the Gsα promoter in imprinted tissues, with little or no expression of either *GNAS* allele in these tissues.

Patients with PHP type 1c have normal Gsα activity and lack identifiable mutations in *GNAS* and are thought to represent a variant of PHP type 1a. PHP type 2 patients have normal cAMP production in response to administered PTH but lack a phosphaturic effect. Little is known about the mutations involved, but because the biochemical picture is similar to that of severe vitamin D deficiency, it may be that most, if not all, cases of PHP type 2 are due to unsuspected vitamin D deficiency.

PTH stimulates the proximal tubule to decrease phosphate reabsorption and increase calcium reabsorption in the distal tubule. In patients with PHP type 1a, the distal tubule phosphaturic effect is blunted, and there is no hypercalciuric effect, so these patients do not form kidney stones as might be expected. Calcium may therefore be supplemented to a greater level than in other causes of hypoparathyroidism without contributing to calcium nephrolithiasis [47].

Hypomagnesemia also causes PTH resistance, and there is often a lag time to normalization of serum calcium levels despite a normal or an increased PTH level after magnesium repletion [15].

Vitamin D-Related Hypocalcemia

Patients with vitamin D deficiency or resistance often develop hypocalcemia. Nutritional vitamin D deficiency may be the most common cause of hypocalcemia throughout the world, resulting from inadequate intake or lack of sunlight exposure [48]. Intestinal malabsorption of vitamin D from many causes may also lead to hypocalcemia. Rare cases of vitamin D resistance, either due to 1α-hydroxylase deficiency or vitamin D receptor mutations, typically present with hypocalcemia. Consequences of hypocalcemia associated with vitamin D deficiency may be severe, including increased risk of hip fracture [49].

Vitamin D Deficiency

Vitamin D2 (ergocalciferol) is normally obtained from plant sources or supplements and vitamin D3 (cholecalciferol) from skin sunlight exposure or supplements. Both forms are transported in the circulation to the liver by vitamin D-binding protein, where they are converted by 25-hydroxylase to 25-hydroxyvitamin D, and then in a smaller amount to the kidneys, where they are 1α-hydroxylated to 1,25-dihydroxyvitamin D. Serum 1,25-dihydroxyvitamin D is the biologically active form of vitamin D in the body because of its 1000-fold higher affinity for the vitamin D receptor than 25-hydroxyvitamin D, and this form normally stimulates the intestine to actively transport calcium and phosphorus from the lumen into the bloodstream by upregulating intestinal transport proteins, particularly when calcium or phosphorus intake is decreased [50]. Serum 1,25-dihydroxyvitamin D also directly suppresses PTH transcription in parathyroid cells, leading to decreased PTH secretion, as well as stimulating osteoclast and osteoblast recruitment and activation in the skeleton. This form of vitamin D feeds back to suppress its own production by renal 1α-hydroxylase and stimulates 24-hydroxylase to increase its own metabolism. Because increased serum PTH, decreased serum calcium, or increased serum phosphorus all normally independently upregulate renal 1α-hydroxylase, hypoparathyroidism leads to reduced renal 1α-hydroxylase activity and decreased 1,25-dihydroxyvitamin D production if serum calcium and phosphorus do not change to accommodate the decreased PTH level.

Illustration: Case 3

A 58-year-old female was seen in hospital after falling at home and sustaining a left hip fracture. Her serum calcium before fracture repair was 7.6 mg/dL (normal, 8.9–10.1 mg/dL), with serum phosphorus 2.3 mg/dL (normal, 2.5–4.5 mg/dL), with her serum creatinine normal at 1.1 mg/dL (normal, 0.6–1.1 mg/dL). Her serum 25-hydroxyvitamin D was very low at 6.6 ng/mL (optimal, 20–50 ng/mL). Her serum PTH was increased at 82 pg/mL (normal, 15–65 pg/mL). Her serum magnesium was normal at 2.2 mg/dL (normal, 1.7–2.3 mg/dL). Her findings indicate that she had significant vitamin D deficiency as the cause of her hypocalcemia and mild hypophosphatemia. Her profound vitamin D deficiency was attributed to lack of sunlight exposure and lack of dietary or supplemental intake of vitamin D. She had been avoiding sunlight to minimize her risk of skin cancer. Vitamin D3 replacement with 50,000 U twice weekly was started after hip surgery for 2 months to replete her vitamin D level.

Any cause of vitamin D deficiency may lead to both hypocalcemia and hypophosphatemia, triggering an increase in PTH that upregulates renal 1α-hydroxylase. Persistent stimulation of PTH secretion by any cause often leads to increased serum total and bone alkaline phosphatase and bone loss over time. If vitamin D deficiency is severe and chronic, this may ultimately lead to excessive production of unmineralized collagenous and noncollagenous matrix in the skeleton, leading to osteomalacia in adults or rickets in children.

It has become appreciated that vitamin D deficiency is common in community-dwelling adults in most countries [51], as well as in hospitalized patients [52], but the prevalence estimate depends on how vitamin D deficiency is defined. Most experts consider serum 25-hydroxyvitamin D to be the best marker of nutritional vitamin D intake currently available, with levels below 10 ng/mL (25 nmol/L) considered deficient because of the increased likelihood of osteomalacia or rickets at this level [53]. Optimal levels associated with nutritional adequacy continue to be debated, with most bone specialists recommending 30 ng/mL (75 nmol/L) for treatment of osteoporosis or metabolic bone disease. The 2011 US Institute of Medicine report concluded that 20 ng/mL (50 nmol/L) was adequate for maintenance of skeletal health in the general population and emphasized that optimal vitamin D levels have not yet been established for most human diseases [54]. In light of the current controversy regarding vitamin D adequacy and optimal levels, vitamin D insufficiency is most often defined as levels between 10 and 20 ng/mL (25–50 nmol/L).

Excessive supplementation with vitamin D by patients is increasingly common, frequently leading to hypercalciuria, but vitamin D toxicity manifested by hypercalcemia remains uncommon. Most bone specialists regard serum 25-hydroxyvitamin D levels above 80 ng/mL (200 nmol/L) with concern, but it is uncommon to see hypercalcemia unless serum 25-hydroxyvitamin D is greater than 150 ng/mL (375 nmol/L).

Any cause that disrupts vitamin D absorption, synthesis, transport, interaction with vitamin D receptors in target tissues, or metabolism may lead to a decrease in vitamin D actions [48]. Inadequate sunlight exposure, especially in the elderly, or those with hyperpigmented skin or using high-grade sunblock to prevent sunburn, may develop vitamin D deficiency. Any cause of malnutrition, intestinal malabsorption, chronic liver disease, or mid- or late-stage chronic kidney disease may lead to inadequate vitamin D absorption or production. Drugs that upregulate cytochrome P450 enzymes that metabolize vitamin D, such as anticonvulsants, including phenytoin, phenobarbital, carbamazepine, or valproate, may lead to vitamin D deficiency if sunlight exposure or dietary or supplemental intake is not sufficient to compensate for increased metabolism [55].

Rare mutations in the CYP27B1 gene affecting the activity of renal 1α-hydroxylase activity give rise to pseudovitamin D deficiency rickets, previously known as vitamin D-dependent rickets type 1 (VDDR1) [56, 57]. This condition results in partial or complete deficiency of the 1α-hydroxylase enzyme, leading to very low levels of 1,25-dihydroxyvitamin D production, with significant hypocalcemia and hypophosphatemia. This condition is diagnosed shortly after birth or in infancy with tetany, seizures, rickets, and failure to thrive. Nutritional vitamin D deficiency causes decreased serum calcium, phosphorus, and 25-hydroxyvitamin D levels, but serum 1,25-dihydroxyvitamin D levels typically remain normal until serum 25-hydroxyvitamin D levels fall to less than 4 ng/mL (10 nmol/L). In this situation, lack of substrate availability leads to a decrease in serum 1,25-dihydroxyvitamin D. In pseudovitamin D deficiency rickets, lack of functional 1α-hydroxylase leads to low serum calcium and phosphorus, increased total and bone alkaline phosphatase, normal 25-hydroxyvitamin D, and very low or undetectable 1,25-dihydroxyvitamin D levels.

Vitamin D-Resistant Rickets

Hereditary vitamin D-resistant rickets is a rare autosomal recessive genetic disorder previously known as VDDR type 2 [58]. This disorder is caused by a mutation in the vitamin D receptor that leads to resistance to the action of 1,25-dihydroxyvitamin D. Mutations have been reported in the ligand-binding domain, DNA-binding domain, and other domains. Resistance to 1,25-dihydroxyvitamin D may be partial or complete. Affected children typically present before age 2 years but occasionally as late as their teens, similar to children with pseudovitamin D deficiency rickets [59], with tetany, seizures, rickets, and failure to thrive. Laboratory assessment shows hypocalcemia, hypophosphatemia, increased alkaline phosphatase, normal 25-hydroxyvitamin D, and increased 1,25-dihydroxyvitamin D. Hyperparathyroidism resulting from the hypocalcemia stimulates renal 1α-hydroxylase production of 1,25-dihydroxyvitamin D. Increased serum 1,25-dihydroxyvitamin D is the main biochemical feature distinguishing this disorder from pseudovitamin D deficiency rickets. Patients have partial or total scalp alopecia in two-thirds of the kindreds reported. The level of hypocalcemia is variable between kindreds as well. Patients do not respond to usual replacement doses of vitamin D or calcium but may respond to pharmacological doses of vitamin D in some cases, depending on residual vitamin D receptor activity. Those with no vitamin D receptor activity usually require treatment with intravenous calcium and/or high-dose oral calcium.

Other Causes of Hypocalcemia

A variety of heterogeneous causes of hypocalcemia exist beyond those commonly recognized to be due to hypoparathyroidism or vitamin D deficiency or resistance.

Hyperphosphatemia of any cause, but commonly due to later stage chronic kidney disease, may reduce serum calcium by complexing to calcium in the circulation and causing soft tissue deposition of calcium phosphate complexes. Renal failure is associated with hyperphosphatemia and decreased 1α-hydroxylase activity, leading to decreased 1,25-dihydroxyvitamin D production. A variety of medications may cause hyperphosphatemia if taken in excessive amounts, including phosphate-containing laxatives or enemas or intravenous phosphorus given to lower serum calcium. Tumor lysis syndrome and rhabdomyolysis may result in acute hyperphosphatemia and lead to acute hypocalcemia.

Transfusions of citrated blood products, usually in large quantities, may cause acute hypocalcemia due to the formation of calcium citrate complexes in the serum. Acute pancreatitis releases lipase into surrounding tissue fluids, which may lead to increased free fatty acids that saponify calcium, resulting in significant hypocalcemia. Excessive uptake of calcium by bone that overwhelms homeostatic mechanisms in place to maintain normal serum calcium will cause hypocalcemia, as seen with "hungry bone" syndrome after surgical cure of severe, long-standing hyperparathyroidism. Older age, higher preoperative serum alkaline phosphatase levels, and larger weight of resected adenoma all predict a higher risk of "hungry bone" syndrome [60]. Rarely, extensive osteoblastic metastases may cause hypocalcemia because of

rapid uptake and formation of new bone. Critical illness is often associated with hypocalcemia because of multiple concurrent causes that may be present [61].

A variety of medications may directly cause hypocalcemia by a variety of mechanisms (Table 21.3). Pseudohypocalcemia may occur within several hours of administration of certain gadolinium-containing contrast agents for magnetic resonance imaging studies [62]. In this situation, spurious critical hypocalcemia of less than 6.0 mg/dL may be found because certain gadolinium agents, but not all, interfere with calcium measurement in certain colorimetric assays. In this case, rechecking serum calcium by a different assay method will usually clarify the diagnosis. Patients reported to have critical hypocalcemia in this setting usually remain asymptomatic, which should raise suspicion regarding the accuracy of the serum calcium level.

With the increasing recognition and treatment of osteoporosis, many patients are treated with antiresorptive agents including oral and intravenous bisphosphonates, denosumab, or raloxifene that may precipitate hypocalcemia [63]. It is prudent to make sure that such patients are treated with adequate vitamin D and calcium before treating these patients to prevent hypocalcemia.

Laboratory Tests and Interpretation

Evaluation of hypocalcemia depends heavily on laboratory studies available to the clinician. Initial laboratory testing should include measurement of serum total calcium, albumin for calculating albumin-corrected serum calcium, ionized calcium if available, magnesium, PTH, and 25-hydroxyvitamin D levels. Serum phosphorus and creatinine should be measured also, as interpretation of the other values is often difficult without knowledge of serum phosphorus or creatinine levels.

Serum 25-hydroxyvitamin D is generally most reliably measured by tandem mass spectroscopy, but this expensive technique is not available in many laboratories. Most clinicians consider serum 25-hydroxyvitamin D less than 10 ng/mL (25 nmol/L) to be deficient because of the increased likelihood of osteomalacia [53]. The Institute of Medicine considers 20 ng/mL (50 nmol/L) an adequate level for skeletal purposes in healthy adults [54]. Serum 25-hydroxyvitamin D between 10 and 20 ng/mL (25–50 nmol/L) is considered by most bone specialists to be insufficient. The upper limit of normal for serum 25-hydroxyvitamin D is considered to be 50 ng/mL (75 nmol/L) by many bone specialists because of the hypercalciuria that may occur above this level. Vitamin D toxicity, with associated hypercalcemia, typically does not occur unless serum 25-hydroxyvitamin D is greater than 150 ng/mL (375 nmol/L) but may rarely occur when above 80 ng/mL (200 nmol/L).

Measurement of intact PTH by a reliable second- or third-generation assay will detect inappropriately low, low–normal, or undetectable values in hypoparathyroid patients. There is less variability in measurement of PTH than 25-hydroxyvitamin D. Serum magnesium deficiency or excess may both limit secretion of PTH [12, 13], so patients with apparent hypoparathyroidism with low serum calcium, increased serum phosphorus, normal creatinine, normal 25-hydroxyvitamin D, and low PTH should always have their serum magnesium checked. Patients with hypoparathyroidism usually have low serum calcium, increased serum phosphorus, normal creatinine, normal 25-hydroxyvitamin D, and low-to-undetectable PTH. Patients with pseudohypoparathyroidism typically have low serum calcium, increased serum phosphorus, normal creatinine, normal 25-hydroxyvitamin D, and increased PTH. Patients with vitamin D deficiency usually have low serum calcium and phosphorus, normal creatinine, and increased PTH.

Measurement of 24-h urine calcium or magnesium may be very important in sorting out the cause of hypocalcemia. Increased 24-h urine calcium may suggest idiopathic hypercalciuria in the untreated patient but is likely due to overtreatment with calcium or vitamin D supplementation in treated hypocalcemic patients. Markedly increased 24-h urinary calcium and asymptomatic mildly decreased serum calcium may be due to autosomal dominant hypocalcemia. Untreated hypocalcemic patients usually have decreased or low–normal 24-h urine calcium. Increased 24-h urine magnesium in the setting of hypomagnesemia strongly suggests renal tubular magnesium wasting, rather than gastrointestinal loss of magnesium.

Management

Treatment of hypocalcemia is intended primarily to improve or eliminate symptoms, reverse skeletal demineralization to the degree it is present, heal osteomalacia if present, maintain acceptable serum total or ionized calcium, and avoid hypercalciuria (24-h urine calcium >300 mg), renal dysfunction, kidney stones, and nephrocalcinosis [64]. Patients who have need for urgent treatment due to symptoms, such as tetany, seizures, laryngospasm, bronchospasm, cardiac rhythm disturbances, altered mental status, or severe hypocalcemia, require intravenous calcium, usually given as calcium gluconate. Typically ten 10-mL ampules of calcium gluconate, with 93 mg elemental calcium per ampule, are added to 900 mL of 5% dextrose and 10 mL infused slowly over 10 min to improve symptoms, with repeat infusion given once or twice more as needed. A maintenance infusion is then typically begun at 10–100 mL/h to control symptoms and improve serum calcium to the lower end of the normal range at around 8.5 mg/dL (2.12 mmol/L), with ionized calcium of around 4 mg/dL (1.0 mmol/L). The infusion rate can be calculated to give 0.3–1.0 mg elemental calcium/kg/h.

After stabilization of the patient, an oral regimen may be started, providing the patient with at least 500 mg elemental calcium three to four times a day. The calcium gluconate infusion is gradually tapered as serum calcium approaches the target level, symptoms improved, and oral calcium supplements are tolerated.

Management of chronic hypocalcemia usually involves oral calcium and vitamin D supplementation, sometimes with thiazide-type diuretics or magnesium supplementation. If serum magnesium levels are decreased, magnesium total body deficits are usually very large, but poorly reflected by the serum magnesium level, because magnesium is mostly located intracellularly. Supplementation with magnesium usually takes months to fully replete body stores. As serum magnesium is gradually repleted, serum calcium and PTH levels return toward normal.

Oral calcium supplements of any type will restore serum calcium toward normal. In general, calcium carbonate or calcium citrate is used most commonly because they are widely available and relatively inexpensive. Calcium carbonate is 40% calcium by weight and calcium citrate 21% calcium by weight. Calcium supplements are usually given in divided doses each day, typically between two and four times a day, with dosing given with meals to enhance absorption. Starting doses are usually 500–1000 mg elemental calcium two or three times each day and titrated upward as needed based on the tolerability, compliance, and clinical target. If calcium supplementation alone is insufficient to achieve serum calcium of 8.0–8.5 mg/dL (2.0–2.13 mmol/L), active vitamin D supplementation is usually started. If renal function is normal, vitamin D2 (ergocalciferol) or D3 (cholecalciferol) may be started at 1000–4000 International Units each day, or alternatively, 50,000 International Units once weekly to several times a week as needed, depending on intestinal absorption efficiency. Severe hypoparathyroidism or PHP typically require higher doses of vitamin D. Care must be taken with these forms of vitamin D, however, as their half-life is prolonged due to storage in body fat, and toxic serum levels of 25-hydroxyvitamin D may take 6–9 months to clear after supplementation is stopped. Because of concerns regarding toxicity, calcitriol (1,25-dihydroxyvitamin D) 0.25 μg once or twice a day is often started in place of vitamin D2 or D3 in the USA, whereas alfacalcidol (1α-hydroxyvitamin D) in low doses is used in Europe. The half-life of these forms of vitamin D is on the order of 1–3 days, so improvement in absorption or offset of action occurs more rapidly. Commercial parenteral vitamin D is no longer available in the USA, but some hospital-compounding pharmacies produce intravenous vitamin D3 based on clinical need.

Patients who develop hypercalciuria while on calcium and vitamin D supplementation, or who are unable to achieve or maintain serum calcium at or near their target range, may require addition of a thiazide-type diuretic to reduce urinary calcium loss. Doses of hydrochlorothiazide or chlorthalidone of 12.5–25 mg each day may be beneficial, but some patients may require as much as 50 or 100 mg to decrease their 24-h urine calcium to less than 300 mg.

Once- or twice-daily injections of PTH 1–34 (teriparatide or other) have been used off-label in short-term trials to normalize serum and urine calcium and phosphorus in patients with hypoparathyroidism [64–66]. This therapy has not been approved by the FDA for treatment of hypoparathyroidism. A pivotal 6-month phase III clinical trial with recombinant human PTH 1–84 (Natpara) was published in 2013 [67], with FDA approval as an adjunct for treatment of hypoparathyroidism in January 2015 and approval in Europe in April 2017. Guidelines for use of recombinant human PTH 1–84 in hypoparathyroidism have recently been published [68, 69].

Parathyroid allograft transplants have been used in a few individuals who either previously or simultaneously have undergone renal transplantation [70, 71]. Advances in stem cell technology may eventually permit stem cells to be used to create new parathyroid tissue in patients where it is lacking.

Patients with pseudovitamin D deficiency rickets (VDDR1) respond to physiologic doses of 1,25-dihydroxyvitamin D3 and calcium and require lifelong therapy. Patients with hereditary vitamin D-resistant rickets (vitamin D-dependent rickets type 2) are challenging to manage, because pharmacologic doses of 1,25-dihydroxyvitamin D3 are usually required to overcome resistance. Calcium supplements of up to 3000 mg elemental calcium may be required. Therapy is continued until undermineralized bones are mineralized, typically within 2–6 months. Close follow-up is necessary to monitor parameters of calcium and mineral metabolism and clinical signs and symptoms. Some cases have failed to respond to this therapy despite 1,25-dihydroxyvitamin D3 levels more than 100 times normal. Long-term calcium infusions in combination with high-dose oral calcium supplements have been used successfully in this situation.

References

1. Shoback D. Clinical practice. Hypoparathyroidism. N Engl J Med. 2008;359:391–403.
2. Shafer AL, Shoback D. Hypocalcemia: definition, etiology, pathogenesis, diagnosis, and management. In: Rosen CJ, editor. Primer on the metabolic bone diseases and disorders of mineral metabolism. 8th ed. Washington, D.C.: American Society for Bone and Mineral Research; 2013. p. 572–8.
3. Mundy GR, Guise TA. Hormonal control of calcium homeostasis. Clin Chem. 1999;45:1347–52.
4. Kantham L, Quinn SJ, Egbuna OI, et al. The calcium-sensing receptor (CaSR) defends against hypercalcemia independently of its regulation of parathyroid hormone secretion. Am J Physiol Endocrinol Metab. 2009;297:E915–23.
5. McGreal GT, Kelly JL, Hehir DJ, Brady MP. Incidence of false positive Chvostek's sign in hospitalised patients. Ir J Med Sci. 1995;164:56.
6. Rehman HU, Wunder S. Trousseau sign in hypocalcemia. CMAJ. 2011;183:E498.
7. Grant CS, Stulak JM, Thompson GB, et al. Risks and adequacy of an optimized surgical approach to the primary surgical management of papillary thyroid carcinoma treated during 1999–2006. World J Surg. 2010;34:1239–46.
8. Lee YS, Nam KH, Chung WY, et al. Postoperative complications of thyroid cancer in a single center experience. J Korean Med Sci. 2010;25:541–5.
9. Edafe O, Antakia R, Laskar N, et al. Systematic review and meta-analysis of predictors of post-thyroidectomy hypocalcaemia. Br J Surg. 2014;101:307–20.
10. Noordzij JP, Lee SL, Bernet VJ, et al. Early prediction of hypocalcemia after thyroidectomy using parathyroid hormone: an analysis of pooled individual patient data from nine observational studies. J Am Coll Surg. 2007;205:748–54.
11. Rude RK, Oldham SB, Singer FR. Functional hypoparathyroidism and parathyroid hormone end-organ resistance in human magnesium deficiency. Clin Endocrinol. 1976;5:209–24.
12. Cholst IN, Steinberg SF, Tropper PJ, et al. The influence of hypermagnesemia on serum calcium and parathyroid hormone levels in human subjects. N Engl J Med. 1984;310:1221–5.
13. Wong ET, Rude RK, Singer FR, et al. A high prevalence of hypomagnesemia and hypermagnesemia in hospitalized patients. Am J Clin Pathol. 1983;79:348–52.
14. Rude RK. Magnesium deficiency: a heterogeneous cause of disease in humans. J Bone Miner Res. 1997;13:749–58.
15. Rude RK. Magnesium depletion and hypermagnesemia. In: Rosen CJ, editor. Primer on the metabolic bone diseases and disorders of mineral metabolism. 7th ed. Washington, D.C.: American Society for Bone and Mineral Research; 2009. p. 325–8.
16. Schlingmann KP, Sassen MC, Weber S, et al. Novel TRPM6 mutations in 21 families with primary hypomagnesemia and secondary hypocalcemia. J Am Soc Nephrol. 2005;16:3061–9.
17. Voets T, Nilius B, Hoefs S, et al. TRPM6 forms the Mg^{2+} influx channel involved in intestinal and renal Mg^{2+} absorption. J Biol Chem. 2004;279:19–25.
18. Toumba M, Sergis A, Kanaris C, et al. Endocrine complications in patients with thalassemia major. Pediatr Endocrinol Rev. 2007;5:642–8.
19. Carpenter TO, Carnes DL Jr, Anast CS. Hypoparathyroidism in Wilson's disease. N Engl J Med. 1983;309:873–7.
20. Goddard CJ. Symptomatic hypocalcaemia associated with metastatic invasion of the parathyroid glands. Br J Hosp Med. 1990;43:72.
21. Pauwels EK, Smit JW, Slats A, Bourguignon M, Overbeek F. Health effects of therapeutic use of 131I in hyperthyroidism. Q J Nucl Med. 2000;44:333–9.
22. Egbuna OI, Brown EM. Hypercalcaemic and hypocalcaemic conditions due to calcium-sensing receptor mutations. Best Pract Res Clin Rheumatol. 2008;22:129–48.
23. Lienhardt A, Bai M, Lagarde J-P, et al. Activating mutations of the calcium-sensing receptor: management of hypocalcemia. J Clin Endocrinol Metab. 2001;86:5313–23.
24. Vargas-Poussou R, Huang C, Hulin P, et al. Functional characterization of a calcium-sensing receptor mutation in severe autosomal

dominant hypocalcemia with a Bartter-like syndrome. J Am Soc Nephrol. 2002;13:2259–66.

25. Michels AW, Gottlieb PA. Autoimmune polyglandular syndromes. Nat Rev Endocrinol. 2010;6:270–7.

26. Shikama N, Nusspaumer G, Hollander GA. Clearing the AIRE: on the pathophysiological basis of the autoimmune polyendocrinopathy syndrome type-1. Endocrinol Metab Clin N Am. 2009;38:273–88.

27. Blizzard RM, Chee D, Davis W. The incidence of parathyroid and other antibodies in the sera of patients with idiopathic hypoparathyroidism. Clin Exp Immunol. 1966;1:119–28.

28. Li Y, Song YH, Rais N, et al. Autoantibodies to the extracellular domain of the calcium sensing receptor in patients with acquired hypoparathyroidism. J Clin Invest. 1996;97:910–4.

29. Brown EM. Anti-parathyroid and anti-calcium sensing receptor antibodies in autoimmune hypoparathyroidism. Endocrinol Metab Clin N Am. 2009;38:437–45.

30. Goldmuntz E. DiGeorge syndrome: new insights. Clin Perinatol. 2005;32:963–78.

31. McDonald-McGinn DM, Sullivan KE. Chromosome 22q11.2 deletion syndrome (DiGeorge syndrome/velocardiofacial syndrome). Medicine (Baltimore). 2011;90:1–18.

32. Bassett AS, Chow EW, Husted J, et al. Clinical features of 78 adults with 22q11 deletion syndrome. Am J Med Genet A. 2005;138:307–13.

33. Parkinson DB, Thakker RV. A donor splice site mutation in the parathyroid hormone gene is associated with autosomal recessive hypoparathyroidism. Nat Genet. 1992;1:149–52.

34. Arnold A, Horst SA, Gardella TJ, et al. Mutation of the signal peptide-encoding region of the preproparathyroid hormone gene in familial isolated hypoparathyroidism. J Clin Invest. 1990;86:1084–7.

35. Thomée C, Schubert SW, Parma J, et al. GCMB mutation in familial isolated hypoparathyroidism with residual secretion of parathyroid hormone. J Clin Endocrinol Metab. 2005;90:2487–92.

36. Baumber L, Tufarelli C, Patel S, et al. Identification of a novel mutation disrupting the DNA binding activity of GCM2 in autosomal recessive familial isolated hypoparathyroidism. J Med Genet. 2005;42:443–8.

37. Van Esch H, Groenen P, Nesbit MA, et al. GATA3 haplo-insufficiency causes human HDR syndrome. Nature. 2000;406:419–22.

38. Ali A, Christie PT, Grigorieva IV, et al. Functional characterization of GATA3 mutations causing the hypoparathyroidism-deafness-renal (HDR) dysplasia syndrome: insight into mechanisms of DNA binding by the GATA3 transcription factor. Hum Mol Genet. 2007;16:265–75.

39. Bowl MR, Nesbit MA, Harding B, et al. An interstitial deletion-insertion involving chromosomes 2p25.3 and Xq27.1, near SOX3, causes X-linked recessive hypoparathyroidism. J Clin Invest. 2005;115:2822–31.

40. Parvari R, Hershkovitz E, Grossman N, et al. Mutation of TBCE causes hypoparathyroidism-retardation-dysmorphism and autosomal recessive Kenny-Caffey syndrome. Nat Genet. 2002;32:448–52.

41. Cassandrini D, Savasta S, Bozzola M, et al. Mitochondrial DNA deletion in a child with mitochondrial encephalomyopathy, growth hormone deficiency, and hypoparathyroidism. J Child Neurol. 2006;21:983–5.

42. Labarthe E, Benoist JF, Brivet M, et al. Partial hypoparathyroidism associated with mitochondrial trifunctional protein deficiency. Eur J Pediatr. 2006;165:389–91.

43. Rubin M, Levine MA. Hypoparathyroidism and pseudohypoparathyroidism. In: Rosen CJ, editor. Primer on the metabolic bone diseases and disorders of mineral metabolism. 7th ed. Washington, D.C.: American Society for Bone and Mineral Research; 2009. p. 354–61.

44. Levine MA. Pseudohypoparathyroidism: from bedside to bench and back. J Bone Miner Res. 1999;14:1255–60.

45. Lui J, Litman D, Rosenberg MJ, Yu S, Biesecker LG, Weinstein LS. A GNAS1 imprinting defect in pseudohypoparathyroidism type 1B. J Clin Invest. 2000;106:1167–74.

46. Brandi ML. Genetics of hypoparathyroidism and pseudohypoparathyroidism. J Endocrinol Investig. 2011;34(7 Suppl):27–34.

47. Mantovani G. Clinical review: Pseudohypoparathyroidism: diagnosis and treatment. J Clin Endocrinol Metab. 2011;96:3020–30.

48. Thacher T, Clarke BL. Vitamin D deficiency. Mayo Clin Proc. 2011;86:50–60.

49. Leboff MS, Kohlmeier L, Franklin J, et al. Occult vitamin D deficiency in postmenopausal U.S. women with acute hip fracture. JAMA. 1999;281:1505–11.

50. Lieben L, Carmeliet G, Masuyama R. Calcemic actions of vitamin D: effects on the intestine, kidney and bone. Best Pract Res Clin Endocrinol Metab. 2011;25:561–72.

51. van Schoor NM, Lips P. Worldwide vitamin D status. Best Pract Res Clin Endocrinol Metab. 2011;25:671–80.

52. Thomas MK, Lloyd-Jones DM, Thadani RI, et al. Hypovitaminosis D in medical inpatients. N Engl J Med. 1998;338:777–83.

53. Priemel M, von Domarus C, Klatte TO, et al. Bone mineralization defects and vitamin D deficiency: histomorphometric analysis of iliac crest bone biopsies and circulating 25-hydroxyvitmain D in 675 patients. J Bone Miner Res. 2010;25:305–12.

54. Institute of Medicine. Dietary reference intakes for calcium and vitamin D. Washington, D.C.: National Academies Press; 2011.

55. Liamis G, Milionis HJ, Elisaf M. A review of drug-induced hypocalcemia. J Bone Miner Metab. 2009;27:635–42.

56. St Arnaud R, Messerlian S, Moir JM, et al. The 25-hydroxyvitamin D 1-alpha-hydroxylase gene maps to the pseudovitamin D-deficiency rickets (PDDR) disease locus. J Bone Miner Res. 1997;12:1552–9.

57. Kitanaka S, Takeyama K, Murayama A, et al. Inactivating mutations in the 25-hydroxyvitamin D_3 1-alpha-hydroxylase gene in patients with pseudovitamin D-deficiency rickets. N Engl J Med. 1998;338:653–61.

58. Brooks MH, Bell NH, Love L, et al. Vitamin D-dependent rickets type II. Resistance of target organs to 1,25-dihydroxyvitamin D. N Engl J Med. 1978;298:996–9.

59. Malloy PJ, Hochber Z, Tiosano D, et al. The molecular basis of hereditary 1,25-dihydroxyvitamin D3 resistant rickets in seven related families. J Clin Invest. 1990;86:2071–9.

60. Brasier AR, Nussbaum SR. Hungry bone syndrome: clinical and biochemical predictors of its occurrence after parathyroid surgery. Am J Med. 1988;84:654–60.

61. Vivien B, Langeron O, Morell E, et al. Early hypocalcemia in severe trauma. Crit Care Med. 2005;33:1946–52.

62. Prince MR, Erel HE, Lent RW, et al. Gadodiamide administration causes spurious hypocalcemia. Radiology. 2003;227:639–46.

63. Rosen CJ, Brown S. Severe hypocalcemia after intravenous bisphosphonate therapy in occult vitamin D deficiency. N Engl J Med. 2003;348:1503–4.

64. Bilezikian JP, Khan A, Potts JT Jr, et al. Hypoparathyroidism: epidemiology, diagnosis, pathophysiology, target organ involvement, treatment, and challenges for future research. J Bone Miner Res. 2011;26:2317–37.

65. Winer KK, Yanovski JA, Cutler GB Jr. Synthetic human parathyroid hormone 1-34 vs calcitriol and calcium in the treatment of hypoparathyroidism. JAMA. 1996;276:631–6.

66. Winer KK, Yanovski JA, Sarani B, Cutler GB. A randomized, cross-over trial of once-daily versus twice-daily parathyroid hormone 1-34 in treatment of hypoparathyroidism. J Clin Endocrinol Metab. 1998;83:3480–6.

67. Mannstadt M, Clarke BL, Vokes T, et al. Efficacy and safety of recombinant human parathyroid hormone (1-84) in hypopara-

thyroidism (REPLACE): a double-blind, placebo-controlled, randomised, phase 3 study. Lancet Diabetes Endocrinol. 2013;1:275–83.

68. Brandi ML, Bilezikian JP, Shoback D, et al. Management of hypoparathyroidism: summary statement and guidelines. J Clin Endocrinol Metab. 2016;101:2273–83.

69. Bollerslev J, Rejnmark L, Marcocci C, et al. European Society of Endocrinology Clinical Guideline: treatment of chronic hypoparathyroidism in adults. Eur J Endocrinol. 2015;173:G1–20.

70. Hasse C, Klock G, Schlosser A, Zimmermann UZ, Rothmund M. Parathyroid allotransplantation without immunosuppression. Lancet. 1997;350:1296–7.

71. Tolloczko T, Wozniewicz B, Gorski A, et al. Cultured parathyroid cells allotransplantation without immunosuppression for treatment of intractable hypoparathyroidism. Ann Transplant. 1996;1:51–3.

Primary Hyperparathyroidism

Francisco Bandeira, Lívia Amaral, Paula Aragão,
and Alyne Layane Pereira Lemos

Epidemiology

Primary hyperparathyroidism is not a rare disease [1–4]. The prevalence ranges from 0.4 to 82 cases per 100,000. In the study by Eufrazino et al., a prevalence of 0.78% was found, of which 81.8% were asymptomatic [5]. In addition, in recent years, there has been an increase in the diagnosis of PHPT, explained in part by the increase in requests for serum PTH. Yeh et al., observed a threefold increase in PHPT prevalence between 1995 and 2010 [6]. It is more common in subjects over 50 years of age and in postmenopausal women.

Etiology

The solitary parathyroid adenoma appears in 85–90% of the cases [3, 7]. Hyperfunction in several parathyroid glands associated with hyperplasia and multiple adenomas occurs in most other cases [1]. In this context, it is important to mention that the disorder in multiple glands represents the most usual finding in subjects who have the primary hyperparathyroidism (PHPT) familial syndromes, corresponding to about 10% of cases [7]. On the other hand, parathyroid carcinoma occurs rarely, accounting for 0.7% of all cases [3]. Furthermore familial PHPT is related to several pathological entities, such as multiple endocrine neoplasia type 1 (MEN1), type 2A (MEN2A), and type 4 (MEN4), familial hypocalciuric hypercalcemia, familial hypercalciuric hypercalcemia, jaw tumor hyperparathyroidism syndrome, familial isolated hyperparathyroidism, and neonatal severe hyperparathyroidism [8–10] (Table 22.1).

MEN1 can be considered a rare cause of PHPT, the incidence of MEN1 being about 2–4% of PHPT cases. However, PHPT is the most common endocrinopathy in the MEN1 syndrome: it is found in almost 100% of the patients over 50 years of age and constitutes the first sign of the disease in most carriers in their 20s [8]. The diagnosis of PHPT in young adults should therefore include the search for MEN1. The search for MEN1 should also be conducted in the immediate family. The prevalence of PHPT in MEN2 is lower than in MEN1 and is found in 20–30% of cases. Furthermore, the majority of patients with PHPT present clinical manifestations that are more discrete than the clinical signs demonstrated by MEN1 carriers [11].

The jaw tumor hyperparathyroidism syndrome is a rare disease. Evidence shows that bone tumors of the jaw related

F. Bandeira
Division of Endocrinology, Agamenon Magalhães Hospital, University of Pernambuco Medical School, Recife, PE, Brazil
e-mail: francisco.bandeira@upe.br

L. Amaral
Universidade Federal de Alagoas (UFAL), Algoas, AL, Brazil

P. Aragão · A. L. P. Lemos (✉)
Division of Endocrinology and Diabetes, Agamenon Magalhães Hospital, University of Pernambuco Medical School, Recife, Pernambuco, Brazil

Table 22.1 The genetic syndromes associated with primary hyperparathyroidism

Familiar syndrome	Clinical features	Genes
Multiple endocrine neoplasia type 1 (MEN1)	PHPT, pituitary adenomas, pancreatic adenoma tumors	*MEN1*
Multiple endocrine neoplasia type 2A (MEN2A)	PHPT, medullary thyroid cancer, pheochromocytoma	*RET*
Multiple endocrine neoplasia type 4 (MEN4)	PHPT, anterior pituitary tumors, pancreatic neuroendocrine tumors	*CDKN1B* (*p27*)
Familial isolated hyperparathyroidism	Isolate PHPT	*MEN1* *CASR* *GCM2*
Hyperparathyroidism—Jaw tumor syndrome	PHPT, often parathyroid carcinoma, jaw tumors	*CDC73*

Adapted from Ref. [9]

© Springer Nature Switzerland AG 2022
F. Bandeira et al. (eds.), *Endocrinology and Diabetes*, https://doi.org/10.1007/978-3-030-90684-9_22

to PHPT can be outlined [12]. Parathyroid cancer has been also detected in more than 15% of cases [12].

Parathyroid carcinoma is a rare disease, accounting for less than 1% of cases. It may occur in young patients and usually presents with severe hypercalcemia and much greater PTH levels when compared to classic primary hyperparathyroidism. Severe disease such as *osteitis fibrosa cystica*, osteoporosis and multiple fractures are common. The histopathological diagnosis is difficult, due to its similarity to the adenoma. Presence of mitoses, cellular pleomorphism, vascular invasion, and invasion of adjacent tissue may facilitate differentiation [9, 10]. The genetic pathogenesis of PHPT is unclear in most cases. Some genes have been identified and are shown in Table 22.1.

Diagnosis

In familial isolated hyperparathyroidism, cases of PHPT are diagnosed in the immediate family in the absence of other endocrinopathies; this characterizes the phenotype as a hidden syndrome, such as MEN1 and MEN2 [1].

Hypercalcemia and an increase in PTH levels constitute the biochemical markers of PHPT. In normal conditions of hypercalcemia, there is an inhibition of the parathyroid glands. This inhibition is translated by low levels of PTH [7].

The majority of patients with PHPT present slightly increased levels of PTH, but up to 10% of the cases can exhibit normal to upper normal levels of PTH [13, 14]. Nevertheless, these levels are inappropriately high because of the hypercalcemia. Hypercalcemia is found in most of the cases of PHPT, but one has to consider the possibility of fluctuations in the levels of serum calcium, which could explain the normal levels of calcemia [13].

Diagnosis includes the evaluation of serum concentrations for calcium, phosphorus, albumin, alkaline phosphatase, intact PTH, 25 (OH)-D vitamin, and renal function [13, 14]. 24-h urinary calcium and the serum levels of creatinine must be evaluated in order to rule out the possibility of familial hypocalciuric hypercalcemia [15, 16].

About 40% of serum calcium is linked to albumin. Serum levels must be adjusted according to the following equation: corrected calcium = serum calcium (mg/dL) + [0.8 × (4 − serum albumin)]. The measurement of the ionized calcium can be useful in specific cases, such as subjects with hyperalbuminemia, thrombocytosis, Waldenstrom's macroglobulinemia, and myeloma, since in these subjects there is hypercalcemia with normal ionized serum calcium (artifactual hypercalcemia) [15, 17].

In a retrospective cohort with 6982 subjects, the serum ionized and total calcium were compared in patients with hypercalcemia. PTH-dependent hypercalcemia was set as total serum calcium (corrected by albumin) equal to or greater than 10.2 mg/dL or ionized calcium (technique of specific ion electrode) equal to or greater than 1.32 mmol/L with the PTH >5 pmol/L (35 pg/mL; reference values 0.9–9 pmol/L). Among these subjects, 343 had high ionized calcium, and 156 (45%) had high total calcium. In a second cohort with 203 subjects, 143 presented histologically confirmed PHPT: high ionized serum calcium was present in 141 cases (98%) and, lastly, increased total serum calcium in 108 (76%), demonstrating a greater diagnostic accuracy when ionized serum calcium was used [18].

A cohort study, based on the population of Tayside in Scotland, used the following criteria to diagnose primary hyperparathyroidism: (1) serum calcium corrected for albumin >10.22 mg/dL (reference values: 8.4–10.22 mg/dL) on at least two occasions, with serum PTH >13.5 ng/L (reference values: 4.5–31.05 ng/L), or (2) serum calcium corrected for serum albumin >10.22 mg/dL on one occasion with serum PTH >31.05 ng/L [19]. These values of serum PTH correspond to 20 pg/mL for assays with reference values between 10 and 65 pg/mL.

The causes of secondary hyperparathyroidism that can increase the serum levels of parathormone, such as the use of thiazide diuretics [14] and lithium, deficiency of vitamin D, and the use of bisphosphonates, must be excluded. Concerning tertiary hyperparathyroidism due to renal failure, genetic causes such as familial hypocalciuric hypercalcemia also need to be sought. The finding of normal levels for calcium corrected by albumin and associated with high serum PTH in the absence of other causes is compatible with normocalcemic PHPT.

Serum PTH and the biochemical markers of the bone remodeling are significantly higher in patients with severe disease. These patients frequently have vitamin D deficiency and easier localization of the parathyroid lesion than asymptomatic patients [3].

The levels of serum phosphorus are usually found to be in the lower normal range. Specific markers of bone modeling (osteocalcin and alkaline phosphatase osteo-specific) or markers of bone resorption (deoxypyridinoline, N-telopeptide, and C-telopeptide) seem to remain either in the high-normal range or slightly above reference values. Hypercalciuria is found in around 30% of asymptomatic patients, in 50% of patients with active urolithiasis, and in 40% with osteitis fibrosa cystica [3, 14]. Patients with severe PHPT have moderate levels of serum calcium and lower levels of serum phosphorus as compared to asymptomatic subjects (14.0 ± 0.7 vs. 10.9 ± 0.4 mg/dL; $p < 0.001$ and 2.0 ± 05 vs. 296 ± 0.2 mg/dL; $p < 0.01$, respectively). In the serum levels of intact PTH, there are greater differences: 1820 ± 349 vs. 133 ± 29 pg/mL; $p < 0.001$ [20].

Serum PTH and the biochemical biomarkers of the bone remodeling are significantly higher in the patients with

Table 22.2 Differential diagnosis of hypercalcemia

1. Malignancies	Solid tumors	Solid tumors	Hematologic malignancies (lymphoma, leukemia, multiple myeloma)	Ectopic production of PTH (thyroid carcinoma, ovarian, lung oat cells)
	Humoral hypercalcemia (carcinomas)	Osteolytic hypercalcemia (breast, lung)		
	Squamous lung, esophagus			
2. PTH-dependent	NEM	PHPT: (a) Adenoma (b) Carcinoma (c) Hyperplasia	Familial hypercalciuric hypercalcemia (FHH)	Treatment with lithium
3. Related to vitamin D	Idiopathic familial hypercalcemia	Granulomatous diseases	Vitamin D intoxication	–
4. Other causes	Milk–alkali syndrome, aluminum intoxication	Endocrine diseases (hyperthyroidism, pheochromocytoma, adrenal insufficiency)	Advanced chronic disease of the liver/kidney	Drugs: Thiazide Theophylline Beryllium

Adapted from Refs. [21, 22]

severe disease, who frequently present vitamin D deficiency and easier localization of the parathyroid lesion than asymptomatic patients [21].

Differential Diagnosis

PHPT needs to be differentiated from other causes of hypercalcemia (Table 22.2), as well as from diseases that can cause osteoporosis, nephrolithiasis, nefrocalcinosis, and hypophosphatemia. PHPT and neoplasia correspond to 90% of hypercalcemia cases. Data from the literature shows that 50–60% of outpatients with hypercalcemia are carriers of the PHPT and about 31% present neoplasia [22].

Hypercalcemia with very low or undetectable PTH plasma levels can be found when the disease is malignant, and, in this case, the PTHrp is responsible for the increase in calcium [12]. Several laboratory characteristics associated with malignity are similar to those of PHPT, such as hypercalcemia, hypophosphatemia, hypercalciuria, and hyperphosphaturia and an increase in the nephrogenic cyclic AMP [23]. However, the difference between primary HPT and the malignant disease with hypercalcemia can be identified without difficulty, based on the clinical history of the patient. The hypercalcemia symptoms of PHPT are manifested over months or years, while in malignancy these symptoms are manifested within weeks and are secondary to the underlying malignant disease. Thus, hypercalcemia in malignant disease is readily revealed and is frequently associated with a survival of about 6 months. Other related symptoms are anemia and weight loss. In general, when hypercalcemia is found, malignancy is clinically revealed by imaging techniques or bone metastasis presented by the patient. In addition to these parameters, persistent hypercalcemia of early onset suggests malignancy, while a mild hypercalcemia lasting for more than 6 months is more likely to be caused by PHPT.

The definitive differential diagnosis is performed by means of serum PTH measurement. In PHPT, when PTH is increased or within normality, the condition may be regarded as PTH-dependent hypercalcemia but is frequently suppressed in malignant disease, which is independent of PTH [17]. In rare cases, PTH can be increased in malignancy due to ectopic production or when parathyroid carcinoma is the cause of the hypercalcemia [24].

Another differential diagnosis that should always be demanded is that of familial hypocalciuric hypercalcemia, which is characterized by a genetic defect in the calcium receptors in the parathyroid glands and kidneys, inherited as a dominant autosomal disorder [8]. The hypercalcemia is mild and followed by hyperphosphatemia, and levels of PTH are normal or slightly increased. The most pronounced laboratory finding is hypocalciuria, which suggests increased tubular resorption of calcium. This diagnosis is considered in young asymptomatic patients that present (1) levels of serum calcium with a slight-to-moderate increase, (2) hypocalciuria, (3) a familial history of hypercalcemia, and (4) a rate of calcium/creatinine clearance of less than 0.01 [2, 9].

Normocalcemic Primary Hyperparathyroidism

Patients that undergo routine evaluations during an investigation for bone loss may have increased levels of PTH, even without hypercalcemia [25].

The term normocalcemic primary hyperparathyroidism (NPHPT) was first used by Wills in 1960, who described a group of patients having characteristics different to those diagnosed with classic PHPT [26].

NPHPT is characterized by levels of serum calcium that remain normal, while PTH levels are high [27–29]. Since there is a greater availability and utilization of assays for the evaluation of this hormone, this condition has been frequently diagnosed. However, examining for other causes of secondary hyperparathyroidism, especially 25-hydroxyvitamin D deficiency, malabsorption syndromes, renal insufficiency, primary hypercalciuria, use of medications such as lithium, thiazide diuretics, and bisphosphonates, is necessary to confirm the diagnosis [13, 28].

Little is known about the epidemiology of NPHPT. In a village in southern Italy, the prevalence of NPHPT in the population above 18 years of age was 0.44% [30]. Another study with 156 female patients diagnosed with osteoporosis was observed in 14% of patients with normocalcemic primary hyperparathyroidism [28]. A pre In Sweden, Lundgren et al. studied 5202 postmenopausal women aged 55–75 years. In the 109 subjects studied, the researchers investigated two indices, observing whether the patients presented hypercalcemia associated with increased levels of PTH and higher levels of either hypercalcemia or PTH. Seventeen (16%) out of the 109 subjects studied had normal levels of serum calcium (<9.9 mg/dL) and increased PTH. This group of 17 subjects included people that had vitamin D deficiency as well as patients with NPHPT [31].

Some complications, such as nephrolithiasis, may be present in some frequency as hypercalcemic PHPT [28, 32, 33].

It remains debatable whether NPHPT incipiently represents classic PHPT or a different spectrum of this pathology [28]. Evidence suggests that patients without secondary causes of hyperparathyroidism may have early-stage PHPT since, if the disease is diagnosed early, it can progress with isolated increased serum PTH, which may or may not be followed by an increase in serum calcium. For these patients, serum calcium should be periodically evaluated during the development of the disease [29, 34].

Skeletal Manifestations

The skeletal complications of PHPT are well-known. Among the classic symptoms, these complications are considered the most familiar consequences of PHPT. The clinical presentation may include focal or widespread bone pain, localized bone edema ("brown tumors"), and fragility fractures [25].

Intense bone demineralization is seen in X-rays of patients with this severe disease. Pathological fractures are frequently seen, especially in the long bones of the lower extremity, and also loss of the lamina dura of the teeth and brain lesions in the salt-and-pepper pattern which refers to the speckled appearance of the tissue. Subperiosteal bone erosions in the distal phalanges and on the edges of the medial phalanges are usually seen as numerous lytic lesions with irregular sclerotic margins, which are more common in the pelvis, long bones, and shoulders. The cortical bone of the long bones is extremely thin and in some patients is almost absent [21].

Bone densitometry is a useful tool for investigating the classic effects of PTH, such as reduction in bone mineral density (BMD) in the distal radius, the site of the cortical bone. The catabolic ability of PTH on the cortical bone is the opposite of its anabolic effect on cancellous bone. In the lumbar spine, the site of cancellous bone, BMD seems to be normal. The hip contains a more uniform mix of cortical and cancellous bone elements, and the BMD is classified as being of an intermediate density between the distal radius and the lumbar spine. Although this classic densitometric profile is usually seen as a distinct pattern characterized by vertebral osteopenia, it can also be seen at the moment of diagnosis. In the more severe types of PHPT, there is an overall decrease in bone density [35].

The prevalence of PHPT and its impact on BMD were evaluated in 3014 men aged 69–81 years in a Swedish cohort, *MrOs*. Subjects with a low glomerular filtration rate (<21 mL/min/1.73 m²) and vitamin D deficiency (<50 nmol/l) were excluded from the study. BMD was compared between patients with and without PHPT. The prevalence of PHPT was estimated to be 0.73%. BMD in the total hip and femur neck was lower among the PHPT group than in the control group. Subjects with high levels of intact PTH were compared with the other subjects from the cohort. For that subgroup, BMD was lower for the total hip and lumbar spine ($p < 0.05$) [36].

A controlled clinical trial compared two groups: (1) carriers of mild PHPT that were submitted to parathyroidectomy ($n = 25$) and (2) patients that had an intact parathyroid ($n = 28$). After 24 months, there was a significant increase in the BMD in the femur neck and total hip, but not in the lumbar spine or forearm of patients submitted to parathyroidectomy when compared with those that did not undergo a parathyroidectomy. There was also a decrease in the biochemical markers of bone remodeling after parathyroidectomy [37]. Another study with 11 patients, including a 5-year follow-up after parathyroidectomy, showed a significant BMD increase in the lumbar spine. However, neither the hip nor the distal radius showed any BMD increase when compared to baseline values. They also observed a reduction in the markers for bone remodeling [38].

Extraskeletal Manifestations

Neuropsychiatric Symptoms

In addition to skeletal manifestations, PHPT may be associated with alterations in other organ systems within the body. Neuropsychiatric symptoms can occur in about 23% of patients with PHPT, such as fatigue, difficulty concentrating, irritability, and mood and sleep disorders [39]. Since few studies have evaluated the prevalence of these manifestations, they remain uncertain [40]. A case–control study compared 39 postmenopausal patients with mild PHPT and 89 women without PHPT. This study revealed a higher prevalence of depression and anxiety and a higher performance on tests for verbal and nonverbal memory in the PHPT carriers. Also observed was the fact that depressive symptoms, nonverbal abstraction, and aspects of the verbal memory were significantly improved after parathyroidectomy [41]. Peripheral neurological alterations, especially sensory–motor polyneuropathy and PHPT, have been suggested by some authors [42, 43]. Recent data report clinical improvement after surgical treatment, which is recommended in patients that have neurological symptoms related to PHPT and do not present any contraindication for surgery [44].

Cardiovascular Symptoms

The literature shows a relationship between PHPT and abnormalities such as arterial hypertension, left ventricular hypertrophy, abnormal heart function, coronary artery disease, vascular abnormalities, conduction disorders, and valvular and myocardial calcification [45]. The mechanism for this aforementioned relationship remains uncertain, but it has been shown that morbidity and the risk of cardiovascular death are greater in PHPT carriers. This is mainly observed in patients with the mild to severe form of the disease [46]. On the other hand, parathyroidectomy decreases cardiovascular risk, as shown in a number of population studies, even with mild forms of the disease. Surgery is therefore indicated in all patients with PHPT and other factors of cardiovascular risk [47, 48].

Renal Manifestations

Nephrolithiasis and nefrocalcinosis are major complications of primary hyperparathyroidism. Hypercalcemia leads to increased filtered calcium load on the glomerulus, leading to hypercalciuria, increasing the risk kidney stones. Although high levels of parathyroid hormone stimulate renal resorption of calcium, renal excretion exceeds resorption. However, hypercalciuria may not be the only factor for the onset of nephrolithiasis. Studies have shown that PTHP patients may present polymorphisms in the gene that encodes the calcium-sensing receptor or CaSR, which is present in the parathyroid glands and in the kidney, modulating PTH actions. CaSR influences renal phosphate homeostasis, urinary acidification, and in urine concentration. This may explain the occurrence of nephrolithiasis in normocalcemic patients [49]. Nefrocalcinosis and nephrolithiasis are also clinical manifestations of asymptomatic and NPHPT. From the experience of our group, a recent study demonstrated an 18.2% rate of nephrolithiasis in NPHPT patients, as well as in the hypercalcemic modality (18.9%), may have shown a non-indolent presentation [50]. A recent study from our group found a prevalence of 20% for occult nephrolithiasis in NPHP patients [32].

Localization of Parathyroid Lesions

Imaging examinations are not indicated for the diagnosis of PHPT. The location of the affected parathyroid is an indication for surgery and can permit the use of less invasive techniques, which is associated with a lower morbidity rate [51]. Ultrasonography and Sestamibi scintigraphy are the most common techniques used for PHPT diagnosis (Figs. 22.1 and 22.2). Cervical ultrasonography is a low-cost examination, as well as noninvasive. When performed by an experienced examiner, it presents a sensitivity and specificity of 88% and 94%, respectively [52]. In cases of ectopic glands or an intrathyroid adenoma, identification and differentiation of thyroid nodules can be difficult. Thus, ultrasonography coupled with 99mTc-labeled Sestamibi scintigraphy increases the chance of identification to almost 100% of the lesions [53]. These two methods are complementary, since ultrasonography provides anatomic information, while the scintigraphy provides functionality data.

Scintigraphy is able to identify the topic and ectopic parathyroid tissues. A study with 64 PHPT patients presented positive scintigraphy in 64% of the patients that had asymptomatic PHPT and 83% of the group that carried nephrolithiasis without bone involvement. That same study showed that 100% of the subjects with the severe disease presented positive scintigraphy as well, but in this case it was characterized by osteitis fibrosa cystica. These results were found when the imaging was evaluated early, which occurred in 70% of the cases analyzed [53] (Fig. 22.3). A small number of patients may have negative imaging, which suggests multiglandular disease. In these cases, the use of the most advanced imaging techniques may be necessary to increase the chances of localizing the affected parathyroid and ectopic tumors and also assist in the decision to proceed with

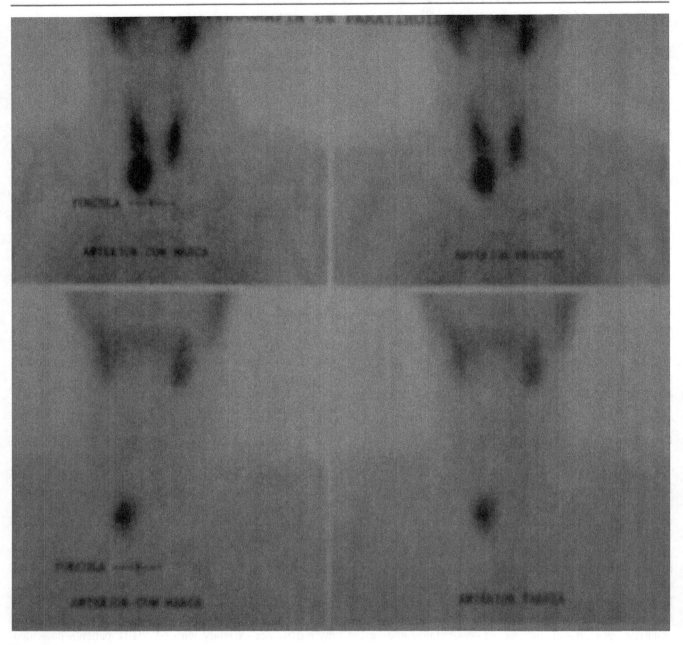

Fig. 22.1 Tc-99-Sestamibi scintigraphy showing a right inferior parathyroid lesion

surgery. Four-dimensional computed tomography was able to localize the adenoma with 82 and 92% sensitivity and specificity, respectively, in 34 PHPT patients [54]. A retrospective trial found almost 100% specificity in the diagnosis of multiglandular disease in 35 patients evaluated; however, the sensibility was much lower (42.9%). As regards the localization of only one lesion, they were able to identify 32 cases with a sensibility of 91% [55]. The preoperative localization of an adenoma allows the use of minimally invasive parathyroidectomy (MIP) with lower morbidity and can be done in an outpatient facility [55].

One of the main disadvantages of imaging examinations is the high incidence of false-positive results due to the size and localization of the parathyroid affected. As a result, fine-needle aspiration of the nodule that was identified by imaging for measurement of PTH in the aspirated material has become an auxiliary method for diagnosing lesions, as shown by a study performed by our group. A group of 15 women without PHPT, who had nodules identified by ultrasonography, showed very high PTH levels, presenting a mean of 4.919 ± 5.124 pg/mL, while the control group had a mean of 10.65 ± 3.49 pg/mL. This tech-

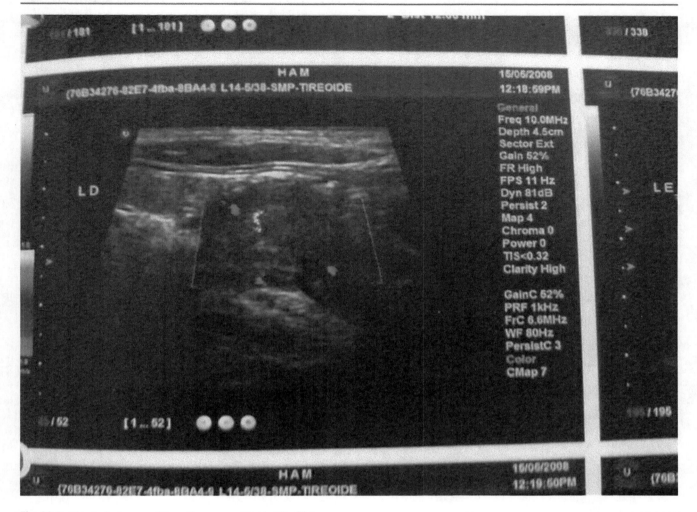

Fig. 22.2 Cervical ultrasound from the same patient in Fig. 23.1

nique showed a greater sensitivity in locating the affected gland than the use of imaging alone [56]. The main methods for locating parathyroid lesions are shown in Table 22.3.

Indications for Parathyroidectomy in PHPT

Parathyroidectomy is the treatment of choice for patients with PHPT, but indicating surgery for subjects in whom a parathyroid lesion was not found may need some criteria. The aim of surgery is to provide treatment by removal of the affected parathyroid. This occurs in 95–98% of the patients operated on by an experienced surgeon, with the number of complications being low. According to the Fourth International Workshop, surgery is indicated for asymptomatic patients if there is a greater benefit than with drug treatment [57, 58]. Table 22.4 lists the conditions in which surgery is particularly indicated.

For patients with normocalcemic primary hyperparathyroidism, surgery is indicated for those, who present with complications such as kidney stones and osteoporosis [58].

With regard to the minimal significant alterations in the bone loss rate during the natural disease progression, asymptomatic PHPT patients who do not meet the criteria for surgery or patients that have some contraindication should have their BMD monitored by biannual bone densitometry (dual-energy X-ray absorptiometry—DXA) [57]. The patients with a vitamin D deficiency (serum levels of 25-OHD below 20 ng/mL) should receive adequate replacement, in accordance with the recommendations for patients without PHPT [46].

Randomized studies [41, 59, 60] have demonstrated the benefits on the quality of life and on BMD of asymptomatic patients submitted to surgery. Even though these studies were randomized, they had a short follow-up period. Finally, another important point about MIP is that this procedure yields excellent t results, produces few complications, and decreases the cost of a surgical procedure [61].

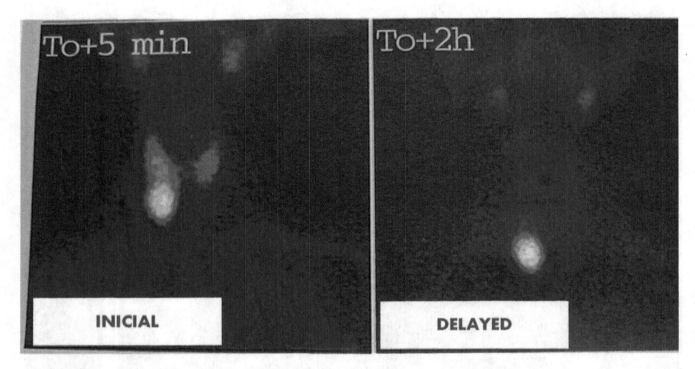

Fig. 22.3 99mTc-Sestamibi scintigraphy showing a large parathyroid adenoma

Table 22.3 Localization procedures for the identification of parathyroid adenoma

Methods	Sensitivity (%)	Specificity (%)
Cervical ultrasonography (US)/ Doppler US	88/97	94/100
Computed tomography fourth dimension	82	92 a 100[a]
Technetium-99 m Sestamibi scintigraphy	90[b]	100
PTH measurement in aspiration fluid (FNA[c])	100	100

Adapted from Refs. [51–54]

[a]The specificity for multiglandular disease is close to 100%

[b]The sensitivity increases in more serious cases being close to 100% in patients with osteitis fibrosa cystica. The accuracy is lower in multiglandular disease

[c]*FNA* fine-needle aspiration

Table 22.4 Surgical indications for asymptomatic primary hyperparathyroidism

Nephrolithiasis
Osteitis fibrosa cystica
Asymptomatic primary hyperparathyroidism associated with one or more of the following conditions:
Serum calcium >1 mg/dL above ULN[a]
Age < 50 years
T-score < −2.5 at the lumbar spine, hip, and/or distal radius
Vertebral fracture by X-ray, CT, MRI, or VFA or deteriorated Trabecular Bone Score
Estimated Glomerular Filtration Rate (Creatinine clearance) <60 mL/min/1,73 m²
24-h urine for calcium>400 mg/d (>10 mmol/d)
Presence of nephrolithiasis or nefrocalcinosis by X-ray, ultrasound, or CT
Patients whose medical monitoring is not possible

Adapted from Refs. [57, 58]

[a]*ULN* upper limit of normality

Surgical Techniques

Bilateral cervical exploration is the traditional surgical technique and consists of the evaluation and removal of the affected parathyroid glands. However, the morbidity, surgical duration, and risks of complications are greater. The early localization of the lesion therefore allows the use of MIP as mentioned above [61].

A prospective, randomized, and blinded study compared MIP with conventional parathyroidectomy in 48 patients with PHPT. In the group submitted to MIP, there was a lower pain intensity in the postoperative period ($p < 0.001$), less use of analgesics ($p < 0.001$), a lower rate of anesthesia procedures ($p < 0.001$), a smaller scar ($p < 0.001$), and greater aesthetic satisfaction postoperatively at 2 days, 1 month ($p < 0.01$), and 6 months ($p < 0.05$); however, 1 year after surgery, aesthetic satisfaction was no longer significantly different in the two groups($p = 0.38$). On the other hand, there was a higher cost with MIP and no significant difference in the quality of life in either group 6 months after the surgical procedure [62].

Intraoperative PTH Monitoring

This procedure is used during MIP for the treatment of PHPT. As regards the time frame for intraoperative PTH monitoring, this is performed after the anesthesia, before the skin incision, and 10 minutes after removal of the enlarged gland [63]. One can observe a fall of less than 50% in the PTH levels, when compared with the baseline values. This fall of less than 50% shows the risk of persistent disease. Several studies have analyzed how useful the intraoperative PTH evaluation can be, and they suggest that this measurement should be indicated in cases (1) that present only an imaging study during preoperative care of positive MIP, (2) when the imaging studies for preoperative localization are discordant, and (3) of reoperation [63–66].

Medical Therapy

Drug therapy is indicated for patients contraindicated for surgical treatment, those with therapy failure, and patients that either do not want the surgical procedure or did not meet the current criteria. Among the options to replace a surgical procedure is cinacalcet, which acts as a calcimimetic and is able to decrease the PTH release. Other options are an antiresorptive agent which inhibits bone remodeling, for example, a bisphosphonate, hormone therapy, and selective modulators of estrogen receptors [46].

Calcimimetic Agents

Calcimimetic agents are drugs that can increase the sensitivity of the calcium-sensing receptor to extracellular calcium, which results in a reduction of PTH. The first calcimimetic developed was a derived phenylalkylamine (R-568); however, it had low availability and a high variability of response. As a result, cinacalcet hydrochloride, with higher availability and a lower pharmacologic variability, was developed [67]. Studies show that cinacalcet decreases PTH levels by up to 50% and is thus able to regulate serum calcium in approximately 80% of treated patients [67]. The recommended starting dose for PHPT is 30 mg once daily which may be adjusted up to 300 mg/day [67].

A multicenter, randomized, double-blind, placebo-controlled study evaluated 78 patients with PHPT to ascertain the long-term ability of cinacalcet to reduce serum calcium and PTH. The patients received a dose starting at 30 mg, twice a day; if there was a persistent hypercalcemia, the dose was increased to 40–50 mg during a 12-week period. The final dose was maintained for 12 weeks, and patients were followed for another 28 weeks. Two doses per day of cinacalcet decreased serum calcium by 0.5 mg/dL or more and normalized (calcium <10.3 mg/dL) in 73% patients treated during a maintenance phase and also decreased levels of PTH by 7.6% over the same period [68]. Serum calcium levels remained normal and PTH remained lowered for up to 52 weeks.

With regard to BMD measured by dual-energy X-ray densitometry (DEXA), no significant changes were found during the 52-week period or the following 5 years [69, 70]. Cinacalcet significantly increased some of the markers of bone remodeling (bone alkaline phosphatase and NTx), and the rate of NTX/urinary creatinine for 52 weeks, when compared with the placebo group, however, remained within the normal range [69].

The use of calcimimetics is indicated for those patients that have hypercalcemia related to renal insufficiency of the tertiary hyperparathyroidism, for those who are carriers of parathyroid carcinoma, or when there is a contraindication for surgery [67].

Hormone Replacement Therapy

The use of estrogens is a therapeutic option for postmenopausal women because it increases BMD in the femoral neck and lumbar spine. This protective effect from fractures was demonstrated in the WHI trial with the use of conjugated estrogens at a dose of 0.625 mg together with a daily 5 mg dose of medroxyprogesterone for 2 years [71]. Nevertheless, their long-term use is not indicated, since they also increase the risk of cardiovascular and breast cancer. Thus one should analyze the risks and benefits before suggesting this therapy [71].

Furthermore, another randomized, double-blind, placebo-controlled study with 42 menopausal women with PHPT over 2 years evaluated the effects of conjugated estrogens at a dose of 0.625 mg, together with a daily 5 mg dose of medroxyprogesterone on BMD, biochemical parameters of bone remodeling, and calcium metabolism. In this study, there was a reduction in total serum calcium, but no changes in the ionized calcium and intact PTH. Regarding the markers of bone remodeling, there was a 22% decrease in alkaline phosphatase, and a 38% decrease in urinary hydroxyproline excretion was also observed. In addition, 60 and 33% reductions were found in N-telopeptide excretion and urinary calcium excretion, respectively [72]. This therapy showed positive effects on the total BMD of the body, lumbar spine, femur, and forearm over the 2 years. These positive effects remained for at least the 4 years of follow-up [73].

Estrogen therapy may thus be the treatment of choice for women that have bone loss and PHPT in the postmenopausal period. This therapy should be indicated if there is no contraindication for its use.

Selective Modulators of Estrogen Receptors (SERMs)

Nowadays, there is little evidence in the literature concerning the selective modulators of estrogen receptors (SERMs). A randomized, double-blind, placebo-controlled investigation,

with 18 patients, demonstrated the efficacy of 60 mg/day raloxifene in reducing both serum calcium levels and markers of bone remodeling (serum NTx and osteocalcin) over an 8-week period. After 4 weeks of treatment with raloxifene, there were no alterations in the calcium and PTH levels. Moreover, during the same period, the markers of bone remodeling returned to baseline values [74].

Bisphosphonates

The bisphosphonates, administered to patients with PHPT, have proven their efficacy in the improvement of bone mass as compared to a placebo, which was measured by DEXA. The use of oral alendronate has been evaluated in 5 studies involving 119 postmenopausal women and 24 men treated for 2 years (Fig. 22.4). The results showed a significant increase in BMD at the lumbar spine and femoral neck, but no substantial change in density of the distal radius. There was also a decrease in the levels of calcium adjusted for albumin and a decrease in PTH and markers of bone turnover [75–79].

Another example [79] is a double-blind, controlled trial with 44 patients who did not undergo parathyroidectomy and used alendronate (10 mg/day) for 2 years. In this case, the study showed a gain in bone mass in the lumbar spine and femoral neck, but there were no changes in calcium or PTH levels. Markers of bone turnover had reduced levels without modifying the risk of fractures.

Jansson and Cols [80] evaluated 21 patients with PHPT who were given 30–40 mg of pamidronate before surgery. A temporary reduction in the levels of serum calcium was

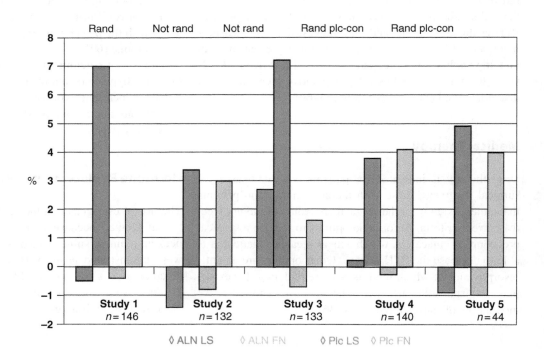

Fig. 22.4 Clinical trials on alendronate therapy for PHPT

observed with the nadir after 6–10 days of infusion, and a return to high levels after this period.

In conclusion, alendronate may represent a therapeutic option and the possibility of bone protection, albeit with no prospect of achieving long-term normocalcemia, and may be associated with increased levels of serum PTH.

References

1. Bilezikian JP, Brandi ML, Rubin M, Silverberg SJ. Primary hyperparathyroidism: new concepts in clinical, densitometric and biochemical features. J Intern Med. 2005;257:6–17.
2. Bandeira F, Graf H, Griz L, Faria M, Lazaretti-Castro M. Endocrinologia e diabetes, vol. 37. 2th ed. Rio de Janeiro: Medbook; 2009. p. 385–93.
3. Bandeira F, Griz L, Caldas G, et al. Characteristics of primary hyperparathyroidism in one institution in Northeast Brazil. Bone. 1998;23(suppl):S380.
4. Mundy GR, Cove DH, Fisken R. Primary hyperparathyroidism: changes in the clinical presentation. Lancet. 1980;1(1):317–20.
5. Eufrazino CSS, Veras A, Bandeira F. Prevalência de hiperparatireoidismo primário em uma grande população atendida em dois centros de referência na cidade do Recife. Arq Bras Endocrinol Metabol. 2010;54:S439.
6. Yeh MW, Ituarte PHG, Zhou HC, Nishimoto S, Amy Liu I-L, Harari A, et al. Incidence and prevalence of primary hyperparathyroidism in a racially mixed population. J Clin Endocrinol Metab. 2013;98(3):1122–9.
7. Rodgers SE, Lew JI, Solórzano CC. Primary hyperparathyroidism. Curr Opin Oncol. 2008;20:52–8.
8. Brandi ML, Falchetti A. Genetics of primary hyperparathyroidism. Urol Int. 2004;72(Suppl 1):11–6.
9. Bilezikian JP, Cusano NE, Khan AA, Liu J-M, Marcocci C, Bandeira F. Primary hyperparathyroidism. Nat Rev Dis Prim. 2016;2:16033.
10. Bandeira L, Bilezikian J. Primary hyperparathyroidism. F1000Research. 2016;5:1–11.
11. Simonds WF, James-Newton LA, Agarwal SK, et al. Familial isolated hyperparathyroidism: clinical and genetic characteristics of thirty-six kindreds. Medicine (Baltimore). 2002;81:1–26.
12. Marx SJ, Simonds SF, Agarwal SK, et al. Hyperparathyroidism in hereditary syndromes: special expressions and special managements. J Bone Miner Res. 2002;17:37–43.
13. Eastell R, Arnold A, Brandi ML, et al. Diagnosis of asymptomatic primary hyperparathyroidism: proceedings of the third international workshop. J Clin Endocrinol Metab. 2009;94:340–50.
14. Andrade LD, Marques TF, Diniz ET, Lucena CS, Griz L, Banderia F. Impact of the use of hydrochlorothiazide in secretion PTH in hypertensive patients. Arq Bras Endocrinol Metabol. 2010;54(Suppl 5):S491.
15. Jacobs TP, Bilezikian JP. Clinical review: rare causes of hypercalcemia. J Clin Endocrinol Metab. 2005;90:66316–22.
16. Pausova Z, Soliman E, Amizuka N, Janicic N, Konrad EM, Arnold A, et al. Role of the RET proto-oncogene in sporadic hyperparathyroidism and in hyperparathyroidism of multiple endocrine neoplasia type 2. J Clin Endocrinol Metab. 1996;81(7):2711.
17. Feder JM, Sirrs S, Anderson D, Sharif J, Khan A. Primary hyperparathyroidism: an overview. Intern J Endocrinol. 2011;2011:251410.
18. Ong GSY, Walsh JP, Stuckey BGA, Brown SJ, Rossi E, Ng JL, et al. The importance of measuring ionized calcium in characterizing calcium status and diagnosing primary hyperparathyroidism. J Clin Endocrinol Metab. 2012;97(9):3138–45.
19. Yu N, Donnan PT, Murphy MJ, Leese GP. Epidemiology of primary hyperparathyroidism in Tayside, Scotland, UK. Clin Endocrinol. 2009;71:485–93.
20. Bandeira F, Caldas G, Freese E, Griz L, Faria M, Bandeira C. Relationship between vitamin D serum status and clinical manifestations of primary hyperparathyroidism. Endocr Pract. 2002;8:266–70.
21. Bandeira FB, Griz L, Caldas G, Bandeira C, Freese E. From mild to severe primary hyperparathyroidism: the Brazilian experience. Arq Bras Endocrinol Metabol. 2006;50(4):657–63.
22. Carroll MF, Schade DS. A practical approach to hypercalemia. Am Fam Physician. 2003;67:1959–66.
23. Bilezikian JP, Silverberg SJ. Normocalcemic primary hyperparathyroidism. Arq Bras Endocrinol Metabol. 2010;54(2):106–9.
24. Guise TA, Mundy GR. Cancer and bone. Endocr Rev. 1998;19(1):18–54.
25. Silverberg SJ, Lewiecki EM, Mosekilde L, et al. Presentation of asymptomatic primary hyperparathyroidism: proceedings of the third international workshop. J Clin Endocrinol Metab. 2009;94:351–65.
26. Silverberg SJ, Bilezikian JP. Primary hyperparathyroidism. Endocrinology. 2001:1075–93.
27. Lowe H, McMahon DJ, Rubin MR, Bilezikian JP, Silverberg SJ. Normocalcemic primary hyperparathyroidism: further characterization of a new clinical phenotype. J Clin Endocrinol Metab. 2007;92:3001–5.
28. Marques TF, Vasconcelos R, Diniz E, Rêgo D, Griz L, Bandeira F. Normocalcemic primary hyperparathyroidism in clinical practice: an indolent condition or a silent threat? Arq Bras Endocrinol Metabol. 2011;55(5):314–7.
29. Tordjman KM, Greenman Y, Osher E, Shenkerman G, Sern N. Characterization of normocalcemic primary hyperparathyroidism. Am J Med. 2004;117:861–3.
30. Vignali E, Certani F, Chiavistelli S, Meola A, Saponaro F, Centoni R. Normocalcemic primary hyperparathyroidism: a survey in a small village of southern Italy. Endocr Connect. 2015;4:1–7.
31. Lundgren E, Hagstrom EG, Lundin J, Winnerback MB, Roos J, Ljunghall S, et al. Primary hyperparathyroidism revisited in menopausal women with serum calcium in the upper normal range at population based screening 8 yrs ago. World J Surg. 2002;26:931–6.
32. Lemos ALP, Andrade SRL, Bandeira E, Bandeira L, Bandeira F. High rate of occult urolithiasis in normocalcemic primary hyperparathyroidism. 101st Annual Meeting of The Endocrine Society 2018, Abstract 2018-A-6003 Endo (accepted).
33. Tuna MM, Çaliskan M, Ünal M, Demirci T, Dogan BA, Küçükler K, et al. Normocalcemic hyperparathyroidism is associated with complications similar to those of hypercalcemic hyperparathyroidism. J Bone Min Metab. 2015;34:331–5.
34. Silverberg SJ, Bilezikian JP. "Incipient" primary hyperparathyroidism: a "forme fruste" of an old disease. J Clin Endocrinol Metab. 2003;88(11):5348–52.
35. Bilezikian JP, Rubin M, Silverberg SJ. Asymptomatic primary hyperparathyroidism. Arq Bras Endocrinol Metabol. 2006;50(4):647–56.
36. Siilin H, Lundgren E, Mallmin H, et al. Prevalence of primary hyperparathyroidism and impact on bone mineral density in elderly men: MrOs Sweden. World J Surg. 2011;35(6):1266–72.
37. Rao DS, Philips ER, Divind GW, Talpos GB. Randomized controlled clinical trial of surgery versus no surgery in patients with mild PHPT. J Clin Endocrinol Metab. 2004;89:5415–22.
38. Tamura Y, Araki A, Chiba Y, Mori S, Hosoi T, Horiuchi T. Remarkable increase in lumbar spine bone mineral density and amelioration in biochemical markers of bone turnover after parathyroidectomy in elderly patients with primary hyperparathyroidism: a 5-year follow-up study. J Bone Miner Metab. 2007;25:226–31.

39. Joborn C, Hetta J, Johansson H, et al. Psychiatric morbidity in primary hyperparathyroidism. World J Surg. 1988;12:476–81.

40. Coker LH, Rorie K, Cantley L, Kirkland K, Stump D, Burbank N, et al. Primary hyperparathyroidism, cognition, and health-related quality of life. Ann Surg. 2005;242(5):642–50.

41. Walker MD, McMahon DJ, Inabnet WB, Lazar RM, Brown I, Vardy S, et al. Neuropsychological features in primary hyperparathyroidism: a prospective study. J Clin Endocrinol Metab. 2009;94(6):1951–8.

42. Eufrazino CSS, Bandeira F, et al. Peripheral polyneuropathy associated with primary hyperparathyroidism. Arq Bras Endocrinol Metabol. 2008;52(6):976.

43. Moskal W. Severe sensorimotor polyneuropathy in primary hyperparathyroidism. Neurol Neurochir Pol. 1999;33(6):1443–7.

44. Chou FF, Sheen-Chen SM, Leong CP. Neuromuscular recovery after parathyroidectomy in primary hyperparathyroidism. Surgery. 1995;117(1):18–25.

45. Hedback M, Odén S, et al. Cardiovascular disease, hypertension and renal function in primary hyperparathyroidism. J Intern Med. 2002;251:476–83.

46. Marcocci C, Cetani F. Primary hyperparathyroidism. N Engl J Med. 2011;365:2389–97.

47. Yu N, Donnan PT, Flynnt RWV, et al. Increased mortality and morbidity in mild primary hyperparathyroid patients. The parathyroid epidemiology and audit research study (PEARS). Clin Endocrinol. 2010;73:30–4.

48. Yu N, Donnan PT, Leeset GP. A record linkage study of outcomes in patients with mild primary hyperparathyroidism: the parathyroid epidemiology and audit research study (PEARS). Clin Endocrinol. 2011;75:160–76.

49. Rejnmark L, Vestergaard P, Mosekilde L. Nephrolithiasis and renal calcifications in primary hyperparathyroidism lars. J Clin Endocrinol Metab. 2015;96:2377–85.

50. Amaral LMB, Queiroz DC, Marques TF, Mendes M, Bandeira F. Normocalcemic versus hypercalcemic primary hyperparathyroidism: more stone than bone? J Osteoporos. 2012;2012:128352.

51. Udelsman R, Pasieka JL, et al. Surgery for asymptomatic primary hyperparathyroidism: proceedings of the third international workshop. J Clin Endocrinol Metab. 2009;94:366–72.

52. Mohammadi A, Moloudi F, Ghasemi-rad M. The role of colour Doppler ultrasonography in the preoperative localization of parathyroid adenomas. Endocr J. 2012;59(5):375–82.

53. Bandeira FAF, Oliveira R, Griz L, Caldas G, Bandeira C. Differences in accuracy of TC 99m – Sestamibi scanning between severe and mild forms of primary hyperparathyroidism. J Nucl Med Technol. 2008;36:30–5.

54. Beland MD, Mayo-Smith WW, Grand DJ, Machan JT, Monchik JM. Dynamic MDCT for localization of occult parathyroid adenomas in 26 patients with primary hyperparathyroidism. AJR Am J Roentgenol. 2011;196(1):61–5.

55. Chazen JL, Gupta A, Dunning A, Phillps CD. Diagnostic accuracy of 4D-CT for parathyroid adenomas and hyperplasia. AJNR Am J Neuroradiol. 2012;33(3):429–33.

56. Carvalho JRP, Diniz ET, Marques TF, Lima TPM, Galamba L, Bandeira F. PTH measurement in the fine-needle aspirates from cervical nodules in primary hyperparathyroidism. Endocr Rev. 2011;32:P1–251.

57. Bilezikian JP, Khan AA, Potts JT. Guidelines for the management of asymptomatic primary hyperparathyroidism: summary statement from the third international workshop. J Clin Endocrinol Metab. 2009;94:335–9.

58. Bilezikian JP, Brandi ML, Eastell R, et al. Guidelines for the management of asymptomatic primary hyperparathyroidism: summary statement from the International Workshop. J Clin Endocrinol Metab. 2014;99(10):3561–9.

59. Rubin MR, Bilezikian JP, McMahon DJ, Jacobs T, Shane E, Siris E, et al. The natural history of primary hyperparathyroidism with or without parathyroid surgery after 15 years. J Clin Endocrinol Metab. 2008;93:3462–70.

60. Bollerslev J, Jansson S, Mollerup CL, Nordenström J, Lundgren E, Tørring O, et al. Medical observation, compared with parathyroidectomy, for asymptomatic primary hyperparathyroidism: a prospective, randomized trial. J Clin Endocrinol Metab. 2007;92(5):1687.

61. Zanocco K, Heller M, Sturgeon C. Cost-effectiveness of parathyroidectomy for primary hyperparathyroidism. Endocr Pract. 2011;17(1):69–74.

62. Slepavicius A, Beisa V, Janusonis V, Strupas K. Focused versus conventional parathyroidectomy for primary hyperparathyroidism: a prospective, randomized, blinded trial. Langenbeck's Arch Surg. 2008;393(5):659–66.

63. Clerici T, Brandle M, Lange J, Doherty GM, Gauger PG. Impact of intraoperative parathyroid hormone monitoring on the prediction of multiglandular parathyroid disease. World J Surg. 2004;28(2):187–92.

64. Barczynski M, Konturek A, Cichon S, Hubalewska-Dydejczyk A, Golkowski F, et al. Intraoperative parathyroid hormone assay improves outcomes of minimally invasive parathyroidectomy mainly in patients with a presumed solitary parathyroid adenoma and missing concordance of preoperative imaging. Clin Endocrinol. 2007;66(6):878–85.

65. Hwang RS, Morris LF, Ro K, Park S, Ituarte PH, Hong JC, et al. A selective, Bayesian approach to intraoperative PTH monitoring. Ann Surg. 2010;251(6):1122–6.

66. Bergenfelz AO, Jansson SK, Wallin GK, Mårtensson HG, Rasmussen L, Eriksson HL, et al. Impact of modern techniques on short-term outcome after surgery for primary hyperparathyroidism: a multicenter study comprising 2,708 patients. Langenbeck's Arch Surg. 2009;394(5):851–60.

67. Miccoli P, Berti P, Materazzi G, Ambrosini CE, Fregoli L, Donatini G. Endoscopic bilateral neck exploration versus quick intraoperative parathormone assay (qPTHa) during endoscopic parathyroidectomy: a prospective randomized trial. Surg Endosc. 2008;22:398–400.

68. Messa P, Alfieri C, Brezzi B. Cinacalcet: pharmacological and clinical aspects. Expert Opin Drug Metab Toxicol. 2008;4(12):1551–60.

69. Peacock M, Bilezikian JP, Klasssen PS, et al. Cinacalcet hydrochloride maintains long-term normocalcemia in patients with primary hyperparathyroidism. J Clin Endocrinol Metab. 2005;90(1):135–41.

70. Peacock M, Bolognese MA, Borofsky M, Scumpia S, Sterling LR, Cheng S. Cinacalcet treatment of primary hyperparathyroidism: biochemical and bone densitometric outcomes in a five-year study. J Clin Endocrinol Metab. 2009;94(12):4860–7.

71. Rossouw JE, Anderson GL, Prentice RL, LaCroix AZ, Kooperberg C, Stefanick ML, et al. Risks and benefits of estrogen plus progestin in healthy postmenopausal women: principal results from the Women's health initiative randomized controlled trial. JAMA. 2002;288(3):321–33.

72. Grey AB, Stapleton JP, Evans MC, Tatnell MA, Reid IR. Effect of hormone replacement therapy on bone mineral density in postmenopausal women with mild primary hyperparathyroidism. Ann Intern Med. 1996;125:360–8.

73. Orr-Walker BJ, Evans MC, Clearwater JM, Horne A, Grey AB, Reid IR. Effect of hormone replacement therapy on bone mineral density in postmenopausal women with primary hyperparathyroidism: four-year follow-up and comparison with healthy postmenopausal women. Arch Intern Med. 2000;160:2161–6.

74. Rubin MR, Lee KH, McMahon DJ, Silverberg SJ. Raloxifene lowers serum calcium and markers of bone turnover in postmenopausal women with primary hyperparathyroidism. J Clin Endocrinol Metab. 2003;88:1174–8.

75. Rossini M, Gatti D, Isaia G, Sartori L, Braga V, Adami S. Effect of oral alendronate in elderly patients with osteoporosis and mild primary hyperparathyroidism. J Bone Miner Res. 2001;16:113–9.

76. Chow CC, Chan WB, Li JK, Chan NN, Chan MH, Ko GT. Oral alendronate increases bone mineral density in postmenopausal women with primary hyperparathyroidism. J Clin Endocrinol Metab. 2003;88:581–7.

77. Parker CR, Blackwell PJ, Fairbairn KJ, Hosking DJ. Alendronate in the treatment of primary hyperparathyroid-related osteoporosis: a 2-year study. J Clin Endocrinol Metab. 2002;87:4482–9.

78. Hershman JM, Hassani S, Braunstein GD, Geola F, Brickman A, Seibel MJ. Bisphosphonate therapy in primary hyperparathyroidism. J Bone Miner Res. 2003;1880:1889.

79. Khan A, Bilezikian JP, Kung AWC, Ahmed MM, Dubois SJ, Ho AY, et al. Alendronate in primary hyperparathyroidism: a double-blind, randomized, placebo-controlled trial. J Clin Endocrinol Metab. 2004;89(7):3319–25.

80. Jansson S, Morgan E. Biochemical effects from treatment with bisphosphonate and surgery in patients with primary hyperparathyroidism. World J Surg. 2004;28:1293–7.

Vitamin D Deficiency

Malachi J. McKenna and Mark Kilbane

Introduction

Vitamin D, which is present in two forms called cholecalciferol (D_3) and ergocalciferol (D_2), is an essential micronutrient and in the bioactive form plays a key role in maintaining bone health [1, 2]. Vitamin D_3 is predominantly derived from skin production by the direct action of ultraviolet light on skin. Alternative sources of D_3 and D_2 are oral intake from natural foodstuffs, fortified foodstuffs, and supplements. Although the principal source is sunlight, oral intake has primacy over sunlight exposure in both the prevention and correction of nutritional vitamin D deficiency [3]. Sunlight exposure can be a cause of skin cancer and for this reason cannot be advocated as a means of preventing vitamin D deficiency. In determining the oral intake that is required to meet the needs both to prevent and to correct vitamin D deficiency, one must consider inadvertent and intentional exposure to sunlight. In other words, the recommended daily allowance for vitamin D as an oral nutrient need only be specified for those who are sun-deprived; those not sun-deprived have lower oral intake requirements [1, 2].

Vitamin D is activated by two hydroxylation steps: first, by 25-hydroxylase (*CYP2R1*) to 25OHD in the liver that is substrate-dependent on sources of parent vitamin D, and then by 1α-hydroxylase (*CYP27B1*) in the kidney to the hormonally active form, 1α,25-dihydroxyvitamin D ($1,25(OH)_2D$) that is tightly regulated by PTH and FGF23 [1]. The hormonal form then circulates to remote sites of action and binds to the vitamin D receptor (VDR), principally at the intestine promoting absorption of calcium and phosphate. The mineral product of calcium and phosphate is essential for the mineralization of newly formed bone matrix at all stages of life. The final activation step occurs also in extrarenal tissues followed by local binding to VDR, which is termed the paracrine/intracrine effect. This effect is not regulated by calciotropic hormones but by tissue-specific cytokines, and it is substrate-dependent. This is a more complicated aspect of vitamin D action, which is the subject of much basic and clinical research over the past three decades.

The IOM 2011 report concluded that there was a well-established causal link between vitamin D intake and skeletal health [1]. Severe vitamin D deficiency leads to rickets in the growing skeleton and osteomalacia in the adult skeleton. In adults, it also predisposes to low bone mass and contributes to bone fragility fractures in the elderly. Deficiencies in the intracrine action may account for associations between vitamin D deficiency and infections, autoimmune disease, cardiovascular disease, diabetes mellitus, falls, and cancer, but the evidence for causality is inconsistent and inconclusive [1, 4]. Mendelian randomization has shown that 25OHD lies in the causal pathway for susceptibility to multiple sclerosis but cannot measure effect size, timing of susceptibility, threshold of susceptibility, and benefit of intervention [5]. Meta-analyses of trials seem to suggest that the risk of non-skeletal disease lies at 25OHD below 30 nmol/L (12 ng/ml) (see below).

Key Points

Definition of Vitamin D Deficiency (Fig. 23.1)

It is probably best for clinicians to divide vitamin D deficiency into two groups: those who have nutritional deficiency and those who have intestinal, liver, or kidney disorders. Nutritional deficiency encompasses the role of both sources of vitamin D: sunlight exposure and oral intake. Based on 25OHD alone, it is incorrect to apply the terms "deficiency"

M. J. McKenna (✉)
Department of Endocrinology, St. Vincent's University Hospital, Dublin, Ireland

UCD School of Medicine and Medical Sciences, University College Dublin, Dublin, Ireland
e-mail: malachi.mckenna@ucd.ie

M. Kilbane
Department of Clinical Chemistry, St. Vincent's University Hospital, Elm Park, Dublin 4, Ireland
e-mail: m.kilbane@svuh.ie

© Springer Nature Switzerland AG 2022
F. Bandeira et al. (eds.), *Endocrinology and Diabetes*, https://doi.org/10.1007/978-3-030-90684-9_23

Fig. 23.1 BMD bone
mineral density; FGF23
fibroblast growth factor 23;
Ca calcium; P phosphate;
25OHD 25-hydroxyvitamin
D; 1,25(OH)₂D 1α,25-
dihydroxyvitamin D

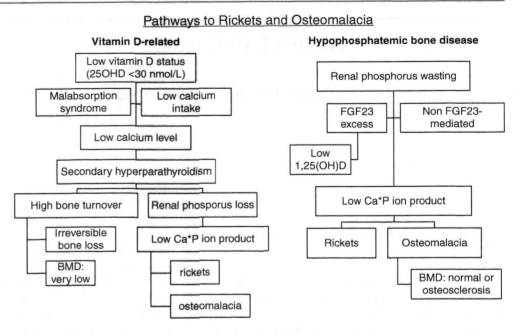

or "insufficiency." Although measuring 25OHD level has a prime role in assessing vitamin D status (see later), it is not a clinical outcome; it is merely a measure of risk of disease [1, 4, 6, 7].

There has been a double paradigm shift since the 1990s: firstly, the term hypovitaminosis D was replaced by the terms "deficiency" and "insufficiency" implying the presence of a disease state; secondly, the 25OHD sufficiency thresholds have steadily increased from 25 nmol/L (10 ng/ml) to 75 nmol/L (30 ng/ml). The IOM 2011 report states that 25OHD is an estimate of risk of clinical outcomes, and that risk of skeletal disease reaches a plateau at 30–40 nmol/L (12–16 ng/ml) [1, 4, 6, 7].

Nutritional vitamin D deficiency is best defined as a clinical, biochemical, radiologic, densitometric, or histomorphometric abnormality that is corrected and prevented by low-dose oral vitamin D supplementation (Fig. 23.1) [8].The natural history of vitamin D-related bone disease at the bone level is a phase of secondary hyperparathyroidism (SHPT) with accelerated irreversible bone loss culminating in a mineralization defect (rickets or osteomalacia) [9]. Once the entire surface of bone is covered by unmineralized bone matrix (osteoid), irreversible bone loss ceases [10]. On the contrary, the natural history for hypophosphatemic bone disease is one of progressive mineralization defect without SHPT [11].

Measuring 25OHD

Serum or plasma 25-hydroxy-vitamin D (25OHD) is the best measure of vitamin D status because its synthesis is substrate-dependent, and it has a long half-life of about 2–3 weeks in vivo [12]. Two types of assay methods predominate for measurement of total 25OHD, 25OHD₃, and 25OHD₂: (1) immunoassays for total 25OHD and (2) liquid chromatography tandem mass spectrometry (LC-MS/MS) for 25OHD₃ and 25OHD₂.

One of the major historical factors contributing to the poor accuracy of 25OHD measurement was the lack of standardization of assay methods [13, 14]. This has been addressed in recent years following the introduction in 2009 of standard reference materials (SRM 972) and solvent-based primary calibrators (SRM 2972) by the American National Institute of Standards and Technology (NIST) in conjunction with the Vitamin D Standardization Program (VDSP). Manufacturers should develop methods traceable to NIST or the University of Ghent reference measurement procedures (RMPs) [15–18]. VDSP advocates that manufacturers should aim to achieve an imprecision of ≤10% and a bias of ≤5% for 25OHD for their methods relative to the RMP [19]. VDSP also includes the retrospective standardization of existing 25(OH)D values collected by epidemiological studies and clinical trials [20]. These developments have had the effect of improving imprecision in 25OHD measurement across methods and between manufacturers. In 1989, interlaboratory CVs (coefficient of variation) for 25OHD methods ranged from 29.3% to 53.7% depending on the concentration measured, compared to 10.3–15.3% in 2017 [21].

Despite the improvements in imprecision, methodological challenges related to 25OHD measurement remain. Most automated immunoassays, which do not have a pre-analytical solvent extraction or protein precipitation step to free 25OHD from vitamin D-binding proteins (DBPs), are subject to DBP matrix interferences [22]. Measurement of the total 25OHD metabolite concentration and equivalent detection of both $25OHD_2$ and $25OHD_3$ by immunoassay is challenging, because binding proteins show a higher affinity for $25OHD_3$ than $25OHD_2$. Cross-reactivity with the metabolite 24,25-dihydroxyvitamin D, which can be present in serum at concentrations of up to 12 nmol/L, can also be a problem for immunoassays [23]. There are limitations associated with 25OHD measurement by LC-MS/MS also. Some LC-MS/MS methods have been shown to suffer from interferences: the C-3 epimer of 25OH D_3 and isobaric substance 7-α-hydroxy-4-cholesten-3-one to name but two [24]. The NIST standard containing 3-epi-25OHD$_3$ (SRM 972 Level 4) allows laboratories to check whether their method suffers from interference from this metabolite. Interferences can be separated by developing novel LC-MS/MS methods that focus on separation of interfering compounds at the liquid chromatography stage. In cases where the patient's result does not fit with the clinical picture, it may be useful to remeasure 25OHD using an alternate method to the primary analysis. Significant differences between results point toward a method-related interference.

It is important for clinical laboratories to provide clinicians with information relating to their 25OHD assays, particularly limitations that address assay traceability, specificity, imprecision, and limit of detection. Participation in a proficiency testing scheme such as the International Vitamin D External Quality Assessment Scheme (DEQAS) by service providers is essential [25]. Clinicians should be alerted to any change of methodology as this could have a significant impact on results, patient classification, and treatment recommendations.

Defining Vitamin D Status and Intake Requirements (Fig. 23.1)

Assessment of vitamin D status should be considered in the light of two governmental reports: the IOM 2011 report, which revised the dietary reference intakes (DRIs) for the USA and Canada, and the Scientific Advisory Committee for Nutrition (SACN) 2016 report, which advised about vitamin D intake in the UK [1, 2]. The 2011 IOM report is now the standard on vitamin D requirement and on vitamin D status because it examined the totality of evidence with respect to harms and benefits for both calcium and vitamin D for the entire population [8]. Using a risk assessment framework, the IOM specified the estimated average requirement (EAR) that meets the need of approximately 50% of the population and the recommended daily allowance (RDA) that meets the need of 97.5% of the population (Fig. 23.1). The EAR is an appropriate estimate when considering intake on a popula-

Table 23.1 Dietary reference intakes for calcium and vitamin D as specified by IOM 2011 report

Life stage group	Calcium mg/d			Vitamin D IU/d		
	EAR	RDA	UL	EAR	RDA	UL
Infants 0–6 months	a	a	1000	b	b	1000
Infants 0–12 months	a	a	1500	b	b	1500
1–3 years old	500	700	2500	400	600	2500
4–8 years old	800	1000	2500	400	600	3000
9–13 years old	1100	1300	3000	400	600	4000
14–18 years old	1100	1300	3000	400	600	4000
19–30 years old	800	1000	2500	400	600	4000
31–50 years old	800	1000	2500	400	600	4000
51–70 years old	800	1000	2000	400	600	4000
51- to 70-year-old females	1000	1200	2000	400	600	4000
71+ years old	1000	1200	2000	400	600	4000
14–18 years old, pregnant/lactating	1100	1300	3000	400	600	4000
19–50 years old, pregnant/lactating	800	1000	2500	400	600	4000

aFor infants, adequate intake is 200 mg/d for 0–6 months of age and 260 mg/d for 6–12 months of age. The adequate intake is used when an EAR/RDA cannot be developed; it is the average intake level based on observed or experimental intakes; and it is likely greater than the needs of most infants
bFor infants, adequate intake is 400 IU/d for 0–12 months of age
EAR estimated average requirement that meets the needs of 50% of the population, *RDA* recommended daily allowance that meets the needs of 97.5% of the population, *UL* upper intake tolerable level

tion basis, whereas the RDA is likely an overestimate of need on an individual basis. The EAR was specified as 10 μg (400 IU) daily corresponding to a 25OHD of 40 nmol/L (16 ng/ml); the RDA was specified as 15 μg (600 IU) daily in those less than 70 years and as 20 μg (800 IU) daily in those over 70 years corresponding a 25OHD of 50 nmol/L (20 ng/ml) (Table 23.1) [6, 7, 26]. SACN also specified a "safe intake" of 10 μg (400 IU) daily but in terms of corresponding 25OHD expressed it differently by advocating from IOM by advocating that 25OHD be maintained above 25 nmol/L (10 ng/ml) throughout the year.

These vitamin D specifications apply to individuals with minimal or no sunlight exposure. This encompasses housebound individuals especially the frail elderly, those who practice concealment for cultural or religious reasons, those with darker skin, those that apply high factor sunscreen, and those residing in high-latitude countries during the months when there is absent skin generation of vitamin D. These otherwise healthy individuals are at risk of reduced vitamin D synthesis [27]. In the USA, the median oral intake of vitamin D is less than 10 μg (400 IU) daily, but the mean 25OHD levels are above 50 nmol/L. The 25OHD level is higher than expected for vitamin D intake; this suggests, not surprisingly, that supply from sunlight exposure, either inadvertent or intentional, contributes substantially to vitamin D status [1]. This reinforces the point that the EAR and RDA apply to sun-deprived individuals.

Regarding terminology, the IOM report considered 25OHD as a "biomarker of exposure" (viz., the best measure of vitamin D supply), but it is not a "biomarker of effect" (viz., it is not a clinical outcome). The report avoided using the terms "vitamin D deficiency" and "vitamin D insufficiency" when defining vitamin D status. Appropriate terms are "hypovitaminosis D" or "low vitamin D status" or "at risk of deficiency" for a result below 30 nmol/L (12 ng/ml) and "range of vitamin D inadequacy" for levels 30–50 nmol/L (12–20 ng/ml). The "tolerable upper intake level (UL)" is defined by the IOM report as the upper level of vitamin D intake beyond which harm could be expected to increase for the general population. The IOM specified the UL as tenfold higher than EAR at 100 µg (4000 IU) daily, corresponding to 25OHD above 125 nmol/L (50 ng/ml). The IOM warned that the UL should not to be considered as a target intake and that striving to achieve 25OHD above the RDA in 97.5% of population means that increasing number will exceed the UL (Fig. 23.2) [7].

Secondary Indices of Vitamin D Deficiency (Fig. 23.3)

If 25OHD is below 30 nmol/L (12 ng/ml), then the clinician should recommend an adequate oral vitamin D intake (see treatment section below) but does not necessarily need to embark on additional investigations. Much lower levels may be associated with clinical features such as proximal myopathy and diffuse bone pain. Secondary biochemical indices include hypocalcemia and hypophosphatemia. Although not calculated in clinical practice, the calcium–phosphate ion product is a measure of the degree of deficiency that links directly with the consequence of a mineralization defect in the bone [28]. Another simple measure that is routinely available is serum total alkaline phosphatase; in the absence of liver disease, it is a direct marker of bone disease.

If the clinician is concerned about vitamin D deficiency, then serum PTH should be measured as part of the assessment because secondary SHPT occurs in response to hypocalcemia. This results in an increase in bone turnover as part of the effort to restore calcium homeostasis. In addition, *CYP27B1* activity is augmented such that $1,25(OH)_2D$ levels may be elevated in vitamin D deficiency; this metabolite is not a measure of vitamin D status. Renal tubular effects of SHPT, such as renal phosphate wasting and renal bicarbonate wasting, may hasten the onset of the mineralization defect in bone. Other factors influence PTH status such as calcium intake, renal function, age, ethnicity, body composition, and geographic location [1, 27]. There is no single threshold level of 25OHD that prevents secondary hyperparathyroidism [29].

An array of bone turnover markers is available for assessing bone status [30]. An increase in bone formation markers may reflect either an increase in bone remodeling activity due to SHPT or a defect in mineralization, whereas increased resorption markers only reflect SHPT. Samples should only be collected in the fasting state; clinicians should obtain protocols from their laboratory service provider for instructions on specimen type required. Formation markers are serum-based: bone specific alkaline phosphatase, procollagen type 1 amino-terminal propeptide and osteocalcin. Resorption markers are either serum-based (beta-C-terminal cross-linking telopeptide of type 1 collagen) or urine-based (amino-terminal cross-linking telopeptide of type 1 collagen).

Specific radiographic changes occur late in vitamin D deficiency. Rickets is a disease of the growing skeleton with radiographic changes being most pronounced at the growth plates in those fastest-growing bones such as around the knee, the distal end of the ulna, the middle ribs, the proximal femur, and the distal tibia. Initially the growth plate widens as a consequence of defective mineralization between epiphysis and metaphysis [31]. Then the metaphyseal surfaces become cupped and irregular. This is accompanied by splaying of the metaphyses and widening of the growth plates that accounts for the classical clinical signs of swelling at the wrists, knees, and anterior ends of the ribs (rickety rosary). Bone deformities occur principally in lower extremities in weight-bearing bones resulting in knock knees, bow-legs, wind-swept legs [32].

Insufficiency-type stress fractures in the setting of osteomalacia are referred to by the eponymous term, Looser zones, which are stress fractures not "pseudofractures" [33]. They are usually multiple in origin and are often symmetric in occurrence. They occur at typical sites in both weight-bearing bones (such as pubic rami, medial aspects of the femur and tibia, and metatarsal bones) and non-weight-bearing bones (such as ribs and medial border of the scapula). Appearances are characteristic in that the fracture appears as a broad rather than a narrow band, margins are parallel, marginal sclerosis is minimal, and callus is usually present, but healing is delayed (Fig. 23.4). Typically, they only occur late as a manifestation of osteomalacia. Traditionally, they were considered to be pathognomic of osteomalacia, but rarely insufficiency-type stress fractures with appearances of Looser zones are described in osteoporosis [34].

Bone mineral density (BMD) should be measured at spine, hip, and forearm (and whole body for those under 20 years) using dual-energy X-ray absorptiometry. While this does not have any discriminant value in diagnostic terms, BMD is a measure of the risk of fragility fracture and is also a baseline measurement to assess the response to treatment.

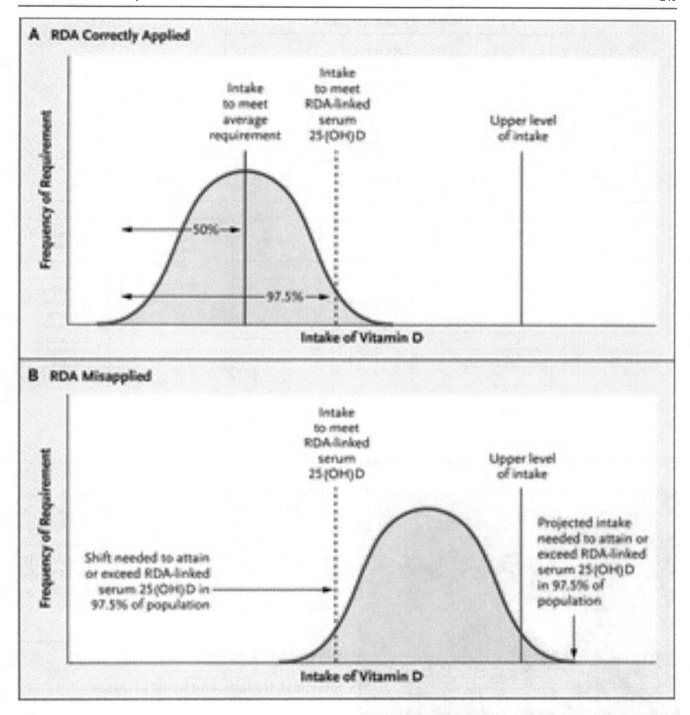

Fig. 23.2 Distribution of vitamin D intake requirements in a healthy population (Panel A) and the upward shift in distribution requirement to attain RDA-linked serum 25OHD concentration in 97.5% of the popu- lation (Panel B). RDA recommended dietary allowance. Reproduced with permission from reference number 7

While correcting vitamin D deficiency in severe cases will result in an improvement in BMD, there is also an irrevers- ible component to the bone loss especially cortical bone that is related to the prolonged phase of SHPT with high bone turnover prior to the onset of the mineralization defect [10]. Hypophosphatemic bone disorders do not have irreversible

PTH-mediated bone loss. In some inherited hypophospha- temic disorders, BMD is increased [35].

Bone histology is rarely performed and rarely needed, especially with the advance in the abovementioned biochem- ical indices. That aside, it is still the gold standard for diag- nosing osteomalacia [11]. There are two principal findings:

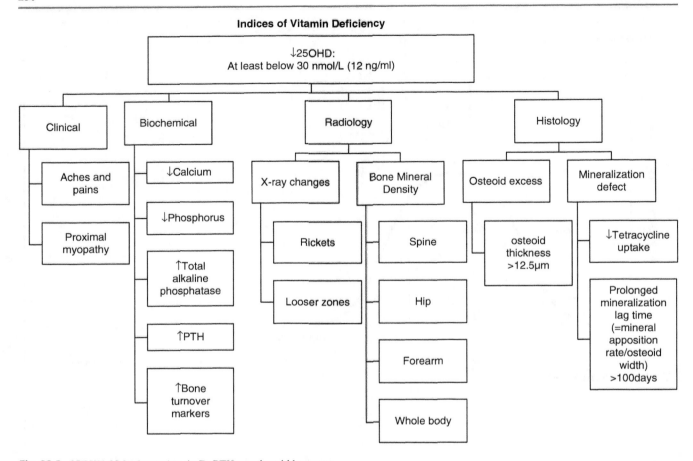

Fig. 23.3 25OHD 25-hydroxyvitamin D, PTH parathyroid hormone

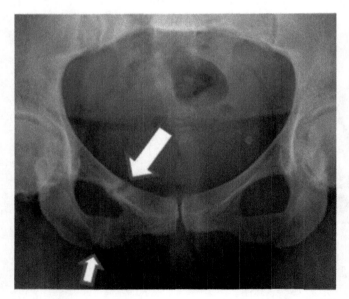

Fig. 23.4 Image of Looser zones in osteomalacia in right superior pubic ramus demonstrating all the characteristics of broad band, minimal callus, transverse and marginal sclerosis in patient with hypophosphatemia due to tumor-induced osteomalacia with elevated FGF23 level. There is also a Looser zone in the right inferior pubic ramus

first, accumulation of unmineralized bone matrix called osteoid and, second, impaired mineralization as measured using tetracycline-based histomorphometry. It is not sufficient to base a diagnosis on osteoid indices alone; any condition that increases bone turnover will also increase the surface extent of osteoid. An osteoid seam width >12.5 μm coupled with a prolonged mineralization lag time >100 days is diagnostic of osteomalacia [11, 36].

Differential Diagnosis (Table 23.2)

Intestinal, Hepatic, and Renal Diseases

Malabsorption of calcium due to disease must be considered and excluded in all cases. Mucosal disorders most notably celiac disease should be considered. Measurement of antibodies to the enzyme tissue transglutaminase and to the endomysium is the best screening test. Diagnosis is confirmed by small bowel histology. Roux-en-Y gastric bypass surgery for obesity leads to a malabsorptive state. Pancreatic insufficiency and cholestatic liver disease, such as primary

Table 23.2 Differential diagnosis of rickets and osteomalacia

1. Vitamin D-related
   (a) Nutritional vitamin D deficiency (combined sun deprivation and inadequate oral intake)
   (b) Disease-specific
   Malabsorption
      Mucosal disorders such as celiac disease
      Pancreatic insufficiency
      Postgastrectomy
      Gastric bypass
   Primary biliary cirrhosis
   Chronic kidney disease
   (c) Inherited
      Loss-of-function mutations of *CYP2R1* (vitamin D-dependent rickets type 1B)
      Loss-of-function mutations of *CYP27B1* (vitamin D-dependent rickets type 1A)
      Nonfunctioning vitamin D receptor (vitamin D-dependent rickets type 2)
2. Deficient calcium intake coupled with high phytate intake
   (a) In Africa and India and in Asian immigrants
3. Hypophosphatemic bone disease due to renal phosphate wasting
   (a) FGF23-mediated
      Inherited
         X-linked hypophosphatemia
         Autosomal dominant hypophosphatemic disease
         Autosomal recessive hypophosphatemic disease
      Acquired
         Tumor-induced osteomalacia
         Post renal transplant hypophosphatemia
   (b) Non-FGF23-mediated
      Fanconi's syndrome
      Drug induced:
         Oral iron chelators
         Antiretrovirals

biliary cirrhosis, are less likely to cause vitamin D-related bone disease. Chronic kidney disease in early stages probably has a higher requirement for substrate vitamin D due to progressive impairment in 1α-hydroxylase. End-stage kidney disease may manifest with osteomalacia as part of mixed bone disease including osteitis fibrosa cystica, adynamic bone disease, and osteosclerosis.

Hypophosphatemic Bone Disease (Table 23.2)

Chronic hypophosphatemia also causes rickets and osteomalacia. It is usually due to a sustained increase in renal phosphate excretion but may also be a consequence of impaired absorption and intake. FGF23 regulates renal phosphate handling by reducing the expression of type 2 sodium-dependent phosphate cotransporters, and it inhibits *CYP27B1* activity. Hypophosphatemic bone disease is divided into two categories: FGF23-mediated and non-FGF23-mediated [35].

In childhood, the commonest cause of inherited renal phosphate wasting is X-linked hypophosphatemia due to inactivating mutations in the PHEX gene that is associated with increased bone expression of FGF23 (OMIM 307800). In adulthood, phosphaturic mesenchymal tumors of mixed connective tissue type that produce an excess of FGF23 that is higher than seen in the inherited conditions leads to severe tumor-induced osteomalacia (TIO) [37]. A number of drugs enhance renal excretion of phosphate resulting in non-FGF23-mediated rickets or osteomalacia such as oral chelators and antiretrovirals [35].

Diagnosis of renal phosphate wasting is straightforward, but it requires measurement of the renal tubular maximum reabsorption of phosphate per unit of glomerular filtrate: TmPO4/GFR. This is conducted by collecting a timed fasting urine and simultaneous blood sample for estimation of phosphate and creatinine in both serum and urine and then by calculating TmPO4/GFR according to a nomogram or an equation [38]. Hypophosphatemia with a low TmPO4/GFR in the absence of hypocalcemia gives a diagnosis of renal phosphate wasting. Serum $1,25(OH)_2D$ levels should be inappropriately low. FGF23 levels can now be measured in specialized laboratories. In childhood, genetic testing for the known mutations should be conducted in hypophosphatemic patients. In adult patients, acquired causes should be sought including TIO, but some of the inherited forms may not present until later in life [35].

Rare Conditions

A few conditions may mimic nutritional vitamin D deficiency. In childhood, there are rare congenital disorders in the metabolism and action of vitamin D that may present as nutritional vitamin D deficiency: loss-of-function mutations of *CYP2R1* (vitamin D-dependent rickets type 1B OMIM 600081), loss-of-function mutations of *CYP27B1* formerly called pseudo-vitamin D deficiency (vitamin D-dependent rickets type 1A, OMIM 264700), and nonfunctioning vitamin D receptor mutations causing hereditary 1,25-dihydroxyvitamin D-resistant rickets (HVDRR, or vitamin D-dependent rickets type 2, OMIM 277440) [39]. These conditions are extremely rare and should only be considered in cases where there is failure to respond to standard intervention (see below).

Calcium deficiency of a severe degree, alone, is now considered to be a cause of rickets that is consistent with the known interdependence of calcium and vitamin D. This has been reported in African children in Nigeria and South Africa who have abundant exposure to sunlight but have extremely low dietary calcium intakes at less than about

200 mg daily on a sustained basis that can be rectified by calcium supplementation [40]. Intake of foods high in phytate and oxalate that chelate calcium may be confounding factors [30]. Similarly, in India where calcium intake is very low and phytate intake is high, rickets and osteomalacia are reported, despite with what would be considered satisfactory vitamin D status in regions where calcium intake is much higher [41, 42].

Hypophosphatasia (OMIM 146300) is a rare heritable form of rickets and osteomalacia with low serum alkaline phosphatase that is caused by loss-of-function mutations in the gene for tissue-nonspecific isoenzyme of alkaline phosphatase (TNSALP) [43]. Inorganic pyrophosphate accumulates that is a potent inhibitor of mineralization. It may manifest in different clinical forms: perinatally with a fatal form, in infancy with severe rickets, in childhood with milder bone disease accompanied by premature loss of teeth, and in adulthood with poorly healing stress fractures. Serum total alkaline phosphatase is low, while calcium, phosphate, 25OHD, and PTH levels are normal. Pyridoxal 5′-phosphate and phosphoethanolamine are usually elevated in serum supporting the diagnosis. Since there is a tendency to hypercalcemia and hyperphosphatemia in childhood presentation, standard treatment for rickets should be avoided; in fact, a restricted calcium intake may be needed to avoid hypercalcemia. For the severe forms of the disease in childhood, they should be treated with asfotase alfa, a hydroxyapatite-targeted recombinant TNSALP, which has been approved for use since 2015 [44].

Chronic metabolic acidosis can cause a mineralization defect. This is seen with renal tubular acidosis because of renal bicarbonate wasting. This is a direct effect of the acidotic state on the bone, which functions as part of the buffering response in the body. Urinary diversion techniques may result in chronic metabolic acidosis, especially ureterosigmoidostomy that was performed in the past and to a lesser extent the extant procedure of uretero-ileostomy. A simple indicant on routine testing is the presence of a normal anion gap metabolic acidosis accompanied by hyperchloremia.

Present and Future Therapies

Vitamin D and Calcium Supplementation

Nutritional vitamin D deficiency is corrected and prevented safely and efficaciously by low-dose vitamin D supplementation. The intake requirements for both vitamin D and calcium as specified by the IOM 2011 report should be followed for all age groups (Table 23.1) [4]. Since 2011, a number

trials have confirmed the accuracy of the simulated vitamin D dose response in all age groups with some nuances with respect to age, ethnicity, obesity, and single gene polymorphisms [45–50]. Vitamin D_3 is favored over D_2 due to the greater potency of the former [51–53]. In view of the interdependence of calcium and vitamin D, the adequacy of calcium intake must be considered in all clinical situations of nutritional vitamin D deficiency, particularly in regions where dietary calcium intake is very low and phytate intake is high [40–42]. A high-calcium intake is better able to compensate for low vitamin D status than a high intake of vitamin D is able to compensate for a low calcium [1].

A recent global consensus on the prevention and management of nutritional rickets has incorporated the findings of the IOM 2011 report providing clinicians with a compendium of advice about vitamin D and calcium requirements across the entire clinical spectrum [54]. This is particularly welcome given the concerns about the rising incidence of rickets and catastrophic hypocalcemia cardiomyopathy in developed countries in conjunction with the great variability in vitamin D status and calcium intakes worldwide.

For adults, the clinician needs to address on an individual basis those cases with diseases that are associated with higher intake requirement of both calcium and vitamin D such as chronic malabsorption. The clinician should be guided by the secondary indices (see above) in order to assess the success of supplemental doses of vitamin D and calcium. Refractory cases may have persistent SHPT that may evolve to tertiary hyperparathyroidism. Rather than opting for high-dose parent vitamin D, one should consider use of activated vitamin D: $1,25(OH)_2D$ or its monohydroxylated analogue 1α-hydroxyvitamin D, which is slightly less potent. Usually, the starting dose is about 0.25 μg twice daily increasing until resolution of the biochemical abnormality. Patients will need frequent monitoring of calcium status, both in serum and urine, as well as all the secondary indices.

Food solutions to vitamin D supply, both traditional fortification and biofortification, improves vitamin D status in the general population, especially during the winter months thereby lessening the need for supplementation [55]. For many decades vitamin D has been added exogenously to milk, to infant formula, and to margarine and more recently to bread and cereals with different practices in different countries [53, 56, 57]. Biofortification is achieved either by addition of vitamin D to animal feeds, exposing animals to ultraviolet light, or exposing mushrooms to ultraviolet light [53, 58, 59]. As the vitamin D health of a nation improves by fortification coupled with increasing supplementation, the risk of hypervitaminosis D escalates [7, 60].

High-Dose Vitamin D Therapy: 25OHD Dose Response and Outcome Response

In evaluating trials of vitamin D therapy, one must understand both the 25OHD dose response and outcome response. High-dose vitamin D therapy may be defined as an oral intake that is a multiple of the intake requirement for adequacy. This should refer to total intake not just supplemental intake. This is achieved by two ways that are not equivalent: high daily dose often ranging from 4000 IU to 10,000 IU (and even higher) or intermittent bolus doses often ranging from 25,000 IU to 500,000 IU given at intervals from 1 month to 1 year.

The lack of equivalence between daily dosing and intermittent bolus dosing is related to the nature of the 25OHD dose response. The IOM 2011 report noted that the 25OHD response was curvilinear in a simulation regression analysis using information from trials conducted during winter months; the mixed effects model with a log transformation of 25OHD yielded the best curvilinear fit: 25OHD in nmol/L = 9.9 ln (total vitamin D intake). This approach shifted the paradigm from supplemental 25OHD dose response to "achieved" 25OHD dose response, now incorporating the influence of all sources of vitamin D intake to 25OHD. The simulated curvilinear dose response in the IOM 2011 report was confirmed by a multidose study ranging trial using seven doses ranging from 400 IU daily to 4800 IU daily, with the best fit for estimating the "achieved" being a quadratic function: 25OHD nmol/L = $54.5 + 24.6*dose/1000 - 2.5*dose^2/1000^2$ [45]. Using either of these equations explains the differences that are seen in comparing linear dose responses with the principal determinant being the baseline 25OHD; it also demonstrates the fallacy of recommending a dose rate constant [61]. In terms of dosing intervals, the 25OHD response is higher in the following rank order – daily, weekly, and monthly – indicating that the 25OHD response is not a simple function of the cumulative dose [62].

Lack of effect and even unexpected harmful outcomes have been demonstrated in randomized control trials of high-dose vitamin D therapy. With falls as a primary outcome, falls were more likely in those high-dose vitamin D groups in three different studies: using 4800 IU daily [63], 60,000 IU monthly [64], and 500,000 yearly [65]. Intramuscular 300,000 IU yearly had a higher hazard ratio of first fracture at both hip and wrist [66]; oral 500,000 IU yearly had a higher rate of all fractures [65]. High-dose vitamin D (50,000 IU monthly) did not improve functional status in postmenopausal women [67]. Maternal administration did not prevent childhood asthma using either 4000 IU daily [68] or 2400 IU daily [69]. Progression to diabetes was not halted by 20,000 IU weekly [70]; insulin resistance was not

improved by 3750 IU daily [71]. The rate of cardiovascular disease was not reduced by high-dose vitamin D over an average of 3.3 years (initial dose of 200,000 IU, followed a month later by monthly doses of 100,000 IU) [72]. Urosepsis was not prevented by 20,000 IU weekly for 5 years [73]. High-dose vitamin D (oral bolus 540,000 IU followed by monthly 90,000 IU for 5 months) did not reduce length of stay in critically ill patients [74]. Administration of oral 100,000 IU every 3–18 months to infants did not prevent first onset of pneumonia, but the rate of repeat pneumonia was significantly higher in the vitamin D therapy group [75]. Meta-analysis of trials using individual level patient data suggests that prevention of respiratory tract infection is most evident in those with 25OHD below 25 nmol/L or in those given daily or weekly doses compared to less frequent bolus doses [76]. In a similar analysis of individual patient data, vitamin D therapy reduced the rate of asthma exacerbation treated with steroids in those with 25OHD below 25 nmol/L but not in those with 25OHD above 25 nmol/L [77].

Future Therapies

While high-dose vitamin D trials have at best had a null effect, the principal research question remains concerning the role of low-dose vitamin supplementation in the prevention of nonskeletal disease, about which the IOM 2011 report and the SACN 2016 report concluded that evidence was inconclusive and inconsistent [1, 2]. To this end, the most important study is the VITamin D and OmegA-3 TriaL (VITAL); this is an ongoing nationwide, randomized, double-blind, placebo-controlled clinical trial [78]. The study population consists of 25,874 US adults without cancer or cardiovascular disease at baseline and over the age of 50 years. It has a two-by-two factorial design, which means from a vitamin D perspective that there will be a group that receives vitamin D alone 50 µg (2000 IU) daily to be compared with a double placebo group. The mean length of the randomized treatment period will be 5 years. Recruitment ran from November 2011 to March 2015, and randomization has been successful with respect to baseline demographic, health, and behavioral characteristics across treatment groups as well with respect to known potential confounders.

Conclusion

Nutritional vitamin D deficiency is common in groups at risk of sun deprivation. It is straight forward to investigate using standard biochemical tests. It is effectively and safely corrected and prevented by following IOM and SACN specified intakes. High-dose vitamin D, daily, and bolus, should be avoided. More severe and refractory cases should be investigated for other causes of vitamin D-related deficiency and for hypophosphatemic bone disease; these conditions are likely to need expert evaluation and pharmacologic intervention with regular supervision of response to intervention.

References

1. Committee to Review Dietary Reference Intakes for Vitamin D and Calcium, Institute of Medicine. Dietary reference intakes for calcium and vitamin D. Washington, DC: The National Academies Press; 2011.
2. Scientific Advisory Committee on Nutrition (2016) Vitamin D and health. Crown.
3. McKenna MJ. Differences in vitamin D status between countries in young adults and the elderly. Am J Med. 1992;93:69–77.
4. Ross AC, Manson JE, Abrams SA, et al. The 2011 report on dietary reference intakes for calcium and vitamin D from the Institute of Medicine: what clinicians need to know. J Clin Endocrinol Metab. 2011;96:53–8.
5. Mokry LE, Ross S, Ahmad OS, Forgetta V, Smith GD, Leong A, Greenwood CMT, Thanassoulis G, Richards JB. Vitamin D and risk of multiple sclerosis: a Mendelian randomization study. PLoS Med. 2015;12:e1001866.
6. Aloia JF. The 2011 report on dietary reference intake for vitamin D: where do we go from here? J Clin Endocrinol Metab. 2011;96:2987–96.
7. Manson JE, Brannon PM, Rosen CJ, Taylor CL. Vitamin D deficiency - is there really a pandemic? N Engl J Med. 2016;375:1817–20.
8. Parfitt AM, Gallagher JC, Heaney RP, Johnston CC, Neer R, Whedon GD. Vitamin D and bone health in the elderly. Am J Clin Nutr. 1982;36:1014–31.
9. McKenna MJ, Freaney R. Secondary hyperparathyroidism in the elderly: means to defining hypovitaminosis D. Osteoporos Int. 1998;8(Suppl 2):S3–6.
10. Parfitt AM, Rao DS, Stanciu J, Villanueva AR, Kleerekoper M, Frame B. Irreversible bone loss in osteomalacia. Comparison of radial photon absorptiometry with iliac bone histomorphometry during treatment. J Clin Invest. 1985;76:2403–12.
11. Parfitt AM. Osteomalacia and related disorders. In: Avioli LV, Krane SM, editors. Metabolic bone disease and clinically related disorders. Third ed. Boston: Academic Press; 1998. p. 327–86.
12. Jones KS, Assar S, Harnpanich D, Bouillon R, Lambrechts D, Prentice A, Schoenmakers I. 25(OH)D2 half-life is shorter than 25(OH)D3 half-life and is influenced by DBP concentration and genotype. J Clin Endocrinol Metab. 2014;99:3373–81.
13. Roth HJ, Schmidt-Gayk H, Weber H, Niederau C. Accuracy and clinical implications of seven 25-hydroxyvitamin D methods compared with liquid chromatography-tandem mass spectrometry as a reference. Ann Clin Biochem. 2008;45:153–9.
14. Farrell CJ, Martin S, McWhinney B, Straub I, Williams P, Herrmann M. State-of-the-art vitamin D assays: a comparison of automated immunoassays with liquid chromatography-tandem mass spectrometry methods. Clin Chem. 2012;58:531–42.
15. Sempos CT, Vesper HW, Phinney KW, Thienpont LM, Coates PM, Vitamin DSP. Vitamin D status as an international issue: national surveys and the problem of standardization. Scand J Clin Lab Invest Suppl. 2012;243:32–40.
16. Binkley N, Sempos CT, Vitamin DSP. Standardizing vitamin D assays: the way forward. J Bone Miner Res. 2014;29:1709–14.
17. Tai SS, Nelson MA, Bedner M, Lang BE, Phinney KW, Sander LC, Yen JH, Betz JM, Sempos CT, Wise SA. Development of standard

18. reference material (SRM) 2973 vitamin D metabolites in frozen human serum (high level). J AOAC Int. 2017;100:1294–303.
18. Stepman HC, Vanderroost A, Van Uytfanghe K, Thienpont LM. Candidate reference measurement procedures for serum 25-hydroxyvitamin D3 and 25-hydroxyvitamin D2 by using isotope-dilution liquid chromatography-tandem mass spectrometry. Clin Chem. 2011;57:441–8.
19. Stockl D, Sluss PM, Thienpont LM. Specifications for trueness and precision of a reference measurement system for serum/plasma 25-hydroxyvitamin D analysis. Clin Chim Acta. 2009;408:8–13.
20. Durazo-Arvizu RA, Tian L, Brooks SPJ, Sarafin K, Cashman KD, Kiely M, Merkel J, Myers GL, Coates PM, Sempos CT. The vitamin D standardization program (VDSP) manual for retrospective laboratory standardization of serum 25-hydroxyvitamin D data. J AOAC Int. 2017;100:1234–43.
21. Carter GD, Berry J, Durazo-Arvizu R, et al. Hydroxyvitamin D assays: an historical perspective from DEQAS. J Steroid Biochem Mol Biol. 2017;177:30–5.
22. Heijboer AC, Blankenstein MA, Kema IP, Buijs MM. Accuracy of 6 routine 25-hydroxyvitamin D assays: influence of vitamin D binding protein concentration. Clin Chem. 2012;58:543–8.
23. Coldwell RD, Trafford DJ, Makin HL, Varley MJ, Kirk DN. Specific estimation of 24,25-dihydroxyvitamin D in plasma by gas chromatography-mass spectrometry. Clin Chem. 1984;30:1193–8.
24. Lensmeyer G, Poquette M, Wiebe D, Binkley N. The C-3 epimer of 25-hydroxyvitamin D(3) is present in adult serum. J Clin Endocrinol Metab. 2012;97:163–8.
25. Carter GD, Berry J, Durazo-Arvizu R, et al. Quality assessment of vitamin D metabolite assays used by clinical and research laboratories. J Steroid Biochem Mol Biol. 2017;173:100–4.
26. Taylor CL, Carriquiry AL, Bailey RL, Sempos CT, Yetley EA. Appropriateness of the probability approach with a nutrient status biomarker to assess population inadequacy: a study using vitamin D. Am J Clin Nutr. 2013;97:72–8.
27. Rosen CJ, Abrams SA, Aloia JF, et al. IOM committee members respond to Endocrine Society Vitamin D guideline. J Clin Endocrinol Metab. 2012;97:1146–52.
28. McKenna MJ, Freaney R, Casey OM, Towers RP, Muldowney FP. Osteomalacia and osteoporosis: evaluation of a diagnostic index. J Clin Pathol. 1983;36:245–52.
29. Sai AJ, Walters RW, Fang X, Gallagher JC. Relationship between vitamin D, parathyroid hormone, and bone health. J Clin Endocrinol Metab. 2011;96:E436–46.
30. Szulc P, Delmas PD. Biochemical markers of bone turnover: potential use in the investigation and management of postmenopausal osteoporosis. Osteoporos Int. 2008;19:1683–704.
31. Adams JE. Radiology of rickets and osteomalacia. In: Feldman D, Pike JW, Adams JS, editors. Vitamin D. Third ed. London: Academic Press; 2011. p. 861–89.
32. Pettifor JM. Vitamin D deficiency and nutritional rickets in children. In: Feldman D, Pike JW, Adams JS, editors. Vitamin D. Third ed. London: Academic Press; 2011. p. 1107–28.
33. McKenna MJ, Heffernan E, Hurson C, McKiernan FE. Clinician approach to diagnosis of stress fractures including bisphosphonate-associated fractures. QJM. 2014;107:99–105.
34. McKenna MJ, Kleerekoper M, Ellis BI, Rao DS, Parfitt AM, Frame B. Atypical insufficiency fractures confused with Looser zones of osteomalacia. Bone. 1987;8:71–8.
35. Imel EA, Econs MJ. Approach to the hypophosphatemic patient. J Clin Endocrinol Metab. 2012;97:696–706.
36. Recker R. Bone biopsy and histomorphometry in clinical practice. In: Rosen CR, editor. Primar on the metabolic bone diseases and disorders of mineral metabolism. Eight ed. Ames: Wiley-Blackwell; 2013. p. 307–16.

37. Lee JC, Su SY, Changou CA, et al. Characterization of FN1-FGFR1 and novel FN1-FGF1 fusion genes in a large series of phosphaturic mesenchymal tumors. Mod Pathol. 2016;29:1335–46.

38. Walton RJ, Bijvoet OL. Nomogram for derivation of renal threshold phosphate concentration. Lancet. 1975;2:309–10.

39. Molin A, Wiedemann A, Demers N, et al. Vitamin D–dependent rickets type 1B (25-hydroxylase deficiency): a rare condition or a misdiagnosed condition? J Bone Miner Res. 2017;32:1893–9.

40. Thacher TD, Smith L, Fischer PR, Isichei CO, Cha SS, Pettifor JM. Optimal dose of calcium for treatment of nutritional rickets: a randomized controlled trial. J Bone Miner Res. 2016;31:2024–31.

41. Aggarwal V, Seth A, Aneja S, Sharma B, Sonkar P, Singh S, Marwaha RK. Role of calcium deficiency in development of nutritional rickets in Indian children: a case control study. J Clin Endocrinol Metab. 2012;97:3461–6.

42. Dhanwal DK, Sahoo S, Gautam VK, Saha R. Hip fracture patients in India have vitamin D deficiency and secondary hyperparathyroidism. Osteoporos Int. 2013;24:553–7.

43. Whyte MP. Hypophosphatasia: an overview for 2017. Bone. 2017;102:15–25.

44. Whyte MP. Hypophosphatasia: enzyme replacement therapy brings new opportunities and new challenges. J Bone Miner Res. 2017;32:667–75.

45. Gallagher JC, Sai A, Templin T, Smith L. Dose response to vitamin D supplementation in postmenopausal women. Ann Intern Med. 2012;156:425–37.

46. Tripkovic L, Wilson LR, Hart K, et al. Daily supplementation with 15 μg vitamin D2 compared with vitamin D3 to increase wintertime 25-hydroxyvitamin D status in healthy South Asian and white European women: a 12-wk randomized, placebo-controlled food-fortification trial. Am J Clin Nutr. 2017;106:481–90.

47. Smith TJ, Tripkovic L, Damsgaard CT, et al. Estimation of the dietary requirement for vitamin D in adolescents aged 14–18 y: a dose-response, double-blind, randomized placebo-controlled trial. Am J Clin Nutr. 2016;104:1301–9.

48. Mortensen C, Damsgaard CT, Hauger H, et al. Estimation of the dietary requirement for vitamin D in white children aged 4-8 y: a randomized, controlled, dose-response trial. Am J Clin Nutr. 2016;104:1310–7.

49. Ohlund I, Lind T, Hernell O, Silverdal SA, Karlsland Akeson P. Increased vitamin D intake differentiated according to skin color is needed to meet requirements in young Swedish children during winter: a double-blind randomized clinical trial. Am J Clin Nutr. 2017;106:105–12.

50. Gaffney-Stomberg E, Lutz LJ, Shcherbina A, Ricke DO, Petrovick M, Cropper TL, Cable SJ, McClung JP. Association between single gene polymorphisms and bone biomarkers and response to calcium and vitamin D supplementation in young adults undergoing military training. J Bone Miner Res. 2017;32:498–507.

51. Oliveri B, Mastaglia SR, Brito GM, Seijo M, Keller GA, Somoza J, Diez RA, Di Girolamo G. Vitamin D3 seems more appropriate than D2 to sustain adequate levels of 25OHD: a pharmacokinetic approach. Eur J Clin Nutr. 2015;69:697–702.

52. Jakobsen J, Andersen E, Christensen T, Andersen R, Bügel S. Vitamin D vitamers affect vitamin D status differently in young healthy males. Nutrients. 2018;10:12.

53. Itkonen ST, Skaffari E, Saaristo P, Saarnio EM, Erkkola M, Jakobsen J, Cashman KD, Lamberg-Allardt C. Effects of vitamin D2-fortified bread v. supplementation with vitamin D2 or D3 on serum 25-hydroxyvitamin D metabolites: an 8-week randomised-controlled trial in young adult Finnish women. Br J Nutr. 2016;115:1232–9.

54. Munns CF, Shaw N, Kiely M, et al. Global consensus recommendations on prevention and management of nutritional rickets. J Clin Endocrinol Metab. 2016;101:394–415.

55. Jaaskelainen T, Itkonen ST, Lundqvist A, et al. The positive impact of general vitamin D food fortification policy on vitamin D status in a representative adult Finnish population: evidence from an 11-y follow-up based on standardized 25-hydroxyvitamin D data. Am J Clin Nutr. 2017;105:1512–20.

56. Bogdan Y, Tornetta P 3rd, Einhorn TA, et al. Healing time and complications in operatively treated atypical femur fractures associated with bisphosphonate use: a multicenter retrospective cohort. J Orthop Trauma. 2016;30:177–81.

57. Akkermans MD, Eussen SR, van der Horst-Graat JM, van Elburg RM, van Goudoever JB, Brus F. A micronutrient-fortified young-child formula improves the iron and vitamin D status of healthy young European children: a randomized, double-blind controlled trial. Am J Clin Nutr. 2017;105:391–9.

58. Hayes A, Duffy S, O'Grady M, et al. Vitamin D–enhanced eggs are protective of wintertime serum 25-hydroxyvitamin D in a randomized controlled trial of adults. Am J Clin Nutr. 2016;104:629–37.

59. Barnkob LL, Argyraki A, Petersen PM, Jakobsen J. Investigation of the effect of UV-LED exposure conditions on the production of vitamin D in pig skin. Food Chem. 2016;212:386–91.

60. McKenna MJ, Murray BF, O'Keane M, Kilbane MT. Rising trend in vitamin D status from 1993 to 2013: dual concerns for the future. Endocr Connect. 2015;4:163–71.

61. McKenna MJ, Murray BF. Vitamin D dose response is underestimated by Endocrine Society's Clinical Practice Guideline. Endocr Connect. 2013;2:87–95.

62. Chel V, Wijnhoven HA, Smit JH, Ooms M, Lips P. Efficacy of different doses and time intervals of oral vitamin D supplementation with or without calcium in elderly nursing home residents. Osteoporos Int. 2008;19:663–71.

63. Smith LM, Gallagher JC, Suiter C. Medium doses of daily vitamin D decrease falls and higher doses of daily vitamin D3 increase falls: a randomized clinical trial. J Steroid Biochem Mol Biol. 2017;173:317–22.

64. Bischoff-Ferrari HA, Dawson-Hughes B, Orav E, et al. Monthly high-dose vitamin d treatment for the prevention of functional decline: a randomized clinical trial. JAMA Intern Med. 2016:1–10.

65. Sanders KM, Stuart AL, Williamson EJ, Simpson JA, Kotowicz MA, Young D, Nicholson GC. Annual high-dose oral vitamin D and falls and fractures in older women: a randomized controlled trial. JAMA. 2010;303:1815–22.

66. Smith H, Anderson F, Raphael H, Maslin P, Crozier S, Cooper C. Effect of annual intramuscular vitamin D on fracture risk in elderly men and women—a population-based, randomized, double-blind, placebo-controlled trial. Rheumatology. 2007;46:1852–7.

67. Hansen KE, Johnson R, Chambers KR, et al. Treatment of vitamin d insufficiency in postmenopausal women: a randomized clinical trial. JAMA Intern Med. 2015;175:1612–21.

68. Litonjua AA, Carey VJ, Laranjo N, et al. Effect of prenatal supplementation with vitamin D on asthma or recurrent wheezing in offspring by age 3 years: the VDAART randomized clinical trial. JAMA. 2016;315:362–70.

69. Chawes BL, Bonnelykke K, Stokholm J, et al. Effect of vitamin D3 supplementation during pregnancy on risk of persistent wheeze in the offspring: a randomized clinical trial. JAMA. 2016;315:353–61.

70. Jorde R, Sollid ST, Svartberg J, Schirmer H, Joakimsen RM, Njolstad I, Fuskevag OM, Figenschau Y, Hutchinson MY. Vitamin D 20,000 IU per week for five years does not prevent progression from prediabetes to diabetes. J Clin Endocrinol Metab. 2016;101:1647–55.

71. El-Hajj Fuleihan G, Baddoura R, Habib RH, et al. Effect of vitamin D replacement on indexes of insulin resistance in overweight elderly individuals: a randomized controlled trial. Am J Clin Nutr. 2016;104:315–23.

72. Scragg R, Stewart AW, Waayer D, Lawes CMM, Toop L, Sluyter J, Murphy J, Khaw KT, Camargo CA Jr. Effect of monthly high-dose

vitamin D supplementation on cardiovascular disease in the vitamin D assessment study: a randomized clinical trial. JAMA Cardiol. 2017;2:608–16.

73. Jorde R, Sollid ST, Svartberg J, Joakimsen RM, Grimnes G, Hutchinson MY. Prevention of urinary tract infections with vitamin D supplementation 20,000 IU per week for five years. Results from an RCT including 511 subjects. Infect Dis (Lond). 2016:1–6.

74. Amrein K. Vitamin D status in critical care: contributor or marker of poor health? Lung India. 2014;31:299–300.

75. Manaseki-Holland S, Maroof Z, Bruce J, Mughal MZ, Masher MI, Bhutta ZA, Walraven G, Chandramohan D. Effect on the incidence of pneumonia of vitamin D supplementation by quarterly bolus dose to infants in Kabul: a randomised controlled superiority trial. Lancet. 2012;379:1419–27.

76. Martineau AR, Jolliffe DA, Hooper RL, et al. Vitamin D supplementation to prevent acute respiratory tract infections: systematic review and meta-analysis of individual participant data. BMJ. 2017;356:i6583.

77. Jolliffe DA, Greenberg L, Hooper RL, et al. Vitamin D supplementation to prevent asthma exacerbations: a systematic review and meta-analysis of individual participant data. Lancet Respir Med. 2017;5(11):881–90.

78. Pradhan AD, Manson JE. Update on the Vitamin D and OmegA-3 trial (VITAL). J Steroid Biochem Mol Biol. 2016;155:252–6.

Postmenopausal Osteoporosis

Patrícia Nunes Mesquita, Juliana Maria Coelho Maia,
Sérgio Ricardo de Lima Andrade, and Francisco Bandeira

Epidemiology

Osteoporosis is a disorder characterized by low bone mass, with microarchitectural disruption and skeletal fragility, resulting in an increased risk of fractures. It is the most common of all osteoid-metabolic disorders and represents a major public health problem worldwide, affecting one in every three women aged 50 and over. Its incidence is most likely associated with the aging of the world's population.

Studies in the USA such as the NHANES III study (Third National Health and Nutritional Examination Survey) have confirmed an elevated occurrence of osteoporosis, with prevalence in the femoral neck of patients over 50 years of age, showing that 20% of women of Caucasian and Hispanic origin, 7% of black women, and 7% of all men are affected [1], which corresponds to around ten million people, 80% of whom are women. Studies indicate that half of all postmenopausal women will have an osteoporotic fracture during their lifetime, with potential consequences that include short-term and long-term morbidity, not to mention the economic aspects involved. Costs related to osteoporosis in 2005 reached approximately $17 billion and could double or triple by 2040. Although medical therapy can reduce the risk of fractures and is cost-effective, osteoporosis often goes undiagnosed and untreated. The US Preventive Services Task Force (USPSTF) therefore recommends that all women 65 and over should be routinely examined [2].

In Brazil there is no concrete data on the occurrence of osteoporotic fractures. It is estimated that around ten million

P. N. Mesquita · J. M. C. Maia
Department of Endocrinology, Agamenon Magalhães Hospital, Recife, Pernambuco, Brazil

F. Bandeira (✉)
Division of Endocrinology, Agamenon Magalhães Hospital, University of Pernambuco Medical School, Recife, PE, Brazil
e-mail: francisco.bandeira@upe.br

S. R. de Lima Andrade
Agamenon Magalhães Hospital, Division of Endocrinology and Diabetes, University of Pernambuco Medical School, Recife, Pernambuco, Brazil

people in the country have osteoporosis and 2.4 million suffer from some type of fracture each year. A study in Recife that evaluated 657 women over 50 years of age found that 29% of them demonstrated the presence of osteoporosis in the lumbar spine and 19% in the femoral neck, with an increased prevalence accompanying the advancement of age [3].

The pathophysiology of osteoporosis is shown in Figs. 24.1 and 24.2. It is important to recognize the problem, along with its risk factors and consequences in order to decrease morbidity, mortality, and the costs associated with the disease.

Risk Factors

Osteoporosis is a multifactorial disease, consisting of some aspects that are potentially modifiable and others that are not. Factors that are genetic, racial, and anthropometric, along with those related to body composition, bone density, diet, physical activity, and other lifestyle factors, are important elements in the predisposition to and development of osteoporosis.

The two major risk determinants for developing osteoporosis are peak bone mass and rate of bone loss. Risk factors that influence these determinants should be evaluated in all postmenopausal women in order to properly estimate the threat of fractures, exclude secondary causes of osteoporosis, identify modifiable risk factors, and determine the appropriate drug therapy for each case [4].

The main risk factors for osteoporosis are listed in Table 24.1.

FRAX

FRAX™ is a tool available online (http://www.shef.ac.uk/FRAX/index.htm) which was developed by the World Health Organization. It is employed to gather independent risk factors for osteoporotic fractures involving individuals over 50 years of age, in order to quantify the probability of

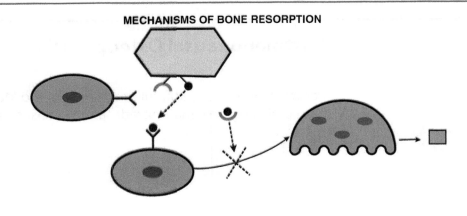

Fig. 24.1 Mechanisms of bone resorption. The stromal cells or osteoblast releases RANKL and osteoprotegerin. RANKL will bind to RANK on the surface of the osteoclast precursor, leading to fusion and differentiation of this cell into mature osteoclasts, which in turn release cathepsin K. When there is increased production of osteoprotegerin, such as in estrogen deficiency, the osteoprotegerin binds to RANKL inhibiting the formation of mature osteoclast

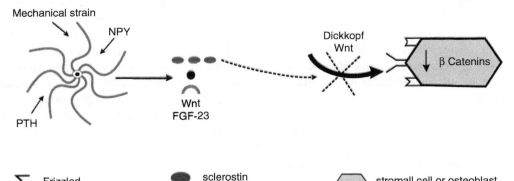

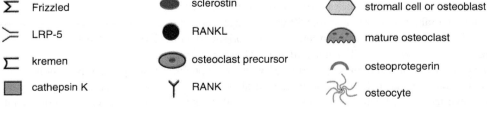

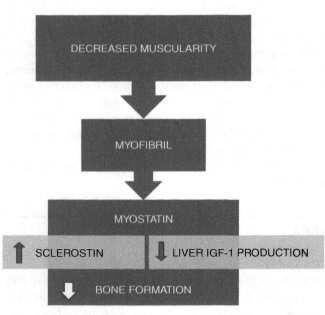

Fig. 24.2 Mechanisms of bone formation. The osteocyte, under the action of PTH, mechanical strain, and NPY, releases sclerostin, which will block the binding of proteins Wnt and Dickkopf to osteoblast receptors, especially the LRP-5

Table 24.1 Risk factors for osteoporosis

Family history of osteoporosis	Cushing syndrome and use of corticosteroids
Advancement of age	Chronic renal failure
Female gender	Celiac disease
Sedentary lifestyle	Hyperthyroidism
Malnutrition	Primary hyperparathyroidism
Low calcium and vitamin D intake	Multiple myeloma
Diabetes mellitus[a]	Time of menopause
Smoking	Low body weight
Alcoholism	Obesity[b]
Personal history of fractures	Deficiency of GH and IGF-1
Delayed puberty and/or hypogonadism	Vitamin D deficiency
Prolonged immobilization	Depression

Data from Ref. [4]
[a]Diabetics show an increase in sclerostin and a decrease in bone mineral density
[b]Obesity increases the risk for some types of fractures

fracture of the femoral neck or other major osteoporotic fractures (vertebral, hip, forearm, and humerus) over the following 10 years.

The variables considered include gender, age, BMI, personal history of fractures after the age of 40, family history of hip fractures, smoking, excessive alcohol consumption, rheumatoid arthritis, use of glucose corticoids, or other secondary causes of osteoporosis [5].

Using population samples from Europe, North America, Asia, and Australia, country-specific data was compiled, allowing calculations based on regional differences. When FRAX is associated with bone mineral density (BMD) testing, it is a more useful tool for predicting fracture risk than the use of either FRAX or BMD alone.

Although its use is not routinely indicated for patients who are already being treated for osteoporosis, a study demonstrated that FRAX may be a useful tool for assessing fracture risk in these patients, pointing to the need to either continue or discontinue medication [6].

Diagnosis

Clinical History and Physical Examination

Through a clinical history and thorough physical examinations, it is possible to detect secondary causes of osteoporosis and risk factors for osteoporosis. In the clinical evaluation of the patient, weight, height, family history of osteoporosis, age, race, nutritional status, calcium and vitamin D intake, thoracic-lumbar pain (chronic or acute), decreased stature, chest deformities, medication use (current and previous), menstrual cycles, time of menopause, history of fractures, and lifestyle habits (smoking, alcohol consumption, and physical activity) should all be taken into consideration.

Most patients with osteoporosis are asymptomatic until the onset of clinical fractures. Vertebral fractures can result in loss of height and/or kyphosis and local pain, due mainly to the shortening and contracture of the paraspinal musculature caused by the reduction of vertebral height [7]. However, most vertebral microfractures are asymptomatic.

Postmenopausal women should also be questioned regarding clinical factors associated with an increased risk of falls, including history of falls, fainting, muscle weakness, problems with coordination and balance, difficulty walking, arthritis in the lower limbs, peripheral neuropathy, and decreased visual acuity.

Laboratory Evaluation

Laboratory tests are important, primarily to exclude secondary causes of osteoporosis. The initial evaluation should include the following: CBC, VHS, 24-h calciuria, calcium, albumin, phosphorus, transaminases, alkaline phosphatase, serum and urine protein electrophoresis, renal function, thyroid function,

Table 24.2 Bone formation and resorption markers

Formation markers	Resorption markers
Alkaline phosphatase	Telopeptides of collagen cross-links
Osteocalcin	Amino-terminal amino-NTX (N-telopeptide)
Pro-peptides of type 2 collagen	Carboxy-terminal—CTX (C-telopeptide)
Amino-terminal (PINP)	Pyridinolines
Carboxy-terminal (PICP)	Hydroxyproline
Osteocalcin (OCN)	Tartrate-resistant phosphatase acid

PTH, and 25 (OH) vitamin D. If any secondary cause is clinically suspected and/or bone loss greater than expected for the age, investigations should be extended to include cortisol after 1 mg of dexamethasone or a 24-h urinary free cortisol, tissue transglutaminase antibodies, bone marrow study, free light chains, free kappa and lambda light chains, serum iron, and ferritin (for suspected hemochromatosis) [8].

Bone Markers

Bone markers are substances released during bone remodeling processes, which can be assayed in serum or urine, and provide dynamic assessment of the activity of the skeleton.

Markers for resorption as well as formation may be utilized (Table 24.2).

These markers should not be used single-handedly for the diagnosis of osteoporosis, nor even to determine which patients require treatment, but they can be useful in predicting bone loss. Studies show that the higher the level of markers, the greater the decrease in bone mass in subsequent years if treatment is not instituted.

The best and most validated use of bone markers is to monitor treatment. Anti-resorptive therapy is associated with the reduction of all resorption markers after 3 months, remaining at these reduced levels while the patient is in treatment. In cases where the response is inadequate and treatment compliance by the patient has been confirmed, the possibility of changing medication or increasing the dosage should be evaluated.

Imaging

Plain Radiography

Plain radiographs demonstrate low sensitivity for the diagnosis of osteoporosis because they show an alteration only when a bone loss of at least 30% already exists. They can be useful for diagnosing fractures, or specialized diagnosis involving other diseases that can affect bone, such as multiple myeloma, osteomalacia, and bone metastases.

Since most vertebral fractures are asymptomatic, several techniques have been studied with the aim of objectively recognizing subclinical vertebral deformities by measuring the height of the vertebral bodies (called morphometric fractures). The semiquantitative score permits a percentage differential evaluation of the anterior, middle, and posterior heights of the vertebral bodies, in order to effectively assess the severity of vertebral fractures [9]:

- 0 Degree—No fracture exists
- 1st Degree—Mild fracture, reduction ranging from 20% to 25% of the vertebral height
- 2nd Degree—Moderate fracture, reduction ranging from 25% to 40% of the vertebral height
- 3rd Degree—Severe fracture, reduction >40% of the vertebral height

Bone Densitometry

Osteoporosis can be diagnosed before the onset of clinical fractures by means of noninvasive methods for determining bone mineral density (BMD), which is the best single predictor of fracture risk [10]. The most accurate noninvasive method is bone densitometry, and the most widely used measure of absorption is dual-energy X-ray absorptiometry (DXA), which measures the area density (grams of mineral per square centimeter of bone; g/cm^2). It can be used at central (lumbar spine and hip) or peripheral (distal radius, heel, and phalanges) sites; however, only central sites are used for diagnosis and monitoring response to treatment.

The World Health Organization (WHO) has defined the diagnosis of low bone mass and osteoporosis, based on the number of standard deviations (SD) below mean BMD detected in normal young adults of the same sex (T-score) [11] (Table 24.3).

The BMD of osteoporotic patients may also be compared with that of a population of corresponding age (Z-score). A Z-score below −2.0 SD is considered below the expected range for the age group [12] and in these cases should be investigated for secondary causes of osteoporosis.

Since all postmenopausal women are at risk of developing osteoporosis, it would be ideal to evaluate the BMD of all of them. As a way of limiting costs, the International Society of Clinical Densitometry (ISCD) suggests screening for osteo-

porosis in women over 65 years of age; those with a history of fractures after minimal or no trauma; in early menopause; with prolonged use of corticosteroids; osteopenia evidenced by plain radiography; a maternal history of osteoporosis or fracture, loss of height, or thoracic kyphosis; underweight (BMI < 19), secondary causes; and the use of medications associated with bone loss [12].

Quantitative Computerized Tomography

This is a technique that measures volumetric density (g/cm^3) at the lumbar spine and peripheral sites using specialized software and standard computerized tomography equipment. It is able to distinguish cortical and trabecular bone compartments and predict fracture risk, as well as DXA, but has a high cost along with limited availability and increased radiation exposure, being used mainly in clinical research.

Ultrasonography

This evaluates the heel bone and the proximal tibia, is practical and inexpensive, and is useful as a method for screening the population at risk for osteoporosis.

Bone Quality

The concept of bone quality has been widely used to justify the occurrence of clinical events not explained by the evaluation of BMD alone. Bone quality takes into consideration the composition and structure of bone, contributing to bone strength regardless of density. Several factors interact to form bone quality, such as bone turnover, geometry, microarchitecture, mineralization, microaggressions, and components of the mineral and bone matrix [13]. The trabecular bone score (TBS) is a bone quality assessment method that analyzes gray tones obtained from two-dimensional image of the lumbar spine acquired by DXA coupled to a software to analyze bone microarchitecture and fracture risk. The more homogenous the color variation of this evaluation, the greater the bone strength and, consequently, the TBS. The reverse is also true. This score is useful for predicting risk of vertebral fractures, hip fractures, and some major osteoporotic fractures in both men and women. TBS alone does not determine therapeutic decision. Associated with FRAX, this score shows increased accuracy for risk of fractures, which may lead to a change in the therapeutic approach. The TBS suffers interference from soft tissue thickness (therefore, this method is only validated for BMI between 15 and 37 kg/m^2), race, and ethnicity. In addition, several conditions usually modify this score, reducing it in older, obese, alcohol, or corticoid users, and patients

Table 24.3 Definition of osteoporosis by the WHO criteria

WHO classification	T-score
Normal	To −1.0 DP
Osteopenia	−1.0 to −2.5 DP
Osteoporosis	<−2.5 DP

Data from Ref. [10]

with type 2 diabetes mellitus, rheumatoid arthritis, or chronic obstructive pulmonary disease, or increasing it in patients with recent treatment for osteoporosis [14, 15].

The evaluation of bone turnover may be conducted through bone marker evaluation and biopsies performed on bone marked with tetracycline [16]. New techniques for bone quality assessment have been developed, such as high-resolution magnetic resonance imaging and high-resolution peripheral quantitative computerized tomography. However, these costly techniques have yet to become readily available.

Treatment

Indication

Many guidelines have been published concerning the management of osteoporosis, in which treatment decisions are based primarily on the results of BMD in combination with patient characteristics.

The FRAX approach developed by the WHO plays a crucial role in guiding treatment recommendations for the management of osteoporosis [17].

The National Osteoporosis Foundation (NOF) recommends treatment of postmenopausal women (and men 50 years or older) with a history of vertebral or hip fracture or osteoporosis based on the measurement of BMD (T-score of −2.5 or less), as well as postmenopausal women with osteopenia, (BMD T-score between −1.0 and − 2.5) associated with a 3% or greater likelihood of hip fracture within 10 years, or a 20% or greater likelihood of osteoporotic fracture calculated by the FRAX approach [18].

The ideal optimal duration of pharmacological treatment for postmenopausal osteoporosis remains controversial. The decision to continue or discontinue therapy should be based on the history and fracture risk, balanced with the risks and benefits of the medication.

Non-pharmacological Treatment

There are three main components in the non-pharmacological therapy of osteoporosis: diet, exercise, and the cessation of smoking. In addition, the patient should also avoid drugs that increase bone loss, such as glucose corticoids.

Calcium/Vitamin D

An optimum diet for the treatment of osteoporosis includes an adequate amount of calories (to prevent malnutrition), along with calcium and vitamin D. Postmenopausal women should have an adequate intake of elemental calcium in divided doses, totaling 1000–1200 mg/day [19].

A recent study with 31,022 patients showed that vitamin D supplementation leads to a less than significant reduction of 10% in the risk of hip fracture (hazard ratio, HR 0.90, CI 95% 0.80–1.01) and a 7% reduction in the risk of non-vertebral fractures (HR 0.93, CI 95% 0.87–0.99) when compared with a control group. When intake levels were differentiated, fracture risk reduction was demonstrated only at the highest level of intake (median, 800 IU per day), with a 30% reduction in the risk of hip fracture (HR 0.70; CI 95% 0.58–0.86) and a 14% reduction in the risk of any type of non-vertebral fracture (HR 0.86, CI 95% 0.76–0.96) [20].

Physical Exercise

Women with osteoporosis should perform physical exercise for at least 30 min three times a week, since exercise has been associated with a reduced risk of hip fracture in older women [21].

A recent meta-analysis of 43 random clinical trials with 4320 postmenopausal women showed a significant positive effect of exercise on the BMD of the lumbar spine and trochanter. The most effective type of exercise for femoral neck BMD was resistance training using progressive force. A combined program that included more than one type of exercise was the most efficient for lumbar spine BMD [22].

Pharmacological Treatment

There are several medications that can be used in the treatment of osteoporosis. The main medications employed are reviewed below (Table 24.4).

Table 24.4 Reduction in fracture incidence

Drugs	Vertebral fracture	Non-vertebral fracture	Hip fracture
Zoledronate	+	+	+
Risendronate	+	+	+
Alendronate	+	+	+
Strontium	+	+	+[a]
Estrogen	+	+	+
Teriparatide	+	+	−
Calcitriol	+	−	−
Ibandronate	+	+	+[a]
Raloxifene	+	−	−
PTH 1–84	+	−	−
Calcitonin	+	−	−
Denosumab	+	+	+
Abaloparatide	+	+	+

Data from Refs. [31, 43–46, 49, 52, 54, 63, 77, 90]
[a]Post hoc subgroup analysis

Estrogens

Several placebo-controlled, randomized studies, including the WHI study and the postmenopausal estrogen/progesterone intervention (PEPI) study, have established that decreases in BMD are attenuated by estrogen, resulting in a lower risk of fracture [23, 24].

In the WHI study, estrogen-progestin therapy was associated with significant reductions in hip fractures (OR 0.7, CI 95% 0.4–1.0 unadjusted; less than five hip fractures per 10,000 person-years), along with vertebral and other osteoporotic fractures (OR 0.7, CI 95% 0.4–1.0 unadjusted, and OR 0.8, CI 95% 0.7–0.9, respectively) [23]. A similar risk reduction for hip fractures was shown using estrogens alone (OR 0.61, 95% CI 0.41–0.91), as were reductions for vertebral fractures (OR 0.62, 95% CI 0.42–0.93) [25].

In a forthcoming sample study, the Million Women Study, current users in postmenopausal therapy were shown to have a significantly lower risk of any fracture when compared to nonusers (RR 0.62, CI 95% 0.58–0.66) [26].

The coadministration of a progestogen, cyclically or continuously, to prevent endometrial hyperplasia does not impair the beneficial effects of estrogen [24].

However, estrogen-progestin therapy is no longer a frontline approach for the treatment of osteoporosis in postmenopausal women, owing to the increased risk of breast cancer, venous thromboembolism, stroke, and perhaps also coronary disease [23].

Tibolone

Tibolone is a synthetic steroid whose metabolites have estrogenic, androgenic, and progestogenic properties. It is used to treat osteoporosis in some countries. In postmenopausal women with osteoporosis, tibolone use has produced a 5–12% increase in lumbar spine BMD within 2 years. However, despite the fact that the LIFT study has reported a reduced risk of vertebral and non-vertebral fractures through the use of tibolone, it was stopped at an early stage because of the unacceptable risk of cerebral stroke [27]. This casts doubt on the drug's safety.

Calcitonin

Using calcitonin for the treatment of osteoporosis, a study that included 5 years of follow-up with 1255 women with T-scores of less than −2 (lumbar spine and at least one vertebral fracture) randomly assigned either a placebo or doses of 100, 200, or 400 IU/day of intranasal calcitonin. A small and inconsistent beneficial effect on the vertebral BMD from nasal calcitonin treatment was found and included a reduction in the risk of vertebral fractures [28].

Data on the effect of calcitonin in locations other than the spinal column are conflicting.

A recent meta-analysis with heterogeneous results, using a limited number of patients, showed calcitonin to be of benefit for the short-term relief of acute pain (less than 10 days) in patients who have suffered a vertebral fracture. In contrast, calcitonin has not proved to be effective for patients with chronic pain (over 3 months) [29].

SERMs (Selective Modulators of Estrogen Receptors)

Selective modulators of estrogen receptors (SERMs) bind with high affinity to the estrogen receptor, having agonist and antagonist properties that vary, depending on the target organ.

Raloxifene is a SERM effective in the treatment of established osteoporosis, which increases BMD in both the lumbar spine and the hip [30–33] and reduces the risk of vertebral fractures [31]. It also appears to reduce the risk of breast cancer without stimulating endometrial hyperplasia or vaginal bleeding but does seem to increase the risk of venous thromboembolism (VTE) [30]. In addition, there are studies that refer to an increased risk of fatal cardiovascular accidents (CVA) [30, 34]. Although serum concentrations of low-density lipoprotein (LDL) cholesterol and total cholesterol decrease, there seems to be no change in the risk of coronary cardiac disease [30].

However, despite the fact that raloxifene reduces vertebral fracture risk in postmenopausal women, it is not clear whether there is a reduction in non-vertebral fractures and therefore seems to be a less potent anti-resorptive agent than alendronate or estrogen [35, 36].

Moreover, unlike the bisphosphonates, SERMs do not appear to have a long-lasting effect on the skeleton and have no residual beneficial effects on BMD after discontinuation of treatment.

In a recent study, raloxifene was shown to decrease the mortality rate from all causes, mainly due to the reduction in non-cardiovascular and non-oncological deaths owing to a mechanism that has yet to be clarified [37].

Tamoxifen, a SERM used most commonly for the treatment of estrogen-dependent breast cancer, also affords some protection against bone loss in postmenopausal women and can be used to treat osteoporosis by reducing fracture rates [38].

Bazedoxifene has also decreased the incidence of new vertebral fractures, but not non-vertebral ones, with common adverse effects that include hot flashes, cramps, low rates of endometrial hyperplasia, cancer, polyps, and slightly higher rates of DVT, effects somewhat similar to those of raloxifene [39].

Lasofoxifene, like raloxifene, reduces the incidence of vertebral fractures but also increases the risk of thromboembolic events, hot flushes, and cramps in the legs. After 5 years of use, lasofoxifene has also been shown to be associated with a decrease in non-vertebral fractures, an effect that raloxifene has not shown. However, none of the SERMs reduce the risk of hip fractures [40].

Bisphosphonates

Bisphosphonates are synthetic analogues of pyrophosphate in which the oxygen bridge is replaced by a carbon atom [41]. They suppress bone resorption mediated by osteoclasts through a mechanism different from other anti-resorptive agents, binding to hydroxyapatite on bone surfaces, particularly those undergoing active resorption. When the osteoclasts begin to reabsorb bone that is impregnated with bisphosphonate, the bisphosphonate released during resorption impairs the ability of osteoclasts to form the wrinkled edge needed to adhere to the bone surface, thereby producing the protons required to continue bone resorption. In addition, they also reduce the activity of the osteoclasts, compromising the development of osteoclast progenitors, along with the recruitment and promotion of apoptosis of the osteoclasts. There also appears to be a beneficial effect on the osteoblasts [42].

Bisphosphonates can be administered orally (alendronate, risedronate, ibandronate) or intravenously (zoledronic acid at a dose of 5 mg every 12 months and ibandronate in a dose of 3 mg every 3 months) [41, 43–46]. They avidly bind to bone minerals, especially to trabecular bone, with a high degree of specificity [47]. However, oral absorption is low (0.6–1.5% of the administered dose). Approximately 40–60% of the dose is distributed in the bone, the remainder being excreted unchanged in the urine without substantial metabolism [41].

Oral bisphosphonates should be taken once a week after fasting, (alendronate in a dose of 70 mg, and risedronate in a 35 mg dose), once a month (ibandronate in a dose of 70 mg or risedronate in a 150 mg dose), or on 2 consecutive days, once a month (risedronate in a dose of 75 mg). The patient must remain upright for at least 30 min after taking the drug in order to minimize gastroesophageal reflux and enhance absorption. Afterward, food, medications, and other liquids should be avoided for at least 30–45 min [43].

Oral and intravenous bisphosphonates are contraindicated in patients who have had previous allergic reactions to any bisphosphonate, or creatinine clearance estimated at 35 ml/min or less, vitamin D deficiency (serum 25 hydroxy-vitamin D less than 30 ng/ml), osteomalacia, or hypocalcemia [43].

Oral bisphosphonates are also contraindicated in patients with impaired swallowing, or esophageal disorders such as achalasia, esophageal varices, and severe gastroesophageal reflux, or those who are unable to sit for at least 30 min after taking the medication [43].

An acute phase reaction (fever, myalgia, bone pain, and weakness) occurs in 20% of patients after an initial intravenous infusion of bisphosphonate and, in a very small number of patients, during oral therapy. Erosive esophagitis, ulceration, and bleeding have been associated with daily oral therapy using alendronate or risedronate but seldom occur with the current regimes (not daily). Heartburn, chest pain, hoarseness, and irritation of the vocal cords can occur with weekly (alendronate or risedronate) or monthly therapy (ibandronate or risedronate) [43].

Osteonecrosis of the jaw is a rare but serious complication of long-term therapy that can appear spontaneously, or after dental surgery. Case reports suggest that atypical fractures of the femur (subtrochanteric and mid-diaphyseal portions) may also occur during prolonged therapy [43, 48].

There are no known interactions between bisphosphonates and other drugs. Evidence of treatment failure with patients adhering properly to a treatment regime indicates the need to change from orally administered bisphosphonate to intravenous zoledronic or another class of drugs, such as anabolic agents (e.g., teriparatide) [43].

Bisphosphonates suppress biochemical indices of bone resorption by around 50% in a month, significantly reducing the incidence of vertebral and non-vertebral fractures, including femoral fractures in patients with osteoporosis within a few months after the start of therapy [47].

BMD increases modestly by around 2–6% during the first year of treatment. In the lumbar spine, it continues to increase slowly for several years, but in the femur, it reaches a plateau after about 2 years. Therapy preserves bone, but does not increase bone volume or restore the bone structure [47].

In the Fracture Intervention Trial (FIT) [44], postmenopausal women with a high risk of fracture, a low BMD in the femoral neck, and at least one vertebral fracture, the alendronate group showed fewer new vertebral fractures ($p = 0.001$) and new hip fractures ($p = 0.05$), when compared with the placebo group [43, 44].

In the vertebral efficacy study with risedronate therapy (VERT) [45], 2.458 postmenopausal women with at least 1 vertebral fracture and lumbar spine T-scores of −2.0 or less, the risedronate group had a lower rate of new vertebral fractures after 3 years when compared to the placebo group. In a subsequent trial, risedronate also proved to be effective in reducing the rate of hip fractures [43, 45].

In the Health Outcomes and Reduced Incidence with Zoledronic Acid Once Yearly study (HORIZON clinical trials), 7765 postmenopausal women suffering from osteoporosis were treated with zoledronic acid (5 mg once a year for

Table 24.5 Reduction in vertebral fracture incidence at pivot trials

Study	Increase in BMD (LS)	Reduction in vertebral Fx[a] (RRR)	Baseline vertebral Fx[a]	ARR / NNT (3 yr)[a]	Drug
FIT II	8.3%	44%	0%	1.7%/59	Alendronate
FIT I	7.9%	47%	100%	7%/15	Alendronate
VERTMN	7.1%	39%	100%	10%/10	Risendronate
VERTNA	5.4%	31%	100%	5%/20	Risendronate
MORE	2.6%	35%	37%	6.5%/16	Raloxifene
BONE	6.0%	52%	100%	4.9%/21	Ibandronate
FPT	14%	65%	100%	9%/12[b]	Teriparatide
HORIZON	7.0%	70%	60%	7.6%/14	Zoledronate
SOTI	14%	41%	100%	11%/9	Strontium Ranelate
FREEDOM	10%	68%	23%	4.8%/21	Denosumab
ACTIVE	11.5%	85%	22%	3.16%/32[c]	Abaloparatide
ACTIVE	11%	77%	22%	2.43%/41[b]	Teriparatide

Data from Refs. [31, 46, 49, 54, 62, 77, 90]

[a]*Fx* fracture, *RRR* relative reduction risk, *ARR* absolute reduction risk, *NNT* number needed to treat

[b]18 months

[c]24 months

3 years). When compared to the placebo group, they showed a significant reduction in the absolute rate of new vertebral fractures as assessed by radiography and also of new hip fractures [43, 47, 49] (Table 24.5).

Other placebo-controlled and randomized oral bisphosphonate studies, including with ibandronate, clodronate, and etidronate, have also shown the efficacy of these medications in reducing the risk of new vertebral fractures. However, these trials were not shown to have the statistical capacity to demonstrate efficacy in the treatment of hip fractures, which makes them less useful clinically. Pamidronate has been used to treat a variety of bone diseases in children and adults, but no studies have evaluated the efficacy of the medication with sufficient capacity to treat hip fractures in postmenopausal women with osteoporoses [43].

The optimal duration for bisphosphonate therapy remains unclear. However, based on available data, it appears likely that discontinuation of therapy after 5 years, at least as a temporary pause for 1–2 years, is not harmful and may indeed be beneficial in patients with low risk for fractures. It could be especially appropriate in patients with an only slightly low BMD, which would imply a lower risk of fractures if bone loss does occur when the person is not receiving treatment [43, 50, 51].

In addition, concern about the occurrence of atypical subtrochanteric fractures and osteonecrosis of the jaw during prolonged bisphosphonate therapy has led the Food and Drug Administration (FDA) to reassess the efficacy of bisphosphonate therapy, with extension of the FLEX study involving alendronate for 5 more years and the HORIZON study with zoledronic acid for 3 more years [52].

This analysis by the FDA revealed little benefit from continued treatment with bisphosphonates beyond 5 years in the final endpoint comprising all vertebral and non-vertebral fractures but was consistent in showing significant reductions in vertebral fracture risk with continued bisphospho-

nate treatment, with no overall reduction in the rate of non-vertebral fractures [52].

Observational studies have shown a greater loss of bone after discontinuation of therapy with risedronate, but there is no data with ibandronate. It is therefore believed that recommendations concerning discontinuation should be limited to alendronate and zoledronic acid [52].

On current evidence, according to ASBMR, it can be concluded that with patients showing *T*-score bone mineral density at the femoral neck below −2.5 after 3–5 years of treatment, it would seem more beneficial to continue with bisphosphonates oral bisphosphonates such as alendronate for up to 10 years and intravenous such as zoledronic acid for up to 6 years [50, 51]. The same applies to patients with existing vertebral fractures and a slightly higher *T*-score, but not above −2.0. In cases involving patients with a *T*-score above −2.0 in the femoral neck, there is a low risk of vertebral fractures, and they are unlikely to benefit from continued treatment [52]. The so-called holiday of the bisphosphonates is the most suitable for such patients, monitoring bone remodeling markers and BMD [50, 51].

In an analysis from data of many clinical trials, Cummings et al. [53] found that the greater increase in *T*-score femoral neck or total femur BMD during treatment, the lower likelihood of fracture at any site.

Denosumab

Denosumab is an IgG2 monoclonal antibody that, similarly to the action of osteoprotegerin (OPG), binds with high affinity and specificity to RANK L, preventing it from activating its receptor (RANK) on the surface of osteoclasts and their precursors. The prevention of the RANKL/RANK interaction inhibits the formation, function, and survival of osteoclasts, thereby decreasing bone resorption.

Denosumab is administered via a subcutaneous injection (SC) of 60 mg every 6 months, requiring no dose adjustment for renal function. Its safety and tolerability have been demonstrated in clinical studies of up to 8 years' duration [54, 55].

Studies have demonstrated that a single dose of denosumab leads to significant suppression of bone turnover. Bone reabsorption markers decrease substantially within 12–24 h after administration of the medication, and this effect has been shown to be reversible upon its clearance [56].

The FREEDOM study (Fracture Reduction Evaluation of Denosumab in Osteoporosis every 6 Months) was a phase III, double-blind, placebo-controlled study lasting 36 months and was designed to analyze the effectiveness of denosumab in reducing vertebral fractures in postmenopausal women. Over 3 years, it evaluated 7808 women with a mean age of 72.3 years and T-scores < -2.5 and demonstrated a significant reduction in the incidence of new vertebral fractures, non-vertebral fractures, and hip fractures, along with a significantly increased BMD in the lumbar spine (9.2%) and total hip (6.0%) when compared to the placebo group ($p < 0.001$). Furthermore, a substudy of FREEDOM ($n = 160$) showed that the medication reduces markers for bone remodeling (sCTx and sP1NP) within the first month [54].

The DECIDE study (Determining Efficacy: Comparison of Initiating Denosumab versus alendronate) was a phase III, multicenter, randomized, double-blind study that compared the efficacy and safety of treatment with denosumab vs. alendronate for 12 months in postmenopausal women with T-scores < -2.0 and minimal or no exposure to bisphosphonates. The women treated with denosumab had significantly greater increases in BMD at all sites when compared with alendronate and greater suppression of bone remodeling markers [57].

The STAND study (Study of Transitioning from Alendronate to Denosumab) compared the efficacy and safety of patients transitioning from alendronate to denosumab during a 1-year period versus patients who continued with alendronate. The study was a multicenter, randomized, double-blind study that included 504 postmenopausal women with T-scores ≤ -2.0 who had been receiving alendronate for at least 6 months. The study showed that the transition from alendronate to denosumab is safe and results in greater increases in BMD in the lumbar spine, femoral neck, and distal radius when compared to the continued use of alendronate ($p \leq 0.0125$). The administration of denosumab further reduced levels of sCTx and P1NP when compared to continued use of alendronate [58].

In the DECIDE and STAND studies combined, approximately 65% of the patients expressed a preference for biannual injections as opposed to daily oral administration [59].

More recently, an extension study evaluated the effects of continued treatment with denosumab over an 8-year period,

showing a constant reduction in bone turnover markers, and continuous increases in BMD, achieving a total gain of 16.5% in the lumbar spine and of 6.8% in the hip [55].

There is evidence of considerable loss of bone mass 1 year after the cessation of denosumab use, even after 7–10 years of treatment, and that this fall is directly proportional to the gain of BMD acquired with the use of this monoclonal antibody. There was an 8% decrease in BMD in LC and total femur and 6% in CF, probably due to the rapid differentiation and activation of neutralized osteoclasts, restarting the bone remodeling process and raising its turnover markers to levels higher than those observed before treatment with denosumab. Patients who participated in the follow-up of the FREEDOM study presented even more significant losses with discontinuation of treatment: a decrease in BMD of 44.6% in CF, 103.3% in total hip, and 8.1% in LC, besides an increase in 13.15% of fractures in weak wrists or vertebrae. Vertebral fractures, inclusive, were the most observed after discontinuation of denosumab, hypothesizing that the trabecular bone is more affected than the cortical. These fractures can be morphometric or clinical, single or multiple. It is not yet known whether the risk of fracture following discontinuation of this human monoclonal antibody increases or returns to pre-treatment values, nor which patients are more likely to have this event, but it is believed that those who have had previous vertebral fractures or during use of denosumab are at greater risk. The use of another anti-resorptive drug such as bisphosphonates after cessation of denosumab contributes to the preservation of bone mass in the same way as in patients who were treated with bisphosphonates before denosumab would have a lower risk of hyperactivation of the RANK-RANKL system with their suspension [60, 61].

Parathyroid Hormone

Despite the well-known deleterious effect of parathyroid hormone (PTH) on bone, the intermittent administration of recombinant human PTH (1–84 or 1–34) is known to stimulate bone formation rather than resorption and is effective in reducing fractures in women with postmenopausal osteoporosis.

PTH 1–34 (Teriparatide, Forteo®) and PTH 1–84 (PreOs) belong to a new class of medications, known as anabolic agents. Teriparatide is available in the USA and Europe for the treatment of severe osteoporosis, and PTH 1–84 has been approved in Europe.

Most of the gain in BMD with the use of PTH occurs within the first few months, although anti-fracture efficacy is evident only after 6 months of treatment. BMD is markedly increased (more than treatment with anti-resorptive agents) at locations predominantly formed of the trabecular bone, such as vertebrae. When the bones are predominantly cortical, such as radius bones, there is no gain. Furthermore, there is evidence that seems to indicate that alterations in BMD from the use of PTH start to diminish after 18 months [62].

So far, teriparatide has proved to be safe and effective for up to 2 years of treatment. The recommended dose is 20 mg daily SC, with no need for dose adjustment due to renal or hepatic impairment, since the drug is rapidly absorbed and eliminated.

The Fracture Prevention Trial (FPT) studied the use of teriparatide (20 mcg or 40 mcg/daily) in 1637 postmenopausal women with prior vertebral fractures, compared with a placebo group [62]. After 18 months of treatment, it was observed that in the group receiving 20 mcg, BMD increased by 9% at the lumbar spine and by 3% in the femoral neck. In the group receiving 40 mcg, BMD increased by 13% at the lumbar spine and 6% in the femoral neck. There was also a significant reduction in the risk of vertebral and non-vertebral fractures when compared to the placebo group, but not in a dose-dependent manner. It was not possible to obtain complete data on hip fractures, since the number of cases was very small.

An extension of the FPT evaluated participants for another 18 months after discontinuation of teriparatide [63] and found that women who used teriparatide showed a small decrease in BMD but that a reduction in vertebral fracture risk persisted (relative risk reduction of 40% when compared to the placebo group).

Similarly, teriparatide and PTH 1–84 showed higher increases in bone remodeling markers between the first and third month of treatment, especially the bone formation markers (sNTx and P1NP). This peak of remodeling markers is associated with greater increases in BMD [64].

The PaTh study evaluated the combination of alendronate with teriparatide in order to determine whether the combination of drugs would decrease the anabolic effect of PTH. The BMD of the lumbar spine, as well as that of the femoral neck, presented greater increases in the group receiving teriparatide alone than in groups that received alendronate alone, or in combination, demonstrating that alendronate reduces the ability of teriparatide to increase BMD [65].

The effects of combination therapy using zoledronic acid with teriparatide in women with postmenopausal osteoporosis were evaluated over a 1-year period, showing a greater and more rapid increase in the lumbar spine and hip BMD than when either of the two drugs was administered alone [66].

Concern exists regarding the potential loss of bone mass that may occur after discontinuation of treatment with PTH. Nonetheless, several studies have shown that treatment with bisphosphonate, estrogen, or raloxifene after discontinuation of PTH preserves the bone mass gain achieved by PTH [67–69].

Parathyroid hormone therapy is indicated in more severe cases of osteoporosis (especially with multiple fractures), very low T-scores (< -3.0) even without fractures in very elderly patients, those with bisphosphonate intolerance, and/or when dealing with fractures potentially affected by anti-resorptive agents.

The main adverse effects of PTH use are nausea, headache, and hypercalcemia and are of more frequent occurrence at higher dose levels. The use of PTH is contraindicated in children and young adults with epiphyses that are still open, tumors or bone metastases, and hypercalcemia. Although the risk is only theoretical and demonstrated only in mice, patients at high risk for osteosarcoma should also avoid using this medication.

Abaloparatide, an analog of PTHrP, a PTH-related protein, composed of 34 amino acids that transiently and potently bind to PTH1 receptors, has a consistent anabolic effect, increasing BMD and reducing fracture risk in all sites [15, 70–72]. This molecule recently approved for use by the FDA presents N-terminal residues common to PTH and PTHrP, binding strongly to the receptor common to these two peptides, predominantly in a conformation that stimulates the RG-ligand, thus leading to an intracellular signaling shorter in relation to teriparatide, which binds in a different conformation with stimulation also of the R0-ligand. Its use promotes a decoupling between the formation and bone resorption processes, causing an increase in P1NP, but a lower elevation in CTX levels, when compared to the use of teriparatide [71]. The ACTIVE study, designed in patients with 22% and 48% of baseline vertebral and non-vertebral fractures, showed a reduction of the risk of vertebral fractures in 86%, non-vertebral fractures in 43%, and osteoporotic fractures in 70% plus a 3.4% increase in BMD in total hip, 2.9% in femoral neck, and 9.2% in lumbar spine after 18 months of using abaloparatide 80 mcg/day subcutaneous compared to teriparatide [70].

A 25-month extension of the ACTIVE study, which observed effects of abaloparatide on BMD and fracture risk, compared the use of this drug for 18 months followed by the use of alendronate for 6 months versus placebo for 18 months followed by alendronate for 6 months. The abaloparatide/alendronate group had a 12.8% increase in BMD in LC, 5.5% in total hip, and 4.5% in CF compared to 3.5%, 1.4%, and 0.5% in these respective sites for the placebo/alendronate group. The abaloparatide group also showed a lower rate of non-vertebral fractures (2.7% vs. 5.6%), as well as a 58% and 45% lower risk of major osteoporotic fractures and clinical fractures, respectively [73].

The 43-month extension of this same study also showed positive results for the user group of abaloparatide for 18 months followed by alendronate for 24 months compared to the group that used 18 months of placebo followed by 24 months of alendronate, an increase of 14.4% in BMD in

LC, 6.4% in total hip, and 5.3% in CF, compared to 6.5%, 2.8%, and 1.6% in these same sites for the placebo/alendronate group [74].

The adverse effects of the use of this new drug are nausea, headache, dizziness, and palpitation. Abaloparatide also offers advantages over teriparatide in terms of storage without the need for refrigeration [71].

Strontium

Strontium ranelate consists of two stable strontium atoms attached to an organic compound, ranelic acid. The exact mechanism of strontium action in humans remains unknown, with some possible mechanisms having been proposed. These include regulation of bone cell differentiation, stimulation of osteoblast proliferation, inhibition of osteoclast formation, activation of calcium receptor sensors, increased expression of OPG, and the stimulated proliferation of pre-osteoblasts [75, 76]. Its use has been approved in Europe, but not in the USA.

In patients taking strontium, the assessment of BMD is not a good indicator of fracture risk reduction, because the medication is incorporated into the bone, thereby weakening DXA ray penetration, since it has an atomic number greater than that of calcium and can cause overestimation of the BMD [76].

Several clinical studies have confirmed the effectiveness of strontium ranelate use for the treatment of postmenopausal osteoporosis. The SOTI (Spinal Osteoporosis Therapeutic Intervention) study [77] evaluated women with previous vertebral fractures, and the use of strontium was associated with a 49% reduced risk of vertebral fractures in the first year and a 41% reduction in risk after 3 years, while the TROPOS (Treatment of Peripheral Osteoporosis) study [78] demonstrated a 16% reduction in the relative risk of all non-vertebral fractures over 3 years. During the studies, increases in markers for bone formation and reductions in markers for resorption were observed, data consistent with the idea that this medicine works by stimulating bone formation and inhibiting bone resorption [77, 78].

A meta-analysis of four studies (including those mentioned above) concluded that evidence exists that strontium ranelate is effective in reducing the risk of vertebral fractures and, to a lesser extent, non-vertebral ones [79].

The main side effects associated with use of the medication are nausea and diarrhea, which occur most frequently during the first 3 months of treatment. Serious adverse effects such as severe skin reactions (Stevens-Johns, toxic epidermal necrolysis, DRESS - drug reaction with eosinophilia and systemic symptoms), in addition to venous thromboembolism, have been reported. However, an extension study lasting 10 years showed that long-term treatment with strontium

is associated with sustained increases in BMD and that it has a good safety profile, showing no cutaneous hypersensibility reactions, and that the annual incidence of venous thromboembolism was only 0.4% [80]. In any case, the medication is not recommended for patients with previous episodes of venous thromboembolism or those who are immobilized and should be discontinued in the case of skin reactions with no resumption of treatment.

Romosozumab

Sclerostin is produced by osteocytes and has an inhibitory effect on bone formation. In animal trials, the administration of a monoclonal anti-sclerostin antibody has resulted in increased bone mass [81, 82]. An example of therapeutic class drugs is romosozumab, not yet approved for use in humans.

In a phase I study, 72 healthy subjects were randomly selected to receive either AMG 785 (an anti-sclerostin monoclonal antibody) or a placebo subcutaneously or intravenously administered in a single dose. AMG 785 was well tolerated, and dose-dependent increases in markers for bone formation, decreased resorption markers, and significant increases in BMD at the lumbar spine (5.3%) and hip (2.8%) were all observed when compared to the placebo group [83].

Romosozumab, a monoclonal anti-sclerostin antibody with high affinity for human sclerostin, is a promising option for the treatment of postmenopausal osteoporosis in FRAME, a phase III study. This study, conducted in patients with vertebral fractures, 18%, and non-vertebral fractures, 22%, tested monthly subcutaneous doses of romosozumab 210 mg for 1 year, followed by the administration of denosumab 60 mg subcutaneously in the following year, comparing results against another group that received placebo in this first year followed by denosumab in the same posology the following year. In the first year, clinical fractures were reduced by 36% and vertebral fractures by 73%, and CM BMD was increased in 13.3%, CF in 5.9%, and total hip in 6.9%. In the second year of FRAME, vertebral fractures were reduced by 75% and clinical fractures by 33%. There was also an early and sustained fall in CTX and a rapid increase in P1NP, which returned to the baseline only 9 months after [84].

The ARCH study, another phase III study in high-risk patients (vertebral fractures and osteoporotic fractures in 96% and 99%, respectively), compared romosozumab for 12 months followed by alendronate for 12 months versus alendronate for 24 months, showing extremely positive results for the romosozumab group. In this group, there was a reduction of vertebral fractures in 48%, non-vertebral fractures in 19%, clinical fractures in 27%, and hip fractures in

38%, in addition to decrease in CTX and increase in P1NP during the 12 months of use of romosozumab [85].

Based on these evidences, we can infer that romosozumab showed a dramatic increase in BMD in the spine and femur, increasing bone formation and mineralization in cortical and trabecular bones, as well as bone strength and microarchitecture without affecting the resorption process. It also reduces the risk of fractures in all osseous sites. Its adverse effects are few and generally mild, such as nasopharyngitis, arthralgia, lower back pain, and site reaction. Osteonecrosis of the mandible and atypical fracture of the femur occurred in one and two cases, respectively, corresponding to less than 0.1% of the casuistry [85].

Cardiovascular and cerebrovascular safety is still debatable and is subject to continuous evaluation due to an increase of 70% in the risk of encephalic vascular accident compared to the alendronate group [85].

Romosozumab has recently been approved for the treatment of postmenopausal osteoporosis in patients with very high risk for fracture [86].

Transdermal Abaloparatide

The routes of oral and transdermal administration of this N-terminal PTHrP 1–34 are currently being evaluated. A phase II study showed that 5 minutes per day of use of abaloparatide patches for 24 weeks was able to significantly increase lumbar spine and total hip BMD in a dose-dependent manner, the best response being obtained at a dose of 80 mcg/day [87].

Oral Calcitonin

An additional treatment option for women with postmenopausal osteoporosis is oral recombinant salmon calcitonin (rsCT) [88, 89]. It acts by inhibiting osteoclastic activity by binding to its receptor. The oral route of administration, available upon formulation of a complex containing 8- (N-2-hydroxy-5-chloro-benzoyl)-aminocaprylic acid (5-CNAC) or a synthetic coating composed of polymers and citric acid in vesicles, which protect the molecule from calcitonin against gastric acidity and intestinal proteolysis, proved to be more effective than intranasal [89]. Oral calcitonin was effective and safe, which was assessed in a phase III study, which showed that oral treatment resulted in an increase from baseline in the lumbar spine BMD greater than that with nasal spray calcitonin or placebo (1.5% ± 3.2% versus 0.78% ± 2.9% and 0.5% ± 3.2%, respectively). Oral rsCT treatment also resulted in greater improvements in trochanteric and total proximal femur BMD and better reductions in bone resorption markers. Oral rsCT was safe and well toler-

ated [88], but a possible increased risk for malignancy and absence of protective evidence against vertebral fractures and frailty make this drug an unpromising option [89]. The main adverse events were in the gastrointestinal system; less than 10% of women experienced a serious adverse event and no deaths occurred in this study [88].

References

1. Ac L, Orwol ES, Jonhston CC, Lindsay RL, Wahner HW, Dunn WL, et al. Prevalence of low femoral bone in older U.S. adults from NHANES III. J Bone Miner Res. 1997;12:1761–8.
2. Nayak S, Roberts MS, Greenspan SL. Cost-effectiveness of different screening strategies for osteoporosis in postmenopausal women. Ann Intern Med. 2011;155(11):751–61. https://doi.org/10.1059/0003-4819-155-11-201112060-00007.
3. Bandeira F, Carvalho EF. Prevalência de osteoporose e fraturas vertebrais em mulheres na pós-menopausa atendidas em serviços de referência. Rev Bras Epidemiol. 2007;10(1):86–98.
4. Management of osteoporosis in postmenopausal women: 2010 position statement of The North American Menopause Society. Menopause. 2010;17(1):25–54.
5. Kanis JA, Johnell O, Oden A, Johansson H, McCloskey EV. FRAX and the assessment of fracture probability in men and women from the UK. Osteoporos Int. 2008;19:385–97.
6. Leslie WD, Lix LM, Johansson H, Oden A, McCloskey E, Kanis JA, et al. Does osteoporosis therapy invalidate FRAX for fracture prediction? J Bone Miner Res. 2012;27(6):1243–51.
7. Siminoski K, Jiang G, Adachi JD, Hanley DA, Cline G, Ioannidis G, et al. Accuracy of height loss during prospective monitoring for detection of incident vertebral fractures. Osteoporos Int. 2005;16(4):403–10.
8. Tarantino U, Iolascon G, Cianferotti L, Masi L, Marcucci G, Giusti F, et al. Clinical guidelines for the prevention and treatment of osteoporosis: summary statements and recommendations from the Italian Society for Orthopaedics and Traumatology. J Orthop Traumatol. 2017;18(1):3.
9. Genant HK, Wu CY, Van Kujik C, Nevitt MC. Vertebral fracture assessment using semiquantitative technique. J Bone Miner Res. 1993;8(9):1137–48.
10. Genant HK, Engelke K, Fuerst T, Glüer CC, Grampp S, Harris ST, et al. Noninvasive assessment of bone mineral and structure: state of the art. J Bone Miner Res. 1996;11(6):707–30.
11. Assessment of fracture risk and its application to screening for postmenopausal osteoporosis. Report of a WHO Study Group. World Health Organ Tech Rep Ser. 1994;843:1–129.
12. Binkley N, Bilezikian JP, Kendler DL, Leib ES, Lewiecki EM, Petak SM. Summary of the International Society For Clinical Densitometry 2005 position development conference. J Bone Miner Res. 2007;22(5):643–5.
13. National Institutes of Health. NIH consensus statement: osteoporosis prevention, diagnosis, and therapy. NIH Consens Statement. 2000;17(1):1–45.
14. Martineau P, Silva BC, Leslie WD. Utility of trabecular bone score in the evaluation of osteoporosis. Curr Opin Endocrinol Diabetes Obes. 2017;24(6):402–10.
15. Bilezikian JP, Hattersley G, Fitzpatrick LA, Harris AG, Shevroja E, Banks K, et al. Abaloparatide-SC improves trabecular microarchitecture as assessed by trabecular bone score (TBS): a 24-week randomized clinical trial. Osteoporos Int. 2017:1–6.
16. Eventov I, Frisch B, Cohen Z, Hammel I. Osteopenia, hematopoiesis, and bone remodelling in iliac crest and femoral biopsies: a

prospective study of 102 cases of femoral neck fractures. Bone. 1991;12(1):1–6.

17. Meadows ES, Mitchell BD, Bolge SC, Johnston JA, Col NF. Factors associated with treatment of women with osteoporosis or osteopenia from a national survey. BMC Womens Health. 2012;12:1.

18. NOF's new clinician's guide to prevention and treatment of osteoporosis. 2008. Available at: http://www.nof.org/professionals/Clinicians_Guide.html. Accessed 22 Aug 2012.

19. Eastell R. Treatment of postmenopausal osteoporosis. N Engl J Med. 1998;338:736.

20. Bischoff-Ferrari HA, Willett WC, Orav EJ, Lips P, Meunier PJ, Lyons RA, et al. A pooled analysis of vitamin D dose requirements for fracture prevention. N Engl J Med. 2012;367:1.

21. Kemmler W, von Stengel S, Engelke K, Häberle L, Kalender WA. Exercise effects on bone mineral density, falls, coronary risk factors, and health care costs in older women: the randomized controlled senior fitness and prevention (SEFIP) study. Arch Intern Med. 2010;170:179.

22. Howe TE, Shea B, Dawson LJ, Downie F, Murray A, Ross C, et al. Exercise for preventing and treating osteoporosis in postmenopausal women. Cochrane Database Syst Rev. 2011;7:CD000333.

23. Rossouw JE, Anderson GL, Prentice RL, LaCroix AZ, Kooperberg C, Stefanick ML, et al. Risks and benefits of estrogen plus progestin in healthy postmenopausal women: principal results from the Women's Health Initiative randomized controlled trial. JAMA. 2002;288(3):321–33.

24. Effects of hormone therapy on bone mineral density: results from the postmenopausal estrogen/progestin interventions (PEPI) trial. The Writing Group for the PEPI. JAMA. 1996;276(17):1389–96.

25. Anderson GL, Limacher M, Assaf AR, Bassford T, Beresford SA, Black H, et al. Effects of conjugated equine estrogen in postmenopausal women with hysterectomy: the Women's Health Initiative randomized controlled trial. JAMA. 2004;291(14):1701–12.

26. Banks E, Beral V, Reeves G, Balkwill A, Balkwill A, Barnes I, Million Women Study Collaborators. Fracture incidence in relation to the pattern of use of hormone therapy in postmenopausal women. JAMA. 2004;291(18):2212–20.

27. Cummings SR, Ettinger B, Delmas PD, Kenemans P, Stathopoulos V, Verweij P, et al. The effects of tibolone in older postmenopausal women. N Engl J Med. 2008;359(7):697–708.

28. Chesnut CH 3rd, Silverman S, Andriano K, Genant H, Gimona A, Harris S, et al. A randomized trial of nasal spray salmon calcitonin in postmenopausal women with established osteoporosis: the prevent recurrence of osteoporotic fractures study. PROOF Study Group. Am J Med. 2000;109(4):267–76.

29. Knopp-Sihota JA, Newburn-Cook CV, Homik J, Cummings GG, Voaklander D. Calcitonin for treating acute and chronic pain of recent and remote osteoporotic vertebral compression fractures: a systematic review and meta-analysis. Osteoporos Int. 2012;23(1):17–38. Epub 2011 Jun 10.

30. Barrett-Connor E, Mosca L, Collins P, Geiger MJ, Grady D, Kornitzer M, et al. Effects of raloxifene on cardiovascular events and breast cancer in postmenopausal women. N Engl J Med. 2006;355(2):125–37.

31. Ettinger B, Black DM, Mitlak BH, Knickerbocker RK, Nickelsen T, Genant HK, et al. Reduction of vertebral fracture risk in postmenopausal women with osteoporosis treated with raloxifene: results from a 3-year randomized clinical trial. Multiple Outcomes of Raloxifene Evaluation (MORE) Investigators. JAMA. 1999;282(7):637–45.

32. Delmas PD, Genant HK, Crans GG, Stock JL, Wong M, Siris E, et al. Severity of prevalent vertebral fractures and the risk of subsequent vertebral and nonvertebral fractures: results from the MORE trial. Bone. 2003;33(4):522–32.

33. Siris ES, Harris ST, Eastell R, Zanchetta JR, Goemaere S, Diez-Perez A, et al. Skeletal effects of raloxifene after 8 years: results from the continuing outcomes relevant to Evista (CORE) study. J Bone Miner Res. 2005;20(9):1514–24. Epub 2005 May 16.

34. Barrett-Connor E, Cox DA, Song J, Mitlak B, Mosca L, Grady D. Raloxifene and risk for stroke based on the Framingham stroke risk score. Am J Med. 2009;122(8):754–61. Epub 2009 Jun 18.

35. Sambrook PN, Geusens P, Ribot C, Solimano JA, Ferrer-Barriendos J, Gaines K, et al. Alendronate produces greater effects than raloxifene on bone density and bone turnover in postmenopausal women with low bone density: results of EFFECT (Efficacy of FOSAMAX versus EVISTA Comparison Trial) International. J Intern Med. 2004;255(4):503–11.

36. Reid IR, Eastell R, Fogelman I, Adachi JD, Rosen A, Netelenbos C, et al. A comparison of the effects of raloxifene and conjugated equine estrogen on bone and lipids in healthy postmenopausal women. Arch Intern Med. 2004;164(8):871–9.

37. Grady D, Cauley JA, Stock JL, Cox DA, Mitlak BH, Song J, et al. Effect of raloxifene on all-cause mortality. Am J Med. 2010;123(5):469.e1–7.

38. Cooke AL, Metge C, Lix L, Prior HJ, Leslie WD. Tamoxifen use and osteoporotic fracture risk: a population-based analysis. J Clin Oncol. 2008;26(32):5227–32. Epub 2008 Oct 6.

39. Archer DF, Pinkerton JV, Utian WH, Menegoci JC, de Villiers TJ, Yuen CK, et al. Bazedoxifene, a selective estrogen receptor modulator: effects on the endometrium, ovaries, and breast from a randomized controlled trial in osteoporotic postmenopausal women. Menopause. 2009;16(6):1109–15.

40. Becker C. Another selective estrogen-receptor modulator for osteoporosis. N Engl J Med. 2010;362(8):752–4.

41. Khosla S, Bilezikian JP, Dempster DW, Lewiecki EM, Miller PD, Neer RM, et al. Benefits and risks of bisphosphonate therapy for osteoporosis. J Clin Endocrinol Metab. 2012;97(7):2272–82. Epub 2012 Apr 20.

42. Plotkin LI, Lezcano V, Thostenson J, Weinstein RS, Manolagas SC, Bellido T. Connexin 43 is required for the anti-apoptotic effect of bisphosphonates on osteocytes and osteoblasts in vivo. J Bone Miner Res. 2008;23(11):1712–21.

43. Favus MJ. Bisphosphonates for osteoporosis. N Engl J Med. 2010;363(21):2027–35.

44. Black DM, Cummings SR, Karpf DB, Cauley JA, Thompson DE, Nevitt MC, et al. Randomised trial of effect of alendronate on risk of fracture in women with existing vertebral fractures. Fracture Intervention Trial Research Group. Lancet. 1996;348(9041):1535–41.

45. Reginster J, Minne HW, Sorensen OH, Hooper M, Roux C, Brandi ML, et al. Randomized trial of the effects of risedronate on vertebral fractures in women with established postmenopausal osteoporosis. Vertebral Efficacy with Risendronate Therapy (VERT) Study Group. Osteoporos Int. 2000;11(1):83–91.

46. Ravn P, Clemmesen B, Riis BJ, Christiansen C. The effect on bone mass and bone markers of different doses of ibandronate: a new bisphosphonate for prevention and treatment of postmenopausal osteoporosis: a 1-year, randomized, double-blind, placebo-controlled dose-finding study. Bone. 1996;19(5):527–33.

47. McClung M. Bisphosphonates: review article. Arq Bras Endocrinol Metab. 2006;50(4):735–44.

48. Carvalho NNC, Voss LA, Almeida MOP, Salgado CL, Bandeira F. Atypical femoral fractures during prolonged use of bisphosphonates: short-term responses to strontium ranelate and teriparatide. J Clin Endocrinol Metab. 2011;96(9):2675–80. Epub 2011 Jul 13.

49. Black DM, Delmas PD, Eastell R, Reid IR, Boonen S, Cauley JA, et al. Once-yearly zoledronic acid for treatment of postmenopausal osteoporosis (HORIZON). N Engl J Med. 2007;356(18):1809–22.

50. Camacho PM, Petak SM, Binkley N, Clarke BL, Harris ST, Hurley DL, et al. American association of clinical endocrinologists and American College of endocrinology clinical practice guidelines

for the diagnosis and treatment of postmenopausal osteoporosis—2016. Endocr Pract. 2016;22(s4):1–42.

51. Adler RA, El-Hajj Fuleihan G, Bauer DC, Camacho PM, Clarke BL, Clines GA, et al. Managing osteoporosis in patients on long-term bisphosphonate treatment: report of a task force of the American Society for Bone and Mineral Research. J Bone Miner Res. 2016;31(1):16–35.

52. Black DM, Bauer DC, Schwartz AV, Cummings SR, Rosen CJ. Continuing bisphosphonate treatment for osteoporosis—for whom and for how long? N Engl J Med. 2012;366(22):2051–3. Epub 2012 May 9.

53. Cummings SR, Cosman F, Lewiecki EM, Schousboe JT, Bauer DC, Black DM, et al. Goal-directed treatment for osteoporosis: a progress report from the ASBMR-NOF working group on goal-directed treatment for osteoporosis. J Bone Miner Res. 2017;32(1):3–10.

54. Cummings SR, San Martin J, McClung MR, Siris ES, Eastell R, Reid IR, et al. Denosumab for prevention of fractures in postmenopausal women with osteoporosis. N Engl J Med. 2009;361(8):756–65.

55. McClung MR, Lewiecki EM, Geller ML, Bolognese MA, Peacock M, Weinstein RL, et al. Effect of denosumab on bone mineral density and biochemical markers of bone turnover: 8-year results of a phase 2 clinical trial. Osteoporos Int. 2013;24(1):227–35. https://doi.org/10.1007/s00198-012-2052-4.

56. Miller PD, Bolognese MA, Lewiecki EM, McClung MR, Ding B, Austin M, et al. Effect of denosumab on bone density and turnover in postmenopausal women with low bone mass after long-term continued, discontinued, and restarting of therapy: a randomized blinded phase 2 clinical trial. Bone. 2008;43(2):222–9.

57. Brown JP, Prince RL, Deal C, Recker RR, Kiel DP, de Gregorio LH, et al. Comparison of the effect of denosumab and alendronate on BMD and biochemical markers of bone turnover in postmenopausal women with low bone mass: a randomized, blinded, phase 3 trial. J Bone Miner Res. 2009;24(1):153–61.

58. Kendler DL, Roux C, Benhamou CL, Brown JP, Lillestol M, Siddhanti S, et al. Effects of denosumab on bone mineral density and bone turnover in postmenopausal women transitioning from alendronate therapy. J Bone Miner Res. 2010;25(1):72–81.

59. Kendler DL, Bessette L, Hill CD, Gold DT, Horne R, Varon SF, et al. Preference and satisfaction with a 6-month subcutaneous injection versus a weekly tablet for treatment of low bone mass. Osteoporos Int. 2010;21(5):837–46.

60. Faienza MF, Chiarito M, D'amato G, Colaianni G, Colucci S, Grano M, Brunetti G. Monoclonal antibodies for treating osteoporosis. Expert Opin Biol Ther. 2018;18(2):149–57. https://doi.org/10.1080/14712598.2018.1401607.

61. Zanchetta MB, Boailchuk J, Massari F, Silveira F, Bogado C, Zanchetta JR. Significant bone loss after stopping long-term denosumab treatment: a post FREEDOM study. Osteoporos Int. 2017:1–7.

62. Neer RM, Arnaud CD, Zanchetta JR, Prince R, Gaich GA, Reginster JY, et al. Effect of parathyroid hormone (1–34) on fractures and bone mineral density in postmenopausal women with osteoporosis. N Engl J Med. 2001;344(19):1434–41.

63. Lindsay R, Scheele WH, Neer R, Pohl G, Adami S, Mautalen C, et al. Sustained vertebral fracture risk reduction after withdrawal of teriparatide in postmenopausal women with osteoporosis. Arch Intern Med. 2004;164(18):2024–30.

64. Bauer DC, Garnero P, Bilezikian JP, Greenspan SL, Ensrud KE, Rosen CJ, et al. Short-term changes in bone turnover markers and bone mineral density response to parathyroid hormone in postmenopausal women with osteoporosis. J Clin Endocrinol Metab. 2006;91(4):1370–5.

65. Finkelstein JS, Wyland JJ, Lee H, Neer RM. Effects of teriparatide, alendronate, or both in women with postmenopausal osteoporosis. J Clin Endocrinol Metab. 2010;95(4):1838–45.

66. Cosman F, Eriksen EF, Recknor C, Miller PD, Guañabens N, Kasperk C, et al. Effects of intravenous zoledronic acid plus subcutaneous teriparatide [rhPTH(1–34)] in postmenopausal osteoporosis. J Bone Miner Res. 2011;26(3):503–11.

67. Black DM, Bilezikian JP, Ensrud KE, Greenspan SL, Palermo L, Hue T, et al. One year of alendronate after one year of parathyroid hormone (1–84) for osteoporosis. N Engl J Med. 2005;353(6):555–65.

68. Adami S, San Martin J, Muñoz-Torres M, Econs MJ, Xie L, Dalsky GP, et al. Effect of raloxifene after recombinant teriparatide [hPTH(1–34)] treatment in postmenopausal women with osteoporosis. Osteoporos Int. 2008;19(1):87–94.

69. Cosman F, Hattersley G, Hu MY, Williams GC, Fitzpatrick LA, Black DM. Effects of abaloparatide-SC on fractures and bone mineral density in subgroups of postmenopausal women with osteoporosis and varying baseline risk factors. J Bone Miner Res. 2017;32(1):17–23.

70. Minisola S, Cipriani C, Occhiuto M, Pepe J. New anabolic therapies for osteoporosis. Intern Emerg Med. 2017;12(7):915–21.

71. Chew CK, Clarke BL. Abaloparatide: recombinant human PTHrP (1–34) anabolic therapy for osteoporosis. Maturitas. 2017;97:53–60.

72. Cosman F, Miller PD, Williams GC, Hattersley G, Hu MY, Valter I, et al. Eighteen months of treatment with subcutaneous abaloparatide followed by 6 months of treatment with alendronate in postmenopausal women with osteoporosis: results of the ACTIVExtend trial. Mayo Clin Proc. Elsevier. 2017;92(2):200–10.

73. Bilizikean JP, Fitzpatrick LA, Williams GC, Hu M, Hattersley G, Rizzoli R. Bone mineral density and bone turnover marker changes with sequential abaloparatide/alendronate: results of ACTIVExtend. J Bone Miner Res. 2017;(Supply 1):S377.

74. Eastell R, Nickelsen T, Marin F, Barker C, Hadji P, Farrerons J, et al. Sequential treatment of severe postmenopausal osteoporosis after teriparatide: final results of the randomized, controlled European Study of Forsteo (EUROFORS). J Bone Miner Res. 2009;24(4):726–36.

75. Bonnelye E, Chabadel A, Saltel F, Jurdic P. Dual effect of strontium ranelate: stimulation of osteoblast differentiation and inhibition of osteoclast formation and resorption in vitro. Bone. 2008;42(1):129–38.

76. Girotra M, Rubin MR, Bilizikian JP. Anabolic skeletal therapy for osteoporosis. Arq Bras Endocrinol Metab. 2006;50(4):745–54.

77. Meunier PJ, Roux C, Seeman E, Ortolani S, Badurski JE, Spector TD, et al. The effects of strontium ranelate on the risk of vertebral fracture in women with postmenopausal osteoporosis. N Engl J Med. 2004;350(5):459–68.

78. Reginster JY, Seeman E, De Vernejoul MC, Adami S, Compston J, Phenekos C, et al. Strontium ranelate reduces the risk of nonvertebral fractures in postmenopausal women with osteoporosis: Treatment of Peripheral Osteoporosis (TROPOS) study. J Clin Endocrinol Metab. 2005;90(5):2816–22.

79. O'Donnell S, Cranney A, Wells GA, Adachi JD, Reginster JY. Strontium ranelate for preventing and treating postmenopausal osteoporosis. Cochrane Database Syst Rev. 2006;3:CD005326.

80. Reginster JY, Kaufman JM, Goemaere S, Devogelaer JP, Benhamou CL, Felsenberg D, et al. Maintenance of antifracture efficacy over 10 years with strontium ranelate in postmenopausal osteoporosis. Osteoporos Int. 2012;23(3):1115–22.

81. Li X, Ominsky MS, Warmington KS, Morony S, Gong J, Cao J, et al. Sclerostin antibody treatment increases bone formation, bone

mass, and bone strength in a rat model of postmenopausal osteoporosis. J Bone Miner Res. 2009;24(4):578–88.

82. Ominsky MS, Vlasseros F, Jolette J, Smith SY, Stouch B, Doellgast G, et al. Two doses of sclerostin antibody in cynomolgus monkeys increases bone formation, bone mineral density, and bone strength. J Bone Miner Res. 2010;25(5):948–59.

83. Padhi D, Jang G, Stouch B, Fang L, Posvar E. Single-dose, placebo-controlled, randomized study of AMG 785, a sclerostin monoclonal antibody. J Bone Miner Res. 2011;26(1):19–26.

84. Bandeira L, Lewiecki EM, Bilezikian JP. Romosozumab for the treatment of osteoporosis. Expert Opin Biol Ther. 2017;17(2):255–63.

85. Saag KG, Petersen J, Brandi ML, Karaplis AC, Lorentzon M, Thomas T, et al. Romosozumab or alendronate for fracture prevention in women with osteoporosis. N Engl J Med. 2017;377(15):1417–27.

86. Paik J, Scott LJ. Romosozumab: A Review in Postmenopausal Osteoporosis. Drugs Aging. 2020;37(11):845–55. https://doi.org/10.1007/s40266-020-00793-8.

87. Dede AD, Makras P, Anastasilakis AD. Investigational anabolic agents for the treatment of osteoporosis: an update on recent developments. Expert Opin Investig Drugs. 2017;26(10):1137–44.

88. Binkley N, Bolognese M, Sidorowicz-Bialynicka A, Vally T, Trout R, Miller C, et al. A phase 3 trial of the efficacy and safety of oral recombinant calcitonin: the oral calcitonin in postmenopausal osteoporosis (ORACAL) trial. J Bone Miner Res. 2012;27(8):1821–9. https://doi.org/10.1002/jbmr.1602.

89. Bandeira L, Lewiecki EM, Bilezikian JP. Pharmacodynamics and pharmacokinetics of oral salmon calcitonin in the treatment of osteoporosis. Expert Opin Drug Metab Toxicol. 2016;12(6):681–9.

90. Miller PD, Hattersley G, Riis BJ, Williams GC, Lau E, Russo LA, et al. Effect of abaloparatide vs. placebo on new vertebral fractures in postmenopausal women with osteoporosis: a randomized clinical trial. JAMA. 2016;316(7):722–33.

Osteoporosis in Men

Luigi Gennari, Leonardo Bandeira, Aline G. Costa,
Natalie E. Cusano, Barbara C. Silva, and John P. Bilezikian

Introduction

Osteoporosis is a growing health economic problem, affecting more than 200 million people worldwide. This disorder occurs as the result of multiple mechanisms that together cause loss of bone mass and strength leading to an increased risk of fractures, most commonly involving the vertebral bodies, the hip, and the forearm. Although osteoporosis has traditionally been considered to be a disease of postmenopausal women, epidemiological data indicate that up to 30–40% of all osteoporotic fractures worldwide occurs in men [1], with an estimated lifetime risk for males aged 50 years or older between 13% and 30% [2, 3], which is greater than his likelihood of developing prostate cancer [4]. Indeed, given the increase in longevity and growth of the population, the number of men with fractures worldwide is likely to increase markedly in the years to come [5].

Importantly, the consequences of osteoporotic fractures in men are more severe than in women, both in terms of morbidity and mortality [3, 6, 7]. For example, hip fracture, which accounts for at least 1/3 of all fractures in men [5], is associated with a threefold higher mortality rate in men than in women [6]. In a large Canadian survey of hip fractures, up to 10% of elderly men died during hospitalization and more than 22 one-third (37.5%) of those who survived to be discharged died within the year [8]. Likewise, men are less likely to return to independent living than women, after a hip fracture has occurred [9]. Moreover, similar to women, the absolute risk of a subsequent fracture in men increases substantially after the first fragility fracture, and this increase is even greater than observed in women [10]. The Australian Dubbo Osteoporosis Study noted that the relative risk of a second fracture after an initial osteoporotic fracture in a cohort of community-dwelling men >60 years old was 3.47 (CI 95%: 2.69–4.48), while for women, the relative risk of the second fragility fracture was 1.97 (CI 95%: 1.71–2.26). Mortality risk was also greater when the second fracture occurred, again with men showing greater mortality [11.3 per 100 person-years (95% CI, 9.8–13.0)] than women [7.8 per 100 person-years (95% CI, 7.1–8.5)] [2]. In MrOs, a large prospective epidemiologic cohort of elderly men, the advent of a rib fracture resulted in a twofold increased risk of future rib, hip, or wrist fracture, independent of BMD or other factors [11].

Despite these points, still a minority of men are screened and treated for osteoporosis and fracture prevention, even after the first fragility fracture has occurred. A recent analyses from Korea, which included 556,410 individuals aged 50 years and older who experienced their first osteoporotic fracture, showed that only 19% of men received anti-osteoporosis therapy after the fracture, a much lower rate than observed among women (42%) [12].

Clinical Case

A 53-year-old male is referred for a diagnostic evaluation of osteoporosis due to the occurrence of a humerus fracture following a minor trauma. There is a strong family history of

L. Gennari
Department of Medicine, Surgery and Neurosciences, University of Siena, Siena, Italy
e-mail: gennari@unisi.it

L. Bandeira
Divison of Endocrinology, Federal University of Sao Paulo, Sao Paulo, SP, Brazil

FBandeira Endocrine Institute, Recife, Brazil
e-mail: leonardo.farias@grupofleury.com.br

A. G. Costa · J. P. Bilezikian (✉)
Metabolic Bone Diseases Unit, Division of Endocrinology, Department of Medicine, College of Physicians and Surgeons, Columbia University, New York, NY, USA
e-mail: jpb2@columbia.edu

N. E. Cusano
Division of Endocrinology, Lenox Hill Hospital, Department of Medicine, New York, NY, USA
e-mail: ncusano@northwell.edu

B. C. Silva
Division of Endocrinology, Felicio Rocho and Santa Casa Hospital, Belo Horizonte, Brazil

© Springer Nature Switzerland AG 2022
F. Bandeira et al. (eds.), *Endocrinology and Diabetes*, https://doi.org/10.1007/978-3-030-90684-9_25

osteoporosis on his paternal side with his father and two uncles all affected. He is otherwise healthy but reports previous wrist and rib fractures in childhood, mainly related to minor trauma during sporting activities. The patient drinks one glass of wine on average per day and is a past smoker (about five to ten cigarettes per day from age 18 to age 37). He is not taking any medication, and there is no previous history of corticosteroid, thyroid hormone, antiseizure, or antidepressive medication use. His diet is relatively poor in calcium-containing foods. His exercise routine, over the past 10–15 years, consists of swimming and playing tennis one to two times per week. There has been no height loss from his peak of 173 cm.

Past medical history Previous rib and wrist fractures during childhood, as noted.

Personal and social history Married, two daughters (23 and 19 years old), both of whom are healthy.

Family history Father died at 77 from myocardial infarction. His mother is 74 years old with hypertension and diabetes. He has no siblings. A strong family history for osteoporosis is as noted.

Physical examination Height 173 cm, weight 65 kg, BMI 21.7 kg/m². Examination of the heart, lungs, and abdomen is normal. There are no physical findings of hypogonadism or other signs suggesting the presence of a secondary cause of osteoporosis.

Laboratory results Calcium, 9.0 mg/dL (nl: 8.9–10.1); phosphorus, 3.7 mg/dL (nl: 2.5–4.5); creatinine, 0.88 mg/dL (nl: 0.76–1.27 mg/dL); PTH, 34 pg/mL (nl: 15–65); 25-hydroxyvitamin D, 23 ng/mL (nl: 30–50 ng/mL); alkaline phosphatase activity, 36 IU/L (nl: 33–96); bone-specific alkaline phosphatase 7 mcg/L (nl: 6–30); and serum C-terminal telopeptide of type 1 collagen 0.334 ng/mL (nl: 0.142–0.522). Total testosterone is 634 ng/dL (nl: 260–1000 ng/dL) with normal FSH and LH levels. Serologies for gluten enteropathy are negative. Liver function is normal. Serum and urine protein electrophoresis is normal. 24-hour urine collection for calcium (180 mg/g creatinine) and cortisol (20 μg) are normal.

Bone Density results Dual-energy X-ray absorptiometry reveals a bone mineral density (BMD) *T*-score of −2.7 in the lumbar spine, −2.4 in the total hip, and −2.6 at the femoral neck.

Summary
The patient has a strong family history for osteoporosis, without any additional risk factors, except for a previous childhood fractures and past smoking. Bone densitometry

confirms the diagnosis of osteoporosis. Without any secondary causes, he would be classified as "idiopathic osteoporosis." The low bone density and recent fragility fracture indicate that he is a candidate for pharmacological therapy.

Key Points to the Diagnosis of Bone Loss in Men

Medical History and Physical Examination

Osteoporosis remains largely underdiagnosed and undertreated in men. Thus, the presence of risk factors (e.g., family history, long-term glucocorticoid therapy) or clinical features like kyphosis, height loss, decreased libido, previous fracture, or back pain should be considered in order to identify men with osteoporosis [13–15]. Medication history should particularly focus upon the use of glucocorticoids, thyroid hormone, antiseizure medications, and serotonin reuptake inhibitors.

The physical examination should always include height so that a comparison can be made with the historical record of peak height. Height loss of more than 5 cm calls for imaging studies such as spinal X-ray or vertebral fracture assessment by dual-energy X-ray absorptiometry (DXA), in order to investigate the possibility of a vertebral fracture. The presence or absence of kyphosis and/or scoliosis should be also considered, as well as an examination of body composition, mobility, and muscle mass, since frailty and sarcopenia are associated with an increased risk of falls and fragility fractures [16–18]. In this respect, hand grip strength analysis and tests of physical performance (e.g., the 6-meter walk test) are helpful tools to identify men at higher risk of falls and fractures [19].

Because secondary osteoporosis is common in men, major signs or symptoms for the following conditions should be sought: hypogonadism (testicular size, hair pattern, decreased libido), hyperthyroidism (neck exam, reflexes, heat intolerance, fatigue, muscle weakness, fine tremors of hands and fingers, Graves' ophthalmopathy), Cushing's syndrome (supraclavicular fat pads, "buffalo" hump, skin thickness, striae rubrae, proximal muscle weakness), chronic obstructive pulmonary disease (anterior-posterior chest diameter, distant breath sounds, breathing difficulty, wheezing, cough, cyanosis), alcoholism (liver size, palmar erythema), and intestinal malabsorption syndromes (leanness, anemia, diarrhea). Any of the above findings can be helpful clues to the differential diagnosis of osteoporosis.

Laboratory Tests

Routine laboratory testing should include serum calcium, phosphate, albumin, creatinine with estimated glomerular filtration rate, alkaline phosphatase activity, liver function tests, complete blood count, and 24-hour urine for calcium excretion [13–15]. Given the widespread prevalence of vitamin D deficiency, serum 25-hydroxyvitamin D levels should also be routinely measured [20, 21].

Depending on the history and the physical examination, further tests such as thyroid function, PTH levels, total and free testosterone (and perhaps also free estradiol), and tissue transglutaminase antibodies should be also investigated in the consideration of a secondary cause of osteoporosis.

Despite the fact that higher levels of bone turnover markers (e.g., the C-terminal telopeptide of type 1 collagen as a marker of bone resorption or the type 1 procollagen amino-terminal-propeptide as a marker of bone formation) are associated with greater bone loss in men, their use for the diagnosis and the follow-up of antiosteoporotic treatment in men remains controversial [22, 23]. Nevertheless, if bone turnover markers are markedly elevated, ongoing bone loss is likely. On the other hand, reduced bone formation markers, indicated low turnover osteoporosis, have been often associated with idiopathic osteoporosis in young or middle-aged men [15].

Bone Mineral Density (BMD)

The measurement of BMD represents a gold standard for the diagnosis of osteoporosis in men for the same reason that it is a diagnostic standard in women. In short, reduced bone density is a very powerful predictor of the fragility fracture. In a prospective analysis of more than 5000 men from the MrOS cohort, hip BMD was even a stronger predictor of hip fracture than what has been established in a comparably large prospective study of women. Per SD reduction in BMD, the increase in fracture risk in men is more than three-fold; in women, it is twofold [24].

The clinical practice guidelines from the Endocrine Society, in agreement with International Society of Clinical Densitometry and the National Osteoporosis Foundation, recommend BMD testing at the hip and spine for all men aged above 70 years (which is considered by itself to be a sufficient risk factor for osteoporosis) or for men aged 50–69 years with a history of fracture or with other risk factors or predisposing conditions [25]. The risk factors included in this latter directive include excessive alcohol intake, smoking, rheumatoid arthritis, glucocorticoid use (>5 mg prednisone or equivalent for >3 months), use of gonadotropin-releasing hormone agonists, low body weight, chronic obstructive pulmonary disease, hyperparathyroidism, hyperthyroidism, hypogonadism, and family history of hip fracture [13–15, 26–28]. Some experts advocate extending this screening window to men with hypercalciuria/nephrolithiasis and those with a history of constitutionally delayed puberty. Importantly, it should be noted that a history of a

fragility fracture, defined as a fracture occurring spontaneously or after minor trauma (e.g., a fall from a standing height), can be considered diagnostic of osteoporosis, irrespective of BMD assessment. In this case, the BMD test is performed not to make the diagnosis but rather to determine the extent of bone loss and its pervasiveness. BMD of spine and hip is the recommended DXA measurement sites. The measurement of forearm BMD (at the distal 1/3 radius) is recommended in men with hyperparathyroidism, those receiving androgen deprivation therapy (ADT) for prostate cancer or when spine and hip BMD cannot be interpreted (e.g., osteoarthritis or hip prosthesis) [25].

As in women, the densitometric diagnosis of osteoporosis is established with a BMD T-score of −2.5 or less (i.e., 2.5 standard deviations below average peak BMD) [29] at the lumbar spine, total hip, or femoral neck. However, in the male population, there is still controversy on whether the young female or male reference ranges should be used to calculate T-scores. The Endocrine Society Guidelines and the International Society of Clinical Densitometry [25, 30] both have recommended the male-specific reference range (25–30 year-old young men who have achieved peak bone mass). Conversely, other organizations, like the International Osteoporosis Foundation, recommend that the reference female database be used for men [31, 32]. The uncertainty over which referent database to use is a result of a differing opinion as to which is more important clinically: absolute fracture risk or relative fracture risk. The argument for using a male referent database for men is that the relationship between BMD and fracture risk is similar among men and women. The relative risk using the male referent database is the same for a T-score of −2.5 as it is for a woman whose T-score is −2.5 using a female referent database. However, even though relative risk is the same, using the gender-specific referent standard, absolute risk is not. A man's T-score of −2.5 confers a lower absolute risk of fracture than a woman's because the risk of fracture is lower in men than in women at any T-score. This latter point has led experts to recommend that the female database be used for both men and women. The absolute risk of fracture is a function of the absolute BMD in g/cm^2, not the T-score. If this approach is taken, however, the diagnosis of osteoporosis in men will be made less frequently and, to a certain extent, will be inconsistent with epidemiological data on fracture incidence in men. Therefore, utilization of the male database seems to make more sense. For example, in the population-based cohort of MrOS, the proportion of men identified as having osteoporosis at baseline was 2.2% using the reference female-specific T-score and 9.4% using the male-specific T-score [33]. Recently, a Spanish cohort of men aged ≥50 years showed that the prevalence of osteoporosis was 1.1% using the female reference database and 13% using the male reference database [34].

Fracture Risk Algorithms

Recently the use of algorithms such as FRAX® or Garvan, incorporating major risk factors for osteoporosis, has been suggested to improve the prediction of fracture risk over simple BMD measurement, as well as for the selection of patients for treatment [35].

The fracture risk calculation tool FRAX® is a country-specific algorithm, applicable to men and women [36, 37], widely used in many countries throughout the world. FRAX® incorporates established clinical risk factors besides BMD (e.g., height, weight, age, sex, family history of hip fracture, glucocorticoid use, rheumatoid arthritis, alcohol intake, smoking, secondary causes of osteoporosis) and calculates a 10-year probability of hip fracture and major osteoporotic fracture (clinical vertebral, hip, forearm, or humerus). Its most important application is to identify those with low bone density, but not osteoporosis, who are at high risk for fracture. In a study of 5891 men of MrOS Study, it was reported that FRAX® predicted hip fracture well, although it performed less well in prediction of other major osteoporotic fractures [38]. In a more recent analysis in 62,275 women and 6455 men from the Manitoba Registry, FRAX was a strong and consistent predictor of major osteoporotic fractures and hip fractures in both genders [39]. In the United States, treatment with a pharmacological agent is recommended if the 10-year fracture risk by FRAX® for a major osteoporotic fracture is ≥20% or for a hip fracture is ≥3% [25].

Differential Diagnosis of Bone Loss in Men

As in women, osteoporosis in men is typically classified into two different categories, primary and secondary. Indeed, secondary causes seem more prevalent in men [13–15], occurring in up to 50% of cases. However, information from population-based studies is limited in this respect, and the observed higher prevalence of secondary osteoporosis in men in clinical practice might reflect less active case finding (e.g., fewer DXA measurements in men outside the context of secondary causes). In other words, it is possible that men are not as likely to be screened for osteoporosis by DXA testing as are women unless they already have been discovered to have risk factors. Moreover, even with a clearly known risk factor, such as use of androgen deprivation therapy, just a minority of the patients seems to undergo DXA, as shown by Kirk et al. [40]. The three most important causes of osteoporosis in men are excessive alcohol intake, hypogonadism (which includes men who have been therapeutically castrated for prostate cancer), and glucocorticoid excess (e.g., endogenous Cushing's syndrome and hypercortisolism or, more commonly, chronic glucocorticoid therapy) [13]. Other

relevant etiologies to be considered include thyroid disorders, gastrointestinal disorders (e.g., celiac disease can be subclinical), hypercalciuria, chronic obstructive pulmonary disease, organ transplantation, neuromuscular disorders, systemic illnesses, and medications. Furthermore, in the setting of a fragility fracture, diagnostic tests to rule out a pathologic condition such as multiple myeloma or skeletal metastases are necessary [13]. An emerging major category of secondary osteoporosis in both genders is represented by type 2 diabetes, which increases bone fragility despite normal or higher than normal BMD levels [41]. In 2018 the International Osteoporosis Foundation (IOF) recommended DXA should be done in all diabetic patients aged 50 years and older. Since bone density is underestimated in these patients, treatment could be considered at a higher T-score (-2 SD) than in non-diabetic patients, and fracture risk should be adjusted by including rheumatoid arthritis on FRAX tool [42].

It is not uncommon that no obvious etiology to the osteoporosis is identified, besides aging itself. In men over the age of 70, it is appropriate to use the term age-related. While diagnostic codes still use the terminology of senile osteoporosis, we prefer the term age-related to avoid the negative connotations of the word "senile." In individuals who are under 70, aging would seem to be an inadequate explanation. Lacking a clear-cut cause in these younger men, osteoporosis in these individuals is often referred to as primary or idiopathic osteoporosis. Although this category is clearly a heterogeneous one, most of the men in this group present a rather typical clinical and histomorphometric phenotype that differs from age-related osteoporosis, namely, decreased bone formation [15, 43]. Most of the structural skeletal abnormalities found in men with primary osteoporosis have been related to alterations in the endocrine system and particularly to impaired IGF-1 and sex hormone action [13–15]. Genetic factors also have a relevant role in primary osteoporosis [44, 45], and either association studies or next-generation sequencing analyses of rare pedigrees with early onset osteoporosis identified polymorphisms or mutations in members of the WNT-LRP5 pathway as a possible cause of bone fragility in young or middle-aged individuals from both genders [46]. Genetic variation of the aromatase CYP19 gene or genes encoding for components of the insulin-like growth factor system may also play a role in some cases [47–49].

Selection of Men for Pharmacological Treatment

At present, there is no universally validated strategy for therapeutic decision making in men. Based on cost-effectiveness analysis in the United States, as recommended by the NOF [50] and subsequently endorsed by the Endocrine Society

[25], pharmacological treatment is recommended under the following conditions: (1) all men with a hip or vertebral fracture occurring without major trauma; (2) men without fragility fractures but whose BMD of the spine and/or hip is −2.5 SD below the mean of normal young males; (3) men who are receiving long-term glucocorticoid treatment with prednisone or equivalent >7.5 mg/dL daily for more than 3 months, also according to the guidelines of the American Society for College of Rheumatology [51]; and (4) men with BMD within the osteopenic range (T-score between −1.0 and −2.5 SD at the spine and/or hip) showing a FRAX-calculated 10-year fracture probability greater than or equal to 3% and 20%, respectively, for hip and major osteoporotic fractures. Generally, the latter indication is not followed in most countries outside United States, where additional region-specific criteria are used.

Approved Treatments for Male Osteoporosis

The management of osteoporosis in men should consist of both general measures and the use of pharmaceuticals with either antiresorptive or anabolic activity on the bone. General measures should include exercise (tailored to the patient's capabilities and possibly including weight-bearing activities), smoking cessation, alcohol restriction (less than 3 units per day), and adequate calcium and vitamin D intake [25]. The recommended amount of daily calcium follows the Institute of Medicine's recommendation of 1000–1200 mg/day, ideally obtained from dietary sources, with the use of calcium supplements only in case of a diet that does not contain the recommended intake. Adequate vitamin D intake varies as a function of the patient's 25-hydroxyvitamin D level which should be between 20 and 50 ng/mL (50–125 nmol/l). This lower limit comes from the Institute of Medicine's guidelines. It should be noted, however, that the IOM did not make recommendations for an osteoporotic population, only for the normal population. Other authoritative organizations, like the Endocrine Society, recommend a higher threshold of 30 ng/mL (75 nmol/l) [25, 52, 53] to define adequacy. Calcium and vitamin D supplementation should be considered as inherent part of all pharmacological approaches to the treatments of osteoporosis in men in the same manner that we emphasize these nutritional elements in women with osteoporosis.

Most of the pharmacologic agents that are currently available for men with osteoporosis have been previously tested much more extensively and approved for women. The studies in men, in general, have not included adequate numbers of patients to ascertain a change in fracture incidence. With only a few exceptions, surrogate endpoints such as increases in BMD and changes in bone turnover markers have been used. On the whole, however, even without fracture end-points, it seems likely that the efficacy of these drugs in men is similar to that in women [25, 54]. Medications available at this time to treat male osteoporosis can be grouped according to their chemical class and function.

Antiresorptive Agents

Bisphosphonates

As in women, aminobisphosphonates are the mainstay of therapy for osteoporosis in men. The current agents approved by the Food and Drug Administration (FDA) for the treatment of male osteoporosis are alendronate or risedronate, as oral regimens, and zoledronic acid, as an intravenous infusion. The oral aminobisphosphonates require morning dosing, on an empty stomach with plain water and waiting approximately 30 minutes before eating, drinking, or taking other medications. Overall, either oral or intravenous aminobisphosphonate regimens for male osteoporosis are generally well tolerated. The most common adverse events include upper gastrointestinal symptoms described with oral regimens and an acute phase reaction (e.g., fever, headache, musculoskeletal pain) described in up to 40% of cases after the first zoledronic acid infusion. Severe adverse events such as osteonecrosis of the jaw (ONJ) and atypical femoral fracture (AFF) are described very rarely in both genders and mostly in case of long-term, continuous treatment regimens. While ONJ and AFF are very serious events, and thus accorded much publicity, it is important to recognize that they occur very rarely. In virtually all analyses that have considered the risk-benefit profile of these drugs, the risk of not treating (i.e., a hip fracture) is always much greater than the risk of either of these rare events.

Alendronate is given weekly (70 mg) although a daily 10 mg formulation is still available. Both the weekly and the daily formulations led to similar BMD increases in men and reduced bone turnover markers [55]. In a first, randomized, placebo-controlled trial, Orwoll and colleagues [56] showed that 2-year alendronate treatment significantly increased lumbar spine (+7.1%), femoral neck (+2.5%) and total body (+2.0%) BMD. The extent was very similar to that seen previously in studies of postmenopausal women. BMD increases were independent of baseline free testosterone, age, baseline BMD T-score, and presence or absence of prevalent vertebral fractures. Of interest, height loss was also reduced in the alendronate-treated group over placebo, as was the incidence of vertebral fractures. The number of nonvertebral fractures was too low to evaluate the effect of alendronate treatment in their prevention. Comparable incremental effects on BMD in men and women with primary and secondary osteoporosis were observed in subsequent studies [57–62] [52–57]. A meta-analysis of randomized controlled trials indicated that alendronate treatment efficiently reduces the risk of vertebral fractures in men with low bone mass or fractures (odds ratio 0.44; 95% CI 0.23–0.83), but there was insufficient evidence to prove a significant effect on nonvertebral fractures (OR 0.60; 95% CI 0.29–1.44) [63]. Of note, the relative risk of vertebral fracture in alendronate-treated men was similar to that previously observed in a meta-analysis of data from postmenopausal women [64].

Risedronate, taken either daily (5 mg), weekly (35 mg) or monthly (150 mg), is effective in the treatment of primary and secondary causes of bone loss in men [65, 66]. In an open-label clinical trial conducted by Ringe et al., daily treatment with risedronate 5 mg for 1 year reduced the incidence of a new vertebral fracture by 60% compared to placebo which was sustained for the second year of treatment and associated with BMD improvements at the lumbar spine (+6.5%), femoral neck (+3.2%), and total hip (+4.4%) [65, 66]. In a 2-year, randomized, double-blind, placebo-controlled study in men with osteoporosis, Boonen et al. demonstrated that weekly risedronate is as effective as daily risedronate in terms of reductions in bone turnover markers and increases in BMD [67]. There were very few fractures in that study, and a difference between placebo and the treatment arms could not be ascertained. In a 2-year open-label extension of this trial, risedronate was associated with further increases in BMD [68]. Risedronate has also been shown to be effective in the treatment of bone loss in men >65 years of age who have sustained a cerebrovascular accident. Although the number of hip fractures was small in that study (ten in the placebo vs two in the risedronate groups), risedronate was associated with a significant reduction in hip fracture incidence [69]. A newer formulation of risedonate (DR 35 mg) is available that can be taken after breakfast [70].

Zoledronic acid is administered intravenously at a dose of 5 mg once yearly for the treatment of osteoporosis. It was as effective as alendronate in increasing BMD and in reducing bone turnover markers in men with idiopathic osteoporosis or osteoporosis due to hypogonadism [71], while it was superior to risedronate in increasing BMD and reducing bone turnover markers in the treatment and prevention of glucocorticoid-induced osteoporosis [72]. Moreover, in the HORIZON Recurrent Fracture Trial (RFT), performed in a mixed male and female sample of patients with a recent low-trauma hip fracture (within 90 days of surgical repair), zoledronic acid lowered the subsequent clinical fracture rate and decreased mortality compared with placebo [73]. A subsequent gender-specific analysis of the same trial showed that the BMD increases in men were of a similar magnitude to those observed in women. However, the male subset was too small to allow a gender-specific analysis of fracture and mortality [74]. Of interest, a placebo-controlled trial was specifically designed to assess fracture endpoints in a large cohort of 1199 men (50–85 years old) with primary or hypogonadism-associated osteoporosis [75]. Zoledronic acid or placebo was administered at baseline and at 1 year. The primary endpoint was the percentage of men who sustained one or more new morphometric vertebral fractures after 24 months. Overall, patients treated with zoledronic acid had a 67% reduction in relative fracture risk after 2 years and a 3.2% reduction in absolute risk (4.9% vs 1.6%; $p = 0.0016$). Furthermore, the group that received active drug experienced fewer moderate to severe vertebral fractures ($p = 0.026$) and less height loss ($p = 0.0002$) in comparison to placebo. Results were similar in men with osteoporosis due to hypogonadism and in men with normal testosterone levels. No difference was seen in serious adverse events between the zoledronic acid and placebo groups [75]. Although the power of the study to detect a reduction in the risk of nonvertebral fracture was modest, rates of nonvertebral fracture were consistently lower with zoledronic acid than placebo and with similar point estimates to that reported in larger studies involving women. This study is a landmark in that it was designed to establish fracture efficacy for a bisphosphonate in men with osteoporosis.

Denosumab

Denosumab is a human IgG antibody that binds to and inactivates RANKL (receptor activator of nuclear factor-kB ligand) [76, 77]. Based on the results of a large phase 3 registration trial with fracture endpoints, this potent antiresorptive therapy was approved for postmenopausal women at high risk for fracture in the United States and Europe in June, 2010. It is administered subcutaneously at a dose of 60 mg every 6 months. Not cleared by renal mechanisms, it has been shown to be efficacious in subjects with creatinine clearance values <30 cc/min, where bisphosphonate treatment is generally contraindicated. In men, the use of denosumab was firstly investigated in a trial of men receiving androgen deprivation therapy (ADT) for nonmetastatic prostate cancer [78]. In that study, the standard dosing regimen of denosumab, 60 mg administered subcutaneously every 6 months, not only reduced bone turnover and increased BMD, but it also significantly reduced the incidence of new vertebral fractures at 36 months (relative risk, 0.38; 95% CIs 0.19 to 0.78; $P = 0.006$). In another highly relevant study, a 12-month, phase 3, randomized controlled trial in men with low BMD showed significant increases in lumbar (5.7%) and femoral (2.4%) BMD versus placebo [79]. These increments were comparable to those reported in the larger trial in postmenopausal women, where efficacy of denosumab on the prevention of vertebral and nonvertebral fractures was demonstrated. On the basis of this additional information, both the FDA and European Medicine Agency (EMA) in 2012 extended the registration of denosumab to all men with osteoporosis at high risk for fracture.

Data in postmenopausal women who used denosumab for 10 years showed that the medication continued to be effective in improving bone mass and reducing fractures, without increasing the incidence of adverse events [80, 81]. However, its discontinuation leads to a rapid increase in BTMs, a reduction in BMD with an increased risk of fractures, especially in patients with a previous history of vertebral fractures. For this reason, if treatment with denosumab needs to be stopped, another medication (e.g., bisphosphonates) should be started [82–84].

Osteoanabolic Agents

These medications have extended our therapeutic options for osteoporosis since they can directly stimulate bone formation over bone resorption and thus, in some instances, they may restore bone quality and quantity to a greater extent that can be obtained with inhibitors of bone resorption. To date, the only available osteoanabolic agent approved worldwide for the treatment of osteoporosis in men is teriparatide, the 1–34 amino terminal fragment of the intact PTH molecule. Teriparatide is administrated as a daily 20 μg subcutaneous injection for no more than 24 months.

In a trial in men with idiopathic osteoporosis or osteoporosis due to hypogonadism Orwoll et al. showed that treatment with teriparatide for 11 months increases BMD to virtually the same extent as in women over that same period of time [85]. Participants were followed for 30 months after the drug was discontinued due to early termination of the trial. Over this period of time, some received antiresorptive therapy. After discontinuation 18 months later, there was an overall reduction in moderate to severe vertebral fractures when the original teriparatide treatment groups (20 and 40 μg) were compared to the original placebo group [86]. In glucocorticoid-induced osteoporosis, a clinical trial in which men were included showed that teriparatide promotes better BMD outcome and lower vertebral fractures when compared with patients treated with alendronate [87, 88]. As shown in the study of Kaufman et al. [86] as well as other studies, discontinuation of teriparatide therapy is associated with rapid reductions in BMD if a bisphosphonate is not used promptly thereafter [89].

In women who have previously been treated with an antiresorptive drug and sequentially with teriparatide, the actions of teriparatide may be delayed [90]. However, effects of prior bisphosphonate therapy are overcome, usually with the first 6 months of PTH treatment. In men, simultaneous therapy with teriparatide and alendronate gave no densitometric advantage over monotherapy with teriparatide alone [91]. Walker et al. reported a randomized, double-blind study to evaluate the combination of teriparatide and risedronate. A total of 29 men, aged 37–81 years, with low BMD at the spine, hip, or distal radius, were enrolled [92]. Patients were randomized to receive risedronate 35 mg weekly plus daily-injected placebo, teriparatide 20 μg sub-cutaneously daily plus weekly oral placebo, or both risedronate plus teriparatide (combination) for 18 months. BMD gains at the lumbar spine were seen in all three groups ($p < 0.05$), but there were no between-group differences. However, total hip BMD increased to a greater extent in the combination group ($3.86 \pm 9.2\%$) versus teriparatide ($0.29 \pm 8.0\%$) or risedronate ($0.82 \pm 8.0\%$; $p < 0.05$ for both). Femoral neck BMD also increased to a greater extent in the combination group ($8.45 \pm 14.1\%$) versus risedronate ($0.50 \pm 12.2\%$; $p = 0.002$), but was not different from teriparatide alone.

The safety of teriparatide has been reviewed with specific reference to reports of osteosarcoma in rats when administered very large doses for a large proportion of a rat's life [93, 94]. The 10-year history of parathyroid hormone as a treatment for osteoporosis does not provide any evidence that osteosarcoma is a risk when teriparatide or PTH(1–84) is used for the treatment of osteoporosis [95, 96]. The drug has now been available for 16 years without any negative signals surfacing in this regard.

Testosterone Replacement

Treatment of male osteoporosis with testosterone focuses upon men with hypogonadism, which is a major cause of secondary osteoporosis in men. There is no rationale for using testosterone in men who are eugonadal. However, despite the well-documented effects of androgen on periosteal bone apposition and the positive results on BMD of testosterone supplementation in hypogonadal men [97], evidence for fracture efficacy is weak [98]. Moreover, concerns about the effect of androgens on the prostate and the cardiovascular system have not been completely ruled out, and the long-term risk to benefit ratio of prolonged testosterone replacement in elderly men has not been well established [99]. Indeed, most of the antiresorptive and osteoanabolic agents available in men have been shown to be effective in preventing bone loss in patients with hypogonadism and low testosterone levels. Therefore, the recommendations of the Endocrine Society emphasize the use of bisphosphonates and other approved therapies for hypogonadal men [25]. This also applies to men at high risk of fracture who are receiving testosterone for hypogonadal symptoms (e.g., low libido, hot flushes, unexplained chronic fatigue). The use of androgen replacement in "lieu of a bone drug" is actually restricted to men with low testosterone levels (<200 ng/dl) who are symptomatic and in whom there are contraindications to the approved pharmacological agents for male osteoporosis. If hypogonadal symptoms are not ameliorated after 6 months of therapy, testosterone should be discontinued, and another therapy should be considered.

Future Therapeutic Approaches

Due to progress in understanding bone biology, novel and promising therapeutic targets for anabolic and antiresorptive treatments for osteoporosis have been recently identified. At the same time given the pivotal role of estrogen on the male skeleton, as established by experimental and clinical observations, the use of compounds targeting the estrogen receptor, such as selective estrogen receptor modulators (SERMS) has been also proposed.

Selective Estrogen Receptor Modulators (SERMs)

The rationale for considering an estrogen-like treatment for osteoporosis in men rests with the studies clearly linking estrogen deficiency to age-related bone loss in men and the pivotal role that estrogen plays in the acquisition of peak bone mass in men [100]. Indeed, while androgen mainly stimulates periosteal cortical apposition and exerts an anabolic effect on muscle mass (thus decreasing the risk of falls in the elderly), estrogen is prominently involved in the regulation of bone turnover and the prevention of bone loss in both genders. Interestingly, in a study in eugonadal osteoporotic men, the increases in BMD and the reduction in bone turnover following testosterone supplementation positively correlated with change in estradiol, but not in testosterone levels [97], providing further rationale for the use of compounds with estrogenic action on bone like selective estrogen receptor modulators (SERMs) to prevent bone loss in males.

In men with hypogonadism induced by androgen deprivation therapy for prostate cancer, either raloxifene or toremifene treatment prevented bone loss in comparison to placebo [101, 102] and, in the case of toremifene, also decreased vertebral fracture risk by 50% [102]. In two small studies, raloxifene was used to treat eugonadal osteoporotic men over a short term, showing a suppressive effect on bone resorption markers only in those cases with low baseline estradiol levels [103, 104]. However, despite these intriguing data, the use of SERMs for male osteoporosis is not recommended.

Selective Androgen Receptor Modulators (SARMs)

This class of compounds includes drugs that activate androgen receptors in a tissue selective manner that might theoretically provide an opportunity to promote the beneficial effects of androgens on bone and muscle with limiting unwanted side effects at the prostate, heart, and liver. Theoretically, SARMs should however be less effective than testosterone on bone if they cannot be converted into estrogen and act on estrogen receptors as testosterone does. Since the discovery of the first SARM in 1990s, some compounds with myo- and osteoanabolic activity in preclinical models have been identified [105], but to date, most, if not all, have failed to advance to clinical development either due to toxicity or lack of efficacy [106, 107].

Abaloparatide

Following the development of teriparatide, different approaches have been employed in order to identify modified PTH or PTH-related peptide (PTHrP) fragments that interact with the PTH receptor (PTHR1) and are endowed with increased activity in bone. Abaloparatide is a 1–34 PTHrP-like molecule in which several amino acids have been modified in order to improve its pharmacokinetics and pharmacodynamic profiles [108]. Based on the results of a large registrative phase 3, double-blind, randomized controlled trial (the ACTIVE trial) in April 2017, subcutaneous abaloparatide (at a daily 80 μg regimen) received approval by the FDA for the treatment of postmenopausal women with osteoporosis at high risk for fracture or patients who have failed or are intolerant to other available osteoporosis therapy. In that study, subcutaneous injections of abaloparatide for 18 months significantly decreased the risk of vertebral (by 86%) and nonvertebral (by 46%) fracture compared with placebo, with a more rapid onset of fracture reduction than teriparatide [109]. The incidence of side effects such as hypercalcemia was also significantly lower with abaloparatide (3.4%) than with teriparatide (6.4%). Similar to teriparatide, the FDA has limited the use of abaloparatide for a cumulative total exposure of 2 years. Studies in men are expected to be forthcoming.

Sclerostin Antibody

Sclerostin, an osteocyte product, plays a key role as a signaling molecule that mediates bone formation, since it acts as a neutralizing factor for the Wnt-LRP5/6-β-catenin pathway, a master promoter of osteoblast differentiation and activity [110]. While Wnt and LRP5/6 regulate relevant aspects of cell growth and differentiation in many tissues so that the generation of specific agonists may lead to unwanted extraskeletal effects, Wnt antagonists, such as sclerostin, are more specific for the skeleton, offering new and potentially safe therapeutic target to stimulate bone formation [111, 112]. Thus, romosozumab, a sclerostin monoclonal antibody has been developed and is currently being clinically tested as a new osteoanabolic agent. Importantly, different preclinical models demonstrated that in different conditions of bone fragility, sclerostin antibody administration is able to improve bone formation and finally bone strength acting through transient stimulation of bone formation coupled with simultaneous suppression of bone resorption, which is unprecedented as a mechanism among therapies for osteoporosis [113]. Consistent with the preclinical reports, in a phase 3 trial on postmenopausal women with osteoporosis who were at high risk for fracture, romosozumab treatment for 12 months followed by alendronate resulted in a significantly lower risk of fracture than alendronate alone [114]. Based on these and the FRAME study data [115], the drug was approved by the FDA and EMA in 2019 for use in postmenopausal women. Due to an imbalance in "serious cardiovascular adverse events" in patients who took romosozumab versus alendronate, the medication should not be used in those who have had a heart attack or stroke within the previous year. Also, healthcare professionals should consider whether the benefits outweigh the risks in those with risk factors for heart disease [116–118]. In men over 55 years old with osteoporosis, the BRIDGE phase 3 trial showed that romosozumab for 12 months increased spine and hip BMD compared with placebo (LS, 12.1 vs 1.2%; TH, 2.5 vs −0.5%) [119].

Monitoring Therapy

The International Society of Clinical Densitometry recommends that patients who are being treated with pharmacological agents should be monitored every 1–2 years with DXA [30]. If BMD stabilizes, the frequency of DXA monitoring can be reduced. Bone turnover markers should be considered as a surrogate tool to assess the status of bone formation and bone resorption and can be useful as early as 3–6 months after initiation of treatment.

Disclosures Dr. Bilezikian is a consultant for Takeda Pharmaceuticals, Japan. No other conflicts of interest are reported.

Funding Source None.

References

1. Johnell O, Kanis JA. An estimate of the worldwide prevalence and disability associated with osteoporotic fractures. Osteoporos Int. 2006;17(12):1726–33.
2. Bliuc D, et al. Mortality risk associated with low-trauma osteoporotic fracture and subsequent fracture in men and women. JAMA. 2009;301(5):513–21.
3. Burge R, et al. Incidence and economic burden of osteoporosis-related fractures in the United States, 2005-2025. J Bone Miner Res. 2007;22(3):465–75.
4. Melton LJ. Epidemiology of fractures. In: Riggs BL, Melton LJ, editors. Osteoporosis: etiology, diagnosis and management. Philadelphia: Lippincott-Raven Publishers; 1995. p. 225–47.
5. Gullberg B, Johnell O, Kanis JA. World-wide projections for hip fracture. Osteoporos Int. 1997;7(5):407–13.
6. Center JR, et al. Mortality after all major types of osteoporotic fracture in men and women: an observational study. Lancet. 1999;353(9156):878–82.
7. Haentjens P, et al. Meta-analysis: excess mortality after hip fracture among older women and men. Ann Intern Med. 2010;152(6):380–90.
8. Jiang HX, et al. Development and initial validation of a risk score for predicting in-hospital and 1-year mortality in patients with hip fractures. J Bone Miner Res. 2005;20(3):494–500.
9. Schurch MA, et al. A prospective study on socioeconomic aspects of fracture of the proximal femur. J Bone Miner Res. 1996;11(12):1935–42.
10. Center JR, et al. Risk of subsequent fracture after low-trauma fracture in men and women. JAMA. 2007;297(4):387–94.
11. Barrett-Connor E, et al. Epidemiology of rib fractures in older men: Osteoporotic Fractures in Men (MrOS) prospective cohort study. BMJ. 2010;340:c1069.
12. Jung Y, et al. Gender differences in anti-osteoporosis drug treatment after osteoporotic fractures. J Bone Miner Metab. 2019;37(1):134–41.
13. Gennari L, Bilezikian JP. Osteoporosis in men. Endocrinol Metab Clin N Am. 2007;36(2):399–419.
14. Khosla S, Amin S, Orwoll E. Osteoporosis in men. Endocr Rev. 2008;29(4):441–64.
15. Gennari L, Bilezikian JP. Idiopathic osteoporosis in men. Curr Osteoporos Rep. 2013;11(4):286–98.
16. Wong AK, et al. Bone-muscle indices as risk factors for fractures in men: the Osteoporotic Fractures in Men (MrOS) Study. J Musculoskelet Neuronal Interact. 2014;14(3):246–54.
17. Cawthon PM, et al. Physical performance and radiographic and clinical vertebral fractures in older men. J Bone Miner Res. 2014;29(9):2101–8.
18. Scott D, et al. Does combined osteopenia/osteoporosis and sarcopenia confer greater risk of falls and fracture than either condition alone in older men? The Concord Health and Ageing in Men Project. J Gerontol A Biol Sci Med Sci. 2019;74(6):827–34.
19. Rosengren BE, et al. Inferior physical performance test results of 10,998 men in the MrOS Study is associated with high fracture risk. Age Ageing. 2012;41(3):339–44.
20. Cauley JA, et al. Serum 25-hydroxyvitamin D and the risk of hip and nonspine fractures in older men. J Bone Miner Res. 2010;25(3):545–53.
21. Orwoll E, et al. Vitamin D deficiency in older men. J Clin Endocrinol Metab. 2009;94(4):1214–22.
22. Szulc P. Biochemical bone turnover markers and osteoporosis in older men: where are we? J Osteoporos. 2011;2011:704015.
23. Bauer DC, et al. Biochemical markers of bone turnover, hip bone loss, and fracture in older men: the MrOS study. J Bone Miner Res. 2009;24(12):2032–8.
24. Cummings SR, et al. BMD and risk of hip and nonvertebral fractures in older men: a prospective study and comparison with older women. J Bone Miner Res. 2006;21(10):1550–6.
25. Watts NB, et al. Osteoporosis in men: an Endocrine Society clinical practice guideline. J Clin Endocrinol Metab. 2012;97(6):1802–22.
26. Geusens P, Sambrook P, Lems W. Fracture prevention in men. Nat Rev Rheumatol. 2009;5(9):497–504.
27. Mackey DC, et al. High-trauma fractures and low bone mineral density in older women and men. JAMA. 2007;298(20):2381–8.
28. Binkley N. A perspective on male osteoporosis. Best Pract Res Clin Rheumatol. 2009;23(6):755–68.
29. Kanis JA, et al. A reference standard for the description of osteoporosis. Bone. 2008;42(3):467–75.

30. Lewiecki EM, et al. The official positions of the International Society for Clinical Densitometry: perceptions and commentary. J Clin Densitom. 2009;12(3):267–71.

31. Kanis J, et al. Diagnostic thresholds for osteoporosis in men. In: Orwoll E, Bilezikian J, Vanderschueren D, editors. Osteoporosis in men. Boston: Academic Press; 2009.

32. Kaufman JM, et al. Treatment of osteoporosis in men. Bone. 2013;53(1):134–44.

33. Ensrud KE, et al. Implications of expanding indications for drug treatment to prevent fracture in older men in United States: cross sectional and longitudinal analysis of prospective cohort study. BMJ. 2014;349:g4120.

34. Olmos JM, et al. Prevalence of vertebral fracture and densitometric osteoporosis in Spanish adult men: the Camargo Cohort Study. J Bone Miner Metab. 2018;36(1):103–10.

35. Sandhu SK, et al. Prognosis of fracture: evaluation of predictive accuracy of the FRAX algorithm and Garvan nomogram. Osteoporos Int. 2010;21(5):863–71.

36. Kanis JA, et al. FRAX and its applications to clinical practice. Bone. 2009;44(5):734–43.

37. Kanis J, on behalf of the World Health Organization Scientific Group. Assessment of osteoporosis at the primary health-care level. Technical report. World Health Organization Collaborating Centre for Metabolic Bone Diseases, University of Sheffield; 2007.

38. Ettinger B, et al. Performance of FRAX in a cohort of community-dwelling, ambulatory older men: the Osteoporotic Fractures in Men (MrOS) study. Osteoporos Int. 2013;24(4):1185–93.

39. Leslie WD, et al. Performance of FRAX in clinical practice according to sex and osteoporosis definitions: the Manitoba BMD registry. Osteoporos Int. 2018;29(3):759–67.

40. Kirk PS, et al. The implications of baseline bone-health assessment at initiation of androgen-deprivation therapy for prostate cancer. BJU Int. 2018;121(4):558–64.

41. Merlotti D, et al. Mechanisms of impaired bone strength in type 1 and 2 diabetes. Nutr Metab Cardiovasc Dis. 2010;20(9):683–90.

42. Ferrari SL, et al. Diagnosis and management of bone fragility in diabetes: an emerging challenge. Osteoporos Int. 2018;29(12):2585–96.

43. Khosla S. Idiopathic osteoporosis – is the osteoblast to blame? J Clin Endocrinol Metab. 1997;82(9):2792–4.

44. Gennari L, Klein R, Ferrari S. The genetics of peak bone mass. In: Orwoll E, Bilezikian J, Vanderschueren D, editors. Osteoporosis in men. Boston: Academic Press; 2009.

45. Van Pottelbergh I, et al. Deficient acquisition of bone during maturation underlies idiopathic osteoporosis in men: evidence from a three-generation family study. J Bone Miner Res. 2003;18(2):303–11.

46. Lara-Castillo N, Johnson ML. LRP receptor family member associated bone disease. Rev Endocr Metab Disord. 2015;16(2):141–8.

47. Bilezikian JP, et al. Increased bone mass as a result of estrogen therapy in a man with aromatase deficiency. N Engl J Med. 1998;339(9):599–603.

48. Gennari L, Nuti R, Bilezikian JP. Aromatase activity and bone homeostasis in men. J Clin Endocrinol Metab. 2004;89(12):5898–907.

49. Kurland ES, et al. Insulin-like growth factor-I in men with idiopathic osteoporosis. J Clin Endocrinol Metab. 1997;82(9):2799–805.

50. Tosteson AN, et al. Cost-effective osteoporosis treatment thresholds: the United States perspective. Osteoporos Int. 2008;19(4):437–47.

51. Buckley L, et al. 2017 American College of Rheumatology guideline for the prevention and treatment of glucocorticoid-induced osteoporosis. Arthritis Rheumatol. 2017;69(8):1095–110.

52. Holick MF, et al. Evaluation, treatment, and prevention of vitamin D deficiency: an Endocrine Society clinical practice guideline. J Clin Endocrinol Metab. 2011;96(7):1911–30.

53. Heaney RP, Holick MF. Why the IOM recommendations for vitamin D are deficient. J Bone Miner Res. 2011;26(3):455–7.

54. Gennari L, Bilezikian JP. New and developing pharmacotherapy for osteoporosis in men. Expert Opin Pharmacother. 2018;19(3):253–64.

55. Miller PD, et al. Weekly oral alendronic acid in male osteoporosis. Clin Drug Investig. 2004;24(6):333–41.

56. Orwoll E, et al. Alendronate for the treatment of osteoporosis in men. N Engl J Med. 2000;343(9):604–10.

57. Ringe JD, Faber H, Dorst A. Alendronate treatment of established primary osteoporosis in men: results of a 2-year prospective study. J Clin Endocrinol Metab. 2001;86(11):5252–5.

58. Weber TJ, Drezner MK. Effect of alendronate on bone mineral density in male idiopathic osteoporosis. Metabolism. 2001;50(8):912–5.

59. Gonnelli S, et al. Alendronate treatment in men with primary osteoporosis: a three-year longitudinal study. Calcif Tissue Int. 2003;73(2):133–9.

60. Ringe JD, et al. Alendronate treatment of established primary osteoporosis in men: 3-year results of a prospective, comparative, two-arm study. Rheumatol Int. 2004;24(2):110–3.

61. Ho YV, et al. Effects of alendronate on bone density in men with primary and secondary osteoporosis. Osteoporos Int. 2000;11(2):98–101.

62. Iwamoto J, et al. Comparison of the effect of alendronate on lumbar bone mineral density and bone turnover in men and postmenopausal women with osteoporosis. Clin Rheumatol. 2007;26(2):161–7.

63. Sawka AM, et al. Does alendronate reduce the risk of fracture in men? A meta-analysis incorporating prior knowledge of anti-fracture efficacy in women. BMC Musculoskelet Disord. 2005;6:39.

64. Cranney A, et al. Meta-analyses of therapies for postmenopausal osteoporosis. II. Meta-analysis of alendronate for the treatment of postmenopausal women. Endocr Rev. 2002;23(4):508–16.

65. Ringe JD, et al. Sustained efficacy of risedronate in men with primary and secondary osteoporosis: results of a 2-year study. Rheumatol Int. 2009;29(3):311–5.

66. Ringe JD, et al. Efficacy of risedronate in men with primary and secondary osteoporosis: results of a 1-year study. Rheumatol Int. 2006;26(5):427–31.

67. Boonen S, et al. Once-weekly risedronate in men with osteoporosis: results of a 2-year, placebo-controlled, double-blind, multicenter study. J Bone Miner Res. 2009;24(4):719–25.

68. Boonen S, et al. Evidence for safety and efficacy of risedronate in men with osteoporosis over 4 years of treatment: results from the 2-year, open-label, extension study of a 2-year, randomized, double-blind, placebo-controlled study. Bone. 2012;51(3):383–8.

69. Sato Y, et al. Risedronate sodium therapy for prevention of hip fracture in men 65 years or older after stroke. Arch Intern Med. 2005;165(15):1743–8.

70. McClung MR, et al. Efficacy and safety of a novel delayed-release risedronate 35 mg once-a-week tablet. Osteoporos Int. 2012;23(1):267–76.

71. Orwoll ES, et al. Efficacy and safety of a once-yearly i.v. Infusion of zoledronic acid 5 mg versus a once-weekly 70-mg oral alendronate in the treatment of male osteoporosis: a randomized, multicenter, double-blind, active-controlled study. J Bone Miner Res. 2010;25(10):2239–50.

72. Sambrook PN, et al. Bisphosphonates and glucocorticoid osteoporosis in men: results of a randomized controlled trial comparing zoledronic acid with risedronate. Bone. 2012;50(1):289–95.

73. Lyles KW, et al. Zoledronic acid and clinical fractures and mortality after hip fracture. N Engl J Med. 2007;357(18):1799–809.

74. Boonen S, et al. Once-yearly zoledronic acid in older men compared with women with recent hip fracture. J Am Geriatr Soc. 2011;59(11):2084–90.

75. Boonen S, et al. Fracture risk and zoledronic acid therapy in men with osteoporosis. N Engl J Med. 2012;367(18):1714–23.

76. Cummings SR, et al. Denosumab for prevention of fractures in postmenopausal women with osteoporosis. N Engl J Med. 2009;361(8):756–65.

77. von Keyserlingk C, et al. Clinical efficacy and safety of denosumab in postmenopausal women with low bone mineral density and osteoporosis: a meta-analysis. Semin Arthritis Rheum. 2011;41(2):178–86.

78. Smith MR, et al. Effects of denosumab on bone mineral density in men receiving androgen deprivation therapy for prostate cancer. J Urol. 2009;182(6):2670–5.

79. Orwoll E, et al. A randomized, placebo-controlled study of the effects of denosumab for the treatment of men with low bone mineral density. J Clin Endocrinol Metab. 2012;97(9):3161–9.

80. Bone H, et al. Ten years of denosumab treatment in postmenopausal women with osteoporosis: results from the FREEDOM extension trial. In: ASBMR 2015 annual meeting. Seattle; 2015.

81. Papapoulos S, et al. The effect of 8 or 5 years of denosumab treatment in postmenopausal women with osteoporosis: results from the FREEDOM Extension study. Osteoporos Int. 2015;26(12):2773–83.

82. Bandeira F, et al. Multiple severe vertebral fractures during the 3-month period following a missed dose of denosumab in a postmenopausal woman with osteoporosis previously treated with alendronate. Int J Clin Pharmacol Ther. 2019;57(3):163–6.

83. Brown JP, et al. Discontinuation of denosumab and associated fracture incidence: analysis from the Fracture Reduction Evaluation of Denosumab in Osteoporosis Every 6 Months (FREEDOM) trial. J Bone Miner Res. 2013;28(4):746–52.

84. McClung MR. Cancel the denosumab holiday. Osteoporos Int. 2016;27(5):1677–82.

85. Orwoll ES, et al. The effect of teriparatide [human parathyroid hormone (1-34)] therapy on bone density in men with osteoporosis. J Bone Miner Res. 2003;18(1):9–17.

86. Kaufman JM, et al. Teriparatide effects on vertebral fractures and bone mineral density in men with osteoporosis: treatment and discontinuation of therapy. Osteoporos Int. 2005;16(5):510–6.

87. Saag KG, et al. Teriparatide or alendronate in glucocorticoid-induced osteoporosis. N Engl J Med. 2007;357(20):2028–39.

88. Saag KG, et al. Effects of teriparatide versus alendronate for treating glucocorticoid-induced osteoporosis: thirty-six-month results of a randomized, double-blind, controlled trial. Arthritis Rheum. 2009;60(11):3346–55.

89. Kurland ES, et al. The importance of bisphosphonate therapy in maintaining bone mass in men after therapy with teriparatide [human parathyroid hormone(1-34)]. Osteoporos Int. 2004;15(12):992–7.

90. Ettinger B, et al. Differential effects of teriparatide on BMD after treatment with raloxifene or alendronate. J Bone Miner Res. 2004;19(5):745–51.

91. Finkelstein JS, et al. The effects of parathyroid hormone, alendronate, or both in men with osteoporosis. N Engl J Med. 2003;349(13):1216–26.

92. Walker MD, et al. Risedronate, teriparatide or their combination in the treatment of male osteoporosis. J Clin Endocrinol Metab. 2012; [In press]

93. Vahle JL, et al. Skeletal changes in rats given daily subcutaneous injections of recombinant human parathyroid hormone (1-34) for 2 years and relevance to human safety. Toxicol Pathol. 2002;30(3):312–21.

94. Jolette J, et al. Defining a noncarcinogenic dose of recombinant human parathyroid hormone 1-84 in a 2-year study in Fischer 344 rats. Toxicol Pathol. 2006;34(7):929–40.

95. Andrews EB, et al. The US postmarketing surveillance study of adult osteosarcoma and teriparatide: study design and findings from the first 7 years. J Bone Miner Res. 2012;27(12):2429–37.

96. Capriani C, Irani D, Bilezikian JP. Safety of osteoanabolic therapy: a decade of experience. J Bone Miner Res. 2012;27(12):2419–28.

97. Anderson FH, et al. Androgen supplementation in eugonadal men with osteoporosis: effects of six months' treatment on markers of bone formation and resorption. J Bone Miner Res. 1997;12(3):472–8.

98. Tracz MJ, et al. Testosterone use in men and its effects on bone health. A systematic review and meta-analysis of randomized placebo-controlled trials. J Clin Endocrinol Metab. 2006;91(6):2011–6.

99. Basaria S, et al. Adverse events associated with testosterone administration. N Engl J Med. 2010;363(2):109–22.

100. LeBlanc ES, et al. The effects of serum testosterone, estradiol, and sex hormone binding globulin levels on fracture risk in older men. J Clin Endocrinol Metab. 2009;94(9):3337–46.

101. Smith MR, et al. Raloxifene to prevent gonadotropin-releasing hormone agonist-induced bone loss in men with prostate cancer: a randomized controlled trial. J Clin Endocrinol Metab. 2004;89(8):3841–6.

102. Smith MR, et al. Toremifene to reduce fracture risk in men receiving androgen deprivation therapy for prostate cancer. J Urol. 2013;189(1 Suppl):S45–50.

103. Doran PM, et al. Effects of raloxifene, a selective estrogen receptor modulator, on bone turnover markers and serum sex steroid and lipid levels in elderly men. J Bone Miner Res. 2001;16(11):2118–25.

104. Uebelhart B, et al. Raloxifene treatment is associated with increased serum estradiol and decreased bone remodeling in healthy middle-aged men with low sex hormone levels. J Bone Miner Res. 2004;19(9):1518–24.

105. Dalton JT, et al. Discovery of nonsteroidal androgens. Biochem Biophys Res Commun. 1998;244(1):1–4.

106. Clarke BL, Khosla S. Modulators of androgen and estrogen receptor activity. Crit Rev Eukaryot Gene Expr. 2010;20(4):275–94.

107. Narayanan R, Coss CC, Dalton JT. Development of selective androgen receptor modulators (SARMs). Mol Cell Endocrinol. 2018;465:134–42.

108. Cosman F. Abaloparatide: a new anabolic therapy on the horizon. Bonekey Rep. 2015;4:661.

109. Miller PD, et al. Effect of abaloparatide vs placebo on new vertebral fractures in postmenopausal women with osteoporosis: a randomized clinical trial. JAMA. 2016;316(7):722–33.

110. Moester MJ, et al. Sclerostin: current knowledge and future perspectives. Calcif Tissue Int. 2010;87(2):99–107.

111. Baron R, Rawadi G. Wnt signaling and the regulation of bone mass. Curr Osteoporos Rep. 2007;5(2):73–80.

112. Papapoulos SE. Targeting sclerostin as potential treatment of osteoporosis. Ann Rheum Dis. 2011;70 Suppl 1:i119–22.

113. Das S, Sakthiswary R. Bone metabolism and histomorphometric changes in murine models treated with sclerostin antibody: a systematic review. Curr Drug Targets. 2013;14(14):1667–74.

114. Saag KG, et al. Romosozumab or alendronate for fracture prevention in women with osteoporosis. N Engl J Med. 2017;377(15):1417–27.

115. Cosman F, et al. Romosozumab treatment in postmenopausal women with osteoporosis. N Engl J Med. 2016;375(16):1532–43.

116. FDA approves new treatment for osteoporosis in postmenopausal women at high risk of fracture. 2019 [cited 2020 Jun-07]; Available from: https://www.fda.gov/news-events/press-announcements/fda-approves-new-treatment-osteoporosis-postmenopausal-women-high-risk-fracture.

117. Evenity. 2019 [cited 2020 Jun-07]; Available from: https://www.ema.europa.eu/en/medicines/human/EPAR/evenity-authorisation-details-section.

118. Amgen and UCB announce increased cardiovascular risk in patients receiving romosozumab, an anti-sclerotin antibody. Rheumatology (Oxford). 2017;56(8):e21.

119. Lewiecki EM, et al. A phase 3 randomized placebo-controlled trial to evaluate efficacy and safety of romosozumab in men with osteoporosis. J Clin Endocrinol Metab. 2018;103(9):3183–93.

Glucocorticoid-Induced Osteoporosis

E. Michael Lewiecki

Introduction

Glucocorticoid excess, whether generated endogenously or administered exogenously, is known to have many adverse effects, including harm to the skeleton. In his seminal report published over 85 years ago, Harvey Cushing analyzed the clinical and pathological findings of 12 patients with pituitary adenomas [1]. In what came to be called "Cushing's disease" (hypercortisolism caused by a pituitary tumor), he described "softening affecting the entire skeleton but more particularly the vertebrae, leading to multiple fractures." Today, hypercortisolism of any cause ("Cushing's syndrome") is most often due to exogenous glucocorticoids prescribed for a wide variety of inflammatory, allergic, and neoplastic conditions. The first clinical use of exogenous glucocorticoids, extracted from whole cattle adrenals, was reported in 1930 [2]. Patients with adrenal insufficiency due to Addison's disease were successfully treated, although transiently, with intravenous infusions of this extract. This was rapidly followed by experiments to isolate individual compounds in the adrenal extract that have biological activity. In 1949, the first clinical use of cortisone was reported [3]. A woman with rheumatoid arthritis (RA) was treated at the Mayo Clinic with cortisone 50 mg intramuscularly (IM) twice daily. RA symptoms improved, but treatment was subsequently discontinued due to development of facial puffiness, hirsutism, acne, and mental disturbances. Soon after, it was reported that orally administered cortisone was as effective as the IM preparation [4]. In 1954, the first analogs of cortisone and hydrocortisone, which were later named prednisone and prednisolone, were used for the treatment of patients with RA [5]. Anti-inflammatory effects were soon enhanced by the development of other glucocorticoids, such as triamcinolone and dexamethasone. However, for use in clinical practice, prednisone and prednisolone emerged as the most commonly used systemic glucocorticoids and remain so in modern times.

Toxic effects of glucocorticoid therapy were easily recognized with the first patient to receive cortisone for RA [3], as they were similar to the effects of endogenous excess seen with Cushing's syndrome. Adverse skeletal effects of chronic glucocorticoid therapy were described as early as 1954 in a report of vertebral fractures with treatment of 3 men with RA and a boy with juvenile polyarthritis [6]. More patients with glucocorticoid-induced osteoporosis (GIO) and vertebral fractures were reported a few years later [7]. It soon became apparent that osteoporosis and fractures were common in patients receiving long-term glucocorticoid therapy. GIO has been estimated to affect about 50% of patients receiving long-term glucocorticoids and may be the most common form of secondary osteoporosis [8]. Despite the availability of many medications to treat GIO [9], many patients who could benefit are not being treated [10].

Patient Case Report

A 72-year-old woman is a former heavy smoker with severe chronic obstructive pulmonary disease (COPD). Treatment includes home oxygen and prednisone 7.5 mg daily for past 12 years, with higher doses required for 2–3 weeks several times each year for exacerbations of COPD. She describes have a well-balanced diet with no vitamin or mineral supplements. She has fallen twice in the past 12 months but has no known fracture. She has never had a bone density test and has never received pharmacological therapy to reduce fracture risk. After hearing from a friend that prednisone can be harmful to bones, she asks her physician whether she needs to be evaluated. Although he does not see the need for this, he makes an appointment for consultation with a physician with expertise in osteoporosis. She is found to weigh 102 pounds (46.3 kg); height is 60.0 inches (152.4 cm) with a wall-mounted stadiometer, which is 2.5 inches (6.4 cm)

E. M. Lewiecki (✉)
New Mexico Clinical Research & Osteoporosis Center, Albuquerque, NM, USA

© Springer Nature Switzerland AG 2022
F. Bandeira et al. (eds.), *Endocrinology and Diabetes*, https://doi.org/10.1007/978-3-030-90684-9_26

shorter than her historical maximum height. Her gait was unstable and she did poorly on balance testing. She has mild kyphosis. There is no spinal process tenderness to palpation. Dual-energy X-ray absorptiometry (DXA) testing shows lumbar spine T-score = −1.9 with the appearance of degenerative arthritis on the spine image and femoral neck T-score = −2.3. Vertebral fracture assessment (VFA) by DXA shows a severe (grade 3) wedge fracture at T12 and moderate (grade 2) fractures at T9 and T10. On laboratory testing there is a low serum 25-hydroxyvitamin D of 12 ng/mL (30 nmol/L) and elevated serum intact parathyroid (PTH) level of 82 pg/mL (8.7 pmol/L). Serum calcium, albumin, magnesium, phosphorus, alkaline phosphatase, and creatinine are normal. The 24-hour urinary calcium is low at 48 mg. After vitamin D replacement, which corrected the abnormal serum 25-hydroxyvitamin D, PTH, and 24-hour urinary calcium, she is started on alendronate 70 mg weekly. She was referred for physical therapy to improve core strength and balance in an effort to reduce fall risk. Continuing efforts were made to minimize her exposure to system glucocorticoids.

Epidemiology

The prevalence of glucocorticoid use in the general community has been estimated to be between 0.5% and 1% [11–14]. In a 5-year longitudinal study of 60,000 postmenopausal women conducted in 10 countries, 4.6% were receiving glucocorticoids at the baseline visit [15]. The most common reasons for taking glucocorticoids are chronic rheumatic inflammatory diseases (e.g., RA, lupus) and chronic lung diseases (e.g., COPD, asthma). Other uses include gastrointestinal disorders (e.g., inflammatory bowel diseases, hepatitis), organ transplantation, and treatment of some malignancies. Over 10% of patients on long-term glucocorticoids have been reported to have clinical fractures, with 30–40% having radiographic vertebral fractures [16, 17]. Risk factors for fracture include low-baseline bone mineral density (BMD), the type of glucocorticoid medication used, the dose and duration of treatment, the underlying disease being treated, age and sex of the patient, menopausal status for women, and previous fracture. A large case-control study of subjects on oral glucocorticoids reported a dose-dependent increase in fracture risk with users of prednisolone, with no increase in risk for users of budesonide or hydrocortisone [18]. A large retrospective cohort study in the UK found rapid onset of increased fracture risk with initiating oral glucocorticoid therapy, rapid return of fracture risk toward baseline with discontinuation, and no dose that was "safe" for skeletal health [19]. Even doses of prednisolone less than 2.5 mg daily were associated with an increase in vertebral fracture risk. Inhaled glucocorticoids can be partially absorbed and may have systemic effects [20]. Use of long-term inhaled glucocorticoids in high doses for patients with COPD has been associated with a modest increase in the risk of hip and upper extremity fractures [21]. Most studies of intranasal glucocorticoids in patients with allergic rhinitis have shown no clinically significant systemic effects in usual doses, although more study is needed, particularly in patients receiving combinations of inhaled and intranasal glucocorticoids [22].

Pathophysiology

The effects of glucocorticoid therapy on BMD are biphasic. There is an initial rapid phase of 6–12% bone loss in the first year of therapy, followed by subsequent bone loss of about 2–3% per year [23]. Trabecular bone is predominately affected, leading to high risk of fractures in the spine, a skeletal site with a high percentage of trabecular bone [8]. There is marked heterogeneity in the skeletal response of individuals to glucocorticoid therapy, perhaps due to polymorphisms of glucocorticoid receptors or variations of enzymes responsible for metabolizing glucocorticoids. There are many direct and indirect effects of glucocorticoids that lead to skeletal fragility and fractures (Fig. 26.1). The dominant effect of glucocorticoids on bone remodeling is to reduce bone formation by decreasing the number, function, and lifespan of osteoblasts, the bone-forming cells. The activity and lifespan of osteocytes, which act as mechanosensors, are also reduced. The effects of glucocorticoids on osteoclasts are complex and controversial. However, the preponderance of evidence suggests that in the first 3–6 months of glucocorticoid therapy, there is an increase in osteoclastic bone resorption, especially in patients with chronic inflammatory diseases, followed by a subsequent decrease in bone resorption. This might explain, at least in part, the biphasic skeletal response to glucocorticoids. The changing pattern of bone remodeling with long-term glucocorticoids (initial suppression of bone formation and increase in bone resorption, followed by suppression of formation and resorption) raises concern regarding the use of potent antiresorptive medications, such as bisphosphonates and denosumab, for treatment of GIO beyond the first several years [24]. The observation that fracture risk for patients on glucocorticoids rises early in the course of exposure and is greater than expected for the level of BMD is consistent with loss of bone strength due to degradation of bone quality (e.g., bone turnover, bone microarchitecture) and osteocyte apoptosis [25]. Long-term glucocorticoids also have nonskeletal consequences (e.g., sarcopenia, falls) that increase fracture risk [26].

Glucocorticoids have indirect negative effects on bone cell activity mediated by growth factors than include insulin-like growth factor I (IGF-I) and sex steroids [8]. Glucocorticoids

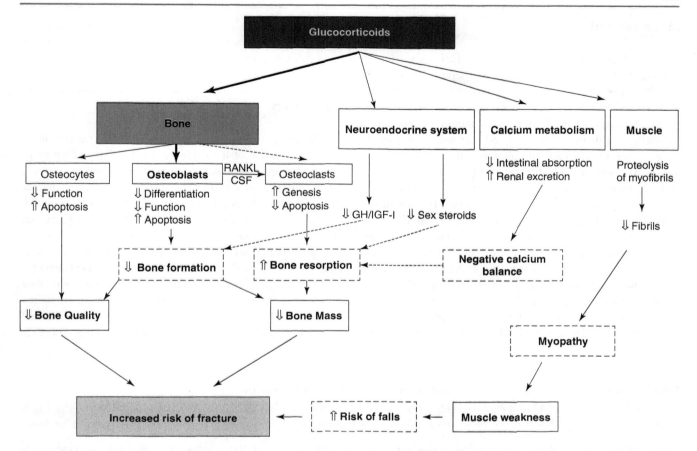

Fig. 26.1 Pathophysiology of GIO [8]. The principal direct skeletal effects of long-term glucocorticoid therapy are due to a decrease in osteoblastic bone formation. Osteocyte function and lifespan is reduced. The effects on osteoclastic bone resorption are biphasic, with an initial transient increase in resorption followed by long-term decrease. Other indirect skeletal effects and nonskeletal effects contribute to high fracture risk with GIO

also reduce intestinal calcium absorption and inhibit renal tubular resorption of calcium. In addition, there are important nonskeletal adverse effects of glucocorticoids that influence fracture risk, such as loss of muscle mass and strength (sarcopenia) that can increase the risk of falls [26].

Assessment of Fracture Risk

Clinicians must be vigilant in assessing fracture risk in patients on systemic glucocorticoids. BMD testing by DXA is useful for all patients initiating treatment that is expected to last for more than 3 months. However, fracture risk may increase soon after starting therapy, especially with high doses, even before there has been a major decline in BMD. The fracture risk algorithm, FRAX [27], assumes an average dose of prednisolone (or prednisone) that is 2.5–7.5 mg daily, or equivalent, for more than 3 months. Fracture risk may be underestimated in patients on doses higher than 7.5 mg daily. It has been recommended to adjust FRAX upward for patients on more than 7.5 mg daily by 20% (e.g., from 2.0% to 2.4%) for 10-year probability of hip fracture and upward by 15% (e.g., from 10% to 11.5%) for the 1-year probability of major osteoporotic fracture [28]. There is limited evidence to suggest that trabecular bone score (TBS), a novel grayscale textural analysis of lumbar spine DXA images, might be helpful as an independent predictor of fracture risk in patients on glucocorticoid therapy [29, 30]. TBS score, if available, can be included as a risk factor in the FRAX calculator. Lateral spine imaging by DXA (vertebral fracture assessment - VFA) or conventional radiography is recommended to evaluate for prevalent vertebral fracture in patients who have received glucocorticoid therapy with prednisone 5 mg or more daily for at least 3 months [31]. The finding of a previously unrecognized vertebral fracture may change diagnostic classification, assessment of fracture risk, and treatment strategies [32].

Management

The initial assessment and treatment of patients starting or continuing long-term glucocorticoid therapy is much the same as for osteoporosis of other causes [33]. This includes a thorough skeletal-related medical history and focused physical examination. The patient should be counseled regarding healthy lifestyle and good nutrition, with particular attention to adequacy of calcium and vitamin D intake and prevention of falls. Fracture risk should be assessed and in appropriately selected patients (see Guidelines) pharmacological therapy to reduce fracture risk should be started. Medications approved for prevention and/or treatment of GIO include alendronate, risedronate, zoledronic acid, denosumab, and teriparatide [34]. Each of these agents increases BMD in patients receiving glucocorticoids, and some have been associated with a reduction in fracture risk [9]. Teriparatide, the only anabolic agent approved for treatment of GIO, reduces vertebral fracture risk more than alendronate [35]. Teriparatide is the only

approved drug that directly addresses the primary mechanism of bone loss with GIO – impairment of osteoblastic bone formation [36].

Guidelines

The American College of Rheumatology (ACR) conducted a systematic review of the evidence for benefits and harms of options for prevention and treatment of GIO and then used a group consensus process to develop clinical practice guidelines [34]. Patients were stratified according to level of fracture risk (low or moderate/high), age (over 40 years or 40 years and older), and childbearing potential. Recommendations for special populations, such as children and people with organ transplantation, were also included. A summary of selected elements of the ACR guidelines and recommendations for a guideline framework from a working group of the International Osteoporosis Foundation and the European Society of Calcified Tissues [37, 38] is provided in Table 26.1. Guidelines can never

Table 26.1 Recommendations for the management of glucocorticoid-induced osteoporosis (GIO)

Category	2017 ACR guidelines [34]	2012 IOF-ECTS framework [37, 38]
Population addressed	Adults and children receiving glucocorticoids (prednisone > 2.5 mg daily) for ≥3 months	Men and women age ≥18 years receiving any dose of oral glucocorticoid therapy for ≥3 months
Initial BMD testing	Adults ≥ age 40 years: as soon as possible when starting glucocorticoids (at least within 6 months) Adults < age 40 years: same as above when fracture risk is high due to previous fracture or osteoporosis risk factors[a] are present	BMD testing for intermediate risk patients when treatment decisions are not clear according to clinical risk factors
Follow-up BMD testing	Adults ≥ age 40 years: every 1–3 years when not treated with osteoporosis medication; every 2–3 years when treated with osteoporosis medication Adults < age 40 years: every 2–3 years when fracture risk is moderate/high[b]	BMD testing at appropriate intervals
FRAX	Adults ≥ age 40 years with adjustment for glucocorticoid dose	Use with adjustment for glucocorticoid dose
Nonpharmacological therapy	Calcium 1000–1200 mg/day, vitamin D 600–800 IU/day with serum level ≥20 ng/mL; lifestyle modifications	Adequate intake of calcium and vitamin D with supplements if needed; lifestyle modifications
Initial pharmacological therapy	Adults (women not of childbearing potential and men) at moderate/high risk[b]: oral bisphosphonate; if not appropriate, consider IV bisphosphonate, teriparatide, denosumab, raloxifene for postmenopausal women (in order of preference) Women of childbearing potential not planning pregnancy during osteoporosis treatment at moderate/high risk[b]: oral bisphosphonate; teriparatide as second-line therapy; when these are not appropriate, IV bisphosphonate, denosumab (in order of preference)	Initiate treatment for postmenopausal women and men ≥ age 50 years according to country-specific thresholds with FRAX with or without BMD. Treatment options include alendronate, etidronate, risedronate, zoledronic acid, and teriparatide. Bone-protective therapy may be appropriate is some premenopausal women and men < age 50 years

These are the highlights of recommendations from two sources [37, 38]. They are similar with many of the essential components in the management of GIO but differ according to many elements, including the time of release and the scope of the recommendations. For details, see the primary references

[a]Risk factors – malnutrition, significant weight loss or low body weight, hypogonadism, secondary hyperparathyroidism, thyroid disease, family history of hip fracture, smoking, alcohol use ≥ units/day

[b]Moderate risk – adults < age 40 years, hip or lumbar spine Z-score <−3.0 or rapid bone loss (≥10% at hip or lumbar spine over 1 year) and continuing glucocorticoid treatment at ≥7.5 mg/day for ≥6 months; adults ≥age 40 years, glucocorticoid-adjusted FRAX major osteoporotic fracture risk 10–19%, hip fracture risk >1%, and <3%; high risk = adults < age 40 years, prior osteoporotic fracture; adults ≥ age 40 years, prior osteoporotic fracture, hip or lumbar spine T-score ≤ −2.5 in men age ≥ 50 years and postmenopausal women, glucocorticoid-adjusted FRAX major osteoporotic fracture risk ≥20%, hip fracture risk ≥3%

ACR American College of Rheumatology, IOF International Osteoporosis Foundation, ECTS European Calcified Tissue Society, IV intravenous, BMD bone mineral density accommodate the many variations of clinical circumstances occurring with individual patients and evolving concepts in the management of skeletal diseases. Concerns regarding the 2017 ACR guidelines have been raised [39]. These include the de-emphasis of the use of anabolic therapy compared with the 2010 ACR guidelines, the recommendation to avoid deno-sumab for renal transplant patients, failure to recommend VFA to evaluate for possible vertebral fracture, and overly stringent criteria for defining treatment failure. As always, treatment decisions in clinical practice should be individualized.

Lessons from the Patient Case Report

Evaluation of skeletal health is mandatory for patients receiving long-term glucocorticoid therapy. Particular attention should be directed to optimizing lifestyle and nutrition, assessing fracture risk, and initiating pharmacological therapy when appropriate. BMD testing by DXA is a useful tool in the assessment of fracture risk, recognizing that these patients may fracture at a higher level of BMD than patients not on glucocorticoids. Vertebral fractures, the most common type of osteoporotic fracture, may not be clinically apparent. Spine imaging by VFA or conventional X-rays may identify previously unrecognized vertebral fractures, which could change diagnostic classification, assessment of fracture risk, and treatment decisions. Vertebral fractures may have adverse effects on pulmonary function, which is especially detrimental to patients with preexisting COPD. While bisphosphonates are the most commonly used medications to treat GIO, there is some evidence suggesting that anabolic therapy is more effective at reducing the risk of vertebral fractures.

Summary

Systemic glucocorticoids are a common cause of drug-induced osteoporosis. Fractures due to GIO can occur early in the course of therapy and may have devastating consequences. Physicians should be vigilant at evaluating patients on glucocorticoids, assessing fracture risk, and initiating countermeasures to reduce fracture risk. Evidence-based guidelines are available to assist physicians in managing patients with GIO. The care of individual patients should be customized according to all available clinical information.

References

1. Cushing H. The basophil adenomas of the pituitary body and their clinical manifestations (pituitary basophilism). Bull Johns Hopkins Hosp. 1932;50:137–95.
2. Rowntree LG, Greene CH, Swingle WW, Pfiffner JJ. The treatment of patients with Addison's disease with the "Cortical Hormone" of Swingle and Pfiffner. Science. 1930;72(1871):482–3.
3. Hench PS, Kendall EC, et al. The effect of a hormone of the adrenal cortex (17-hydroxy-11-dehydrocorticosterone; compound E) and of pituitary adrenocorticotropic hormone on rheumatoid arthritis. Proc Staff Meet Mayo Clin. 1949;24(8):181–97.
4. Freyberg RH, Traeger CT, Adams CH, Kuscu T, Wainerdi H, Bonomo I. Effectiveness of cortisone administered orally. Science. 1950;112(2911):429.
5. Bunim JJ, Pechet MM, Bollet AJ. Studies on metacortandralone and metacortandracin in rheumatoid arthritis; antirheumatic potency, metabolic effects, and hormonal properties. J Am Med Assoc. 1955;157(4):311–8.
6. Curtiss PH Jr, Clark WS, Herndon CH. Vertebral fractures resulting from prolonged cortisone and corticotropin therapy. JAMA. 1954;156(5):467–9.
7. Howell DS, Ragan C. The course of rheumatoid arthritis during four years of induced hyperadrenalism (IHA). Medicine (Baltimore). 1956;35(2):83–119.
8. Canalis E, Mazziotti G, Giustina A, Bilezikian JP. Glucocorticoid-induced osteoporosis: pathophysiology and therapy. Osteoporos Int. 2007;18(10):1319–28.
9. Whittier X, Saag KG. Glucocorticoid-induced osteoporosis. Rheum Dis Clin N Am. 2016;42(1):177–89.
10. Curtis JR, Westfall AO, Allison JJ, Becker A, Casebeer L, Freeman A, et al. Longitudinal patterns in the prevention of osteoporosis in glucocorticoid-treated patients. Arthritis Rheum. 2005;52(8):2485–94.
11. Fardet L, Petersen I, Nazareth I. Monitoring of patients on long-term glucocorticoid therapy: a population-based cohort study. Medicine (Baltimore). 2015;94(15):e647.
12. Fardet L, Petersen I, Nazareth I. Prevalence of long-term oral glucocorticoid prescriptions in the UK over the past 20 years. Rheumatology (Oxford). 2011;50(11):1982–90.
13. Soucy E, Bellamy N, Adachi JD, Pope JE, Flynn J, Sutton E, et al. A Canadian survey on the management of corticosteroid induced osteoporosis by rheumatologists. J Rheumatol. 2000;27(6):1506–12.
14. Overman RA, Yeh JY, Deal CL. Prevalence of oral glucocorticoid usage in the United States: a general population perspective. Arthritis Care Res (Hoboken). 2013;65(2):294–8.
15. Silverman S, Curtis J, Saag K, Flahive J, Adachi J, Anderson F, et al. International management of bone health in glucocorticoid-exposed individuals in the observational GLOW study. Osteoporos Int. 2015;26(1):419–20.
16. Curtis JR, Westfall AO, Allison J, Bijlsma JW, Freeman A, George V, et al. Population-based assessment of adverse events associated with long-term glucocorticoid use. Arthritis Rheum. 2006;55(3):420–6.
17. Angeli A, Guglielmi G, Dovio A, Capelli G, de Feo D, Giannini S, et al. High prevalence of asymptomatic vertebral fractures in postmenopausal women receiving chronic glucocorticoid therapy: a cross-sectional outpatient study. Bone. 2006;39(2):253–9.
18. Vestergaard P, Rejnmark L, Mosekilde L. Fracture risk associated with different types of oral corticosteroids and effect of termination of corticosteroids on the risk of fractures. Calcif Tissue Int. 2008;82(4):249–57.
19. van Staa TP, Leufkens HGM, Abenhaim L, Zhang B, Cooper C. Use of oral corticosteroids and risk of fractures. J Bone Miner Res. 2000;15:993–1000.
20. Lipworth BJ. Systemic adverse effects of inhaled corticosteroid therapy, a systematic review and meta-analysis. Arch Intern Med. 1999;159:941–55.
21. Gonzalez AV, Coulombe J, Ernst P, Suissa S. Long-term use of inhaled corticosteroids in COPD and the risk of fracture. Chest. 2018;153(2):321–8.
22. Bensch GW. Safety of intranasal corticosteroids. Ann Allergy Asthma Immunol. 2016;117(6):601–5.
23. LoCascio V, Bonucci E, Imbimbo B, Ballanti P, Adami S, Milani S, et al. Bone loss in response to long-term glucocorticoid therapy. Bone Miner. 1990;8(1):39–51.

24. Teitelbaum SL. Glucocorticoids and the osteoclast. Clin Exp Rheumatol. 2015;33(4 Suppl 92):S37–9.

25. Weinstein RS. Clinical practice. Glucocorticoid-induced bone disease. N Engl J Med. 2011;365(1):62–70.

26. Klein GL. The effect of glucocorticoids on bone and muscle. Osteoporos Sarcopenia. 2015;1(1):39–45.

27. University of Sheffield. FRAX fracture risk assessment tool. Available from http://www.shef.ac.uk/FRAX/. Accessed 27 Nov 2017.

28. Kanis JA, Johansson H, Oden A, McCloskey EV. Guidance for the adjustment of FRAX according to the dose of glucocorticoids. Osteoporos Int. 2011;22(3):809–16.

29. Harvey NC, Gluer CC, Binkley N, McCloskey EV, Brandi ML, Cooper C, et al. Trabecular bone score (TBS) as a new complementary approach for osteoporosis evaluation in clinical practice. Bone. 2015;78:216–24.

30. Choi YJ, Chung YS, Suh CH, Jung JY, Kim HA. Trabecular bone score as a supplementary tool for the discrimination of osteoporotic fractures in postmenopausal women with rheumatoid arthritis. Medicine (Baltimore). 2017;96(45):e8661.

31. Shepherd JA, Schousboe JT, Broy SB, Engelke K, Leslie WD. Executive summary of the 2015 ISCD position development conference on advanced measures from DXA and QCT: fracture prediction beyond BMD. J Clin Densitom. 2015;18(3):274–86.

32. Lewiecki EM, Laster AJ. Clinical applications of vertebral fracture assessment by dual-energy X-ray absorptiometry. J Clin Endocrinol Metab. 2006;91(11):4215–22.

33. Lewiecki EM. Evaluation of the patient at risk for osteoporosis. In: Marcus R, Feldman D, Dempster DW, Luckey M, Cauley JA, editors. Osteoporosis. 2. Fourth ed. Waltham: Elsevier; 2013. p. 1481–504.

34. Buckley L, Guyatt G, Fink HA, Cannon M, Grossman J, Hansen KE, et al. 2017 American College of Rheumatology Guideline for the prevention and treatment of glucocorticoid-induced osteoporosis. Arthritis Rheumatol. 2017;69(8):1521–37.

35. Saag KG, Shane E, Boonen S, Marin F, Donley DW, Taylor KA, et al. Teriparatide or alendronate in glucocorticoid-induced osteoporosis. N Engl J Med. 2007;357(20):2028–39.

36. Amgen. FDA accepts supplemental biologics license application for Prolia® (Denosumab) in glucocorticoid-induced osteoporosis 2017. Available from https://www.amgen.com/media/news-releases/2017/10/fda-accepts-supplemental-biologics-license-application-for-prolia-denosumab-in-glucocorticoidinduced-osteoporosis/. Accessed 26 Nov 2017.

37. Lekamwasam S, Adachi JD, Agnusdei D, Bilezikian J, Boonen S, Borgstrom F, et al. An appendix to the 2012 IOF-ECTS guidelines for the management of glucocorticoid-induced osteoporosis. Arch Osteoporos. 2012;7:25–30.

38. Lekamwasam S, Adachi JD, Agnusdei D, Bilezikian J, Boonen S, Borgstrom F, et al. A framework for the development of guidelines for the management of glucocorticoid-induced osteoporosis. Osteoporos Int. 2012;23(9):2257–76.

39. Maricic M, Deal C, Dore R, Laster A. Comment on 2017 American College of Rheumatology Guideline for the prevention and treatment of glucocorticoid-induced osteoporosis. Arthritis Care Res (Hoboken). 2018;70(6):949–50.

Metabolic Bone Diseases Other Than Osteoporosis

Manoel Aderson Soares Filho, Natália Rocha da Silva, Vanessa Leão de Medeiros Fabrino, and Francisco Bandeira

Osteogenesis Imperfecta

Osteogenesis imperfecta (OI) is a hereditary disorder of the connective tissue. It is caused by qualitative or quantitative abnormalities involving type I collagen, with varied phenotypic presentations. Patients who are affected may suffer multiple fractures, at times with little or no trauma. In more serious cases, death may occur during the neonatal period. Mild and moderate forms can manifest as premature osteoporosis or severe mineral loss in the bones during postmenopause. Some patients also exhibit blue sclera. The incidence of OI is approximately 1 in every 20,000–25,000 live births in the USA [1].

Pathophysiology

Type I collagen is a structural protein important to the bones, tendons, ligaments, skin, and sclera. OI is commonly caused by mutations in genes forming the code in the alpha-1 and alpha-2 chains within type I collagen, or proteins involved in the formation of type I collagen. The fibrils of type I collagen are composed of polymers of tropocollagen molecules that form a triple helix containing portions of an alpha-1 chain and two alpha-2 chains [2, 3].

M. A. S. Filho
Department of Endocrinology, Agamenon Magalhães Hospital, Division of Endocrinology and Diabetes, University of Pernambuco Medical School, Recife, Pernambuco, Brazil

N. R. da Silva (✉)
Department of Endocrinology, Agamenon Magalhães Hospital, Division of Endocrinology, Recife, Pernambuco, Brazil

V. L. de Medeiros Fabrino
Instituto de Medicina Professor Fernando Figueira (IMIP), Department of Pediatric Endocrinology, Recife, Pernambuco, Brazil

F. Bandeira
Division of Endocrinology, Agamenon Magalhães Hospital, University of Pernambuco Medical School, Recife, PE, Brazil

Most patients with OI exhibit a dominant autosomal mutation in COL1A1 (located at 17q21.31-q22) or COL1A2 (located at 7q22.1) that affects the structure of one of the two alpha chains of type I collagen. The clinical severity depends on the effect of the mutation. Mutations that lead to reduction in the amount of collagen result in less severe phenotypes (OI type I), in contrast to mutations that disrupt the formation of triple-helix collagen that lead to lethal forms (type II OI). Ten percent of patients have a recessive autosomal genetic defect, as with normal COL1A1 and COL1A2 genes.

Mutations in the gene of the FK506-binding protein (FKBP10 or FKBP65), located at 17q21, were identified in samples from five consanguineous families from Turkey and Mexican families with hereditary characteristics causing moderate-to-severe OI [4]. Mutations in the FKBP10 protein, which affect the secretion of type I procollagen, in addition to causing type III OI, may result in a severe form of isolated type IV OI that begins during the prenatal stage [5].

The recessive form of osteogenesis is caused by a deficiency or a mutation in one of the three components of the 3-prolyl hydroxylation complex that modifies the structure of type I collagen and can cause severe to lethal forms of the disease [6]. Mutations causing severe recessive forms can be identified in other genes that encode proteins involved in bone formation and homeostasis, including SERPINH1 (located in t 11q13.5), SERPINF1 (located in 17p13.3), and SP7/OSX (located in 12q13.13) [7, 8]. The presence of abnormal protein structure determines bone fragility.

Disorganized bone structure can be observed histologically, in many cases with normal mineralization, but with significant reduction in cortical thickness, cancellous bone volume, and the number and thickness of trabeculae. A cross-sectional study compared the microstructure and bone density in 39 patients with type I OI with 39 controls. Twenty-seven patients had been treated with bisphosphonates. High-resolution computerized tomography was performed on the distal radius and tibia, as well as bone densitometry (BMD) of the lumbar spine and femoral neck. Patients with OI were shorter in stature but with similar body weight. BMD values were lower for the hip and lumbar spine in OI patients when compared with control patients. The bone area in the radius was 5% lower in patients with OI and 18% lower in the cortical bone, and the trabecular number was significantly lower in patients than in controls [9].

Clinical Manifestations

The clinical features (Table 27.1) range from intrauterine fractures to fractures that normally occur only in adolescence and adult life. Fractures are the result of minimal trauma and bone deformities may occur. Family members with the same mutation may exhibit differing degrees of severity, most likely resulting from defects affecting other components of the connective tissue.

The types of OI can be divided according to their severity (Table 27.2):

- Mild (type I): Patients with type I OI suffer from few or no fractures before puberty, or sometimes numerous fractures throughout their lives. The deformities are minimal, and the individuals usually have lower than normal stature. Frequently, no fractures occur before the child begins to walk. The long bones of the arms, legs, and ribs are most often affected, as well as the small bones of the hands and feet. The frequency of fractures decreases after puberty. In adults there is premature osteoporosis and early hearing loss.
- Moderate to severe (types III–IX): These children have a high frequency of fractures, moderate-to-severe bone deformities, kyphoscoliosis, short stature, and progressive hearing loss, with some children unable to move around. Adults exhibit early osteoporosis and hearing loss, more severe when compared with the mild form. Pregnant women exhibit accelerated bone loss during pregnancy and breastfeeding. Hypermobility of the joints can lead to pain and diminished function.
- Lethal form (type II): Patients with the lethal perinatal form usually have intrauterine death or die during early childhood. Fractures and respiratory insufficiency are frequent causes of death. In such cases, genetic counseling should be provided for families affected.

Diagnosis

A diagnosis of OI should be considered in any child with recurrent fractures from minimal trauma [3]. Family history, clinical examination, and radiological findings are important for diagnostic confirmation. The clinical picture is not always characteristic. Extra-skeletal manifestations may be subclinical (hearing loss), nonspecific, or more common at some ages (dentinogenesis imperfecta is most notable in the first dentition).

- Imaging studies: X-rays of long bones and the spine may show fractures, bone calluses, or deformities, and the X-rays of the skull may reveal the presence of wormian bones.
- Laboratory: Assessment of calcium metabolism (serum calcium, phosphorus, alkaline phosphatase, and PTH) is useful to rule out any preexisting hypocalcaemia or hyperparathyroidism. In cases involving OI, the parameters are usually normal. In type VI OI, increases in alkaline phosphatase may occur. Hypercalciuria is common in children with OI, and the magnitude of the urinary calcium loss reflects the severity of bone disease (shorter height, and higher rate of fracture). Bone formation markers are usually low and markers for bone resorption (CTX) usually high, especially in the more severely affected patient [10, 11].

Table 27.1 Osteogenesis imperfecta symptoms

Osteogenesis imperfecta symptoms		
Atypical fractures	Short stature	Scoliosis
Blue sclera	Hearing loss	Dentinogenesis imperfecta
Laxity of the ligaments	Wormian bones	Laxity of the skin

Table 27.2 Clinical characteristics according to the type of OI

Types of OI	Severity of fractures	Stature	Sclera	Hearing loss	Dentinogenesis imperfecta
I	Slight (<100)	Normal–slightly lower	Blue	Present in 50%	Rarely
II	Perinatal death—multiple	Severely low stature	Blue	–	Yes
III	Severe—multiple	Very low	Blue at birth	Frequent	Yes
IV	Mild to moderate	Variable	Normal	Sometimes	Sometimes
V	Moderate—multiple	Variable	Normal	No	No
VI	Moderate	Slightly lower	Normal—discretely blue	No	No
VII	Moderate	Slightly lower	Normal—discretely blue	No	No
VIII	Severe/lethal	Short members dwarfism	Normal	Not related	No
IX	Severe/lethal	Short limbs	Blue	No	Yes

Differential Diagnosis

Child victims of trauma, as well as patients with severe OI, may exhibit multiple fractures at different stages of fusion. In a study involving 39 children (older than 1 year of age) with fractured collarbones, 82% were considered to be the result of child abuse, 8% accidental injury, and 8% bone fragility, and in one case fractures were the result of osteogenesis imperfect itself [12].

Another study evaluated 61 children victims of child abuse. After reviewing the medical records, 33 cases were confirmed as OI. The median age at examination was 7.1 months. All patients had fractures, 14 exhibited pain, 7 swelling, 5 showed limited movements, and 2 showed an abnormal position of their limbs. Radiographic findings consistent with OI were found in 19 of 33 patients (58%); clinical findings were present in 23 of 33 patients (70%) and a family history of OI in 55% [13]. Therefore, in cases where child abuse is suspected, OI should always be considered, since any error in diagnosis can lead to serious consequences for the children and their families.

The clinical picture of OI is not always characteristic. Patients with mild OI exhibit no fractures until they start to move around. Retinal hemorrhage, subdural hematoma, and bruising may also occur as indirect signs of trauma.

Rickets may cause slow growth, bone deformities, elevated alkaline phosphatase, defects in bone mineralization, and, in some cases, abnormal formation of the teeth. Abnormalities in the sclera and hearing loss typically do not occur, and on X-rays, epiphyseal plate enlargement is present. In the adult patient, osteomalacia may cause bone pain, fractures, and elevated alkaline phosphatase, also without causing hearing loss or blue sclera. Radiological findings include decreased bone density, pseudofractures, and loss of trabecular definition.

Other rare skeletal syndromes causing bone fragility and deformities should also be considered in the differential diagnosis of OI, and these include Bruck syndrome, osteoporosis pseudoglioma syndrome, polyostotic fibrous dysplasia, and juvenile Paget's disease, hypophosphatasia, and idiopathic juvenile osteoporosis.

Treatment

The focus of treatment should be multidisciplinary in order to oversee early care and minimize complications. The objective is to reduce the rate of fractures, prevent deformities, decrease chronic pain, and improve functional capacity.

Bisphosphonates are the main therapeutic agents used to prevent fractures in most forms (except for type VI) although none have been approved specifically for use in children and

Table 27.3 Administration of pamidronate in children with OI

Age	Dose of pamidronate	Frequency
<2 years	0.5 mg/kg/day for 3 days	2/2 months
Between 2 and 3 years	0.75 mg/kg/day for 3 days	3/3 months
>3 years	1.0 mg/kg/day for 3 days	4/4 months

adults with OI. Bisphosphonates are stable pyrophosphate analogues and are potent inhibitors of bone reabsorption and bone turnover.

The majority of studies was conducted in children and did not include control groups. Observed benefits included an increase in bone mineral density, reduced fracture rate, and improvement in mobility and pain [14]. Pamidronate is administered intravenously during consecutive 3-day cycles, with 2- to 4-month intervals, using 0.5 mg/kg/day up to 1 mg/kg/day depending on the age (Table 27.3).

Short-term adverse effects on bone quality and fracture healing are not present, despite the significant reduction in bone turnover with bisphosphonate treatment [15]. Linear growth does not appear to be affected and the greatest benefit seems to occur within the first 2–4 years of therapy. It is prudent to reserve pamidronate for patients in whom the clinical benefits outweigh the risks (deformity of long bones, vertebral compression fractures, and three or more fractures per year) since the long-term effects as yet are not well understood [16].

In a meta-analysis, oral risedronate (35 mg per week) for 24 weeks led to bone mineral density increases by 3.9% at the lumbar spine without statistical significance in the total hip measurements. Bone pain did not improve significantly, and the fracture rate remained high [17].

A randomized, placebo-controlled clinical trial measured serum sclerostin levels in adults with OI and evaluated the effects of teriparatide on osteoanabolic therapy. Compared with control participants matched to age and sex, mean levels of sclerostin were lower in those with type I or type III/VI OI. Sclerostin levels increased in the group of patients with type I OI during therapy with teriparatide. This study suggested that regulation of sclerostin is altered in osteogenesis imperfecta and that serum sclerostin may help predict the response to anabolic therapies in OI [18].

In most cases, orthopedic care focuses on fractures but also should be considered for the correction and prevention of deformities, especially in the lower limbs, including surgical treatment.

Osteomalacia

Osteomalacia is not a common metabolic bone disease but is often neglected especially in its early stages because of the nonspecific nature of symptoms such as vague bone pain and muscle weakness [19]. The disease is characterized by a generalized weakening of bone, leading to deformity, and it is often caused by defects occurring at any step of the metabolism or action of vitamin D [20]. It occurs mostly due to dietary deficiency and exposure to sunlight but can also be due to intestinal malabsorption, chronic kidney failure, or vitamin D resistance [19] (Table 27.4). Osteomalacia can also occur in patients with primary hypophosphatasia (Table 27.5) due to one of the syndromes of hereditary hypophosphatemia (X-linked, autosomal dominant and with hypercalciuria) or oncogenic due to fibroblastic growth factor-23 (FGF-23) secretion by the tumor [21, 22].

There is an increasing prevalence of vitamin D deficiency in many countries, even in those close to the equator, and those with abundant sunlight [23]. The at-risk population includes the elderly with little exposure to sunlight as well as patients with poor absorption including those with celiac disease and those submitted to gastrointestinal bypass surgery. Likewise, individuals living in cold weather climates, as well as women who wear clothes that cover almost the entire body area, are also predisposed to hypovitaminosis D [20].

The main histological findings are an excessive accumulation of bone matrix that is not, or only poorly, mineralized, decreased bone volume, increased accumulation of osteoid, and increases in the osteoid thickness of bones and the surface area [24].

Clinical Manifestations

Osteomalacia may be asymptomatic. When symptomatic, general symptoms include chronic bone and muscle pain, weakness, fatigue, difficulty in walking, and a high risk of fractures due to bone fragility. Deformities related to the softening of the adult skeleton include kyphosis, pectus carinatum, a decrease in stature, genu varum, and acetabular protrusion [25].

Bone pain seems to be caused by hydration of the demineralized bone matrix beneath the periosteum, which is extended, causing compression of nerve terminals. It is usually persistent, diffuse, and symmetrical, starting in the lower back and spreading to the pelvic girdle, hip, and ribs. Pain on palpation of these sites is an important clinical sign. Muscle weakness is usually proximal and associated with hypotonia, atrophy, and discomfort during movement [19].

Diagnosis

The most characteristic laboratory findings are a lower serum calcium level, a decrease in urinary calcium levels, hypophosphatemia, and increased levels of alkaline phosphatase (ALP) (Table 27.6). Increased ALP activity is the most frequent and earliest marker for osteomalacia and reflects the activity of the osteoblast, which forms the demineralized matrix [25]. The key test for the diagnosis of vitamin D deficiency is the demonstration of decreases in serum 26OHD [26].

PTH may be typically increased. As vitamin D deficiency increases, the hypersecretion of PTH leads to bone remodeling and endocortical bone reabsorption, resulting in cortical bone loss and increased risk of fractures. In addition, biochemical markers for bone turnover may be increased [19].

On X-rays, the most characteristic feature is the Looser's zone, a band adjacent to the periosteum which represents a stress fracture (cracks without repetitive posttraumatic displacement). It occurs most commonly in the ribs, pubis, and scapula (Fig. 27.1). This is in contrast to the fissures that occur in the long bones in Paget's disease [26]. Bone scintigraphy usually shows areas of focal increases in MDP uptake (Fig. 27.2). Bone mineral density is usually decreased, mainly in the cortical [19].

Although the diagnosis of osteomalacia can be carried out on the basis of clinical and laboratory findings, transiliac bone biopsy, with tetracycline labeling, can help make a definitive diagnosis. This takes less than 30 min, under local anesthesia, with minimal discomfort to the patient. The specimen should be stored in 70% alcohol and sent to a specialized laboratory for histomorphometric studies. The characteristic finding is impaired mineralization with an absent two-band tetracycline label [27].

Table 27.4 Etiology of osteomalacia

Causes of osteomalacia
Vitamin D deficiency
Lack of sunlight
Malabsorption syndrome
Liver diseases
Chronic renal insufficiency
Anticonvulsants
Reduced calcium intake
Heavy metals: aluminum, lead, cadmium

Table 27.5 Etiology of hypophosphatemic osteomalacia

Causes of hypophosphatemic osteomalacia
X-linked
Autosomal dominant
With hypercalciuria
Oncogenic osteomalacia

Table 27.6 Laboratory findings in nutritional osteomalacia

Laboratory results for osteomalacia	
Elevated PTH	100%
25 (OH) vitamin D <15 ng/ml	100%
Elevated alkaline phosphatase	95%
Low urinary calcium	87%
Low calcium and phosphate levels	27%

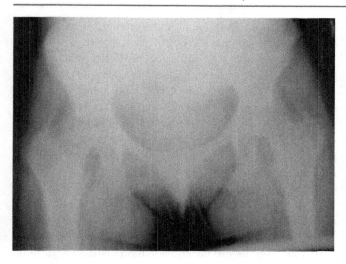

Fig. 27.1 Looser's zone at the right pubis in a 32-year-old woman with hypophosphatemic osteomalacia

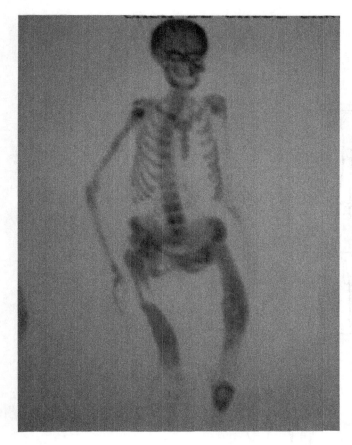

Fig. 27.2 Bone scintigraphy in a 52-year-old woman with primary hyperparathyroidism and osteomalacia. Serum 25OHD: 8 ng/ml

Low serum 25OHD levels, increased FGF-23 levels, and the presence of hypophosphatemia are reliable biomarkers for tumor-induced osteomalacia (TIO). FGF-23 is normally secreted by osteocytes and is an important regulator of phosphate homeostasis due to its action in the kidneys. It may

also be secreted ectopically by mesenchymal tumors which are usually benign, typically very small, and difficult to locate. In fact patients with hypophosphatemic osteomalacia who have no family history for the disease should be screened for TIO. Whole-body Tc-99 sestamibi or I-111-pentetreotide scintigraphy as well as FGD-PET or scintigraphy may be employed, followed by computerized tomography (CT) and/ or magnetic resonance imaging (MRI) of the suspected lesions in an attempt to localize the tumor [28].

Selective venous sampling for FGF-23 measurements may be needed as a localizing procedure especially when multiple sites are identified by imaging examinations. It is also useful when a high degree of certainty is necessary for the location of the tumor before surgery [29].

The differential diagnosis should also be made as shown in Table 27.7 [30].

Treatment

Vitamin D is effective in the treatment of nutritional osteomalacia, or for malabsorption.

In general, 50,000 units of cholecalciferol (vitamin D3) are given once a week for 8 weeks, followed by an adjustment based on 25OHD levels. Bone biopsy may be performed to confirm that osteomalacia has been cured before starting antiresorptive or anabolic agents used for treating residual associated osteoporosis [31].

TIO is treated with a phosphate supplement (1–3 g/day of elemental phosphorus), along with vitamin D, until the tumor has been identified and excised [28]. There are reports of successful treatment of TIO with percutaneous, CT-guided, ethanol, and cryoablation [32].

Paget's Disease of Bone

Paget's disease of bone (PDB) was first described in 1877 by an English physician, Sir James Paget. It is a chronic skeletal disease characterized by increased osteoclastic activity that leads to increased bone reabsorption [33]. There

Table 27.7 Differential diagnosis

Differential diagnosis
Polymyalgia rheumatica
Polymyositis
Fibromyalgia
Bone metastases
Multiple myeloma
Osteoporosis
Paget's disease
Myeloproliferative syndromes
Renal osteodystrophy

is a compensatory increase in the rate of newly formed bone. The rate of change in skeletal remodeling leads to architectural modifications characterized by nonlamellar excessive more vascularized bone formation which is less compact than normal bone. This disease may be localized, monostotic, or polyostotic, and the main sites affected are the vertebrae, long bones of the lower limbs, pelvis, and skull (see Fig. 27.3) [34].

Pathogenesis

Osteoclasts are derived from mononuclear precursor cells of monocytic-macrophage lineage, which fuse to form multinucleated osteoclasts, and are then activated to carry out bone resorption. Both local and systemic factors in the bone microenvironment are important for regulating the formation and activation of osteoclasts. In particular, the receptor activator of the nuclear factor-kB ligand (RANKL), a member of TNF superfamily, is an important regulator of osteoclast differentiation. Most of the factors, including $1.25-(OH)_2D_3$, IL-1, IL-11, and the parathyroid hormone, promote indirect osteoclast activation by binding to stromal marrow cells and inducing the expression of RANK in its ligand [35, 36].

There are at least seven mapped genetic loci associated with Paget's disease; the best documented is the mutation in the P392L in SQSTM1 (PDB3 gene map locus 5q35) [37].

Patients without mutations in the SQSTM1 gene seem to have a susceptibility to genetic polymorphisms in regions of

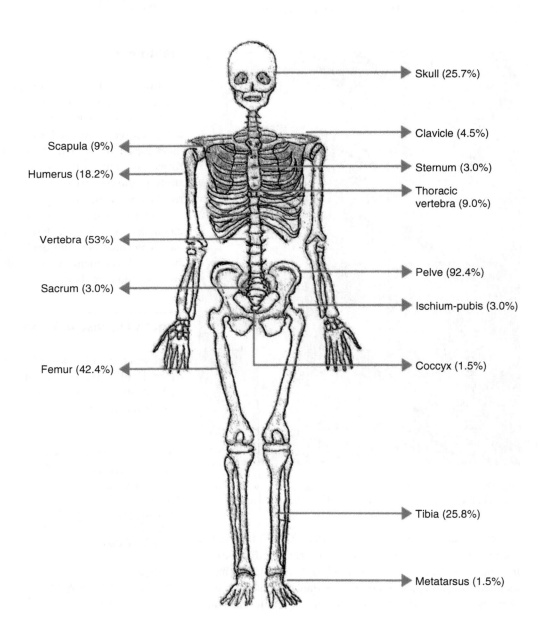

Fig. 27.3 Sites of bone involvement in PDB. PDB Paget's disease of bone. (Data from reference [37])

Skull (25.7%)

Clavicle (4.5%)

Scapula (9%)

Humerus (18.2%)

Sternum (3.0%)

Thoracic vertebra (9.0%)

Vertebra (53%)

Pelve (92.4%)

Sacrum (3.0%)

Ischium-pubis (3.0%)

Coccyx (1.5%)

Femur (42.4%)

Tibia (25.8%)

Metatarsus (1.5%)

the following genes: CaSR, ESR1, TNFRSF11B (OPG), TNFRSF11A (RANK), CSF1 (M-CSF), OPTN, TM7SF4 (DC-STAMP), VCP, NUP205, RIN3, PML, and GOLGA6A, resulting in increased risk for development of PDB. The nature of these genes shows that Paget's disease is caused by the deregulation of osteoclastogenesis [38].

In situ hybridization studies and immune-histochemical analysis suggest the possibility of infection of osteoclasts by a virus, particularly paramyxovirus, as a contributor etiological factor of PDB [34]. The identification of genetic mutations involved in osteoclastogenesis, and characterization of the nongenetic factors that may be involved, appears to be important in developing ways to understand and control the exaggerated bone remodeling in Paget's disease.

Histopathology

Osteoclasts with Paget's disease are multinucleated and excessive in numbers. Increased bone turnover results in abnormal deposition of lamellar bone inserted into the bone tissue. The bone looks disorganized, with thickened trabeculae surrounded by numerous enlarged and multinucleated osteoclasts. The disorganization of the bone tissue leads to increased bone volume, resulting in the manifold complications of the disease. The normal bone marrow is replaced by a large amount of vascular tissue.

Epidemiology

Geographical distribution is variable, the disease being more common in England, the USA, Australia, and New Zealand, but rare in Scandinavia and Asia (see Fig. 27.4). In Brazil, it is found predominantly in locations with a long-standing history of European colonization as in the city of Recife. In this location the prevalence reaches 0.7% in people over 45 years of age [34, 39].

Clinical Manifestations

Paget's disease is usually asymptomatic and discovered incidentally. The main clinical manifestations are bone pain, fractures, skeletal deformities, and secondary arthritis. In most cases, PDB may be diagnosed from the combination of symptoms, radiological findings, and increased concentration of biochemical markers for bone remodeling.

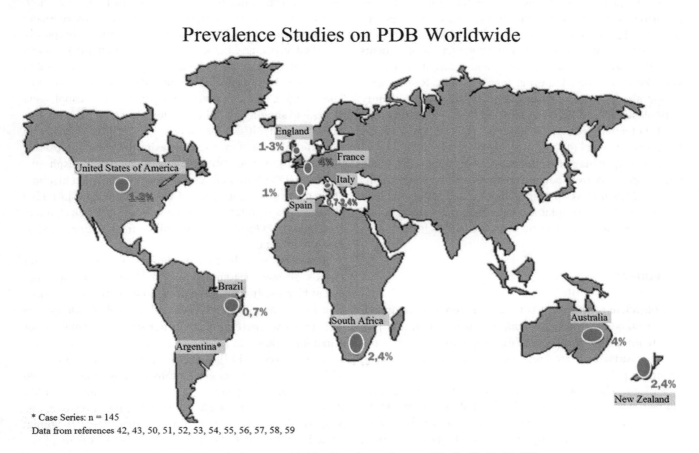

Prevalence Studies on PDB Worldwide

England 1-3%
France 4%
United States of America 1-2%
Italy
Spain 1% 0,7-3,4%
Brazil 0,7%
South Africa 2,4%
Argentina*
Australia 4%
New Zealand 2,4%

* Case Series: n = 145
Data from references 42, 43, 50, 51, 52, 53, 54, 55, 56, 57, 58, 59

Fig. 27.4 Geographical distribution of Paget's disease worldwide. (Data from references [42, 43, 50–54, 55–59])

Juvenile Paget's disease is an extremely rare autosomal recessive disease, characterized by deafness in infancy, fractures, and deformities as the result of generalized bone turnover, normally due to deficiencies in osteoprotegerin (the decoy receptor for the RANK) gene [34].

Diagnosis

PDB can be diagnosed when high serum ALP activity is found, or by routine X-ray examination [40].

Other bone turnover markers are often elevated in active disease, such as serum C-telopeptide (CTx) or urinary N-telopeptide (NTx). Serum calcium and phosphorus are normal in most patients. Hypercalcemia or hypercalciuria can occur in immobilizations or fractures [41].

Plain radiography and bone scintigraphy are useful in patients suspected of having PDB. The radiological findings may be diagnostic, showing typical irregular areas of osteosclerosis with adjacent areas of osteolysis, reflecting abnormal bone turnover characteristic of the disease. The osteolytic lesion that is seen in the skull in the early stages of the disease is known as *osteoporosis circumscripta*. Bone scintigraphy may be more sensitive, albeit less specific, than plain X-rays, especially early in the disease. Computed tomography and magnetic resonance imaging may be useful in unusual lesions, when the diagnosis of malignancy is likely [42].

It is important to obtain a baseline bone scan in all patients with PDB to document the extent and location of lesions, since the sites involved rarely change over time. Radiography should also be performed on the involved sites to identify musculoskeletal consequences of the disease, such as fractures, potentially malignant lesions, osteoarthritis, or other bone abnormalities [43].

Bone biopsy may be useful in atypical cases, as in young adults especially from countries with a low prevalence of the disease. Nonetheless, in suspected localized lesions without characteristic radiographic findings, bone aspiration sometimes shows the characteristic giant osteoclasts [43].

Treatment

The objective of treatment is to relieve pain, restore normal bone metabolism, decrease bone vascularization, and prevent future complications such as bone deformities, secondary osteoarthritis, fractures, and compression of nerve structures [44].

Patients whose symptoms are caused by active Paget's disease (often associated with elevated ALP) should be treated. The most common symptom is bone pain in Pagetic sites, causing headache, or pain in the back, joints, or limbs.

Asymptomatic PDB is detected in imaging studies performed for other reasons (e.g., nephrolithiasis) or by the observation of elevated levels of ALP. The main indication for treatment of asymptomatic patients is biochemically active disease at sites where complications may occur (e.g., skull, spine, and bones adjacent to joints). In other sites, consider treatment if the AP is two to four times above the upper limit of normal. Other indications for treatment of asymptomatic patients include planned surgery for active Pagetic sites (for the purpose of reducing bone turnover and vascularization, thus minimizing blood loss during the procedure) and the rare development of hypocalcaemia in association with the immobilization of patients with polyostotic disease. If such asymptomatic patients do not meet the above criteria for treatment, they should be followed up annually to assess disease progression [45].

Calcitonin was the first inhibitor of osteoclast activity to be used in the treatment of PDB. Nowadays it is used infrequently. It suppresses bone turnover and relieves pain but is more expensive and less effective and presents more side effects (nausea, metallic taste, and flushing) than bisphosphonates. The initial dose is 100 units/day, subcutaneously tapering to 50 units/day.

Bisphosphonates are considered the treatment of choice for PDB. They bind to bone surfaces in regions of high resorption, reducing osteoclastic activity, thereby reducing the bone turnover. When taken orally, they are poorly absorbed, especially in the presence of food in the stomach. They should therefore be taken when fasting, with water, 30–60 min before meals, or any other medications [44]. They may cause heartburn, dyspepsia, and esophageal ulcers and should be used with caution in patients with gastritis or duodenitis. More rarely, they can also cause an acute febrile reaction, uveitis, rash, and osteonecrosis of the jaw [46]. Normal serum levels of calcium, phosphorus, and 25OHD should preferentially be present when bisphosphonate therapy is initiated. Calcium should be provided (1200 mg/day, preferably through a nutritional diet), along with vitamin D (800–2000 units/day), in all patients undergoing treatment.

Etidronate was the first bisphosphonate to be used for Paget's disease, beginning in 1971. The newer and more potent bisphosphonates have proven more effective, leading to a longer period of remission [44]. Oral alendronate is more effective than etidronate. In a regimen of 40 mg/day for 6 months, it leads to a 77% decrease in ALP levels, versus 44% for etidronate [47]. Risedronate leads to similar results, with 30 mg daily doses given orally for 2 months. It should not be used in patients with CrCl<30 ml/min [48]. Pamidronate is well tolerated and easily administered in hospitals or clinics, using 2- to 6-h IV infusions of 30–90 mg, diluted in 500 ml of 0.9% saline or 5% glucose solution [49].

Zoledronic acid (zoledronate) has proven to be the most potent bisphosphonate for the treatment of PDB. It is 10,000 times more potent than etidronate and 100 times more potent than pamidronate [50]. It can be administered in 5 mg, IV infusions, for a shorter time (15–30 min) and in a smaller volume of at least 100 ml (saline or glucose). Hypophosphatemia, hypocalcaemia, and hypokalemia, as with other IV bisphosphonates, may occur, especially in patients with vitamin D deficiency at the time of infusion, as well as fever, chills, myalgia, and arthralgia [50, 51]. Zoledronic acid should also not be used in patients with severe renal impairment creatinine clearance (<30 ml/min) [46] (Table 27.8). In clinical trials comparing oral and intravenous bisphosphonates, side effects, mainly gastrointestinal, were more prevalent when the oral route was used [50].

Indications for restart treatment with bisphosphonates depend on increasing evidence of abnormal bone metabolism, determined by serial measurements of ALP, radiological progression of the disease, or recurrent pain. Increased ALP alone is not always an indication for retreatment. For retreatment, the dose and duration of therapy are the same as the initial treatment [45, 52].

It has been suggested that normalization of bone turnover may improve the clinical outcome in Paget's disease, preventing complications such as fractures and development of osteoarthritis [53]. The PRISM trial evaluated the long-term efficacy of intensive treatment with bisphosphonates versus symptomatic treatment. Initially, the main results of an intention-to-treat analysis showed that intensive bisphosphonate therapy was more effective at normalizing ALP than symptomatic therapy, with 81% of patients receiving intensive care reaching normalized ALP levels at 2 years.

However, there was no significant difference between the groups in terms of fracture, quality of life, or pain [54]. The study extension concluded that long-term intensive bisphosphonate therapy did not confer a clinical benefit in comparison with symptomatic treatment and was associated with a nonsignificant increase in the risk of fractures, orthopedic events, and serious adverse events. The results of this study suggest that, in patients with an established diagnosis of Paget's disease, bisphosphonate therapy should focus on symptom control rather than suppression of bone turnover [53].

Table 27.8 Bisphosphonate regimen Paget's disease

Medication	Dosage	Time period
Etidronate	400 mg/day (oral)	6 months
Alendronate	40 mg/day (oral)	6 months
Risedronate	30 mg/day (oral)	2 months
Pamidronate	60–90 mg/dose (IV)	Every 3 months
Zoledronate	5 mg (IV)	Single injection

References

1. Rauch F, Glorieux FH. Osteogenesis imperfecta. Lancet. 2004;363:1377–85.
2. Gajko-Galicka A. Mutations in type I collagen genes resulting in osteogenesis imperfecta in humans. Acta Biochim Pol. 2002;49:433.
3. Khandanpour N, Connolly D, Raghavan A, Griffiths PD, Hoggard N. Craniospinal abnormalities and neurologic complications of osteogenesis imperfecta: imaging overview. Radiographics. 2012;32:2101–12.
4. Alanay Y, Avaygan H, Camacho N, Utine EG, Boduroglu K, Aktas D, et al. Mutations in the gene encoding the RER protein FKBP65 cause autosomal-recessive osteogenesis imperfecta. Am J Hum Genet. 2010;86:551.
5. Schwarze U, Cundy T, Pyott SM, et al. Mutations in FKBP10, which result in Bruck syndrome and recessive forms of osteogenesis imperfecta, inhibit the hydroxylation of telopeptide lysines in bone collagen. Hum Mol Genet. 2013;22(1):1–17. https://doi.org/10.1093/hmg/dds371.
6. Forlino A, Cabral WA, Barnes AM, Marini JC. New perspectives on osteogenesis imperfecta. Nat Rev Endocrinol. 2011;7(9):540–57.
7. Christiansen HE, Schwarze U, Pyott SM, AlSwaid A, Al Balwi M, Alrasheed S, et al. Homozygosity for a missense mutation in SERPINH1, which encodes the collagen chaperone protein HSP47, results in severe recessive osteogenesis imperfecta. Am J Hum Genet. 2010;86:389.
8. Becker J, Semler O, Gilissen C, Li Y, Bolz HJ, Giunta C, et al. Exome sequencing identifies truncating mutations in human SERPINF1 in autosomal-recessive osteogenesis imperfecta. Am J Hum Genet. 2011;88:362.
9. Folkestad L, Hald JD, Hansen S, Gram J, Langdahl B, Abrahamsen B, et al. Bone geometry, density, and microarchitecture in the distal radius and tibia in adults with osteogenesis imperfecta type I assessed by high-resolution pQCT. J Bone Miner Res. 2012;27:1405–12.
10. Chines A, Boniface A, McAlister W, Whyte M. Hypercalciuria in osteogenesis imperfecta: a follow-up study to assess renal effects. Bone. 1995;16:333.
11. Lund AM, Hansen M, Kollerup G, Juul A, Teisner B, Skovby F. Collagen-derived markers of bone metabolism in osteogenesis imperfecta. Acta Paediatr. 1998;87:1131.
12. Bulloch B, Schubert CJ, Brophy PD, Johnson N, Reed HM, Shapiro RA. Cause and clinical characteristics of rib fractures in infants. Pediatrics. 2000;105:E48.
13. Singh Kocher M, Dichtel L. Osteogenesis imperfecta misdiagnosed as child abuse. J Pediatr Orthop B. 2011;20(6):440–3.
14. Salehpour S, Tavakkoli S. Cyclic pamidronate therapy in children with osteogenesis imperfecta. J Pediatr Endocrinol Metab. 2010;23:73–5.
15. Pizones J, Plotkin H, Parra-Garcia JI, Alvarez P, Gutierrez P, Bueno A, et al. Bone healing in children with osteogenesis imperfecta treated with bisphosphonates. J Pediatr Orthop. 2005;25:332.
16. Rauch F, Glorieux FH. Bisphosphonate treatment of osteogenesis imperfecta: which drug, for whom, for how long? Ann Med. 2005;37:295–8.
17. Bradbury LA, Barlow S, Geoghegan F, Hannon RA, Stuckey SL, Wass JA, et al. Risedronate in adults with osteogenesis imperfecta type I: increased bone mineral density and decreased bone turnover, but high fracture rate persists. Osteoporos Int. 2012;23(1):285–94.
18. Nicol L, Wang Y, Smith R, Sloan J, Nagamani SC, Shapiro J, Lee B, Orwoll E. Serum sclerostin levels in adults with osteogenesis imperfecta: comparison with normal individuals and response to teriparatide therapy. J Bone Miner Res. 2017. https://doi.org/10.1002/jbmr.3312.

19. Bhan A, Rao AD, Rao DS. Osteomalacia as a result of vitamin D deficiency. Endocrinol Metab Clin N Am. 2010;39(2):321–31.

20. Thacher TD, Clarke BL. Vitamin D insufficiency. Mayo Clin Proc. 2011;86(1):50–60.

21. Khaliq W, Cheripalli P, Tangella K. Tumor-induced osteomalacia (TIO): atypical presentation. South Med J. 2011;104(5):348–50.

22. Ruppe MD, Jan de Beur SM. Tumor-induced osteomalacia. Primer on the metabolic bone diseases and disorders of mineral metabolism. 7th ed. Philadelphia: Lippincott Williams & Wilkins; 2008.

23. Bandeira F, Griz L, Dreyer P, Eufrazino C, Bandeira C, Freese E. Vitamin D deficiency: a global perspective. Arq Bras Endocrinol Metabol. 2006;50:640–6.

24. Russell LA. Osteoporosis and osteomalacia. Rheum Dis Clin N Am. 2010;36(4):665–80.

25. Bingham CT, Fitzpatrick LA. Noninvasive testing in the diagnosis of osteomalacia. Am J Med. 1993;95:519.

26. Scharla S. Diagnosis of disorders of vitamin D-metabolism and osteomalacia. Clin Lab. 2008;54(11–12):451–9.

27. Recker RR. Bone biopsy and histomorphometry in clinical practice. In: Rosen CJ, editor. Primer on the metabolic bone diseases and disorders of mineral metabolism. 7th ed. Washington, DC: American Society of Bone and Mineral Research; 2008. p. 180.

28. Chong WH, Molinolo AA, Chen CC, Collins MT. Tumor-induced osteomalacia. Endocr Relat Cancer. 2011;18:R53–77.

29. Andreopoulou P, Dumitrescu CE, Kelly MH, Brillante BA, Peck CMC, Wodajo FM, et al. Selective venous catheterization for the localization of phosphaturic mesenchymal tumors. J Bone Miner Res. 2011;26(6):1295–302.

30. Reuss-Borst M. Metabolische Knochenkrankheit Osteomalazie. Z Rheumatol. 2014;73:316–22.

31. Pepper KJ, Judd SE, Nanes MS, et al. Evaluation of vitamin D repletion regimens to correct vitamin D status in adults. Endocr Pract. 2009;15:95–103.

32. Tutton S, Olson E, King D, Shaker JL, et al. Successful treatment of tumor-induced osteomalacia with CT-guided percutaneous ethanol and cryoablation. J Clin Endocrinol Metab. 2012;97:3421–5.

33. Dickson D, Camp J, Ghormley R. Osteitis deformans: Paget's disease of the bone. Radiology. 1945;44:449–70.

34. Griz L, Caldas G, Bandeira C, Assunção V, Bandeira F. Paget's disease of bone. Arq Bras Endocrinol Metabol. 2006;50:814–22.

35. Whyte MP. Paget's disease of bone, and genetic disorders of RANKL/OPG/NF-kappaB signaling. Ann N Y Acad Sci. 2006;1068:143.

36. Michou L, Collet C, Laplanche JL, Orcel P, Cornélis F. Genetics of Paget's disease of bone. Joint Bone Spine. 2006;73:243.

37. Chung PY, Beyens G, Boonen S, et al. The majority of the genetic risk for Paget's disease of bone is explained by genetic variants close to the CSF1, OPTN, TM7SF4, and TNFRSF11A genes. Hum Genet. 2010;128:615.

38. Chung PY, Van Hul W. Paget's disease of bone: evidence for complex pathogenetic interactions. Semin Arthritis Rheum. 2012;41(5):619–41.

39. Bandeira F, Assunção V, Diniz ET, Lucena CS, Griz L. Characteristics of Paget's disease of bone in the city of Recife, Brazil. Rheumatol Int. 2010;30(8):1055–61.

40. Reis RL, Poncell MF, Diniz ET, Bandeira F. Epidemiology of Paget's disease of bone in the city of Recife, Brazil. Rheumatol Int. 2012;32(10):3087–91.

41. Naot D. Paget's disease of bone: an update. Curr Opin Endocrinol Diabetes Obes. 2011;18(6):352–8.

42. Cortis K, Micallef K, Mizzi A. Imaging Paget's disease of bone—from head to toe. Clin Radiol. 2011;66(7):662–72.

43. Ito A, Yajima A. Is bone biopsy necessary for the diagnosis of metabolic bone diseases? Necessity of bone biopsy. Clin Calcium. 2011;21(9):1388–92.

44. Griz L, Colares V, Bandeira F. Treatment of Paget's disease of bone: importance of the zoledronic acid. Arq Bras Endocrinol Metabol. 2006;50:845–51.

45. Siris ES, Lyles KW, Singer FR, Meunier PJ. Medical management of Paget's disease of bone: indications for treatment and review of current therapies. J Bone Miner Res. 2006;21 Suppl 2:P94.

46. Ferrugia MC, Summerlin DJ, Kroviak E, Huntley T, Freeman S, Borrowdale R, et al. Osteonecrosis of mandible/maxilla and use of new bisphosphonates. Laryngoscope. 2006;116:115–20.

47. Siris ES, Weinstein RS, Altman R, Conte JM, Favus M, Lombardi A, et al. Comparative study of alendronate and etidronate for the treatment of Paget's disease of bone. J Clin Endocrinol Metab. 1996;81:961–7.

48. Singuer FR, Clemens TL, Eusebio RA, Bekker PJ. Risedronate, a highly effective oral agent in the treatment of patients with severe Paget's disease. J Clin Endocrinol Metab. 1998;83(6):1906–10.

49. Walsh JP, Ward LC, Stewart GO, Will RK, Criddle RA, Prince RL, et al. A randomized clinical trial comparing oral alendronate and intravenous pamidronate for the treatment of Paget's disease of bone. Bone. 2004;34:747.

50. Merlotti D, Gennari L, Martini G, Vallegi F, De Paola V, Avanzati A, et al. Comparison of different intravenous bisphosphonate regimens for Paget's disease of bone. J Bone Miner Res. 2007;22:1510.

51. Reid IR, Lyles K, Su G, Brown JP, Walsh JP, Pino-Montes J, et al. A single infusion of zoledronic acid produces sustained remissions in Paget disease: data to 6.5 years. J Bone Miner Res. 2011;26:2261–70.

52. Michou L, Brown JP. Emerging strategies and therapies for treatment of Paget's disease of bone. Drug Des Devel Ther. 2011;5:225–39.

53. Tan A, Goodman K, Walker A, Hudson J, MacLennan GS, Selby PL, Fraser WD, Ralston SH, for the PRISM-EZ Trial Group. Long-term randomized trial of intensive versus symptomatic management in Paget's disease of bone: the PRISM-EZ study. J Bone Miner Res. 2017;32:1165–73.

54. Langston AL, Campbell MK, Fraser WD, MacLennan GS, Selby PL, Ralston SH. Randomized trial of intensive bisphosphonate treatment versus symptomatic management in Paget's disease of bone. J Bone Miner Res. 2010;25:20–31.

55. Cook SJ, Wall C. Paget's disease of bone: A clinical update. Aust J Gen Pract. 2021;50(1–2):23–9. https://doi.org/10.31128/AJGP-10-20-5690.

56. Makaram NS, Ralston SH. Genetic Determinants of Paget's Disease of Bone. Curr Osteoporos Rep. 2021;19(3):327–37. https://doi.org/10.1007/s11914-021-00676-w.

57. Miladi S, Rouached L, Maatallah K, et al. Complications of Paget Bone Disease: A Study of 69 Patients. Curr Rheumatol Rev. 2021;17(4):390–6. https://doi.org/10.2174/1573397117666210908102615.

58. Nakatsuji Y, Miyashita M, Kadoya M, Nakatsuchi Y. Paget's Disease of the Skull. Intern Med. 2021. https://doi.org/10.2169/internalmedicine.7696-21.

59. Walker JA, Tuck SP. Paget's Disease of the Bone: Patterns of Referral to Secondary Care Following Diagnosis on X-rays. Calcif Tissue Int. 2021;108(5):634–9. https://doi.org/10.1007/s00223-020-00800-5.

Classification and Laboratory Diagnosis of Diabetes Mellitus

28

Matthew J. L. Hare and Duncan J. Topliss

Abbreviations

2hPG	2-hour plasma glucose
ADA	American Diabetes Association
BMI	Body mass index
DKA	Diabetic ketoacidosis
DM	Diabetes mellitus
FPG	Fasting plasma glucose
GAD	Glutamic acid decarboxylase
GDM	Gestational diabetes mellitus
HbA1c	Hemoglobin A1c
IADPSG	International Association of Diabetes and Pregnancy Study Groups
ICA	Islet cell antibody
IFG	Impaired fasting glycemia
IGT	Impaired glucose tolerance
LADA	Latent autoimmune diabetes of adulthood
MODY	Maturity-onset diabetes of the young
OGTT	Oral glucose tolerance test
WHO	World Health Organization

Introduction

Diabetes mellitus is a metabolic disorder of various etiologies, characterized by chronic hyperglycemia and disruption to carbohydrate, protein, and fat metabolism. Diabetes results from impairment of insulin secretion, insulin action,

M. J. L. Hare (✉)
Department of Endocrinology and Diabetes, The Alfred, Melbourne, VIC, Australia
e-mail: m.hare@alfred.org.au

D. J. Topliss
Department of Endocrinology and Diabetes, The Alfred, Melbourne, VIC, Australia

Department of Medicine, Monash University, Clayton, VIC, Australia
e-mail: duncan.topliss@monash.edu

or usually a combination of the two. The long-term complications of these metabolic derangements are a major cause of morbidity and mortality. The prevalence of diabetes is increasing globally and the associated economic burden is significant. The sequelae of diabetes include the microvascular complications of retinopathy, neuropathy and nephropathy, as well as the macrovascular complications of ischemic heart disease, stroke, and peripheral vascular disease. Cardiovascular disease is the leading cause of mortality in diabetes.

Diabetes can present with classic symptoms of polyuria, polydipsia, blurred vision, and weight loss or with a potentially fatal hyperglycemic emergency such as diabetic ketoacidosis or hyperosmolar hyperglycemic state. However, in many cases it is detected in asymptomatic individuals. Diagnosis is thus often very reliant on biochemical testing. It is important that clinicians have a working understanding of the different etiologies of diabetes as well as an appreciation of the various diagnostic measures employed and how they developed.

Part II: Classification of Diabetes Mellitus

The World Health Organization (WHO) and American Diabetes Association (ADA) classify diabetes into four main categories (Table 28.1) [1, 2]:

- Type 1
- Type 2
- Gestational
- Other specific types

Type 1 accounts for about 5–10% of cases and is characterized by insulin deficiency largely due to autoimmune pancreatic beta cell destruction [2]. There are also rare cases of "idiopathic" type 1 diabetes, predominantly seen in people of African and Asian ancestry, in which no known autoimmune marker is detected, but patients are insulinopenic and

© Springer Nature Switzerland AG 2022
F. Bandeira et al. (eds.), *Endocrinology and Diabetes*, https://doi.org/10.1007/978-3-030-90684-9_28

303

Table 28.1 Etiologic classification of diabetes mellitus

Type 1
  Autoimmune
  Idiopathic
Type 2
Gestational
Other specific types
  Genetic defects of β-cell function:
    MODY types 1–6, 9, 10
    Mitochondrial DNA
  Genetic defects in insulin action:
    Type A insulin resistance
    Leprechaunism
    Lipoatrophic diabetes
    Rabson–Mendenhall syndrome
  Disorders of the exocrine pancreas:
    Pancreatitis
    Pancreatic neoplasm
    Pancreatic surgery
    Cystic fibrosis
    Hemochromatosis
  Endocrinopathies:
    Cushing's syndrome
    Acromegaly
    Pheochromocytoma
    Hyperthyroidism
    Glucagonoma
    Somatostatinoma
  Medication-induced:
    Glucocorticoids
    Checkpoint inhibitor immunotherapy
    Nicotinic acid
    Calcineurin inhibitors
    Pentamidine
    Diazoxide
    Phenytoin
    β-Adrenergic agonists
    Thiazides
    α-Interferon
  Posttransplantation
  Infections:
    Congenital rubella
    Cytomegalovirus
  Uncommon forms of immune-mediated diabetes:
    "Stiff-man" syndrome
    Anti-insulin receptor antibodies
  Other genetic syndromes sometimes associated with diabetes:
    Down syndrome
    Klinefelter syndrome
    Turner syndrome
    Wolfram syndrome
    Friedreich ataxia
    Huntington chorea
    Laurence–Moon–Biedl syndrome
    Myotonic dystrophy
    Prader–Willi syndrome
    Porphyria cutanea tarda

prone to ketoacidosis. Type 2 accounts for 90–95% of all diabetes and includes people with peripheral insulin resistance and relative insulin deficiency. Multiple factors contribute to the development of type 2, and in general the etiology is not well understood. It is often associated with overweight and obesity.

Gestational diabetes mellitus (GDM) incorporates diabetes that is first diagnosed in the second or third trimester of pregnancy where testing does not clearly indicate preexisting type 1 or type 2 diabetes. Other specific types of diabetes include cases due to another particular cause such as known genetic disorders, diseases of the exocrine pancreas, and adverse effects of medication.

Historical Perspective on Diabetes Nomenclature

Though diabetes mellitus was recognized several centuries ago, it was Himsworth who first proposed that diabetes could be differentiated into insulin-sensitive and insulin-insensitive types in 1936 [3]. Bornstein and Lawrence found insulin bioactivity in the plasma of people with maturity-onset but not juvenile-onset diabetes [4]. Berson and Yalow conclusively demonstrated this distinction by developing an insulin radioimmunoassay [5]. This formed the basis of the initial classification of diabetes. During that time, patients with diabetes were classified according to the age of onset into juvenile-onset and maturity-onset subtypes, juvenile-onset being insulin-sensitive, and maturity-onset being insulin-insensitive. In 1980, recognizing that age of onset did not necessarily correlate with insulin dependency, the WHO Expert Committee on Diabetes removed age of onset from the classification, instead using the terms: insulin-dependent (type 1) and non-insulin-dependent (type 2) [6]. In 1997, an international expert committee recommended removal of the terms insulin-dependent and non-insulin-dependent given that many patients with type 2 diabetes have progressive beta cell failure and subsequently require insulin therapy. This was adopted by the ADA that year and by the WHO in 1999 [7, 8].

There have been substantive changes over the years in the classification of GDM also. As early as the 1940s, it was noted that women who were diagnosed with diabetes years after pregnancy had had higher rates of fetal loss and neonatal mortality with prior pregnancies [9]. The first oral glucose tolerance test (OGTT) criteria for diagnosis of gestational diabetes were put forward by O'Sullivan and Mahan in 1964 [10]. Until relatively recently, GDM incorporated any degree of glucose intolerance first recognized during pregnancy [7]. Given the increasing prevalence of impaired glucose regulation at earlier ages, current guidelines use the terms "overt diabetes" or "diabetes in pregnancy" for women meeting standard OGTT cut points for diabetes, using the term GDM for lesser degrees of glucose intolerance [11, 12].

Case Examples Illustrating Different Classifications of Diabetes

Diabetes is a heterogenous disease; clinical presentation and disease progression can vary greatly between individuals. Assigning a type of diabetes to a patient frequently depends on his/her phenotype and the circumstances present at the time of diagnosis. Sometimes, the type may not be evident at diagnosis, and many patients do not easily fit into a single class. Usually, the diagnosis becomes more clear over time. These cases discussions illustrate some of the different types of diabetes and the challenges that can exist in determining the specific diagnosis.

Case 1

A 19-year-old student with no past medical history was admitted for diabetic ketoacidosis (DKA), precipitated by urinary tract infection. She had been lethargic, with weight loss, polydipsia, and polyuria for 2 months. Prior to her admission, she complained of 3 days' history of fever, dysuria, frequency, and abdominal pain. She did not have any family history of diabetes. She was of slim build, with a body mass index (BMI) of only 17.3 kg/m².

Laboratory investigations on admission:

- *Total white cell count: 16.4 × 10³ U/L (4–10)*
- *Serum sodium: 128 mmol/L (135–145)*
- *Serum glucose: 34.5 mmol/L (3.1–7.8)*
- *Serum bicarbonate: 13.8 mmol/L (19–31)*
- *Serum creatinine: 171 µmol/L (65–125)*
- *Arterial blood pH: 7.23 (7.35–7.45)*
- *Serum ketones: 4.6 mmol/L (<0.6)*
- *Glycated HbA1c: 9.2%*
- *Glutamic acid decarboxylase (GAD) antibody: 117.4 U/ mL (0–0.8)*
- *Islet cell antibody (ICA): negative*
- *Urine microscopy: 450 white blood cells*

This is a typical case of a newly diagnosed type 1 diabetes, presenting with DKA. Type 1 DM is usually diagnosed before 30–40 years of age, most commonly during childhood or adolescence. However, it can occur throughout life and is sometimes misdiagnosed as type 2 DM when it presents in older age groups. The lean body habitus of Case 1 is also typical of a patient with type 1 DM. Type 1 DM is usually

characterized by the presence of anti-GAD (glutamic acid decarboxylase), anti-islet cell (ICA), or anti-insulin antibodies, which reflect the autoimmune processes that cause β-cell destruction. Patients with type 1 DM require insulin for survival and to prevent DKA.

Case 2

A 26-year-old man was diagnosed with diabetes 5 years ago during a routine health screen. Both his parents developed diabetes in their 40s. He was overweight with a BMI of 28.3 kg/m² and waist circumference of 110 cm. He is currently on two oral hypoglycemic agents (metformin and sitagliptin). He does not suffer from any macrovascular or microvascular complications of DM.

Laboratory investigations during his latest outpatient clinic review:

- *HbA1c: 7.6%*
- *Triglycerides: 2.0 mmol/L (<1.7)*
- *Low-density lipoprotein (LDL): 3.2 mmol/L (<2.6)*
- *High-density lipoprotein (HDL): 0.9 mmol/L (1–1.6)*

This is a case of a relatively young patient with type 2 DM. Most people with type 2 DM are overweight or obese. Adiposity contributes to insulin resistance. Though type 2 DM was traditionally described in older individuals, there is a growing incidence of type 2 DM in young adults and even children, which is thought to largely relate to increasing rates of obesity. More than in type 1 DM, type 2 DM shows strong familial aggregation. DKA seldom occurs in this type of diabetes unless there is a significant precipitating illness such as infection. Type 2 diabetes is usually diagnosed late as it develops gradually and patients remain asymptomatic during the initial stages. Lifestyle modification and weight reduction can decrease insulin resistance in these patients. Initial treatment usually involves oral hypoglycemic agents. The UK Prospective Diabetes Study (UKPDS) [13] showed that, over time, despite lifestyle modification and pharmacotherapy, there is progressive loss in β-cell function, and insulin may ultimately be needed for control of these patients' glycemic deterioration (Table 28.2, differences between type 1 DM and type 2 DM).

Case 3

A 40-year-old man with generalized vitiligo was diagnosed with diabetes 2 years ago when he was admitted to hospital for lower limb cellulitis. There was no family history. He was of slim build with a BMI of 18.6 kg/m². His physician started him on metformin and gliclazide with improvement in his glycemic control. However, despite compliance to diet and increasing doses of his medication, he was unable to keep his

Table 28.2 Differences between type 1 DM and type 2 DM

	Type 1 DM	Type 2 DM
Frequency	5–10% of all DM	>90% of all DM
Etiology	Immune-mediated islet cell destruction, leading to absolute insulin deficiency; can be idiopathic	Insulin resistance with relative insulin deficiency
Age at presentation	Usually during childhood or adolescence	Usually after middle age
Body habitus	Usually slim	Usually overweight
Family history of DM	Usually no	Usually yes
Treatment	Need insulin at diagnosis	Usually treated with lifestyle modification and oral hypoglycemic agents but may require insulin later

HbA1c below a target of 7% (53 mmol/mol). His fasting C-peptide was 0.1 nmol/L, indicating inadequate pancreatic β-cell reserve. His anti-GAD antibodies and ICA were both positive. He was started on insulin 15 months after his presentation, with prompt improvement in his glycemic control.

The age of Case 3 at presentation and initial lack of insulin dependence pointed toward a diagnosis of type 2 DM. However, he had several features more typical of type 1 DM, including his lean body mass, lack of family history of diabetes, and subsequent rapid progression to insulin dependency. The diagnosis was confirmed by the presence of GAD and ICA antibodies. The presence of vitiligo also suggested a predisposition for autoimmunity. This is an atypical form of diabetes known as latent autoimmune diabetes of adult onset (LADA). LADA is defined by three features, including adult age at diagnosis (usually above the age of 30), the presence of diabetes-associated autoantibodies, and a delay in the progression to insulin dependency (more than 6 months, up to 10–12 years) [14]. Case 3 fulfilled all these three criteria. Studies have shown that among patients with phenotypic type 2, LADA occurs in 10% of people above 35 years old and 25% below that age [15]. It is important to distinguish patients with LADA from type 2 DM, as treatment of choice is early insulin therapy to prevent the progression to complete β-cell failure from glucose toxicity. Sulfonylureas, which are commonly used to treat type 2 DM, have been thought to promote β-cell failure due to their stimulatory effect of insulin secretion by the pancreas and should generally be avoided in LADA [16].

Case 4

A 36-year-old overweight man of African-American ethnicity, diagnosed with type 2 diabetes 3 years ago (anti-GAD and ICA negative, HbA1c 8.5% (69 mmol/mol)), noncompliant to his treatment with metformin and gliclazide, was admitted to the hospital with DKA. There was no evidence of infection or other precipitants for his DKA. He was switched to biphasic insulin (30 units pre-breakfast and 20 units pre-dinner) before his discharge from hospital. However, he started experiencing hypoglycemic events at home which persisted even after he had progressively reduced the dosage of biphasic insulin to 18 units pre-breakfast and 8 units pre-dinner. His fasting C-peptide was 0.8 nmol/L, indicating presence of sufficient pancreatic reserve. He was subsequently switched back to sustained release metformin 1000 mg twice daily and gliclazide 60 mg once daily. His hypoglycemic episodes resolved, and his overall glycemic control improved with his HbA1c dropping to 7.2%.

This illustrates a seemingly typical case of type 2 DM in an overweight individual. However, it is unusual for patients with type 2 DM to develop DKA, particularly in the absence of precipitants. This is an example of another atypical form of diabetes, known as ketosis-prone type 2 DM. It is more common in African-American and Hispanic patients. Hence, it is also known as Flatbush diabetes, in recognition of the place from where many of the first-described cases came from [17]. Patients with ketosis-prone type 2 are usually young to middle-aged overweight individuals with a history of acute, unprovoked episodes of DKA. Unlike in type 1 DM, DKA in these patients is not due to irreversible β-cell damage but hypothesized to be due to increased susceptibility to β-cell desensitization due to glucose toxicity [18]. Upon reversal of glucose toxicity with insulin therapy, the β-cell function partially recovers. Basal and stimulated C-peptide levels of more than 0.33 nmol/L and 0.5 nmol/L, respectively, shortly after presentation of DKA, as well as more than 0.5 nmol/L and 0.75 nmol/L, respectively, during follow-up, have been shown to be good predictors of remissions [17–19]. It is advisable to keep patients with ketosis-prone type 2 DM on oral hypoglycemic agents (usually low-dose sulfonylurea and metformin), as normoglycemic remission periods are significantly shortened (to within 2 years) if they are treated with diet control alone after discontinuation of insulin therapy [19–21].

Case 5

A 19-year-old student presented with a few months of polydipsia and polyuria and was diagnosed with diabetes. In view of his young age and lean build (BMI 19.8 kg/m²), he was treated as having type 1 DM and was commenced on subcutaneous insulin therapy. During one of his outpatient reviews, it was realized that he had a very significant family history of young-onset diabetes (Fig. 28.1, family tree showing affected individuals). He underwent genetic testing for maturity-onset diabetes of the young (MODY) which confirmed mutation in HNF1α, one of the transcription factors

Fig. 28.1 Family tree showing people with DM in Case 5's family. Note: The numbers indicate the age of onset of DM in affected family members

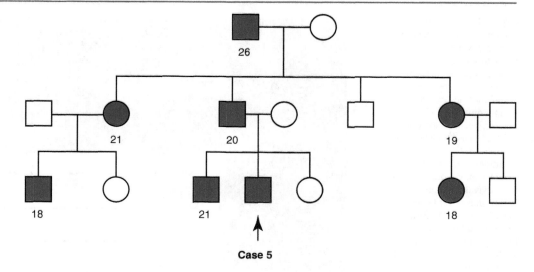

Case 5

that affect β-cell development and function. He was switched to gliclazide and has maintained satisfactory glycemic control since then.

MODY is the most common form of monogenic diabetes. It is characterized by early age of onset (typically less than 25 years), initial non-insulin dependence and an autosomal dominant pattern of inheritance [22]. Several different genetic abnormalities have been identified. The most commonly affected genes are those encoding for glucokinase (GCK) and three transcription factors: hepatic nuclear factor 1 alpha (HNF1A), hepatic nuclear factor 4 alpha (HNF4A), and hepatic nuclear factor 1 beta (HNF1B). In predominantly Europid populations, MODY accounts for between 1.2% and 3.0% of diabetes cases diagnosed in childhood [22].

Clinical presentation (including age of onset, severity and progression of hyperglycemia) varies greatly depending on the underlying genetic mutation, but affected patients are non-insulin-dependent at the onset of the disease. In addition, they are usually of lean body habitus with no or minimal insulin resistance. Patients with glucokinase dysfunction MODY have mild fasting hyperglycemia (fasting plasma glucose, FPG, 5.5–8.0 mmol/L) from birth. Their glycemic excursion during an OGTT is often also very mild (increment of less than 4.6 mmol/L) [23]. As their hyperglycemia is mild, they generally do not have symptoms, do not require treatment, or develop microvascular complications. However, insulin treatment may be required during pregnancy but is often of limited efficacy [24]. In contrast, patients with transcription factor MODY (of which HNF1A is most common) are usually born with normal glucose regulation but develop progressive β-cell dysfunction leading to diabetes onset between the age of 10–30 years old. At presentation, they usually have normal fasting plasma glucose but markedly elevated glucose excursion during an OGTT. Patients with HNF1A and HNF4A–MODY tend to respond well to low-dose sulfo-

nylurea therapy, whereas those with HNF1B–MODY generally require insulin therapy [22].

MODY should be considered in patients with diabetes diagnosed before 25 years old, who do not fully fit into the phenotypes of type 1 or type 2 DM and who have a strong family history of young-onset diabetes. A MODY probability calculator has been developed and validated. It is available online and as a smart phone application [25]. Differentiating MODY from type 1 DM is particularly important as these patients can often be effectively treated without insulin therapy. Genetic testing is important, not only to guide appropriate treatment and predict clinical course but also to provide genetic counseling for their families, since there is a 50% risk of first-degree relatives having the same gene mutation due to its autosomal dominant inheritance.

Part II: Clinical Stages of Diabetes

Patients who ultimately develop diabetes typically pass through a spectrum of clinical stages during its progression (Fig. 28.2). Initially, glucose regulation is normal, and patients remain normoglycemic even if they are subjected to an OGTT. This stage is followed by a variable period of intermediate hyperglycemia, sometimes referred to as "prediabetes." This can be defined as impaired fasting glycemia (IFG) using FPG criteria or impaired glucose tolerance (IGT) using 2-hour plasma glucose (2hPG) criteria. The ADA, but not the WHO, also recognized an intermediate range of HbA1c. Even intermediate hyperglycemia is associated with increased cardiovascular risk and retinopathy. Patients with intermediate hyperglycemia have a 5–10% risk of progression to actual diabetes annually, compared to 0.7% in normoglycemic people [26]. It is also possible for people with intermediate hyperglycemia to regress back to normoglyce-

Fig. 28.2 Disorders of glycemia: clinical stages and etiologic types. *Even after being treated for a hyperglycemic emergency, patients with type 1 and rarely type 2 diabetes can, for a period, return to normoglycemia (sometimes referred to as "honeymoon" remission); **in rare situations, other types of diabetes may require insulin for survival. (Adapted with permission from: Definition and diagnosis of diabetes mellitus and intermediate hyperglycemia—Report of a WHO/IDF consultation. 2006; Page 38 Appendix 4)

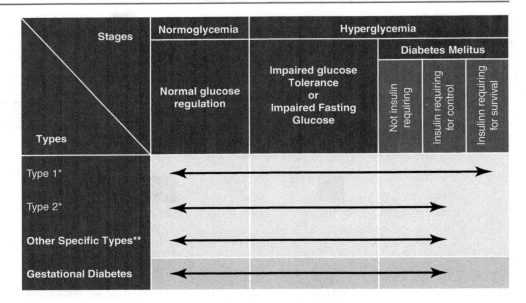

mia. Once diabetes develops, lifestyle modification or oral hypoglycemic agents may be sufficient for some patients, depending on the type of diabetes. On the other hand, some may require insulin for survival or control.

Separate staging of type 1 DM has also been proposed based around worsening dysglycemia and reduction in functioning ß-cell mass through the stages [27]:

- Stage 1: ß-cell autoimmunity with normoglycemia and pre-symptomatic
- Stage 2: ß-cell autoimmunity with dysglycemia but pre-symptomatic
- Stage 3: ß-cell autoimmunity with dysglycemia and symptomatic

Part III: Laboratory Diagnosis of Diabetes Mellitus

Since the twentieth century, the diagnosis of all types of diabetes mellitus has been based on detection of hyperglycemia. Prior to the development of methodologies for quantifying blood glucose levels, the diagnosis was largely based on the detection of glycosuria in a patient with the appropriate clinical syndrome. At present, in the setting of marked symptomatic hyperglycemia or a hyperglycemic crisis, a single elevated random plasma glucose level above 11.1 mmol/L can be considered diagnostic of diabetes. However, diabetes is commonly diagnosed in asymptomatic individuals, particularly with type 2 DM and GDM. In these cases, the diagnosis is essentially biochemical and relies on accepted diagnostic thresholds. Three measures are currently accepted diagnostic tests for diabetes: FPG, OGTT, and hemoglobin

A1c (HbA1c). A patient with an elevated diagnostic marker should have the same test repeated on a separate occasion to confirm the diagnosis of diabetes.

Determining Diagnostic Thresholds

Over time, two main approaches have been utilized for determining diagnostic cut points for diabetes (Fig. 28.3). In some populations, a bimodal distribution of glycemia has been found, suggesting a "normal" and an "abnormal" population. The intersection between the two curves can be used as a point of differentiation between those with diabetes and those without. Such distributions were observed in the 1970s in populations with high prevalence of diabetes, such as the Pima Indians and the Micronesian population of Nauru. These data formed the basis of the 1979 National Diabetes Data Group (NDDG) criteria and subsequent 1980 WHO criteria for the diagnosis of diabetes [28]. These criteria remained as the foundation for the diagnosis of type 2 diabetes for almost two decades.

The second approach is to examine the relationship between a diagnostic marker and a significant clinical outcome to see if there is a threshold value at which the risk of the clinical outcome increases above the baseline population risk. To an extent, such threshold values are seen with retinopathy and glycemia, whether measured with FPG, 2hPG, or HbA1c [29]. Such data form the basis of current ADA and WHO diagnostic criteria [28]. It should be noted that the relationship between cardiovascular risk and glycemia is approximately linear. Similarly, in pregnancy, the relationship between glycemia and adverse outcomes such as macrosomia, requirement for C-section, and neonatal hypoglycemia are essentially linear [30]. Therefore, the diagnostic cut

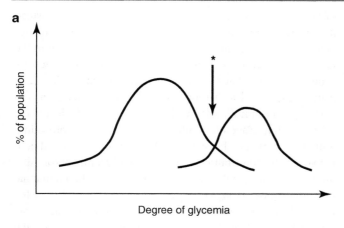

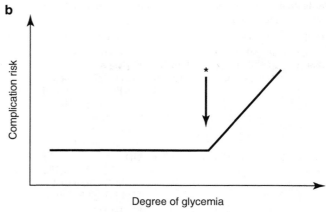

Fig. 28.3 Determining diagnostic thresholds. Graph **a** shows a bimodal distribution of glycemia in a population, as is seen for plasma glucose levels in some high-risk groups. The asterisk indicates the intersection of the two apparent curves, which can be used as a threshold level to differentiate between "normal" and "diabetes." Graph **b** shows an example of a nonlinear association between risk of a particu-lar complication and degree of glycemia, somewhat like the relation-ship between prevalent retinopathy and plasma glucose levels. Again the asterisk depicts a threshold value at which the risk of this complica-tion begins to rise above the baseline population risk. This could also be used a diagnostic cut point

points for diabetes are somewhat arbitrary, dichotomizing degrees of glycemia into two groups: those with diabetes and those without.

Tests of Glycemia for Diabetes Diagnosis

Among the diagnostic armamentarium used for diabetes, OGTT has traditionally been the test of choice. However, current international criteria allow for the use of either FPG, 2hPG, or HbA1c in diabetes diagnosis. The same tests are used to identify patients with intermediate hyperglycemia, although there is some disagreement about the use of HbA1c for this purpose and it is not recognized by the WHO. The current ADA and WHO criteria are presented in Table 28.3. The criteria are much the same, aside from different thresholds to define impaired fasting glycemia (IFG). In 2003, the ADA reduced the threshold for IFG to 5.6 mmol/L to improve the correlation with impaired glucose tolerance (IGT) and to improve the sensitivity and specificity for predicting future diabetes [31].

Criteria for the diagnosis of GDM have been the source of considerable debate and discussion in recent years. Current WHO guidelines recommend the OGTT for the diagnosis of gestational diabetes [11]. It is generally only performed once as a screening test in the third trimester, and a repeat test is not considered necessary to confirm the diagnosis. Additional first trimester screening is recommended for women with risk factors for type 2 diabetes. The ADA guidelines still accommodate the option of a two-step screening process in which women undergo a 1-hour 50 g glucose challenge test and then, if positive, proceed to a 2-hour 75 g glucose toler-ance test. HbA1c is not recommended for GDM diagnosis

Table 28.3 Current ADA and WHO criteria for diabetes and interme-diate hyperglycemia [1, 2]

	ADA	WHO
Diabetes mellitus		
FPG[a]	≥7.0	≥7.0
2hPG[b]	≥11.1	≥11.1
HbA1c[c]	≥6.5 (48)	≥6.5 (48)
Intermediate hyperglycemia		
IFG[d]	5.6–6.9	6.1–6.9
IGT[e]	≥7.8 and <11.1	≥7.8 and <11.1
Defined by HbA1c[c]	5.7–6.4 (38–46)	*NA*

[a]FPG, fasting venous plasma glucose, mmol/L
[b]2hPG, 2-hour plasma glucose, (venous plasma glucose 2 hours after 75 g glucose load), mmol/L
[c]HbA1c, hemoglobin A1c,% (mmol/mol)
[d]IFG, impaired fasting glucose, defined using fasting plasma glucose, mmol/L
[e]IGT, impaired glucose tolerance, defined using 2hPG, expressed in mmol/L

due to changes in red cell turnover in pregnancy. The original OGTT criteria for GDM were determined on the basis of the mother's risk of subsequent type 2 diabetes. The specific cut points were adjusted over the years due to changes in assay methodology, particularly with the move from whole blood glucose to plasma glucose levels. The 1999 WHO guidelines recommended the use of the same criteria for GDM as for all other forms of impaired glucose regulation, creating signifi-cant discordance between various criteria around the world.

In 2010, the International Association of Diabetes and Pregnancy Study Groups published recommendations for standardizing the approach to GDM diagnosis using OGTT criteria based on outcome data from the observational Hyperglycemia and Adverse Pregnancy Outcomes (HAPO) study [12]. These recommendations have been adopted by

Table 28.4 IADPSG recommendations for screening and diagnosis of diabetes in pregnancy

Timing	Tests	Criteria
1st antenatal visit	If risk factors for diabetes, check FPG, random PG, or HbA1c	Overt/preexisting diabetes if: FPG ≥7.0 mmol/L RPG ≥11.1 mmol/L HbA1c ≥6.5% GDM if: FPG ≥ 5.1 but <7.0 mmol/L
24- to 28-week gestation	75 g OGTT	GDM if: FPG ≥5.1 mmol/L 1hPG ≥10 mmol/L 2hPG ≥8.5 mmolL Overt diabetes if: FPG ≥7.0 mmol/L
6–8 weeks post-partum	75 g OGTT for women with GDM	Usual WHO/ADA diagnostic criteria for diabetes

the WHO and variably by other national organizations (Table 28.4). The lowered glycemic thresholds for diagnosis have led to significant increases in rates of GDM.

Serum Glucose and OGTT

The test for FPG requires patients to be fasted for minimum of 8 h. It is a simple and economical test. However, the blood specimen must be spun down quickly in the laboratory as there is steady loss of glucose with time even if fluoride blood tubes are used due to ongoing glycolysis. This is because glucose consumption takes place within blood cells shortly after sampling, but fluoride inhibits glycolysis only in its more distal steps [32]. It has been estimated that glucose concentration decreases 5–7% (i.e., around 0.5 mmol/L) per hour [32, 33]. This rate may increase further in the setting of high ambient temperature [32, 33]. The pre-analytical variability of FPG is around 5–10% [29]. In addition, there can be significant intra-individual variability in FPG due to factors other than diabetes, such as concurrent illness (e.g., sepsis).

OGTT also requires patients to be fasted for 8 h. A blood sample is taken at baseline for plasma glucose before giving a glucose load (75 g of glucose in 300 ml of water to be consumed over 5 min). Plasma glucose is repeated after 120 min (2hPG). The use of a standard 75 g glucose load in all individuals irrespective of age, body habitus, or other factors has been questioned. There is some evidence that differences in 2hPG between men and women are explained by height [34].

Glycated Hemoglobin (HbA1c)

HbA1c is a molecule of normal adult hemoglobin (HbA) with glucose bound at the N-terminal valine. The glycation

of hemoglobin is a nonenzymatic process, which is instead driven by blood glucose concentrations. It was first recognized as a component of human hemoglobin by Allen in the late 1950s and subsequently associated with diabetes by Rahbar a decade later [35]. The concentration of HbA1c is usually expressed as a proportion of HbA (either as a percentage or in mmol/mol). An individual's HbA1c level correlates with average blood glucose levels over the preceding 3 months, which is the average life span of a red blood cell. However, the contribution of preceding glycemia across that 3-month period is not equal. Tahara et al. have shown that the immediate past 30 days of glycemia accounts for 50% of the HbA1c level, the next 30 days (30–60 days before) accounts for 25%, and then 60–120 days before accounts for the remaining 25% [36].

HbA1c has been a cornerstone of diabetes management over the past few decades as a marker of glycemic control, guiding treatment decisions. As early as the 1980s, it was suggested that HbA1c could be a valuable marker for the diagnosis of diabetes. However, its restricted availability and lack of assay standardization prevented its introduction. Over the following decades, significant progress was made, particularly by the National Glycohemoglobin Standardization Program (NGSP) which originated in the USA [37]. This program utilized a direct comparison method, standardizing assays to the reference assay used in the seminal Diabetes Control and Complications Trial (DCCT). Since then an international reference system has been developed by the International Federation of Clinical Chemistry and Laboratory Medicine (IFCC) [38]. This system standardizes assays to a highly specific reference method using high performance liquid chromatography and either spray mass spectrometry or capillary electrophoresis. Assays calibrated to these highly specific methods produce lower HbA1c values due to less interference. Therefore, HbA1c is now reported in three different units: the standard international units of mmol/mol, NGSP/DCCT equivalent values (%), and estimated average glucose. The estimated average glucose (eAG) can also be derived from HbA1c (%) using this formula [39]: $eAG\ (mmol/L) = (HbA1c \times 1.59) - 2.59$.

In 2009 an expert committee recommended the inclusion of HbA1c into diagnostic criteria for diabetes at a cut point of 6.5% (48 mmol/mol) [31]. This recommendation was subsequently adopted by the ADA and WHO [2, 40]. More and more clinicians are using HbA1c for diagnosis because it is convenient to perform as patients do not need to be fasted. There is greater pre-analytical stability (compared to plasma glucose testing) and less variation with factors such as stress and illness [41]. HbA1c correlates well with microvascular (and to a lesser extent, macrovascular) complications of diabetes. On the other hand, HbA1c is a costlier test and may not be available in certain developing countries. In addition, care must be taken in the interpretation of HbA1c results, as

Table 28.5 Conditions associated with falsely low/high HbA1c levels

Falsely low HbA1c	Falsely high HbA1c
Associated with increased erythrocyte turnover:	*Associated with decreased erythrocyte turnover:*
Hemolysis	Iron-deficiency anemia
Hemorrhage	Postsplenectomy
Venesection	
Hypersplenism	
Treatment of iron-deficiency anemia	
G6PD deficiency (with or without hemolysis)	
Drugs, e.g., antiretrovirals, ribavirin, dapsone, erythropoietin	
Pregnancy	
Hemoglobinopathies, e.g., beta-thalassemia	

they can be misleading in patients with anemia, hemoglobinopathies, or other causes of abnormal red cell turnover, as well as following blood transfusions (Table 28.5) [35].

Case 6

A 28-year-old primigravida, who was diagnosed with diabetes at 26-week gestation, had been overweight since childhood. Her prepregnancy BMI was 29.4 kg/m². Both her parents were diagnosed with type 2 DM in their 50s. Her fasting plasma glucose (FPG) done during her first antenatal consultation was 4.9 mmol/L. OGTT done at 26-week gestation showed an elevated 2-h plasma glucose of 9.2 mmol/L. She was started on insulin therapy for her GDM and subsequently delivered a healthy 3.2 kg baby boy at 38-week gestation. Results of the OGTT performed 8 weeks postpartum were normal.

The woman in this example had risk factors for type 2 DM and was thus screened for preexisting diabetes in the first trimester. Her first trimester FPG was normal. However, she subsequently developed GDM which was diagnosed on OGTT at 26 weeks. Women with GDM have a 35–60% risk of developing type 2 DM; hence an OGTT should be repeated 6–8 weeks postpartum [42]. While Case 6 had a normal repeat OGTT, she continues to be at higher risk of developing GDM in any subsequent pregnancies and for type 2 DM in future.

Case 7

A 62-year-old man with end-stage renal failure on hemodialysis was found on routine blood tests during dialysis, to have random blood glucose ranging from 10.6 to 14.1 mmol/L. He did not have any osmotic symptoms such as polydipsia and polyuria. His HbA1c was 5.6%, but OGTT showed elevated FPG and 2hPG readings of 7.4 mmol/L and 12.8 mmol/L, respectively.

This is a case with discordant HbA1c and OGTT results. HbA1c is an unreliable test in patients with significant renal impairment due to a few factors. The presence of carbamylated hemoglobin in patients with renal failure can interfere with some of the HbA1c assays, giving rise to falsely high HbA1c levels [43, 44]. On the other hand, uremia causes loss of erythrocyte surface lipids, leading to reduced deformability and shorter survival and hence falsely low HbA1c levels. This is particularly so in patients on hemodialysis [45]. In addition, many patients with renal failure are on erythropoietin therapy, and this causes erythrocytosis which also gives rise to falsely low HbA1c levels. In view of these factors, plasma glucose is a more suitable test to use for the diagnosis of diabetes in patients with renal failure. On the same note, regular self-monitoring of capillary blood glucose is also more reliable in the assessment of glycemic control in these patients, compared to HbA1c. So this case does have diabetes despite normal HbA1c.

Tests to Aid Determination of Diabetes Type

C-Peptide

Like insulin, connecting peptide (C-peptide) is a cleaved product of proinsulin. It is secreted in equimolar concentrations with insulin into the circulation but has no definite effects on carbohydrate metabolism. Its plasma half-life is 30 min, much longer than that of insulin (around 4 min). Unlike insulin, it is not extracted by the liver and is excreted almost entirely by the kidneys. It also has constant peripheral clearance at different plasma concentrations and during changes in plasma glucose concentrations. C-peptide is not a diagnostic test for diabetes, but in view of the characteristics mentioned above, it is commonly used as a marker of β-cell function or reserve, as it reflects endogenous insulin production of the pancreatic islet cells. A fasting C-peptide of <0.2 nmol/L has been shown to reflect severe insulin deficiency, indicating the need for exogenous insulin therapy [46]. C-peptide can be stimulated by the administration of 1 mg of glucagon intravenously. Its levels are measured at baseline and 6 and 10 min after intravenous glucagon. Normal stimulation of C-peptide is a 150–300% elevation over basal levels [47]. A stimulated C-peptide of <0.5 nmol/L is suggestive of severe insulin deficiency [46]. Even though C-peptide cannot be used in diagnosis, it is useful in cases where the type of diabetes is not clear as it can help clinicians decide if these patients require insulin therapy. This has been illustrated in Cases 3 and 4 earlier in this chapter.

Autoantibodies

There are four main autoantibodies associated with type 1 DM, namely, islet cell autoantibodies (ICA), glutamic acid decarboxylase autoantibodies (GAD), islet antigen-2 autoantibodies, and insulin autoantibodies [48]. Again, these are not diagnostic tests for diabetes but can help to differentiate type 1 DM from other types of diabetes. Up to 90% of patients with type 1 DM have at least one positive autoantibody. However, the prevalence of positive autoantibodies is dependent on ethnicity, with the highest prevalence among Caucasians. In certain non-white populations, the prevalence of known autoantibodies may be as low as 40–50% [49].

Autoantibodies against GAD are most commonly to the GAD65 isoform (GAD65Ab). GAD65Ab are more sensitive than ICA autoantibodies. Unlike ICA autoantibodies, they remain detectable for many years even after substantial loss of β-cell function [50]. In addition, their detection rate increases with age in new-onset type 1 DM. This is in contrast to insulin autoantibodies whose predictive value for type 1 DM seems to be higher among younger children, possibly due to a higher rate of β-cell destruction. Insulin autoantibodies are detectable in 90% of children who have type 1 DM before the age of 5, compared to only 40–50% of adolescents older than 15 years old [51]. Islet antigen-2 autoantibodies are detected in about 60–70% of patients with new-onset type 1 DM [52]. They are often preceded by insulin autoantibodies, GAD65Ab and ICA autoantibodies, respectively [53], and the frequency decreases with increasing age of onset.

Conclusion

Diabetes mellitus is a heterogeneous collection of disorders of various etiologies, characterized by hyperglycemia due to impairment of insulin action and secretion. It is important to ascertain the etiology behind each patient's diabetes in order to understand and predict its clinical course as well as guide management. Age at onset, clinical presentation, phenotype, medical history, and family history all play important roles in helping to determine the diagnosis. Measurement of C-peptide and autoantibodies can also be of assistance.

Though OGTT was traditionally used as the gold-standard diagnostic test for diabetes, more clinicians are now switching to HbA1c or FPG, largely for convenience. It is of value for clinicians to understand how the various diagnostic criteria were developed and the potential factors, other than glycemia, which may affect the different tests.

References

1. World Health Organization. Definition and diagnosis of diabetes mellitus and intermediate hyperglycemia. Report of a WHO/IDF consultation. Geneva; 2006.
2. American Diabetes Association. 2. Classification and diagnosis of diabetes: standards of medical care in diabetes-2018. Diabetes Care. 2018;41(supp 1):S13–27.
3. Himsworth HP. Diabetes mellitus: its differentiation into insulin-sensitive and insulin-insensitive types. Lancet. 1936;1:117.
4. Bornstein J, Lawrence RD. Plasma insulin in human diabetes mellitus. Br Med J. 1951;2:1541–4.
5. Berson SA, Yalow RS. Immunoassay of endogenous plasma insulin in man. J Clin Invest. 1960;39:1157–75.
6. World Health Organization. Second report of the WHO expert committee on diabetes mellitus. Technical report series no. 646. Geneva; 1980.
7. World Health Organization. Definition, diagnosis and classification of diabetes mellitus and its complications—report of a WHO consultation 1999 (WHO/NCD/NCS 99.2). Geneva; 1999.
8. American Diabetes Association Expert Committee. Report of the expert committee on the diagnosis and classification of diabetes mellitus. Diabetes Care. 1997;20:1183–97.
9. Miller HC. The effect of diabetic and prediabetic pregnancies on the fetus and newborn infant. J Pediatr. 1946;26:455–61.
10. O'Sullivan JB, Mahan CM. Criteria for the oral glucose tolerance test in pregnancy. Diabetes. 1964;13:278–85.
11. World Health Organization. Diagnostic criteria and classification of hyperglycaemia first detected in pregnancy. Geneva; 2013.
12. IADPS. International association of diabetes and pregnancy study groups recommendations on the diagnosis and classification of hyperglycemia in pregnancy. Diabetes Care. 2010;33(3):676–82.
13. UKPDS. Overview of six years' therapy of type 2 diabetes—a progressive disease. Diabetes. 1995;44:1248–58.
14. Leslie RD, Williams R, Pozzilli P. Clinical review: type 1 diabetes and latent autoimmune diabetes in adults: one end of the rainbow. J Clin Endocrinol Metab. 2006;91:1654–9.
15. Stenstrom G, Gottsater A, Bakhtadz E, Berger B, Sundkvist G. Latent autoimmune diabetes in adults. Diabetes. 2005;54:S68–72.
16. Pozzilli P, Di Mario U. Autoimmune diabetes not requiring insulin at diagnosis (latent autoimmune diabetes of the adult): definition, characterization, and potential prevention. Diabetes Care. 2001;24:1460–7.
17. Umpierrez GE, Smiley D, Kitabchi AE. Narrative review: ketosis-prone type 2 diabetes mellitus. Ann Intern Med. 2006;144: 350–7.
18. Mauvais-Jarvis F, Sobngwi E, Porcher R, Riveline J-P, Kevorkian J-P, Vaisse C, et al. Ketosis-prone type 2 diabetes in patients of sub-Saharan African origin: clinical pathophysiology and natural history of β-cell dysfunction and insulin resistance. Diabetes. 2004;53:645–53.
19. Umpierrez GE, Casals MM, Gebhart SP, Mixon PS, Clark WS, Phillips LS. Diabetes ketoacidosis in obese African-Americans. Diabetes. 1995;44:790–5.
20. Banerji MA, Chaiken RL, Lebovitz HE. Long-term normoglycemic remission in black newly diagnosed NIDDM subjects. Diabetes. 1996;45:337–41.
21. Umpierrez GE, Clark WS, Steen MT. Sulphonylurea treatment prevents recurrence of hyperglycemia in obese African-American patients with a history of hyperglycemic crises. Diabetes Care. 1997;20:479–83.
22. Hattersley AT, Patel KA. Precision diabetes: learning from monogenic diabetes. Diabetologia. 2017;60(5):769–77.
23. Misra S, Hattersley AT. Chapter 18: monogenic causes of diabetes. In: Textbook of diabetes. 5th ed. UK: Wiley-Blackwell; 2016.
24. Chakera AJ, Steele AM, Gloyn AL, Shepherd MH, Shields B, Ellard S, Hattersley AT. Recognition and management of individuals with hyperglycemia because of a heterozygous glucokinase mutation. Diabetes Care. 2015;38(7):1383–92.
25. DiabetesGenes.org, MODY Probability Calculator, Accessed via: www.diabetesgenes.org/content/mody-probability-calculator/. Accessed on: 28th December 2017.
26. Aroda VR, Ratner R. Approach to the patient with prediabetes. J Clin Endocrinol Metab. 2008;93:3259–65.

27. Insel RA, Dunne JL, Atkinson MA, Chiang JL, Dabelea D, Gottlieb PA, et al. Staging presymptomatic type 1 diabetes: a scientific statement of JDRF, the Endocrine Society, and the American Diabetes Association. Diabetes Care. 2015;38(10):1964–74.

28. Hare MJL, Shaw JE, Zimmet PZ. Diagnosing diabetes mellitus in the twenty-first century – what is the role of haemoglobin A1c? Hamdan Med J. 2012;5:123–30.

29. Colagiuri S, Lee CM, Wong TY, Balkau B, Shaw JE, Borch-Johnsen K, et al. Glycemic thresholds for diabetes-specific retinopathy: implications for diagnostic criteria for diabetes. Diabetes Care. 2011;34(10):145–50.

30. The HAPO Study Cooperative Research Group. Hyperglycemia and adverse pregnancy outcomes. N Eng J Med. 2008;358(18):1991–2002.

31. International Expert Committee. International Expert Committee report on the role of the A1C assay in the diagnosis of diabetes. Diabetes Care. 2009;32:1327–34.

32. Mikesh LM, Bruns DE. Stabilization of glucose in blood specimens: mechanism of delay in fluoride inhibition of glycolysis. Clin Chem. 2008;54:930–2.

33. Bruns DE, Knowler WC. Stabilization of glucose in blood samples: why it matters. Clin Chem. 2009;55:850–2.

34. Sicree RA, Zimmet PZ, Dunstan DW, Cameron AJ, Welborn TA, Shaw JE. Differences in height explain gender differences in the response to the oral glucose tolerance test – the AusDiab study. Diabet Med. 2008;25:296–302.

35. Hare MJL, Shaw JE, Zimmet PZ. Current controversies in the use of haemoglobin A1c. J Intern Med. 2012;271(3):227–36.

36. Tahara Y, Shima K. The response of glycated hemoglobin to stepwise plasma glucose change over time in diabetic patients. Diabetes Care. 1993;16:1313–4.

37. Little RR, Rohlfing CL, Wiedmeyer HM, Myers GL, Sacks DB, Goldstein DE. The national glycohemoglobin standardization program: a five-year progress report. Clin Chem. 2001;47:1985–92.

38. Hoelzel W, Weykamp C, Jeppsson JO, Miedema K, Barr JR, Goodall I, et al. IFCC reference system for measurement of hemoglobin A1c in human blood and the national standardization schemes in the United States, Japan, and Sweden: a method-comparison study. Clin Chem. 2004;50:166–74.

39. Nathan DM, Kuenen J, Borg R, Zheng H, Schoenfeld D, Heine RJ. Translating the AIC assay into estimated average glucose values. Diabetes Care. 2008;31(8):1473–8.

40. World Health Organization. Use of glycated hemoglobin (HbA1c) in the diagnosis of diabetes mellitus—abbreviated report of a WHO consultation. Geneva; 2011.

41. Bonora E, Tuomilehto J. The pros and cons of diagnosing diabetes with A1c. Diabetes Care. 2011;34 Suppl 2:S184–90.

42. Centers for Disease Control and Prevention: national diabetes fact sheet: general information and national estimates on diabetes in the United States, 2011. Atlanta: U.S. Department of Health and Human Services, Centers for Disease Control and Prevention; 2011.

43. Casparie AF, Miedema K. Glycosylated hemoglobin in diabetes and renal failure. Lancet. 1977;2(8041):758–9.

44. De Boer MJ, Miedema K, Casparie AF. Glycosylated hemoglobin in renal failure. Diabetologia. 1980;18(6):437–40.

45. Eschbach JW Jr, Funk D, Adamson J, Kuhn I, Scribner BH, Finch CA. Erythropoiesis in patients with renal failure undergoing chronic dialysis. N Engl J Med. 1967;276:653–8.

46. Diabetes Control and Complications Trial Research Group. The effect of intensive treatment of diabetes on the development and progression of long-term complications in insulin-dependent diabetes mellitus. N Engl J Med. 1993;329:977–86.

47. Desimone ME, Weinstock RS. Endotext, diabetes and carbohydrate metabolism chapter 11: pancreatic islet function tests. Updated 29 October 2015. Accessed 27 Dec 2017.

48. Delli AJ, Larsson HE, Ivarsson SA, Lernmark AK, Kong APS, Chan JCN. Type 1 diabetes. In: Textbook of diabetes. 4th ed. UK: Wiley-Blackwell. p. 141–52.

49. Lee YS, Ng WY, Thai AC, Lui KF, Loke KY. Prevalence of ICA and GAD antibodies at initial presentation of type 1 diabetes mellitus in Singapore children. J Pediatr Endocrinol Metab. 2001;14:767–72.

50. Sanjeev CB, Hagopian WA, Landin-Olsson M, Kockum I, Woo W, Palmer JP, et al. Association between autoantibody markers and subtypes of DR4 and DR4-DQ in Swedish children with insulin-dependent diabetes reveals closer association of tyrosine pyrophosphatase autoimmunity with DR4 than DQ8. Tissue Antigens. 1998;51:281–6.

51. Vardi P, Ziegler AG, Mathews JH, Dib S, Keller RJ, Ricker AT, et al. Concentration of insulin autoantibodies at onset of type 1 diabetes: inverse log-linear correlation with age. Diabetes Care. 1988;11:736–9.

52. Graham J, Hagopian WA, Kockum I, Li LS, Sanjeevi CB, Lowe RM, et al. Genetic effects on age-dependent onset and islet cell autoantibody markers in type 1 diabetes. Diabetes. 2002;51:1346–55.

53. Barker JM, Barriga KJ, Yu LP, Miao DM, Erlich HA, Norris JM, et al. Prediction of autoantibody positivity and progression to type 1 diabetes: diabetes autoimmunity study in the young (DAISY). J Clin Endocrinol Metab. 2004;89:3896–902.

Gestational Diabetes

H. David McIntyre and Jeremy J. N. Oats

Diagnosis of Gestational Diabetes

The diagnosis and indeed the existence of gestational diabetes mellitus (GDM) have been debated for many years. Historically, the first description of diabetes that had its onset during and symptomatically disappeared after the pregnancy was made by Bennewitz in 1824 [1]. However, it was not the 1940s when Miller documented the increased frequency of prior adverse obstetric outcomes in women who later developed diabetes that recognition of GDM as an entity began to gain credence [2]. At that stage, it was considered to be a pregnancy-limited condition which resolved in the postpartum period [3]. Its importance as a form of "prediabetes" was recognized by O'Sullivan and Mahan in 1964 [4]. They identified GDM as a precursor and predictor of later permanent diabetes. These two important strands of the epidemiologic importance of GDM have become increasingly interwoven since that time.

Current understanding of the pathophysiology of GDM includes two key components. These are the existence of pancreatic β-cell dysfunction (generally inferred to be present before pregnancy) and the unmasking of this problem by the development of insulin resistance during pregnancy, which requires enhanced insulin production to maintain normoglycemia. The etiologic factors underlying GDM, namely, β-cell dysfunction and insulin resistance, are not routinely measured in routine clinical practice, which relies on identification of their major consequence, hyperglycemia, for diagnosis of GDM. This is generally measured under the additional stress of an oral glucose load, in the form of an oral glucose tolerance test (OGTT), which serves to unmask more subtle degrees of hyperglycemia. The major effects of maternal hyperglycemia are seen through stimulation of fetal growth by mild fetal hyperglycemia and consequent fetal hyperinsulinemia as outlined by Pedersen and refined by Freinkel to include the role of other nutrients [5]. The Pedersen hypothesis and modifications are represented in Fig. 29.1.

Prior diagnostic pathways and nomenclature for diagnosis of GDM have been heterogeneous. However, the recently published results of the Hyperglycemia and Adverse Pregnancy Outcome (HAPO) study [6] and subsequent consensus development process organized by the International Association of Diabetes in Pregnancy Study Groups (IADPSG) [7] have led to a clearer and more uniform approach, grounded primarily in the risk of adverse pregnancy outcomes associated with mild hyperglycemia in pregnancy. The IADPSG criteria [7], now also endorsed by the World Health Organization [8] and the International Federation of Gynecology and Obstetrics (FIGO) [9], provide the primary point of reference for diagnosis of GDM in this paper.

The HAPO study [6] demonstrated a continuous and essentially linear relationship between maternal glycemia, measured during a three sample (fasting, 1 hour, 2 hours) 75 gram OGTT performed between 24- and 32-week gestation and a series of clinically important pregnancy complications, including excessive fetal growth (both large for gestational age babies and those with excess body fat), risk of neonatal hyperinsulinemia, primary caesarean section, and risk of pre eclampsia. Similar associations were also seen with a range of secondary outcomes including neonatal hypoglycemia, premature birth, shoulder dystocia and birth trauma, hyperbilirubinemia, and need for intensive neonatal care.

The independent associations of glucose with these outcomes persisted after adjustment for multiple potential confounders, including maternal body mass index (BMI) [6, 10].

H. D. McIntyre (✉)
Department of Obstetric Medicine, Mater Health Services and Mater Clinical Unit, University of Queensland, South Brisbane, QLD, Australia
e-mail: David.mcintyre@mater.org.au

J. J. N. Oats
School of Population and Global Health, University of Melbourne, Carlton, VIC, Australia

© Springer Nature Switzerland AG 2022
F. Bandeira et al. (eds.), *Endocrinology and Diabetes*, https://doi.org/10.1007/978-3-030-90684-9_29

Fig. 29.1 The Pedersen
hypothesis. "Maternal
hyperglycemia begets fetal
macrosomia" Modified by
Freinkel to include nutrients
other than glucose (lipids and
amino acids)

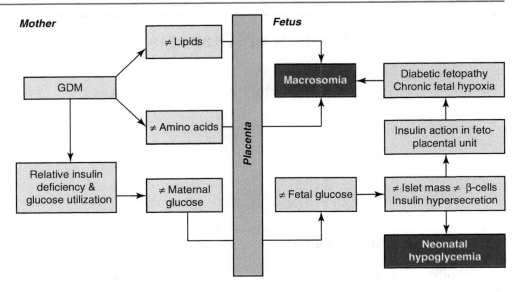

Fig. 29.2 IADPSG
recommended diagnostic
pathway for overt diabetes in
pregnancy and gestational
diabetes

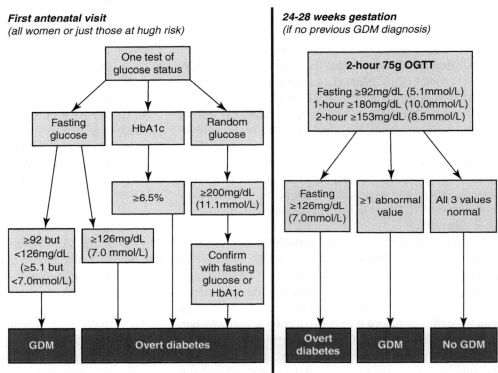

HAPO also considered the potential role of glycosylated hemoglobin (HbA1c) in the detection of GDM but concluded that HbA1c was not sufficiently discriminatory to be of value in this setting. Further, HAPO confirmed the Pedersen hypothesis [11] by clearly demonstrating the association between even mild degrees of maternal hyperglycemia and the fetal consequences of LGA, increased adiposity, and hyperinsulinemia.

Importantly, the HAPO study demonstrated no threshold for glucose associations with adverse outcomes, suggesting that new diagnostic criteria for GDM would need to be developed through a consensus process, a conclusion reached one and a half decades previously by Sacks et al. [12]. The consensus process organized by IADPSG subsequently developed a two-stage protocol for diagnosis of GDM and related disorders, summarized in Fig. 29.2. The recommended diagnostic values for GDM were determined by consensus and are by definition arbitrary. They were based on the risks of fetal outcomes related to maternal glycemia, specifically LGA, neonatal adiposity (body fat >90th centile), and neonatal hyperinsulinemia. The diagnostic glucose thresholds chosen (fasting, 1 hour or 2 hour at 75 gram OGTT) were those associated in continuous statistical models with odds ratios of 1.75 compared to the HAPO cohort mean for the three outcomes mentioned above, after extensive adjustment for other confounders [7].

In recognition of the increasing prevalence of prepregnancy diabetes (principally Type 2 diabetes) and obesity in women of reproductive age across many populations, IADPSG recommended early pregnancy testing for undiagnosed, severe hyperglycemia in early pregnancy. Implementation of early pregnancy testing on a universal or selective (risk factor based) basis was left open in the IADPSG recommendations due to the lack of firm data in this field and the widely varying diabetes prevalences in different populations around the world. The IADPSG Guidelines recommend that testing be undertaken using any of the following: fasting glucose, HbA1c, or random glucose (with confirmation), and that the results should be assessed using existing non pregnancy specific diagnostic criteria (see Fig. 29.2). Subsequently, the WHO recommendations introduced the term "Diabetes in Pregnancy" to characterize hyperglycemia, first noted in pregnancy, that would have been consistent with a diagnosis of diabetes if detected prior to pregnancy [8].

Importantly, hyperglycemia of this severity, if detected in early pregnancy, is likely to have antedated the diagnosis of pregnancy. Clinically, these women have been shown to have high rates of established microvascular diabetes complications [13] and thus demand urgent attention, both for their pregnancy care and for management of their diabetes and associated complications.

The IADPSG and WHO recommend that all women not previously identified as having abnormal glucose metabolism should undergo a formal 75 gram OGTT at 24- to 28-week gestation. Non-fasting glucose challenge tests, favored in some previous diagnostic algorithms, are not recommended due to limited sensitivity [14] and lack of clear associations with pregnancy outcomes. Following the IADPSG/WHO criteria, GDM is diagnosed if any one of the three relevant glucose values (fasting, 1 hour or 2 hour post 75 gram glucose load) equals or exceeds the thresholds noted in Fig. 29.1. If a fasting test is performed in early pregnancy, some women may be diagnosed as GDM at this stage. Otherwise, the diagnosis would generally be made at 24–28 weeks.

Given the fine distinctions to be drawn between normal and abnormal results, standardization and calibration of glucose measurements at the OGTT and at other testing points in pregnancy are critical. Venous plasma glucose should be used for all measures, and laboratories should pay careful attention to methodology and quality control [7].

Differential Diagnosis/Other Considerations

Since GDM is most commonly an asymptomatic condition diagnosed on the basis of glucose concentrations during the exogenous stress of an OGTT, differential diagnosis is not generally an important clinical consideration. However, it is important to consider other aspects of the condition including (1) other specific forms of abnormal glucose metabolism which may present as GDM and (2) important maternal and pregnancy factors which predispose to GDM.

Monogenic causes of diabetes are increasingly recognized, and though they tend to comprise only a small proportion of cases, they may be first detected in pregnancy due to increased glucose testing. Autosomal mutations causing diabetes are commonly grouped under the heading of maturity-onset diabetes of the young (MODY). Collectively, MODY variants may account for up to 10% of cases of GDM [15].

The example of glucokinase gene (GCK) mutations causing MODY2 [16] is particularly instructive. GCK mutations in the mother are associated with mild fasting hyperglycemia, generally without other abnormalities on the oral glucose tolerance test. If the fetus carries the same mutation, birthweight tends to be normal as both mother and fetus are adapted to "sensing" glucose at the same level. By contrast, if the mother carries the GCK mutation (and therefore is mildly hyperglycemic) and the fetus is normal, birthweight is increased. Conversely, if the mother is normal and the fetus carries the GCK mutation, birthweight is reduced. This elegant experiment of nature demonstrates the potential importance of both genes and environment in determining fetal growth.

Autoimmune diabetes, including early Type 1 diabetes and Latent Autoimmune Diabetes of Adult Life (LADA) may also be detected due to glucose testing in pregnancy. The definitive diagnosis is not always clear in this instance. In a recent case series from France, this form of diabetes, described as "Type 1 diabetes masquerading as GDM" was associated with pregnancy complications [17]. Prevalence of GAD or islet cell antibodies has been reported to be as high as 6% in some GDM cohorts [18] and is associated with a higher incidence of progression to overt diabetes postpartum.

The use of clinical risk factors for prediction of GDM is of limited utility, and this forms one argument in favor of universal diagnostic testing in pregnancy. Increased placental size, as seen in multiple pregnancies, is associated with a higher risk of GDM in some studies [19]. While a number of demographic and anthropometric factors, such as maternal age, ethnicity, body mass index, and previous history of GDM or macrosomia, are associated with higher risk of GDM, no one factor or combination of factors offers sufficient discriminatory power to eliminate the need for biochemical assessment.

Reported recurrence rates of GDM in subsequent pregnancies vary from 36% to 69% [20]. Recurrence risk appears higher in the presence of maternal obesity, early diagnosis of GDM in the index pregnancy, and excessive inter pregnancy weight gain. It remains unclear why recurrence rates for GDM are not higher than observed, given that women are by definition older and frequently heavier at the time of subsequent pregnancies. This observation does suggest that variability in the interaction between a woman and a particular fetus (or fetoplacental unit) may play a role in the etiology of GDM.

Current and Future Therapies

Current therapy for GDM is largely "glucocentric." The major therapeutic goal is achievement of glucose levels as close to normal pregnancy values as possible. Our discussion will include the current definition of normoglycemia in pregnancy, evidence favoring treatment, available therapeutic modalities, recent evidence for the use of ultrasound estimation of fetal growth to guide the intensity of treatment, and decisions regarding the mode and timing of delivery. Postpartum follow-up for the woman with GDM will also be addressed.

Normoglycemia in pregnancy The definition of normal pregnancy glucose levels, both fasting and in the postprandial state, has been investigated by a variety of methods, including detailed hospital inpatient studies, ambulatory studies using capillary glucose meters and continuous glucose monitoring (CGMS) over many years. A comprehensive analysis of this literature was published by Hernandez et al. in 2011 [21] and concluded that mean glucose levels in normal weight pregnant women were lower than previously described (mean ± SD fasting 71 ± 8 mg/dL or 3.9 ± 0.4 mmol/L; 1 hour post-meal 109 ± 10 mg/dL or 6.1 ± 0.6 mmol/L; 2 hours post-meal 99 ± 10 mg/dL or 5.5 ± 0.6 mmol/L). The commonly used statistical upper limits of these observations (mean + 2 SD) are also substantially lower than current, largely empirical, glucose treatment targets advocated in GDM [22–27] (Table 29.1) . The determination of optimal glucose targets remains contentious, although the current recommendations of major professional bodies are largely congruent. The values mentioned in Table 29.1 are the maximal glucose values in the fasting and postprandial states considered acceptable by the relevant organizations, or reported as treatment targets by the randomized controlled trials. The abbreviations and data sources for Table 29.1 are as follows: ADA, American Diabetes Association [23]; ADIPS, Australasian Diabetes in Pregnancy Society [27]; ACOG, American College of Obstetricians and Gynecologists [23]; NICE, National Institute of Clinical

Table 29.1 Glucose targets recommended by major national organizations in gestational diabetes or reported in major randomized controlled trials

Organization	Fasting (≤)	1 hour post-meal (≤)	2 hours post-meal (≤)
ADA	95 mg/dL 5.3 mmol/L	140 mg/dL 7.8 mmol/L	120 mg/dL 6.7 mmol/L
ADIPS	90 mg/dL 5.0 mmol/L	133 mg/dL 7.4 mmol/L	120 mg /dL 6.7 mmol/L
ACOG	95 mg/dL 5.3 mmol/L	130 mg /dL 7.2 mmol/L	
NICE	106 mg/dL 5.9 mmol/L		140 mg/dL 7.8 mmol/L
DIPSI	90 mg/dL 5.0 mmol/L		120 mg/dL 6.7 mmol/L
CDA	95 mg/dL 5.3 mmol/L	140 mg/dL 7.8 mmol/L	120 mg/dL 6.7 mmol/L
Trial			
ACHOIS	99 mg/dL 5.5 mmol/L		126 mg /dL 7.0 mmol/L
MFMN	95 mg/dL 5.3 mmol/L		120 mg/dL 6.7 mmol/L

Excellence (UK) [23]: DIPSI, Diabetes in Pregnancy Society India [24]: CDA, Canadian Diabetes Association [26]; ACHOIS, Australian Carbohydrate Intolerance Study [28]; and MFMN, Maternal Fetal Medicine Networks study [29].

Evidence for treatment of GDM Although the clinical importance of treating GDM was hotly debated for many years, two large randomized controlled trials have now been conducted, with largely congruent results. The ACHOIS study [28], conducted principally in Australia, randomized 490 women to an intervention including dietary advice, home blood glucose monitoring, and insulin therapy as required and compared them to 510 women assigned to standard care. The primary composite outcome of serious perinatal complications (death, shoulder dystocia, bone fracture, or nerve palsy) was reduced from 4% to 1% ($p = 0.01$) with intervention. Only 20% of women required adjunctive insulin treatment. The rates of LGA and macrosomia (defined as birthweight ≥4000 grams) were also reduced, with no increase in small for gestational age (SGA) babies. Quality of life was improved with treatment, and hypertensive complications of pregnancy were less frequent. Treated women had higher rates of induction of labor but similar rates of caesarean delivery. Admission of neonates to the neonatal nursery was more frequent with intervention, possibly related to hospital policies.

The US-based Maternal-Fetal Medicine Units Network trial of the treatment of mild GDM [29] randomly assigned 485 women to intervention vs. 473 assigned to standard care. This study excluded women with fasting glucose ≥95 mg/dL (5.3 mmol/L) but required them to have 2/3 other OGTT values in excess of ADA thresholds for the diagnosis of gestational diabetes [23]. The composite outcome used in this trial included both perinatal mortality and neonatal outcomes associated with maternal hyperglycemia (hypoglycemia, hyperbilirubinemia, hyperinsulinemia, and birth trauma). The vast majority (92%) of treated women were managed by lifestyle interventions, with only 37/485 or 7.6% needing adjunctive insulin therapy. As with the ACHOIS study, the rates of LGA and macrosomia were reduced with treatment as was neonatal fat mass. Hypertensive disorders of pregnancy, caesarean section, maternal weight gain from enrolment, and shoulder dystocia were all reduced by active intervention. The composite neonatal outcome did not differ between the treatment groups.

Both of these studies demonstrate that active treatment of women with GDM reduces serious pregnancy complications including hypertensive disorders of pregnancy and excessive fetal growth and its consequences. Thus, after many years of debate, active treatment of GDM appears justified.

Current therapy of GDM Lifestyle modification, including medical nutrition therapy and encouragement of physical activity, forms the primary mode of therapy for GDM. As noted above, such therapy proved sufficient in 80–90% of women enrolled in the two major randomized trials. The American Dietetic Association evidence-based nutrition practice guidelines for GDM [30] provide a sound overall framework for nutritional interventions. They advocate review by a registered dietitian within 1 week of GDM diagnosis and a minimum of two follow-up visits. While dietary recommendations are individualized, the general guidance favors mild energy restriction to approximately 70% of recommended daily intake for overweight/obese women and reduction of total carbohydrate intake to less than 45% of total caloric intake. Other recent studies have specifically examined the role of glycemic index in nutritional therapy for GDM [31] and have suggested that this may enhance the effects of standard treatment and assist some women in meeting glycemic targets and obviating the need for pharmacotherapy, although overall pregnancy outcomes have been reported as similar to those achieved with a high-fiber diet [32].

Insulin therapy remains the cornerstone of treatment for women who fail to meet glycemic goals after lifestyle modification. The glucose targets currently recommended by various international organizations and those used in the two major randomized trials are listed in Table 29.1. The choice of insulin regimen for an individual woman depends on the pattern of elevated glucose readings seen on home glucose monitoring. Women with predominant fasting hyperglycemia may respond well to a single evening injection of intermediate (NPH) or long-acting (glargine or detemir) insulin. Those with predominant elevation of postprandial glucose are generally treated with soluble insulin or a rapid acting analogue (aspart or lispro) insulin prior to meals. Women with a mixed pattern of elevated glucose readings may also be treated with premixed insulins, generally twice daily at breakfast and dinner time. A recent detailed review [33] has concluded that there is minimal evidence available to choose between specific insulin regimens.

Other therapeutic options Oral hypoglycemic agents, principally glibenclamide (glyburide in the USA) and metformin, have also been trialled in gestational diabetes. The first major randomized controlled trial of glyburide, conducted by Langer and colleagues [34], reported equivalent glucose control and no substantial differences in outcomes in women treated with glyburide as compared to insulin after failure of lifestyle management. Langer's study was not powered to examine major pregnancy outcomes. Subsequently, a systematic review of this and subsequent randomized trials [35] reported no differences in terms of glycemic control or pregnancy outcomes when comparing glyburide and insulin therapy. However, a large recent (non-randomized) cohort study of 10,682 women from the "Sweet Success" program in California reported increased rates of LGA and neonatal intensive care unit admission in those women treated with glyburide [36], and a more recent systematic review has concluded that glyburide is inferior to metformin and insulin in the treatment of GDM [37].

Metformin has also been evaluated in the large "metformin in gestational diabetes (MiG)" study [38] and two smaller randomized trials [39, 40]. These studies included women who failed to meet glycemic targets after lifestyle interventions for GDM. They demonstrated very similar glucose control and pregnancy outcomes with metformin therapy when compared to standard insulin treatment. The rate of supplemental insulin therapy was high overall – 46% in the MiG study and 32% in the Finnish report, but surprisingly no patients in the study from New Mexico USA required supplemental insulin therapy. Patient preferences were clearly in favor of metformin therapy.

Uncontrolled reports suggested that metformin reduces pregnancy complications in women with polycystic ovarian syndrome treated during pregnancy [41–43], but a recent randomized trial failed to confirm any benefit [44].

Two randomized trials [45, 46] comparing metformin with glyburide/glibenclamide in the treatment of GDM have shown somewhat discordant results. In a report from Brazil [45, 47], Silva et al. reported comparable efficacy between these two medications, with supplemental insulin required in around 25% of each group. In contrast, Moore et al. [46] reported that 35% of metformin-treated women required supplemental insulin as compared to 16% of those treated with glyburide.

The use of oral hypoglycemic agents in the treatment of GDM varies widely on a country by country basis, with glyburide favored in the USA [48], while metformin is recommended more widely in the UK and Australasia [49–51]. Some practitioners remain concerned by the possibility of adverse fetal effects of oral drugs. Glyburide was initially reported to be absent or at very low levels in cord blood, due to limited transplacental passage and active counter transport [52, 53]. However, a more recent report using a more sensitive assay describes variable transplacental transport with cord blood levels higher than maternal plasma concentrations in 37% of cases [54]. Metformin crosses the placenta readily [55–57] but has shown no adverse fetal or early childhood effects to date [58, 59].

As noted above, many of the adverse effects of GDM relate to excessive fetal growth, driven by nutrient excess and consequent fetal hyperinsulinism as outlined in the Pederson hypothesis [11] and its subsequent modification by Freinkel and Metzger [5]. These have also been presented in Fig. 29.1. Direct assessment of amniotic fluid insulin concentrations, pioneered by Weiss et al. [60] demonstrated that fetal hyperinsulinemia was associated with increased risks of pregnancy complications. In turn, Schafer Graf et al. [61] noted that fetal abdominal circumference (AC) on ultrasound could be used to noninvasively predict fetal hyperinsulinism and identify those babies most at risk of diabetic fetopathy.

Subsequently, an alternative approach to treatment of GDM, based on ultrasound assessment of fetal growth, in particular fetal AC, has been proposed and evaluated in four randomized studies [62–66]. According to this approach, summarized by Kjos et al. [64], glucose-lowering treatment may be intensified in those pregnancies where the fetus shows evidence of accelerated growth, generally determined by fetal AC > 75th centile for gestational age on ultrasonographic assessment. These protocols suggest that "low-risk" pregnancies, as defined by normal (<75th centile) fetal AC, may require less stringent glycemic control and conversely that detection of an increased AC should lead to intensification of glucose-lowering therapy.

A summary of the traditional (glucocentric) and alternative (USS-guided) pathways for GDM therapy is presented in Fig. 29.3.

Fetal surveillance and timing of delivery Despite a lack of high-level evidence of definite benefit, fetal ultrasound is frequently used to assess fetal well-being and to estimate fetal weight to assist in determining the timing and mode of delivery. Most units have extrapolated their practices in this area from those developed for pregestational or preexisting diabetes.

The experience reported by the Diabetes Unit at the National Maternity Hospital Dublin in1983 and again in 1992 is particularly instructive [67]. They noted that the only deaths in normally formed infants occurred when there was clinical (rather than ultrasonographic) evidence of fetal macrosomia, polyhydramnios, or poor metabolic control. Consequently in their absence, this group of experienced clinicians allowed the otherwise uncomplicated pregnancies to go to full term (40 completed weeks of gestation) [68]. This noninterventionist approach produced a caesarean section rate of 7%, and vaginal delivery was achieved in 90% of women!

The widespread practice of cardiotocographic fetal monitoring in GDM in the absence of other obstetric indications such as fetal growth restriction and the hypertensive disorders is likewise poorly supported by evidence. The current protocols are largely empiric and driven by expert opinion. The report of Landon et al. [69], which considered women with Type 1 diabetes, noted that fetal surveillance most commonly led to intervention in women with associated vascular disease, such as hypertension or nephropathy.

Gabbe and colleagues recommended that in uncomplicated GDM pregnancies, CTG monitoring should be commenced after 40-week gestation while awaiting spontaneous onset of labor [70]. However, there is again a paucity of high-level evidence in this area to guide the clinician.

A 2001 Cochrane review [71] found that there was only one randomized controlled trial [72] comparing planned elective delivery at 38-week gestation vs. expectant management (awaiting the onset of spontaneous labor up to 42-week gestation, with twice weekly CTG and amniotic fluid volume surveillance). This trial included a range of insulin treated women, rather than simply women with gestational diabetes. The review concluded that induction at 38 weeks did not result in an increase in caesarean section RR 0.81 (95% CI 0.52–1.26). However, the risk of macrosomia (birthweight ≥4000 g) was lessened in the elective delivery group RR 0.56 (95% CI 0.32–0.98), and there were three cases of mild shoulder dystocia in the expectant group. The authors concluded that there was insufficient evidence to make a conclusive recommendation. Similar conclusions were reached by Witkop et al. in 2009 [73].

Mode of delivery The major concern regarding vaginal delivery in women with gestational diabetes is the potential risk of shoulder dystocia and in particular resultant brachial plexus palsy. Ultimately, the relative size of the fetal shoulders and the maternal pelvis, the strength of the uterine contractions and the mother's expulsive efforts, and the fetal diameters determine the likelihood of successful vaginal delivery. None of these can be reliably measured and/or predicted.

Although increasing fetal weight is positively associated with an increasing risk of shoulder dystocia, many cases

Fig. 29.3 Treatment pathways for GDM – "glucocentric" pathway including treatment with insulin and oral hypoglycemic agents and alternative "USS-guided" pathway. For details see text

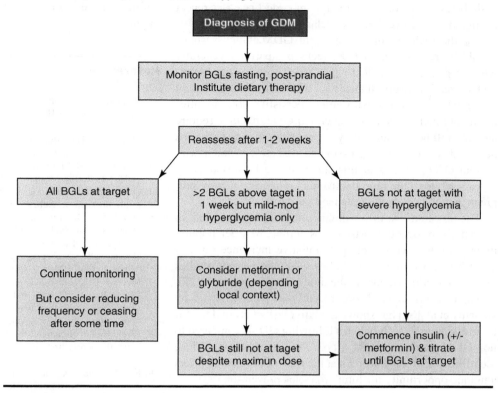

'Glucocentric' pathway: insulin and oral hypoglycemics

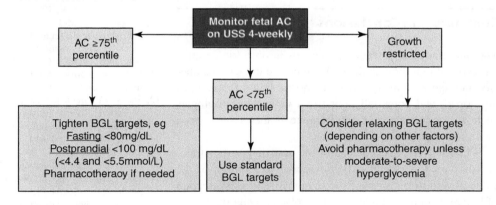

Alternative USS-guided pathway (in addition to above)

occur in babies with birthweight less than 4000 g as those who are classified as being macrosomic (i.e., birthweight >4000 g). Furthermore 50% of cases of brachial plexus palsy occur in the absence of shoulder dystocia, suggesting that ante- and intrapartum factors also play an important etiological role in its genesis [74].

Despite overall uncertainties, it is common practice to offer elective caesarean delivery if the estimated fetal weight is 4000 g or 4250 g or more [75].

Postpartum follow-up The diagnosis of GDM carries long-term health implications for both mother and baby. In particular, the risk of future diabetes for the mother is sub-

stantial, and the diagnosis of GDM offers an opportunity for diabetes prevention. While the fetal/neonatal effects for GDM are important, we consider them to be outside the scope of the current discussion.

Women with GDM should be encouraged to breast feed. In addition to benefits for their offspring [76], there is evidence that this may reduce their own risk of progression to diabetes [77, 78].

In the immediate postnatal period, maternal glycemia returns to normal in most cases. However, women first detected as having "diabetes in pregnancy" clearly require close monitoring as they are likely to have ongoing hyperglycemia. For many of these women, the clinical diagnosis of diabetes will be obvious, though in borderline cases repeat testing may improve diagnostic clarity.

For the majority of women with GDM, glucose status should be re assessed at 6–8 weeks postpartum, generally with a repeat 75 gram OGTT [79, 80]. Those women identified as having overt diabetes at this time clearly require immediate care. Those with milder persisting abnormalities in glucose metabolism (IGT and/or IFG) at this time require annual follow-up and may benefit from interventions designed to prevent progression to diabetes. Women with normal OGTT results at this stage should be tested every 2 years while in the reproductive age range and ideally pre-pregnancy for any further planned gestations [79, 80].

The absolute risk of a woman with GDM progressing to overt diabetes over time varies substantially between populations, with Kim et al. noting cumulative incidence rates of Type 2 DM varying from 2.6% to 70% in various studies [81], with fasting glucose at the time of the diagnostic OGTT a major determinant. More recently, a meta-analysis by Bellamy et al. [82] has shown a relative risk of around ten for progression to Type 2 diabetes following GDM (compared to non-GDM women) across a broad range of studies. Thus, identification of these women at the time of pregnancy offers a unique opportunity for future diabetes prevention [83].

Summary and Conclusions

The importance of gestational diabetes in obstetric practice has evolved rapidly with the global increase in maternal obesity and age at delivery. New diagnostic criteria have been developed, and potentially important underlying etiologies such as monogenic and autoimmune diabetes have been identified in particular populations.

While universal acceptance of the new diagnostic strategies has yet to be achieved, widespread recognition of the value of a uniform approach to diagnosis and classification of hyperglycemia in pregnancy is evolving. Ongoing points of contention in treatment of GDM include the potential role of oral hypoglycemic agents and the use of "customized" glycemic treatment targets adjusted according to assessments of fetal growth.

Many aspects of therapy of GDM remain steeped in tradition, but high-level evidence is slowly accumulating to guide future practice. Evidence in the area of optimal fetal surveillance, timing, and mode of delivery remains sparse, with clinical decisions based more on local preferences and protocols than on high-level evidence.

A diagnosis of GDM identifies a pregnant woman as being at risk of future diabetes and offers the opportunity for prevention of this potentially devastating disease. It may also serve to identify "at-risk" families and offer broader opportunities for prevention of obesity and Type 2 diabetes in her offspring.

References

1. Hadden DR, Hillebrand B. The first recorded case of diabetic pregnancy (Bennewitz HG, 1824, University of Berlin). Diabetologia. 1989;32(8):625.
2. Miller HC. The effect of diabetic and prediabetic pregnancies on the fetus and newborn infant. J Pediatr. 1946;29(4):455–61.
3. Carrington ER, Shuman CR, Reardon HS. Evaluation of the prediabetic state during pregnancy. Obstet Gynecol. 1957;9(6):664–9.
4. O'Sullivan JB, Mahan CM. Criteria for the oral glucose tolerance test in pregnancy. Diabetes. 1964;13:278–85.
5. Freinkel N. Banting lecture 1980. Of pregnancy and progeny. Diabetes. 1980;29(12):1023–35.
6. Metzger BE, Lowe LP, Dyer AR, Trimble ER, Chaovarindr U, Coustan DR, et al. Hyperglycemia and adverse pregnancy outcomes. N Engl J Med. 2008;358(19):1991–2002.
7. Metzger BE, Gabbe SG, Persson B, Buchanan TA, Catalano PA, Damm P, et al. International association of diabetes and pregnancy study groups recommendations on the diagnosis and classification of hyperglycemia in pregnancy. Diabetes Care. 2010;33(3):676–82.
8. World Health Organization. Diagnostic criteria and classification of hyperglycaemia first detected in pregnancy. Geneva: WHO Press; 2013.
9. Hod M, Kapur A, Sacks DA, Hadar E, Agarwal M, Di Renzo GC, et al. The International Federation of Gynecology and Obstetrics (FIGO) initiative on gestational diabetes mellitus: a pragmatic guide for diagnosis, management, and care. Int J Gynaecol Obstet. 2015;131 Suppl 3:S173–211.
10. Catalano PM, McIntyre HD, Cruickshank JK, McCance DR, Dyer AR, Metzger BE, et al. The hyperglycemia and adverse pregnancy outcome study: associations of GDM and obesity with pregnancy outcomes. Diabetes Care. 2012;35:780–6.
11. Pedersen J, Bojsen-Moller B, Poulsen H. Blood sugar in newborn infants of diabetic mothers. Acta Endocrinol. 1954;15(1):33–52.
12. Sacks DA, Greenspoon JS, Abu-Fadil S, Henry HM, Wolde-Tsadik G, Yao JF. Toward universal criteria for gestational diabetes: the 75-gram glucose tolerance test in pregnancy. Am J Obstet Gynecol. 1995;172(2 Pt 1):607–14.
13. Omori Y, Jovanovic L. Proposal for the reconsideration of the definition of gestational diabetes. Diabetes Care. 2005;28(10):2592–3.
14. van Leeuwen M, Louwerse MD, Opmeer BC, Limpens J, Serlie MJ, Reitsma JB, et al. Glucose challenge test for detecting gestational diabetes mellitus: a systematic review. BJOG. 2012;119(4):393–401.
15. Buchanan TA, Xiang AH. Gestational diabetes mellitus. J Clin Invest. 2005;115(3):485–91.
16. Hattersley AT, Beards F, Ballantyne E, Appleton M, Harvey R, Ellard S. Mutations in the glucokinase gene of the fetus result in reduced birth weight. Nat Genet. 1998;19(3):268–70.
17. Wucher H, Lepercq J, Carette C, Colas C, Dubois-Laforgue D, Gautier JF, et al. Poor prognosis of pregnancy in women with autoimmune type 1 diabetes mellitus masquerading as gestational diabetes. Diabetes Metab. 2011;37(1):47–51.
18. Nilsson C, Ursing D, Torn C, Aberg A, Landin-Olsson M. Presence of GAD antibodies during gestational diabetes mellitus predicts type 1 diabetes. Diabetes Care. 2007;30(8):1968–71.
19. Rauh-Hain JA, Rana S, Tamez H, Wang A, Cohen B, Cohen A, et al. Risk for developing gestational diabetes in women with twin pregnancies. J Matern Fetal Neonatal Med. 2009;22(4):293–9.

20. Ben-Haroush A, Yogev Y, Hod M. Epidemiology of gestational diabetes mellitus and its association with type 2 diabetes. Diabet Med. 2004;21(2):103–13.

21. Hernandez TL, Friedman JE, Van Pelt RE, Barbour LA. Patterns of glycemia in normal pregnancy: should the current therapeutic targets be challenged? Diabetes Care. 2011;34(7):1660–8.

22. American Diabetes A. Standards of medical care in diabetes--2011. Diabetes Care. 2011;34 Suppl 1:S11–61.

23. Simmons D, McElduff A, McIntyre HD, Elrishi M. Gestational diabetes mellitus: NICE for the U.S.? A comparison of the American Diabetes Association and the American College of Obstetricians and Gynecologists guidelines with the U.K. National Institute for Health and Clinical Excellence guidelines. Diabetes Care. 2010;33(1):34–7.

24. Seshiah V, Das AK, Balaji V, Joshi SR, Parikh MN, Gupta S, et al. Gestational diabetes mellitus--guidelines. J Assoc Physicians India. 2006;54:622–8.

25. Canadian Diabetes A, Dietitians of C, Diabete Q, Ordre professionnel des dietetistes du Q. Recommendations for nutrition best practice in the management of gestational diabetes mellitus. Executive summary (1). Can J Diet Pract Res. 2006;67(4):206–8.

26. Canadian Diabetes Association. Canadian Diabetes Association 2008 clinical practice guidelines for the prevention and management of diabetes in Canada. Can J Diabetes. 2008;32:S168–S81.

27. Nankervis A, McIntyre HD, Moses RG, Ross GP, Callaway LK. Testing for gestational diabetes mellitus in Australia. Diabetes Care. 2013;36(5):e64.

28. Crowther CA, Hiller JE, Moss JR, McPhee AJ, Jeffries WS, Robinson JS. Effect of treatment of gestational diabetes mellitus on pregnancy outcomes. N Engl J Med. 2005;352(24):2477–86.

29. Landon MB, Spong CY, Thom E, Carpenter MW, Ramin SM, Casey B, et al. A multicenter, randomized trial of treatment for mild gestational diabetes. N Engl J Med. 2009;361(14):1339–48.

30. Reader D, Splett P, Gunderson EP, Diabetes C, Education Dietetic Practice G. Impact of gestational diabetes mellitus nutrition practice guidelines implemented by registered dietitians on pregnancy outcomes. J Am Diet Assoc. 2006;106(9):1426–33.

31. Moses RG, Brand-Miller JC. The use of a low glycaemic index diet in pregnancy: an evolving treatment paradigm. Diabetes Res Clin Pract. 2011;91(1):13–4.

32. Louie JC, Markovic TP, Perera N, Foote D, Petocz P, Ross GP, et al. A randomized controlled trial investigating the effects of a low-glycemic index diet on pregnancy outcomes in gestational diabetes mellitus. Diabetes Care. 2011;34(11):2341–6.

33. McElduff A, Moses RG. Insulin therapy in pregnancy. Endocrinol Metab Clin North Am. 2012;41(1):161–73.

34. Langer O, Conway DL, Berkus MD, Xenakis EM, Gonzales O. A comparison of glyburide and insulin in women with gestational diabetes mellitus. N Engl J Med. 2000;343(16):1134–8.

35. Dhulkotia JS, Ola B, Fraser R, Farrell T. Oral hypoglycemic agents vs insulin in management of gestational diabetes: a systematic review and metaanalysis. Am J Obstet Gynecol. 2010;203(5):457 e1–9.

36. Cheng YW, Chung JH, Block-Kurbisch I, Inturrisi M, Caughey AB. Treatment of gestational diabetes mellitus: glyburide compared to subcutaneous insulin therapy and associated perinatal outcomes. J Matern Fetal Neonatal Med. 2012;25(4):379–84.

37. Balsells M, Garcia-Patterson A, Sola I, Roque M, Gich I, Corcoy R. Glibenclamide, metformin, and insulin for the treatment of gestational diabetes: a systematic review and meta-analysis. BMJ. 2015;350:h102.

38. Rowan JA, Hague WM, Gao W, Battin MR, Moore MP. Metformin versus insulin for the treatment of gestational diabetes. N Engl J Med. 2008;358(19):2003–15.

39. Moore LE, Briery CM, Clokey D, Martin RW, Williford NJ, Bofill JA, et al. Metformin and insulin in the management of gestational diabetes mellitus: preliminary results of a comparison. J Reprod Med. 2007;52(11):1011–5.

40. Ijas H, Vaarasmaki M, Morin-Papunen L, Keravuo R, Ebeling T, Saarela T, et al. Metformin should be considered in the treatment of gestational diabetes: a prospective randomised study. BJOG. 2011;118(7):880–5.

41. Jakubowicz DJ, Iuorno MJ, Jakubowicz S, Roberts KA, Nestler JE. Effects of metformin on early pregnancy loss in the polycystic ovary syndrome. J Clin Endocrinol Metab. 2002;87(2):524–9.

42. De Leo V, Musacchio MC, Piomboni P, Di Sabatino A, Morgante G. The administration of metformin during pregnancy reduces polycystic ovary syndrome related gestational complications. Eur J Obstet Gynecol Reprod Biol. 2011;157(1):63–6.

43. Glueck CJ, Wang P, Kobayashi S, Phillips H, Sieve-Smith L. Metformin therapy throughout pregnancy reduces the development of gestational diabetes in women with polycystic ovary syndrome. Fertil Steril. 2002;77(3):520–5.

44. Vanky E, Stridsklev S, Heimstad R, Romundstad P, Skogoy K, Kleggetveit O, et al. Metformin versus placebo from first trimester to delivery in polycystic ovary syndrome: a randomized, controlled multicenter study. J Clin Endocrinol Metab. 2010;95(12):E448–55.

45. Silva JC, Fachin DR, Coral ML, Bertini AM. Perinatal impact of the use of metformin and glyburide for the treatment of gestational diabetes mellitus. J Perinat Med. 2012;40(3):225–8.

46. Moore LE, Clokey D, Rappaport VJ, Curet LB. Metformin compared with glyburide in gestational diabetes: a randomized controlled trial. Obstet Gynecol. 2010;115(1):55–9.

47. Silva JC, Pacheco C, Bizato J, de Souza BV, Ribeiro TE, Bertini AM. Metformin compared with glyburide for the management of gestational diabetes. Int J Gynaecol Obstet. 2010;111(1):37–40.

48. Ogunyemi DA, Fong A, Rad S, Fong S, Kjos SL. Attitudes and practices of healthcare providers regarding gestational diabetes: results of a survey conducted at the 2010 meeting of the International Association of Diabetes in Pregnancy Study Group (IADPSG). Diabet Med. 2011;28(8):976–86.

49. Simmons D, Walters BNJ, Rowan JA, McIntyre HD. Metformin therapy and diabetes in pregnancy. Med J Aust. 2004;180(9):462–4.

50. Goh JE, Sadler L, Rowan J. Metformin for gestational diabetes in routine clinical practice. Diabet Med. 2011;28(9):1082–7.

51. Gandhi P, Bustani R, Madhuvrata P, Farrell T. Introduction of metformin for gestational diabetes mellitus in clinical practice: has it had an impact? Eur J Obstet Gynecol Reprod Biol. 2012;160(2):147–50.

52. Cygalova LH, Hofman J, Ceckova M, Staud F. Transplacental pharmacokinetics of glyburide, rhodamine 123, and BODIPY FL prazosin: effect of drug efflux transporters and lipid solubility. J Pharmacol Exp Ther. 2009;331(3):1118–25.

53. Hemauer SJ, Patrikeeva SL, Nanovskaya TN, Hankins GD, Ahmed MS. Role of human placental apical membrane transporters in the efflux of glyburide, rosiglitazone, and metformin. Am J Obstet Gynecol. 2010;202(4):383 e1–7.

54. Schwartz RA, Rosenn B, Aleksa K, Koren G. Glyburide transport across the human placenta. Obstet Gynecol. 2015;125(3):583–8.

55. Charles B, Norris R, Xiao X, Hague W. Population pharmacokinetics of metformin in late pregnancy. Ther Drug Monit. 2006;28(1):67–72.

56. Kovo M, Haroutiunian S, Feldman N, Hoffman A, Glezerman M. Determination of metformin transfer across the human placenta using a dually perfused ex vivo placental cotyledon model. Eur J Obstet Gynecol Reprod Biol. 2008;136(1):29–33.

57. Kovo M, Kogman N, Ovadia O, Nakash I, Golan A, Hoffman A. Carrier-mediated transport of metformin across the human placenta determined by using the ex vivo perfusion of the placental cotyledon model. Prenat Diagn. 2008;28(6):544–8.

58. Rowan JA, Rush EC, Obolonkin V, Battin M, Wouldes T, Hague WM. Metformin in gestational diabetes: the offspring follow-up

(MiG TOFU): body composition at 2 years of age. Diabetes Care. 2011;34(10):2279–84.

59. Glueck CJ, Salehi M, Sieve L, Wang P. Growth, motor, and social development in breast- and formula-fed infants of metformin-treated women with polycystic ovary syndrome. J Pediatr. 2006;148(5):628–32.

60. Weiss PA, Hofmann HM, Winter RR, Lichtenegger W, Purstner P, Haas J. Diagnosis and treatment of gestational diabetes according to amniotic fluid insulin levels. Arch Gynecol. 1986;239(2):81–91.

61. Schaefer-Graf UM, Kjos SL, Buhling KJ, Henrich W, Brauer M, Heinze T, et al. Amniotic fluid insulin levels and fetal abdominal circumference at time of amniocentesis in pregnancies with diabetes. Diabet Med. 2003;20(5):349–54.

62. Buchanan TA, Kjos SL, Montoro MN, Wu PY, Madrilejo NG, Gonzalez M, et al. Use of fetal ultrasound to select metabolic therapy for pregnancies complicated by mild gestational diabetes. Diabetes Care. 1994;17(4):275–83.

63. Kjos SL, Schaefer-Graf U, Sardesi S, Peters RK, Buley A, Xiang AH, et al. A randomized controlled trial using glycemic plus fetal ultrasound parameters versus glycemic parameters to determine insulin therapy in gestational diabetes with fasting hyperglycemia. Diabetes Care. 2001;24(11):1904–10.

64. Kjos SL, Schaefer-Graf UM. Modified therapy for gestational diabetes using high-risk and low-risk fetal abdominal circumference growth to select strict versus relaxed maternal glycemic targets. Diabetes Care. 2007;30 Suppl 2:S200–5.

65. Schaefer-Graf UM, Kjos SL, Fauzan OH, Buhling KJ, Siebert G, Buhrer C, et al. A randomized trial evaluating a predominantly fetal growth-based strategy to guide management of gestational diabetes in Caucasian women. Diabetes Care. 2004;27(2):297–302.

66. Bonomo M, Cetin I, Pisoni MP, Faden D, Mion E, Taricco E, et al. Flexible treatment of gestational diabetes modulated on ultrasound evaluation of intrauterine growth: a controlled randomized clinical trial. Diabetes Metab. 2004;30(3):237–44.

67. Drury MI, Stronge JM, Foley ME, MacDonald DW. Pregnancy in the diabetic patient: timing and mode of delivery. Obstet Gynecol. 1983;62(3):279–82.

68. Rasmussen MJ, Firth R, Foley M, Stronge JM. The timing of delivery in diabetic pregnancy: a 10-year review. Aust N Z J Obstet Gynaecol. 1992;32(4):313–7.

69. Landon MB, Langer O, Gabbe SG, Schick C, Brustman L. Fetal surveillance in pregnancies complicated by insulin-dependent diabetes mellitus. Am J Obstet Gynecol. 1992;167(3):617–21.

70. Gabbe S, Hill L, Schmidt L, Schulkin J. Management of diabetes by obstetrician-gynecologists. Obstet Gynecol. 1998;91(5 Pt 1):643–7.

71. Boulvain M, Stan C, Irion O. Elective delivery in diabetic pregnant women. Cochrane Database Syst Rev. 2001;(2):CD001997.

72. Kjos SL, Henry OA, Montoro M, Buchanan TA, Mestman JH. Insulin-requiring diabetes in pregnancy: a randomized trial of active induction of labor and expectant management. Am J Obstet Gynecol. 1993;169(3):611–5.

73. Witkop CT, Neale D, Wilson LM, Bass EB, Nicholson WK. Active compared with expectant delivery management in women with gestational diabetes: a systematic review. Obstet Gynecol. 2009;113(1):206–17.

74. Gherman RB, Ouzounian JG, Miller DA, Kwok L, Goodwin TM. Spontaneous vaginal delivery: a risk factor for Erb's palsy? Am J Obstet Gynecol. 1998;178(3):423–7.

75. Hod M, Bar J, Peled Y, Fried S, Katz I, Itzhak M, et al. Antepartum management protocol. Timing and mode of delivery in gestational diabetes. Diabetes Care. 1998;21 Suppl 2:B113–7.

76. Crume TL, Ogden LG, Mayer-Davis EJ, Hamman RF, Norris JM, Bischoff KJ, et al. The impact of neonatal breast-feeding on growth trajectories of youth exposed and unexposed to diabetes in utero: the EPOCH Study. Int J Obes (Lond). 2012;36(4):529–34. https://doi.org/10.1038/ijo.2011.254. Epub 2 Jan 31.

77. O'Reilly M, Avalos G, Dennedy MC, O'Sullivan EP, Dunne FP. Breast-feeding is associated with reduced postpartum maternal glucose intolerance after gestational diabetes. Ir Med J. 2012;105(5 Suppl):31–6.

78. Gunderson EP, Hedderson MM, Chiang V, Crites Y, Walton D, Azevedo RA, et al. Lactation intensity and postpartum maternal glucose tolerance and insulin resistance in women with recent GDM: the SWIFT cohort. Diabetes Care. 2012;35(1):50–6. Epub 2011 Oct 19.

79. Hoffman L, Nolan C, Wilson JD, Oats JJ, Simmons D. Gestational diabetes mellitus--management guidelines. The Australasian Diabetes in Pregnancy Society. Med J Aust. 1998;169(2):93–7.

80. Oats JJ, McIntyre HD. Revision of guidelines for the management of gestational diabetes mellitus. Med J Aust. 2004;181(6):342.

81. Kim C, Newton KM, Knopp RH. Gestational diabetes and the incidence of type 2 diabetes: a systematic review. Diabetes Care. 2002;25(10):1862–8.

82. Bellamy L, Casas JP, Hingorani AD, Williams D. Type 2 diabetes mellitus after gestational diabetes: a systematic review and meta-analysis. Lancet. 2009;373(9677):1773–9.

83. Bentley-Lewis R. Gestational diabetes mellitus: an opportunity of a lifetime. Lancet. 2009;373(9677):1738–40.

Oral Therapies for Type 2 Diabetes

30

Josivan Gomes de Lima, Lúcia Helena Coelho Nóbrega, and Natalia Nobrega de Lima

Introduction

Diabetes is an important health problem not only in the USA but all over the world. It is responsible for numerous complications, such as blindness, amputation, and kidney disease. Various studies have demonstrated the importance of glycemic control to avoid developing these chronic complications [1]. More recently, the concept of glycemic memory has been implicated to highlight the need for better glycemic control since the diagnosis [2].

In recent years, several new drugs have become available for the treatment of type 2 diabetes. Not only are these therapies new, but they also act by new mechanisms, thus targeting several defects involved in the pathophysiology of diabetes. In addition to newer therapeutics, older drugs such as metformin are still available and used to achieve glycemic control. Furthermore, several additional drugs are in development, some of which will likely be available in the future. In this chapter, we will discuss the mechanisms of action, doses, side effects, efficacy, indications, and contraindications of the available oral drugs for type 2 diabetes. Injection drugs and insulin will be discussed elsewhere in this book.

Present and Future Therapies

Insulin resistance in the liver and muscle and β-cell failure in the pancreas are the traditional pathophysiologic defects of type 2 diabetes. Metformin, which acts primarily in the liver; thiazolidinediones, which primarily acts in the muscle; and sulfonylureas, which increase β-cell secretion of insulin, are examples of drugs that are used to correct or minimize these defects. Incretin deficiency and resistance, which can be treated by DPP-4 inhibitors, are also observed in diabetes. DPP-4 inhibitors improve α-cell function and

decrease hyperglucagonemia, which contributes to hyperglycemia. Fast-acting bromocriptine is available to treat insulin resistance in the brain [3]. α-Glucosidase inhibitors decrease the intestinal absorption of glucose [4], whereas reabsorption of glucose in the kidney can be inhibited by SGLT2 inhibitors [5].

Metformin

Metformin is a biguanide drug. Because insulin resistance is considered the main defect in type 2 diabetes, metformin is considered a first-line drug in the management of hyperglycemia [6, 7]. If there is no contraindication to metformin, it is considered by several guidelines to be a first-line treatment option immediately after diagnosis [6, 8]. *History.* Metformin was first synthesized in the 1920s but, due to the discovery and availability of insulin at the same time, it was not studied in clinical trials until the 1950s, when the first trial was published [8]. Together with phenformin, metformin was introduced into clinical practice in 1957 [9]. Phenformin was later withdrawn from the market due to an association with lactic acidosis. Although there was an initial delay in the approval of metformin in the USA (1995), it is currently the most prescribed antidiabetic drug in the USA and around the world. *Mechanism of action.* Metformin acts by different mechanisms and can be used to both prevent and to treat diabetes. Its main target is the liver, where it decreases basal hepatic glucose output, activates AMPK (AMP-activated protein kinase), and inhibits gluconeogenesis [8, 9]. Its action in the skeletal muscle is not as significant. There are some observational data that suggest that metformin may protect against cancer [10]. *Pharmacokinetics.* Metformin is absorbed in the small intestine and reaches its maximal concentration (Cmax) 1–2 hours after ingestion, with a half-life ranging between 1.5 and 4.9 hours. Unlike sulfonylureas, metformin is not bounded to plasma proteins [9]. It is eliminated primarily (90%) by the kidney via glomerular filtration or tubular

J. G. de Lima (✉) · L. H. C. Nóbrega · N. N. de Lima
Departamento de Medicina Clinica, Hospital Universitaro Onofre Lopes, Natal, RN, Brazil

© Springer Nature Switzerland AG 2022
F. Bandeira et al. (eds.), *Endocrinology and Diabetes*, https://doi.org/10.1007/978-3-030-90684-9_30

secretion. *Administration*. Metformin should initially be administered in small doses (500 mg or 850 mg after the largest meal of the day) to minimize the occurrence of gastrointestinal adverse effects. Afterward, the dose should be increased, with increments of one tablet every week until the maximal dose of 2550 mg/day is achieved. The extended-release formulation is generally administered once per day during the evening meal and also requires titration. Metformin is also available in combination with glipizide, glyburide, pioglitazone, repaglinide, and sitagliptin. *Efficacy*. Metformin decreases HbA1c by 1.5% and fasting glycemia by approximately 20% [11]. The typical effective dose is 1500–2000 mg/day. *Adverse effects*. Nausea, vomiting, flatulence, anorexia, and diarrhea are the most frequent adverse effects observed with metformin. These effects can be avoided if the dose is adequately titrated, as described above. Approximately 3% of patients experience a metallic taste; this effect usually resolves spontaneously. Lactic acidosis can occur because metformin blocks gluconeogenesis, resulting in the accumulation of lactate. However, this complication is very rare (1 case/100,000 person-years of exposure), as long as the drug is not administered to those with contraindications. Lactic acidosis is an extremely serious condition with a mortality rate of up to 50%. Symptoms, such as nausea, vomiting, abdominal pain, anorexia, and hypotension, are nonspecific. Metformin reduces intestinal absorption of vitamin B_{12}, and inadequate levels of this vitamin have been shown to occur in less than 10% of patients [12]. This deficiency rarely causes megaloblastic anemia and usually reverses after discontinuation of metformin. Measurements of serum vitamin B_{12} every 2–3 years may be useful to prevent complications due to B_{12} deficiency. *Contraindications*. Any condition in which the risk of acidosis is increased contraindicates the use of metformin. These conditions include congestive heart failure class 3 or 4, renal disease (men with a serum creatinine ≥ 1.5 mg/dl or women ≥ 1.4 mg/dl), impaired hepatic function, acute myocardial infarction, septicemia, cardiovascular collapse, and age > 80 years (unless creatinine clearance is adequate). If the patient requires any radiological studies with iodinated contrast, metformin should be discontinued temporarily 48 hours before and after the procedure because the contrast agent can cause renal dysfunction. Metformin should also be discontinued for any major surgery. *Advantages and disadvantages*. Metformin does not cause weight gain and can cause weight loss. It acts directly on the main defect of type 2 diabetes (insulin resistance) and also affects lipid metabolism, decreasing triglycerides and LDL. It can be used in combination with many other oral drugs, as well as with insulin. It is considered a nonexpensive drug. The only disadvantage is the possibility of adverse events, mainly gastrointestinal side effects.

Sulfonylureas

Despite some disadvantages, sulfonylureas have been used to manage type 2 diabetes for more than 50 years and, together with metformin, are the most widely used class of drugs for the treatment of type 2 diabetes. There are six sulfonylureas currently available in the USA: first-generation chlorpropamide, tolbutamide, and tolazamide, and second-generation glyburide (glibenclamide), glipizide, and glimepiride. *Mechanism of action*. Sulfonylureas target the receptor SUR, which is found on the surface of β cells. This receptor is one of two subunits in the ATP-dependent potassium channel (the other subunit is the channel itself). After binding to the SUR receptor, sulfonylureas cause the ATP-dependent potassium channel to close, resulting in an accumulation of potassium inside the β cell and a subsequent influx of calcium, ultimately leading to depolarization of the cell. Higher concentrations of intracellular calcium stimulate the migration of insulin granules to the cell surface, where they fuse to the membrane and release insulin into the bloodstream. Sulfonylureas do not seem to have a direct effect on the liver, peripheral tissues, or muscle. Instead, the effects on these tissues are realized via increased insulin secretion. *Pharmacokinetics*. After oral administration, sulfonylureas are almost completely absorbed and metabolized by the liver. First-generation sulfonylureas are extensively protein bound and excreted exclusively by the kidney. Second-generation sulfonylureas do not bind to circulating proteins and are excreted in different proportions in the urine and feces (glipizide 80% urine and 20% feces; glyburide 50% urine and 50% feces; glimepiride 60% urine and 40% feces). The onset and duration of action differ among the different drugs. All sulfonylurea agents except chlorpropamide have a short plasma half-life (4–10 hours). The half-life of chlorpropamide is longer than 24 hours. *Administration*. Usually, sulfonylureas are not prescribed first line. Instead, they are commonly used in combination with other drugs. The combination with metformin can decrease the possibility of weight gain. Thiazolidinediones, α-glucosidase inhibitors, and insulin can also be given in combination with sulfonylureas. Due to the risk of hypoglycemia, patients should be started on a low dose of sulfonylurea, which should be increased gradually every 7 days depending on the level of glycemia. If the patient adheres to his/her diet and/or loses weight, it is likely that the dose can be decreased. Chlorpropamide is administered once daily due to its longer half-life, whereas tolbutamide is administered two to three times a day, due to its very short half-life. Second-generation drugs can usually be given once a day, but maximal doses must sometimes be given in two daily doses. *Efficacy*. Sulfonylureas can decrease HbA1c by 1–2%. Like other antidiabetic drugs, the poorer the glycemic control, the greater the improvement. Glimepiride and glyburide have the highest affinity for the SUR receptor and are the most potent sulfonylureas. Tolbutamide seems to be the least potent. The best candidate to receive a prescription of a sulfonylurea is a patient who is insulin-deficient with sufficient residual β-cell secretion capacity. UKPDS and other studies have shown that the response to sulfonylureas diminishes over time, most likely because of the progressive decline in β-cell function. Monitoring glycemia and HbA1c are important to change treatment as soon as needed to avoid clinical inertia and the deterioration of diabetes control. Weight gain, poor compliance, a sedentary lifestyle, intercurrent illness (surgery, infection, and trauma), and inadequate dosage can also interfere with the efficacy. *Adverse effects.* Hypoglycemia is the most serious adverse event of sulfonylureas, and doctors and patients have to be aware of and watchful for this possibility [13]. Age, concomitant use of some drugs (β-blockers, coumarins, chloramphenicol, probenecid, inhibitors of MAO), impaired liver or kidney function, alcohol use, combined use with insulin, and prolonged exercise are risk factors for hypoglycemia. The risk of hypoglycemia is higher with glyburide than with glimepiride or gliclazide [14]. Weight gain can occur, as well as headache, asthenia, dizziness, and nausea. Hematological complications (hemolytic anemia, agranulocytosis, and thrombocytopenia) are rare and less likely to occur with second-generation sulfonylureas. Chlorpropamide can lead to hyponatremia due to water retention. Tolbutamide and chlorpropamide can cause flush if the patient drinks alcohol. Because ATP-dependent potassium channels are also present in cardiac cells and coronary vessels, sulfonylureas may decrease vasodilatation during myocardial infarction and cause more severe myocardial damage [15]. Gliclazide is more selective for pancreatic receptors and seems to have less cardiac adverse effects [15, 16]. Recently, the TOSCA IT trial showed similar long-term cardiovascular effects of sulfonylureas versus pioglitazone, given in addition to metformin, although a higher incidence of hypoglycemia with sulfonylureas [17]. *Contraindications.* Sulfonylureas cannot be used during pregnancy, and there are no studies establishing safety and effectiveness in pediatric patients. Because sulfonylureas are metabolized in the liver, they should be avoided in patients with hepatic dysfunction. Kidney dysfunction is also a relative contraindication, mainly to first-generation drugs that are excreted in the urine. *Advantages and disadvantages.* Understanding the mechanism of sulfonylureas can also shed light on sulfonylureas as a secretagogue class. On the one hand, sulfonylureas increase insulin secretion and decrease glycemia. On the other hand, long-term use could increase the possibility of β-cell failure. Furthermore, the increase in insulin secretion is independent of the level of glycemia and raises the risk for

hypoglycemia. Another disadvantage of this class is the possibility of weight gain.

Thiazolidinediones (TZD)

Thiazolidinediones activate peroxisome proliferator-activated receptor gamma (PPAR-γ) and improve insulin resistance, primarily in muscle [18, 19]. PPAR-γ is a nuclear receptor that triggers various downstream effects. While the three drugs in this class have common effects, they also have unique effects [20]. Troglitazone (Rezulin), the first PPAR-γ agonist, is no longer available due to concerns with hepatotoxicity. Rosiglitazone (Avandia) and pioglitazone (Actos) are currently on the market, but adverse cardiovascular outcomes have been observed with rosiglitazone [21, 22]. Pioglitazone, on the other hand, has a better activity on lipid metabolism, and the PROACTIVE study [23] showed some cardiovascular benefits with this drug [18, 24, 25]. The IRIS (Insulin Resistance Intervention after Stroke) trial showed pioglitazone in nondiabetic patients with insulin resistance (HOMA-IR > 3.0), and previous stroke or transient ischemic attack decreased the chance of a new event by 24% [26]. *Mechanism of action.* Classically, TZDs are insulin sensitizers that primarily act on muscle insulin resistance, in contrast to metformin, which primarily acts on the liver. Activation of PPAR-γ by TZDs can stimulate expression of several genes, including those responsible for production of glucose transporters (GLUT). These changes improve insulin activity. Decreases in TNF-α and hepatic glucokinase help to lower hyperglycemia. TZDs can also modulate lipid metabolism and adipocyte differentiation. Different affinities for PPAR-α and PPAR-δ can explain the different clinical effects of the TZDs [24]. *Pharmacokinetics.* The main structure (thiazolidine-2-4-dione) of TZDs is common to all drugs in this class, and modifications in the side chain are responsible for differences in pharmacokinetics. TZDs are extensively bound to serum protein (>99%). Cytochrome P450 enzymes are important for the metabolism of rosiglitazone (CYP2C8 and CYP2C9) and pioglitazone (CYP3A4). *Administration.* TZDs can be taken without regard to meals. They can be prescribed as monotherapy or in combination with metformin, DPP-IV inhibitors, sulfonylureas, or insulin [27]. Rosiglitazone is available in 2, 4, and 8 mg tablets to be given once or twice a day. There are 15, 30, and 45 mg tablets of pioglitazone and should always be taken once daily. Although no studies have demonstrated alterations in liver function tests, as was observed with troglitazone, it is recommended to measure liver function prior to initiating therapy and periodically thereafter. Dose adjustments are not needed in patients with kidney dysfunction, but if there is any active liver disease or if serum ALT levels are >2.5 times the upper limit of normal, TZDs should not be prescribed. *Efficacy.* TZDs can decrease HbA1c by between 0.5 and 1.5%. This decrease is similar for both pioglitazone and rosiglitazone [25, 28]. Because pioglitazone has a higher affinity for PPAR-α, it has a better lipid profile and has been shown to lower triglyceridemia and increase HDL [24, 25]. *Adverse effects.* Weight gain (1–4 kg) can occur due to changes in adipocyte differentiation. Metabolically, this increase in weight is not a large problem, because it generally correlates with a decrease in visceral fat and an increase in subcutaneous fat and a reduction in the number of large adipocytes and an increase in the small adipocytes, which results in lowering free fatty acids and reducing insulin resistance. The activation of PPAR-γ can increase adipocyte formation rather than osteoblasts, which can increase the risk of osteoporosis and fractures [21, 26]. Hypoglycemia is not a concern with TZDs but may be in patients taking a TZD with a sulfonylurea or a TZD and insulin. Due to volume expansion, edema, anemia, and heart failure can occur [22, 26]. Edema generally occurs if TZDs are combined with insulin. There are some data suggesting that pioglitazone may increase the risk of bladder cancer [24], but this is still controversial, and a recent meta-analysis did not show this association [29]. *Contraindications.* TZDs can exacerbate heart failure and should be avoided in patients with NYHA class 3 or 4. *Advantages and disadvantages.* TZDs are good options for the treatment of type 2 diabetes. They are generally not used as monotherapy but can add benefits if prescribed in combination with others drugs. Anemia, heart failure, and osteoporosis, as well as controversy regarding cardiovascular risk, are some limitations of this class. Pioglitazone is a good choice for patients who need to improve their lipid profile (triglycerides and HDL) [30].

DPP-4 Inhibitors

In the last few years, a better understanding of the effects of incretin has identified new targets for diabetes treatment [31]. Glucose-dependent insulinotropic polypeptide (GIP) and glucagon-like peptide 1 (GLP-1) are incretins produced by intestinal K and L cells. Their activity in islets cells depends on glycemia. During hyperglycemia, they can stimulate β cell and inhibit α-cell function, thus increasing insulin and decreasing glucagon, resulting in normal glycemia. During hypoglycemia, insulin secretion decreases and glucagon increases to restore normoglycemia. The major problem to using GIP and GLP-1 in the treatment of diabetes is the fact that they are degraded by the DPP-4 enzyme and, consequently, have very short half-lives. GLP-1 agonists/analogs

with longer half-lives or DPP-4 inhibitors can be used as clinical tools [31]. Sitagliptin, linagliptin, and saxagliptin are DPP-4 inhibitors available in the USA. Vildagliptin is available in other countries around the world. *Mechanism of action.* Oral intake of glucose can induce a higher increase in insulin secretion than venous glucose administration. This is called the incretin effect and is mediated by intestinal hormones, mainly GIP and GLP-1. Gliptins act by inhibiting the enzymatic breakdown of GIP and GLP-1, thereby prolonging their effects in several tissues. *Pharmacokinetics.* Gliptins are quickly absorbed after oral administration. Sitagliptin is metabolized in the liver by CYP3A4, and 79% is excreted unchanged in the urine. Patients with kidney failure need dosage adjustments of saxagliptin, sitagliptin, and vildagliptin. There is no clinically relevant interaction with other drugs. *Administration.* Oral administration with or without food is recommended [saxagliptin (2.5 or 5.0 mg/day), linagliptin (5 mg/day), alogliptin (25, 12.5, or 6.25 mg/day), and sitagliptin (100, 50, or 25 mg/day)], except if given in combination with metformin, when the dose is divided and taken twice daily. Vildagliptin 50 mg is given twice daily. In patients with kidney failure, dosage adjustments must be made for saxagliptin (2.5 mg/day if GFR <50 mL/min/1.73 m^2), alogliptin (12.5 mg if GFR 30 to 60 mL/min/1.73 m^2 and 6.25 mg if <30 ml/min/1.73 m^2), sitagliptin (50 mg if GFR 30 to 50 mL/min/1.73 m^2 and 25 mg if <30 ml/min/1.73 m^2), and vildagliptin. *Efficacy.* These drugs cause a modest decrease in HbA1c (0.4–0.9%) [32], and all the DPP-4 inhibitors appear to have similar efficacy [33]. The decrease in postprandial glycemia is more prominent than in fasting glycemia. For this reason, combination of DPP-4 inhibitors with metformin is a good option because metformin decreases nocturnal hepatic glucose output, whereas gliptin decreases postprandial increments. The unique mechanism of action, which does not promote hypoglycemia, weight gain or serious adverse effects [32], and the possibility (not yet proven in humans) of β-cell proliferation or protection make this class quite useful. *Adverse effects.* Patients taking gliptin usually do not complain about side effects [31]. DPP-4 is not specific for GLP-1, and, while the effects of DPP-4 inhibition on other DPP-4 substrates are unknown, they do not seem to be clinically relevant. Effects on immune function remain a concern; in clinical trials, nasopharyngitis, upper respiratory tract infection, and headaches occurred more often in patients treated with DPP-4 inhibitors [34]. When administered as monotherapy, the incidence of hypoglycemia with DPP-4 inhibitors was similar to that of placebo, but if administered in combination with a sulfonylurea, it is important to remember that sulfonylureas have a higher probability to cause hypoglycemia. If DPP-4 inhibitors are combined with metformin or pioglitazone, there is no additional risk of hypoglycemia. Cases of acute pancreatitis have been reported in patients on sitagliptin [35] as well as in patients treated with exenatide, but upon reviewing these cases, the incidence is similar to that in the diabetic control group [36]. *Safety*. Saxagliptin (SAVOR-TIMI 53), linagliptin (EXAMINE), and sitagliptin (TECOS) have already published trials evaluating cardiovascular events [37–39]. None of these drugs increase or decrease the risk of major adverse cardiovascular events. Saxagliptin increase the rate of heart failure hospitalization [39]. *Advantages and disadvantages*. The major advantage of the DPP-4 inhibitors is achieving good glycemic control without hypoglycemia. Effects beyond glycemia are still being studied and need to be confirmed. Preservation of β-cell function is also a possible advantage. The small decrease in HbA1c and the high cost are disadvantages. DPP-4 inhibitors are commonly used in combination with metformin and most of the other types of antidiabetic drugs, but if there is intolerance or any contraindication to metformin, pioglitazone, or sulfonylureas, the gliptins can be used as monotherapy.

α-Glucosidase Inhibitors

Some studies have suggested that post-prandial glycemia (PPG) is a better predictor of cardiovascular risk than fasting glycemia [40]. In this context, the α-glucosidase inhibitors offer the possibility to decrease PPG while decreasing cardiovascular risk. This class was first available to reduce PPG, but due to the adverse gastrointestinal effects and the availability of DPP-4 inhibitors, it is not commonly used. These drugs are a third-line choice for treating diabetes. There are two medications available: acarbose (Precose) and miglitol (Glyset). *Mechanism of action*. α-Glucosidase inhibitors reversibly bind to α-glucosidases (sucrase, maltase, glucoamylase, isomaltase) found in the brush border and delay the absorption of carbohydrates in the small intestine, decreasing the PPG peak [4]. These enzymes assist in the digestion of oligosaccharides and disaccharides into monosaccharides. *Pharmacokinetics*. Acarbose only acts in the small intestine and is not absorbed, while miglitol is almost entirely absorbed and could have some additional extraintestinal effects, decreasing hepatic glycogenolysis (in vitro *studies*). Approximately 1–2% of active acarbose is absorbed, and, after metabolism in the liver, it is excreted by the kidneys. The bioavailability of miglitol ranges from 50% to 100%, and absorption does not affect the hypoglycemic effectiveness. Miglitol is not metabolized and is excreted unchanged by the kidneys or, if not absorbed, in the feces. *Administration*. These drugs must be given with each meal, and, because of the gastrointestinal side effects, patients

should gradually increase the dose to maximize effectiveness and decrease side effects. For example, patients can start with 25 mg tid and slowly increase the dose to 50–100 mg tid. Some patients will need to begin with a once-daily dose. Because the drugs only work in the presence of dietary carbohydrate, the doses should be given with the first bite of each meal. Acarbose is approved as monotherapy or in combination with metformin, sulfonylureas, or insulin. Miglitol is approved as monotherapy or in combination with sulfonylureas. *Efficacy*. There is a modest decrease in HbA1c (0.5 a 1.0%) with these drugs [4]. The improvement in PPG (40–50 mg/dl) is better than the improvement in fasting glycemia (25–30 mg/dl). There is no head-to-head comparative study of the two α-glucosidase inhibitors, but the efficacies of acarbose and miglitol seem to be similar. *Adverse effects*. Side effects are mainly gastrointestinal and depend on the correct administration and titration of the dose. Because these drugs delay the absorption of carbohydrates, production of gas by the natural flora of the large intestine can lead to flatulence, abdominal distention, and diarrhea [41]. These side effects are usually transient but can occur in up to 60% of patients and are one limitation to the use of this class. During clinical trials, elevation in liver enzymes occurred in patients taking doses of 200–300 mg tid of acarbose, and the manufacturer recommends measuring liver function every 3 months during the first year [42]. The α-glucosidase inhibitors do not cause hypoglycemia but can do so if used in combination with sulfonylureas or insulin. If a patient taking combination therapy experiences an episode of hypoglycemia, he needs to use glucose tablets or a glucagon injection instead of food because complex carbohydrate absorption will be blocked. Neither acarbose nor miglitol caused weight loss. The ACE (Acarbose Cardiovascular Evaluation) trial studied patients with impaired glucose tolerance and coronary heart disease, comparing acarbose 50 mg three times a day or matched placebo. After almost 6 years, there was no significant cardiovascular difference between groups [43]. *Contraindications*. Because miglitol is eliminated by the kidney, it should not be used if creatinine clearance is lower than 25 ml/min/1.73 m^2 or if plasma creatinine is higher than 2.0 mg/dl. Both acarbose and miglitol are contraindicated in pregnancy and nursing as well as in diabetic ketoacidosis, inflammatory bowel disease, intestinal obstruction, colonic ulceration, and hypersensitivity to acarbose or miglitol.

Glinides

The only glinides currently available are nateglinide and repaglinide. Glinides are secretagogue agents such as sulfonylureas, but they have a reduced risk of hypoglycemia due to their short half-life and can be taken only when the patient eats. *Mechanism of action.* Like sulfonylureas, glinides bind to a membrane receptor found in β cells and close the ATP-dependent potassium channel, resulting in depolarization of the cell and opening of calcium channels [44]. The influx of calcium induces insulin secretion. Although their mechanism is very similar to that of sulfonylureas, the onset is faster, and the duration is shorter (fast on, fast off). *Pharmacokinetics.* Inactive metabolites of repaglinide are excreted in the feces after metabolization via oxidative biotransformation. Nateglinide is metabolized in the liver by CYP3A4 (30%) and CYP2C9 (70%), and approximately 16% is excreted unchanged by the kidneys. *Administration.* Repaglinide is available in tablets of 0.5, 1, and 2 mg, and nateglinide is available in 60 and 120 mg tablets. Administration with food does not affect the bioavailability of repaglinide but decreases that of nateglinide. Repaglinide can be taken at the start of each meal or 15–30 minutes before, while nateglinide is better taken 1–30 minutes before each meal [45]. If a meal is skipped or added, a dose of repaglinide must be skipped or added. *Efficacy.* Glinides act mainly on postprandial glycemia, and reduction of HbA1c is between 0.7 and 1.5% [46]. Glinides can be used with other antidiabetic drugs, except for sulfonylureas. Because the efficacy and action are similar to that of sulfonylureas, if a patient is already on sulfonylureas, there is no advantage to change to glinides. *Adverse effects.* Like sulfonylureas, hypoglycemia can occur but is less frequent. Weight gain can occur because glinides increase insulin secretion. Other adverse effects such as headache, arthralgia, nausea, upper respiratory infections, and constipation are rare. *Contraindications.* Glinides cannot be used during pregnancy or by nursing mothers. There are no studies in children, and the use of glinides in this population is not recommended. *Advantages and disadvantages.* Because of the lower incidence of hypoglycemia, older patients can experience some benefits with the glinides. The efficacy and action are similar to sulfonylureas, but because there is no sulfa moiety, patients with allergies to sulfa can use these drugs. The administration immediately before each meal is also an advantage for patients who do not eat at regular times throughout the day. Higher cost and lower HbA1c reduction than sulfonylureas are some disadvantages. No dose adjustment is necessary for patients with moderate renal failure. Nateglinide can also be used without adjustment in patients with moderate hepatic failure, but the dose of repaglinide may need to be reduced.

Bromocriptine

Bromocriptine mesylate quick release was approved by FDA in May 2009 and is the only antidiabetic drug that acts not in the pancreas, liver, or muscle but in the hypothalamus. *Mechanism of action.* Bromocriptine is an ergot derivate sympatholytic D2-dopamine agonist that acts centrally to modulate glucose and energy pathways, resulting in an increase in hypothalamic dopamine and inhibition of sympathetic and serotonergic activities. As a result, hepatic glucose output, insulin resistance, free fat acids, triglyceridemia, and glycemia are reduced. *Pharmacokinetics.* After oral administration, 65–95% of an administered dose is absorbed, but only 7% reaches the systemic circulation after first-pass hepatic metabolism. Bromocriptine is metabolized by CYP3A4 and excreted primarily in the bile, with only 2–6% excreted in the urine. *Administration.* The quick-release bromocriptine is administered once daily, 2 hours after waking, in the morning, with food to reduce the possibility of nausea. Patients start with one tablet (0.8 mg) and increase the dose by one tablet/week as needed, until the maximal dose of six tablets (4.8 mg) is reached. *Efficacy.* Bromocriptine reduces HbA1c by 0.4–0.8% and can be used alone or in combination with any other antidiabetic drug [47]. *Adverse effects.* Nausea is the most common adverse effect (32%) and can be reduced with dose titration. Asthenia, constipation, dizziness, and rhinitis can occur [47]. *Contraindications.* There are no studies in patients with renal or hepatic failure. Bromocriptine quick release is different from the 2.5–5.0 mg bromocriptine that is used for pituitary adenomas. Psychosis, type 1 diabetes and syncopal attacks are contraindications. *Advantages and disadvantages.* The mechanism of action is different from all other drugs used to type 2 diabetes. Therefore, bromocriptine can be an option for patients already on other drugs who are not able to achieve glycemic control. Bromocriptine can also reduce weight, and a study has shown that it may also reduce cardiovascular events [3]. Adverse effects, mainly nausea, can limit its use.

Gliflozins

The gliflozins, also known as SGLT2 (sodium-glucose cotransporter-2) inhibitors, are a new class antihyperglycemic agents. There are three drugs currently approved by the FDA to treat type 2 diabetes: empagliflozin (approved in August 2014), canagliflozin (approved in March 2013), and dapagliflozin (approved in January 2014). *Mechanism of action.* The SGLT2 proteins are located in renal tubules and are responsible for reabsorbing glucose and sodium back into the blood. The gliflozins inhibit those proteins, increasing the excretion of glucose and sodium. As a result, they lower glucose levels and blood pressure and cause weight loss, because of the calories lost as glucose. The mechanism of action does not depend on beta-cell function and insulin secretion, and the risk of hypoglycemia is very low. *Pharmacokinetics.* Gliflozins are quickly absorbed after oral administration, and peak plasma concentration occurs within 1–2 hours post-dose. Patients with kidney failure cannot use this class of drugs because it will not be effective, due to its renal mechanism of action. Coadministration of these drugs with diuretics can increase urine volume and enhance the potential for volume depletion, and coadministration with insulin or sulfonylureas can increase the risk of hypoglycemia, which can be minimized by lowering the dose of the insulin/sulfonylureas. Glycemic control with 1,5-anhydroglucitol assay is not recommended because SGLT2 inhibitors can interfere with the results. *Administration.* Oral administration with or without food is recommended: dapagliflozin (5 or 10 mg/day), empagliflozin (10 or 25 mg/day), and canagliflozin (100 or 300 mg/day). In patients with kidney failure, no dosage adjustments are necessary, but the drug will not be effective, due to its renal action. Canagliflozin should not be initiated if glomerular filtration rate (GFR) < 45 ml/min/1.73 m^2, and its dose should be limited to 100 mg/day if GFR between 45 and 60 ml/min/1.73 m^2. Dapagliflozin should not be used if GFR < 60 ml/min/1.73 m^2 and empagliflozin if GFR < 45 ml/min/1.73 m^2. *Efficacy.* These drugs cause a modest decrease in HbA1c (0.7–1.0%) after 24 weeks of usage. Safety and effectiveness in pediatric patients have not been evaluated. In patients with high cardiovascular risk, empagliflozin had a lower rate of death for cardiovascular causes (38% risk relative reduction), hospitalization for heart failure (35% risk relative reduction), and death from any cause (32% risk relative reduction) [48]. Cardiovascular effects with canagliflozin have also been studied: the risk of major adverse cardiovascular events (MACE) decreased by 13% compared to placebo [49]. *Adverse effects.* Some of the adverse effects are common to all of the drugs in this class, such as symptomatic hypotension, increase in creatinine and decrease in GFR, hypoglycemia if associated with insulin or secretagogues, genital mycotic and urinary tract infections, and LDL increase. The symptomatic hypotension occurs due to

the intravascular volume contraction. It can occur particularly in patients with impaired renal function, elderly, and patients using loop diuretics, so these symptoms must be monitored especially in these groups. They also can increase serum creatinine and decrease GFR, so the renal function should be evaluated before initiating the therapy and monitored periodically, especially in patients with moderate renal impairment and in the elderly. The FDA has warned of the risk of acute renal failure with canagliflozin and dapagliflozin. Patients with decreased blood volume, chronic kidney insufficiency, congestive heart failure, or taking other medications such as diuretics, angiotensin-converting enzyme inhibitors, angiotensin receptor blockers, and nonsteroidal anti-inflammatory drugs are more predisposed [50]. Patients with previous history of genital mycotic infections are more likely to develop this condition when using the gliflozins. Urinary tract infections are less frequent. Inhibitors of SGLT2 can increase glucagon and cause euglycemic diabetic ketoacidosis (DKA), especially in patients with insulin-deficient diabetes [51]. So if a patient has clinical symptoms of DKA, it should be suspected and treated appropriately, and the gliflozin must be suspended until the resolution of this condition. Canagliflozin use doubles leg and foot amputations [49], but this was not observed with empagliflozin [52]. *Contraindications.* The gliflozins should not be prescribed if there is severe renal impairment and end-stage renal disease or patients are on dialysis. This class is pregnancy category C. *Advantages and disadvantages.* These drugs have a completely new mechanism of action that consists in increasing renal elimination of glucose and sodium. Therefore, it can also decrease blood pressure control and body weight, with a low risk of hypoglycemia. Empagliflozin and canagliflozin decrease the risk of cardiovascular events in patients with elevated risk.

Conclusion

Some years ago we did not have so many drugs to treat diabetic patients. Currently, we have several options (Table 30.1). A thorough understanding of the mechanism of action of each drug, as well their advantages, contraindications, and side effects, is essential to choosing the best drug or combination of drugs to achieve good glycemic control with minimal side effects, thus preventing acute and chronic complications of type 2 diabetes.

Table 30.1 Oral drugs to treat type 2 diabetes

Drug	Daily dose	Reduction in HbA1c	Side effects	Contraindications
Metformin (500 mg, 850 mg, 1000 mg. Extended-release: 500 mg/750 mg, 1000 mg)	Initial small dose and titrate. Max 2550 mg/day	1–2%	Nauseas, vomiting, flatulence, anorexia, abdominal pain, diarrhea	Congestive heart failure (class 3 or 4), serum creatinine ≥1.5 mg/dl (man) ≥ 1.4 mg/dl (woman), impaired hepatic function, acute myocardial infarction, septicemia
Chlorpropamide (Diabinese) 100 mg, 250 mg	Initial: 250 mg. Max: 750 mg	1–2%	Hypoglycemia, weight gain, photosensitivity	Type 1 diabetes; pregnancy and nursing
Glimepiride (Amaryl) 1 mg, 2 mg, 4 mg	Initial: 1–2 mg.Max: 8 mg			
Glyburide (Diabeta) 1.25 mg, 2.5 mg, 5 mg	Initial: 2.5–5 mg. Max: 20 mg			
Glipizide 5 mg, 10 mg. Extended-release 2.5 mg, 5 mg, 10 mg	Initial: 5 mg Max: 20 mg			
Pioglitazone (Actos) 15 mg, 30 mg, 45 mg	Initial: 15–30 mg. Max: 45 mg	0,5–1,5%	Weight gain, osteoporosis/fracture, bladder cancer (pioglitazone), cardiovascular event (rosiglitazone)	Heart failure NYHA classes 3 and 4
Rosiglitazone (Avandia) 2 mg, 4 mg, 8 mg	Initial: 2 mg bid or 4 mg qd. Max: 8 mg			
Sitagliptin (25 mg, 50 mg, 100 mg); saxagliptin (2.5 mg, 5 mg), linagliptin (5 mg), alogliptin (25 mg, 12.5 mg, 6.25 mg).	According to renal function (except linagliptin)	0.4–0.9%	Increase heart failure hospitalization (saxagliptin)	–
Acarbose (Precose) 25 mg, 50 mg, 100 mg	Initial: 25 mg tid. Max: >60 kg–100 mg tid; <60 kg–50 mg tid	0.4–1.0%	Flatulence, abdominal distention, diarrhea. If in combination with other drug and patient develop mild hypoglycemia, use dextrose, not sucrose (cane sugar) to treat	Renal failure (clearance Cr < 25 ml/min or creatinine >2 mg/dl. Ketoacidosis, bowel disease, colonic ulceration
Miglitol (Glyset) 25 mg, 50 mg, 100 mg	Initial: 25 mg tid. Max: 100 mg tid			
Nateglinide (Starlix) 60 mg, 120 mg	Initial/Max: 120 mg tid	0.7–1.5%	Hypoglycemia, headache, arthralgia, nausea, upper respiratory infections, constipation	Children, pregnancy, nursing, type 1 diabetes, ketoacidosis
Repaglinide (Prandin) 0.5 mg, 1 mg, 2 mg	Initial (depends on HbA1c): 0.5–1 mg tid. Max: 16 mg/day			
Bromocriptine (Cycloset) 0.8 mg	Initial: 0.8 mg 2 h after waking in the morning. Max: 4.8 mg	0.4–0.8%	Nausea, fatigue, constipation, dizziness, rhinitis, headache	Renal and hepatic failure, psychosis, type 1 diabetes, syncopal attacks, migraine headache
Dapagliflozin (Farxiga); canagliflozin (Invokana); empagliflozin (Jardiance)	Dapagliflozin 5 mg, 10 mg Canagliflozin 100 mg, 300 mg Empagliflozin 10 mg, 25 mg	0.7–1.0%	Genital and urinary tract infections, hypotension, increase of LDL, euglycemic diabetic ketoacidosis	Severe renal impairment

References

1. Intensive blood-glucose control with sulphonylureas or insulin compared with conventional treatment and risk of complications in patients with type 2 diabetes (UKPDS 33). UK Prospective Diabetes Study (UKPDS) Group. Lancet. 1998;352:837–53.
2. Effects of intensive glucose lowering in type 2 diabetes. N Engl J Med. 2008;358:2545–59.
3. Gaziano JM, Cincotta AH, O'Connor CM, Ezrokhi M, Rutty D, Ma ZJ, Scranton RE. Randomized clinical trial of quick-release bromocriptine among patients with type 2 diabetes on overall safety and cardiovascular outcomes. Diabetes Care. 2010;33:1503–8.
4. Holman RR, Cull CA, Turner RC. A randomized double-blind trial of acarbose in type 2 diabetes shows improved glycemic control over 3 years (U.K. Prospective Diabetes Study 44). Diabetes Care. 1999;22:960–4.
5. Bolinder J, Ljunggren O, Kullberg J, Johansson L, Wilding J, Langkilde AM, Sugg J, Parikh S. Effects of dapagliflozin on body weight, total fat mass, and regional adipose tissue distribution in patients with type 2 diabetes mellitus with inadequate glycemic control on metformin. J Clin Endocrinol Metab. 2012;97:1020–31.
6. Nathan DM, Buse JB, Davidson MB, Ferrannini E, Holman RR, Sherwin R, Zinman B. Medical management of hyperglycemia in type 2 diabetes: a consensus algorithm for the initiation and adjustment of therapy: a consensus statement of the American

Diabetes Association and the European Association for the Study of Diabetes. Diabetes Care. 2009;32:193–203.

7. Handelsman Y, Mechanick JI, Blonde L, Grunberger G, Bloomgarden ZT, Bray GA, Dagogo-Jack S, Davidson JA, Einhorn D, Ganda O, Garber AJ, Hirsch IB, Horton ES, Ismail-Beigi F, Jellinger PS, Jones KL, Jovanovic L, Lebovitz H, Levy P, Moghissi ES, Orzeck EA, Vinik AI, Wyne KL. American Association of Clinical Endocrinologists Medical Guidelines for Clinical Practice for developing a diabetes mellitus comprehensive care plan. Endocr Pract. 2011;17 Suppl 2:1–53.

8. Viollet B, Guigas B, Sanz Garcia N, Leclerc J, Foretz M, Andreelli F. Cellular and molecular mechanisms of metformin: an overview. Clin Sci (Lond). 2012;122:253–70.

9. Bailey CJ. Biguanides and NIDDM. Diabetes Care. 1992;15:755–72.

10. Libby G, Donnelly LA, Donnan PT, Alessi DR, Morris AD, Evans JM. New users of metformin are at low risk of incident cancer: a cohort study among people with type 2 diabetes. Diabetes Care. 2009;32:1620–5.

11. DeFronzo RA, Goodman AM. Efficacy of metformin in patients with non-insulin-dependent diabetes mellitus. The Multicenter Metformin Study Group. N Engl J Med. 1995;333:541–9.

12. de Jager J, Kooy A, Lehert P, Wulffele MG, van der Kolk J, Bets D, Verburg J, Donker AJ, Stehouwer CD. Long term treatment with metformin in patients with type 2 diabetes and risk of vitamin B-12 deficiency: randomised placebo controlled trial. BMJ. 2010;340:c2181.

13. Shorr RI, Ray WA, Daugherty JR, Griffin MR. Individual sulfonyl-ureas and serious hypoglycemia in older people. J Am Geriatr Soc. 1996;44:751–5.

14. Gangji AS, Cukierman T, Gerstein HC, Goldsmith CH, Clase CM. A systematic review and meta-analysis of hypoglycemia and cardiovascular events: a comparison of glyburide with other secre-tagogues and with insulin. Diabetes Care. 2007;30:389–94.

15. Schramm TK, Gislason GH, Vaag A, Rasmussen JN, Folke F, Hansen ML, Fosbol EL, Kober L, Norgaard ML, Madsen M, Hansen PR, Torp-Pedersen C. Mortality and cardiovascular risk associated with different insulin secretagogues compared with met-formin in type 2 diabetes, with or without a previous myocardial infarction: a nationwide study. Eur Heart J. 2011;32:1900–8.

16. Lee TM, Lin MS, Tsai CH, Huang CL, Chang NC. Effects of sul-fonylureas on left ventricular mass in type 2 diabetic patients. Am J Physiol Heart Circ Physiol. 2007;292:H608–13.

17. Vaccaro O, Masulli M, Nicolucci A, Bonora E, Del Prato S, Maggioni AP, Rivellese AA, Squatrito S, Giorda CB, Sesti G, Mocarelli P, Lucisano G, Sacco M, Signorini S, Cappellini F, Perriello G, Babini AC, Lapolla A, Gregori G, Giordano C, Corsi L, Buzzetti R, Clemente G, Di Cianni G, Iannarelli R, Cordera R, La Macchia O, Zamboni C, Scaranna C, Boemi M, Iovine C, Lauro D, Leotta S, Dall'Aglio E, Cannarsa E, Tonutti L, Pugliese G, Bossi AC, Anichini R, Dotta F, Di Benedetto A, Citro G, Antenucci D, Ricci L, Giorgino F, Santini C, Gnasso A, De Cosmo S, Zavaroni D, Vedovato M, Consoli A, Calabrese M, di Bartolo P, Fornengo P, Riccardi G. Effects on the incidence of cardiovascular events of the addition of pioglitazone versus sulfonylureas in patients with type 2 diabetes inadequately controlled with metformin (TOSCA. IT): a randomised, multicentre trial. Lancet Diabetes Endocrinol. 2017;5:887–97.

18. Yki-Jarvinen H. Thiazolidinediones. N Engl J Med. 2004;351:1106–18.

19. Park KS, Ciaraldi TP, Abrams-Carter L, Mudaliar S, Nikoulina SE, Henry RR. PPAR-gamma gene expression is elevated in skeletal muscle of obese and type II diabetic subjects. Diabetes. 1997;46:1230–4.

20. Vidal-Puig AJ, Considine RV, Jimenez-Linan M, Werman A, Pories WJ, Caro JF, Flier JS. Peroxisome proliferator-activated recep-tor gene expression in human tissues. Effects of obesity, weight loss, and regulation by insulin and glucocorticoids. J Clin Invest. 1997;99:2416–22.

21. Home PD, Pocock SJ, Beck-Nielsen H, Curtis PS, Gomis R, Hanefeld M, Jones NP, Komajda M, McMurray JJ. Rosiglitazone evaluated for cardiovascular outcomes in oral agent combination therapy for type 2 diabetes (RECORD): a multicentre, randomised, open-label trial. Lancet. 2009;373:2125–35.

22. Lipscombe LL, Gomes T, Levesque LE, Hux JE, Juurlink DN, Alter DA. Thiazolidinediones and cardiovascular outcomes in older patients with diabetes. JAMA. 2007;298:2634–43.

23. Dormandy JA, Charbonnel B, Eckland DJ, Erdmann E, Massi-Benedetti M, Moules IK, Skene AM, Tan MH, Lefebvre PJ, Murray GD, Standl E, Wilcox RG, Wilhelmsen L, Betteridge J, Birkeland K, Golay A, Heine RJ, Koranyi L, Laakso M, Mokan M, Norkus A, Pirags V, Podar T, Scheen A, Scherbaum W, Schernthaner G, Schmitz O, Skrha J, Smith U, Taton J. Secondary prevention of macrovascular events in patients with type 2 diabetes in the PROactive Study (PROspective pioglitAzone Clinical Trial In macroVascular Events): a randomised controlled trial. Lancet. 2005;366:1279–89.

24. Friedland SN, Leong A, Filion KB, Genest J, Lega IC, Mottillo S, Poirier P, Reoch J, Eisenberg MJ. The cardiovascular effects of peroxisome proliferator-activated receptor agonists. Am J Med. 2012;125:126–33.

25. Chiquette E, Ramirez G, Defronzo R. A meta-analysis comparing the effect of thiazolidinediones on cardiovascular risk factors. Arch Intern Med. 2004;164:2097–104.

26. Kernan WN, Viscoli CM, Furie KL, Young LH, Inzucchi SE, Gorman M, Guarino PD, Lovejoy AM, Peduzzi PN, Conwit R, Brass LM, Schwartz GG, Adams HP Jr, Berger L, Carolei A, Clark W, Coull B, Ford GA, Kleindorfer D, O'Leary JR, Parsons MW, Ringleb P, Sen S, Spence JD, Tanne D, Wang D, Winder TR. Pioglitazone after ischemic stroke or transient ischemic attack. N Engl J Med. 2016;374:1321–31.

27. Fonseca V, Rosenstock J, Patwardhan R, Salzman A. Effect of metformin and rosiglitazone combination therapy in patients with type 2 diabetes mellitus: a randomized controlled trial. JAMA. 2000;283:1695–702.

28. Aronoff S, Rosenblatt S, Braithwaite S, Egan JW, Mathisen AL, Schneider RL. Pioglitazone hydrochloride monotherapy improves glycemic control in the treatment of patients with type 2 diabetes: a 6-month randomized placebo-controlled dose-response study. The Pioglitazone 001 Study Group. Diabetes Care. 2000;23:1605–11.

29. Filipova E, Uzunova K, Kalinov K, Vekov T. Pioglitazone and the risk of bladder cancer: a meta-analysis. Diabetes Ther. 2017;8:705–26.

30. Goldberg RB, Kendall DM, Deeg MA, Buse JB, Zagar AJ, Pinaire JA, Tan MH, Khan MA, Perez AT, Jacober SJ. A comparison of lipid and glycemic effects of pioglitazone and rosiglitazone in patients with type 2 diabetes and dyslipidemia. Diabetes Care. 2005;28:1547–54.

31. Drucker DJ, Nauck MA. The incretin system: glucagon-like pep-tide-1 receptor agonists and dipeptidyl peptidase-4 inhibitors in type 2 diabetes. Lancet. 2006;368:1696–705.

32. Richter B, Bandeira-Echtler E, Bergerhoff K, Lerch CL. Dipeptidyl peptidase-4 (DPP-4) inhibitors for type 2 diabetes mellitus. Cochrane Database Syst Rev. 2008:CD006739.

33. Scheen AJ, Charpentier G, Ostgren CJ, Hellqvist A, Gause-Nilsson I. Efficacy and safety of saxagliptin in combination with metformin compared with sitagliptin in combination with metformin in adult patients with type 2 diabetes mellitus. Diabetes Metab Res Rev. 2010;26:540–9.

34. Amori RE, Lau J, Pittas AG. Efficacy and safety of incretin therapy in type 2 diabetes: systematic review and meta-analysis. JAMA. 2007;298:194–206.

35. Elashoff M, Matveyenko AV, Gier B, Elashoff R, Butler PC. Pancreatitis, pancreatic, and thyroid cancer with glucagon-like peptide-1-based therapies. Gastroenterology. 2011;141:150–6.

36. Garg R, Chen W, Pendergrass M. Acute pancreatitis in type 2 diabetes treated with exenatide or sitagliptin: a retrospective observational pharmacy claims analysis. Diabetes Care. 2010;33:2349–54.

37. Green JB, Bethel MA, Armstrong PW, Buse JB, Engel SS, Garg J, Josse R, Kaufman KD, Koglin J, Korn S, Lachin JM, McGuire DK, Pencina MJ, Standl E, Stein PP, Suryawanshi S, Van de Werf F, Peterson ED, Holman RR. Effect of sitagliptin on cardiovascular outcomes in type 2 diabetes. N Engl J Med. 2015;373:232–42.

38. White WB, Cannon CP, Heller SR, Nissen SE, Bergenstal RM, Bakris GL, Perez AT, Fleck PR, Mehta CR, Kupfer S, Wilson C, Cushman WC, Zannad F. Alogliptin after acute coronary syndrome in patients with type 2 diabetes. N Engl J Med. 2013;369:1327–35.

39. Scirica BM, Bhatt DL, Braunwald E, Steg PG, Davidson J, Hirshberg B, Ohman P, Frederich R, Wiviott SD, Hoffman EB, Cavender MA, Udell JA, Desai NR, Mosenzon O, McGuire DK, Ray KK, Leiter LA, Raz I. Saxagliptin and cardiovascular outcomes in patients with type 2 diabetes mellitus. N Engl J Med. 2013;369:1317–26.

40. Glucose tolerance and mortality: comparison of WHO and American Diabetes Association diagnostic criteria. The DECODE study group. European Diabetes Epidemiology Group. Diabetes Epidemiology: Collaborative analysis Of Diagnostic criteria in Europe. Lancet. 1999;354:617–21.

41. Chiasson JL, Josse RG, Hunt JA, Palmason C, Rodger NW, Ross SA, Ryan EA, Tan MH, Wolever TM. The efficacy of acarbose in the treatment of patients with non-insulin-dependent diabetes mellitus. A multicenter controlled clinical trial. Ann Intern Med. 1994;121:928–35.

42. Carrascosa M, Pascual F, Aresti S. Acarbose-induced acute severe hepatotoxicity. Lancet. 1997;349:698–9.

43. Holman RR, Coleman RL, Chan JCN, Chiasson JL, Feng H, Ge J, Gerstein HC, Gray R, Huo Y, Lang Z, McMurray JJ, Ryden L, Schroder S, Sun Y, Theodorakis MJ, Tendera M, Tucker L, Tuomilehto J, Wei Y, Yang W, Wang D, Hu D, Pan C. Effects of acarbose on cardiovascular and diabetes outcomes in patients with coronary heart disease and impaired glucose tolerance (ACE): a randomised, double-blind, placebo-controlled trial. Lancet Diabetes Endocrinol. 2017;5:877–86.

44. Fuhlendorff J, Rorsman P, Kofod H, Brand CL, Rolin B, MacKay P, Shymko R, Carr RD. Stimulation of insulin release by repaglinide and glibenclamide involves both common and distinct processes. Diabetes. 1998;47:345–51.

45. Schmitz O, Lund S, Andersen PH, Jonler M, Porksen N. Optimizing insulin secretagogue therapy in patients with type 2 diabetes: a randomized double-blind study with repaglinide. Diabetes Care. 2002;25:342–6.

46. Wolffenbuttel BH, Landgraf R. A 1-year multicenter randomized double-blind comparison of repaglinide and glyburide for the treatment of type 2 diabetes. Dutch and German Repaglinide Study Group. Diabetes Care. 1999;22:463–7.

47. Cincotta AH, Meier AH, Cincotta M Jr. Bromocriptine improves glycaemic control and serum lipid profile in obese type 2 diabetic subjects: a new approach in the treatment of diabetes. Expert Opin Investig Drugs. 1999;8:1683–707.

48. Zinman B, Wanner C, Lachin JM, Fitchett D, Bluhmki E, Hantel S, Mattheus M, Devins T, Johansen OE, Woerle HJ, Broedl UC, Inzucchi SE. Empagliflozin, cardiovascular outcomes, and mortality in type 2 diabetes. N Engl J Med. 2015;373:2117–28.

49. Neal B, Perkovic V, Mahaffey KW, de Zeeuw D, Fulcher G, Erondu N, Shaw W, Law G, Desai M, Matthews DR. Canagliflozin and cardiovascular and renal events in type 2 diabetes. N Engl J Med. 2017;377:644–57.

50. FDA Drug Safety Communication: FDA strengthens kidney warnings for diabetes medicines canagliflozin (Invokana, Invokamet) and dapagliflozin (Farxiga, Xigduo XR) [article online]. 2016. Available from https://www.fda.gov/Drugs/DrugSafety/ucm505860.htm. Accessed 12/18/2017.

51. Fralick M, Schneeweiss S, Patorno E. Risk of diabetic ketoacidosis after initiation of an SGLT2 inhibitor. N Engl J Med. 2017;376:2300–2.

52. Inzucchi SE, Iliev H, Pfarr E, Zinman B. Empagliflozin and assessment of lower-limb amputations in the EMPA-REG OUTCOME trial. Diabetes Care. 2018;41:e4–5.

GLP-1 Receptor Agonists for the Treatment of Type 2 Diabetes

Francisco Bandeira, Fábio Moura, Bruna Burkhardt Costi, and Ana Carolina S. M. Cardoso

The Incretin Effect

The observation that the insulin secretion response was approximately two to three times greater with an oral glucose intake in comparison with the same amount administered intravenously gave rise to the term "incretin effect" [1].

Incretin hormones are "derived" from the intestine and belong to the glucagon superfamily. Two hormones are related to the incretinic effect: glucose-dependent insulinotropic polypeptide (GIP) and GLP-1. The GIP is produced by K cells in the distal ileum and colon, while GLP-1 is secreted in L cells in the distal jejunum, ileum, and colon. Both are released in response to food intake and two- to threefold increases in plasma levels, with peak values dependent on the amount and type of food [2]. The GLP1 plasma levels increase a few minutes after the ingestion of food, suggesting that neural and endocrine mechanisms stimulate GLP-1 secretion even before L-cell stimulation by nutrients [3]. The incretins are rapidly degraded by the DPP-IV enzyme found on the surface of epithelial and endothelial cells, as well as in plasma [4]. The half-life of GLP-1 is less than 2 minutes, while that of the GIP is around 5–7 minutes [2]. The action of incretin occurs through its binding to specific receptors distributed systemically (pancreatic cells, gastrointestinal tract, central nervous system, heart, lungs, and kidneys) [2–5].

Biological Effects of GLP-1

Pancreatic Effects

GLP1 binds to specific receptors on pancreatic beta (β) cells and stimulates insulin-glucose production in a glucose-dependent manner [6]. It also regulates the production of other β-cell substances such as glucokinase and type 2 glucose transporter (GLUT-2) that enhance cell sensitivity to β glucose [7].

It has also been demonstrated that GLP-1 stimulates the differentiation of precursor cells into mature β cells, promotes their proliferation, and increases their resistance to apoptosis [8, 9]. However, it is important to remember that these effects were demonstrated by short-term studies. More data are needed to confirm whether chronic therapy with GLP-1 promotes sustained improvement in the quantity and function of the pancreatic β cells [10].

GLP-1 acts on alpha (α) cells by inhibiting pancreatic glucagon secretion, also in a glucose-dependent manner [10]. More importantly, the counter-regulatory mechanisms are not affected, as a result of which glucagon release in the presence of hypoglycemia is preserved [11].

Extra-Pancreatic Effects

Due to the broad distribution of GLP-1 receptors on various tissues, their activation is associated with a variety of extra-pancreatic effects, some of which are essential for glycemic control [10].

In animal models, GLP-1 inhibits hepatic glucose production and increases the production of glycogen [12]. There is an improvement in hepatic insulin sensitivity and reversal of hepatic steatosis. In humans, there is an enhancement of the markers of hepatic damage [13, 14].

GLP-1 and GLP1 agonists exert their inhibitory actions on acid secretion and delay postprandial gastric emptying in a dose-dependent manner. The mechanisms involved in

F. Bandeira (✉)
Division of Endocrinology, Agamenon Magalhães Hospital, University of Pernambuco Medical School, Recife, PE, Brazil

F. Moura
Endocrinology and Metabolism, Osvaldo Cruz Hospital—University of Pernambuco, Recife, PE, Brazil

B. B. Costi
Endocrinology, Agamenon Magalhaes Hospital, Jaboatao dos Guararapes, Recife, PE, Brazil

A. C. S. M. Cardoso
Agamenon Magalhaes Hospital, Department of Endocrinology and Metabolism, Recife, PE, Brazil

© Springer Nature Switzerland AG 2022
F. Bandeira et al. (eds.), *Endocrinology and Diabetes*, https://doi.org/10.1007/978-3-030-90684-9_31

gastrointestinal effects are complex and have yet to be fully clarified. The decrease in the rate of gastric emptying is associated with lower levels of postprandial glucose and insulin, thus having an important impact on the normalization of glycemia [15].

The GLP-1 molecules are small, so they can cross the blood-brain barrier and activate specific brain receptors, particularly at the hypothalamic nucleus. Their actions in the central nervous system (CNS) include increased satiety and appetite suppression, resulting in weight loss [2]. Complementary mechanisms are suggested, such as vagal inhibition, induced gastric distension, and an increased feeling of fullness, contributing to the inhibition of hunger and weight loss [2, 5].

The cardiovascular effects of GLP-1 are probably cardioprotective, with actions such as a significant reduction of the cardiac infarct area, an improvement in glucose uptake by the myocardium, and an improved left ventricular function [16]. GLP-1 also results in an improvement in endothelial dysfunction and attenuation of atherosclerotic plaque progression [17]. The effects on blood pressure are still uncertain, with some studies reporting small decreases in systolic and diastolic pressures and others showing no benefits [10].

In relation to lipid metabolism, GLP-1 and GLP1 RA may have minor benefits, with a small reduction in LDL cholesterol and triglycerides and a moderate increase in HDL, probably related to weight loss [10].

The Incretin Effect on Type 2 Diabetes

Unlike what was observed in healthy individuals, in diabetic patients, there are no significant differences in C-peptide concentration (indirect measure of insulin production) between oral and intravenous glucose administrations [1]. This finding led to the conclusion that the incretin effect was absent or markedly reduced in type 2 diabetes and that this mechanism might be involved in the disease's pathophysiology and progression.

There have been many studies of GIP secretion in diabetic patients, and although no changes in its plasma concentration have been found, there is a clear reduction in the capacity to stimulate insulin secretion in DM2 [18]. There is a lot of controversy regarding changes to the GLP-1 in diabetic patients. Most studies indicate no reduction in the levels of GLP-1 in this population, but some subgroups, especially those with long-standing diabetes, may have changes in the postprandial secretion of this polypeptide [18].

Exenatide

In the 1990s, certain molecules that could cause hypoglycemia were described in the saliva of venomous lizards of the *helodermatideum* family. Those molecules were called "exendins." Exendin-3 was present in the saliva of *Heloderma horridum* (lizard) and exandin-4 in that of *Heloderma suspectum* (Gila monster). The molecules were nearly identical in their chemical structure, differing only in two amino acids. From the standpoint of biological activity, both acted on pancreatic acini, leading to cAMP production, but, unlike exendin-3, exendin-4 did not stimulate amylase or VIP release [19]. The therapeutic potential of these drugs has now begun to be considered. Exenatide is a synthetic version of exendin-4 [20, 21]. It is a peptide containing 39 amino acids and shares 53% homology with native GLP1. It was the first drug of a new class of anti-hyperglycemic drugs known as GLP1 RA which, together with the DPP-IV inhibitors, are known as "incretinomimetics" [22]. Exenatide has the same affinity for the GLP1 receptor as the native GLP1, but is much more resistant to degradation by the DPP-IV enzyme, and its presence can be detected in circulation 10 h after administration, while GLP1 is inactivated after 2 min [21–23]. This mechanism of exenatide allows it to be used twice daily.

It is marketed under the name *Byetta* [20], with 5 and 10 mcg doses. It was recently marketed as an extended-release preparation, under the brand name *Bydureon*, 2 mg with the same pharmacological properties. This is administered at weekly intervals [24].

The biological actions of exenatide are [21–23]:

1. Stimulating the production of insulin—Exenatide stimulates insulin secretion in a glucose-dependent manner recovering both first-phase (rapid initial 10–15 min) and second-phase insulin secretion. However, as previously mentioned, its insulinotropic effect is suppressed when blood glucose approaches 72 mg/dL, so the risk of hypoglycemia is very low, a property that clearly differentiates this class of drug from other hypoglycemic drugs.
2. Suppression of glucagon secretion—Glucagon secretion is inappropriately elevated in type 2 diabetes and is deleted in a glucose-dependent manner by exenatide. In other words, when the patient has hyperglycemia, glucagon secretion is suppressed, while in the presence of hypoglycemia, it is stimulated, enhancing the counter-regulatory response.
3. Delayed gastric emptying.
4. Reduction in food intake.
5. Reduction in body weight
6. Beta-cell proliferation—In animal models, exenatide stimulated beta-cell proliferation and neogenesis.
7. Possible cardiovascular benefits (see extra-pancreatic effects of the GLP1 agonist)—Exenatide is administered subcutaneously 30–60 min before meals, with an interval of 6 h between doses. Following subcutaneous administration, the median concentration of exenatide was 211 pg/mL, and the area under the curve was 1036 pg.h/mL. Its half-life was 2.5 h, and the drug was detectable

in the circulation 10 h after dosing. There was no difference in drug bioavailability whether injected in the arms, abdomen, or thighs. Likewise age, gender, weight, and ethnicity apparently did not significantly alter the kinetics of the drug. Elimination occurred predominantly by glomerular filtration followed by subsequent proteolytic degradation.

The slow-release exenatide (*Bydureon*) consists of microspheres of exenatide associated with a biodegradable polymer—"poly" (lactide-co-glycolide). The miscrospheres undergo a process of erosion, allowing a slow and continuous release of the drug. Its administration is weekly, and the dose is 2 mg [23, 24].

Side Effects

Gastrointestinal effects—nausea, vomiting, and diarrhea—usually mild, were the most common side effects observed in clinical trials with exenatide, especially in the first month of treatment. Starting with low doses and gradually increasing the dose minimizes the frequency and intensity of symptoms [21, 23].

The risk of hypoglycemia was low when exenatide was used in isolation or associated with insulin sensitizers such as metformin or glitazones [25, 26]. Its use concomitantly with sulfonylureas increased the risk of hypoglycemia. When this association is the therapeutic option, the dose of sulfonylurea should always be decreased [27, 28].

An increase in reported cases of pancreatitis, in both its edematous and hemorrhagic forms, was associated with exenatide [29], but large recent databases did not confirm this association. It is well established that obesity and type 2 diabetes are risk factors for pancreatitis. Moreover, in this group of patients, the presence of comorbidities such as hypertriglyceridemia and gallstones, other classic risk factors for pancreatitis, is quite common. That is, this population is already at high risk for the condition. There is, however, a possible mechanism by which obesity and diabetes increase the risk of pancreatitis, namely, the replication of pancreatic microduct stimulation, which triggers the formation of partially obstructed and distorted ducts, with flow obstruction, leading to inflammation and pancreatitis [30]. Since 2008, the FDA has been warning that patients on exenatide who experience abdominal pain, nausea, or vomiting should always be investigated for this condition [20, 22, 23].

In mice, an increased incidence of medullary thyroid carcinoma, hitherto not understood in humans, was described. This finding could be explained by an increase in the GLP1 receptors of C cells in mice, which is about 10–12 times higher than that found in humans, which leads to the possibility of this effect being specific to mice [20, 21, 29].

Between 2005 and 2008, 78 cases of kidney failure associated with exenatide were reported, which generated an alert about the use of the drug in high-risk populations and pre-existing renal disease, especially for patients with CrCl between 30 and 60 ml/min/m². The drug is contraindicated in patients with CrCl below 30 ml/min/m² [21, 23].

Approximately 45% of patients who used exenatide developed antibodies against the molecule. The clinical significance of this finding is not yet fully understood. The occurrence of headache has also been more frequent with the use of exenatide [21, 23, 24]. To date, there is no evidence that exenatide increases cardiovascular risk [31]. In fact, it seems that the drug has cardio-protective effects: some animal studies have shown an improvement in cardiac output, an increase in left ventricle ejection fraction, a decreased mean arterial pressure, increases in nitric oxide production with better myocardial perfusion, and a diminished ischemic area. There are ongoing clinical studies designed to test this hypothesis. A meta-analysis published in *The American Journal of Cardiology* assessing the cardiovascular risk associated with the use of DPP-IV inhibitors, another class of drugs that also acts primarily in the "incretin system," suggested cardiovascular protection [32].

Exenatide Twice Daily and Extended Release

In a head-to-head comparison between exenatide 10 mcg twice daily and extended-release exenatide, 2 mg once a week, with 295 patients with type 2 diabetes, lasting 30 weeks, there were more patients with adequate control defined as HbA1c <7% in the extended-release arm than in the conventional arm (two daily applications), with no differences in relation to the risk of hypoglycemia or weight loss [33].

Exenatide caused greater reductions in HbA1c than glimepiride, sitagliptin, and glitazone when used in combination with metformin. Again, additional benefits were evidenced, such as weight loss and a low risk of hypoglycemia. Furthermore, side effects, especially gastrointestinal ones, were more frequent with exenatide, and there were more dropouts in the group of patients who used the drug. Nevertheless, despite the greater number of dropouts, there were no observed differences regarding the occurrence of serious adverse effects [25–28, 34] (Tables 31.1 and 31.2).

Compared with insulin glargine and premixed insulin, exenatide was no less effective in achieving good glycemic control, with the best results in terms of hypoglycemia risk and weight loss. Once again, the patients using exenatide showed more side effects, especially nausea and vomiting [35–37].

A small trial evaluated the possibility of replacing glargine insulin with exenatide in type 2 diabetes patients. 61% of patients who switched drugs were able to maintain good

Table 31.1 Exenatide plus another T2DM drug: results of main trials

Drug	Rationale	Study design	Follow-up	Main results	Side effects
Metformin [25]	Metformin plus placebo × metformin plus exenatide	Cohort. $N = 150$	82 weeks	Lower Hba1c and weight reduction with exenatide	More nausea and vomiting with exenatide
Sulfonylurea [27]	Sulfonylurea plus placebo × sulfonylurea plus exenatide	Randomized, double-blind. $N = 337$	30 weeks	Lower Hba1c and weight reduction with exenatide	More nausea, vomiting, diarrhea, and dose-dependent hypoglycemia with exenatide
Glitazones [34]	Exenatide plus glitazones × exenatide or glitazones plus metformin	Randomized, open. $N = 137$	20 weeks	Lower HbA1c and improved insulin sensitivity with exenatide plus glitazone	More nausea and vomiting with exenatide
Glargine insulin [36]	Exenatide × glargine insulin plus metformin or pioglitazone	Randomized, double-blind. $N = 262$	24 weeks	Weight loss and no hypoglycemia with exenatide: no HbA1c differences	More nausea, vomiting, diarrhea with exenatide

Table 31.2 Head-to-head trials: exenatide × other drugs for T2DM

Drug	Rationale	Study design	Follow-up	Main results	Side effects
Sulfonylurea [28]	Exenatide × sulfonylurea plus metformin	Randomized, single-blind. $N = 1029$	236 weeks	Lower Hba1c, weight loss, and less hypoglycemia with exenatide	More nausea, vomiting, diarrhea, and dropouts with exenatide
Pioglitazone [26]	Exenatide plus metformin × pioglitazone plus metformin	Randomized, double-blind. $N = 491$	26 weeks	Lower Hba1c and weight loss with exenatide	More nausea and diarrhea with exenatide
Sitagliptin [26]	Exenatide plus metformin × sitagliptin plus metformin	Randomized, double-blind. $N = 491$	26 weeks	Lower Hba1c and weight loss with exenatide	More nausea and diarrhea with exenatide
Insulin, glargine [35]	Exenatide plus metformin × glargine insulin plus metformin	Randomized, single-blind. $N = 69$	52 weeks	No differences in HbA1c between drugs. Weight loss and improved insulin secretion with exenatide	More nausea, vomiting, diarrhea with exenatide
Insulin, glargine [38]	Switching glargine insulin plus metformin for exenatide plus metformin	Randomized, open. $N = 49$	16 weeks	61% patients could maintain a good glycemic control after switching from glargine insulin to exenatide	More nausea and vomiting with exenatide
Premixed insulin [37]	Exenatide plus metformin × premixed insulin plus metformin	Randomized, open. $N = 501$	52 weeks	No differences in HbA1c between drugs. Weight loss and less hypoglycemia with exenatide	More nausea, vomiting, diarrhea, and dropouts with exenatide

glycemic control. A shorter duration of type 2 diabetes and the use of low doses of insulin were significantly associated with a greater chance of success [38].

Liraglutide

Liraglutide was the second GLP-1 RA approved for use in type 2 diabetes. The native hormone has been modified to develop a compound with pharmacokinetic properties suitable for once-daily administration.

It is available for subcutaneous use in a single daily dose. It exhibits a 97% structural similarity to endogenous GLP-1 and has a half-life of approximately 13 h. This pharmacokinetic profile is due to the combination of prolonged absorption at the site of injection, a rate of albumin binding greater than 98%, and a high resistance to degradation by DPP-IV [39].

The trials for the approval of liraglutide comprised the LEAD (Liraglutide Effect and Action in Diabetes) program,

which included 6 large randomized controlled trials, with a total of over 4000 patients, conducted in over 600 centers in 40 countries [40–45]. The objectives of the LEAD studies were to evaluate the efficacy and safety of liraglutide and compare it with other treatments available for type 2 diabetes. The summary of the studies is found in Table 31.3.

In relation to glycemic control, a significant and sustained HbA1c reduction of around 1.1–1.5% was obtained in all studies. Liraglutide also showed a lower risk of hypoglycemia. All the LEAD studies showed a significant reduction in body weight of approximately 1.0–3.2 kg. A reduction in systolic blood pressure of about 2.1–6.7 mmHg was also observed. The possibility of an improvement in metabolic control associated with decreased body weight is of paramount importance in the current scenario of a growing global prevalence of obesity and the forecast significant increase in the number of diabetics.

Liraglutide is, in general, well tolerated. The most common adverse events were related to the gastrointestinal tract, including nausea, vomiting, and diarrhea, occurring in

Table 31.3 Summary of LEAD trials

Trial	Liraglutide-associated drug	Comparison	Study design	Main end point/follow-up	Summary
LEAD 1 [42]	Glimepiride	Liraglutide versus rosiglitazone or placebo plus glimepiride	Double-blind, randomized. N = 1041	HbA1c—26 weeks	Lower HbA1c with liraglutide (1.2 or 1.8 mg) than placebo or rosiglitazone when added to glimepiride
LEAD 2 [40]	Metformin	Liraglutide plus metformin versus metformin plus glimepiride	Randomized, controlled, open. N = 1091	HbA1c—26 weeks	Lower HbA1c with liraglutide than glimepiride when added to metformin
LEAD 3 [43]	Placebo	Glimepiride 8 mg versus liraglutide 1.2 or 1.8 mg plus placebo	Double-blind, randomized. N = 746	HbA1c—52 weeks	Lower HbA1c and with liraglutide than glimepiride. More side effects with liraglutide
LEAD 4 [45]	Metformin plus rosiglitazone	Liraglutide 1.2/1.8 mg versus placebo metformin, plus rosiglitazone and metformin	Double-blind, randomized. N = 533	HbA1c—26 weeks	Lower HbA1c, increase in C peptide, and dose-dependent weight loss with liraglutide than placebo
LEAD 5 [44]	Metformin plus glimepiride	Liraglutide versus placebo versus glargine insulin plus metformin and glimepiride	Randomized, open, multicenter. N = 581	HbA1c—26 weeks	Lower HbA1c, more weight loss, and less hypoglycemia with liraglutide. More side effects with liraglutide
LEAD 6 [41]	Metformin, glimepiride, or both drugs	Liraglutide versus exenatide plus metformin, glimepiride, or both drugs	Randomized, open, multicenter. N = 464	HbA1c—26 weeks	Liraglutide reduced mean HbA1c significantly more than exenatide

10–40% of patients participating in the studies cited above. Most cases were mild and transient, occurring early in treatment and rarely resulting in discontinuation of the medication.

The effect on thyroid C cell in humans is unclear, since there are fewer C thyroid cells than in mice and the expression of GLP-1 receptors on those cells is very low [46]. A study was carried out to compare the levels of plasma calcitonin in humans using liraglutide versus a control group, and after 2 years of follow-up, there were no consistent differences between the two groups, supporting the hypothesis that this drug does not increase the risk of follicular thyroid carcinoma in humans [47]. Until more definite data become available, the US Food and Drug Administration (FDA) does not recommend its use in patients with a past or family history of medullary carcinoma of the thyroid or multiple endocrine neoplasia (MEN) type 2A or 2B.

Among the LEAD studies, there were 7 cases of pancreatitis reported in 4257 patients using liraglutide, while in the comparator group, there were 2 cases. The small number of events hinders a proper conclusion involving causality. As previously mentioned, it is well established that diabetic patients show an increased risk of pancreatitis, a risk that can be three times higher than in the nondiabetic population, complicating data interpretation. The current recommendation of the FDA is to monitor the occurrence of abdominal pain and to immediately suspend the use of liraglutide use if pancreatitis is suspected.

In the LEAD studies, liraglutide was associated with a lower rate of major cardiovascular events compared with other therapies which served as comparators. It is possible that the beneficial effects of liraglutide on glycemic control, weight loss, and reduction in systolic blood pressure contributed to this result, but long-term studies are still being conducted to establish whether there are any real cardiovascular benefits.

Liraglutide is used initially at a dose of 0.6 mg, with progression to 1.2 mg. This gradual progression helps to minimize the side effects. To achieve a better glycemic control, it can be used at a dose of 1.8 mg. There is no need for dose adjustment according to age, gender, or ethnicity. It should be used with caution in patients with liver and kidney failure, although its pharmacokinetics do not change significantly in the presence of advanced renal failure.

In the SCALE program, studies with liraglutide 3.0 mg, along with diet and physical activity, induced significant weight loss vs placebo, regardless of BMI, diabetic or pre-diabetic. In addition, there was an improvement in glycemic parameters, blood pressure, lipid profile, cardiovascular risk markers, and quality of life (including mental health). The liraglutide dose of 3.0 mg was well tolerated. The most common adverse events were nausea, diarrhea, and constipation, usually mild-moderate and transient. However, even the events of pancreatitis and gallbladder disorders were low. There was a higher frequency in this dosage [48].

Dulaglutide

Dulaglutide is a long-acting GLP-1 for its resistance to degradation by DPP-IV, and due to the increased size, it has its reabsorption in the gastrointestinal tract and renal excretion delayed. Because of these characteristics, it has a prolonged half-life of about 5 days, making weekly administration possible [49–51].

Table 31.4 Summary of AWARD trials

Trial	Dulaglutide-associated drug	Comparison	Study design	Main end point/follow-up	Summary
AWARD-1	Metformin Pioglitazone	Dulaglutide versus exenatide or placebo	Randomized, multicenter. $N = 976$	HbA1c—52 weeks	Lower HbA1c with Dulaglutide (0.75 or 1.5 mg) than exenatide or placebo
AWARD-3	Placebo	Dulaglutide versus metformin	Randomized, double-blind. $N = 807$	HbA1c—52 weeks	Lower HbA1c, more weight loss with liraglutide than metformin
AWARD-5	Metformin	Dulaglutide and metformin versus sitagliptin and metformin	Multicenter, randomized. $N = 657$	HbA1c—104 weeks	Lower HbA1c, more weight loss with liraglutide 1.5 mg

Table 31.5 Summary of SUSTAIN trials [58–65]

Trial	Semaglutide-associated drug	Comparison	Study design	Main end point/follow-up	Summary
SUSTAIN 1	Placebo	Semaglutide versus placebo	Randomized, double-blind $N = 388$	HBA1c—30 weeks	Semaglutide significantly improved HbA1c and body weight in patients with type 2 diabetes compared with placebo
SUSTAIN 2	Sitagliptin	Semaglutide versus sitagliptin	Randomized, double-blind $N = 1231$	HBA1c—56 weeks	The weekly semaglutide was superior to sitagliptin in improving glycemic control and reducing body weight in participants with type 2 diabetes
SUSTAIN 3	Exenatide ER	Semaglutide versus exenatide ER	Randomized, double-blind $N = 813$	HbA1c—56 weeks	Semaglutide 1.0 mg was superior to exenatide ER 2.0 mg in improving glycemic control and reducing body weight
SUSTAIN 4	Insulin glargine	Semaglutide versus insulin glargine	Randomized, double-blind $N = 1809$	HbA1c—30 weeks	Compared to insulin glargine, semaglutide resulted in greater reductions in HbA1c and in weight, with fewer hypoglycemic episodes
SUSTAIN 5	Basal insulin and placebo	Semaglutide versus basal insulin + placebo	Randomized, double-blind $N = 601$	HbA1c—56 weeks	Semaglutide was well tolerated. Significantly reduced HbA1c and body weight versus basal insulin and placebo
SUSTAIN 6	Placebo	Semaglutide versus placebo	Randomized, double-blind $N = 3297$	Cardiovascular risk—104 weeks	Reduction of cardiovascular outcomes with non-fatal AMI and stroke. There was no difference between groups in cardiovascular mortality
SUSTAIN 7	Dulaglutide	Semaglutide versus dulaglutide	Randomized, open-label, active-controlled, parallel group $N = 1201$	Cardiovascular risk, HbA1c—40 weeks	At low and high doses, semaglutide was superior to dulaglutide in improving glycemic control and reducing body weight

According to the AWARDS studies (Table 31.4), dulaglutide showed a significant reduction of glycemic levels, with HBA1c falling from 0.71% to 1.5%. A modest reduction of SBP was also seen, but with a slight increase in heart rate without hemodynamic repercussions. There was a loss of 1.3–3 kg with use of this drug. Beta-cell function and insulin sensitivity have increased in these studies.

Total and LDL cholesterol levels decreased without alterations in HDL. Adverse events were the same in the other GLP-1 with gastrointestinal symptoms being the most commonly reported such as nausea, vomiting, and diarrhea being the most mild to moderate and transitory. It can be given in doses of 0.75 and 1.5 mg weekly subcutaneous.

Semaglutide

Semaglutide is a GLP-1 analog with a prolonged half-life of approximately 1 week, allowing its administration at the dose of 1 mg weekly subcutaneously. The SUSTAIN study evaluated cardiovascular outcomes in type 2 diabetic subjects in long-term use of semaglutide (Table 31.5). The result of this study presented a reduction in the risk for primary outcome of death from cardiovascular causes (non-fatal AMI and non-fatal stroke) without significant difference in the rate of cardiovascular deaths. The systolic blood pressure presented a reduction ranging from 1.3 to 2.6 mmHg. The mean level of HBA1c reduction was 1.1% to 1.4%. There was a loss of body weight around 3.6 to 4.9 kg. Patients presented a lower risk of new or worsening nephropathy, according to differences in macroalbuminuria. However, there was a higher risk of complications of diabetic retinopathy than those receiving placebo [52].

The Role of GLP1 RA in the Modern Treatment of T2DM

At the 2012 ADA/EASD position statement, the indications for incretin-based therapies were greatly expanded in comparison with the previous document. In patients poorly controlled despite a proper diet, physical activity, and monotherapy with metformin, if the main objectives are to achieve good glycemic control with a low risk of hypoglycemia and leading to weight loss, GLP1 RA should be the first choice, although the costs and potential side effects should always be taken into consideration [53].

GLP-1 RA in the Treatment of Obesity

The World Health Organization estimates that the worldwide prevalence of overweight is 1.5 million adults, while 500 million are believed to be obese. It is known that the risk of developing T2DM is directly proportional to excessive body weight, increasing approximately 3-fold in overweight patients and 20-fold in obese ones when compared to individuals with a normal body mass index (BMI) [54]. Obesity, particularly when associated with increased visceral adipose tissue, is an independent risk factor for coronary heart disease, contributing to a substantial increase in cardiovascular morbidity and mortality. Considering that there is a global trend toward an increased prevalence of obesity and T2DM and that the therapies most widely available for T2DM induce weight gain (insulins, thiazolidinediones, sulfonylureas), the prospect of drugs that act in glycemic control, leading to a better metabolic profile, is quite encouraging.

Studies with GLP-1 in diabetic patients showed metabolic benefits, including weight loss, with a negligible risk of hypoglycemia when used as monotherapy, due to glucose-dependent insulin release. The proposed mechanisms to induce weight loss involve delayed emptying gastric, leading to early satiety and appetite suppression at the level of the CNS. Such features have raised the possibility of using these agents for treating obesity in nondiabetic patients, driven by the limited therapeutic arsenal currently used for this purpose.

A meta-analysis of 21 studies involving GLP-1 analogs in obese or overweight diabetic and nondiabetic patients was performed, and it was found that there was a weight loss in all studies [55]. The mean weight reduction obtained with the highest dose of GLP-1 RA ranged from −0.2 to −7.2 kg. Patients without diabetes had a greater weight loss than diabetics (mean, −3.2 kg versus 2.8 kg). There were no differences in change in body weight between exenatide and liraglutide or between short-acting exenatide and slow-release exenatide. The results suggest that treatments with GLP-1 agonists are an effective intervention for overweight or obese patients, irrespective of the presence of T2DM.

The study on long-term safety, tolerability, and sustained weight loss with liraglutide in nondiabetics was reported after 2 years of follow-up [56]. The patients studied were obese (BMI 30–40), nondiabetic, aged 18–65, and enrolled in a program of diet and exercise associated with liraglutide (2.4/3.0 mg), placebo, or orlistat. Weight loss with liraglutide was 7.8 kg, which is better than placebo and orlistat, and sustained over 2 years. Over 70% of patients taking liraglutide maintained a weight loss greater than 5% relative to baseline, which was associated with an improvement in cardiovascular risk factors and metabolic changes. There were an improvement in systolic blood pressure, a decreased prevalence of diabetes (over 50%), and an improvement in body composition, with loss of adipose tissue and decreased waist circumference. Tolerability was good, and adverse events were mostly mild or moderate, in particular nausea and vomiting, which were much more common than with placebo, as described in other studies. There was no decrease in adherence due to the fact that it is an injectable medication. The results of this study are very important in corroborating the safety and efficacy of liraglutide.

Lixisenatide

Lixisenatide is a GLP-1 receptor agonist derived from exenatide which is available in Europe for clinical use [57]. It has a more pronounced effect on PPG, mainly after the first meal of the day, and is labeling for once-daily 20 micrograms subcutaneous injections. The effects on decreasing HbA1c and body weight however are less than with liraglutide administration. Lixisenatide is undergoing clinical development as a combination product with insulin glargine. This treatment combination has been shown to substantially improve HbA1c, without significant weight gain, in the GetGoal-L, the GetGoal-L-Asia, and the GetGoal-Duo 1 studies. At present, unless lixisenatide is priced lower than the already available GLP-1RA alternatives, it appears that the main place in therapy for lixisenatide is in the combination with insulin glargine. There is also an ongoing multicenter study for the evaluation of cardiovascular outcomes in patients with type 2 diabetes after acute coronary syndrome during treatment with lixisenatide.

References

1. Nauck MA, Stöckmann F, Ebert R, Creutzfeldt W. Reduced incretin effect in type 2 (non-insulin-dependent) diabetes. Diabetologia. 1986;29:46–52.

2. Baggio LL, Drucker DJ. Biology of incretins: GLP-1 and GIP. Gastroenterology. 2007;132:2131–57.

3. Drucker DJ, Nauck MA. The incretin system: glucagon-like peptide-1 receptor agonists and dipeptidyl peptidase-4 inhibitors in type 2 diabetes. Lancet. 2006;368:1696–705.

4. Hansen L, Deacon CF, Orskov C, Holst JJ. Glucagon-like peptide-1-(7–36)amide is transformed to glucagon-like peptide-1-(9–36)amide by dipeptidyl peptidase IV in the capillaries supplying the L cells of the porcine intestine. Endocrinology. 1999;140:5356–63.

5. Abu-Hamdah R, Rabiee A, Meneilly GS, Shannon RP, Andersen DK, Elahi D. Clinical review: the extrapancreatic effects of glucagon-like peptide-1 and related peptides. J Clin Endocrinol Metab. 2009;94:1843–52.

6. Perfetti R, Merkel P. Glucagon-like peptide-1: a major regulator of pancreatic beta-cell function. Eur J Endocrinol. 2000;143:717–25.

7. Wang Y, Perfetti R, Greig NH, Holloway HW, DeOre KA, et al. Glucagonlike peptide-1 can reverse the age-related decline in glucose tolerance in rats. J Clin Invest. 1997;99:2883–9.

8. Xu G, Stoffers DA, Habener JF, Bonner-Weir S. Exendin-4 stimulates both beta cell replication and neogenesis, resulting in increased beta-cell mass and improved glucose tolerance in diabetic rats. Diabetes. 1999;48:2270–6.

9. Li Y, Hansotia T, Yusta B, Ris F, Halban PA, Drucker DJ. Glucagon-like peptide-1 receptor signaling modulates beta cell apoptosis. J Biol Chem. 2003;278:471–8.

10. Cernea S, Raz I. Therapy in the early stage: incretins. Diabetes Care. 2011;34:S264–71.

11. Nauck MA, Heimesaat MM, Behle K, Holst JJ, Nauck MS, et al. Effects of glucagon-like peptide 1 on counterregulatory hormone responses, cognitive functions, and insulin secretion during hyperinsulinemic, stepped hypoglycemic clamp experiments in healthy volunteers. J Clin Endocrinol Metab. 2002;87:1239–46.

12. Lee YS, Shin S, Shigihara T, Hahm E, Liu MJ, et al. Glucagonlike peptide-1 gene therapy in obese diabetic mice results in long-term cure of diabetes by improving insulin sensitivity and reducing hepatic gluconeogenesis. Diabetes. 2007;56:1671–9.

13. Klonoff DC, Buse JB, Nielsen LL, Guan X, Bowlus CL, et al. Exenatide effects on diabetes, obesity, cardiovascular risk factors and hepatic biomarkers in patients with type 2 diabetes treated for at least 3 years. Curr Med Res Opin. 2008;24:275–86.

14. Ding X, Saxena NK, Lin S, Gupta NA, Anania FA. Exendin-4, a glucagon-like protein-1 (GLP-1) receptor agonist, reverses hepatic steatosis in ob/ob mice. Hepatology. 2006;43:173–81.

15. Marathe CS, Rayner CK, Jones KL, Horowitz M. Effects of GLP-1 and incretin-based therapies on gastrointestinal motor function. Exp Diabetes Res. 2011;2011:279530.

16. Timmers L, Henriques JP, de Kleijn DP, Devries JH, Kemperman H, et al. Exenatide reduces infarct size and improves cardiac function in a porcine model of ischemia and reperfusion injury. J Am Coll Cardiol. 2009;53:501–10.

17. Arakawa M, Mita T, Azuma K, Ebato C, Goto H, et al. Inhibition of monocyte adhesion to endothelial cells and attenuation of atherosclerotic lesion by a glucagon-like peptide-1 receptor agonist, exendin-4. Diabetes. 2010;59:1030–7.

18. Meier JJ. The contribution of incretin hormones to the pathogenesis of type 2 diabetes. Best Pract Res Clin Endocrinol Metab. 2009;23:433–41.

19. Eng J, Kleinman WA, Singh L, Singh G, Raufman JP. Isolation and characterization of exendin-4, an exendin-3 analogue, from helo-derma suspectum venom. Further evidence for an exendin receptor on dispersed acini from guinea pig pancreas. J Biol Chem. 1992;267:7402–6.

20. http://www.fda.gov/drugs/drugsafety/postmarket. Accessed 21 Jul 2012.

21. Iltz JL, Baker DE, Setter SM, Keith CR. Exenatide: an incretin mimetic for the treatment of type 2 diabetes mellitus. Clin Ther. 2006;28:S56–8.

22. Unger JE. Incretins: clinical perspectives, relevance, and applications for the primary care physician in the treatment of patients with type 2 diabetes mellitus. Mayo Clin Proc. 2010;85:S38–49.

23. Parkes DG, Pittner R, Jodka C, Smith P, Young A. Insulinotropic actions of exendin-4 and glucagon-like peptide-1 in vivo and in vitro. Metabolism. 2001;50:583–9.

24. http://www.fda.gov/drus/drugssafety/UCM289869. Accessed 21 Jul 2012.

25. Ratner RE, Maggs D, Nielsen LL, Stonehouse AH, Poon T, et al. Long-term effects of exenatide therapy over 82 weeks on glycaemic control and weight in over-weight metformin-treated patients with type 2 diabetes mellitus. Diabetes Obes Metab. 2006;8:419–28.

26. Bergenstal RM, Wysham C, Macconell L, Malloy J, Walsh B, et al. Efficacy and safety of exenatide once weekly versus sitagliptin or pioglitazone as an adjunct to metformin for treatment of type 2 diabetes (DURATION-2): a randomised trial. Lancet. 2010;376:431–9.

27. Buse JB, Henry RR, Han J, Kim DD, Fineman MS, et al. Effects of exenatide (exendin-4) on glycemic control over 30 weeks in sulfonylurea-treated patients with type 2 diabetes. Diabetes Care. 2004;27:2628–35.

28. Gallwitz B, Guzman J, Dotta F, Guerci B, Simó R, et al. Exenatide twice daily versus glimepiride for prevention of glycaemic deterioration in patients with type 2 diabetes with metformin failure (EUREXA): an open-label, randomised controlled trial. Lancet. 2012;379:2270–8.

29. Elashoff M, Matveyenko AV, Gier B, Elashoff R, Butler PC. Pancreatitis, pancreatic, and thyroid cancer with glucagon-like peptide-1-based therapies. Gastroenterology. 2011;141:150–6.

30. Butler PC, Dry S, Elashoff R. GLP-1-based therapy for diabetes: what you do not know can hurt you. Diabetes Care. 2010;33:453–5.

31. Ussher JE, Drucker JE. Cardiovascular biology of the incretin system. Endocr Rev. 2012;33:187–215.

32. Patil HR, Al Badarin FJ, Al Shami HA, Bhatti SK, Lavie CJ, et al. Meta-analysis of effect of dipeptidyl peptidase-4 inhibitors on cardiovascular risk in type 2 diabetes mellitus. Am J Cardiol. 2012;110:826–33.

33. Blevins T, Pullman J, Malloy J, Yan P, Taylor K, et al. DURATION-5: exenatide once weekly resulted in greater improvements in glycemic control compared with exenatide twice daily in patients with type 2 diabetes. J Clin Endocrinol Metab. 2011;96:1301–10.

34. De Fronzo RA, Triplitt C, Qu Y, Lewis M, Maggs D, Glass LC. Effects of exenatide plus rosiglitazone on β-cell function and insulin sensitivity in subjects with type 2 diabetes on metformin. Diabetes Care. 2010;33(5):951–7.

35. Bunck MC, Diamant M, Cornér A, Eliasson B, Malloy JL, et al. One-year treatment with exenatide improves β-cell function, compared with insulin glargine, in metformin-treated type 2 diabetic patients a randomized, controlled trial. Diabetes Care. 2009;32:762–8.

36. Buse JB, Bergenstal RM, Glass LC, Heilmann CR, Lewis MS, et al. Use of twice-daily exenatide in basal insulin–treated patients with type 2 diabetes: a randomized. Controlled Trial Ann Intern Med. 2011;154:103–12.

37. Nauck MA, Duran S, Kim D, Johns D, Northrup J, et al. A comparison of twice-daily exenatide and biphasic insulin aspart in patients with type 2 diabetes who were suboptimally controlled with sulfonylurea and metformin: a non-inferiority study. Diabetologia. 2007;50:259–67.

38. Davis SN, Johns D, Maggs D, Xu H, Northrup JH, Brodows RG. Exploring the substitution of exenatide for insulin in patients with type 2 diabetes treated with insulin in combination with oral anti-diabetes agents. Diabetes Care. 2007;30:2767–72.

39. Russell-Jones D. Molecular, pharmacological and clinical aspects of liraglutide, a once-daily human GLP-1 analogue. Mol Cell Endocrinol. 2009;297:137–40.

40. Nauck M, Frid A, Hermansen K, Shah NS, Tankova T, et al. Efficacy and safety comparison of liraglutide, glimepiride, and placebo, all in combination with metformin, in type 2 diabetes: The LEAD (liraglutide effect and action in diabetes)-2 study. Diabetes Care. 2009;32:84–90.

41. Buse JB, Rosenstock J, Sesti G, Schmidt WE, Montanya E, et al. Liraglutide once a day versus exenatide twice a day for type 2 diabetes: A 26-week randomised, parallel-group, multinational, open-label trial (LEAD-6). Lancet. 2009;374:39–47.

42. Marre M, Shaw J, Brändle M, Bebakar WM, Kamaruddin NA, et al. Liraglutide, a once-daily human GLP-1 analogue, added to a sulphonylurea over 26 weeks produces greater improvements in glycaemic and weight control compared with adding rosiglitazone or placebo in subjects with Type 2 diabetes (LEAD-1 SU). Diabet Med. 2009;26:268–78.

43. Garber A, Henry R, Ratner R, Garcia-Hernandez PA, Rodriguez-Pattzi H, et al. Liraglutide versus glimepiride monotherapy for type 2 diabetes (LEAD-3 Mono): a randomised, 52-week, phase III, double-blind, parallel-treatment trial. Lancet. 2009;373:473–81.

44. Russell-Jones D, Vaag A, Schmitz O, Sethi BK, Lalic N, et al. Liraglutide vs insulin glargine and placebo in combination with metformin and sulfonylurea therapy in type 2 diabetes mellitus (LEAD-5 met + SU): a randomised controlled trial. Diabetologia. 2009;52:2046–55.

45. Zinman B, Gerich J, Buse JB, Lewin A, Schwartz S, et al. Efficacy and safety of the human glucagon-like peptide-1 analog liraglutide in combination with metformin and thiazolidinedione in patients with type 2 diabetes (LEAD-4 Met + TZD). Diabetes Care. 2009;32:1224–30.

46. Bjerre Knudsen L, Madsen LW, Andersen S, Almholt K, de Boer AS, et al. Glucagon-like Peptide-1 receptor agonists activate rodent thyroid C-cells causing calcitonin release and C-cell proliferation. Endocrinology. 2010;151:1473–86.

47. Hegedüs L, Moses AC, Zdravkovic M, Le Thi T, Daniels GH. GLP-1 and calcitonin concentration in humans: lack of evidence of calcitonin release from sequential screening in over 5000 subjects with type 2 diabetes or nondiabetic obese subjects treated with the human GLP-1 analog, liraglutide. J Clin Endocrinol Metab. 2011;96:853–60.

48. Pi-Sunyer X, Astrup A, Fujioka K. et al; SCALE Obesity and Prediabetes NN8022-1839 Study Group. A randomized, controlled trial of 3.0 mg of liraglutide in weight management. N Engl J Med. 2015;373(1):11–22.

49. Wysham C, Blevins T, Arakaki R, et al. Efficacy and safety of dulaglutide added onto pioglitazone and metformin versus exenatide in type 2 diabetes in a randomized controlled trial (AWARD-1). Diabetes Care. 2014;37:2159.

50. Umpierrez G, Tofé Povedano S, Pérez Manghi F, et al. Efficacy and safety of dulaglutide monotherapy versus metformin in type 2 diabetes in a randomized controlled trial (AWARD-3). Diabetes Care. 2014;37:2168.

51. Weinstock RS, Guerci B, Umpierrez G, et al. Safety and efficacy of once-weekly dulaglutide versus sitagliptin after 2 years in metformin-treated patients with type 2 diabetes (AWARD-5): a randomized, phase III study. Diabetes Obes Metab. 2015;17:849.

52. Marso SP, Bain SC, Consoli A, Daniels GH, Brown-Frandsen K. Semaglutide and cardiovascular outcomes in patients with type 2 diabetes. N Engl J Med. 2017;2017(376):890–2.

53. Inzucchi SE, Bergenstal RM, Buse JB, Diamant M, Ferrannini E, et al. Management of hyperglycemia in type 2 diabetes: a patient-centered approach position statement of the American diabetes association (ADA) and the European association for the study of diabetes (EASD). Diabetes Care. 2012;35:1364–79.

54. Field AE, Coakley EH, Must A, Spadano JL, Laird N, et al. Impact of overweight on the risk of developing common chronic diseases during a 10-year period. Arch Intern Med. 2001;161:1581–6.

55. Vilsboll T, Christensen M, Junker AE, Knop FK, Gluud LL. Effects of glucagon-like peptide-1 receptor agonists on weight loss: systematic review and meta-analyses of randomised controlled trials. BMJ. 2012;344:d7771.

56. Astrup A, Carraro R, Finer N, Harper A, Kunesova M, et al. Safety, tolerability and sustained weight loss over 2 years with the once-daily human GLP-1 analog, liraglutide. Int J Obes (Lond). 2012;36:843–54.

57. Petersen AB, Christensen M. Clinical potential of lixisenatide once daily treatment for type 2 diabetes mellitus. Diabetes Metab Synd Obes. 2013;6:217–31.

58. Sorli C, Harashima S-I, Tsoukas GM, Unger J, Karsbøl JD, Hansen T, et al. Efficacy and safety of once-weekly semaglutide monotherapy versus placebo in patients with type 2 diabetes (SUSTAIN 1): a double-blind, randomised, placebo-controlled, parallel-group, multinational, multicentre phase 3a trial. Lancet Diabetes Endocrinol. 2017;5(4):251–60.

59. Ahrén B, Masmiquel L, Kumar H, Sargin M, Karsbøl JD, Jacobsen SH, et al. Efficacy and safety of once-weekly semaglutide versus once-daily sitagliptin as an add-on to metformin, thiazolidinediones, or both, in patients with type 2 diabetes (SUSTAIN 2): a 56-week, double-blind, phase 3a, randomised trial. Lancet Diabetes Endocrinol. 2017;5(5):341–54.

60. Ahmann AJ, Capehorn M, Charpentier G, Dotta F, Henkel E, Lingvay I, et al. Sustain 3. 2017:1–9.

61. Aroda VR, Bain SC, Cariou B, Piletič M, Rose L, Axelsen M, et al. Efficacy and safety of once-weekly semaglutide versus once-daily insulin glargine as add-on to metformin (with or without sulfonylureas) in insulin-naive patients with type 2 diabetes (SUSTAIN 4): a randomised, open-label, parallel-group, multicentre, multinational, phase 3a trial. Lancet Diabetes Endocrinol. 2017;5(5):355–66.

62. Rodbard H, Lingvay I, Reed J, et al. Efficacy and safety of semaglutide once-weekly vs placebo as add-on to basal insulin alone or in combination with metformin in subjects with type 2 diabetes (SUSTAIN 5) ‖ePoster #766. 2016 [cited 2016 Nov 5]. Available from: http://www.easdvirtualmeeting.org/resources/efficacy-and-safety-of-semaglutide-once-weekly-vs-placebo-as-add-on-to-basal-insulin-alone-or-in-combination-with-metformin-in-subjects-with-type-2-diabetes-sustain-5-871c6042-fbff-48ef-aec0-e9b358e10195

63. Kaul S. Mitigating cardiovascular risk in type 2 diabetes with anti-diabetes drugs: a review of principal cardiovascular outcome results of EMPA-REG OUTCOME, LEADER, and SUSTAIN-6 trials. Diabetes Care. 2017;40(7):821–31.

64. Pratley RE, Aroda VR, Lingvay I, Lüdemann J, Andreassen C, Navarria A, et al. Semaglutide versus dulaglutide once weekly in patients with type 2 diabetes (SUSTAIN 7): a randomised, open-label, phase 3b trial. Lancet Diabetes Endocrinol [Internet]. 2018;8587(Sustain 7):1–12. Available from: http://linkinghub.elsevier.com/retrieve/pii/S221385871830024X

65. Marso SP, Bain SC, Consoli A, Eliaschewitz FG, Jódar E, Leiter LA, et al. Semaglutide and cardiovascular outcomes in patients with type 2 diabetes. N Engl J Med [Internet]. 2016;375(19):1834–44. Available from: http://www.nejm.org/doi/10.1056/NEJMoa1607141.

Insulin Therapy

Balduino Tschiedel and Marcia Puñales

Insulin Therapy in Type 1 Diabetes and Type 2 Diabetes Inpatient

The benefits achieved in the long term, with a more rigorous metabolic control in preventing and reducing chronic complications of diabetes mellitus (DM), were strongly established in both type 1 (T1D) and type 2 (T2D) diabetes. Large prospective studies, such as the Diabetes Control and Complications Trial (DCCT) and the United Kingdom Prospective Diabetes Study (UKPDS), about the influence of metabolic control on the incidence of microvascular and macrovascular chronic complications of diabetes published in the 1990s, established that a reduction of 1% of the glycated hemoglobin (HbA1c) levels influences significantly the protection of microangiopathy and neuropathy [1, 2].

Insulin Therapy in Type 1 Diabetes

The aim of the treatment of type 1 diabetes (T1D), both at onset and years after the diagnosis, is the maintenance of near-normoglycemia to prevent the onset and/or delay the progression of long-term complications [1, 3, 4]. The data from the Diabetes Control and Complications Trial (DCCT) suggested that the residual b-cell function is associated with improved outcomes, with better glycemic control and lower risk for hypoglycemia and less long-term chronic complications [5].

The beneficial and protective effects achieved with intensified insulin control in the prospective DCCT study were clear and remained in the Epidemiology of Diabetes Interventions and Complications (EDIC) study, despite the augment of HbA1c levels, over the follow-up period. However, there is still a gap between evidence and clinical medical practice, since the majority of diabetes patients do not achieve the optimal goal. In 2009, DCCT/EDIC study demonstrated that 81–87% of patients with diabetes had glycated hemoglobin HbA1c levels >7.0% [6], and these results were also showed in UK study where 74% of patients have HbA1c >7.5% [7]. This fact emphasizes that glycemic control is still not satisfactory, in part due to less than optimal insulin therapy.

The recommended therapy for T1D consists of intensive insulin treatment, using multiple daily insulin injections (three to four injections per day of basal and prandial insulin) or continuous subcutaneous insulin infusion (CSII) therapy, matching of prandial insulin to carbohydrate intake, blood glucose tests, and physical activity. The goal of the T1D treatment is to keep blood glucose levels throughout the day near normal limits, avoiding hypoglycemia and glucose variability [8–11].

The American Diabetes Association (ADA) recommends, in adults and non-pregnant woman, glycemic targets of fasting and preprandial capillary blood glucose between 80 and 130 mg/dL and 1–2 h postprandial <180 mg/dL and HbA1c <7.0%, or <6.5% in a selected population, avoiding hypoglycemia [11]. In children and adolescents, it is recommended to achieve blood glucose between 90 and 130 mg/dL before meals and 90 and 150 mg/dL at bedtime and overnight and HbA1c <7.5%. A lower level of HbA1c (<7.0%) can be achieved without hypoglycemia [12]. The International Society for Pediatric and Adolescent Diabetes (ISPAD) recommends for children and adolescents to maintain as optimal fasting or preprandial blood glucose levels between 70 and 145 mg/dL, postprandial between 90 and 180 mg/dL, at bedtime between 120 and 180 mg/dL, and overnight between 80 and 162 mg/dL [13, 14], although the treatment goals should be individualized, taking into account the patient's age and the risk of hypoglycemia, especially nocturnal and unawareness. Recently, ISPAD published a guideline for managing diabetes in preschool children, and it is recommended to maintain before meals blood glucose between 90

B. Tschiedel (✉)
Instituto da Criança com Diabetes, Grupo Hospitalar Conceição, Porto Alegre, RS, Brazil

M. Puñales
Instituto da Criança com Diabetes and Hospital Criança Conceição, Grupo Hospitalar Conceição, Porto Alegre, RS, Brazil

© Springer Nature Switzerland AG 2022
F. Bandeira et al. (eds.), *Endocrinology and Diabetes*, https://doi.org/10.1007/978-3-030-90684-9_32

and 130 mg/dL and at bedtime/overnight between 90 and 150 mg/dL and HbA1c <7.5% [15].

Less rigorous HbA1c target (<8%) may be indicated in elderly patients and those with a history of severe hypoglycemia, advanced microvascular or macrovascular diabetes complications, extensive comorbid pathologies, or long diabetes duration [11, 16]. Pregnant women should maintain lower blood glucose levels, between 60 and 90 mg/dL if fasting and preprandial and <120 mg/dL postprandial, and normal HbA1c [11, 17].

Different therapeutic schedules have been used over the years in the management of patients with T1D [18–20]. Due to the pharmacokinetic profile of the intermediate-acting neutral protamine Hagedorn (isophane insulin; NPH), the conventional treatment with NPH once or twice a day does not mimic the physiology pattern of the endogenous basal insulin secretion and may cause hypoglycemia during its peak of action and hyperglycemia 10–14 h after its administration.

The physiologic insulin replacement attempts to mimic normal insulin secretion. Generally, physiologic regimens replace basal and prandial insulin (often referred to as "bolus") separately. The basal insulin is responsible for avoiding lipolysis and hepatic glucose release in the inter-digestive period; a prandial insulin and additional doses of insulin are responsible to correct the preprandial hyperglycemia or those that occur during the inter-food period. The prandial insulin mimics the response of endogenous insulin secretion to food intake. This physiological response induces a rapid and intense insulin secretion (first phase) followed by a more prolonged secretion into the portal circulation (second stage).

The total daily insulin dose for patients with newly onset of T1D or recent diagnosis of ketoacidosis recommended varies from 0.5 to 1.0 U/kg/day. However, sometimes higher doses of insulin are required to recover metabolic balance [21–25]. The total daily insulin dose depends on age, body weight, pubertal stage, duration and stage of diabetes, local insulin administration, carbohydrate intake, self-monitoring and HbA1c levels, daily routine, and presence of acute complications, as infections or sick days [26]. At the partial remission phase, the daily total insulin dose is generally <0.5 U/kg/day, and subsequently, after this phase, the daily requirement of insulin increases from 0.7 to 1.0 U/kg/day in prepubertal children and can reach 1.0–2.0 U/kg/day during puberty [26] or at stress situation (physical or emotional) from 1.2 to 1.5 U/kg/day. These data are summarized in Table 32.1.

Usually, in the first 6 months of the T1D diagnosis, denominated "honeymoon period," characterized by the normalization of blood glucose levels, it is recommended to maintain small amounts of insulin during this period, since it lasts from several weeks to months [21–25]. There is evidence that in

Table 32.1 Insulin doses at different ages and periods

	Dose (U/kg/day)
Honeymoon period	<0.5
At diagnosis or after ketoacidosis	0.5–1.0
Prepubertal	0.7–1.0
Pubertal	1.0–2.0
Sick days	1.2–1.5
Basal insulin	30–50%

young T1D adults, the initial phase of the disease is progressive and characterized by a slow decline of beta-cell function compared to children and adolescents [27]. Interesting data were also obtained from the DCCT study, suggesting that the persistence of residual beta-cell function is associated with better outcomes, such as improved glycemic control, lower risk of hypoglycemia, and less long-term chronic complications [1, 5, 28, 29], indicating intensive treatment (basal-bolus) since the beginning of the diagnosis.

The intensive insulin treatment is achieved by using multiple daily insulin injections (MDI): three to four injections per day of basal and prandial insulin or continuous subcutaneous insulin infusion (CSII) therapy (insulin pump) [21–25]. The metabolic control (HbA1c) obtained with CSII is slightly better than multiple daily injections; however, both are appropriate and effective [30–32], primarily if associated with continuous glucose monitoring system [33–35].

MDI treatment can be obtained using NPH insulin (two to four times a day: before breakfast and bedtime, or before breakfast, lunch, and bedtime, or before breakfast, lunch, dinner, and bedtime) or insulin glargine (once daily: before breakfast or lunch or dinner or bedtime) or insulin detemir (once or twice a day: before breakfast and/or dinner and/or bedtime) or insulin degludec (once daily: before breakfast or lunch or dinner or bedtime) or glargine U300 (>18 years, once daily: before breakfast or lunch or dinner or bedtime) associated with fast-acting insulin (regular) administered half an hour before meals or fast-acting insulin analogues (lispro, aspart, or glulisine) administered before meals or even after meals [21–25, 36, 37]. The effectiveness of these analogues after meals is at least comparable with the administration of regular insulin before meal [38–40], making it possible to administer in young children just after the carbohydrate ingestion. When regular insulin is administered 5 min before meals, it is less effective than 10–40 min before because of its profile action.

As regards long-acting insulin analogues, glargine was approved for use in children with at least 2 years of age, and detemir and degludec were approved for use in children with ≥1 year of age [41–46]. The only long-acting insulin analogue that is not yet approved for children and adolescents <18 years of age is glargine U-300.

The comparison of multiple daily NPH insulin with glargine in patients 5–16 years showed that patients treated with insulin glargine had a lower fasting glucose, with similar HbA1c levels. Perhaps, the most important benefit of using long-acting insulin analogues is the reduction of the hypoglycemic events, mainly nocturnal hypoglycemia. Moreover, it has been reported that the use of these analogues reduces the occurrence of severe hypoglycemia (seizures, loss of consciousness, or need of assistance of another person to give carbohydrate). The use of long-acting analogues is associated with lower frequency of hypoglycemia, so they are recommended in younger children, who are under neurodevelopment growth, and the harmful effects of the recurrence of severe hypoglycemia may cause permanent damages to the central nervous system [44, 47–49].

Classically, the intensive treatment is obtained by the administration of NPH insulin twice a day, using around 70% in the morning and 30% at bedtime, associated with three daily applications of fast-acting human insulin or fast-acting analogues. Another form of treatment is to administer NPH insulin three times per day, about 50% by morning (70% NPH and 30% fast-acting), approximately 25% at lunch (60% NPH and 40% fast-acting), and the remaining 25% at bedtime [50–53]. It is also possible to administer NPH insulin four times per day, about 30% of the dose by morning (70% NPH and 30% fast-acting), approximately 30% at lunch (60% NPH and 40% fast-acting), 20% at dinner (90% NPH and 10% fast-acting), and the remaining 20% at bedtime (NPH at bedtime only) or approximately 0.2 U/kg. Nevertheless, it is important to remember that insulin pump treatment has contributed to understanding basal-bolus regimen, and today it is recommended that the percentage of basal and bolus insulin should be similar, being recommended that the basal insulin dose should be 30–50% of the total dose prescribed.

Intensive treatment can also be achieved by replacing the NPH insulin to glargine (once daily), detemir (once or twice daily) insulin, degludec (once daily), or glargine U-300 (>18 years, once daily). The replacement of NPH insulin to glargine, glargine U-300, or degludec is performed by reducing the basal dose of insulin by 20% and was subsequently adjusted depending on the results of fasting blood glucose [44]. The replacement of NPH to insulin detemir requires no decrease in insulin dose previously used, but may require two applications per day [43, 44].

The administration of long-acting insulin analogues before breakfast, dinner, or bedtime had been compared, and data showed lower episodes of nocturnal hypoglycemia when the administration was before breakfast, despite the association to a slight increase of fasting glucose.

Hypoglycemia is the most common adverse effect of intensive insulin therapy and is defined by a glucose value <70 mg/dL. In the Diabetes Control and Complications Trial, intensive therapy increased the risk of severe hypoglycemia. The events were reported by 26% of patients with a mean of 1.9 episodes per patient per year, and 43% of episodes occurred nocturnally.

The insulin adjustment is held from fasting plasma glucose and self-monitoring blood glucose, preprandial and postprandial [21–24]. All patients with T1D should perform the self-monitoring of blood glucose tests, and the American Diabetes Association suggests three or more tests per day [54]. The dose of NPH insulin at bedtime is adjusted according to the blood glucose tests at fasting and the other doses by the preprandial results, adjusted every 3 or 4 days. The adjustments of insulin long-acting analogues are done by the fasting blood glucose levels and at least every 5–7 days. The fast-acting human insulin and analogue doses are adjusted by the results of the blood glucose tests 2 h post-meals, considering the sensibility factor and the carbohydrate intake.

Intensive treatment can also be obtained with biphasic insulin, but its use in T1D presents some drawbacks due to lack of flexibility of better adjustments, leading to greater risk of hypoglycemia. However, the use of biphasic insulin may be useful in patients with visual or motor restrictions or those denying multiple daily injections [55].

There are different strategies for the management of insulin and blood glucose control during physical activity [56, 57].

The reduction of the basal insulin or the fast-acting insulin pre-exercise, extra carbohydrate ingestion, and the reduction of basal insulin after exercise are strategies that can be implemented and have advantages and disadvantages. Reducing the NPH or long-acting analogue doses in 20–60% and reducing fast-acting insulin by 30–50% pre-exercise may be necessary, depending on the intensity of the exercise, and this reduction can reach even up to 90% [56].

There are many barriers in order to achieve adequate glycemic control in T1D, including the occurrence and fear of hypoglycemic events, complexity of the day-to-day management, and, particularly, the need for self-monitoring and frequent insulin adjustments. These challenges cause a large impact on the quality of life of patients and considerable costs to health [58]. It is expected that in some years we will be able to prevent these conditions with advances in new techniques and therapeutic agents. However, at the present, the most important issue is to help patients with T1D deal with their disease properly, reducing the occurrence of acute and chronic complications and improving their quality of life.

Insulin Therapy in Type 2 Diabetes

Randomized controlled clinical trials that compared intensive to conventional treatment in T2D, such as the United Kingdom Prospective Diabetes Study (UKPDS) and the Kumamoto Study, established glycemic targets of diabetes treatment associated with better long-term outcomes. Although these studies present different epidemiological data, clinical interventions, and outcomes, all agree with the fact that the reduction of blood glucose is effective in decreasing microvascular and neuropathic chronic complications.

The UKPDS study, which evaluated 5112 T2D patients during 20 years, demonstrated a decrease in chronic complications with intensive treatment, with a reduction of approximately 1% in HbA1c levels (7.9–7.0%), resulting in a 25% reduction of the risk of microvascular complications and 16% of acute myocardial infarction in 10 years [2]. Additionally, it demonstrated benefits of the intensive blood pressure control [59].

Another study (STENO-2), with T2D in intensive care, with HbA1c goals of <6.5%, blood pressure <130/80 mmHg, statin use (total cholesterol <180 mg/dL and LDL <100 mg/dL), and inhibitors of angiotensin-converting enzyme (in cases of persistent microalbuminuria), showed a 53% reduction in the risk of cardiovascular events [60].

The DECODE study showed that postprandial hyperglycemia is an independent risk factor for mortality [61]. Mainly, the prevention of microvascular and macrovascular complications in T2D patients requires tight control of fasting, preprandial and postprandial blood glucose, HbA1c, lipids, and blood pressure. However, in older patients with previous cardiovascular disease and longstanding diabetes, the glycemic control may not be so strict, as demonstrated by the ACCORD study, which showed an increase in cardiovascular mortality and other causes in T2D patients in intensive care [62].

The ADA recommends as targets for T2D treatment preprandial glucose between 90 and 130 mg/dL and HbA1c levels <7.0% [63, 64]. However, the American Association of Clinical Endocrinologists (AACE) [65] and the International Diabetes Federation (IDF) [66] suggest HbA1c levels <6.5%. To achieve these goals, the proper maintenance of fasting glucose, in addition to postprandial glucose through basal-bolus insulin, is an important factor in the treatment of subjects with T2D [67].

The pathophysiology of pharmacological treatment of subjects with T2D depends on various aspects contributing to hyperglycemia. The peripheral insulin resistance (adipocytes and skeletal muscle), presented in 85–90% of the cases [67], the deficiency of the insulin production by the beta cell, and the excessive hepatic glucose production caused by the insulin resistance are all contributor factors to the onset of hyperglycemia. As shown in UKPDS, the persistence of elevated levels of HbA1c leads to the progressive loss of beta-cell function in secreting insulin [2].

The metabolic abnormalities associated with T2D deteriorate with the increase of age. The sooner the treatment is initiated in T2D patients, when mild levels of HbA1c occur, the better the improvement of the metabolic control and the decrease of the long-term complications.

The T2D treatment begins with monotherapy, and subsequently a second drug is added, and, if necessary, a third oral drug or insulin is implemented. However, different societies recommend that insulin might be implemented earlier, shortly after oral monotherapy. This treatment initially begins by changes in lifestyle (diet, cholesterol control, weight reduction, blood pressure control, physical activity, and tobacco control) associated with metformin [68–70]. If these interventions are not effective in reducing HbA1c levels <7.0%, another approach must be implemented 3 months after the initiation of metformin. However, there is no consensus on the second drug used, being insulin, sulfonylurea, thiazolidinedione (pioglitazone), glucagon-like peptide-1 (GLP-1) agonists, alpha-glucosidase inhibitors, sodium-glucose co-transporter 2 (SGLT2) inhibitors, or dipeptidyl peptidase-4 (DPP-4) inhibitors [68–70].

Although insulin therapy for T2DM treatment has conventionally been postponed as the latest therapeutic option, different diabetes guidelines and consensus suggest considering insulin as the first line of treatment. Therefore, insulin could be indicated as a second drug added after metformin, when the patient presents intense clinical evidence (polyuria, polydipsia, polyphagia, weight loss) of glucotoxicity, severe hyperglycemia with ketonuria, decompensation, and/or HbA1c ≥8.5%. However, if the clinical evidence is less intense, and/or HbA1c levels <8.5%, another oral drug can be added before using insulin.

To start insulin therapy in T2D patients, it is recommended to start with 10 U (or 0.2 U/kg of body weight) of a basal insulin (NPH, glargine, detemir, degludec, or glargine U-300) at bedtime, maintaining the oral antidiabetic agents already being used [71–76].

In a study comparing the use of glimepiride associated with insulin glargine in the morning or at bedtime or bedtime NPH insulin in 695 patients with T2D, HbA1c levels decreased 1.24% with glargine in the morning, 0.96% using glargine at bedtime, and 0.84% using NPH insulin at bedtime [77]. The improvement in HbA1c was more evident with glargine in the morning than at bedtime ($p = 0.008$) and than NPH at bedtime ($p = 0.001$).

The randomized treat-to-target study, which compared insulin glargine or human NPH insulin to oral therapy in subjects with T2D, showed similar results of HbA1c levels (6.96% vs. 6.97%) and fasting glucose (117 mg/dL vs. 120 mg/dL) [78]. The insulin adjustment was performed every 3 days, according to the blood glucose tests. In the LANMET study, with T2D patients with inadequate glycemic control, on use of oral antidiabetics (90% with sulfonylureas associated with metformin), and without previous treatment with insulin, 110 subjects were randomized to receive insulin glargine at bedtime plus metformin or NPH insulin plus metformin for 36 weeks [79]. The initial dose of insulin was 10 U for those using previously only metformin and 20 U for those using metformin associated with sulfonylurea. The individuals randomized to receive insulin glargine showed lower fasting plasma glucose than NPH group (103.5 mg/dL vs. 107.3 mg/dL, $p < 0.001$) [79]. In this study, the insulin dose was increased by 2 U every 3 days if the fasting plasma glucose (FPG) ≥ 100 mg/dL within 3 days and 4 U if FPG ≥ 180 mg/dL in the same period and successively. The patient was responsible for his insulin adjustment or self-titration, maintaining their optimal dose without endocrinologist visits and telephone calls.

In the UKPDS, patients with T2D receiving insulin therapy had lower HbA1c levels, but 1.0–2.0% more patients receiving insulin reported at least one episode of severe hypoglycemia per year than those patients receiving other therapies. Intensive therapy, with oral medications or insulin, has been shown to increase the risk of episodes of hypoglycemia.

The GOAL study, involving 7893 patients with T2D, uncontrolled on oral antidiabetics randomized to 4 treatment groups with long-acting insulin analogue glargine, involving different forms of titration and different ways of measuring HbA1c, found significant reductions in HbA1c and blood glucose in all groups ($p < 0.0001$) [59]. However, the group with active titration showed a greater reduction in HbA1c than those with usual titration (1.5% vs. 1.3%, $p < 0.0001$), and a greater proportion of patients achieved an HbA1c <7.0% (38% vs. 30%, $p < 0.0001$) [80].

In patients with T2D using only one dose of NPH at bedtime, it is possible to use twice a day (morning and bedtime) when goals are not being achieved, before starting to use fast-acting insulin. When the basal insulin at bedtime or twice a day associated with oral antidiabetics is no longer sufficient to maintain HbA1c levels <7.0%, it is necessary to intensify insulinization. This means starting with fast-acting insulin (human or analogues), maintaining the basal or biphasic insulin. When insulinization is intensified, oral insulin secretagogues (sulfonylurea, glinides) must be suspended, but metformin is maintained.

In T2D, a study using insulin glargine as basal insulin demonstrated that a fast-acting insulin could be started initially at the main meal, as it causes the greatest increase in postprandial glycemia or results in the highest elevation of premeal glucose, and then this insulin could be extended to the other meals, if necessary, to achieve HbA1c goal [81].

In a study with T2D uncontrolled patients at diagnosis, which compared the use of NPH insulin at bedtime plus regular insulin before meals and NPH plus lispro, the use of the insulin analogue showed to be superior in achieving metabolic control, with suppression of glucagon secretion and reduction of the glucotoxicity [82]. Another study also observed that use of insulin lispro in patients with T2D, administered before meals, was more effective in reducing HbA1c than the use of metformin or NPH insulin at bedtime. In a study comparing the insulin analogues lispro and aspart, the results evidenced that both have the same effectiveness in controlling postprandial glucose excursions [83]. The administration of insulin aspart 15 min after the meal is as or more effective in controlling postprandial hyperglycemia than implementing the regular insulin before meals [38]. Greater predictability of action and lower glycemic variation with the use of these analogues have also been described in individuals with T2D [84]. Individuals with T2D treated for 26 weeks with the long-acting analogue insulin detemir associated with aspart insulin before meals showed glycemic control comparable to those treated with NPH and aspart. However, as demonstrated in other studies, there were less variability between individuals and less weight gain with insulin detemir [85, 86].

In a study including 7637 T2D patients randomized to receive either insulin degludec (3818 patients) or insulin glargine U-100 (3819 patients) once daily between dinner and bedtime in a double-blind, treat-to-target and evaluation of cardiovascular outcome, of those randomized 6509 (85.2%) had already cardiovascular disease established, chronic kidney disease, or both. At baseline, the mean age was 65.0 years, duration of T2D 16.4 years, and HbA1c $8.4 \pm 1.7\%$; 83.9% of the T2D were receiving insulin. The primary outcome occurred in 325 patients (8.5%) of degludec group and in 356 (9.3%) of glargine group. After 24 months of treatment, the mean HbA1c was $7.5 \pm 1.2\%$ in both groups, and the mean fasting plasma glucose level was significantly lower in the degludec group (128 ± 56 vs. 136 ± 57 mg/dL, $p < 0.001$). Severe hypoglycemia happened in 187 degludec patients (4.9%) and in 252 glargine patients (6.6%), $p < 0.001$. Rates of adverse events did not differ between the two groups [45].

Regarding the use of biphasic insulin in subjects with T2D, studies demonstrated that the biphasic analogues are more effective in reducing the postprandial hyperglycemia than those containing NPH and regular, without significant reduction of HbA1c [87, 88]. However, the improvement of postprandial hyperglycemia and glycemic variability reduction, despite HbA1c levels, may be important factors in reducing the risk of onset and progression of microvascular and macrovascular chronic complications. The use of biphasic insulins (premix) may be recommended for those patients with the greatest difficulty in assimilating the basal-bolus regimen, considered apparently to be more convenient because the doses are already previously divided on a fixed percentage of basal and fast-acting insulin analogues 70/30, 75/25, or 50/50.

In T2D patients who need to use basal-bolus regimen, due to severe insulinopenia, glucose variability occurs frequently, and continuous subcutaneous insulin infusion can be indicated.

Insulin Therapy Inpatient

Hyperglycemia is a common acute complication of critically ill patients, during hospitalization at intensive care units (ICUs). Some studies demonstrated that the presence of hyperglycemia, in particular severe hyperglycemia, is associated with increased morbidity and mortality in some patients, but some clinical and randomized trials evaluating the effects of tighter glucose on the mortality of critically ill patients showed conflicting data.

Despite these conflicting evidences, the American Diabetes Association, the American Association of Clinical Endocrinologists, the Brazilian Diabetes Society, and other professional organizations recommend intensive insulin therapy as the standard of care for critically ill patients [69, 89–92].

The main barrier to implement a tight glucose control in critically ill patients during hospitalization is the increased risk of severe hypoglycemia that has been described to be associated with increased mortality. Because of these aspects and risks or benefits, the tight glucose control is used infrequently by some clinicians. The Normoglycemia in Intensive Care Evaluation—Survival Using Glucose Algorithm Regulation (NICE-SUGAR) study, an international multicenter trial involving 6104 patients and the largest randomized clinical trial of intensive insulin therapy, evidenced that blood glucose target ≤180 mg/dL is associated with lower mortality than did a target of 81–108 mg/dL [93].

It is recommended that all clinicians assess all patients admitted to the hospital for a history of diabetes. When present, this diagnosis should be clearly identified in the medical record. All patients, independent of a prior diagnosis of diabetes, have laboratory blood glucose (BG) testing on hospital admission. The patients without a history of diabetes with BG greater than 7.8 mmol/L (140 mg/dL) should be monitored with bedside capillary BG testing for at least 24–48 h. Those with BG greater than 7.8 mmol/L require appropriate therapeutic intervention [89].

The inpatient care of individuals with diabetes and hyperglycemia is complex, involving multiple providers with varying degrees of expertise who are dispersed across many different areas of the hospital. Multidisciplinary local protocols should guide safe glycemic control, hypoglycemia prevention, and patient preparation for care transitions. Poor coordination of glucose monitoring, meal delivery, and insulin administration is a common barrier to optimal care of the patients during the hospitalization period.

Protocol for Insulin Therapy in Critically Ill Patients

The most efficient and safe therapeutic option to treat critically ill patients is by continuous intravenous insulin pump infusion [69, 92, 94]. It is recommended preferably to use regular human insulin than fast-acting analogues, in solutions containing 100 U diluted in 100 mL of 0.9% saline solution (1 U/mL).

Some authors recommend an initial intravenous bolus of insulin before starting the infusion, to reduce the glucotoxicity if glycemia is greater than 300 mg/dL, using a standard formula to correct the hyperglycemia (glycemia ÷ 100 = insulin dose). The initial infusion rate can be calculated by rate infusion (mL/h) = current glycemia − minimal glycemia × correction factor (CF). The minimal of blood glucose depends on each case and may be established at 100 mg/dL. The CF depends on the patient's estimated insulin resistance; it is common to start with a factor of 0.02, rising 0.03–0.05 in those with more insulin resistance or reducing to 0.01 in patients more sensitive to insulin.

The infusion rate should be adjusted to maintain blood glucose at target, noting that the prompt glucose decline should be avoided, reducing the rate of insulin infusion, and, in the presence of hyperglycemia, the rate must be accelerated. Thus, the dynamic behavior of glycemia analyzed the last three measures, and it is important to adjust the rate of insulin infusion. Glucose measurements during insulin infusion should be performed initially every hour and in those with glycemic control at target every 2 or 3 h.

It is important to avoid glycemic variability in these critically ill patients, because there is an increase of the mortality, independent of the glucose variation, induced by the cellular oxidative stress during this period.

Protocol for Insulin Therapy in Non-critically Ill Patients

Some studies demonstrated that the presence of hyperglycemia in non-critically ill patients also increases morbidity and mortality [69, 89–91].

It is recommended that only patients with well-controlled T2D maintain oral antidiabetic agents and the others should discontinue oral diabetes drugs and non-insulin injectable diabetes medications upon hospital admission.

To start insulinization in these patients, the dose could be calculated at a total daily dose of 0.2–0.3 U/kg of body weight in patients with aged ≥70 years and/or glomerular filtration rate less than 60 mL/min or 0.4 U/kg of body weight per day for patients not meeting the criteria above who have BG concentrations of 7.8–11.1 mmol/L (140–200 mg/dL) or 0.5 U/kg of body weight per day for patients not meeting the criteria above when BG concentration is 11.2–22.2 mmol/L (201–400 mg/dL).

The total calculated dose is distributed approximately as 50% basal insulin and 50% prandial insulin. If the basal insulin is glargine or detemir give it once a day or twice if detemir or NPH is given, at the same time each day, and the fast-acting (prandial) insulin should be given in three equally

Table 32.2 Supplemental doses of insulin according to BG and insulin sensitivity

BG (mg/dL)	Insulin-sensitive	Usual	Insulin-resistant
>141–180	2	4	6
181–220	4	6	8
221–260	6	8	10
261–300	8	10	12
301–350	10	12	14
351–400	12	14	16
>400	14	16	18

divided doses before each meal. If the patient is not able to eat, it is necessary to hold prandial insulin, maintaining basal insulin at a lower percentage (40%).

The prandial insulin doses are adjusted according to the results of bedside BG measurements. The supplemental (correction) fast-acting insulin analogue or regular insulin is required if the patient is able and expected to eat all or most of the meals. Give regular insulin or fast-acting insulin analogue before each meal following Table 32.2. If a patient is not able to eat or is receiving enteral nutrition, give regular insulin every 6 h or fast-acting insulin analogue every 4–6 h. In patients receiving parenteral nutrition, it is recommended to use continuous endovenous insulin infusion.

If fasting and premeal plasma glucose are persistently above 7.8 mmol/L (140 mg/dL) in the absence of hypoglycemia, increase insulin scale of insulin from the insulin-sensitive to the usual or from the usual to the insulin-resistant column. If a patient develops hypoglycemia (BG <3.8 mmol/L or 70 mg/dL) or acts in the opposite way, decrease the regular insulin or fast-acting insulin analogue from the insulin-resistant to the usual column or from the usual to the insulin-sensitive column.

References

1. The effect of intensive treatment of diabetes on the development and progression of long-term complications in insulin-dependent diabetes mellitus. The diabetes control and complications trial research group. N Engl J Med. 1993;329(14):977–86.
2. Intensive blood-glucose control with sulphonylureas or insulin compared with conventional treatment and risk of complications in patients with type 2 diabetes (UKPDS 33). UK Prospective Diabetes Study (UKPDS) Group. Lancet. 1998;352(9131):837–53.
3. Effect of intensive therapy on the microvascular complications of type 1 diabetes mellitus. JAMA. 2002;287(19):2563–9.
4. Epidemiology of diabetes interventions and complications (EDIC). Design, implementation, and preliminary results of a long-term follow-up of the diabetes control and complications trial cohort. Diabetes Care. 1999;22(1):99–111.
5. Effect of intensive therapy on residual beta-cell function in patients with type 1 diabetes in the diabetes control and complications trial. A randomized, controlled trial. The Diabetes Control and Complications Trial Research Group. Ann Intern Med. 1998;128(7):517–23.
6. Nathan DM, Zinman B, Cleary PA, Backlund JY, Genuth S, Miller R, et al. Modern-day clinical course of type 1 diabetes mellitus after 30 years' duration: the diabetes control and complications trial/epidemiology of diabetes interventions and complications and Pittsburgh epidemiology of diabetes complications experience (1983–2005). Arch Intern Med. 2009;169(14):1307–16.
7. Calvert M, Shankar A, McManus RJ, Lester H, Freemantle N. Effect of the quality and outcomes framework on diabetes care in the United Kingdom: retrospective cohort study. BMJ. 2009;338:b1870.
8. Standards of medical care in diabetes-2017: summary of revisions. Diabetes Care. 2017;40(Suppl 1):S4–5.
9. Consensus statement on the worldwide standardization of the hemoglobin A1C measurement: the American Diabetes Association, European Association for the Study of Diabetes, International Federation of Clinical Chemistry and Laboratory Medicine, and the International Diabetes Federation. Diabetes Care. 2007;30(9):2399–400.
10. Rodbard HW, Blonde L, Braithwaite SS, Brett EM, Cobin RH, Handelsman Y, et al. American Association of Clinical Endocrinologists medical guidelines for clinical practice for the management of diabetes mellitus. Endocr Pract. 2007;13 Suppl 1:1–68.
11. Glycemic targets: standards of medical care in diabetes-2018. Diabetes Care. 2018;41(Suppl 1):S55–S64.
12. Children and adolescents: standards of medical care in diabetes-2018. Diabetes Care. 2018;41(Suppl 1):S126–S36.
13. Rewers M, Pihoker C, Donaghue K, Hanas R, Swift P, Klingensmith GJ. Assessment and monitoring of glycemic control in children and adolescents with diabetes. Pediatr Diabetes. 2009;10 Suppl 12:71–81.
14. Rewers M, Pihoker C, Donaghue K, Hanas R, Swift P, Klingensmith GJ. Assessment and monitoring of glycemic control in children and adolescents with diabetes. Pediatr Diabetes. 2007;8(6):408–18.
15. Sundberg F, Barnard K, Cato A, de Beaufort C, DiMeglio LA, Dooley G, et al. ISPAD guidelines. Managing diabetes in preschool children. Pediatr Diabetes. 2017;18(7):499–517.
16. Older adults: standards of medical care in diabetes-2018. Diabetes Care. 2018;41(Suppl 1):S119–S25.
17. Management of diabetes in pregnancy: standards of medical care in diabetes-2018. Diabetes Care. 2018;41(Suppl 1):S137–S43.
18. Ludvigsson J, Bolli GB. Intensive insulin treatment in diabetic children. Diabetes Nutr Metab. 2001;14(5):292–304.
19. White NH, Cleary PA, Dahms W, Goldstein D, Malone J, Tamborlane WV. Beneficial effects of intensive therapy of diabetes during adolescence: outcomes after the conclusion of the Diabetes Control and Complications Trial (DCCT). J Pediatr. 2001;139(6):804–12.
20. Pesic M, Zivic S, Radenkovic S, Velojic M, Dimic D, Antic S. Comparison between basal insulin glargine and NPH insulin in patients with diabetes type 1 on conventional intensive insulin therapy. Vojnosanit Pregl. 2007;64(4):247–52.
21. Gerich JE. Novel insulins: expanding options in diabetes management. Am J Med. 2002;113(4):308–16.
22. Dunn CJ, Plosker GL, Keating GM, McKeage K, Scott LJ. Insulin glargine: an updated review of its use in the management of diabetes mellitus. Drugs. 2003;63(16):1743–78.
23. Skyler JS. Intensive insulin therapy: a personal and historical perspective. Diabetes Educ. 1989;15(1):33–9.
24. Hirsch IB, Farkas-Hirsch R, Skyler JS. Intensive insulin therapy for treatment of type I diabetes. Diabetes Care. 1990;13(12):1265–83.
25. Bolli GB. Insulin treatment in type 1 diabetes. Endocr Pract. 2006;12 Suppl 1:105–9.
26. Bangstad HJ, Danne T, Deeb L, Jarosz-Chobot P, Urakami T, Hanas R. Insulin treatment in children and adolescents with diabetes. Pediatr Diabetes. 2009;10 Suppl 12:82–99.

27. Bruno G, Cerutti F, Merletti F, Cavallo-Perin P, Gandolfo E, Rivetti M, et al. Residual beta-cell function and male/female ratio are higher in incident young adults than in children: the registry of type 1 diabetes of the province of Turin, Italy, 1984–2000. Diabetes Care. 2005;28(2):312–7.

28. Nathan DM, Cleary PA, Backlund JY, Genuth SM, Lachin JM, Orchard TJ, et al. Intensive diabetes treatment and cardiovascular disease in patients with type 1 diabetes. N Engl J Med. 2005;353(25):2643–53.

29. White NH, Sun W, Cleary PA, Danis RP, Davis MD, Hainsworth DP, et al. Prolonged effect of intensive therapy on the risk of retinopathy complications in patients with type 1 diabetes mellitus: 10 years after the diabetes control and complications trial. Arch Ophthalmol. 2008;126(12):1707–15.

30. Raskin P, Holcombe JH, Tamborlane WV, Malone JI, Strowig S, Ahern JA, et al. A comparison of insulin lispro and buffered regular human insulin administered via continuous subcutaneous insulin infusion pump. J Diabetes Complications. 2001;15(6):295–300.

31. Maiorino MI, Bellastella G, Casciano O, Cirillo P, Simeon V, Chiodini P, et al. The effects of subcutaneous insulin infusion versus multiple insulin injections on glucose variability in young adults with type 1 diabetes: the 2-year follow-up of the observational METRO study. Diabetes Technol Ther. 2018.

32. Karges B, Schwandt A, Heidtmann B, Kordonouri O, Binder E, Schierloh U, et al. Association of insulin pump therapy vs insulin injection therapy with severe hypoglycemia, ketoacidosis, and glycemic control among children, adolescents, and young Adults with type 1 diabetes. JAMA. 2017;318(14):1358–66.

33. Matejko B, Skupien J, Mrozinska S, Grzanka M, Cyganek K, Kiec-Wilk B, et al. Factors associated with glycemic control in adult type 1 diabetes patients treated with insulin pump therapy. Endocrine. 2015;48(1):164–9.

34. Picard S, Hanaire H, Baillot-Rudoni S, Gilbert-Bonnemaison E, Not D, Reznik Y, et al. Evaluation of the adherence to continuous glucose monitoring in the management of type 1 diabetes patients on sensor-augmented pump therapy: the SENLOCOR study. Diabetes Technol Ther. 2016;18(3):127–35.

35. Thabit H, Hovorka R. Continuous subcutaneous insulin infusion therapy and multiple daily insulin injections in type 1 diabetes mellitus: a comparative overview and future horizons. Expert Opin Drug Deliv. 2016;13(3):389–400.

36. Skyler JS, Cefalu WT, Kourides IA, Landschulz WH, Balagtas CC, Cheng SL, et al. Efficacy of inhaled human insulin in type 1 diabetes mellitus: a randomised proof-of-concept study. Lancet. 2001;357(9253):331–5.

37. Skyler JS, Jovanovic L, Klioze S, Reis J, Duggan W. Two-year safety and efficacy of inhaled human insulin (Exubera) in adult patients with type 1 diabetes. Diabetes Care. 2007;30(3):579–85.

38. Brunner GA, Hirschberger S, Sendlhofer G, Wutte A, Ellmerer M, Balent B, et al. Post-prandial administration of the insulin analogue insulin aspart in patients with type 1 diabetes mellitus. Diabet Med. 2000;17(5):371–5.

39. Schernthaner G, Wein W, Sandholzer K, Equiluz-Bruck S, Bates PC, Birkett MA. Postprandial insulin lispro. A new therapeutic option for type 1 diabetic patients. Diabetes Care. 1998;21(4):570–3.

40. Danne T, Aman J, Schober E, Deiss D, Jacobsen JL, Friberg HH, et al. A comparison of postprandial and preprandial administration of insulin aspart in children and adolescents with type 1 diabetes. Diabetes Care. 2003;26(8):2359–64.

41. Campbell RK, White JR, Levien T, Baker D. Insulin glargine. Clin Ther. 2001;23(12):1938–57; discussion 23.

42. Monami M, Marchionni N, Mannucci E. Long-acting insulin analogues vs. NPH human insulin in type 1 diabetes. A meta-analysis. Diabetes Obes Metab. 2009;11(4):372–8.

43. Robertson KJ, Schoenle E, Gucev Z, Mordhorst L, Gall MA, Ludvigsson J. Insulin detemir compared with NPH insulin in children and adolescents with type 1 diabetes. Diabet Med. 2007;24(1):27–34.

44. Tumini S, Carinci S. Unmet needs in children with diabetes: the role of basal insulin. Minerva Pediatr. 2017;69(6):513–30.

45. Marso SP, McGuire DK, Zinman B, Poulter NR, Emerson SS, Pieber TR, et al. Efficacy and safety of degludec versus glargine in type 2 diabetes. N Engl J Med. 2017;377(8):723–32.

46. Thalange N, Deeb L, Iotova V, Kawamura T, Klingensmith G, Philotheou A, et al. Insulin degludec in combination with bolus insulin aspart is safe and effective in children and adolescents with type 1 diabetes. Pediatr Diabetes. 2015;16(3):164–76.

47. Rovet JF, Ehrlich RM, Hoppe M. Intellectual deficits associated with early onset of insulin-dependent diabetes mellitus in children. Diabetes Care. 1987;10(4):510–5.

48. Naguib JM, Kulinskaya E, Lomax CL, Garralda ME. Neurocognitive performance in children with type 1 diabetes--a meta-analysis. J Pediatr Psychol. 2009;34(3):271–82.

49. Rovet JF, Ehrlich RM, Hoppe M. Specific intellectual deficits in children with early onset diabetes mellitus. Child Dev. 1988;59(1):226–34.

50. Instituto da Criança com Diabetes: http://www.icdrs.org.br/conduta.php.

51. Lalli C, Ciofetta M, Del Sindaco P, Torlone E, Pampanelli S, Compagnucci P, et al. Long-term intensive treatment of type 1 diabetes with the short-acting insulin analog lispro in variable combination with NPH insulin at mealtime. Diabetes Care. 1999;22(3):468–77.

52. Rossetti P, Pampanelli S, Fanelli C, Porcellati F, Costa E, Torlone E, et al. Intensive replacement of basal insulin in patients with type 1 diabetes given rapid-acting insulin analog at mealtime: a 3-month comparison between administration of NPH insulin four times daily and glargine insulin at dinner or bedtime. Diabetes Care. 2003;26(5):1490–6.

53. Bolli GB, Di Marchi RD, Park GD, Pramming S, Koivisto VA. Insulin analogues and their potential in the management of diabetes mellitus. Diabetologia. 1999;42(10):1151–67.

54. Standards of medical care in diabetes--2012. Diabetes Care. 2012;35 Suppl 1:S11–63.

55. Hirsch IB. Insulin analogues. N Engl J Med. 2005;352(2):174–83.

56. Macknight JM, Mistry DJ, Pastors JG, Holmes V, Rynders CA. The daily management of athletes with diabetes. Clin Sports Med. 2009;28(3):479–95.

57. Riddell MC, Gallen IW, Smart CE, Taplin CE, Adolfsson P, Lumb AN, et al. Exercise management in type 1 diabetes: a consensus statement. Lancet Diabetes Endocrinol. 2017;5(5):377–90.

58. Economic costs of diabetes in the U.S. In 2007. Diabetes Care. 2008;31(3):596–615.

59. Tight blood pressure control and risk of macrovascular and microvascular complications in type 2 diabetes: UKPDS 38. UK Prospective Diabetes Study Group. BMJ. 1998;317(7160):703–13.

60. Gaede P, Vedel P, Larsen N, Jensen GV, Parving HH, Pedersen O. Multifactorial intervention and cardiovascular disease in patients with type 2 diabetes. N Engl J Med. 2003;348(5):383–93.

61. Glucose tolerance and mortality: comparison of WHO and American Diabetes Association diagnostic criteria. The DECODE study group. European Diabetes Epidemiology Group. Diabetes epidemiology: collaborative analysis of diagnostic criteria in Europe. Lancet. 1999;354(9179):617–21.

62. Gerstein HC, Miller ME, Byington RP, Goff DC Jr, Bigger JT, Buse JB, et al. Effects of intensive glucose lowering in type 2 diabetes. N Engl J Med. 2008;358(24):2545–59.

63. Standards of medical care in diabetes--2006. Diabetes Care. 2006;29 Suppl 1:S4–42.

64. Standards of medical care in diabetes--2010. Diabetes Care;33 Suppl 1:S11–61.

65. American College of Endocrinology and American Diabetes Association consensus statement on inpatient diabetes and glycemic control. Endocr Pract. 2006;12(4):458–68.

66. A desktop guide to type 2 diabetes mellitus. European Diabetes Policy Group 1999. Diabet Med. 1999;16(9):716–30.

67. Garber AJ. The metabolic syndrome. Med Clin North Am. 2004;88(4):837–46, ix.

68. Pharmacologic approaches to glycemic treatment: standards of medical care in diabetes-2018. Diabetes Care. 2018;41(Suppl 1):S73–S85.

69. Diretrizes da Sociedade Brasileira de Diabetes 2017–18; 2017.

70. Khamseh ME, Yousefzadeh G, Banazadeh Z, Ghareh S. Practical focus on American Diabetes Association/European Association for the study of diabetes consensus algorithm in patients with type 2 diabetes mellitus: timely insulin initiation and titration (Iran-AFECT). Diabetes Metab J. 2017;41(1):31–7.

71. DeWitt DE, Hirsch IB. Outpatient insulin therapy in type 1 and type 2 diabetes mellitus: scientific review. JAMA. 2003;289(17):2254–64.

72. Kumar S, Jang HC, Demirag NG, Skjoth TV, Endahl L, Bode B. Efficacy and safety of once-daily insulin degludec/insulin aspart compared with once-daily insulin glargine in participants with type 2 diabetes: a randomized, treat-to-target study. Diabet Med. 2016;34(2):180–8.

73. Freemantle N, Chou E, Frois C, Zhuo D, Lehmacher W, Vlajnic A, et al. Safety and efficacy of insulin glargine 300 u/mL compared with other basal insulin therapies in patients with type 2 diabetes mellitus: a network meta-analysis. BMJ Open. 2016;6(2):e009421.

74. Zinman B, DeVries JH, Bode B, Russell-Jones D, Leiter LA, Moses A, et al. Efficacy and safety of insulin degludec three times a week versus insulin glargine once a day in insulin-naive patients with type 2 diabetes: results of two phase 3, 26 week, randomised, open-label, treat-to-target, non-inferiority trials. Lancet Diabetes Endocrinol. 2016;1(2):123–31.

75. Rodbard HW, Bode BW, Harris SB, Rose L, Lehmann L, Jarlov H, et al. Safety and efficacy of insulin degludec/liraglutide (IDegLira) added to sulphonylurea alone or to sulphonylurea and metformin in insulin-naive people with type 2 diabetes: the DUAL IV trial. Diabet Med. 2017;34(2):189–96.

76. Stailey M, Conway SE. Review of the next generation of long-acting basal insulins: insulin degludec and insulin glargine. Consult Pharm. 2017;32(1):42–6.

77. Fritsche A, Schweitzer MA, Haring HU. Glimepiride combined with morning insulin glargine, bedtime neutral protamine hagedorn insulin, or bedtime insulin glargine in patients with type 2 diabetes. A randomized, controlled trial. Ann Intern Med. 2003;138(12):952–9.

78. Riddle MC, Rosenstock J, Gerich J. The treat-to-target trial: randomized addition of glargine or human NPH insulin to oral therapy of type 2 diabetic patients. Diabetes Care. 2003;26(11):3080–6.

79. Yki-Jarvinen H, Kauppinen-Makelin R, Tiikkainen M, Vahatalo M, Virtamo H, Nikkila K, et al. Insulin glargine or NPH combined with metformin in type 2 diabetes: the LANMET study. Diabetologia. 2006;49(3):442–51.

80. Kennedy L, Herman WH, Strange P, Harris A. Impact of active versus usual algorithmic titration of basal insulin and point-of-care versus laboratory measurement of HbA1c on glycemic control in patients with type 2 diabetes: the Glycemic Optimization with Algorithms and Labs at Point of Care (GOAL A1C) trial. Diabetes Care. 2006;29(1):1–8.

81. Lankisch MR, Ferlinz KC, Leahy JL, Scherbaum WA. Introducing a simplified approach to insulin therapy in type 2 diabetes: a comparison of two single-dose regimens of insulin glulisine plus insulin glargine and oral antidiabetic drugs. Diabetes Obes Metab. 2008;10(12):1178–85.

82. Murase Y, Yagi K, Sugihara M, Chujo D, Otsuji M, Muramoto H, et al. Lispro is superior to regular insulin in transient intensive insulin therapy in type 2 diabetes. Intern Med. 2004;43(9):779–86.

83. Plank J, Wutte A, Brunner G, Siebenhofer A, Semlitsch B, Sommer R, et al. A direct comparison of insulin aspart and insulin lispro in patients with type 1 diabetes. Diabetes Care. 2002;25(11):2053–7.

84. Rosenfalck AM, Thorsby P, Kjems L, Birkeland K, Dejgaard A, Hanssen KF, et al. Improved postprandial glycaemic control with insulin Aspart in type 2 diabetic patients treated with insulin. Acta Diabetol. 2000;37(1):41–6.

85. Haak T, Tiengo A, Draeger E, Suntum M, Waldhausl W. Lower within-subject variability of fasting blood glucose and reduced weight gain with insulin detemir compared to NPH insulin in patients with type 2 diabetes. Diabetes Obes Metab. 2005;7(1):56–64.

86. Rosenstock J, Park G, Zimmerman J. Basal insulin glargine (HOE 901) versus NPH insulin in patients with type 1 diabetes on multiple daily insulin regimens. U.S. Insulin Glargine (HOE 901) Type 1 Diabetes Investigator Group. Diabetes Care. 2000;23(8):1137–42.

87. Koivisto VA, Tuominen JA, Ebeling P. Lispro Mix25 insulin as premeal therapy in type 2 diabetic patients. Diabetes Care. 1999;22(3):459–62.

88. Kilo C, Mezitis N, Jain R, Mersey J, McGill J, Raskin P. Starting patients with type 2 diabetes on insulin therapy using once-daily injections of biphasic insulin aspart 70/30, biphasic human insulin 70/30, or NPH insulin in combination with metformin. J Diabetes Complications. 2003;17(6):307–13.

89. Umpierrez GE, Hellman R, Korytkowski MT, Kosiborod M, Maynard GA, Montori VM, et al. Management of hyperglycemia in hospitalized patients in non-critical care setting: an endocrine society clinical practice guideline. J Clin Endocrinol Metab. 2012;97(1):16–38.

90. Moghissi ES, Korytkowski MT, DiNardo M, Einhorn D, Hellman R, Hirsch IB, et al. American Association of Clinical Endocrinologists and American Diabetes Association consensus statement on inpatient glycemic control. Endocr Pract. 2009;15(4):353–69.

91. SBD. Controle da hiperglicemia intra-hospitalr em pacientes críticos e não críticos Posicionamento Oficial SBD. 2011;11.

92. Diabetes Care in the Hospital: standards of medical care in diabetes-2018. Diabetes Care. 2018;41(Suppl 1):S144–S51.

93. Finfer S, Chittock DR, Su SY, Blair D, Foster D, Dhingra V, et al. Intensive versus conventional glucose control in critically ill patients. N Engl J Med. 2009;360(13):1283–97.

94. Smiley D, Rhee M, Peng L, Roediger L, Mulligan P, Satterwhite L, et al. Safety and efficacy of continuous insulin infusion in noncritical care settings. J Hosp Med. 2012;5(4):212–7.

Diabetic Ketoacidosis and Hyperosmolar Hyperglycemic State

Fernanda Moura Victor, Sérgio Ricardo de Lima Andrade, and Francisco Bandeira

Introduction

Diabetic ketoacidosis (DKA) and hyperosmolar hyperglycemic state (HHS) are serious acute metabolic complications that occur in patients with type 1 diabetes mellitus (T1DM) and type 2 diabetes mellitus (T2DM), representing two extremes in the decompensation spectrum of disease [1].

DKA is the most common acute hyperglycemic complication of diabetes, with an estimated annual incidence of 4 to 8 episodes per 1000 admissions of patients with diabetes. The SEARCH study [2] evaluated the prevalence of DKA in young diabetics aged 0–19 years and reported it to be present in 25–30% of cases of type 1 diabetes and in 4–29% of young people with type 2 diabetes at the time of the diagnosis. A recent systematic review to better clarify the epidemiological data of DKA in adults with T1DM provided an overall prevalence of DKA ranging from approximately 50 to 100 annual events per 1000 patients [3]. HHS is less common than DKA, accounting for less than 1% of all diabetes-related admissions, but has a much higher mortality rate, currently in the order of 11% in the United States, but reaching more than 40% in some series compared to a rate of less than 5% in patients with DKA [4, 5]. Most cases of HHS are seen in elderly patients with type 2 diabetes mellitus, and the prognosis is determined by the severity of dehydration, presence of comorbidities, and advanced age [6].

F. M. Victor (✉)
Division of Endocrinology, Agamenon Magalhães Hospital, Recife, PE, Brazil

S. R. de Lima Andrade
Agamenon Magalhães Hospital, Division of Endocrinology and Diabetes, University of Pernambuco Medical School, Recife, Pernambuco, Brazil

F. Bandeira
Division of Endocrinology, Agamenon Magalhães Hospital, University of Pernambuco Medical School, Recife, PE, Brazil
e-mail: francisco.bandeira@upe.br

The management of these diabetic emergencies represents a substantial economic burden. In the United States, the average cost of DKA management is $17,500 per patient, totaling an annual cost of $2.4 billion [1]. In 2014, a total of 14.2 million visits to the emergency department were registered in patients with diabetes, with 207 thousand visits due to hyperglycemic crises (9.5 per 1000 people with diabetes) [7].

DKA is characterized by a triad of increased *total body ketone concentration*, metabolic acidosis, and uncontrolled hyperglycemia, whereas HHS is characterized by severe hyperglycemia, hyperosmolality, and dehydration in the absence of significant ketoacidosis. The term "hyperglycemic hyperosmolar state" has been adopted by several authors, since patients may present a low level of ketosis, and coma does not occur in all cases of HHS [4, 5]. Patients have some degree of impairment of consciousness (somnolence, drowsiness, and numbness), but only about 30–50% progress to a state of coma. Thus, the use of the terms "hyperosmolar coma," "non-ketotic hyperosmolar hyperglycemic coma," and "non-ketotic hyperosmolar hyperglycemic state" has been avoided [5].

These metabolic disorders result from the combination of absolute or relative insulin deficiency and an increase in counterregulatory hormones (glucagon, catecholamines, cortisol, and growth hormone) [1, 6]. Most DKA patients have type 1 diabetes; however, patients with type 2 diabetes suffering from catabolic stress such as trauma, surgery, or infection are also at risk for DKA [4].

Diabetic ketoacidosis is the initial presentation in 20 to 30% of patients with T1DM, while the main precipitating causes of DKA in patients with known diabetes are infection and omission or inadequate insulin administration. Other causes include silent myocardial infarction, pancreatitis, stroke, trauma, and drugs that affect the metabolism of carbohydrates, such as glucocorticoids, sympathomimetics, and atypical antipsychotics [4, 8] (Table 33.1). In addition, an association has been reported between the use of sodium-glucose cotransporter-2 (SGLT-2) inhibitors and the development of DKA among patients with T1DM and T2DM [9].

© Springer Nature Switzerland AG 2022
F. Bandeira et al. (eds.), *Endocrinology and Diabetes*, https://doi.org/10.1007/978-3-030-90684-9_33

Table 33.1 Risk factors for DKA and HHS

Infection
Low adherence to insulin therapy or omission of treatment (insulin/ oral hypoglycemic agents)
Recent diabetes diagnosis
Acute conditions (acute myocardial infarction, stroke, pancreatitis, trauma)
Difficulty in accessing health services
Drugs (atypical antipsychotics, glucocorticoids, sympathomimetic agents, thiazides, phenytoin, SGLT-2 inhibitors, etc.)

On the other hand, HHS occurs more commonly in elderly patients with T2DM. Infection is the main aggravating factor in almost all series and occurs in 40–60% of patients, with pneumonia (40–60%) and urinary tract infection (5–16%) being the most commonly detected infections. Up to 20% of cases do not have a previous diagnosis of diabetes [10, 11]. Underlying medical disease such as stroke, myocardial infarction, and trauma, resulting in the release of counterregulatory hormones and/or compromising access to water, can result in severe dehydration and HHS. In most patients, restricted water intake is due to the fact that the patient is bedbound and is exacerbated by the altered thirst response in the elderly. Some medications are associated with metabolic decompensation and HHS, such as glucocorticoids, thiazide diuretics, phenytoin, beta-blockers, and atypical antipsychotics [6].

Pathophysiology

The combination of absolute or relative insulinopenia and high concentrations of counterregulatory hormones results in an accelerated catabolic state with increased production of glucose by the liver and kidney (via glycogenolysis and gluconeogenesis) and, at the same time, restricts the use of peripheral glucose, leading to hyperglycemia and hyperosmolality [12]. Due to osmotic diuresis, there are still dehydration and electrolyte disturbances [1, 4].

Acute and chronic hyperglycemias are proinflammatory states. There is two- to threefold increase in the levels of proinflammatory cytokines (TNFα, 1Lβ, 1 L6, and 1 L8), cardiovascular risk markers, and products of reactive oxygen species, in addition to cortisol, growth hormone, and free fatty acids, in patients with hyperglycemic crises in the absence of apparent infection or cardiovascular disorders, with normalization after institution of insulin therapy and resolution of hyperglycemia [13]. These events are also associated with increased levels of counterregulatory hormones and leukocytosis. In addition, procoagulant and inflammatory states may be nonspecific phenomena due to stress and may partially account for the association of hyperglycemic crises with hypercoagulability [8].

Diabetic Ketoacidosis

Hyperglycemia develops as a result of three processes: increased hepatic gluconeogenesis, accelerated glycogenolysis, and impaired glucose utilization by peripheral tissues [1, 4]. These processes promote the excessive release of free fatty acids and glycerol in the circulation from lipolysis by increasing lipase activity, with subsequent hepatic oxidation in ketone bodies (β-hydroxybutyrate and acetoacetate) by the predominant glucagon stimulus, resulting in ketonemia. With the accumulation of ketone bodies, metabolic acidosis sets in [14]. In the DKA state, metabolism and clearance of ketone bodies are decreased. Both hyperglycemia and high levels of ketone bodies cause osmotic diuresis, leading to hypovolemia and decreased glomerular filtration rate, which contribute to the aggravation of the hyperglycemia [1, 4, 5].

Hyperosmolar Hyperglycemic State

The pathogenesis of HHS is not as well understood as that of DKA, but a greater degree of dehydration and differences in insulin availability distinguish it from DKA [15]. Patients with HHS are also insulin-deficient. However, they exhibit higher insulin concentrations (demonstrated by basal and stimulated C-peptide levels) than patients with DKA. Insulin levels in HHS are relatively insufficient to facilitate the use of glucose by tissues, but are sufficient to prevent lipolysis and subsequent ketogenesis. In addition, patients with HHS have lower concentrations of free fatty acids, cortisol, growth hormone, and glucagon [4, 16].

Diagnosis

Patients with DKA usually develop polyuria, polydipsia, and weight loss within hours. Nausea, vomiting, and abdominal pain are detected in 40–75% of cases [17, 18]. Physical examination reveals signs of dehydration, changes in mental status, hypothermia, and ketone breath in the patient's breathing. A rapid and deep breathing pattern (Kussmaul respiration) is observed in patients with severe metabolic acidosis, due to the stimulation of the respiratory centers by the increase of pCO2 [1, 18]. Although infection is a common precipitating factor for DKA and HHS, patients may be normothermic or even hypothermic, mainly due to peripheral vasodilation. Severe hypothermia, when present, is a sign of a poor prognosis [19].

The condition can be classified as mild, moderate, or severe, depending on the extent of metabolic acidosis and changes in the level of consciousness. The key diagnostic criterion is an elevation in serum concentration of ketone bodies. Although most patients with DKA have high plasma glucose levels, this does not determine severity [1, 20]. Confirmation of increased ketone body production is performed using either the nitroprusside reaction or the direct measurement of β-hydroxybutyrate. The nitroprusside reaction provides a semiquantitative estimate of acetoacetate and acetone levels in plasma or urine, but does not detect the presence of β-hydroxybutyrate, which is the predominant ketone among DKA patients. Despite presenting a higher cost, direct measurement of β-hydroxybutyrate is the preferred option for diagnosing ketoacidosis (≥3 mmol/l), as well as for following the patient's response to treatment [15, 21].

The current American Diabetes Association (ADA) diagnostic criteria for DKA are a glucose concentration greater than 13.9 mmol/L (250 mg/dL, the "D" of DKA), the presence of ketones (either in the urine or in the blood, "K"), and metabolic acidosis ("A"), with a pH lower than 7.30 (measured in arterial or venous blood) and a serum bicarbonate concentration of 18.0 mmol or less/L [4]. The ADA guideline therefore suggests a glucose concentration limit ≥13.9 mmol/L (250 mg/dL) to diagnose DKA; however, many patients have a lower increase in plasma glucose concentration after retention or decreased insulin dose in the presence of disease or reduced food intake [22].

In contrast, the insidious onset of HHS (several days) versus DKA (<1–2 days) results in more severe manifestations of hyperglycemia, dehydration, and plasma hyperosmolality, which correlate with lowering of the level of consciousness [1] (Table 33.2). Focal neurological signs (hemianopia and hemiparesis) and seizures (focal or generalized) may also be present in the clinical spectrum of HHS [15].

Currently, ADA and international guidelines include, as diagnostic criteria for HHS, a plasma glucose level >33.3 mmol/L (600 mg/dl), an effective serum osmolality $(2 \times [Na^+ \text{ in mEq/L}]) + \text{glucose in mmol/L}]/18) > 320$ mmol/kg, and the absence of appreciable metabolic acidosis and

ketonemia [4, 6]. The guidelines also recommend disregarding urea from the calculation of effective serum osmolality since it is equally distributed in all body compartments and its accumulation does not induce an osmotic gradient across cell membranes [15]. Encephalopathy symptoms are usually present when serum sodium levels exceed 160 mmol/L and when the effective osmolality is >320 mmol/kg. Estimates suggest that approximately 20–30% of patients with HHS present with metabolic acidosis due to an increase in anion gap as a result of concomitant ketoacidosis alone or in combination with increased levels of lactate [1].

In 1973, Munro et al. [23] reported that in 211 DKA episodes, 16 (7.6%) had a blood glucose concentration lower than 11.1 mmol/L (200 mg/dL), a condition referred to as euglycemic DKA (euDKA). This presentation is also seen in pregnant women with diabetes, in patients with impaired gluconeogenesis due to alcohol abuse, and more recently in patients treated with sodium and glucose cotransporter-2 (SGLT-2) inhibitors [22]. SGLT-2 inhibitors are a class of anti-diabetic agents that reduce blood glucose levels by blocking glucose reabsorption in the proximal convoluted tubule of the kidney, causing glycosuria [24].

In October 2015, the American Association of Clinical Endocrinologists (AACE)/American College of Endocrinology (ACE) convened a conference of experts from Europe and the United States to evaluate the reported cases by balancing the scientific evidence for the association between therapy with SGLT-2 inhibitors (iSGLT-2) and DKA, as well as to provide recommendations for the care of affected patients and to publish an official position on the subject (Table 33.3). SGLT-2 inhibitors are not approved for use in T1DM. However, AACE/ACE encourages the continuation of ongoing studies, as early results reveal that SGLT-2 inhibitors have a promising impact on glycemic regulation in this population. It is also suggested that, in future trials with T1DM, lower doses of SGLT-2 inhibitors should be considered and the insulin dose should not be routinely reduced when the medication is started [16]. In addition, the CANVAS study, comprising 10,142 subjects, reported no significant differences in DKA between the placebo and canagliflozin

Table 33.2 Clinical aspects of DKA and HSS

DKA	HHS
Patients diagnosed with DM or first manifestation of DM	Usually in patients diagnosed with DM
Start <1–2 days	Slow start (several days)
Hyperglycemia, polyuria, polydipsia, weight loss	More severe manifestations of hyperglycemia, dehydration, plasma hyperosmolality, and lowering of the level of consciousness
Nausea, vomiting, abdominal pain	
Hypothermia	
Plasma hyperosmolality and lowering of the level of consciousness variables	
Metabolic acidosis	
Breath of Kussmaul	

Table 33.3 Recommendations to minimize the risk of euglycemic DKA with iSGLT-2

Avoid stopping insulin or excessively reducing the dose
Immediately stop drug use and provide appropriate clinical care in emergency surgeries or extreme stress events
Measure ketonemia, rather than measuring urine ketones, in symptomatic patients with DKA diagnosis
Avoid excessive consumption of alcoholic beverages and ketogenic diets in patients using iSGLT-2
Suspend iSGLT-2 24 hours before elective surgeries, invasive procedures, and intense exercise

arms (0.3 and 0.6 events per thousand patients/yr., respectively). Likewise, the EMPA-REG outcome trial, in which 7020 patients were treated with empagliflozin or placebo, showed similar incidences for DKA, less than 1%, between the placebo and empagliflozin arms [25, 26].

The laboratory evaluation of patients with hyperglycemic crises should include plasma glucose, renal function and electrolytes (for the calculation of anion gap), plasma osmolality, urine ketones by dipstick and serum ketones (if urine ketones are present), and arterial blood gases, complete with differential and urine summary. Additional investigations include electrocardiogram, chest X-ray, and cultures [4, 8]. The diagnostic criteria for DKA and HHS are shown in Table 33.4.

Although most patients with HHS present a pH of 7.30 and a level of bicarbonate greater than 18 mEq/L on admission, mild ketonemia may also be part of the clinical picture, and a significant overlap between DKA and HHS is observed in more than one third of patients. Clinically, HHS presents lower ketosis and higher hyperglycemia than DKA [4]. On the other hand, the determination of elevation ketonemia or ketonuria represents the main diagnostic resource in DKA. The nitroprusside reaction measures the levels of acetoacetic acid in blood and urine, but its use is not recommended to follow the resolution of the clinical picture, since this method is not able to recognize β-hydroxybutyrate, the main metabolite produced in DKA that is converted to acetoacetate during therapy, and the ketone test can show high values, mistakenly suggesting a deterioration of ketonemia and indicating a false clinical worsening of the patient. Another source of error is drugs, such as angiotensin-converting enzyme inhibitors (captopril, e.g.), which have sulfhydryl groups potentially capable of interacting with the reagent in the nitroprusside test and yielding false-positive results [27].

As an alternative to pH and β-hydroxybutyrate measurement, serum bicarbonate and calculated anion gap (AG) can be monitored. The anion gap $[AG = Na^+ - (HCO_3^- + Cl^-)]$ provides an estimate of the major unmeasured anions in plasma which, in DKA, are mainly ketoacids. AG normalization reflects the correction of ketoacidosis as the ketoacids are removed from the blood [8]. Most DKA patients have AG >20 mEq/L, but occasionally they may develop hyperchloremic metabolic acidosis without a significant change in the anion gap [28].

Leukocytosis is common in both conditions and may be related to increased levels of cortisol and catecholamines secondary to the stress of hyperglycemia and dehydration. Values above 25,000 leukocytes/mm³ require screening for a possible triggering infection. Dehydration may also favor hemoconcentration [8, 20]. Initial serum sodium is generally low due to the osmotic movement of water from intracellular to extracellular space secondary to hyperglycemia. Therefore, the presence of hypernatremia and hyperglycemia indicates severe dehydration [8]. High blood glucose levels may mistakenly lower plasma sodium results, suggesting the use of the formula proposed by Katz for sodium correction: corrected Na^+ = measured Na^+ + [(1.6 × (glycemia - 100)]/100 [29]. In patients with severe hypertriglyceridemia, pseudohyponatremia may occur in DKA [5].

The state of insulinopenia can elevate the serum potassium due to the exit of potassium to the extracellular location. The presence of a normal or downright low kalemia on admission of patients with DKA suggests a severe potassium deficit, usually around 3 to 5 mEq/kg of body weight. In this case, a more potent potassium replacement should be instituted, along with cardiac monitoring for possible arrhythmias [8, 30]. An electrocardiogram may also be useful to rule out the possibility of a silent infarction, especially in patients with T2DM. In addition to the laboratory changes described, nonspecific elevations of amylase and lipase may be observed in 16–25% of DKA cases. Elevation of amylase correlates with pH and serum osmolality, but lipase elevation is related only to serum osmolality, and the diagnosis of acute pancreatitis based on isolated elevation of pancreatic enzymes is not justifiable [31].

Table 33.4 Diagnostic criteria for DKA, according to severity classification, and HHS

| | DKA | | | |
Parameters	Light	Moderate	Severe	HHS
Glucose (mg/dl)	>250	>250	>250	>600
Bicarbonate (mmol/L)	15–18	10–14	<10	>15
Arterial or venous pH	7.25–7.30	7.00–7.24	<7.00	>7.30
Acetoacetate in blood or urine	Positive	Positive	Positive	Negative or light +
β-Hydroxybutyrate in blood or urine (mmol/L)	>3	>3	>3	<3
Effective serum osmolality (mmol/kg)	Variable	Variable	Variable	>320
Anion gap[a] (mmol/L)	>10	>12	>12	<12
Impairment of consciousness	Alert	Alert or sleepy	Stupor/coma	Stupor/coma

[a]Anion gap = $[Na^+ - (HCO_3^- + Cl^-)]$

Differential Diagnosis

Other conditions that occur with metabolic acidosis and an increase in the anion gap should be considered in the differential diagnosis of DKA.

Lactic acidosis usually manifests itself as a result of tissue hypoperfusion, resulting in the non-oxidative metabolism of glucose to lactic acid. The presentation is similar to that of DKA. In pure lactic acidosis, hyperlactatemia predominates, but blood glucose and ketones must be normal. In situations of prolonged fasting or ketogenic diets, ketosis is caused by insufficient carbohydrate availability, resulting in physiological lipolysis and ketone production to provide fuel substrates for the tissues. Blood glucose is usually normal. Urine may have large amounts of ketones, but rarely is there ketonemia [4, 32, 33].

In alcoholic ketoacidosis, the appropriate ketogenic response to poor carbohydrate intake is potentiated through the effects of alcohol on the liver. Metabolic acidosis is usually mild to moderate, with anion gap characteristically high, identifying ketonemia and ketonuria, with an even higher proportion of β-hydroxybutyrate to acetoacetate than DKA, as well as a negative or weak positive nitroprusside method [15, 34].

Severe chronic renal failure may trigger uremic acidosis, characterized by a significant change in renal function and normoglycemia. PH and anion gap are usually discretely abnormal, and dialytic therapy needs to be instituted in most cases [32]. Acidosis related to drug intoxication, such as salicylates, ethylene glycol, and methanol, is also described and should be investigated. In salicylate poisoning, blood glucose is low or normal, osmolality is normal, and ketones are negative, with the possibility of detecting the drug in the urine or blood [35].

Treatment

The initial step of DKA or HHS treatment is aggressive volume replacement with isotonic crystalloid solution, 500–1000 mL/h in 1–2 hours or 15–20 mL/kg in the first hour. This fluid therapy is responsible for restoring intravascular, intracellular, and interstitial volumes, reestablishing renal and tissue perfusion, decreasing hyperglycemia and ketogenesis, and reducing the release of counterregulatory hormones [1]. If the patient is still hemodynamically unstable after this initial hydration, volume resuscitation can be continued by tapping an amount of volume to be infused so as not to render the patient congested [4]. While this vigorous expansion is proceeding, serum measurements of potassium, sodium, blood glucose, urea, creatinine, and diuresis should be taken [1]. It is worth mentioning that patients with HHS usually require more vigorous hydration than those with DKA due to the water deficit being practically double in patients with HHS [1, 4].

After this first step, corrected sodium should be calculated, using the formula corrected Na$^+$ = measured Na$^+$ + [1.6 × (glycemia - 100)]/100. If the corrected sodium is between 135 and 145 mEq/L or >145 mEq/L, hydration should be continued using hypotonic solution composed of equal proportions of saline solution and distilled water at an infusion rate of 250–500 mL each hour, also guided by the volume status of the patient. If corrected sodium is between <135 mEq/L, the use of 250–500 mL saline is continued every hour, monitoring blood volume and diuresis. When capillary blood glucose (CBG) reaches 200 mg/dl in DKA or 300 mg/dl in HHS, infusion of hypotonic solution plus glucose to a final concentration of 5% dextrose solution is initiated at an infusion rate of 150–250 mL/h to maintain CBG between 150 and 200 mg/dL until resolution of the acidosis [1, 4]. Serum glycoside 5% 1000 mL plus 20% NaCl 20 mL may be prescribed to arrive at this solution.

The other pillar of DKA/HHS treatment is potassium testing and its replacement, if necessary, prior to the initiation of insulin infusion, the main measure for correction of acidosis. In the case of serum potassium of 3.3 to 5.0 mEq/L, 20–30 mEq/L of potassium is added to the hydration to maintain a stable serum level of this ion [4] and regular insulin 0.1 U/Kg IV bolus, followed by infusion of regular insulin solution at a dose of 0.1 U/kg/hr. [1, 4]. The use of the standard solution composed of saline 0.9% 100 mL + regular insulin 100 U in continuous insulin infusion (CII) intravenous is recommended if the patient is hospitalized in an intensive care setting. Intravenous insulin is the first choice for patients with severe DKA/HHS who are admitted to the intensive care unit, presenting hypovolemic shock, poor peripheral perfusion, or anasarca [1, 4, 22]. Previous bolus administration of this same insulin 0.1 U/kg remains controversial, since there were no significant differences in the treatment or risk of hypoglycemia [1, 4]. If this bolus is not done, increase the administration of intravenous insulin to 0.14 U/kg/hr. to suppress the production of ketone bodies [4].

If potassium is less than 3.3 mEq/L, administer 20–30 mEq/h of this electrolyte to reach a potassium level of 3.3 mEq/L, thus preventing hypokalemia resulting from insulin administration and fluid therapy. In the case of serum potassium above 5.0 mEq/L, infusion of insulin can be initiated without potassium replacement [1, 4].

Subcutaneous insulin may be used instead of intravenous for correction of acidosis in mild to moderate and uncomplicated cases [1, 4]. These cases can be managed in an intermediate care unit, provided there is a trained team available. Lispro or aspart insulins are used at the initial 0.2–0.3 U/kg dose, followed by maintenance at a dose 0.1 U/kg/h or 0.2 U/kg every 2 hours [1, 22]. The subcutaneous and muscular routes are just as effective as the intravenous route [1, 4, 22], and the intramuscular one has the disadvantage of being more painful and can cause hematomas in users of anticoagulants [1]. Insulin therapy by any route of administration is capable of suppressing lipolysis and ketogenesis, decreasing hepatic gluconeogenesis, and restoring cellular metabolism [1].

Following the administration of insulin, capillary blood glucose is monitored every hour. When this parameter reaches 200–250 mg/dl in DKA or 300 mg/dl in HHS, the supply should be reduced to 50% of the dose, maintaining capillary blood glucose between 150 and 200 mg/dl in the DKA [1, 4] or 200 and 300 mg/dl in HHS until resolution of the clinical picture [1]. Acidosis resolution is considered when arterial or venous pH reaches values greater than or equal to 7.3, bicarbonate equal to or greater than 18 mmol/L, normal gap anion, and CBG below 200 mg/dl for DKA [4] or serum osmolarity below 310 mmOsm/kg [1, 4], CBG below 300 mg/dL, and recovery of the level of consciousness for HHS [1, 4, 22]. Generally, hyperglycemia takes about 6 hours to reach such levels, while the production of ketone bodies ceases only after 12 hours of therapy [4].

When the patient is able to ingest food, if intravenous insulin is used and if the condition is in resolution [1, 4, 22], the administration of subcutaneous insulin at a dose of 0.5–0.7 U/Kg/day [1] should be started, preferably using analogues of insulin in a basal-bolus regimen, concomitant with the food supply. The use of insulin glargine and glulisine reduced episodes of hypoglycemia to 15% when compared to NPH and regular insulin, responsible for 41% of such episodes. Insulin infusion should be switched off 2 hours after the first subcutaneous injection. If the patient was on insulin

prior to hospitalization uses, he or she can return to the previous regimen [1, 4] (Fig. 33.1).

In contrast, for the treatment of euglycemic ketoacidosis, which usually presents with blood glucose levels lower than 200 mg/dl, vigorous hydration should be prioritized and the use of ultra-rapid subcutaneous insulin preferred (Fig. 33.2).

Although the main action for the correction of acidosis is the use of insulin, bicarbonate should be replaced when the pH is ≤6.9. To do this, use 50–100 mmol of 8.4% sodium bicarbonate diluted in 200 ml of sterile water [4] or in 0.45% saline 500 ml in 2 hours until pH >7.0 [1]. If it is difficult to reverse the acidosis, the administration of bicarbonate [1, 4] may be repeated, and conditions associated with this state such as hypovolemia and infections should be ruled out [1]. The use of intravenous bicarbonate does not present any benefits in recovering from severe acidosis. It may also increase the risk of hypokalemia, paradoxal central nervous system acidosis [1, 4], and decreased tissue oxygenation. Bicarbonate should not be used in HHS or if pH >7.0 [1].

Phosphate deficiency is uncommon and usually arises only after the onset of insulin therapy. Phosphate replacement should only be indicated when serum levels are lower than 1.0 mg/dl or in the presence of muscle weakness, heart or respiratory depression, or anemia. A solution containing 20–30 mEq/L of potassium phosphate [1, 4] may be used. In the case of mild depletions, the correction occurs through food intake [1]. Administration of intravenous phosphate may lead to hypocalcemia, and most studies have failed to demonstrate any benefits from this replacement [1, 4, 22].

In order to monitor the patient with DKA/HHS, venous blood gases should be requested, less painful to the patient,

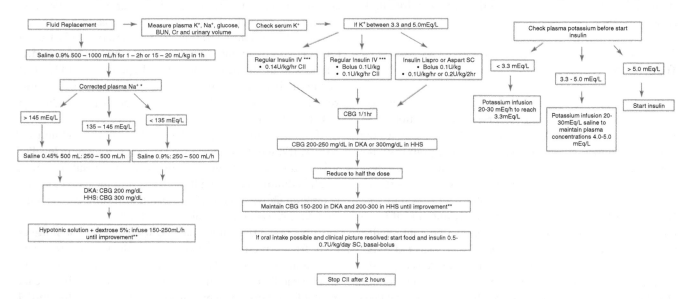

Fig. 33.1 Algorithm for the therapeutic management of DKA and HHS. (*Corrected Na⁺ = measured Na⁺ + [1,6 x (measured blood glucose – 100)]/100; **Plasma bicarbonate >18 mmol/L, pH ≥7.3, and glucose <200 mg/dL; ***CII: Saline 0.9% 100 mL + regular insulin 100 U (1 mL = 1 U))

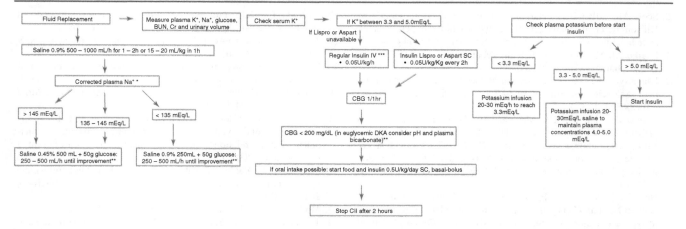

Fig. 33.2 Euglycemic DKA management. (*Corrected Na + = measured Na+ + [1,6 x (measured blood glucose – 100)]/100; **Plasma bicarbonate >18 mmol/L, pH ≥7.3, and glucose <200 mg/dL (not valid for euglycemic DKA. Consider pH and plasma bicarbonate); ***CII: Saline 0.9% 100 mL + regular insulin 100 U (1 mL = 1 U))

and equally effective for the evaluation of metabolic parameters, serum potassium, and plasma glucose every 2 to 4 hours until the patient attains stability [4].

The possible complications of DKA/HHS treatment are hypoglycemia secondary to the use of insulin, which may manifest without adrenergic symptoms; hypokalemia, which may be worsened by the administration of bicarbonate; and cerebral edema. The latter complication, rare in adults and with 0.3–1.0% incidence in children, should be suspected if the patient presents a headache, a diminished level of consciousness, pupillary alterations, bradycardia, papilledema, sphincter incontinence, elevated blood pressure, or respiratory arrest. Blood glucose should be maintained between 200 and 300 mg/dl until osmolarity is corrected, which is unlikely to be rapid, and hyperhydration avoided. If cerebral edema occurs, use mannitol and mechanical ventilation in an attempt to reverse this condition [4].

References

1. Umpierrez G, Korytkowski M. Diabetic emergencies-ketoacidosis, hyperglycaemic hyperosmolar state and hypoglycaemia. Nat Rev Endocrinol. 2016;12(4):222–32.
2. Dabelea D, Rewers A, Stafford JM, Standiford DA, Lawrence JM, Saydah S, et al. Trends in the prevalence of ketoacidosis at diabetes diagnosis: the SEARCH for diabetes in youth study. Pediatrics. 2014;133(4):e938–45.
3. Farsani SF, Brodovicz K, Soleymanlou N, Marquard J, Wissinger E, Maiese BA. Incidence and prevalence of diabetic ketoacidosis (DKA) among adults with type 1 diabetes mellitus (T1D): a systematic literature review. BMJ Open. 2017;7(7)
4. Kitabchi AE, Umpierrez GE, Miles JM, Fisher JN. Hyperglycemic crises in adult patients with diabetes. Diabetes Care. 2009;32(7):1335–43.
5. Kitabchi AE, Umpierrez GE, Murphy MB, Kreisberg RA. Hyperglycemic crises in adult patients with diabetes: a consensus statement from the American Diabetes Association. Diabetes Care. 2006;29(12):2739–48.
6. Pasquel FJ, Umpierrez GE. Hyperosmolar hyperglycemic state: a historic review of the clinical presentation, diagnosis, and treatment. Diabetes Care. 2014;37(11):3124–31.
7. Control C for D, Prevention. National Diabetes Statistics Report: Estimates of Diabetes and Its Burden in the United States. Atlanta, GA: Centers for Disease Control and Prevention; 2014. US Dep Heal Hum Serv. 2017;(CDC):2009–12.
8. Kitabchi AE, Fisher J. Hyperglycemic crises: diabetic ketoacidosis (DKA) and hyperglycemic hyperosmolar state (HHS). Diabetes Care. 2009.
9. Peters AL, Buschur EO, Buse JB, Cohan P, Diner JC, Hirsch IB. Euglycemic diabetic ketoacidosis: a potential complication of treatment with sodium-glucose cotransporter 2 inhibition. Diabetes Care. 2015;38(9):1687–93.
10. Wachtel TJ. Predisposing factors for the diabetic hyperosmolar state. Arch Intern Med. 1987;147(3):499.
11. Umpierrez G, Kelly J, Navarrete J, Casals M, Kitabchi A. Hyperglycemic crises in urban blacks. Arch Intern Med. 1997;157:669–75.
12. Zabar B. Diabetic ketoacidosis and hyperglycemic hyperosmolar state. Pract Emerg Resusc. Crit Care. 2013:389–96.
13. Stentz FB, Umpierrez GE, Cuervo R, Kitabchi AE. Proinflammatory cytokines, markers of cardiovascular risks, oxidative stress, and lipid peroxidation in patients with hyperglycemic crises. Diabetes. 2004;1(21):2079–86.
14. Miles JM, Haymond MW, Nissen SL, Gerich JE. Effects of free fatty acid availability, glucagon excess, and insulin deficiency on ketone body production in postabsorptive man. J Clin Invest. 1983;71(6):1554–61.
15. Kitabchi A, Umpierrez GE, Murphy MB, Barrett EJ, Wall BM. Management of Hyperglycemic Crises in patients with diabetes. Diabetes Care. 2001;24:131–53.
16. Handelsman Y, Henry RR, Bloomgarden ZT, Dagogo-Jack S, DeFronzo RA, Einhorn D, et al. American Association of Clinical Endocrinologists and American College of endocrinology position statement on the Association of Sglt-2 inhibitors and diabetic ketoacidosis. Endocr Pract. 2016;22(6):753–62.
17. Umpierrez G, Freire AX. Abdominal pain in patients with hyperglycemic crises. J Crit Care. 2002;17(1):63–7.
18. Mauvais-Jarvis F, Riveline J, Kevorkian J, Vaisse C, Charpentier G, Guillausseau P, et al. Ketosis-prone type 2 diabetes in patients of sub-Saharan African origin. Diabetes. 2004;53:645–53.
19. Matz R. Hypothermia in diabetic acidosis. Hormones. 1972;3:36–41.

20. Scott AR, Allan B, Dhatariya K, Flanagan D, Hammersley M, Hillson R, et al. Management of hyperosmolar hyperglycaemic state in adults with diabetes. Diabet Med. 2015;32(6):714–24.

21. Sheikh-Ali M. Can serum B-hydroxybutyrate be used to diagnose DKA? Diabetes Care. 2008;31(4):643–7.

22. Dhatariya KK, Umpierrez GE. Guidelines for management of diabetic ketoacidosis: time to revise? Lancet Diabetes Endocrinol. 2017;5(5):321–3.

23. Munro JF, Campbell IW, McCuish AC, Duncan L. Euglycaemic diabetic ketoacidosis. Br Med J. 1973;2:578–80.

24. Burke KR, Schumacher C, Spencer H. SGLT2 inhibitors: a systematic review of diabetic ketoacidosis and related risk factors in the primary literature. ARPN J Eng Appl Sci. 2017;12(10): 3218–21.

25. Neal B, Perkovic V, Mahaffey KW, De Zeeuw D, Fulcher G, Erondu N, et al. Canagliflozin and cardiovascular and renal events in type 2 diabetes. N Engl J Med. 2017; https://doi.org/10.1056/NEJMoa1611925.

26. Zinman B, Wanner C, Lachin JM, Fitchett D, Bluhmki E, Hantel S, et al. Empagliflozin, cardiovascular outcomes, and mortality in type 2 diabetes. N Engl J Med. 2015;373(22):2117–28.

27. Csako G, Elin RJ. Unrecognized false-positive ketones from drugs containing free-sulfhydryl groups. JAMA. 1993;269:1634.

28. Adrogué HJ. Plasma Acid-Base patterns in diabetic ketoacidosis. N Engl J Med. 1982;307:1603–10.

29. Katz MA. Hyperglycemia-induced hyponatremia - calculation of expected serum sodium depression. N Engl J Med. 1973;289:843–4.

30. Beigelman PM. Potassium in severe diabetic ketoacidosis. Am J Med. 1973;54(4):419–20.

31. Yadav D, Nair S, Norkus EP, Pitchumoni CS. Nonspecific hyperamylasemia and hyperlipasemia in diabetic ketoacidosis: incidence and correlation with biochemical abnormalities. Am J Gastroenterol. 2000;95(11):3123–8.

32. Maletkovic J, Drexler A. Diabetic ketoacidosis and hyperglycemic hyperosmolar state. Endocrinol Metab Clin North Am [Internet]. 2013;42(4):677–95.

33. Madias NE. Lactic acidosis. Kidney Int. 1986;29(3):752–74.

34. Tanaka M, Miyazaki Y, Ishiwana S, Matsuyama K. Alcoholic ketoacidosis associated with multiple complications: report of 3 cases. Intern Med. 2004;43(10):955–9.

35. Brenner BE, Simon RR. Management of Salicylate Intoxication. Drugs. 1982;24(4):335–40.

Hypoglycemia in the Non-diabetic Patient

Maria Daniela Hurtado and Adrian Vella

Hypoglycemia is frequent in clinical practice. However, in contrast to patients with diabetes, true hypoglycemia is uncommon in non-diabetic patients [1]. The definition of hypoglycemia differs in patients with and without diabetes. In patients with diabetes, hypoglycemia is defined as any abnormally low plasma glucose concentration, with or without symptoms, that exposes an individual to potential harm [2]. In non-diabetic individuals, hypoglycemia is defined as a low plasma glucose concentration that causes symptoms and/or signs, including brain function impairment [3].

Clinical Presentation

Hypoglycemic symptoms and signs are the result of the activation of the counter-regulatory cholinergic and adrenergic nervous systems (autonomic symptoms) and functional brain impairment from glucose depravation (neuroglycopenic symptoms). Autonomic symptoms and signs include diaphoresis, tremors or shakiness, palpitations or pounding of the heart, anxiety or nervousness, increased hunger, and paresthesia [4]. Neuroglycopenic symptoms and signs include fatigue, behavioral changes, cognitive impairment – from confusion to seizures, and coma [5]. Autonomic symptoms usually occur at a threshold of 60 mg/dl, whereas neuroglycopenic symptoms occur at a threshold of 50 mg/dl. Glycemic thresholds are dynamic. For instance, if hypoglycemia is recurrent, the plasma glucose concentration threshold at which symptoms occur decreases [6].

Pathophysiology

In normal subjects, glucose supply is tightly controlled by the dynamic regulation of glucose production and usage. In the postprandial state, rising plasma glucose concentrations stimulate insulin secretion to restore euglycemia. Insulin suppresses glycogenolysis and gluconeogenesis and increases glucose uptake in the muscle and adipose tissue. During the fasting state, in order to provide a continuous glucose flux to the brain, glucose is released from the liver and to a lesser extent the kidney. There are several glucose counter-regulatory mechanisms that come into play to prevent hypoglycemia. Each occurs at different thresholds [7]. First, as plasma glucose concentration falls and reaches a threshold of ~80 mg/dL, insulin secretion declines, thereby decreasing peripheral glucose disposal. Insulin secretion is completely suppressed only when glucose levels reach a threshold of 55–60 mg/dL. Second, at a glucose threshold of 65 to 70 mg/dl, glucagon secretion increases to stimulate gluconeogenesis and glycogenolysis. At the same threshold, the third mechanism, increased epinephrine secretion, comes into play. Epinephrine impairs peripheral glucose uptake and increases delivery of gluconeogenic substrates to the liver. If all the aforementioned mechanisms are not sufficient to maintain euglycemia, cortisol and growth hormone are released to enhance hepatic glucose production and to limit glucose utilization [7, 8]. However, because of the time-dependent nature of their actions on glucose metabolism, it is unlikely that cortisol and GH have any meaningful effect on counter-regulation [9, 10].

Behavioral counter-regulatory mechanisms are as important as the hormonal ones. Symptoms of hypoglycemia, which occur at a plasma glucose concentration of <60 mg/dL, trigger food ingestion which is an important behavioral defense. The disruption or dysregulation of any of these physiological mechanisms may lead to hypoglycemia.

M. D. Hurtado · A. Vella (✉)
Division of Endocrinology, Diabetes, Metabolism & Nutrition, Mayo Clinic, Rochester, MN, USA
e-mail: hurtado.mariadaniela@mayo.edu; vella.adrian@mayo.edu

© Springer Nature Switzerland AG 2022
F. Bandeira et al. (eds.), *Endocrinology and Diabetes*, https://doi.org/10.1007/978-3-030-90684-9_34

Differential Diagnosis

The differential diagnosis of hypoglycemia depends on the context in which it occurs. The likely causes of hypoglycemia differ significantly in otherwise well patients compared to hospitalized, chronically ill individuals. The characterization of hypoglycemic disorders by the timing of symptoms in relation to food intake has been challenged and largely abandoned because some conditions can cause hypoglycemia in both the fasting and postprandial states [11], and often it is difficult to reliably differentiate the timing of symptoms.

In seemingly well patients, hyperinsulinemic hypoglycemia that is not caused by medication is most commonly due to insulinoma. On the other hand, underlying systemic disease, medication side effects, medication-disease interactions, and other iatrogenic factors are more likely in hospitalized patients. In this chapter, we will also discuss genetic conditions and drugs that predispose to hypoglycemia, as well as the etiology of non-insulin-mediated hypoglycemia.

The Healthy Patient: Hyperinsulinemic Hypoglycemia

Endogenous hyperinsulinemic hypoglycemia was first described at the Mayo Clinic in 1926 when an orthopedic surgeon presented with hypoglycemic episodes and was found to have a metastatic pancreatic islet cell tumor [12]. Extracts from the liver metastases obtained at the time of abdominal exploration led to hypoglycemia in laboratory animals. These observations established the clinical entity of insulinoma. Besides insulinoma, other causes of endogenous hyperinsulinism include functional β-cell disorders (non-insulinoma pancreatogenous hypoglycemia and post-bariatric bypass hypoglycemia), insulin autoimmune hypoglycemia syndrome due to insulin and (more rarely) insulin receptor antibodies, and hypoglycemia due to the (inappropriate) use of insulin secretagogues or insulin.

Insulinoma

Insulinomas are rare functional neuroendocrine tumors with an incidence of 1 in 250,000 person-years [11]. Despite their relative rarity, insulinomas represent the most common functional neuroendocrine tumor and are also the most common cause of endogenous hyperinsulinemic hypoglycemia. Insulinomas occur in people of all ethnicities and have a slight predominance for men. The majority of insulinomas are less than 2 cm in size, benign, solitary, and sporadic [13]. Less than 10% of patients present with multifocal disease and/or are part of a genetic syndrome such as multiple endocrine neoplasia syndrome 1 (MEN1).

Insulinomas classically present with hypoglycemia in the fasting state although hypoglycemia can also occur in the postprandial state [14]. Patients are usually healthy, except for experiencing periods of neuroglycopenia [15]. The 72-hour fast, discussed later in this chapter, is often used to document Whipple's triad and elucidate the mechanism of hypoglycemia. Lesions are usually identified on imaging studies, and surgical enucleation or resection is the treatment of choice.

Malignant insulinomas account for less than 10% of insulinomas [13, 16]. Presentation is similar to that of other hypoglycemic disorders. Malignant tumors are differentiated from benign tumors based on the presence of extrapancreatic disease whether as local soft tissue invasion or as distant metastases. Insulinomas have a high cure rate and, in the case of sporadic insulinomas, low risk of recurrence [13, 16, 17]. Malignant insulinomas have a poorer prognosis with a 15-year survival rate of 29% [18].

Non-insulinoma Pancreatogenous Hypoglycemia Syndrome (NIPHS)

NIPHS was first described at the Mayo Clinic in 1999 by FJ Service and colleagues. Service et al. reported five cases of postprandial hyperinsulinemic hypoglycemia that were not due to insulinomas and had a positive selective arterial calcium stimulation test. All patients underwent partial pancreatectomy. The pathology of the resected pancreata revealed pancreatic islet cell hypertrophy and nesidioblastosis. No mutations in Kir6.2 and SUR1 genes were present. Mutations in both genes have previously been associated with familial persistent hyperinsulinemic hypoglycemia of infancy [19].

NIPHS is rare and typically characterized by hypoglycemia in the postprandial state – usually between 2 and 4 hours following a meal, negative imaging studies, abnormal selective arterial calcium stimulation test in those who undergo surgery, and nesidioblastosis or occult islet tumor on histology [19–21]. The mixed meal test can help confirm hypoglycemia in the postprandial state but does not establish a diagnosis.

Post-Bariatric Surgery Hypoglycemia

Bariatric surgery patients may present with multiple nonspecific symptoms in the postoperative period that are not necessarily due to hypoglycemia. Post-bariatric surgery hypoglycemia has an estimated incidence of 2–4% in patients who have undergone Roux-en-Y gastric bypass [22, 23]. Most commonly, hypoglycemia occurs in the postprandial state, develops months to years following surgery, and has a female predominance [23, 24]. Symptoms are frequently provoked by high intake of simple sugars. The mixed meal test can be used to document postprandial hypoglycemia. If positive, it is followed by invasive testing and treatment.

Although NIPHS and post-bariatric surgery hypoglycemia share underlying physiopathology and clinical presentation, they are considered two different entities. Post-bariatric surgery hypoglycemia is more common than NIPHS.

Insulin Antibody-Mediated Hypoglycemia

Insulin antibodies can develop after exposure to exogenous insulin (more common with porcine and bovine insulin) administration or arise spontaneously. Insulin antibodies are not infrequent in patients receiving insulin and are more common in those in whom insulin therapy was initiated prior to the era of highly purified insulins [25, 26]. These antibodies rarely cause hypoglycemia. It has been postulated that these antibodies may have a higher affinity for insulin and result in limited insulin dissociation. However, this has been disputed [27]. It is now believed that these antibodies are less likely to cause hypoglycemia, because once insulin is released, its action (in diabetic patients) is impaired by hyperglycemia and decreased insulin action.

On the other hand, insulin antibodies, spontaneously generated in the absence of prior insulin exposure, lead to hypoglycemia more frequently. It is thought that the unregulated release of insulin, regardless of the plasma glucose concentration, in combination with normal glucose metabolism and normal insulin action, predisposes to more frequent symptomatic hypoglycemia. This condition is known as insulin autoimmune syndrome. Insulin autoimmune syndrome is a rare disorder first described in 1970. It is more commonly seen in Asians of Korean or Japanese descent [28, 29]. Patients often have a history of other autoimmune disorders and/or exposure to sulfhydryl-containing drugs such as methimazole [29]. Symptoms of hypoglycemia may range from mild to severe and can occur in the fasting and postprandial states.

Diagnosis can be challenging. Insulin antibody measurement may be of diagnostic utility only in patients with no history of insulin use. In this population, the presence of antibodies does not exclude the possibility of surreptitious insulin use.

The Ill Patient

Hypoglycemia, both spontaneous and secondary to treatment with insulin or other medications that cause hypoglycemia, is a frequent finding in the ICU and has been linked to a poor prognosis with increased mortality in critically ill patients [30, 31]. Critically ill patients not only have decreased glycogen storage in the setting of decreased oral intake but also have impaired gluconeogenesis and altered peripheral glucose utilization [32–34].

In patients with and without diabetes mellitus, besides insulin therapy to manage hyperglycemia, the most frequently underlying diseases associated with hypoglycemia include malignancies, cerebrovascular disease, sepsis, pneumonia, alcohol dependence, liver disease, renal failure, heart failure, and self-harm with hypoglycemic agents [1, 35]. In patient with diabetes alone, suspension of nutritional therapy while on insulin therapy is a frequent cause of hypoglycemia as well.

The underlying mechanisms of hypoglycemia in the critically ill have not been fully elucidated. In the setting of sepsis, it has been shown that endotoxins impair hepatic gluconeogenesis in a rat model [36]. In the setting of hepatic failure, hypoglycemia ensues when hepatocytes are not able to mobilize glycogen storages during the fasting state. Alcohol and other toxins can also alter intrahepatic pathways that are vital for normal gluconeogenesis and glycogenolysis [37]. Hypoglycemia due to renal failure is thought to be multifactorial due to impaired gluconeogenesis secondary to deficiency of amino acid precursors, particularly alanine; decreased insulin clearance; and poor nutrition and muscle wasting with impaired glycogenesis [38].

Genetic Causation and Predisposition to Hypoglycemia

Advances in the areas of molecular biology and genomics have provided a deeper mechanistic understanding of the endocrine and metabolic pathways that regulate glucose homeostasis. Defects in genes encoding for proteins that are integral to these pathways can result in hypoglycemia in the neonatal period or at an early age in childhood. For instance, congenital hyperinsulinism can be caused by mutations in key genes that regulate insulin secretion (GCK, HNF4A, HNF1A, and UCP2 defects). Other genetic abnormalities affect transcription factors or regulatory genes that can result in deficiency of counter-regulatory hormones. These include congenital hypopituitarism (PIT-1 mutation), isolated ACTH deficiency (POMC and TPIT mutations), isolated GH deficiency (SOX3 mutations), primary adrenal insufficiency-isolated or, as part of type 1 autoimmune polyendocrinopathy syndrome (AIRE mutation), dopamine b-hydroxylase deficiency (DBH mutation), and other rarer disorders [39].

Rarely, defects that affect hepatic glycogen synthesis, gluconeogenesis, and galactose and amino acid metabolism can also cause hypoglycemia. Some examples of diseases caused by alterations in these pathways are:

- Glycogen storage disease (GDS) I, the most common GSD, results from defects in either glucose-6-phosphatase (chromosome 17q21) or glucose-6-phosphate translocase (chromosome 11q23.3). These proteins are essential in the final steps of glycogenolysis and gluconeogenesis.

- Hereditary fructose intolerance is caused by aldolase B deficiency (chromosome 9q22.3). This enzyme is a crucial link between fructose metabolism and gluconeogenesis.
- Galactosemia results from abnormalities of enzymes that regulate galactose conversion into glucose. Defects in this pathway result in neonatal hypoglycemia after newborns are breastfed.
- Maple syrup urine disease is due to a defect in the degradation of branched amino acids which, as a result, cannot enter gluconeogenesis [39].

Lastly, some genetic syndromes can present with hypoglycemia in some but not all children that are affected. For example, Beckwith-Wiedemann syndrome, Laron syndrome, or primary growth hormone resistance may cause hypoglycemia. Similarly, extreme insulin resistance syndromes such as leprechaunism and Rabson-Mendenhall syndrome that are due to genetic mutations of the insulin receptor gene may also result in hypoglycemia [40]. In these cases, permanently high insulin concentration can limit mobilization of free fatty acids from adipose tissue resulting in impaired β-oxidation to ketones during fasting, resulting in hypoglycemia.

MEN1 is a rare genetic syndrome that may predispose to hypoglycemia in adulthood. The mutation affects the genome location that encodes for the menin protein, a tumor suppressor protein, on chromosome 11 (11q13) [41]. MEN1 is an autosomal dominant hereditary disorder characterized by an increased predisposition to tumors of the pituitary, parathyroid glands, and pancreatic islet cells [42]. Functioning neuroendocrine tumors occurs in one to two thirds of the patients affected with MEN1. Insulinomas are rare and affect only 10% of the patients with MEN1 and enteropancreatic tumors. Unlike patients with sporadic insulinoma, MEN1 patients with these tumors tend to be younger at the time of diagnosis, have multiple tumors, and have a higher recurrence rate [18, 42].

Drug-Induced Hypoglycemia

Drugs are the most common cause of hypoglycemia. Antidiabetic agents, particularly insulin and sulfonylureas, are the leading cause of drug-induced hypoglycemia [43]. However, non-antidiabetic drugs either can also cause hypoglycemia per se or can enhance the hypoglycemic effect of diabetic drugs. Commonly used non-diabetic drugs that can induce hypoglycemia are salicylates (e.g., aspirin),cardiac medications (e.g., amiodarone, hydralazine, β-blockers, and ACE inhibitors), antibiotics (e.g., ceftriaxone, ciprofloxacin, doxycycline, and piperacillin-tazobactam), anti-malaric agents (e.g., hydroxychloroquine, mefloquine, and quinine), HIV medications (e.g., entecavir, stavudine, zidovudine, zal-

citabine), antifungals (e.g., ketoconazole and voriconazole), anti-epileptic (e.g., gabapentin, phenytoin), and psychiatric medications (e.g., chlorpromazine, haloperidol, and sertraline) [44]. This is a non-exhaustive list.

Pathophysiologic mechanisms for drug-induced hypoglycemia include enhanced insulin secretion, improved insulin action, or decreased insulin clearance; however, usually the mechanisms behind drug-induced hypoglycemic effects are not clear. Mechanisms by which drugs can enhance insulin secretion include increased pancreatic blood flow (e.g., ACE inhibitors), alteration of β-cell membrane channels (e.g., fluoroquinolones and antiarrhythmic and antimalarial drugs), and decreased insulin degradation [45–47]. Other medications can decrease renal blood flow and hence decrease insulin and other antidiabetic drugs.

In the healthy, non-diabetic patient, the clinician should have a high suspicion for factitious hypoglycemia [48]. This is typically seen in patients who have access to medical supplies such as healthcare workers or those who have sick relatives [49].

Non-insulin-Mediated Hypoglycemia

Non-islet cell tumor-induced hypoglycemia is a rare paraneoplastic syndrome most commonly described in patients with large, slow-growing tumors particularly of mesenchymal origin [50]. Although it was initially attributed to increased glucose utilization by large and highly metabolic tumors, it is now recognized that the underlying physiopathology mechanism is a paraneoplastic phenomenon. These tumors, benign or malignant, produce large amounts of "big" insulin growth factor 2 (IGF-2). "Big" IGF-2 is the result of incomplete and abnormally processed pro-IGF-2 and has insulin-like activity like other insulin growth factors. The activation of insulin receptors by IGF-2 promotes continuous glucose uptake by the muscles, decreased lipolysis by adipocytes, and impaired glucagon release. High concentrations of IGF-2 also result in low plasma growth hormone and IGF-1 due to negative feedback on the pituitary gland. All these factors increase the vulnerability to hypoglycemia. Biochemical workup reveals low plasma glucose concentration with suppressed insulin, proinsulin, betahydroxybutyrate and C-peptide. Also, plasma glucose concentration increases >25 mg/dl after glucagon administration.

Hypoglycemia Evaluation

It is important to decide which patients require hypoglycemia evaluation to avoid unnecessary testing and expense. A thorough history, physical examination, and review of laboratory data are important, particularly if the patient describes symptoms that are suggestive of neuroglycopenia. The diagnostic approaches may differ depending on the clinical situation, i.e., ill, and hospitalized patients versus healthy patients without significant comorbidities.

Establishing a Diagnosis of Hypoglycemia

In the ill, hospitalized patient, clinicians should focus on identifying a possible underlying condition. A particular attention should be paid to the possibility of adrenal insufficiency. Clinicians should also review the list of medications thoroughly.

In the seemingly well patient, since workup is completed generally in the outpatient setting, it is not always possible for the patient to obtain the necessary laboratory tests at the time when the symptoms occur. If the history and laboratory data are suggestive of a hypoglycemic disorder but Whipple's triad has not been documented, the clinician should aim to provoke a hypoglycemic episode. A 72-hour fast or a mixed meal study, if symptoms are suggestive of fasting or postprandial hypoglycemia, respectively, should be the initial tests. Fig. 34.1 is a decision tree for the initial diagnosis and evaluation of a patient with hypoglycemic symptoms.

Seventy-Two-Hour Fast

The 72-hour fast consists of a prolonged withholding of food and caloric fluids until Whipple's triad is documented. Normal individuals will not develop hypoglycemia after a prolonged fast due to activation of glycogenolysis and gluconeogenesis. Hypoglycemia only ensues if there is a defect in endogenous glucose production. For instance, in the case of an insulinoma, continuous insulin secretion prevents the physiologic endogenous glucose production

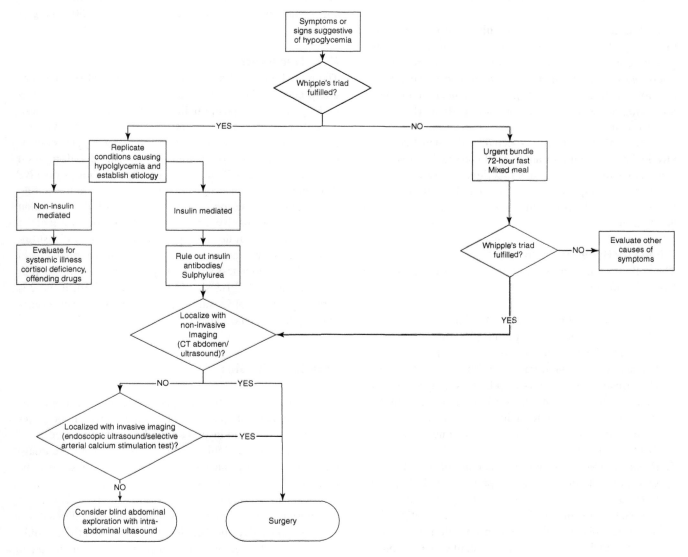

Fig. 34.1 Decision tree for the diagnosis and workup of hypoglycemic disorders

increase that is expected in the fasting state. The 72-hour fast should be undertaken by a center that is experienced in performing the test. The fast can be initiated in the outpatient setting as 35% of patients will have a positive test within the first 12 hours. If hypoglycemia does not occur in the first 12 hours, individuals should be admitted to an inpatient ward to complete the fast. Ninety-three percent of patients will likely have a positive fast by 48 hours of fasting and 99% by 72 hours [16].

While patients undergo the 72-hour fast, the test should only be terminated if one of the following criteria is met:

1. Documentation of Whipple's triad.
2. Plasma glucose concentration <45 mg/dL.
3. Plasma glucose concentration <55 mg/dl with previous documentation of Whipple's triad.
4. Progressive increase in β-hydroxybutyrate.
5. After 72 hours if no symptoms occur.

Ending the fast may be a difficult decision, especially in the setting of nonspecific symptoms with low normal plasma glucose concentration near the hypoglycemic threshold. It is important to keep in mind that low plasma glucose may be physiological, and plasma glucose concentration in the 40–50 mg/dl range is not uncommon, particularly in young lean women.

If neuroglycopenia is suspected, a detailed history and physical exam are important to establish the diagnosis. Tests can include those of cognitive function, for example, serial 7 subtractions. Frequent reevaluation may be required, including the need for bedside glucose testing if laboratory values are delayed.

Criteria for Hyperinsulinemia

The following laboratory findings confirm the presence of hyperinsulinemia:

1. Plasma insulin concentration ≥3 μU/ml.
2. Plasma C-peptide concentration ≥200 pmol/l.
3. Plasma proinsulin concentration ≥5 pmol/l.
4. Plasma β-hydroxybutyrate concentration ≤2.7 mmol/l. Hyperinsulinemia results in β-hydroxybutyrate suppression. A β-hydroxybutyrate concentration >2.7 mmol/l, or if two consecutive values at least 6 hours apart exceed the value at hour 18 of the fast, suggests a negative 72-hour fast test [51].
5. Plasma glucose concentration increase of >25 mg/dl after glucagon administration. In patients with hyperinsulinemia, liver glycogen stores are maintained in the fasting state (insulin has an anti-glycogenolytic effect); therefore, plasma glucose concentration increases in response to the glycogenolytic effect of glucagon. Normal

individuals will have used all glycogen stored in the liver after a prolonged fast and will not respond to glucagon stimulation.
6. Negative sulfonylurea and meglitinide screen. Both types of medications can cause an identical laboratory profile to an insulinoma. Therefore, these should be measured using liquid chromatographic tandem mass spectrography.
7. Absence of insulin antibodies. The presence of insulin antibodies is only of utility in patients with no history of insulin use. If antibodies are present, the clinician should consider the possibility of insulin antibody-mediated hypoglycemia or surreptitious insulin use.

The interpretation of insulin, C-peptide, and proinsulin concentrations during the prolonged supervised fast depends on the concomitant plasma glucose concentration. The normal overnight fasting ranges for these polypeptides do not apply when the plasma glucose concentration is 50–55 mg/dl or lower.

Mixed Meal Test

The mixed meal test does not have established standards of interpretation. This study is generally performed in patients with symptoms of postprandial hypoglycemia. For the test, patients consume a non-liquid meal and are observed for 5 hours following food ingestion [52]. Plasma glucose, insulin, C-peptide, and proinsulin are measured before food ingestion and every 30 minutes thereafter. The test is positive if patients develop neuroglycopenic symptoms in the setting of a plasma glucose concentration ≤ 50 mg/dl. It is important to note that a positive test only confirms the presence of Whipple's triad but does not provide a diagnosis. If insulinoma is still suspected in a patient with a positive mixed meal study, the 72-hour fast should be performed. If the 72-hour fast is negative, NIPHS should be suspected [19]. If there is a history of bariatric surgery, then post-bariatric surgery hypoglycemia is more likely.

Localizing Studies

Localizing studies are only performed once endogenous hyperinsulinemic hypoglycemia with negative hypoglycemic agent screen and insulin antibodies is documented.

Insulinomas are highly vascularized, and therefore imaging techniques are successful in localizing these lesions. Imaging not only can identify the primary tumor, but it also allows for the evaluation of metastatic lesions. Localization is important as it will prevent morbidity and mortality associated with extensive abdominal explorations and the possible need for repeat surgeries. Surgical cure depends on the accurate localization of the tumor. There are noninvasive and invasive techniques available.

Noninvasive Radiologic Studies

The advantages of noninvasive techniques are lower expense and fewer complications. The size of the tumor and the patient's body habitus can limit the diagnostic utility of non-invasive techniques. Dynamic computed tomography has an excellent sensitivity >90%, transabdominal ultrasonography is operator dependent and therefore has a variable sensitivity, and magnetic resonance imaging has a variable sensitivity with an average of 70% [13].

Imaging characteristics of CT typically involve enhancing and vascular lesions visualized during both arterial and portal venous phases, although smaller lesions are better seen during the arterial phase (Figs. 34.2 and 34.3). Lesions do not classically alter the natural contour of the pancreas.

Invasive Techniques

If computed tomography, magnetic resonance imaging, and transabdominal ultrasonography fail to localize the source of endogenous hyperinsulinemia, more invasive procedures may be needed. Alternatives include endoscopic ultrasonography (sensitivity 95–100%) and arteriography (sensitivity <70%) [13]. Arteriography is now only limited to selective arterial calcium stimulation test in our practice. Intraoperative ultrasound has a high sensitivity if performed by experienced providers and is particularly helpful in detecting lesions in MEN1.

The decision about which study to perform will depend on the center's experience and expertise.

If more invasive procedures fail to localize the source of insulin, selective arterial calcium stimulation is indicated. It is important to keep in mind that negative imaging does not exclude insulinoma.

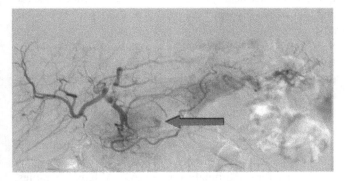

Fig. 34.2 Contrast-enhanced computed tomography of the abdomen including triphasic imaging through the pancreas of a 38-year-old male with endogenous hyperinsulinemic hypoglycemia. A subtle, rounded, 1.8-cm nodule in the neck of the pancreas slightly enhances on the late arterial phase, concerning for an insulinoma

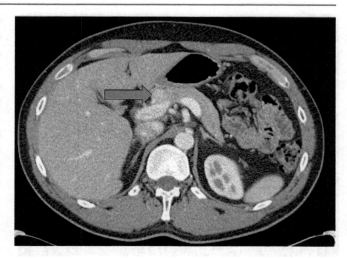

Fig. 34.3 Contrast-enhanced computed tomography of the abdomen including triphasic imaging through the pancreas of a 48-year-old female with endogenous hyperinsulinemic hypoglycemia reveals a 7-mm nodule in the posterior tail of the pancreas, concerning for an insulinoma

Selective Arterial Calcium Stimulation

Selective arterial calcium stimulation is reserved for patients with negative radiologic localizing studies. It guides not only insulinoma management but also NIPHS and post-bariatric surgery hypoglycemia management. Although pancreatic islet cell hypertrophy due to NIPHS and post-bariatric surgery hypoglycemia is a diffuse process, insulin response to calcium injection often localizes to one arterial domain. Interestingly, selective arterial calcium stimulation can distinguish between an insulinoma and a more diffuse process such as seen in NIPHS or in post-bariatric surgery hypoglycemia [53]. Insulinomas cause significantly higher absolute and relative hepatic venous insulin concentrations.

The sensitivity of this technique is higher than 90% [54, 55]. The procedure involves catheterization of the right hepatic vein via the inferior vena cava. Calcium gluconate is selectively and sequentially injected into the gastroduodenal artery, superior mesenteric artery, and splenic artery. After selective injection into each artery, insulin concentration is measured in hepatic venous effluent samples collected at 20, 40, and 60 seconds following the calcium gluconate infusion. A two- to threefold rise in insulin concentration in any of these samples reveals the area of the pancreas where excess insulin is coming from. If hepatic vein insulin concentration increases after selective calcium gluconate injection into the gastroduodenal artery, then the insulinoma or tissue hyperplasia is located in the head of the pancreas, whereas if hepatic vein insulin concentration increases after selective calcium gluconate injection into the superior mesenteric or splenic arteries, the dysfunctional tissue is located in the uncinated process or the body or tail of the pancreas,

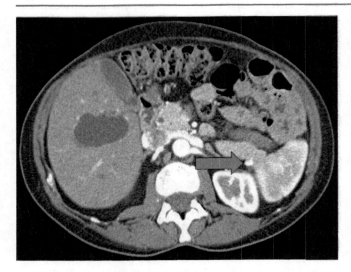

Fig. 34.4 A 53-year-old female with endogenous hyperinsulinemic hypoglycemia. Arteriogram after calcium gluconate infusion into the superior mesenteric artery, gastroduodenal artery, and splenic artery reveals a vascular "blush" in the gastroduodenal artery region

Table 34.1 Calcium stimulated hepatic venous sampling showing a sixfold increase in venous insulin concentration in the arterial domain of the gastroduodenal artery at 40 seconds, corresponding to the abnormal arteriogram. Stimulated insulin after concentrations in the superior mesenteric and splenic arteries remains flat

Venous insulin (mcIU/ml)	Superior mesenteric artery	Gastroduodenal artery	Splenic artery
Systemic insulin	20.1	9.7	7.3
Hepatic (baseline)	14	10	7.7
Insulin 20 s	13.8	30.7	8.2
Insulin 40 s	15.5	64.6	8.5
Insulin 60 s	12.7	44	7.8

respectively. Fig. 34.4 and Table 34.1 show the arteriogram after selective arterial calcium stimulation and corresponding hepatic vein insulin concentration in a 53-year-old female with endogenous hyperinsulinemic hypoglycemia with negative imaging.

Selective arterial calcium stimulation test may be used as a diagnostic tool in patients with renal failure, when plasma β-cell polypeptide concentrations are unreliable [56].

Treatment

Treatment is directed to the specific etiology.

Insulinomas

The gold standard of care for insulinomas is surgical resection. The surgical approach, open surgery versus laparos-

copy, depends on the tumor size, localization, focality, and invasion. Very deep lesions may require segmental resection, but solitary and superficial lesions can be managed with enucleation. Malignant insulinomas require more extensive resection. Importantly, surgeons should aim to preserve endocrine and exocrine function if possible. Surgical cure rate is above 90% [57]. Non-malignant insulinomas have a good prognosis with survival that is no different from that expected for the population [13, 16, 17]. Malignant insulinomas, on the other hand, have a survival rate of 29% at 15 years following diagnosis [18]. Roughly 7% of sporadic insulinomas recur. Recurrence rate is much higher in patients with MEN1.

Medical therapy is expensive and carries significant adverse events. It is only indicated in patients who are not good surgical candidates or those who have unresectable disease. Among the medications used, diazoxide, which inhibits insulin release from β-cells, achieves symptomatic control in roughly 50% of patients at the expense of side effects (fluid retention, weight gain, nausea, and/or hirsutism) [58, 59].

Somatostatin analogues, such as octreotide and lanreotide, have been shown to have a variable effect on the symptomatic management of insulinomas. A beneficial effect may be limited to insulinomas expressing somatostatin receptor-2 [60]. Activation of such receptors mediates somatostatin-induced insulin suppression and glucagon release. Somatostatin analogues have also been shown to have an anti-proliferative effect and are considered first-line therapy in inoperable malignant insulinomas [61].

Cytotoxic chemotherapy has variable effects on tumor progression and symptoms. It is limited to patients with highly and rapidly progressive tumors given the high toxicity. Novel therapies including everolimus, an mTOR inhibitor, and sunitinib, a tyrosine kinase inhibitor, have been used in the treatment of advanced neuroendocrine tumors. Everolimus has been proven to stabilize advanced disease and to improve glycemic control but at the expense of severe adverse events, including severe pulmonary toxicity. Sunitinib is anti-angiogenic and also has anti-tumor activity. It has demonstrated to increase progression-free survival in patients with pancreatic neuroendocrine tumors. However, there is some evidence that it can worsen hypoglycemia so its utility in the treatment of insulin-producing neuroendocrine tumors remains to be determined [62].

Cytoreductive therapy with ethanol, delivered through endoscopic ultrasonography or intraoperatively, may be effective for symptomatic control [63]. Ablative therapies, such as ethanol ablation and arterial embolization, should only be considered in patients with extensive disease and/or in poor surgical candidates in combination with medical therapy, for symptomatic control only and not with curative intent.

NIPHS and Post-Bariatric Surgery Hypoglycemia

Most patients achieve symptomatic control with diet modification. Reports suggest that diazoxide, acarbose, verapamil, and octreotide may improve hypoglycemic symptoms [64–67]. Partial pancreatectomy is considered in those who fail medical therapy but has poor long-term outcomes in terms of symptom resolution; 90% of patients who have undergone extended distal pancreatectomy develop recurrence of symptoms [68].

In the case of post-bariatric surgery hypoglycemia, more aggressive therapies include enteral feeding and reversal of the surgical procedure. The latter has not always resulted in hypoglycemia resolution [69, 70].

Non-islet Cell Tumor Hypoglycemia

Tumor resection is the mainstay treatment for non-islet cell tumor hypoglycemia. Other therapeutic options include localized anti-tumor therapy, glucagon infusion (most useful during acute hypoglycemia), and growth hormone at supraphysiological doses. Octreotide has limited utility [50].

Iatrogenic

Offending drugs should be eliminated. When insulin is used to treat hyperglycemia, enteral/parental feeding interruptions should be minimized. Hypoglycemia in the setting of underlying systemic disease should be rapidly identified and prevented.

Future Therapies

Several potential therapies are currently being investigated as treatment modalities for more severe cases of endogenous hyperinsulinemic hypoglycemia. Most of these therapies have been used in very few patients, and further studies will be needed to prove their efficacy and assess their adverse event profile.

- Pasireotide is a novel multi-receptor somatostatin analogue with higher affinity to somatostatin receptor-5, which selectively modulates insulin secretion. It has been used effectively for the treatment of Cushing's disease and acromegaly. Significant side effects include a high incidence of hyperglycemia and diabetes. Two case reports using pasireotide have demonstrated symptomatic efficacy in the treatment of refractory hypoglycemia in malignant insulinoma. Further studies will be needed to assess its anti-proliferative effect [71, 72].
- Several case reports have suggested beenfit of exendin (9–39), a GLP-1 receptor antagonist, which is now being studied as a therapy for post-bariatric surgery hypoglycemia. In one small study, nine patients with recurrent symptomatic hypoglycemia after Roux-en-Y gastric bypass received exendin (9–39) during an OGTT. Exendin (9–39) prevented hyperinsulinemic hypoglycemia and improved symptoms [73].
- Nuclear therapy using peptide receptor radionucleotides linked to somatostatin analogues has resulted in increased progression-free survival for neuroendocrine tumors [74]. Two small case series in patients with insulinoma have demonstrated that this therapy may be effective in controlling symptoms despite of having no effect on tumor progression [75, 76].

Conclusion

Hypoglycemia is life-threatening. If neuroglycopenia is suspected, a full evaluation should ensue. The diagnostic approach includes a 72-hour fast or a mixed meal study to document Whipple's triad. Hyperinsulinemic hypoglycemia most commonly occurs in healthy patients, with insulinoma predominating as the etiology. NIPHS is a relatively newer clinical entity characterized by β-cell hypertrophy and hyperplasia. Similar pancreatic changes have also been described in bariatric surgery patients who develop hypoglycemia postoperatively. In contrast, ill patients tend to have multifactorial hypoglycemia from an underlying systemic disease and/or iatrogenic factors. In both healthy and ill patients, drug-induced hypoglycemia should be excluded. Treatment of hypoglycemia includes relief of neuroglycopenia. Additional therapies should be directed at the underlying disorder.

References

1. Nirantharakumar K, Marshall T, Hodson J, Narendran P, Deeks J, Coleman JJ, et al. Hypoglycemia in non-diabetic in-patients: clinical or criminal? PLoS One. 2012;7(7):e40384.
2. Seaquist ER, Anderson J, Childs B, Cryer P, Dagogo-Jack S, Fish L, et al. Hypoglycemia and diabetes: a report of a workgroup of the american diabetes association and the endocrine Society. Diabetes Care. 2013;36(5):1384–95.
3. Cryer PE, Axelrod L, Grossman AB, Heller SR, Montori VM, Seaquist ER, et al. Evaluation and management of adult hypoglycemic disorders: an endocrine society clinical practice guideline. J Clin Endocrinol Metabol. 2009;94(3):709–28.
4. Towler DA, Havlin CE. Craft S, Cryer P. Mechanism of awareness of hypoglycemia. Perception of neurogenic (predominantly cholinergic) rather than neuroglycopenic symptoms. Diabetes. 1993;42(12):1791–8.

5. Cryer PE. Hypoglycemia, functional brain failure, and brain death. J Clin Invest. 2007;117(4):868–70.

6. Amiel SA, Sherwin RS, Simonson DC, Tamborlane WV. Effect of intensive insulin therapy on glycemic thresholds for counterregulatory hormone release. Diabetes. 1988;37(7):901–7.

7. Cryer PE. Glucose counterregulation: prevention and correction of hypoglycemia in humans. Am J Phys Anthropol. 1993;264(2 Pt 1):E149–55.

8. Moller N, Jorgensen JO. Effects of growth hormone on glucose, lipid, and protein metabolism in human subjects. Endocr Rev. 2009;30(2):152–77.

9. Gerich J, Cryer P, Rizza R. Hormonal mechanisms in acute glucose counterregulation: the relative roles of glucagon, epinephrine, norepinephrine, growth hormone, and cortisol. Metabolism. 1980;29(11 Suppl 1):1164–75.

10. Dinneen S, Alzaid A, Miles J, Rizza R. Effects of the normal nocturnal rise in cortisol on carbohydrate and fat metabolism in IDDM. Am J Phys Anthropol. 1995;268(4 Pt 1):E595–603.

11. Service FJ. Hypoglycemic disorders. N Engl J Med. 1995;332(17):1144–52.

12. Wilder RM, Allan FN, Power MH, Robertson HE. Carcinoma of the islands of the pancreas: Hyperinsulinism and hypoglycemia. J Am Med Assoc. 1927;89(5):348–55.

13. Mehrabi A, Fischer L, Hafezi M, Dirlewanger A, Grenacher L, Diener MK, et al. A systematic review of localization, surgical treatment options, and outcome of insulinoma. Pancreas. 2014;43(5):675–86.

14. Kar P, Price P, Sawers S, Bhattacharya S, Reznek RH, Grossman AB. Insulinomas may present with normoglycemia after prolonged fasting but glucose-stimulated hypoglycemia. J Clin Endocrinol Metab. 2006;91(12):4733–6.

15. Dizon AM, Kowalyk S, Hoogwerf BJ. Neuroglycopenic and other symptoms in patients with insulinomas. Am J Med. 1999;106(3):307–10.

16. Service FJ, Dale AJ, Elveback LR, Jiang NS. Insulinoma: clinical and diagnostic features of 60 consecutive cases. Mayo Clin Proc. 1976;51(7):417–29.

17. Hochwald SN, Zee S, Conlon KC, Colleoni R, Louie O, Brennan MF, et al. Prognostic factors in pancreatic endocrine neoplasms: an analysis of 136 cases with a proposal for low-grade and intermediate-grade groups. J Clin Oncol: Official J Am Soc Clin Oncol. 2002;20(11):2633–42.

18. Service FJ, McMahon MM, O'Brien PC, Ballard DJ. Functioning insulinoma--incidence, recurrence, and long-term survival of patients: a 60-year study. Mayo Clin Proc. 1991;66(7):711–9.

19. Service FJ, Natt N, Thompson GB, Grant CS, van Heerden JA, Andrews JC, et al. Noninsulinoma pancreatogenous hypoglycemia: a novel syndrome of hyperinsulinemic hypoglycemia in adults independent of mutations in Kir6.2 and SUR1 genes. J Clin Endocrinol Metab. 1999;84(5):1582–9.

20. Thompson GB, Service FJ, Andrews JC, Lloyd RV, Natt N, van Heerden JA, et al. Noninsulinoma pancreatogenous hypoglycemia syndrome: an update in 10 surgically treated patients. Surgery. 2000;128(6):937–44;discussion 44–5.

21. Anlauf M, Wieben D, Perren A, Sipos B, Komminoth P, Raffel A, et al. Persistent hyperinsulinemic hypoglycemia in 15 adults with diffuse nesidioblastosis: diagnostic criteria, incidence, and characterization of beta-cell changes. Am J Surg Pathol. 2005;29(4):524–33.

22. Marsk R, Jonas E, Rasmussen F, Naslund E. Nationwide cohort study of post-gastric bypass hypoglycaemia including 5,040 patients undergoing surgery for obesity in 1986–2006 in Sweden. Diabetologia. 2010;53(11):2307–11.

23. Michaels AD, Hunter Mehaffey J, Brenton French W, Schirmer BD, Kirby JL, Hallowell PT. Hypoglycemia following bariatric surgery: our 31-year experience. Obes Surg. 2017:1–6.

24. Service GJ, Thompson GB, Service FJ, Andrews JC, Collazo-Clavell ML, Lloyd RV. Hyperinsulinemic hypoglycemia with nesidioblastosis after gastric-bypass surgery. N Engl J Med. 2005;353(3):249–54.

25. Wredling R, Lins PE, Adamson U. Prevalence of anti-insulin antibodies and its relation to severe hypoglycaemia in insulin-treated diabetic patients. Scand J Clin Lab Invest. 1990;50(5):551–7.

26. Schernthaner G. Immunogenicity and allergenic potential of animal and human insulins. Diabetes Care. 1993;16(Suppl 3):155–65.

27. Goldman J, Baldwin D, Rubenstein AH, Klink DD, Blackard WG, Fisher LK, et al. Characterization of circulating insulin and proinsulin-binding antibodies in autoimmune hypoglycemia. J Clin Invest. 1979;63(5):1050–9.

28. Basu A, Service FJ, Yu L, Heser D, Ferries LM, Eisenbarth G. Insulin autoimmunity and hypoglycemia in seven white patients. Endocr Pract. 2005;11(2):97–103.

29. Lichtman MA, Balderman SR. Unusual manifestations of essential monoclonal gammopathy. II. Simulation of the insulin autoimmune syndrome. Rambam Maimonides Med J. 2015;6(3).

30. Krinsley JS, Grover A. Severe hypoglycemia in critically ill patients: risk factors and outcomes. Crit Care Med. 2007;35(10):2262–7.

31. Hermanides J, Bosman RJ, Vriesendorp TM, Dotsch R, Rosendaal FR, Zandstra DF, et al. Hypoglycemia is associated with intensive care unit mortality. Crit Care Med. 2010;38(6):1430–4.

32. Mizock BA. Alterations in carbohydrate metabolism during stress: a review of the literature. Am J Med. 1995;98(1):75–84.

33. Vary TC, Drnevich D, Jurasinski C, Brennan WA, Jr. Mechanisms regulating skeletal muscle glucose metabolism in sepsis. Shock (Augusta, Ga). 1995;3(6):403–10.

34. Chambrier C, Laville M, Rhzioual Berrada K, Odeon M, Bouletreau P, Beylot M. Insulin sensitivity of glucose and fat metabolism in severe sepsis. Clin Sci (London, England: 1979). 2000;99(4):321–8.

35. Sako A, Yasunaga H, Matsui H, Fushimi K, Hamasaki H, Katsuyama H, et al. Hospitalization for hypoglycemia in Japanese diabetic patients. Medicine (United States). 2015;94(25):e1029.

36. Tanaka H, Nishikawa Y, Fukushima T, Taniguchi A, Fujita Y, Tsuda K, et al. Lipopolysaccharide inhibits hepatic gluconeogenesis in rats: The role of immune cells. J Diabetes Invest. 2017;

37. Bernal W, Wendon J. Acute Liver Failure. N Engl J Med. 2013;369(26):2525–34.

38. Arem R. Hypoglycemia associated with renal failure. Endocrinol Metab Clin N Am. 1989;18(1):103–21.

39. Hussain FYaK. Genetic Disorders Leading to Hypoglycaemia. J Genetic Syndromes Gene Therapy 2013.

40. Kapoor RR, James C, Hussain K. Hyperinsulinism in developmental syndromes. Endocr Dev. 2009;14:95–113.

41. Chandrasekharappa SC, Guru SC, Manickam P, Olufemi SE, Collins FS, Emmert-Buck MR, et al. Positional cloning of the gene for multiple endocrine neoplasia-type 1. Science (New York, NY). 1997;276(5311):404–7.

42. Thakker RV, Newey PJ, Walls GV, Bilezikian J, Dralle H, Ebeling PR, et al. Clinical practice guidelines for multiple endocrine neoplasia type 1 (MEN1). J Clin Endocrinol Metab. 2012;97(9):2990–3011.

43. U.K. Prospective Diabetes Study 16: Overview of 6 Years' Therapy of Type II Diabetes: A Progressive Disease. Diabetes. 1995;44(11):1249.

44. Ben Salem C, Fathallah N, Hmouda H, Bouraoui K. Drug-induced hypoglycaemia: an update. Drug Saf. 2011;34(1):21–45.

45. Huang Z, Jansson L, Sjoholm A. Vasoactive drugs enhance pancreatic islet blood flow, augment insulin secretion and improve glucose tolerance in female rats. Clinical science (London, England: 1979). 2007;112(1):69–76.

46. Davis TM, Dembo LG, Kaye-Eddie SA, Hewitt BJ, Hislop RG, Batty KT. Neurological, cardiovascular and metabolic effects of mefloquine in healthy volunteers: a double-blind, placebo-controlled trial. Br J Clin Pharmacol. 1996;42(4):415–21.

47. Blazar BR, Whitley CB, Kitabchi AE, Tsai MY, Santiago J, White N, et al. In vivo chloroquine-induced inhibition of insulin degradation in a diabetic patient with severe insulin resistance. Diabetes. 1984;33(12):1133–7.

48. Marks V, Teale JD. Hypoglycemia: factitious and felonious. Endocrinol Metab Clin N Am. 1999;28(3):579–601.

49. Grunberger G, Weiner JL, Silverman R, Taylor S, Gorden P. Factitious hypoglycemia due to surreptitious administration of insulin: Diagnosis, treatment, and long-term follow-up. Ann Intern Med. 1988;108(2):252–7.

50. Bodnar TW, Acevedo MJ, Pietropaolo M. Management of non-islet-cell tumor hypoglycemia: a clinical review. J Clin Endocrinol Metab. 2014;99(3):713–22.

51. Service FJ, O'Brien PC. Increasing serum betahydroxybutyrate concentrations during the 72-hour fast: evidence against hyperinsulinemic hypoglycemia. J Clin Endocrinol Metab. 2005;90(8):4555–8.

52. Service FJ. Diagnostic approach to adults with hypoglycemic disorders. Endocrinol Metab Clin N Am. 1999;28(3):519–32. vi

53. Thompson SM, Vella A, Thompson GB, Rumilla KM, Service FJ, Grant CS, et al. Selective arterial calcium stimulation with hepatic venous sampling differentiates insulinoma from nesidioblastosis. J Clin Endocrinol Metab. 2015;100(11):4189–97.

54. Guettier JM, Kam A, Chang R, Skarulis MC, Cochran C, Alexander HR, et al. Localization of insulinomas to regions of the pancreas by intraarterial calcium stimulation: the NIH experience. J Clin Endocrinol Metab. 2009;94(4):1074–80.

55. Thompson SM, Vella A, Service FJ, Grant CS, Thompson GB, Andrews JC. Impact of variant pancreatic arterial anatomy and overlap in regional perfusion on the interpretation of selective arterial calcium stimulation with hepatic venous sampling for preoperative localization of occult insulinoma. Surgery. 2015;158(1):162–72.

56. Basu A, Sheehan MT, Thompson GB, Service FJ. Insulinoma in chronic renal failure: a case report. J Clin Endocrinol Metab. 2002;87(11):4889–91.

57. Richards ML, Thompson GB, Farley DR, Kendrick ML, Service JF, Vella A, et al. Setting the bar for laparoscopic resection of sporadic insulinoma. World J Surg. 2011;35(4):785–9.

58. Gill GV, Rauf O, MacFarlane IA. Diazoxide treatment for insulinoma: a national UK survey. Postgrad Med J. 1997;73(864):640–1.

59. Goode PN, Farndon JR, Anderson J, Johnston IDA, Morte JA. Diazoxide in the management of patients with insulinoma. World J Surg. 1986;10(4):586–91.

60. Vezzosi D, Bennet A, Courbon F, Caron P. Short- and long-term somatostatin analogue treatment in patients with hypoglycaemia related to endogenous hyperinsulinism. Clin Endocrinol. 2008;68(6):904–11.

61. Baldelli R, Barnabei A, Rizza L, Isidori AM, Rota F, Di Giacinto P, et al. Somatostatin analogs therapy in gastroenteropancreatic neuroendocrine tumors: current aspects and new perspectives. Front Endocrinol. 2014;5:7.

62. Brown E, Watkin D, Evans J, Yip V, Cuthbertson DJ. Multidisciplinary management of refractory insulinomas. Clinical Endocrinology. n/a-n/a.

63. Levy MJ, Thompson GB, Topazian MD, Callstrom MR, Grant CS, Vella A. US-guided ethanol ablation of insulinomas: a new treatment option. Gastrointest Endosc. 2012;75(1):200–6.

64. Spanakis E, Gragnoli C. Successful medical management of status post-Roux-en-Y-gastric-bypass hyperinsulinemic hypoglycemia. Obes Surg. 2009;19(9):1333–4.

65. Moreira RO, Moreira RB, Machado NA, Goncalves TB, Coutinho WF. Post-prandial hypoglycemia after bariatric surgery: pharmacological treatment with verapamil and acarbose. Obes Surg. 2008;18(12):1618–21.

66. Nadelson J, Epstein A. A rare case of noninsulinoma pancreatogenous hypoglycemia syndrome. Case Rep Gastrointest Med. 2012;2012:164305.

67. Mathavan VK, Arregui M, Davis C, Singh K, Patel A, Meacham J. Management of postgastric bypass noninsulinoma pancreatogenous hypoglycemia. Surg Endosc. 2010;24(10):2547–55.

68. Vanderveen KA, Grant CS, Thompson GB, Farley DR, Richards ML, Vella A, et al. Outcomes and quality of life after partial pancreatectomy for noninsulinoma pancreatogenous hypoglycemia from diffuse islet cell disease. Surgery. 2010;148(6):1237–45; discussion 45–6.

69. Campos GM, Ziemelis M, Paparodis R, Ahmed M, Davis DB. Laparoscopic reversal of Roux-en-Y gastric bypass: technique and utility for treatment of endocrine complications. Surg Obesity Relat Dis: Official J Am Soc Bariatric Surg. 2014;10(1):36–43.

70. Lee CJ, Brown T, Magnuson TH, Egan JM, Carlson O, Elahi D. Hormonal response to a mixed-meal challenge after reversal of gastric bypass for hypoglycemia. J Clin Endocrinol Metab. 2013;98(7):E1208–12.

71. Hendren NS, Panach K, Brown TJ, Peng L, Beg MS, Weissler J, et al. Pasireotide for the treatment of refractory hypoglycaemia from malignant insulinoma. Clin Endocrinol (Oxf). 2017.

72. Tirosh A, Stemmer SM, Solomonov E, Elnekave E, Saeger W, Ravkin Y, et al. Pasireotide for malignant insulinoma. Hormones (Athens, Greece). 2016;15(2):271–6.

73. Craig CM, Liu LF, Nguyen T, Price C, Bingham J, McLaughlin TL. Efficacy and pharmacokinetics of subcutaneous exendin (9–39) in patients with post-bariatric hypoglycaemia. Diabetes Obes Metab. 2017;

74. Strosberg J, El-Haddad G, Wolin E, Hendifar A, Yao J, Chasen B, et al. Phase 3 trial of 177Lu-dotatate for midgut neuroendocrine tumors. N Engl J Med. 2017;376(2):125–35.

75. Makis W, McCann K, McEwan AJ. Metastatic insulinoma pancreatic neuroendocrine tumor treated with 177Lu-DOTATATE induction and maintenance peptide receptor radionuclide therapy: a suggested protocol. Clin Nucl Med. 2016;41(1):53–4.

76. Challis BG, Powlson AS, Casey RT, Pearson C, Lam BY, Ma M, et al. Adult-onset hyperinsulinaemic hypoglycaemia in clinical practice: diagnosis, aetiology and management. Endocrine Connections. 2017;6(7):540–8.

Hypoglycaemia in Diabetes

Elaine Y. K. Chow and Simon Heller

Introduction

It is well established that intensive glucose control in patients with type 1 and type 2 diabetes reduces microvascular complications in the long term [1, 2]. However, this continues to be achieved at the expense of increased risk of hypoglycaemia. Current insulin secretagogues or conventional subcutaneous insulin delivery cannot replace the physiology of the β cell. As a result, insulin concentrations are often inappropriately raised. Hypoglycaemia thus remains a common side effect of diabetes treatment and one that is most feared by patients. Hypoglycaemia is not only an unpleasant experience but is associated with potentially serious physical and psychological consequences. It remains the main limiting factor in achieving optimal glucose control in patients with insulin- or sulphonylurea-treated diabetes [3]. Furthermore, post hoc analyses from clinical trials have suggested that hypoglycaemia is associated with increased mortality [4, 5].

Definition

A clinical definition based on Whipple's triad (decreased blood glucose, symptoms compatible with hypoglycaemia which resolves with consumption of carbohydrate) remains relevant in day-to-day practice [6]. Hypoglycaemia can be further classified according to severity, and the broad definitions have been widely adopted both clinically and in research settings. A mild/moderate episode is one in which the person is able to self-treat. A severe hypoglycaemic episode is where the person requires external assistance to recover. It has been more difficult to agree biochemical thresholds for hypoglycaemia despite recent attempts [7]. The varying definitions and self-reported nature of hypoglycaemic episodes have made it difficult to compare incidence between studies. The International Hypoglycaemia Study Group has recommended that a glucose concentration of <3.0 mmol/L (<54 mg/dL), which is considered to be clinically significant biochemical hypoglycaemia, be reported in clinical trials [8]. Their position statement was initially adopted by both the ADA and EASD, but other organisations including the International Society for Pediatric and Adolescent Diabetes, Juvenile Diabetes Research Foundation, Advanced Technologies & Treatments for Diabetes and European Medicines Agency have adopted this new classification as well as many pharmacological companies.

Based on observational data, it is estimated that most patients with type 1 diabetes will experience 1–2 mild hypoglycaemic episodes per week and 1–2 episodes of severe hypoglycaemia per year [9]. One in ten severe episodes will involve contact with the emergency services. The risk of hypoglycaemia is lower in type 2 diabetes compared with type 1 diabetes, because when endogenous insulin secretion is relatively intact, counterregulatory responses are preserved (see below). A prospective study of patients attending hospital clinics in the UK has estimated the risk of severe hypoglycaemia at around 0.1 episodes per patient per year in patients taking sulphonylureas [10]. Rates of severe hypoglycaemia were no higher in patients with type 2 diabetes recently started on insulin compared to those taking sulphonylureas. The incidence of hypoglycaemia is highly skewed, with a large number of events concentrated in a small proportion of at-risk patients.

E. Y. K. Chow
Phase 1 Clinical Trial Centre, Department of Medicine and Therapeutics, Prince of Wales Hospital, The Chinese University of Hong Kong, Hong Kong, SAR, China
e-mail: e.chow@cuhk.edu.hk

S. Heller (✉)
Academic Unit of Diabetes, Endocrinology and Metabolism, School of Medicine and Biomedical Sciences, Sheffield, UK
e-mail: s.heller@sheffield.ac.uk

© Springer Nature Switzerland AG 2022
F. Bandeira et al. (eds.), *Endocrinology and Diabetes*, https://doi.org/10.1007/978-3-030-90684-9_35

Morbidity and Mortality Associated with Hypoglycaemia

Acute Effects of Hypoglycaemia

Even mild hypoglycaemia which leads to symptoms and cognitive side effects impacts the lives of patients. It has been estimated some individuals take around half a day to recover from a non-severe episode [11]. Patients who have suffered nocturnal hypoglycaemia are less able to function normally the next day [11]. Severe hypoglycaemia can lead to loss of consciousness and seizures resulting in physical injuries [12], and in the elderly, hypoglycaemic events are associated with increased fall-related fractures [13]. Road traffic accidents as a result of hypoglycaemia are relatively uncommon, but consequences can be lethal [12].

The number of deaths directly attributed to hypoglycaemia is difficult to estimate. Hypoglycaemia is often unrecognised, and post-mortem changes in blood glucose can prevent confirmation of a suspected hypoglycaemic death. In young adults with type 1 diabetes, it has been estimated the proportion of deaths caused by hypoglycaemia is between 7 and 10% [14, 15], slightly lower than that associated with ketoacidosis. Death due to acute hypoglycaemia may be preceded by permanent brain damage and myocardial or cerebral infarction or related to secondary complications due to convulsion and injury. Hypoglycaemia has also been linked to the "dead-in-bed syndrome". This describes a scenario in type 1 diabetic patients with no macrovascular complications, who go to bed apparently well and are found dead in an undisturbed bed in the next morning [16]. Commonly, the cause of death cannot be established at autopsy, and our group have hypothesised that nocturnal hypoglycaemia, in vulnerable individuals, might precipitate fatal arrhythmias [17].

Long-Term Effects of Hypoglycaemia

The long-term emotional consequences of hypoglycaemia can be devastating. The loss of control and independence may lead to constant fear of a hypoglycaemic episode. Many patients rate fear of hypoglycaemia as much as developing long-term complications. Risk of hypoglycaemia presents a major barrier to some in maintaining tight glycaemic control, while individuals prone to recurrent hypoglycaemia are a constant source of anxiety to family and carers [18].

There is ongoing debate as to whether repeated episodes of severe hypoglycaemia can cause cumulative deterioration in cognitive function. Earlier retrospective, cross-sectional studies suggested that recurrent severe hypoglycaemia led to moderate cognitive decrements [19]. However, prospective data from the Diabetes Control and Complications Trial (DCCT) showed no apparent deterioration in cognitive function in patients with recurrent hypoglycaemia over 18 years [20]. Several large-scale studies have highlighted a possible association between hypoglycaemia and dementia in elderly patients with type 2 diabetes [21]. However, it is difficult to determine the direction of causality, as cognitively impaired patients are also more vulnerable to hypoglycaemia.

A further controversy has recently emerged as to whether hypoglycaemia can increase mortality in individuals with type 2 diabetes. Three large-scale randomised controlled trials have explored the effect of intensive glycaemic control on macrovascular disease, in established type 2 diabetic patients with cardiovascular risk. Intensive control increased the risk of hypoglycaemia but failed to reduce macrovascular events significantly in two studies [22, 23] and in the ACCORD study appeared to increase mortality [4]. Post hoc analyses reported a history of preceding hypoglycaemia as a strong independent predictor of death [23]. Overall mortality was twofold to threefold higher and cardiovascular mortality, threefold higher in those who have experienced hypoglycaemia [5, 24]. Interestingly, during trials of intensive insulin therapy in non-diabetic critically ill patients, the risk of death in patients who experienced hypoglycaemia was twofold higher compared to those without [25]. In the absence of a direct link between hypoglycaemia and death, it is not possible to confirm causality. The association might also be the result of confounding, in that patients experiencing hypoglycaemia are more likely to die [5]. However, hypoglycaemia generates pathophysiological changes particularly those due to activation of the sympathoadrenal system which have the potential to aggravate ischemic heart disease. Experimental studies have shown that hypoglycaemia produces abnormalities in cardiac repolarisation, reduces myocardial perfusion and exerts acute pro-inflammatory and pro-thrombotic effects [26]. In experimental studies of type 2 diabetes patients, the pro-thrombotic effects were not limited to the acute episode but extended up to 7 days after the event [27]. Thus, although the precise morbid effects of hypoglycaemia are still to be established, there is a clinical imperative in minimising its frequency and effects.

Presentation

A complex hierarchy of autonomic and neuroendocrine defences ensures that the glucose supply to the brain (its prime metabolic substrate) is maintained. In a non-diabetic individual, pancreatic insulin secretion is suppressed when glucose falls to around 80 mg/dl (4.5 mmol/l) [28]. At lower glucose concentrations, of around 65–70 mg/d (3.6–3.9 mmol/l), the counterregulatory hormones, glucagon and catecholamines are released which stimulates glycogenolysis and gluconeogenesis while reducing peripheral glucose uptake. However, in those with established type 1 diabetes (who have lost the ability to regulate release of insulin from the β cells), glucagon release from α cells, which is mediated by adjacent β cells, is progressively impaired [29]. Thus, within a few years of diagnosis, individuals with type 1 diabetes are particularly dependent on the catecholamine response as a primary defence against hypoglycaemia. During prolonged hypoglycaemia, release of cortisol and growth hormone may also contribute to glucose recovery, although release of these hormones during hypoglycaemia is also diminished with increased duration of disease [30] (Fig. 35.1).

Activation of the sympathetic neural system also contributes to the generation of peripheral symptomatic responses to hypoglycaemia. Early after diagnosis, adults characteristically experience tremor, palpitations, anxiety, sweating, hunger and paraesthesiae at glucose concentrations of around 65 mg/dl (3.5 mmol/l). These "autonomic" symptoms alert individuals and prompt them to consume carbohydrate. Additional symptoms ("neuroglycopenic") generally develop at 50–54 mg/dl (2.8–3.0 mmol/l). These include confusion, drowsiness, odd behaviour, speech difficulties and in-coordination. Elderly patients may experience an additional group of neurological symptoms that can be confused for a cerebrovascular event [31]. Diagnosis is usually straightforward where a concomitant blood glucose is measured at the time of presentation. However, patients often treat themselves when symptomatic before checking their blood glucose.

If glucose levels fall to 35 mg/dl (2 mmol/l) or below, this usually produces profound neurological impairment which may include focal and generalised seizures. Seizures are often mistaken for idiopathic epilepsy (and, rarely, vice versa) since EEG changes can be similar. In rare cases where blood glucose is less than <20 mg/dl (1.0 mmol/l) for a protracted period, irreversible neuronal damage can occur. Magnetic resonance imaging typically shows lesions in the cerebral cortex and hippocampus with sparing of hindbrain structures. Some patients may survive but remain in a persistent vegetative state [32].

Symptoms of hypoglycaemia can vary between and even within individuals. Factors which may modulate symptoms and awareness include sex, age, diurnal effects, prevalent glycaemic control and previous hypoglycaemic episodes. In adults with type 1 diabetes, symptoms are often reset to develop at lower glucose thresholds compared to non-diabetic individuals, particularly in those with tight glycaemic control or long-duration diabetes. However, in those with type 2 diabetes, thresholds are often set at higher glucose levels, even on occasions in the normal range (above 70 mg/dl or 4 mmol/l) [33].

Diminished or absent warning symptoms of hypoglycaemia are major factors contributing to the risk of further severe episodes. A useful clinical "rule of thumb" is to describe patients whose warning symptoms develop at or below 55 mg/dl (3 mmol/l), around the threshold for onset of cognitive dysfunction, as having impaired awareness. Experimental studies involving non-diabetic individuals

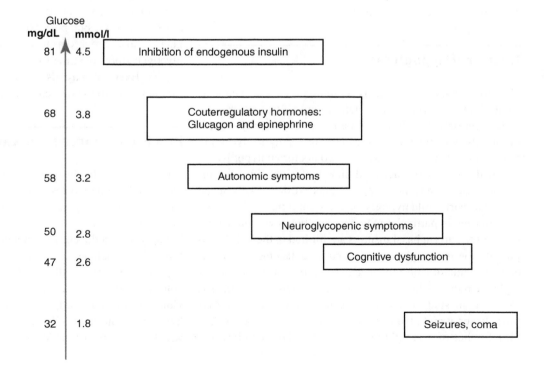

Fig. 35.1 Thresholds to hormonal, symptomatic and neurological responses to hypoglycaemia in non-diabetic adults. (Modified from Chap. 7 Impaired Awareness of Hypoglycaemia, p. 142, Fisher and Frier 2007 Hypoglycemia in Clinical Diabetes, John Wiley and Sons, with permission)

have demonstrated that counterregulatory and symptomatic responses to hypoglycaemia can be attenuated by antecedent hypoglycaemia on the previous day [34]. Some responses, such as sweating, may be depressed for as long as 8 days [35]. These observations have been confirmed in both individuals with type 1 and type 2 diabetes [36, 37]. Thus, patients may enter a vicious cycle where hypoglycaemia begets more hypoglycaemia. Subsequent studies have demonstrated reduced hypoglycaemic awareness can be reversed (at least in part) by scrupulous avoidance of hypoglycaemia for 2–3 weeks although this sometimes occurred even without restoration of counterregulatory hormone release [38–40].

Causes of Hypoglycaemia

As described above, hypoglycaemia arises where there is an excess of insulin compared to circulating blood glucose. In the clinical situation, it is frequently possible to establish a contributory cause which can be assigned one of the following categories [28]:

- Excess exogenous insulin (or insulin secretagogue)—wrong dose, wrong time or formulation.
- Increased insulin sensitivity—e.g. nighttime, post-exercise, weight loss, early pregnancy.
- Decreased exogenous carbohydrate intake—e.g. missed meal, vomiting, fasting, malabsorption.
- Decreased endogenous glucose production—e.g. alcohol which depresses hepatic gluconeogenesis.
- Increased glucose utilisation—e.g. exercise.

Nocturnal Hypoglycaemia

Nocturnal hypoglycaemia is common—in the Diabetes Control and Complications Trial, around half of severe episodes occurred at night [41]. In a more recent study involving adults with type 1 diabetes aiming for tight glycaemic targets, most participants experienced nocturnal hypoglycaemia with low glucose detected on 8% of nights by continuous glucose monitoring [42]. Patients are less likely to be alerted by early/mild hypoglycaemic symptoms while asleep, and children in particular may go many hours without eating overnight. Current basal insulins are limited in their ability to provide continuous physiological basal replacement. Further, counterregulatory hormonal and symptomatic responses at night are reduced due to both the effect of supine posture and sleep. In one study, epinephrine responses were three to four times lower at night while asleep compared with when awake [43]. Studies of overnight monitoring in children with type 1

diabetes have reported frequent, prolonged nocturnal episodes, lasting more than 3 hours [44], presumably due to the combined contribution of the factors identified above.

Alcohol

Alcohol has been implicated in up to a fifth of severe hypoglycaemic episodes requiring hospital admission [45]. Alcohol impairs both awareness of hypoglycaemia [46] and the ability of the person to self-treat due both to its inebriating effects and by suppressing gluconeogenesis. Alcohol also has a delayed effect on hypoglycaemia, often described as the "morning after the night before" phenomenon. Alcohol suppresses lipolysis which in turn suppresses hepatic glucose output [47], an effect which may extend into the following day. In one study of adults with type 1 diabetes, alcohol doubled the risk of hypoglycaemia in the following 24 h [48].

Exercise

Exercise has clear cardiovascular benefits in both types of diabetes and is encouraged. However, it can increase the risk of hypoglycaemia due to increase in insulin sensitivity and exercise-mediated activation of glucose utilisation in skeletal muscle. In non-diabetic individuals, exercise stimulates sympathetic activation to inhibit insulin secretion and stimulate hepatic output of glucose via glycogenolysis. In insulin-treated diabetic patients, the prevailing insulin levels are independent of and cannot be suppressed by exercise [49]. This contributes to a fall in glucose and acute hypoglycaemia during exercise, but post-exercise hypoglycaemia (6–15 h later) is also a risk due to preferential repletion of muscle glycogen stores over the liver and an increase in insulin sensitivity. Exercise may also blunt subsequent counterregulatory defences to hypoglycaemic episodes [50].

Risk Factors for Hypoglycaemia

Much of the pathophysiology described is common to most individuals with diabetes, yet for some individuals, hypoglycaemia is extremely rare, while others experience multiple, disruptive and severe events. The likelihood of developing hypoglycaemia depends upon a number of contributory factors. These include those that determine the physiological capacity to counterregulate and generate awareness, pharmacology of glucose-lowering agents, the ability of the individual to self-manage their diabetes and recognise and treat hypoglycaemia as well as psychological characteristics, which remain poorly understood.

Long Duration of Diabetes

One of the most important contributors to hypoglycaemic risk is duration of diabetes. In an observational UK study, adults with a duration of type 1 diabetes for over 15 years were three times more likely to experience severe hypoglycaemia compared to those with diabetes for less than 5 years [10]. This presumably reflects loss of beta-cell function and counterregulatory defences with type 1 diabetes. In advanced type 2 diabetes, glucagon responses to hypoglycaemia are also progressively impaired as patients become insulin deficient [51]. The risk has been shown to be highest in those using insulin for over 5 years as rates of severe hypoglycaemia approach those of individuals with newly diagnosed type 1 diabetes [10].

Hypoglycaemia Unawareness

Nearly 20% of patients with type 1 diabetes develop reduced awareness of hypoglycaemia, the prevalence increasing with duration of diabetes [52]. A recent study also suggests that around 10% of adults with type 2 diabetes also have difficulty recognising hypoglycaemia [53]. A number of scoring systems have been developed to quantify awareness of hypoglycaemia, with the Gold [54] and Clarke scores [55] being the most widely adopted. Impaired hypoglycaemia awareness has been shown to increase the risk of severe hypoglycaemia by fivefold to sixfold in prospective surveys [54, 55]. One of the ironical consequences is that individuals with unawareness are often excluded from trials of new therapy such as insulin analogues or continuous glucose monitoring which have the potential to reduce the risk of hypoglycaemia.

Renal Failure

Renal failure is often under-recognised as a contributor to hypoglycaemia. Renal failure reduces metabolism of insulin and clearance of metabolites of drugs such as sulphonylureas. It also affects reabsorption of filtered glucose as well as gluconeogenesis (the kidneys provide as much as 30% of glucose production due to gluconeogenesis). In type 2 diabetes, it is estimated that the risk of severe hypoglycaemia is increased by twofold to threefold in those with eGFR <60 ml/min 1.73 m^2 [56]. Management of diabetic patients with end-stage renal failure on dialysis is particularly challenging. It usually necessitates major reductions in insulin doses and avoidance of sulphonylureas [57].

Treatment Factors

Insulin and insulin secretagogues unsurprisingly are far more likely to cause hypoglycaemia. Insulin "sensitisers" such as metformin and thiazolidinones have a minimal risk of hypoglycaemia. In the UK Prospective Diabetes Study, the rate of self-reported hypoglycaemia was 0.3% in patients on metformin monotherapy in the first 6 years of diagnosis [58]. Emerging data on the incretin-based therapies dipeptidyl peptidase-4 (DPP-4) inhibitors and glucagon-like peptide-1 (GLP-1) analogues indicate that the risk of significant hypoglycaemia is also very low [59], unless patients are being treated concurrently with sulphonylureas or insulin.

It has been estimated that 39% of patients on sulphonylureas alone will experience mild hypoglycaemia and severe hypoglycaemia will occur in 0.8% each year [10]. The third-generation sulphonylureas (gliclazide, glimepiride) and meglitinides have a lower risk of hypoglycaemia compared to older drugs such as glyburide (glibenclamide), presumably due to shorter duration of action. The risk is increased when sulphonylureas are part of combination therapy, particularly with insulin [60].

Insulin analogues have a pharmacokinetic profile that should lower the potential for hypoglycaemia compared to human insulins. The rapid-acting insulin analogues (aspart, lispro, glulisine) separate into single molecules more readily and hence are less likely to accumulate. In a meta-analysis comparing lispro with regular human insulin, the frequency of hypoglycaemia was modestly reduced (3.1% versus 4.4%) [61]. The first-generation long-acting analogues also confer a slightly lower risk for hypoglycaemia compared with isophane insulins [62]. The second-generation basal insulin analogues have been shown to further reduce hypoglycaemia. Insulin degludec, as compared with insulin glargine 100 units/ml, was associated with lower overall symptomatic hypoglycaemia rates in type 1 and type 2 diabetes patients [63, 64]. Similar benefits have been observed with insulin glargine 300 units/ml as compared with first-generation glargine 100 units/ml in adults with type 2 diabetes [65]. Most if not all the benefit is generally observed for nocturnal episodes, and troublesome nocturnal hypoglycaemia is a robust indication for the use of insulin analogues. Differences also exist according to the type of insulin regimen. In the 4 T study, once-daily basal insulin, when initiated in type 2 diabetic patients, was associated with the lowest risk of hypoglycaemia. The risk of hypoglycaemia was higher with twice-daily biphasic regimes and highest in those on prandial-basal regimes; however, fewer reached HbA1c targets in the biphasic group [66].

Psychosocial Factors

The risk of hypoglycaemia is clearly affected by the ability of the patient to recognise and self-treat an episode. This applies particularly to the elderly and cognitively impaired. In trials of intensive glycaemic control in type 2 diabetes, patients with cognitive impairment were at higher risk of hypoglycaemia requiring assistance [67], and similar findings have been reported in community studies [68]. In a German study, one-third of type 2 diabetic patients who experienced severe hypoglycaemia lived in a nursing home or were cared for by a home care service [69]. Patients with type 2 diabetes are more likely to require hospital care for hypoglycaemia compared with type 1 diabetic patients.

Probably one of the most important and least studied contributing areas is the contribution of psychological factors which drive patients to maintain tight glycaemic targets despite the obvious risks even in those with major recurrent episodes [70]. There is some evidence that identifying these factors and addressing them specifically can reduce hypoglycaemic risk. However, much further work needs to be undertaken in understanding this important area and developing interventions to address it.

Clinical Assessment

Assessment of hypoglycaemia should be a part of every diabetes review. The clinician should establish (1) the frequency and nature of hypoglycaemic episodes and (2) the overall risk of hypoglycaemia. Fig. 35.2 illustrates key points to clinical assessment. Part of this should include their daily insulin administration routine. The timing of prandial doses is important. Delayed or missed meals can result in the peak of insulin action coinciding with having little food in the system. Alternatively, patients who prefer to inject postprandially may experience episodes if the insulin peaks in the post-absorptive phase. Recurrent hypoglycaemia can also occur if patients administer boluses of short-acting insulin too close together, sometimes known as insulin "stacking". This tends to occur where patients over-correct high glucose values by repeated insulin boluses and is a particular concern in those using insulin pumps. Injecting into areas of lipohypertrophy can lead to unpredictable absorption.

Hypoglycaemia awareness should be assessed (Fig. 35.2), and corroboration from a relative or partner is often useful [71]. Diabetes duration, treatment regime and overall glycaemic control will help to determine a patient's risk of hypoglycaemia. However, if there is a sudden increase in hypoglycaemia that appears out of proportion to the diabetes history, other medical causes should be sought such as renal failure, hepatic failure, malabsorption, hyperthyroidism or

Clinical information:
Type 1 or 2 diabetes
Duration of diabetes
Duration of insulin treatment
Hypoglycemic potential of diabetic treatment: insulin/sulphonylureas (high) vs metformin/DPP-4 inhibitors/GLP-1 analogues/thiazolediones (low)
Other drugs (e.g. quinine, trimethoprim, salicylates)
Psychosocial risk factors e.g. living alone, cognitive impairment

Enquire:
Hypoglycemia
- Frequency
- Severity: self-treated, requiring assistance of family or paramedics
- Timing: nocturnal, relation to meals, exercise, alcohol
Review glucose monitoring diary

Assess hypoglycemia awareness:
- At what blood sugar level do you start noticing symptoms of hypos?
- Have there been times when your blood sugar is below 3mmol without any warnings?
- Are there episodes of hypoglycemia that others have noticed before you?

Impact of hypoglycemia on lifestyle:
Driving, high-risk occupations
Explore fear/anxiety surrounding hypoglycemia

Examine:
Injection site for lipohypertrophy

Laboratory tests:
Renal function
Liver function
Consider the following if unexplained increase in hypoglycemia
Thyroid function test
9am cortisol or short synacthen test
Coeliac screen
Insulin binding antibodies

Fig. 35.2 Clinical assessment of patients with hypoglycaemia

adrenal insufficiency. Certain drugs can also increase the potential for hypoglycaemia on their own or through interactions with glucose-lowering agents (Fig. 35.2).

Management

Treatment of Acute Hypoglycaemia

All episodes of hypoglycaemia should be treated promptly. Mild hypoglycaemic episodes in a conscious, cooperative patient can be easily treated by rapid-acting carbohydrate (15–20 g). Fig. 35.3 lists some examples of suitable treatments that are accessible and portable. Patients are often tempted to "over-treat" hypoglycaemia with excessive carbohydrate, but this can lead to rebound hyperglycaemia and worsen glucose control. Rapid-acting carbohydrate should be repeated if blood glucose remains low, and patients should be instructed to check their blood glucose 10–15 min later.

Immediate management of acute hypoglycemia

- *Conscious, co-operative, able to swallow*
  15-20 g rapid acting carbohydrate
  e.g. 150-200ml pure fruit juice
      90-120ml Lucozade
      5-6 glucose tablets
      3-4 heaped teaspoons of sugar

- *Conscious, uncooperative, still able to swallow*
  1.5-2 tubes oral dextrose gel

- *Unconscious, seizures*
  Glucagon 1mg IM
      or
  10% Dextrose IV (150ml) or 20% dextrose IV
  (75ml) over 10-15min

Repeat rapid acting glucose if blood glucose less
than 70mg/dL (<4mmol/l) after 15 minutes. Seek
further medical help if blood glucose remains low
after 3 cycles.

Recovery:
- Follow up with long acting carbohydrate (e.g. 2
  biscuits, 1 slice of toast) unless meal within 1
  hour
- Review diabetic treatment regime

Fig. 35.3 Acute management of diabetic hypoglycaemia

Once blood glucose is restored to the normal range, this
should be followed up with long-acting carbohydrate if a
meal is not due within 1 h. In patients who are un-cooperative
but able to swallow, oral glucose gels can be used.
Unconscious patients should be treated with intramuscular
glucagon or intravenous glucose with repeated doses of 10%
glucose solution now replacing the injection of 50% glucose
which was particularly likely to cause thrombophlebitis. In
patients who are malnourished or alcohol-dependent, liver
glycogen stores are depleted, and glucagon may be ineffective. Intravenous glucose is preferable if venous access is
available.

Prevention of Hypoglycaemia

It is clearly important to avoid recurrent hypoglycaemic episodes, and a previous history of hypoglycaemia strongly predicts future risk [72]. Education is the key to effective
self-management. In type 2 diabetes, a review of treatment
regimens and glycaemic targets can reduce hypoglycaemia
in many cases. In type 1 diabetes patients with long disease
duration and multiple risk factors, a combination of strategies, including the use of newer insulin delivery/glucose
monitoring technologies, may be required, such as low glucose suspend pumps.

Education

Many cases of hypoglycaemia are attributed to errors in insulin usage (see above) and can be addressed by educating
patients about the correct time and site of insulin administration. Specific strategies may be adopted to reduce hypoglycaemia associated with alcohol and exercise. Patients should
have sufficient carbohydrate prior to alcohol, and insulin
may need to be reduced. The effect of exercise on glucose is
affected by the duration and intensity of physical activity,
and often a suitable regimen can only be determined with
trial and error. Patients may need to consume extra carbohydrate prior to exercise to allow for a margin for glucose to
fall. Rapid-acting or background insulin may need to be
reduced depending on their exercise regime. Patients should
also avoid exercising at the peak of insulin action and injecting in the exercising muscle.

Structured education programmes that integrate education on carbohydrate estimation and insulin dose adjustment,
as well as hypoglycaemia advice, can make a major difference to reducing hypoglycaemia. The Insulin Treatment and
Training Programmes developed in Germany and its British
adaptation, the Dose Adjustment for Normal Eating
(DAFNE) programme, offering flexible insulin training for
type 1 diabetic patients, have reported reduced rates of severe
hypoglycaemia [73] and improved hypoglycaemia recognition in nearly half of those who were unaware [74]. Blood
Glucose Awareness Training (BGAT) has been shown to
reduce severe hypoglycaemic episodes through teaching
patients to identify their individual symptoms (internal cues)
and how to anticipate blood glucose extremes based on food,
exercise and insulin regimes (external cues) [75]. It may also
owe its success at least in part to the training in self-
management which accompanies it. The psychological
effects of hypoglycaemia are complex and to successfully
prevent hypoglycaemia require a multifaceted approach.
Biopsychosocial interventions such as the HyPOS programme, which addresses dysfunctional beliefs about the
causes and consequences of hypoglycaemia, have also been
effective [76].

Individualised Glycaemic Targets

There is a consistent relationship between intensive glycaemic targets and increased risk of hypoglycaemia in clinical
trials [77], although the relationship is less clear in observational studies of clinical practice [72]. The risk and benefits
of intensive glycaemic control in preventing complications
versus risk of hypoglycaemia need to be weighed for individual patients and discussed with them. The American

Diabetes Association and European Association for the Study of Diabetes have advocated an individualised approach to glycaemic targets [78]. A HbA1c of <7% remains the recommended goal for the majority of patients. However, in those with a history of severe hypoglycaemia, limited life expectancy, extensive comorbidities and glucose targets which result in HbA1c concentrations of 7.5–8% may be safer and more appropriate [78, 79].

Glucose-Lowering Agents with Lower Hypoglycaemic Potential

The choice of treatment regimen should also involve a risk-benefit assessment. In patients with type 2 diabetes, hypoglycaemic risk can be lowered through the use of insulin sensitisers and incretin-based therapies as opposed to insulin secretagogues. Clinicians should be cautious when introducing add-on therapy as the risk is cumulative. Dose reductions may be necessary, and some agents, particularly sulphonylureas, may need to be stopped. Switching to analogue insulins can also reduce the risk of hypoglycaemia particularly at night. The second-generation analogue insulins have been associated with a further risk reduction in hypoglycaemia, particularly at night [63–65]. Analogue insulins may not be cost-effective in all patients, but are indicated in those at high risk of hypoglycaemia.

Continuous Subcutaneous Insulin Therapy

Continuous subcutaneous insulin therapy (CSII) has the advantage over multiple daily injections in its ability to vary basal insulin delivery rates over short intervals. This may be particularly useful in the management of nocturnal hypoglycaemia. Basal rates can be reduced in the early hours of the morning when risk is the highest. Some early studies reported surprisingly little effect on hypoglycaemia, perhaps because of a failure to train patients in the essential related skills of carbohydrate and insulin dose adjustment. In a recent meta-analysis of CSII versus standard multiple daily injections in individuals reporting hypoglycaemic problems, CSII reduced severe hypoglycaemia by threefold to fourfold [80].

Continuous Glucose Monitoring

Continuous glucose monitoring (CGM) has emerged as an alternative technology to conventional self-monitoring of blood glucose (SMBG). Most CGM systems measure interstitial glucose every few minutes via a subcutaneous sensor which displays the prevalent glucose via a portable device or mobile phone. There are various forms of CGM, blinded or

professional CGM, where the profiles may be available for retrospective review and treatment adjustment by healthcare professionals. Flash, or intermittently scanned (isCGM), displays current sensor glucose values only upon scanning of the reader, but without predictive alerts or alarms. Full real-time CGM systems (rtCGM) will display sensor glucose values continuously and activate alarms when the glucose falls too low or is too high. Furthermore, these devices contain predictive algorithms which can warn patients of impending hypoglycaemia or hyperglycaemia. In the randomised controlled study to evaluate the Impact of Novel Glucose Sensing Technology on Hypoglycaemia in Type 1 Diabetes (IMPACT) trial, use of the isCGM system was associated with a 38% reduction in the time spent in hypoglycaemia [81]. A recent randomised controlled trial using a crossover design evaluated the impact of rtCGM versus SMBG use in T1D patients with impaired hypoglycaemia awareness and found that rtCGM use significantly reduced severe hypoglycaemia in this high-risk population [82]. There are also inherent limitations in CGM technology. There is a lag between interstitial and blood glucose which is exaggerated during rapid glucose fluctuations. CGM also has lower accuracy in the extreme hypoglycaemic range. As with any technology, effectiveness of CGM relies heavily on patient adherence and sensor use [83] and so may be most useful in motivated patients.

Sensor-Augmented Pumps and Closed-Loop Systems

Insulin pump devices have been combined with rtCGM monitoring systems in the form of sensor-augmented pump (SAP) systems. In the STAR-3 study where SAP were compared with multiple daily injections and conventional blood glucose monitoring, overall HbA1c was improved with SAP, but rates of severe hypoglycaemia were not significantly different [84]. The "low glucose suspend" technology, such that basal insulin is automatically suspended when interstitial glucose falls below a defined threshold, has shown encouraging results in reducing the duration and severity of hypoglycaemia at night [85] and throughout the day [86].

The holy grail of insulin delivery systems, or the "artificial pancreas", is one which can automatically adjust rates of insulin delivery based on real-time glucose values. Earlier closed-loop systems have been compared against CSII in randomised controlled trial in children and adolescents, where time spent in hypoglycaemia was halved [87]. The first hybrid closed-loop system which automatically adjusts basal insulin based on CGM glucose was approved by FDA in 2016, with several other systems under development. In clinical trials, closed-loop systems have been shown to reduce hypoglycaemia and increase time in range (3.9–10 mmol/L) from 60 to 67% [88]. The next challenge is the fully automated closed loop, which is capable of automating meal-time insulin and changes relating to exercise.

Hypoglycaemia in type 1 diabetes is not only the consequence of iatrogenic hyperinsulinaemia but is also a consequence of defective glucagon counterregulation. Bihormonal pumps are currently in development which can not only switch off insulin but also release glucagon in the event of low glucose. A bihormonal closed-loop system has been tested in six patients with type 1 diabetes without any endogenous insulin secretion, which showed minimal hypoglycaemia throughout the 2-day use, even following exercise [89]. A larger trial of 43 type 1 diabetes showed lower rates of CGM glucose <3.3 mmol (0.6% versus 1.9%) while on the bionic pancreas during home use for a period of 11 days [90]. Clearly, new insulin delivery/glucose sensing technologies offer promising solutions to preventing hypoglycaemia, although most still require patient input and collaboration, dealing with alarms and wearable components, and will not be the answer for all.

Islet Cell and Pancreatic Transplant

Islet cell transplantation is a treatment option in type 1 diabetic patients who suffer disabling hypoglycaemia despite best medical therapy. Pancreatic transplantation has been practiced since the 1960s. However, successful islet transplantation has only recently been possible following refined cell isolation and immunosuppression protocols pioneered by the Edmonton group [91]. Islet cell transplantation restores the major physiological defence of automatic inhibition of endogenous insulin and may also restore glucagon secretion during hypoglycaemia, at least in part [92]. Although one of the benefits of islet cell transplantation is insulin independence, the benefits of protection from severe hypoglycaemia even apply to those who remain insulin dependent. Based on data from the UK programme, it is estimated that 90%, 75% and 50% of transplanted patients will be free from severe hypoglycaemia at 1, 3 and 5 years, respectively [93]. Pancreatic transplantation can offer similar protection from hypoglycaemia and higher rates of insulin independence, but the operation carries greater morbidity and mortality.

Lifestyle Implications

The risk of hypoglycaemia in individuals with diabetes has led to major restrictions on different aspects of their lives, including employment, recreational and daily activities. One key restriction concerns driving. Studies employing driving simulators have reported impaired performance on certain components such as braking and speeding at glucose levels as high as 70 mg/dl (4 mmol/l) in those with type 1 diabetes. Participants were also slow to recognise and correct a low glucose [94]. Current guidance recommends that patients should always check their blood glucose to be a minimum of 90 mg/dl (5 mmol/l) or above before driving [94]. Rapid-acting and more substantial carbohydrate should always be available in the vehicle. For longer journeys, glucose should be checked two hourly. If patients experience hypoglycaemia while driving, in the UK, they are required to remove themselves from the driver's seat and not drive for 45 min after glucose levels are restored to allow for full recovery of cognitive function. In patients who have experienced recurrent severe hypoglycaemia or absent hypoglycaemia awareness, patients are required to inform vehicle licencing authorities, who will generally withdraw their driving licence. It is the responsibility of the clinician to make an assessment of fitness to drive and advise patients to inform the vehicle licencing authorities as appropriate.

Conclusion

Hypoglycaemia is a common and major side effect of insulin and sulphonylurea treatment that remains a formidable barrier to optimal glucose control, even in the modern era of intensive glycaemic therapy. Physical and psychological consequences of hypoglycaemia are substantial for patients and their families, which extend beyond the acute episode. The burden of hypoglycaemia in elderly patients with type 2 diabetes is also considerable.

A recent focus in developing agents with lower hypoglycaemic potential may benefit individuals with type 2 diabetes. For people with type 1 diabetes, technological advances have begun to enable better detection of hypoglycaemia and more physiological replacement of insulin and/or other counterregulatory hormones, although the technology is expensive and not available to all. There will be a time when hypoglycaemia will no longer figure so prominently in the lives of individuals with diabetes. However, as we approach 100 years after the discovery of insulin, it remains a major side effect of treatment and arguably is the major factor preventing those with insulin-treated diabetes from achieving glucose targets.

References

1. Nathan DM, Cleary PA, Backlund JY, Genuth SM, Lachin JM, Orchard TJ, et al. Intensive diabetes treatment and cardiovascular disease in patients with type 1 diabetes. N Engl J Med. 2005;353:2643–53.
2. Holman RR, Paul SK, Bethel MA, Matthews DR, Neil HA. 10-year follow-up of intensive glucose control in type 2 diabetes. N Engl J Med. 2008;359:1577–89.

3. Cryer PE. Hypoglycemia: still the limiting factor in the glycemic management of diabetes. Endocr Pract. 2008;14:750–6.

4. Gerstein HC, Miller ME, Byington RP, Goff DC Jr, Bigger JT, Buse JB, et al. Effects of intensive glucose lowering in type 2 diabetes. N Engl J Med. 2008;358:2545–59.

5. Zoungas S, Patel A, Chalmers J, de Galan BE, Li Q, Billot L, et al. Severe hypoglycemia and risks of vascular events and death. N Engl J Med. 2010;363:1410–8.

6. Cryer PE, Axelrod L, Grossman AB, Heller SR, Montori VM, Seaquist ER, et al. Evaluation and management of adult hypoglycemic disorders: an Endocrine Society Clinical Practice Guideline. J Clin Endocrinol Metab. 2009;94:709–28.

7. Hypoglycemia ADA Working Group. Defining and reporting hypoglycemia in diabetes: a report from the American Diabetes Association Workgroup on Hypoglycemia. Diabetes Care. 2005;28:1245–9.

8. International Hypoglycemia Study Group. Glucose Concentrations of Less than 3.0mmol/L (54 mg/dL) should be reported in clinical trials: A joint Position Statement of the American Diabetes Association and the European Association for the Study of Diabetes. Diabetes Care. 2017;40(1):155–7.

9. Strachan MW. Frequency, causes and risk factors for hypoglycaemia in type 1 diabetes. In: Frier BM, Fisher BM, editors. Hypoglycaemia in clinical diabetes. Chichester, England: John Wiley & Sons; 2007. p. 49–82.

10. UK Hypoglycaemia Study Group. Risk of hypoglycaemia in types 1 and 2 diabetes: effects of treatment modalities and their duration. Diabetologia. 2007;50:1140–7.

11. Brod M, Christensen T, Bushnell DM. The impact of non-severe hypoglycemic events on daytime function and diabetes management among adults with type 1 and type 2 diabetes. J Med Econ. 2012;15:869–77.

12. MacLeod KM, Hepburn DA, Frier BM. Frequency and morbidity of severe hypoglycaemia in insulin-treated diabetic patients. Diabet Med. 1993;10:238–45.

13. Johnston SS, Conner C, Aagren M, Ruiz K, Bouchard J. Association between hypoglycaemic events and fall-related fractures in Medicare-covered patients with type 2 diabetes. Diabetes Obes Metab. 2012;14:634–43.

14. Skrivarhaug T, Bangstad HJ, Stene LC, Sandvik L, Hanssen KF, Joner G. Long-term mortality in a nationwide cohort of childhood-onset type 1 diabetic patients in Norway. Diabetologia. 2006;49:298–305.

15. Feltbower RG, Bodansky HJ, Patterson CC, Parslow RC, Stephenson CR, Reynolds C, et al. Acute complications and drug misuse are important causes of death for children and young adults with type 1 diabetes: results from the Yorkshire Register of diabetes in children and young adults. Diabetes Care. 2008;31:922–6.

16. Tattersall RB, Gill GV. Unexplained deaths of type 1 diabetic patients. Diabet Med. 1991;8:49–58.

17. Heller SR. Abnormalities of the electrocardiogram during hypoglycaemia: the cause of the dead in bed syndrome? Int J Clin Pract Suppl. 2002;129:27–32.

18. Barnard K, Thomas S, Royle P, Noyes K, Waugh N. Fear of hypoglycaemia in parents of young children with type 1 diabetes: a systematic review. BMC Pediatr. 2010;10:50.

19. Deary IJ, Crawford JR, Hepburn DA, Langan SJ, Blackmore LM, Frier BM. Severe hypoglycaemia and intelligence in adult patients with insulin-treated diabetes. Diabetes. 1993;42:341–4.

20. Jacobson AM, Musen G, Ryan CM, Silvers N, Cleary P, Waberski B, et al. Long-term effect of diabetes and its treatment on cognitive function. N Engl J Med. 2007;356:1842–52.

21. Aung PP, Strachan MW, Frier BM, Butcher I, Deary IJ, Price JF. Severe hypoglycaemia and late-life cognitive ability in older people with Type 2 diabetes: the Edinburgh Type 2 Diabetes Study. Diabet Med. 2012;29:328–36.

22. Patel A, MacMahon S, Chalmers J, Neal B, Billot L, Woodward M, et al. Intensive blood glucose control and vascular outcomes in patients with type 2 diabetes. N Engl J Med. 2008;358:2560–72.

23. Duckworth W, Abraira C, Moritz T, Reda D, Emanuele N, Reaven PD, et al. Glucose control and vascular complications in veterans with type 2 diabetes. N Engl J Med. 2009;360:129–39.

24. Bonds DE, Miller ME, Bergenstal RM, Buse JB, Byington RP, Cutler JA, et al. The association between symptomatic, severe hypoglycaemia and mortality in type 2 diabetes: retrospective epidemiological analysis of the ACCORD study. BMJ. 2010;340:b4909.

25. Finfer S, Liu B, Chittock DR, Norton R, Myburgh JA, McArthur C, et al. Hypoglycemia and risk of death in critically ill patients. N Engl J Med. 2012;367:1108–18.

26. Wright RJ, Newby DE, Stirling D, Ludlam CA, Macdonald IA, Frier BM. Effects of acute insulin-induced hypoglycemia on indices of inflammation: putative mechanism for aggravating vascular disease in diabetes. Diabetes Care. 2010;33:1591–7.

27. Chow E, Iqbal A, Walkinshaw E, Phoneix F, Macdonald IA, Storey RF, Ajjan R, Heller SR. Prolonged prothrombotic effects of antecedent hypoglycaemia in individuals with Type 2 diabetes. Diabetes Care. 2018;41(12):2625–33.

28. Cryer PE, Davis SN, Shamoon H. Hypoglycemia in diabetes. Diabetes Care. 2003;26:1902–12.

29. Bolli GB, De Feo P, Compagnucci P, Cartechini MG, Angeletti G, Santeusanio F, et al. Abnormal glucose counterregulation in IDDM. Interaction of anti- insulin antibodies and impaired glucagon and epinephrine secretion. Diabetes. 1983;32:134–41.

30. Macdonald IA, King P. Normal glucose metabolism and responses to hypoglycaemia. In: Frier BM, Fisher BM, editors. Hypoglycaemia in clinical diabetes. Chichester, England: John Wiley & Sons; 2007. p. 1–24.

31. Jaap AJ, Jones GC, McCrimmon RJ, Deary IJ, Frier BM. Perceived symptoms of hypoglycaemia in elderly type 2 diabetic patients treated with insulin. Diabet Med. 1998;15:398–401.

32. Fujioka M, Okuchi K, Hiramatsu KI, Sakaki T, Sakaguchi S, Ishii Y. Specific changes in human brain after hypoglycemic injury. Stroke. 1997;28:584–7.

33. Spyer G, Hattersley AT, MacDonald IA, Amiel S, MacLeod KM. Hypoglycaemic counter-regulation at normal blood glucose concentrations in patients with well controlled type-2 diabetes. Lancet. 2000;356:1970–4.

34. Heller SR, Cryer PE. Reduced neuroendocrine and symptomatic responses to subsequent hypoglycemia after one episode of hypoglycemia in non-diabetic humans. Diabetes. 1991;40:223–6.

35. George E, Harris N, Bedford C, Macdonald IA, Hardisty CA, Heller SR. Prolonged but partial impairment of the hypoglycaemic physiological response following short-term hypoglycaemia in normal subjects. Diabetologia. 1995;38:1183–90.

36. Dagogo-Jack SE, Craft S, Cryer PE. Hypoglycemia-associated autonomic failure in insulin-dependent diabetes mellitus. J Clin Invest. 1993;91:819–28.

37. Davis SN, Mann S, Briscoe VJ, Ertl AC, Tate DB. Effects of intensive therapy and antecedent hypoglycemia on counterregulatory responses to hypoglycemia in type 2 diabetes. Diabetes. 2009;58:701–9.

38. Fanelli CG, Epifano L, Rambotti AM, Pampanelli S, Di Vincenzo A, Modarelli F, et al. Meticulous prevention of hypoglycemia normalizes the glycemic thresholds of most of neuroendocrine responses to, symptoms of, and cognitive function during hypoglycemia in intensively treated patients with short-term IDDM. Diabetes. 1993;42:1683–9.

39. Cranston I, Lomas J, Maran A, Macdonald IA, Amiel SA. Restoration of hypoglycaemia unawareness in patients with long-duration insulin-dependent diabetes. Lancet. 1994;344:283–7.

40. Dagogo-Jack SE, Rattarasarn C, Cryer PE. Reversal of hypoglycemia unawareness, but not counterregulation, in IDDM. Diabetes. 1994;43:1426–34.

41. The Diabetes Control and Complications Trial Research Group. Epidemiology of severe hypoglycemia in the Diabetes Control and Complications Trial. Am J Med. 1999;90:450–9.

42. Juvenile Diabetes Foundation Continuous Glucose Monitoring Study Group. Prolonged nocturnal hypoglycemia is common during 12 months of continuous glucose monitoring in children and adults with type 1 diabetes. Diabetes Care. 2010;33:1004–8.

43. Jones TW, Porter P, Sherwin RS, Davis EA, O'Leary P, Frazer F, et al. Decreased epinephrine responses to hypoglycemia during sleep. N Engl J Med. 1998;338:1657–62.

44. Matyka KA, Crowne EC, Havel PJ, Macdonald IA, Matthews D, Dunger DB. Counterregulation during spontaneous nocturnal hypoglycemia in prepubertal children with type 1 diabetes. Diabetes Care. 1999;22:1144–50.

45. Hart SP, Frier BM. Causes, management and morbidity of acute hypoglycaemia in adults requiring hospital admission. QJM. 1998;91:505–10.

46. Kerr D, Macdonald IA, Heller SR, Tattersall RB. Alcohol intoxication causes hypoglycaemia unawareness in healthy volunteers and patients with Type 1 (insulin-dependent) diabetes. Diabetologia. 1990;33:216–21.

47. Avogaro A, Beltramello P, Gnudi L, Maran A, Valerio A, Miola M, et al. Alcohol intake impairs glucose counterregulation during acute insulin-induced hypoglycemia in IDDM patients. Evidence for a critical role of free fatty acids. Diabetes. 1993;42:1626–34.

48. Richardson T, Thomas P, Ryder J, Kerr D. Influence of caffeine on frequency of hypoglycemia detected by continuous interstitial glucose monitoring system in patients with long-standing type 1 diabetes. Diabetes Care. 2005;28:1316–20.

49. Frier BM. Living with Hypoglycaemia. In: Frier BM, Fisher BM, editors. Hypoglycaemia in clinical diabetes. Chichester, England: John Wiley & Sons; 2007. p. 309–32.

50. Galassetti P, Tate D, Neill RA, Morrey S, Wasserman DH, Davis SN. Effect of sex on counterregulatory responses to exercise after antecedent hypoglycemia in type 1 diabetes. Am J Physiol Endocrinol Metab. 2004;287:E16–24.

51. Segel SA, Paramore DS, Cryer PE. Hypoglycemia-associated autonomic failure in advanced type 2 diabetes. Diabetes. 2002;51:724–33.

52. Geddes J, Schopman JE, Zammitt NN, Frier BM. Prevalence of impaired awareness of hypoglycaemia in adults with type 1 diabetes. Diabet Med. 2008;25:501–4.

53. Schopman JE, Geddes J, Frier BM. Prevalence of impaired awareness of hypoglycaemia and frequency of hypoglycaemia in insulin-treated type 2 diabetes. Diabetes Res Clin Pract. 2010;87:64–8.

54. Gold AE, MacLeod KM, Frier BM. Frequency of severe hypoglycemia in patients with type I (insulin dependent) diabetes with impaired awareness of hypoglycemia. Diabetes Care. 1994;17:697–703.

55. Clarke WL, Cox DJ, Gonder-Frederick LA, Julian D, Schlundt D, Polonsky W. Reduced awareness of hypoglycemia in adults with IDDM. A prospective study of hypoglycemic frequency and associated symptoms. Diabetes Care. 1995;18:517–22.

56. Davis TM, Brown SG, Jacobs IG, Bulsara M, Bruce DG, Davis WA. Determinants of severe hypoglycemia complicating type 2 diabetes: the Fremantle diabetes study. J Clin Endocrinol Metab. 2010;95:2240–7.

57. Park J, Lertdumrongluk P, Molnar MZ, Kovesdy CP, Kalantar-Zadeh K. Glycemic control in diabetic dialysis patients and the burnt-out diabetes phenomenon. Curr Diab Rep. 2012;12:432–9.

58. Prospective UK. Diabetes Study Group. Effect of intensive blood-glucose control with metformin on complications in overweight patients with type 2 diabetes (UKPDS 34). UK Prospective Diabetes Study (UKPDS) Group. Lancet. 1998;352:854–65.

59. Tschope D, Bramlage P, Binz C, Krekler M, Deeg E, Gitt AK. Incidence and predictors of hypoglycaemia in type 2 diabetes—an analysis of the prospective DiaRegis registry. BMC Endocr Disord. 2012;12:23.

60. Fonseca V, Gill J, Zhou R, Leahy J. An analysis of early insulin glargine added to metformin with or without sulfonylurea: impact on glycaemic control and hypoglycaemia. Diabetes Obes Metab. 2011;13:814–22.

61. Brunelle BL, Llewelyn J, Anderson JHJ, Gale EA, Koivisto VA. Meta-analysis of the effect of insulin lispro on severe hypoglycemia in patients with type 1 diabetes. Diabetes Care. 1998;21:1726–31.

62. Monami M, Marchionni N, Mannucci E. Long-acting insulin analogues vs. NPH human insulin in type 1 diabetes. A meta-analysis. Diabetes Obes Metab. 2009;11:372–8.

63. Lane W, Bailey TS, Gerety G, Gumprecht J, Phillis-Tsimikas A, Hansen CT, et al. Effect of Insulin Degludec versus Insulin glargine U100 on hypoglycemia in patients with type 1 diabetes. The SWITCH 1 Randomized Clinical Trial. JAMA. 2017;318(1):33–4.

64. Wysham C, Bhargava A, Chaykin L, et al. Effect of Insulin Degludec versus Insulin glargine U100 on hypoglycemia in Patients with Type 2 diabetes: The SWITCH 2 Randomized clinical trial. JAMA. 2017;318(1):45–56.

65. Riddle MC, Bolli GB, Zieman M, Muelen-Bartmer I, Bizet F, Home PD, et al. New insulin glargine 300 units/ml versus glargine 100 units/ml in people with type 2 diabetes using basal and mealtime insulin: glucose control and hypoglycemia in a 6-month randomized controlled trial (EDITION 1). Diabetes Care. 2014;37(10):2755–62.

66. Holman RR, Thorne KI, Farmer AJ, Davies MJ, Keenan JF, Paul S, et al. Addition of biphasic, prandial, or basal insulin to oral therapy in type 2 diabetes. N Engl J Med. 2007;357:1716–30.

67. Punthakee Z, Miller ME, Launer LJ, Williamson JD, Lazar RM, Cukierman-Yaffee T, et al. Poor cognitive function and risk of severe hypoglycemia in type 2 diabetes: post hoc epidemiologic analysis of the ACCORD trial. Diabetes Care. 2012;35:787–93.

68. Bruce DG, Davis WA, Casey GP, Clarnette RM, Brown SG, Jacobs IG, et al. Severe hypoglycaemia and cognitive impairment in older patients with diabetes: the Fremantle Diabetes Study. Diabetologia. 2009;52:1808–15.

69. Holstein A, Plaschke A, Egberts EH. Clinical characterisation of severe hypoglycaemia—a prospective population-based study. Exp Clin Endocrinol Diabetes. 2003;111:364–9.

70. Rogers HA, de Zoysa N, Amiel SA. Patient experience of hypoglycaemia unawareness in Type 1 diabetes: are patients appropriately concerned? Diabet Med. 2012;29:321–7.

71. Heller S, Chapman J, McCloud J, Ward J. Unreliability of reports of hypoglycaemia by diabetic patients. BMJ. 1995;310:440.

72. Donnelly LA, Morris AD, Frier BM, Ellis JD, Donnan PT, Durrant R, et al. Frequency and predictors of hypoglycaemia in Type 1 and insulin-treated Type 2 diabetes: a population-based study. Diabet Med. 2005;22:749–55.

73. Samann A, Muhlhauser I, Bender R, Kloos C, Muller UA. Glycaemic control and severe hypoglycaemia following training in flexible, intensive insulin therapy to enable dietary freedom in people with type 1 diabetes: a prospective implementation study. Diabetologia. 2005;48:1965–70.

74. Hopkins D, Lawrence I, Mansell P, Thompson G, Amiel S, Campbell M, et al. Improved biomedical and psychological outcomes 1 year after structured education in flexible insulin therapy for people with type 1 diabetes: the U.K. DAFNE experience. Diabetes Care. 2012;35:1638–42.

75. Schachinger H, Hegar K, Hermanns N, Straumann M, Keller U, Fehm-Wolfsdorf G, et al. Randomized controlled clinical trial of

Blood Glucose Awareness Training (BGAT III) in Switzerland and Germany. J Behav Med. 2005;28:587–94.

76. Hermanns N, Kulzer B, Krichbaum M, Kubiak T, Haak T. Long-term effect of an education program (HyPOS) on the incidence of severe hypoglycemia in patients with type 1 diabetes. Diabetes Care. 2010;33:e36.

77. Turnbull FM, Abraira C, Anderson RJ, Byington RP, Chalmers JP, Duckworth WC, et al. Intensive glucose control and macrovascular outcomes in type 2 diabetes. Diabetologia. 2009;52:2288–98.

78. Inzucchi SE, Bergenstal RM, Buse JB, Diamant M, Ferrannini E, Nauck M, et al. Management of hyperglycaemia in type 2 diabetes: a patient-centered approach. Position statement of the American Diabetes Association (ADA) and the European Association for the Study of Diabetes (EASD). Diabetologia. 2012;55:1577–96.

79. Montori VM, Fernandez-Balsells M. Glycemic control in type 2 diabetes: time for an evidence-based about-face? Ann Intern Med. 2009;150:803–8.

80. Pickup JC, Sutton AJ. Severe hypoglycaemia and glycaemic control in Type 1 diabetes: meta-analysis of multiple daily insulin injections compared with continuous subcutaneous insulin infusion. Diabet Med. 2008;25:765–74.

81. Bolinder J, Antuna R, Geelhoed-Dujivestjin P. Novel glucose-sensing technology and hypoglycaemia in type 1 diabetes: a multicenter, non-masked, randomized controlled trial. Lancet. 2016;388:2254–63.

82. Van Beers CA, DeVries JH, Klejer SJ, et al. Continuous glucose monitoring for patients with type 1 diabetes and impaired awareness of hypoglycaemia (IN CONTROL): a randomized open-label, cross over trial. Lancet Diabetes Endocrinol. 2016;4:893–902.

83. Langendam M, Luijf YM, Hooft L, Devries JH, Mudde AH, Scholten RJ. Continuous glucose monitoring systems for type 1 diabetes mellitus. Cochrane Database Syst Rev. 2012;1:CD008101.

84. Bergenstal RM, Tamborlane WV, Ahmann A, Buse JB, Dailey G, Davis SN, et al. Effectiveness of sensor-augmented insulin-pump therapy in type 1 diabetes. N Engl J Med. 2010;363:311–20.

85. Choudhary P, Shin J, Wang Y, Evans ML, Hammond PJ, Kerr D, et al. Insulin pump therapy with automated insulin suspension in response to hypoglycemia: reduction in nocturnal hypoglycemia in those at greatest risk. Diabetes Care. 2011;34:2023–5.

86. Garg S, Brazg RL, Bailey TS, Buckingham BA, Slover RH, Klonoff DC, et al. Reduction in duration of hypoglycemia by automatic suspension of insulin delivery: the in-clinic ASPIRE study. Diabetes Technol Ther. 2012;14:205–9.

87. Hovorka R, Allen JM, Elleri D, Chassin LJ, Harris J, Xing D, et al. Manual closed-loop insulin delivery in children and adolescents with type 1 diabetes: a phase 2 randomised crossover trial. Lancet. 2010;375:743–51.

88. Garg SJ, Weinzimer SA, Tamborlane WV, Buckingham BA, Bode B, et al. Glucose Outcomes with In-home use of a hybrid closed-loop insulin delivery system in adolescents and adults with Type 1 diabetes. Diabetes Technol Ther. 2017;19:155–63.

89. Russell SJ, El-Khatib FH, Nathan DM, Magyar KL, Jiang J, Damiano ER. Blood glucose control in type 1 diabetes with a bihormonal bionic endocrine pancreas. Diabetes Care. 2012;35:2148–55.

90. El-Khatib FH, Balliro C, Hillard MA, Magyar KL, Ehkaspour, Sinha M et al. Home use of a bihormonal bionic pancreas versus insulin pump therapy in adults with type 1 diabetes: a multicenter randomized crossover trial. Lancet. 2017;89(10067):369–80.

91. Shapiro AM, Ricordi C, Hering BJ, Auchincloss H, Lindblad R, Robertson RP, et al. International trial of the Edmonton protocol for islet transplantation. N Engl J Med. 2006;355:1318–30.

92. Rickels MR. Recovery of endocrine function after islet and pancreas transplantation. Curr Diab Rep. 2012;12:587–96.

93. Choudhary P, Parrot NR, Birtles L, Rutter MK. Islet cell transplantation: current status in the UK. Pract Diabetes. 2012;29:280–5.

94. Cox DJ, Gonder-Frederick LA, Kovatchev BP, Julian DM, Clarke WL. Progressive hypoglycemia's impact on driving simulation performance. Occurrence, awareness and correction. Diabetes Care. 2000;23:163–70.

The Diabetic Neuropathies

36

Ana Carla Montenegro, Luiz Griz, and Francisco Bandeira

Introduction

The diabetic neuropathies are heterogeneous disorders which present with variable clinical manifestations affecting different parts of the nervous system [1] (Table 36.1). Involvement of the peripheral and autonomic nervous systems is probably the most common complication of diabetes. The duration and severity of hyperglycemia are major risk factors for the development of diabetic neuropathy in patients with type 1 or type 2 diabetes [2]. The UK Prospective Diabetes Study showed that other factors, including dyslipidemia and hypertension as part of the metabolic syndrome, are instrumental in the onset and progression of diabetic neuropathy in patients with type 2 diabetes [3].

The pathogenesis of the diabetic neuropathy is complex. The implicated metabolic factors include the following: accumulation of advanced glycosylation end products, accumulation of sorbitol, disruption of the hexosamine pathway, disruption of the protein kinase C pathway, activation of the poly(ADP-ribose) polymerase pathway, and increased oxidative stress. This occurs in a fiber-selective pattern that preferentially affects distal sensory and autonomic fibers, leading to the progressive loss of sensation that underlies the clinical manifestations of diabetic polyneuropathy [4].

Clinical diabetic neuropathy is categorized into distinct syndromes according to the neurologic distribution. There are many forms of diabetic neuropathy including symmetric polyneuropathy, autonomic neuropathy, radiculopathies, and focal and multifocal neuropathies. Clinical and subclini-

Table 36.1 Classification of diabetic neuropathy

Diabetic neuropathies
Diffuse neuropathy
DSPN (distal symmetric polyneuropathy)
Primarily small-fiber neuropathy
Primarily large-fiber neuropathy
Mixed small-and large-fiber neuropathy (most common)
Autonomic
Cardiovascular
Reduced HRV
Resting tachycardia
Orthostatic hypotension
Sudden death (malignant arrhythmia)
Gastrointestinal
Diabetic gastroparesis (gastropathy)
Diabetic enteropathy
Colonic hypomotility (constipation)
Urogenital
Diabetic cystopathy (neurogenic bladder)
Erectile dysfunction
Female sexual dysfunction
Sudomotor dysfunction
Distal hypohidrosis/anhidrosis
Gustatory sweating
Hypoglycemia unawareness
Abnormal pupillary function
Mononeuropathy (mononeuritis multiplex) (atypical forms)
Isolated cranial or peripheral nerve (e.g., CN III, ulnar, femoral, peroneal)
Mononeuritis multiplex (if confluent may resemble polyneuropathy)
Radiculopathy or polyradiculopathy (atypical forms)
Radiculoplexus neuropathy (aka lumbosacral polyradiculopathy, proximal motor amyotrophy)
Thoracic radiculopathy
Nondiabetic neuropathies common in diabetes
Pressure palsies
Chronic inflammatory demyelinating polyneuropathy
Radiculoplexus neuropathy
Acute painful small-fiber neuropathies (treatment-induced)

cal neuropathy has been estimated to occur in 10–100% of diabetic patients, depending upon the diagnostic criteria and patient populations examined. Prevalence is a function of disease duration, about 50% of patients with diabetes will

A. C. Montenegro (✉)
Internal Medicine and Endocrinology, IMIP—Instituto de Medicina Integral de Pernambuco, Recife, Pernambuco, Brazil

L. Griz
School of Medicine, University of Pernambuco, Recife, Pernambuco, Brazil

F. Bandeira
Division of Endocrinology, Agamenon Magalhães Hospital, University of Pernambuco Medical School, Recife, PE, Brazil

© Springer Nature Switzerland AG 2022
F. Bandeira et al. (eds.), *Endocrinology and Diabetes*, https://doi.org/10.1007/978-3-030-90684-9_36

develop neuropathy, and about 25% of those patients will experience no pain at all [5]. Most common among the neuropathies are chronic sensorimotor distal symmetric polyneuropathy [1]. The chronic sensorimotor distal polyneuropathy represents a diffuse symmetric and length-dependent injury to peripheral nerves that has major implications on quality of life, morbidity, and costs from a public health perspective [1, 6]. Diabetic neuropathy can affect any part of the nervous system. Painful diabetic neuropathy (PDN) affects 16% of patients with diabetes, and it is frequently unreported (12.5%) and more frequently untreated (39%) [7].

Diabetic neuropathy should be suspected in all patients with type 2 diabetes and in patients who have had type 1 diabetes for more than 5 years [2]. In some instances, patients with diabetic neuropathy have few complaints, but their physical examination reveals mild to moderately severe sensory loss [1, 2]. Ten to eighteen percent of patients have evidence of nerve damage at the time their diabetes is diagnosed, suggesting that even early impairment of glucose handling, classified as prediabetes, may be associated with neuropathy. Up to 50% of diabetic peripheral neuropathies may be asymptomatic. If not recognized and if preventive foot care is not implemented, patients are at risk for injuries to their insensate feet [8].

The early recognition and appropriate management of neuropathy in the patient with diabetes are important for several reasons, nondiabetic neuropathies may be present in diabetic patients, a number of treatment options exist for symptomatic diabetic neuropathy, autonomic neuropathy may involve every system in the body, and autonomic neuropathy may cause substantial morbidity and increased mortality, particularly if cardiovascular autonomic neuropathy is present. Because >80% of amputations follow a foot ulcer or injury, early recognition of at-risk patients and providing education and appropriate care may reduce ulceration and amputation [1, 8].

Distal Symmetric Polyneuropathy

This is the most common presentation of neuropathy in the diabetic patient, accounting for about 75% of diabetic neuropathies [8]. The DCCT/EDIC suggests that DSPN occurs in at least 20% of people with type 1 diabetes after 20 years of disease duration and 10–15% of newly diagnosed patients with type 2 diabetes, with rates increasing to 50% after 10 years of disease duration [9]. There is emerging evidence that DSPN, especially the painful small-fiber neuropathy subtype, may be present in 10–30% of subjects with impaired glucose tolerance, also known as prediabetes [10] or metabolic syndrome [11]. Up to 50% of patients may experience symptoms. Patients may not volunteer symptoms but on inquiry admit that feet feel numb or dead. Patients with pre-

diabetes may present with intense painful feet. The diabetic polyneuropathy is frequently insidious in onset and can lead to formation of foot ulcers and muscle and joint disease and is the most important cause of Charcot neuropathy (CN).

The more advanced small- and large-fiber dysfunction, with loss of sensory, proprioception, temperature discrimination, and pain, all are also a contributor to fall and fractures [12].

When to Suspect and Main Characteristics of Diabetic Polyneuropathy

Diabetic neuropathy should be suspected in any patient with type 1 diabetes for more than 5 years in duration and in all patients with type 2 diabetes. In patients with prediabetes presenting with "idiopathic" painful neuropathy, diabetic neuropathy should be suspected [1, 2]. Risk factors to DSPN are glycemia, height (perhaps as a proxy for nerve length), smoking, blood pressure, weight, and lipid measures [8].

Symptoms vary according to the class of sensory fibers involved (Table 36.2). The most common early symptoms are induced by the involvement of small fibers and include pain and dysesthesias (unpleasant sensations of burning) [9]. Neuropathic pain may be the first symptom that prompts patients to seek medical care and is present in up to 25% of individuals with DSPN measures [8].

The diabetic polyneuropathy can be defined as the presence of symptoms and/or signs of peripheral nerve dysfunction in people with diabetes after exclusion of other causes [9]. The neuropathy pain is typically worse at night, and symptoms are most commonly experienced in the feet more than calves and lower limbs, although in some cases the hands may be affected. The physical examination may be helpful and usually reveals sensory loss of vibration, pain, temperature perception, and loss of deep tendon reflexes [10].

Table 36.2 Symptoms and signs of DSPN

	Large myelinated nerve fibers	Small myelinated fibers
Function	Pressure, balance	Nociception, protective sensation
Symptom[a]	Numbness, tingling, poor balance	Pain: burning, electric shocks, stabbing
Examination (clinically diagnostic)	Ankle reflexes: reduced/absent Vibration perception: reduced/absent 10-g monofilament: reduced/absent Proprioception: reduced/absent	Thermal (cold/hot) discrimination: reduced/absent[b] Pinprick sensation: reduced/absent[b]

[a]To document the presence of symptoms for diagnosis
[b]Documented in symmetrical, distal to proximal pattern

Table 36.3 Symptoms of diabetic neuropathy

Sensorimotor neuropathy

Muscular symptoms: muscle weakness (not fatigue), atrophy, balance problems, ataxic gait

Sensory symptoms: pain, paresthesia, numbness, paralysis, cramping, nighttime falls, antalgic gait

Autonomic neuropathy

Cardiovascular symptoms: exercise intolerance, fatigue, sustained heart rate, syncope, dizziness, lightheadedness, balance problems

Gastrointestinal symptoms: dysphagia, bloating, nausea and vomiting, diarrhea, constipation, loss of bowel control

Genitourinary symptoms: loss of bladder control, urinary tract infection, urinary frequency or dribbling, erectile dysfunction, loss of libido, dyspareunia, vaginal dryness, anorgasmia

Sudomotor (sweat glands) symptoms: pruritus, dry skin, limb hair loss, calluses, reddened areas

Endocrine symptoms: hypoglycemic unawareness

Other symptoms: difficulty driving at night, depression, anxiety, sleep disorders, cognitive changes

The diabetic patients should be screened annually (Table 36.3) by examining pinprick, temperature (small-fiber function) and vibration perception (using a 128 Hz tuning fork), 10 g monofilament pressure sensation at the distal halluces and ankle reflexes (large-fiber function). Combinations of more than one test have 87% sensitivity in detecting polyneuropathy. Loss of 10 g monofilament perception and reduced vibration perception predict foot ulcers [1, 10]. The feet should be examined for ulcers, calluses, and deformities, and footwear should be inspected.

The diagnosis of diabetic polyneuropathy is based on the interpretation of a constellation of symptoms and signs such as loss of vibratory or light touch sensation and reduced or absent ankle tendon reflexes [1, 11]. The symptoms most frequently found are burning pain, electrical or stabbing sensations, paresthesia, or dysesthesias in the lower extremities. Accurate assessment of symptoms in diabetic neuropathy is known to be difficult. Symptoms do not always indicate underlying neuropathy, as absence of symptoms should never be assumed to indicate an absence of signs. Therefore, we should rely on clinical signs to diagnose diabetic neuropathy. Confirmation can be made with and quantitative electrophysiology [11] (Table 36.4).

Screening Tests

The need to identify simplified criteria has resulted in the development of at least two simple screening test scores: one is the UK screening score (Table 36.5) [12] and the other is the Michigan screening score (Table 36.6) [13].

In the UK score, the peripheral neuropathy is considered to be present if there are moderate or severe signs (≥6 points),

Table 36.4 Evaluation for diabetic neuropathy

History

Screen for symptoms of diabetic neuropathy (see also Table 36.3)

Review diabetes history, disease management, daily glycemic records, and previous hemoglobin A1C levels

Identify any family history of diabetes or neuropathy

Review medication history (including use of over-the-counter products and herbal or homeopathic products) and environmental exposures

Review for other causes of neuropathy, including vitamin B12 deficiency, alcoholism, toxic exposures, medications, cancers, and autoimmune disease

Physical examination

Vital signs and pain index

Supine and standing blood pressure for postural hypotension

Cardiovascular examination to look for arrhythmias, absent or diminished pulses, edema, or delayed capillary refilling

Cutaneous examination to look for extremity hair loss, skin or nail changes (including callus), and pretrophic (red) areas, especially between toes

Neurologic examination using the 5.07 Semmes-Weinstein (10-g) nylon filament test (10-g monofilament test)

Inspection of feet for asymmetry, loss of arch height, or hammer toes

Evaluation of all positive screening findings

Table 36.5 UK screening score [12]

Symptoms

What is the sensation felt? Maximum is 2 points

　Burning, numbness, or tingling in the feet (2 points);

　Fatigue, cramping, or aching (1 point)

What is the location of symptoms? Maximum is 2 points

　Feet (2 points)

　Calves (1 points)

　Elsewhere (0 points)

Have the symptoms ever awakened you at night?

　Yes (1 point)

What is the timing of symptoms? Maximum is 2 points

　Worse at night (2 points)

　Present day and night (1 point)

　Present only during the day (0 points)

How are symptoms relieved? Maximum is 2 points

　Walking around (2 points)

　Standing (1 point)

　Sitting or lying or no relief (0 points)

0–2 points, normal; 3–4 points, mild neuropathy; 5–6 points, moderate neuropathy; 7–9 points, severe neuropathy

Table 36.6 Michigan neuropathy screening score [13]

Do the feet show dry skin, callus, fissure, infection, or deformities? The presence of any of these indicators of neuropathy is scored as 1 point, and an additional point is added if an ulcer is present

What is the vibration sense on the dorsum of the great toes?

Reduced (0, 5 points); absent (1 point)

What is the Achilles tendon reflex?

Absent (1 point); present with reinforcement (0, 5 points)

>2 points—neuropathy

even in the absence of symptoms, or if there are at least mild signs (≥3 points) in the presence of moderate symptoms (≥5 points). A neurologic sign score of 8 or more indicates that the patent's feet are at high risk for ulceration.

Differential Diagnosis

Other causes of neuropathy in a diabetic patient should be considered if there is any aspect of history or clinical presentation suggesting features atypical of diabetic neuropathy.

The chronic inflammatory demyelinating polyneuropathy and neuropathy due to vitamin B12 deficiency, hypothyroidism, and uremia occur more frequently in patients with diabetes than in the general population [1, 14].

Acute Sensory Neuropathy and How to Distinguish from Chronic Sensorimotor Diabetic Polyneuropathy

Acute sensory neuropathy may occur after periods of poor metabolic control (e.g., ketoacidosis) or sudden change in glycemic control, also called insulin neuritis [15]. It presents few signs on physical examination. It is a rare condition and is characterized by the acute onset of severe sensory symptoms with marked nocturnal exacerbation [15]. There are other types of acute diabetic neuropathy, diabetic neuropathic cachexia and diabetic anorexia, when severe weight loss unintended and intentional, respectively, occurs [1].

Treatment

There are three main elements in the treatment of diabetic polyneuropathy: glycemic control, foot care, and treatment of pain.

The Role of Glycemic Control

The Diabetes Control and Complications Trial (DCCT) has shown that in type 1 diabetic patients, the risk of diabetic polyneuropathy and autonomic neuropathy can be reduced with improved blood glucose control [1, 2]. The occurrence of diabetic neuropathy was reduced by 60% over a 10-year period with rigorous blood glucose control. Similar findings were noted in the Stockholm Diabetes Intervention Study [16, 17]. The importance of glycemic control in type 2 diabetic patients is less strong.

The importance of intensive control glycemic in established neuropathy is unclear. Uncontrolled studies suggest that neuropathy symptoms may improve with intensive antidiabetic therapy [15–18]. Although controlled trial evidence is lacking, several observational studies suggest that neuropathic symptoms improve not only with optimization of control but also with the avoidance of extreme blood glucose fluctuations [1, 16].

Lifestyle Modifications

The Italian supervised treadmill study and the University of Utah type 2 diabetes study, recently reports nerve fiber regeneration in patients with type 2 diabetes engaged an exercise program compared with loss of nerve fibers in those who only followed standard of care [19]. The Diabetes Prevention Program (DPP) reported benefits of lifestyle intervention on measures of autonomic cardiovascular and DSNP; this trial did not include subjects with established diabetes [8].

Foot Care

Once a patient has diabetic neuropathy, foot care is even more important to prevent ulceration, infection, and amputation. The lifetime risk of a foot ulcer for diabetic patients may be as high as 25% [20]. The diabetic patients need to inspect their feet for the presence of dry or cracking skin, fissures, plantar callus formation, and signs of early infection between the toes and around the toe nails. Foot amputations are an important cause of morbidity in patients with diabetes mellitus [19, 20]. Several risk factors are predictive of ulcers and amputation. Foot amputations are preventable with early recognition and therapy of risk factors. The most important are previous foot ulceration, sensitive neuropathy (it promotes ulcer formation by decreasing pain sensation and perception of pressure), foot deformity, and vascular disease [16, 20]. Other factors have to be considered such as duration of diabetes, glycemic control, presence of claudication, and history of cigarette smoking. Systematic screening examinations for neuropathic and vascular involvement of the lower extremities and careful inspection of feet may substantially reduce morbidity from foot problems [1, 16].

Pathogenetic Therapies

There remains a lack of treatment options that effectively target the natural history of DSNP once established. The evidence from randomized clinical trials is very limited [1, 21].

Painful Diabetic Neuropathy

Only a small fraction of patients with diabetic polyneuropathy have painful symptoms. There are many treatment options available; however, before initiating therapy, it is important to confirm that the pain is due to diabetic polyneuropathy. A disc lesion should be considered if the pain has development in relation to recent trauma or its onset is abrupt. Peripheral vascular disease should be considered [1, 21, 22].

A rational approach to treating the patient with painful diabetic neuropathy requires a systematic, stepwise approach. There are pharmacological and nonpharmacological therapies to reduce pain and improve physical function [23].

The pharmacological agents include anticonvulsants, antidepressants, opioids, anti-arrhythmics, cannabinoids, cannabinoids, aldose reductase inhibitors, protein kinase C beta inhibitors, antioxidants (alpha-lipoic acid), transketolase activators (thiamines and allithiamines), and topical medications (analgesic patches, anesthetic patches, capsaicin cream, clonidine) [1, 22–25] (Table 36.7).

Pregabalin and duloxetine have received regulatory approval for the treatment of neuropathic pain in diabetes by the US Food and Drug Administration (FDA), Health Canada, and the European Medicines Agency. The opioid, tapentadol, has regulatory approval in the USA and Canada, but the evidence of its use is weaker [26].

The nonpharmacologic modalities are infrared therapy, shoe magnets, exercise, acupuncture, external stimulation (transcutaneous electrical nerve stimulation), spinal cord stimulation, biofeedback and behavioral therapy, surgical decompression, and intrathecal baclofen [27, 28].

Table 36.7 Drug therapy for painful diabetic neuropathy

Anticonvulsants
Pregabalin—300–600 mg/day
Gabapentin—900–3600 mg/day
Valproate—500–1200 mg/day
Antidepressants
Duloxetine—60–120 mg/day
Venlafaxine—75–225 mg/day
Amitriptyline—25–100 mg/day
Opioids
Tramadol—210 mg/day
Oxycodone—37–120 mg/day
Morphine sulfate–titrated to 120 mg/day
Dextromethorphan—400 mg/day
Others
Capsaicin—0.075% QID
Isosorbide dinitrate spray
Electrical stimulation percutaneous nerve stimulation × 3–4 weeks

Antidepressants

Based on randomized controlled trials, the antidepressants amitriptyline, venlafaxine, and duloxetine are beneficial for reducing pain associated with diabetic neuropathy [16, 29]. Dates are insufficient to recommend one of these agents over the others. A systematic review found that tricyclic antidepressants were more effective for short-term pain relief than traditional or newer-generation anticonvulsants [30, 31]. The therapeutic effect usually occurs sooner (within 6 weeks) and at lower doses than is typical when these drugs are given for the treatment of depression.

Duloxetine is probably effective in lessening the pain of diabetic neuropathy [16, 30]. Duloxetine showed rapid onset of action and sustained benefit, and it was also effective in relieving pain at night. Amitriptyline appears to be effective as duloxetine for the treatment of painful diabetic neuropathy and is less expensive [16].

The efficacy of venlafaxine was evaluated for two studies. In a randomized controlled trial, venlafaxine at higher doses was associated with significant benefit in pain relief compared with placebo [28]. In a study, venlafaxine plus gabapentin showed 18% more relief than with placebo plus gabapentin [30, 31].

There is insufficient evidence to support or refute the use of imipramine, nortriptyline, or fluoxetine.

Tricyclic agents such as amitriptyline and desipramine (mainly amitriptyline) are recommended in patients with severe pain. Side effects of tricyclic antidepressants include dry mouth, somnolence, and urinary retention. This class of drugs can be added to anticonvulsants, but not duloxetine. Amitriptyline is contraindicated in patients with cardiac disease; they should be given duloxetine or venlafaxine.

Anticonvulsants

Pregabalin and valproate may be useful for treating painful diabetic neuropathy. The effectiveness of pregabalin for the treatment of painful diabetic neuropathy was evaluated in seven randomized clinical trials. All studies found that pregabalin relieved pain, but the effect size was small relative to placebo. There were a clear dose-related increase in effectiveness and an increase in the incidence of most adverse events. The most common adverse events were dizziness, somnolence, and peripheral edema. It can cause sedation and confusion. Two small studies evaluated the efficacy of valproate. Both studies were conducted at the same center, [30].

The role of gabapentin for the treatment of painful diabetic neuropathy is controversial [6, 31]. A small randomized trial found that gabapentin was not superior to placebo. The major side effects of gabapentin are somnolence, dizziness, and ataxia [30].

There is insufficient evidence to support or refute the use of topiramate and carbamazepine for the treatment of painful diabetic neuropathy [16].

Other Agents

Alpha-lipoic acid, a potent antioxidant, has been associated with some benefit for symptomatic diabetic neuropathy. Its use may be recommended in patients with who are refractory to or intolerant of antidepressants or anticonvulsants [16, 32]. However, there remains a lack of treatment options that effectively target the natural history of DSNP once established. The evidence from randomized clinical trials is very limited [16, 32].

Capsaicin cream causes analgesia through the local depletion of substance P; it is a component of hot peppers. Studies of capsaicin showed modest but statistically significant improvement in pain compared with placebo [6, 33]. Capsaicin can be added for patients with pain who are refractory to or intolerant of antidepressant or anticonvulsants. A side effect is burning pain, which is exacerbated by contact with warm water and hot weather.

One trial showed that lidocaine patches significantly improved pain and quality of life in 56 patients with painful diabetic neuropathy [33, 34].

Opioids have been studied for the treatment of painful diabetic neuropathy. Tramadol and oxycodone were more effective than placebo for relieving pain. However, the trials supporting the efficacy of opioids such as tramadol and oxycodone are all limited by short-term follow-up [16, 23, 26].

Several other agents have been tested in patients with painful diabetic neuropathy. Acetyl-L-carnitine, the acetylated ester of the amino acid L-carnitine, was associated with significant improvement in pain scores [1, 16, 34, 35]. Isosorbide dinitrate topical spray showed a moderate effect in lessening the pain relative to placebo [6]. Nonsteroidal anti-inflammatory drugs (NSAIDs) ibuprofen and sulindac can lead to substantial pain relief in patients with diabetic neuropathy; however, they should be used with caution because of concerns that they may impair nerve circulation and worsen nerve injury due to the inhibition of prostacyclin synthesis [16] and also because of the risk of renal damage.

Nonpharmacological Therapy

Percutaneous electrical nerve stimulation may be effective for pain relief in diabetic neuropathy [6, 16]. However, the percutaneous techniques evaluated in trials are not widely available in clinical practice.

One study using pulsed electromagnetic fields compared with a sham device failed to demonstrate an effect in patients with painful diabetic neuropathy. Likewise, Reiki therapy and laser treatment did not show any effect as well [6].

Finally, sorbitol accumulation may play a role in diabetic neuropathy, but the use of aldose reductase inhibitors to prevent sorbitol formation has so far failed to show clinical benefits.

Autonomic Neuropathy

Autonomic neuropathies affect the autonomic neurons (parasympathetic, sympathetic, or both) and are associated with a variety of site-specific symptoms [8, 16, 36].

The symptoms of autonomic dysfunction should be elicited accurately during consultation of a diabetic patient. There are a large number of symptoms affecting many different organ systems, including cardiovascular, gastrointestinal, genitourinary, pupillary, sudomotor, and neuroendocrine systems. Major clinical manifestations of diabetic autonomic neuropathy include resting tachycardia, exercise intolerance, orthostatic hypotension, constipation, gastroparesis, erectile dysfunction, and hypoglycemic autonomic failure [1, 16, 36, 37].

Cardiovascular Autonomic Neuropathy

Diabetic autonomic neuropathy is associated with significant morbidity and mortality in some patients with diabetes. It is classified as subclinical or clinical depending upon the presence or absence of symptoms [1, 38–40].

Cardiovascular autonomic neuropathy is defined as the impairment of autonomic control of the cardiovascular system. It is the most studied and clinically important form of diabetic autonomic neuropathy. The prevalence of cardiovascular autonomic neuropathy varies widely depending on the cohort studied and the tests used, diagnostic criteria, and the population studied [39–41].

The cardiovascular autonomic neuropathy may be subclinical; in this case, the disease is defined by cardiovascular reflex testing, which may have prognostic implications. Clinically, it is associated with resting tachycardia (>100 bpm). Persistent sinus tachycardia can occur, and there may be no variation in heart rate during activities that normally increase parasympathetic vagal tone, such as deep breathing and Valsalva maneuver. Other manifestations are exercise intolerance, orthostatic hypotension, and intraoperative cardiovascular instability [1, 41].

Cardiac denervation can occur in diabetic patients with autonomic neuropathy. It is associated with silent myocardial infarction and ischemia and increased mortality [40]. Hypotension and hypertension after vigorous exercise are more likely to develop in patients with autonomic neuropathy, particularly when starting an exercise program. Cardiac autonomic function testing should be performed when planning an exercise program for individuals with diabetes about to embark on a moderate- to high-intensity exercise program [1, 41].

The presence of cardiovascular autonomic neuropathy may be associated with adverse renal and cerebrovascular outcomes [41].

A patient's history and physical examination are ineffective for the early detection of subclinical autonomic neuropathy. It may only be detected by using cardiovascular reflex tests or tests of peripheral sympathetic function [30, 42]. There are many tests that assess parasympathetic integrity, including cardiovascular tests of heart rate response, orthostatic hypotension test, QT interval, ambulatory blood pressure monitoring for dipping status, heart rate variability, and time and frequency domain indices. These tests are relatively insensitive to sympathetic deficits. The choice of tests remains debatable and dependent upon the indication. Of these tests, heart rate variability in response to deep breathing has the greatest specificity (approximately 80%). Regular tests for heart rate variability provide early detection and thereby promote timely diagnostic and therapeutic interventions. These tests may also facilitate differential diagnosis and attribution of symptoms (e.g., erectile dysfunction, dyspepsia, and dizziness) to autonomic dysfunction [42].

Direct assessment of cardiac sympathetic integrity has become possible with the introduction of radiolabeled analogues of norepinephrine, which are actively taken up by the sympathetic nerve terminals of the heart. These tests have limited clinical utility because they are expensive and not widely available [1, 41].

At the time of diagnosis of type 2 diabetes and although CAN prevalence is very low in newly diagnosed patients with type 1 diabetes, within 5 years after diagnosis of type 1 diabetes, patients should be screened for cardiovascular autonomic neuropathy [1].

Exercise program can improve both early and more advanced cardiovascular autonomic neuropathy. There are general recommendations: making changes in posture slowly and tensing the legs by crossing them while actively standing on both legs. It can minimize postural symptoms. It is important the discontinuation of aggravating drugs (e.g., tranquilizers, antidepressants, and diuretics) [42].

Fludrocortisone (0.1–0.4 mg/day) and salt diet may be helpful in severe cases but can cause hypertension or peripheral edema. The somatostatin analogue, octreotide (50 mcg three times daily), may be helpful in diabetic patients with refractory and symptomatic postural. It may exacerbate bowel dysfunction and cause fluctuations in glycemic control [1, 16, 41].

Gastrointestinal Autonomic Neuropathy

Any section of the gastrointestinal tract may be affected. The symptoms of gastrointestinal autonomic neuropathy vary with the site of involvement. Gastroparesis should be suspected in patients with erratic glucose control. Evaluation of gastric emptying should be done if the patients have anorexia, nausea, vomiting, early satiety, and postprandial fullness. Barium studies or referral for endoscopy may be required [1, 16]. The patients with esophageal motility disorders have dysphagia and retrosternal pain. Other symptoms are constipation, diarrhea, or even incontinence.

The treatment of gastroparesis varies with the type of symptoms. Must be guided frequent small meals, prokinetic agents (metoclopramide, domperidone, erythromycin) [1].

Autonomic diarrhea is often nocturnal and alternating with constipation and incontinence. The treatment varies with the causative factors responsible for the diarrhea: antibiotics for bacterial overgrowth, loperamide for aberrant motility, and biofeedback for anorectal dysfunction. When the diarrhea is intractable, octreotide is an alternative [16].

Genitourinary Autonomic Neuropathy

The genitourinary tract disturbances are associated with bladder and/or sexual dysfunction. Diabetic bladder dysfunction initially presents as a decrease in the ability to sense a full bladder, and it results in incomplete emptying. These abnormalities can result in recurrent urinary tract infections and overflow incontinence. In men, the genitourinary autonomic neuropathy may cause loss of penile erection and/or retrograde ejaculation. Women can have decreased libido and reduced vaginal lubrication [43].

Treatment consists of a strict voluntary urination schedule coupled with bethanechol (10–30 mg three times daily). More advanced cases require intermittent catheterization or resection of internal sphincter at the bladder neck. Sexual dysfunction must be treated with sex therapy, psychological counseling, and treatment with type 5 phosphodiesterase inhibition [1, 16, 43, 44].

The Effect on Diabetes Control

Episodes of hypoglycemia may be more common in patients with autonomic neuropathy. Several factors may account for this, such as diabetic gastroparesis and alterations in neuroendocrine responses, including a reduction in glucagon and epinephrine secretion in response to hypoglycemia [1, 44].

Focal and Multifocal Neuropathies

- The most common peripheral mononeuropathy in diabetic patients is median mononeuropathy.
- Cranial neuropathies are extremely rare.
- Electrophysiological is suggestive of demyelination and axonal degeneration.

The diabetic mononeuropathy affects the median nerve (the most common), ulnar, radial, and peroneal. The cranial mononeuropathies are rare and occur in those nerves which supply the extraocular muscle (cranial nerves III, VI, and IV) [1]. Others are diabetic amyotrophy and thoracic polyradiculopathy [5, 45].

The diagnosis of diabetic mononeuropathy can be done through clinical careful evaluation and electrophysiological studies. The electrophysiological studies show a reduction in nerve conduction and amplitude suggestive of underlying demyelination and axonal degeneration. Many of these patients complain acute, asymmetric, focal pain followed by weakness involving the proximal leg and, after careful clinical and electrodiagnostic examinations, are found to have a high lumbar radiculopathy (diabetic amyotrophy) [1, 46]. Another cause of pain in diabetics is thoracic polyradiculopathy; the patients present with severe abdominal pain, and the differential diagnostic is done with gastrointestinal causes.

General Recommendations

- Tight glycemic control can prevent, delay, or slow the progression of diabetic neuropathy in patients with type 1 diabetes.
- Patients with diabetes should be educated about proper foot care and should check their feet daily.
- All patients with diabetes should have an annual foot examination by a healthcare professional.

References

1. Boulton AJ, Vinik AL, Arezzo JC, Bril V, Feldman EL, Freeman R, et al. Diabetic neuropathies: a statement by the American Diabetes Association. Diabetes Care. 2005;28:956–62.
2. The Diabetes Control and Complications Trial Research Group. The effect of intensive treatment of diabetes on the development and progression of long-term complications in insulin-dependent diabetes mellitus. N Engl J Med. 1993;329:977–86.
3. UK Prospective Diabetes Study (UKPDS) Group. Intensive blood blood-glucose control with sulphonylureas or insulin compared with conventional treatment and risk of complications in patients with type 2 diabetes (UKPDS 33). Lancet. 1998;352:837–53.
4. Edwards JL, Vincent AM, Cheng HT, Feldman EL. Diabetic neuropathy: mechanisms to management. Pharmacol Ther. 2008;120:1–34.
5. Dyck PJ, Kratz KM, Karnes JL, Litchy WJ, Klein R, Pach JM, et al. The prevalence by staged severity of various types of diabetic neuropathy, retinopathy, and nephropathy in a population-based cohort: The Rochester Diabetic Neuropathy Study. Neurology. 1993;43:817–24.
6. Bril V, England J, Franklin GM, Backonja M, Cohen J, Del Toro D, et al. Evidence-based guideline: treatment of painful diabetic neuropathy: report of the American Academy of Neurology, the American Association of Neuromuscular and Electrodiagnostic Medicine, and the American Academy of Physical Medicine and Rehabilitation. Neurology. 2011;76:1758–65.
7. Dousi C, MacFarlane IA, Woodward A, Nurmikko TJ, Bundred PE, Benbow SJ. Chronic painful peripheral neuropathy in an urban community: a controlled comparison of people with and without diabetes. Diabet Med. 2004;21:976–82.
8. Pop-Busui R, Boulton AJM, Feldman EL, Bril V, Freeman R, Malik RA, et al. Diabetic neuropathy: a position statement by the American Diabetes Association. Diabetes Care. 2017;40:136–54.
9. Freeman R, Baron R, Bouhassira D, Cabrera J, Emir B. Sensory profiles of patients with neuropathic pain based on the neuropathic pain symptoms and signs. Pain. 2014;155:367–76.
10. Ziegler D, Keller J, Maier C, Pannek J. German diabetes association diabetic neuropathy. Exp Clin Endocrinol Diabetes. 2014;122:406–15.
11. Callaghan BC, Xia R, Banerjee M, et al. Health ABC Study. Metabolic syndrome components are associated with symptomatic polyneuropathy independent of glycemic status Diabetes Care 2016;39:801–7.
12. Boulon AJM, Cries FA, Jervell JA. Guidelines for diagnosis and outpatients management diabetic peripheral neuropathy. Diabet Med. 1998;15:508–14.
13. Young MJ, Boulton AJ, MacLeod AF, Wiliiams DR, Sonksen PH. A multicentre study of the prevalence of diabetic peripheral neuropathy in the United Kingdom hospital clinic population. Diabetologia. 1993;36:150–4.
14. Ang L, Jaiswal M, Martin C, Po-Busui R. Glucose control and diabetic neuropathy: lessons from recent large clinical trials. Curr Diab Rep. 2014;14:528.
15. Dabby R, Sadeh M, Lampl Y, Gilad R, Watemberg N. Acute painful neuropathy induced by rapid correction of glucose levels in diabetic patients. Biomed Pharmacother. 2009;63:707–9.
16. Pop-Busui R, Boulton AJM, Felman EL, Brill V, Freeman R, Malik RA, Sosenko JM, Ziegler D. Diabetic neuropathy: a position statement by the American Diabetes Association. Diabetes Care. 2017;40:136–54.
17. Reichard P, Berglund B, Britz A, Nilsson BY, Rosenqvist U. Intensified conventional insulin treatment retards the microvascular complications of insulin-dependent diabetes mellitus (IDDM): the Stockholm Diabetes Intervention Study (SDIS) after 5 years. J Intern Med. 1991;230:101–8.
18. Boulton AJ, Drury J, Clarke B, Ward JD. Continuous subcutaneous insulin infusion in the management of painful diabetic neuropathy. Diabetes Care. 1982;5:386–90.
19. Singleton JR, Marcus RL, Jackson JE, Lessard MK, Graham TE, Smith AG. Exercise increase cutaneous nerve density in diabetic patients without neuropathy. Ann Clin Transl Neurol. 2014;1:844–9.
20. Abbou CA, Carrington AL, Ashe H, Sath S, Every LC, Griffiths J, et al. The North-West Diabetes Foot Care Study: incidence of, and risk factors for, new diabetes foot ulceration in a community-based patient cohort. Diabet Med. 2002;19:377–84.

21. Feldman EL, Stevens MJ, Thomas PK, Brown MB, Canal N, Greene DA. A practical two-step quantitative clinical and electrophysiological assessment for the diagnosis and stating of diabetic neuropathy. Diabetes Care. 1994;17:1281–9.

22. Brown SJ, Handsaker JC, Bowling FL, Boulton AJ, Reeves ND. Diabetic peripheral neuropathy compromises balance during daily activities. Diabetes Care. 2015;38:1116–22.

23. Wong MC, Chung JW, Wong TK. Effects of treatments for symptoms of painful diabetic neuropathy: systematic review. BMJ. 2007;335:87.

24. Ziegler D, Low PA, Litchy WJ, et al. Efficacy and safety of antioxidant treatment with a-lipoic acid over 4 years in diabetic polyneuropathy: the NATHAN 1 trial. Diabetes Care. 2011;34:2054–60.

25. Rowbotham MC, Goli V, Kunz NR, Lei D. Venlafaxine extended release in the treatment of painful diabetic neuropathy: a double-blind, placebo-controlled study. Pain. 2004;110:697–706.

26. Chou R, Ballantyne JC, Fanciullo GJ, Fine PG, Miaskowsk C. Research gaps on use of opioids for chronic noncancer pain: findings from a review of the evidence for an American Pain Society and American Academy of Pain Medicine clinical practice guideline. J Pain. 2009;10:147–59.

27. Greene DA, Borwn MJ, Braunstein SN, Shwartz SS, Asbury AK, Winwgrad AI. Comparison of clinical cause and sequential electrophysiological tests in diabetics with symptomatic polyneuropathy and its implications for clinical trials. Diabetes. 1981;30:139–47.

28. Bosi E, Conti M, Vermigli C, Cazzetta E, Peretti MC, Cordoni G, et al. Effectiveness of frequency-modulated electromagnetic neural stimulation in the treatment of painful diabetic neuropathy. Diabetologia. 2005;48:817–23.

29. Simpson DA. Gabapentin and venlafaxine for the treatment of painful diabetic neuropathy. J Clin Neuromuscul Dis. 2001;3:53–62.

30. Backonja M, Beydoun A, Edwards KR, Schwartz SL, Fonseca V, Hes M, et al. Gabapentin for the symptomatic treatment of painful neuropathy in patients with diabetes mellitus: a randomized controlled trial. JAMA. 1998;280:1831–6.

31. Kochar DK, Jain N, Agarwal RP, Srivastava T, Agarwal P, Gupta S. Sodium valproate in the management of painful neuropathy in type 2-a randomized placebo controlled study. Acta Neurol Scand. 2002;106:248–52.

32. Ziegler D, Nowak H, Kempler P, Vargha P, Low PA. Treatment of symptomatic diabetic polyneuropathy with the antioxidant alpha-lipoic acid: a meta analysis. Diabet Med. 2004;21:114–21.

33. Tandan R, Lewis GA, Krusinski PB, Badger GB, Fries TJ. Topical capsaicin in painful diabetic neuropathy. Controlled study with long-term follow-up. Diabetes Care. 1992;15:8–14.

34. Barbano RL, Herrmann DN, Hart-Gouleau S, Penella-Vaughan J, Lodewick PA, Dworkin RH. Effectiveness, tolerability, and impact on quality of life of the 5% lidocaine patch in diabetic polyneuropathy. Arch Neurol. 2004;61:914–8.

35. Sima AA, Calvani M, Mehra M, Amato A. Acetyl-l-carnitine improves pain, nerve regeneration, and vibratory perception in patients with chronic diabetic neuropathy: an analysis of two randomized placebo-controlled trials. Diabetes Care. 2005;28:89–94.

36. Vinik AI, Ziegler D. Diabetic cardiovascular autonomic neuropathy. Circulation. 2007;115(3):387–97.

37. Ziegle D. Cardiovascular autonomic neuropathy: clinical manifestations and measurement. Diabetes Rev. 1999;7:342–57.

38. Cohen JA, Estacio RO, Lundgren RA, Esler AL, Schrier RW. Diabetic autonomic neuropathy is associated with an increased incidence of strokes. Auton Neurosci. 2003;108:73–8.

39. Spallone V, Ziegler D, Freeman R, Bernardi L, Frontoni S, Pop-Busui R, et al. Cardiovascular autonomic neuropathy in diabetes: clinical impact, assessment, diagnosis, and management. Diabetes Metab Res Rev. 2011;27(7):639–53; (Epub ahead of print)

40. Howorka K, Pumpria J, Haber P, Koller-Strametz J, Mondrzyk J, Shabmann A. Effects of physical training on heart rate variability in diabetic patients with various degrees of cardiovascular autonomic neuropathy. Cardiovasc Res. 1997;34:206–14.

41. Pagkalos M, Koutlianos N, Kouidi E, Pagkalos E, Mandroukas K, Deliagiannis A. Heart rate variability modifications following exercise training in type 2 diabetic patients with definite cardiac autonomic neuropathy. Br J Sports Med. 2008;42:47–54.

42. Stevens MJ, Edmonds ME, Mathias CJ, Watkins PJ. Disabling postural hypotension complicating diabetic autonomic neuropathy. Diabet Med. 1989;8:870–4.

43. Brown JS, Wessells H, Chancellor MB, Howards SS, Stamm WE, Steers WD. Urologic complications of diabetes. Diabetes Care. 2005;28:177–85.

44. Asghar O, Petropoulos IN, Alam U, et al. Cornel confocal microscopy defects neuropathy in subjects with impaired glucose tolerance. Diabetes Care. 2014;37:2643–6.

45. Kikta DG, Breuer AC, Wibourn AJ. Thoracic root pain in diabetes: the spectrum of clinical and electromyographic findings. Ann Neurol. 1982;11:80–5.

46. Franse LV, Valk GD, Dekker JH, Heine RJ, van Eijk JT. "Numbness of feet" is a poor indicator for polyneuropathy in type 2 diabetic patients. Diabet Med. 2000;17:105–10.

Diabetic Nephropathy

Maria Elba Bandeira de Farias, Deborah Cristina de Lemos Araújo Queiroz, and Fernanda Moura Victor

Introduction

Diabetic nephropathy (DN) occurs in 20–40% of patients with diabetes and is a major cause of morbidity and mortality. It occurs not only in persons with type 1 (T1) and type 2 (T2) diabetes mellitus (DM) but also in diabetes of exocrine pancreas, previously called secondary pancreatic DM or type 3c diabetes forms of DM, which results from a disruption of the global architecture or physiology of the pancreas caused by a process such as inflammation, neoplasia, or surgical resection [1, 2].

The number of individuals known to have end-stage renal disease (ESRD) worldwide is growing rapidly, as a result of improved diagnostic capabilities, the global epidemic of type 2 diabetes (T2DM), and other causes of chronic kidney disease (CKD) [3]. CKD is mainly related to diabetes and/or hypertension. About one out of three adults with diabetes and one out of five adults with hypertension have CKD [4]. Diabetes is the most frequent cause of severe CKD [1] and in Western countries is the leading cause of ESRD [5]. Nowadays, it's estimated that 40–50% of patients with T2DM and 30–33% with T1DM will develop kidney disease. The amount of people with CKD and ESRD is increasing in consonance with the rising incidence of diabetes [6, 7].

In the United States, 2011–2012, the estimated prevalence of CKD (stages 1–4) in adults with 20 years of age or more and diagnosis of diabetes was 36.5% (CI 95%, 32.2–40.8%). In 2014, a total of 52,159 people developed ESRD with diabetes as the main cause of renal disease, and the prevalence ratio adjusted for age, sex, and ethnicity was 154.4 per million inhabitants [7, 8].

The progression to ESRD is similar in type 1 and type 2 diabetes. However, as T2DM is more prevalent, the majority of patients with ESRD are type 2 diabetics. The tenth edition of the International Diabetes Federation (IDF) Diabetes Atlas reported an estimated increase of 46% on world prevalence of diabetes. This means an estimated raise from 537 million in 2021 to 783 million in 2045, on the number of diabetic patients [9, 10]. The prevalence of diabetic nephropathy has increased [3] because of the epidemic of diabetes, longer periods of disease without a good glycemic control, and improvements in the treatment of hypertension and coronary heart disease, which have prolonged the lifespan of patients with T2DM and increased the risk of developing complications such as nephropathy and ESRD. The end-stage renal disease (ESRD) is up to ten times more prevalent in people with diabetes [9–11].

However, a greater number of patients with diabetes are in developing countries [9], which do not have sufficient resources or a health infrastructure that would enable them to provide universal renal replacement therapy. Furthermore, even in developed countries, fewer than 1 in 20 patients with DM and CKD survives to ESRD, succumbing to cardiovascular disease (CVD), heart failure, or infection, and the severity of diabetic renal disease significantly contributes to this outcome [3]. The number of deaths related to CKD associated with diabetes increased 94% between 1990 and 2012, and the great majority was mainly related to cardiovascular disease [7]. Hence, it is of great importance to obtain an early diagnosis, appropriate management, and the development of new strategies of treatment, particularly those related to the control of glycemia, blood pressure, and other comorbidities associated with diabetes, that may lead to better outcomes.

Diagnosis

The term diabetic nephropathy is used to describe a specific renal condition caused by diabetes, characterized by hyperfiltration; persistent albuminuria, with a continuous decline in the glomerular filtration rate (GFR); raised arterial blood

M. E. B. de Farias (✉)
Division of Endocrinology and Diabetes, University of Pernambuco Medical School, Agamenon Magalhães Hospital, State Department of Health/SUS/UPE, Recife, Pernambuco, Brazil

D. C. de Lemos Araújo Queiroz · F. M. Victor
Endocrinology, Agamenon Magalhães, Recife, Pernambuco, Brazil

© Springer Nature Switzerland AG 2022
F. Bandeira et al. (eds.), *Endocrinology and Diabetes*, https://doi.org/10.1007/978-3-030-90684-9_37

pressure (BP); and enhanced cardiovascular morbidity and mortality [11] (Table 37.1). Diabetic kidney disease (DKD), diabetic nephropathy, is clinically diagnosed based on the presence of persistent albuminuria (>30 mg/g creatinine) and/or reduced eGFR in the absence of signs or symptoms of other primary causes of kidney damage [12].

Albuminuria, urinary albumin excretion rates (UAE), can be measured easily by albumin-to-creatinine ratio (ACR) in a random spot collection, but also in 24-h or timed collections, which are less predictive and accurate [13]. If albuminuria is abnormal, the test should be confirmed by two or three samples within 3 or 6 months, 4–6 weeks apart, due to the variability in albumin excretion. Albumin excretion may rise due to exercise within 24 h of sampling, infection, fever, congestive heart failure (CHF), marked hyperglycemia, hypercholesterolemia, and high blood pressure. Persistent albuminuria ≥30 mg/g creatinine indicates microalbuminuria and requires treatment with ACE inhibitor or ARB, even in the absence of hypertension [14].

The glomerular filtration rate is estimated using validated formulae (eGFR). The Chronic Kidney Disease Epidemiology Collaboration (CKD-EPI) equation and the Modification of Diet in Renal Disease (MDRD) Study equation are recommended in most guidelines, and eGFR is considered abnormal when below 60 mL/min/1.73 m^2. CKD-EPI is generally preferred [4, 13].

Persistent albuminuria in the range of 30–299 mg/g Cr (microalbuminuria) is considered the earliest stage of DN in type 1 diabetes (T1DM) and a marker for development of nephropathy in T2DM and for increased CVD risk [15].

The pathophysiological mechanisms in the development of DN are multifactorial. Hyperglycemia is related to structural and functional changes such as glomerular hyperfiltration, glomerular and tubular epithelial hypertrophy, and microalbuminuria, followed by the development of glomerular basement membrane (GBM) thickening, accumulation of mesangial matrix, evident proteinuria, and eventually glomerulosclerosis and ESRD. Nevertheless, intensive therapy to improve glycemic control is able to attenuate the development of nephropathy, as assessed by urinary albumin excretion (UAE), but not fully prevent it [16] (Fig. 37.1).

Hemodynamic and metabolic pathways are involved in the development of DN. Hyperfiltration and hyperperfusion injuries occur very early in DN and are glomerular hemodynamic changes related to the decrease of arteriolar resistance, more evident on the afferent side, which lead to a rise in glomerular capillary pressure. In addition to hyperglycemia, other factors, such as prostanoids, angiotensin II (ANGII), nitric oxide (NO), atrial natriuretic factor, growth hormone, glucagon, and insulin, may be related to the increase in filtration and perfusion. Vascular endothelial growth factor (VEGF) and cytokines such as transforming growth factor-beta (TGF-β) increase NO production and mediate hyperfiltration. Glomerulosclerosis occurs as a result of high intraglomerular pressure, an increase in mesangial cell matrix production, and GBM thickening [17, 18].

Hyperglycemia augments the oxidative stress and overproduction of reactive oxygen species (ROS) that stimulate protein kinase C (PKC) pathways, advanced glycosylation end product (AGE) formation, TGF-β, and ANG-II [17].

Glucose transporter-1 (GLUT-1) regulates the entry of glucose into the kidney cell, and glucose activates the metabolic pathways. Nonenzymatic glycosylation of glucose produces AGE, activates PKC, and accelerates the polyol pathway; hemodynamic changes activate VEGF, TGF-β, interleukin-1 (IL-1), IL-6, IL-18, and tumor necrosis factor alpha (TNFα) and together increase albumin permeability in GBM and extracellular matrix accumulation, leading to elevated proteinuria, glomerulosclerosis, and tubulointerstitial fibrosis [18].

Pathologic abnormalities in the kidneys occur before the onset of microalbuminuria. The hallmark of DN is a nodular glomerulosclerosis, the Kimmelstiel-Wilson lesion [19], but less than one-third of diabetic patients with microalbuminuria have the typical glomerulopathy [20]. The earliest changes are an increase in the extracellular matrix and mesangial cell hypertrophy. There is an increased deposition of type 4 collagen in GBM, and the thickening may start as early as 1 year after the onset of T1DM, and later in glomerulosclerosis, the deposition of collagen types 1 and 3 also occurs. Hyperglycemia impairs integrin expression and the structure and function of the podocytes, which are glomerular epithelial cells that cover the GBM. Hyperglycemia also reduces the number of podocytes, which is related to proteinuria, although this decrease is observed even in the absence of proteinuria and occurs before the development of glomerulosclerosis and tubulointerstitial damage [18] (Fig. 37.2).

Recent data suggest that epigenetic modifications may be involved on the pathogenesis of diabetic nephropathy. Hyperglycemia and other factors, such as inflammation, hypoxia, and cytokines, may induce aberrant DNA methylation leading to fibroblast proliferation and fibrosis and regulating other genes associated with DN. Some other epigenetic processes may also have a role on DN such as noncoding RNA and histone modifications. The importance of identifying epigenetic changes relies on the fact that they are reversible changes which may enable therapeutic devel-

Table 37.1 Laboratory tests for the screening and diagnosis of diabetic nephropathy

Albuminuria—albumin/creatinine ratio
Serum creatinine
[a]eGFR-MDRD or CKD-EPI

[a]eGFR estimated glomerular filtration rate, MDRD Modification of Diet in Renal Disease, CKD-EPI Chronic Kidney Disease Epidemiology Collaboration—equation

Fig. 37.1 Kidney alterations of diabetic nephropathy

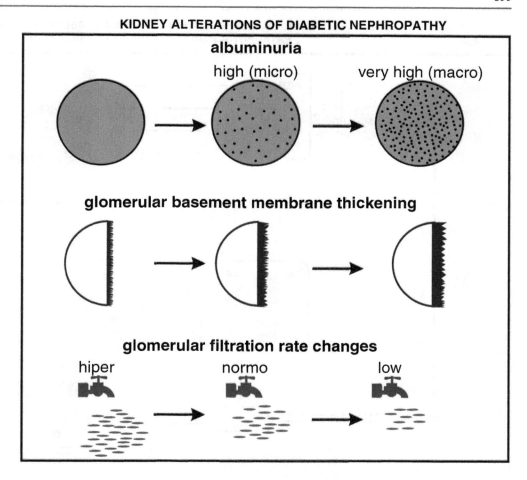

KIDNEY ALTERATIONS OF DIABETIC NEPHROPATHY

albuminuria

high (micro) → very high (macro)

glomerular basement membrane thickening

glomerular filtration rate changes

hiper → normo → low

opment. Nevertheless, these mechanisms are not fully understood and need further researches [6].

In view of the heterogeneity of kidney lesions and the complexity of the natural history of DN, Tervaert et al., in 2010, defined four classes of DN according to the glomerular lesions found on electron microscopy that can be applied in both type 1 and type 2 diabetes [21]. In this classification, class I is identified by an isolated GBM thickening (>430 nm in males over 9 years of age and >395 nm in females), with no evidence of mesangial expansion, increased mesangial matrix, or global glomerulosclerosis involving more than 50% of the glomeruli, and glomeruli lesions then increase progressively to class IV, which is characterized by advanced diabetic sclerosis (>50% global glomerulosclerosis).

The "conventional" natural history of DN was defined in the 1980s, based on longitudinal studies of patients with type 1 and type 2 diabetes, and divided DN into five stages [22] as follows: stage 1 with a reversible glomerular hyperfiltration; stage 2 with normal GFR and normoalbuminuria; stage 3 GFR still normal but associated with microalbuminuria (5–10 years after diagnosis of DM); stage 4, in which proteinuria appears and may reach nephrotic range levels (after 10–20 years of diabetes progression); and stage 5, characterized by a GFR slope below 10 ml/min/year and CKD, leading to ESRD.

Information on the likelihood of passing from one stage to another in newly diagnosed patients was provided by the findings of the UK Prospective Diabetes Study (UKPDS) [23]. However, the study also emphasized that the risk of mortality increased in parallel with the worsening of renal disease. After 10 years of diagnosis, 25% of the patients with T2DM developed microalbuminuria and 5% macroalbuminuria, and in the latter, the death rate exceeded the rate of progression to an advanced stage of nephropathy [24].

The Diabetes Control and Complications Trial (DCCT) showed that less than 2% of patients on intensive treatment developed renal failure after 30 years of diagnosis. The development of microalbuminuria in patients with T1DM usually begins 5–15 years after the onset of diabetes and increases progressively. Patients without proteinuria after 20–25 years have an approximately 1% per year risk of developing clinical renal disease [16].

Nevertheless, another natural history of DN has been identified, particularly in type 1 and type 2 diabetic patients, although it is not clear why some patients develop the "clas-

**METABOLIC AND HEMODYNAMIC PATHWAYS RELATED TO THE
PATHOPHYSIOLOGY OF DIABETIC NEPHROPATHY**

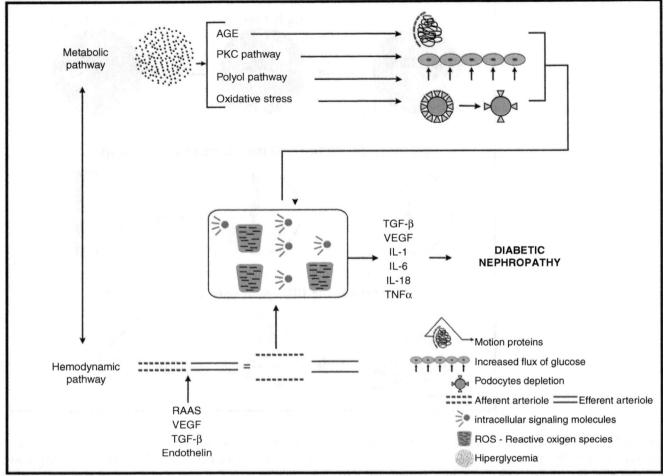

AGE : Advance Glycosylation Products; **PKC** : Protein Kinase C; **TGF-β** : Transforming Growth Factor β; **VEGF** : Vascular Endothelial Growth Factor;
IL-1,6,18 - Interleukin 1,6,18 - **TNFα** - Tumor Necrosis Factor α; **RAAS** - Renin Angiotensin Aldosterone System

Fig. 37.2 Metabolic and hemodynamic pathways related to the pathophysiology of diabetic nephropathy. (AGE advanced glycosylation products, PKC protein kinase C, TGF-β transforming growth factor, VEGF vascular endothelial growth factor, IL-1,6,18 interleukin-1,6,18, TNFα tumor necrosis factor α, RAAS renin-angiotensin-aldosterone system)

sical" DN with significant proteinuria, while others have impaired renal function associated with very low levels of proteinuria that may persist until the ESRD [16, 22].

It would be useful to identify individuals, still normo-albuminuric, whose likelihood of progression to microalbuminuria is increased, but this is not yet possible. In addition to environmental influences, there is evidence in support of genetic susceptibility to microvascular complications of nephropathy in diabetic patients. Earlier investigations that focused on genetic mapping have generally yielded conflicting results, probably because, like other human diseases or syndromes, DN can develop from the interactions of several genes that in isolation would have no effect but which, when subtly altered, could predispose to DN [25].

Hence, it is important to enquire about the family history of DN and to screen periodically all diabetic patients. Microalbumin and serum creatinine (SCr) tests are valuable laboratory markers used to detect early signs of kidney damage [9, 11]. A recent study that evaluated the risk stratification of kidney disease emphasized that both the urine microalbumin level and urine albumin/creatinine ratio tests are needed to fully assess kidney disease and its associated risks of death and progression to ESRD [26] (Table 37.2).

"Kidney Disease: Improving Global Outcomes" (KDIGO) conducted a meta-analysis of nine cohorts from the general population and another eight cohorts with a high risk for CKD, which confirmed that lower eGFR and higher albuminuria are risk factors for ESRD, acute kidney injury, and progressive CKD in both the general and high-risk popula-

Table 37.2 Treatment targets of glycemia, blood pressure, and dyslipidemia

Glycemic control	HbA1C < 7.0% < 6.5%	Caution with patients with advanced kidney disease and high-risk CVD[a]
BP[b] control	≤130 × 80 mmHg	Caution with patients with high-risk CVD
LDL[c]	CVD risk <100/dl, <70 mg/dl	Stage 5 of kidney disease: start statin only if specific CVD risk

[a]CVD cardiovascular disease
[b]BP blood pressure
[c]LDL cholesterol low-density lipoprotein

tions, independent of each other and irrespective of cardiovascular risk factors [27].

The gold standard for GFR measurement is urinary clearance of an exogenous filtration marker, which is expensive and troublesome, and in addition to which it varies during the day. In clinical practice, SCr is used to estimate GFR, applying the modification of diet in real disease (MDRD) and/or CKD Epidemiology Collaboration (CKD-EPI) equations [28], which use clinical variables as substitutes for unmeasured non-GFR determinants and provide more accurate estimates than SCr alone. Estimates of the CKD burden depend in part on the equation used to define the eGFR: when the more recent CKD-EPI equation is used, the prevalence of eGFR below 60 ml/min/1.73 m^2 is lowered by a factor of 0.88 (6.9 versus 7.8%), compared with the estimate from the older MDRD study equation [9].

In patients with T1DM, the first screening is recommended at 5 years after the diagnosis [29], but it is suggested that patients with poor metabolic control be evaluated at the onset of puberty, which is an independent risk factor for microalbuminuria [30]. On the other hand, as about 7% of the patients with type 2 diabetes will already have microalbuminuria at the time of diagnosis of diabetes, the screening must be started by then. If microalbuminuria is absent, the screening must be repeated annually for both type 1 and 2 diabetic patients [24].

In general, the medical societies recommend that an assessment of UAE be performed annually [14, 31], starting at the diagnosis of T2DM and 5 years after that for T1DM, in combination with a measurement of SCr in order to estimate GFR and determine the stage of CKD.

Kidney disease is classified in five stages [31] according to the GFR (ml/min per 1.73 m^2 body surface area), considering kidney damage as abnormalities on pathologic, urine, blood, or imaging tests. Stage 1 is characterized by kidney damage with normal or increased GFR (≥90), stage 2 also by kidney damage associated with mildly decreased GFR (60–89), stage 3 by a moderately decreased GFR (30–59), stage 4 by a severely decreased GFR [15–28], and stage 5 as kidney failure defined as GFR below 15 or dialysis.

In February 2007, a consensus conference in the United Kingdom [32] approved the division of stage 3 CKD into stage 3A (eGFR 45–59) and stage 3B (eGFR 30–44) and added the suffix "p" to the GFR-based stage for patients with proteinuria (random urine protein/creatinine ratio >100 mg/mmol). These changes have been endorsed by the National Institute for Health and Care Excellence (NICE), the Scottish Intercollegiate Guidelines Network (SIGN), and the National Kidney Foundation Kidney Disease Outcomes Quality Initiative (NKF-KDOQI). Patients at stages 1–3 are considered to have early CKD.

Differential Diagnosis

Very often clinicians tend to attribute proteinuria and renal impairment to DM, but that is not the only renal abnormality found in diabetics [33]. Other causes of CKD should be considered in patients that present with an absence of diabetic retinopathy, low or rapidly decreasing GFR, rapidly progressive proteinuria or nephrotic syndrome, refractory hypertension, presence of active urinary sediment, signs or symptoms of other systemic disease, or a reduction in GFR of more than 30% within 2–3 months after starting angiotensin-converting enzyme inhibitors (ACEi) or angiotensin receptor blockers (ARBs) [31]. Moreover, in some patients, the DN may be associated with other kidney diseases.

Nondiabetic renal disease (NDRD) includes a heterogeneous mixture of the following glomerular and nonglomerular conditions [33]:

1. Glomerular disease other than diabetic nephropathy: immunoglobulin A nephropathy, focal and segmental glomerular sclerosis, microvascular complications of diabetes, membraneous glomerulonephritis, membranoproliferative glomerulonephritis, pauci-immune, systemic lupus erythematosus, and others
2. Nonglomerular renal disease: macrovascular (renovascular), acute kidney injury (acute interstitial nephritis, e.g., contrast nephropathy, sepsis, and ACEI/ARBs/direct renin inhibitor (DRI) induced, and acute tubular necrosis, e.g., sepsis and diuretic toxicity), electrolyte abnormality, urinary tract infection, etc.

Nevertheless, no consensus classification is available at the moment for kidney biopsy in a diabetic patient with any pathological condition.

Treatment (Table 37.2)

Interventions that have been reported to be useful in preventing or retarding the progression of DN include the following: good glycemic and blood pressure control, treatment of hyperlipidemia, cessation of smoking, and restriction of protein intake. Patients who develop ESRD will require renal replacement therapy. Thus, when the patient has an eGFR <30 mL/min/1.73 m², he/she should be referred to evaluation of specialist for renal replacement treatment [15, 34].

Blood pressure and glycemic control represent the major cornerstones for preventing and treating diabetic nephropathy [16]. The DCCT reported that any decrease in hemoglobin A1C (HbA1C) was strongly associated with a reduction in the risk of developing microalbuminuria and progression to overt nephropathy [16], and UKPDS clearly demonstrated a role for intensified glycemic control in subjects newly diagnosed with T2DM, in whom treatment led to a fall in HbA1C from 7.9% to 7.0% [35].

To reduce the risk or slow the progression of nephropathy, the American Diabetes Association (ADA) recommends the optimization of glucose and control of blood pressure. The ADVANCE study demonstrated that the decrease in HbA1C to a mean of 6.5% was associated with a further reduction in renal events, as assessed by the development and progression of microalbuminuria [36]. However, the findings of the ACCORD study [37] led to controversy regarding the appropriate HbA1C target for reducing macrovascular disease.

The major risk of reaching HbA1C levels below 7.0% is the increased likelihood of developing hypoglycemia. For people with decreased kidney function (CKD stages 3–5), hypoglycemia is a major concern because it impairs the clearance of insulin and a number of oral agents used to treat diabetes, as well as reduces kidney gluconeogenesis [31]. Drug adjustments must be made to prevent or, at least, reduce the risk of hypoglycemia.

Sulfonylureas in general have predominantly renal elimination and are not recommended for patients with creatinine clearance (CrCl) below 50 ml/min, except for glipizide, which has hepatic elimination of inactive metabolites and should be interrupted when CrCl falls below 30 ml/min. Malnutrition, acute illness, liver disease, and alcoholism are risk factors for hypoglycemia. Meglitinides are oxidized by the liver but still entail a risk of hypoglycemia because active metabolites may accumulate in renal dysfunction, repaglinide being the one that accumulates the smallest amount of metabolites. Metformin is eliminated unchanged by the kidneys; NKF-KDOQI contraindicated its use with a serum creatinine over 1.5 mg/dl in males and 1.4 mg/dl in women due to the risk of lactic acidosis, although NICE recommends that it should be used with care for patients with an eGFR below 45 ml/min/1.73 m² and discontinued if the eGFR falls below 30 ml/min/1.73 m². Acarbose is not rec-

ommended if CrCl is below 25 ml/min, and miglitol produces renal elimination, but as there are no studies in patients with kidney disease, FDA does not recommend either of them if serum creatinine is ≥2 mg/dl. The risk of side effects when using thiazolidinediones increases with renal disease [31, 38].

Exenatide and its formulation with extended release are eliminated by renal filtration and need no adjustment with CrCl above 50 ml/min. Increases in the dosage from 5 to 10 µg should be applied with care if CrCl is 30–50 ml/min, and, according to FDA, when CrCl is below 30 ml/min, it should be stopped. Liraglutide should be used with care when CrCl is below 60 ml/min, and when below 30 ml/min, its side effects increase, but experience of its use is still limited in CKD. It's not necessary to adjust dulaglutide dosage in patients with mildly to moderately decreased eGFR, but it shouldn't be used when the eGFR is below 30 ml/min/1.73 m². The usage of SGLT-2 inhibitor does not require dose adjustment with mild kidney dysfunction (eGFR ≥ 60 mL/min/1.73 m²), but as it depends on the kidney's ability to filtrate glucose, it's not recommended when the eGFR is below 45 ml/min/1.73 m² [39].

The dipeptidyl peptidase-4 (DPP4) inhibitor agents need no adjustment if CrCl ≥ 50 ml/min; sitagliptin should be reduced to 50 mg/d if it is 30–50 ml/min and to 25 mg if <30 and saxagliptin to 2.5 mg if <50 ml/min. Linagliptin is fecally eliminated unchanged, so it may be safely used in patients with CKD. Colesevelam and bromocriptine need no adjustments. As up to 50% of insulin is eliminated by the kidney, it is recommended that it be reduced by 25% when CrCl is 10–50 ml/min and by 50% if it falls below 10 ml/min [31, 38].

In addition to the importance of glycemic control, it has been shown that a more aggressive BP reduction reduces the progression of DN. The mechanism of hypertension in DN is complex and not fully understood, being related to excessive sodium retention, activation of the sympathetic nervous system (SNS) and the renin-angiotensin-aldosterone system (RAAS), augmented oxidative stress, and endothelial cell dysfunction (ECD) [40].

The UKPDS provided strong evidence that control of BP can slow the development of nephropathy [41]. Treatment using angiotensin-converting enzyme inhibitors (ACEi) retards the progression from micro- to macroalbuminuria and can slow the reduction of the GFR in patients with macroalbuminuria [42, 43]. In T2DM with hypertension and normoalbuminuria, renin-angiotensin system (RAS) inhibition has been shown to delay the onset of microalbuminuria [44, 45]. The evidences suggest that ACE inhibitors [46] have renoprotective actions in addition to their antihypertensive effects for primary prevention [47].

Angiotensin receptor blockers have also been shown to reduce the rate of progression from micro- to macroalbuminuria, as well as ESRD, in patients with T2DM. The Irbesartan in Diabetic Nephropathy Trial (IDNT) [48] and Reduction of Endpoints in Non-Insulin-Dependent Diabetes Mellitus (NIDDM) study, as well as the Angiotensin Antagonist Losartan (RENAAL) studies, have reported the efficacy of ARBs in nephropathy [37].

The ROADMAP trial investigators evaluated type 2 diabetics with normoalbuminuria and reported that olmesartan was associated with a delayed onset of microalbuminuria, with BP control according to the current standards ($<130 \times 80$ mmHg), but there was a higher rate of fatal cardiovascular events with olmesartan among patients with preexisting CVD [45].

It is not known whether the RAS blockade reduced progression to microalbuminuria in normotensive T2DM. Mauer et al. reported that the early blockade of the RAS in patients with T1DM did not slow progression of nephropathy [49].

Furthermore, as it is not yet possible to predict the patients at risk of developing nephropathy, present evidence does not support the use of RAS blockade for the primary prevention of DN [25].

Some reports show that the risk of progressive DN continues to decrease with falls in BP even below the normal range, and such reductions are associated with better clinical outcomes. A recent subanalysis from the BP arm of the ADVANCE study suggested that optimal BP control is less than 125/75 mmHg, particularly in those patients with overt nephropathy [50].

The ideal BP goal in diabetic patients with nephropathy remains questionable, and currently the recommended target is considered to be the same as that for the general diabetic population [51]. An ACE inhibitor or an ARB, usually in combination with a diuretic, should be used to treat hypertensive diabetics if CKD is at stages 1–4 with the target of <130/80 mmHg [31].

As the ACEi and ARB are individually renoprotective, questions have arisen regarding the usefulness of combined therapy. The suggestion that a more complete inhibition of angiotensin II, through non-ACE pathways, would improve the results stimulated some trials, the older ones, that studied combinations of ACEi and ARB reported effects that were promising, with significant reductions in albuminuria and/or BP and a good tolerability. Nevertheless, the Candesartan and Lisinopril Microalbuminuria (CALM II) [52] study reported that after 12 months of treatment, the effect of the combined therapy was no different from the maximization of each therapy alone in relation to BP or albuminuria. Concerns about this strategy came up with the Ongoing Telmisartan Alone and in Combination with Ramipril Global Endpoint Trial (ONTARGET) [53]. This study tested patients at high risk for a CV event with an ACEi and/or ARB and observed no differences between groups at the primary endpoint, comprising stroke, myocardial infarction, and sudden cardiac death. However, those patients randomized to combination therapy had higher rates of renal impairment and hyperkalemia, a more rapid decline in eGFR, and a greater need for dialysis for acute renal failure episodes during the trial.

The Combination Angiotensin Receptor Blocker and Angiotensin-Converting Enzyme Inhibitor for Treatment of Diabetic Nephropathy VA NEPHRON-D (Veterans Affairs Nephropathy in Diabetes) Study: Nephropathy iN Diabetes Study (VA NEPHRON) study is a multicenter, prospective, randomized parallel group trial which tested the efficacy and safety of ACEi (lisinopril)/ARB (losartan) versus ARB on the composite endpoint of reduction in GFR to 30 ml/min (if GFR >60 ml/min), reduction in GFR by 50% (if GFR <60 ml/min), ESRD, or death in patients with DM2 and nephropathy. The results of this trial confirmed that the dual blockade with ACEi and ARB had no significant benefit in the primary endpoints of renal disease progression or death [54].

Other drugs, such as diuretics, calcium channel blockers, and β-blockers, should be used as additional therapy to further lower blood pressure in patients already treated with ACE inhibitors or ARBs or as alternative therapy for individuals unable to tolerate those classes of drug. What is generally recommended is the combination of an ACEi or ARB with another class of drug, preferably a diuretic, and calcium channel blockers [31, 42].

ACEi/ARBs are recommended for people with diabetes, proteinuria, CKD, and ACR over 2.5 mg/mmol (men) or 3.5 mg/mmol (women), irrespective of the presence of hypertension or stage of CKD, and should be titrated to the maximum tolerated therapeutic dose before the addition of a second-line agent, with monitoring of the eGFR and serum potassium [42]. An established clinical strategy is the association of mineralocorticoid receptor (MR) antagonists to control blood pressure. A recent randomized clinical trial supports the beneficial use of Finerenone on CKD and CVD outcomes in people with type 2 diabetes, already in treatment with an ACE inhibitor or ARB. Treatment with Finerenone in a median follow-up of 2.6 years reduced in 18% the death from renal causes and the decline above 40% in eGFR. https://doi.org/10.1056/NEJMoa2025845 [55].

The treatment of other comorbidities such as obesity and dyslipidemia should also be considered in patients with DN. Obesity is associated with glomerular hyperfiltration and an increase in transcapillary hydraulic pressure, hemodynamic changes that may accelerate the development and progression of CKD [36]. Weight loss ameliorates obesity-induced glomerular hyperfiltration and decreases proteinuria, in addition to its beneficial effects on BP and diabetes control [56].

Dyslipidemia is a risk marker for progressive kidney injury and a risk factor for CVD. However, the evidence that the treatment of dyslipidemia reduces CKD progression is mostly restricted to post hoc subgroup analyses from large cardiovascular clinical trials, such as the Heart Protection Study and the Cholesterol and Recurrent Events (CARE) study. Results from the Study of Heart and Renal Protection (SHARP) trial showed no significant differences in the number of patients with CKD suffering from kidney failure. People with DM and nondialysis CKD should be treated according to current guidelines for high-risk groups [56]. All guidelines agree that statins are the best choice to start the treatment of dyslipidemia in patients with T2DM, and most continue to recommend a low-density lipoprotein cholesterol (LDL-C) target <70 mg/dL (1.8 mmol/L) in people with T2DM and established CVD or at a high risk based on the estimated 10-year risk calculated with the UK Prospective Diabetes Study (UKPDS) risk engine or the Atherosclerotic Cardiovascular Disease (ASCVD) pooled equation. And the LDL-C target for those without established CVD and without a high 10-year CVD risk should be <100 mg/dL (2.6 mmol/L) [13].

For patients on dialysis, it is more complex, and the guidelines recommend not to initiate lipid-lowering therapy in dialysis patients and to keep incident dialysis patients on their preexisting lipid-lowering treatment. However, some data suggest that high-risk patients with high baseline LDL-C may benefit from treatment, particularly, with statin/ezetimibe combination [57, 58].

Further studies are needed to evaluate the extent of CVD benefits associated with the use of new lipid-modifying agents, proprotein convertase subtilisin/kexin type 9 (PCSK9) inhibitors, and cholesteryl ester transfer protein (CETP) inhibitors in patients with DKD. And the trials should be designed to compare effects on the profile of lipid abnormalities observed in CKD or dialysis populations [59].

The target for low-density lipoprotein cholesterol (LDL-C) in people with DM and CKD stages 1–4 should be below 100 mg/dl, but may be considered to be below 70 mg/dl, while patients whose level is above the target should be treated with a statin, which is the preferred therapy [14, 31]. However, a statin should only be started in patients on hemodialysis therapy if there is a specific cardiovascular indication.

No adjustment of dosage is necessary for bile acid sequestrants, niacin, ezetimibe, atorvastatin, or pravastatin. The dosage of rosuvastatin should not exceed 10 mg if CrCl is below 30 ml/min/1.73 m^2 and the patient is not on hemodialysis; it is recommended that simvastatin therapy be started at 5 mg daily in patients with severe kidney disease; daily doses of lovastatin above 20 mg should be used with care if CrCl is below 30 ml/min, while fluvastatin may be used with care in patients with severe kidney disease, but there are no studies using doses greater than 40 mg. The dose of gemfibrozil should be decreased or alternative therapy considered in patients with SCr over 2 mg/dl. Therapy with fenofibrate

should be started at 54 mg daily; its effects on kidney function and lipid concentrations should be assessed and the dose reduced in patients with CrCl below 50 ml/min [31].

Smoking has also been shown to increase the risk of progression of CKD to end-stage renal disease (ESRD) irrespective of the primary renal disease; hence, the indication is a total cessation of smoking.

A diet therapy with protein restriction is recommended for patients with CKD as it has a great impact on this population. Although dietary protein is limited, adequate caloric intake should be maintained by increasing calories from carbohydrates and/or fats, and the qualitative and quantitative aspects of proteins, carbohydrates, and fats should also be taken into consideration.

A reduction in protein intake to 0.8–1.0 g/kg body wt/day in individuals at the earlier stages of CKD and below 0.8 g/kg body wt/day at the later stages of CKD may improve the results of renal function as assessed by UAE rate and GFR [31]. For adults with eGFR < 45 mL/min/1.73 m^2 and for the management of substantial proteinuria (urinary protein excretion, >0.3 g/day), 0.6–0.8 g/kg body wt/day is the most frequently recommended [60]. Nevertheless, reducing the amount of dietary protein below 0.8 g/kg/day does not alter glycemic control, cardiovascular risk measures, or the course of GFR decline. On the other hand, it's recommended to avoid high-protein intake (>1.3 g/kg/day) in adults with CKD at risk of progression [61]. However, in patients on dialysis, it's commonly observed protein energy wasting, and increased dietary protein intake may be necessary to help preserve muscle mass [62].

An intake of 800–1000 mg of elemental calcium per day (20–25 mmol per day) is suggested for people with stage 3 or 4 chronic kidney disease, as studies report that this procedure can result in a stable calcium balance. It is also recommended to supplement vitamin D when serum level is documented as low [60]. The KDIGO suggests avoiding hypercalcemia in adult patients with CKD stages 3a–5D and supports that patients on treatment with calcimimetic who develop hypocalcemia should require intense calcium treatment. However, the Work Group recommend an individualized approach on hypocalcemia treatment due to unproven benefits and potential risk for harm [63].

The optimal time for the initiation of chronic dialysis remains unknown. There is a trend in the nephrology literature toward an earlier initiation of dialysis. However, prospective data that could guide physicians are not yet available [64].

Patients with CKD stage 4 should be referred to a nephrologist. Late nephrology referral before dialysis initiation is associated with increased morbidity and mortality [65].

Kidney transplantation provides high-quality life years for patients with ESRD. The largest numbers of transplants are performed in the United States, China, Brazil, and India, and the countries whose populations have the greatest access to transplantation are Austria, the United States, Croatia, Norway, Portugal, and Spain. However, access to transplantation is still considerably limited across the globe [5].

Guidelines [14, 31] recommend that all patients be evaluated annually with the measurement of creatinine, UAE, and potassium and that those whose GRF is 45–60 be referred to a nephrologist if a nondiabetic kidney disease is suspected. The eGFR should be monitored every 6 months and bicarbonate, hemoglobin, calcium, phosphorus, and parathyroid hormone at least once a year; ensure vitamin D sufficiency and consider bone density testing due to the relation between nephropathy and bone disease. The need for dose adjustment of medications should be evaluated and the patient referred for diet counseling. If the GFR is 30–44, the eGFR should be monitored every 3 months and electrolytes, bicarbonate, calcium, phosphorus, parathyroid hormone, hemoglobin, albumin, and weight every 3–6 months; dose adjustment of medications should be considered, and if GFR is below 30, the patient should be referred to a nephrologist.

Hemoglobin A1C (A1C) remains a widely used and trusted tool for assessing glycemic control in patients without advanced nephropathy or anemia, but there are conflicting data as to what A1C level should be targeted to prevent complications, especially cardiovascular ones, in patients with nephropathy. A lower value of A1C for similar glucose levels is seen in patients with DN than for those without nephropathy. This observation may reflect a shortened erythrocyte survival. The accuracy of the A1C assay is diminished by uremia, and unadjusted A1C results are not the optimal assay for patients on hemodialysis or peritoneal dialysis treatment as it may underestimate glycemic control in those patients [31, 66].

It is reported that glycated albumin (GA) more accurately reflects recent glucose control, but it is still necessary to prospectively assess the impact of GA on patient survival and hospitalizations. GA has also been considered a useful glycemic index, especially, in patients with diabetes and CKD, because it is not influenced by erythrocyte lifespan, uremia, or blood transfusions, all of which can interfere in HbA1C measurements. Freedman et al. reported that for each 5% increase in GA, the risk of death increased by 14% in patients under dialysis treatment, and A1C and casual serum glucose did not predict survival. Glycated albumin may be influenced by albuminuria, cirrhosis, thyroid dysfunction, and smoking and A1C not only by advanced nephropathy but also by a rapid change in diabetes control; severe anemia; hemolytic anemia; iron deficiency; recent blood transfusion; HIV positivity treated with antiretroviral therapy, erythropoietin, and other drugs interacting with erythropoiesis; and chronic alcohol abuse. However, until the GA assay is available, frequent measurements of serum glucose appear more valuable

than A1C in patients on dialysis to evaluate glycemic control [66, 67]. GA was considered a better predictor and could be a useful marker to predict early DN in T2DM patients, as it was reported that higher GA levels were significantly associated with increased risk of early DN development, independent of A1C [68].

Novel Therapies

Some trials have reported that new groups of medication, recently developed for glycemic control in patients with T2DM, namely, dipeptidyl peptidase-4 (DPP4) inhibitor, glucagon-like peptide-1 (GLP-1) receptor agonist, and sodium-glucose cotransporter-2 (SGLT-2) inhibitors, possess renoprotective effects [69].

The SAVOR-TIMI trial showed that saxagliptin, a DPP-4 inhibitor, caused an improvement or less deterioration in albumin-to-creatinine ratio, but with no changes in eGFR [70]. Liraglutide, a GLP-1 receptor agonist, was tested on LEADER Trial with reported lower incidence of nephropathy, evaluated as new-onset albuminuria, doubling of SCr and CrCl below 45 ml/min/1.73m^2, need for renal replacement therapy, and death related to renal causes (1.5 number of events per 100 patients per year versus 1.9 number of events per 100 patients per year; p 0.003) [71].

The EMPA-REG OUTCOME trial evaluated empagliflozin, a SGLT-2 inhibitor, and reported relative risk (RR) reduction of doubling of SCr (RR: 44%, 1.5% versus 2.6%), progression to macroalbuminuria (RR: 38%, 11.2% versus 16.2%), and initiation of renal replacement therapy (RR: 55%, 0.3% versus 0.6%) and also slowed GFR decline (annual decrease 0.1960.11 versus 1.6760.13 ml/min per 1.73 m^2; p 0.001) [72].

The CANVAS Program Report which combines the data from two trials, CANVAS and CANVAS Renal, evaluated the safety and effect of canagliflozin (SGLT-2 inhibitor), on the occurrence of cardiovascular and renal events in patients with T2DM, and indicated a class effect in the reduction of cardiovascular and renal events when the SGLT-2 inhibitor was used in higher-risk diabetic patients with T2DM [72, 73]. The CREDENCE (Canagliflozin and Renal Events in Diabetes with Established Nephropathy Clinical Evaluation) trial was a randomized, double-blind, placebo-controlled trial with canagliflozin in patients with type 2 diabetes, which primary outcome was a composite of end-stage kidney disease (dialysis, transplantation, or a sustained estimated GFR. It was early terminated because it showed a 30% lower relative risk of reaching the primary endpoint. The relative risk of the renal-specific composite of end-stage kidney disease, a doubling of the creatinine level, or death from renal causes was lower by 34% (hazard ratio, 0.66; 95% CI, 0.53

to 0.81; P < 0.001), and the relative risk of end-stage kidney disease was lower by 32% (hazard ratio, 0.68; 95% CI, 0.54 to 0.86; P = 0.002)> <0.001). Moreover, the relative risk of end-stage kidney disease was lower by 32% (hazard ratio, 0.68; 95% CI, 0.54 to 0.86; P = 0.002). It also showed a lower risk of cardiovascular death, myocardial infarction, or stroke, hospitalization for heart failure, and no significant difference in the risk of fracture and amputation between canagliflozin and placebo groups. https://doi.org/10.1056/NEJMoa1811744 [74] DAPA-CKD (Dapagliflozin And Prevention of Adverse Outcomes in Chronic Kidney Disease) another multicentre, double-blind, placebo-controlled, randomized trial in which primary outcome was a composite of sustained decline in eGFR of at least 50%, end-stage kidney disease, or kidney-related or cardiovascular death. Secondary efficacy outcomes were a kidney-specific composite (the same as the primary outcome but excluding cardiovascular death), a composite of cardiovascular death or hospitalization for heart failure (HHF), and all-cause mortality, it included about two-thirds of participants with type 2 diabetes and about one-third did not, with background ACE inhibition/ ARB treatment. Dapagliflozin significantly reduced the risk of a sustained decline in eGFR, progression to ESRD, death from renal or cardiovascular causes, and a 29% reduction in risk of death from cardiovascular causes or HHF irrespective of diabetes status. Additionally, dapagliflozin demonstrated a reduction in all-cause mortality (31% relative risk reduction with a 2.9% absolute risk reduction, hazard ratio [HR] 0.69, 95% CI 0.53–0.88, P = 0.0035). https://doi.org/10.1016/S2213-8587(20)30369-7 [75, 76]

Table 37.3 SGLT2 Inhibitors and Dose for Glycaemic control according to glomerular filtration rate

SGLT2 Inhibitor// eGFR, 3mL/min/1.73 m²	≥ 60	45–60	30 to <45
Empaglifozin [77]	10mg–25 mg once daily	10mg – 25 mg once daily	Do not initiate; Discontinue
Dapaglifozin [78]	5 mg–10 mg once daily	5 mg – 10 mg once daily	No dose adjustment
Canaglifozin	100 mg–300 mg once daily	100 mg once daily 100 mg once daily	Do not initiate, but patient may continue if albuminuria > 300 mg/day

Rosenwasser RF, Sultan S, Sutton D, Choksi R, Epstein BJ. SGLT-2 inhibitors and their potential in the treatment of diabetes. Diabetes Metab Syndr Obes. 2013;6:453–467 [77]
AstraZeneca. Farxiga (dapagliflozin) prescribing information, 2020. Available from https://den8dhaj6zs0e.cloudfront.net/50fd68b9-106b-4550-b5d0-12b045f8b184/0be9cb1b-3b33-41c7-bfc2-04c9f718e442/0be9cb1b-3b33-41c7-bfc2-04c9f718e442_viewable_rendition__v.pdf. Accessed 11 December 2021 [78]
Boehringer Ingelheim. Invokana (canagliflozin) prescribing information, 2020. Available from https://docs.boehringer-ingelheim.com/Prescribing%20 Information/PIs/Jardiance/jardiance.pdf. Accessed 11 December 2021 [79]

The AWARD-7 study in patients with type 2 diabetes and moderate to severe CKD showed a steeper decline in eGFR (-3.3 mL/ min/1.73 m²) with insulin compared to dulaglutide, with an eGFR decline of -0.7 mL/min/1.73 m² for both low-dose (0.75 mg weekly and high-dose (1.5 mg weekly) groups over one year. The gradients of eGFR decline between the groups were maintained even among patients with a urine albumin-to-creatinine ratio >300 mg/g creatinine, with eGFR declines of -0.7 and -0.5 mL/min/1.73 m² for dulaglutide 1.5 mg and 0.75 mg, respectively, compared to -5.5 mL/min/1.73 m² for insulin. More patients on insulin reached the composite renal endpoint of ESRD or >40% decline in eGFR than the patients on high dose dulaglutide (10.8 vs. 5.2%, P <0.038). https://doi.org/10.1016/S2213-8587(18)30104-9 [80]. And recently, it released data from clinical trials of semaglutide, another GLP-1 receptor agonist, that show reduced risk of albuminuria onset and progression. The SUSTAIN-6 (Trial to Evaluate Cardiovascular and Other Long-term Outcomes with Semaglutide in Subjects with Type 2 Diabetes) [81], and also the LEADER (Liraglutide Effect and Action in Diabetes: Evaluation of Cardiovascular Outcome Results) [82], and REWIND (Researching Cardiovascular Events With a Weekly Incretin in Diabetes) [80] placebo-controlled trials reported significant risk reductions of 36, 22, and 15%, respectively, in secondary composite renal end-points (new onset of macroalbuminuria, doubling of serum creatinine, sustained 45% reduction in eGFR, RRT, or renal death), with macroalbuminuria reduction. https://doi.org/10.1016/S0140-6736(19)31150-X The consistency of these recent data across glucagon-like peptide-1 receptor agonists suggests a class effect of protection from DKD [83].

These studies suggest that GLP-1 receptor agonists may have similar efficacy as SGLT2 inhibitors for reducing cardiorenal risk, particularly for patients with a lower renal reserve who have a higher risk for DKD progression. The ongoing EMPA-SEMA (Renal Effects of Treatment with Empagliflozin Alone or in Combination with Semaglutide in Patients with Type 2 Diabetes and Albuminuria) trial was designed to determine whether GLP-1 receptor agonists and SGLT2 inhibitors act synergistically to optimize renal outcomes. ClinicalTrials.gov. Renal effects of treatment with empagliflozin alone or in combination with semaglutide in patients with type 2 diabetes and albuminuria (EmpaSema). Available from https://clinicaltrials.gov/ct2/show/NCT04061200. Accessed 11 December 2021 [84].

The mechanisms involved in injury to the kidney glomerular, interstitial, and vascular functions consist of inflammation, oxidative stress, endothelial dysfunction, and accelerated fibrosis, as described above. Endothelium dysfunction consists of the impairment of many aspects of endothelial functions, including the anti-inflammatory, antiproliferative ones and vasodilatation. Vascular inflammation is a result of a combination of an impaired vasomotor response, an increase in cell proliferation and platelet aggregation, and vascular permeability.

Extensive research is currently underway in this field, and several new pathogenic mediators for DN have been discovered, including renin, AGE, PKC, transforming growth factor-beta1 (TGF-β1), NO, VEGF, and oxidative stress.

Studies have focused on the role of these mediators and possible novel treatments using these approaches, and the following new classes of treatment are under investigation: protein kinase C-inhibitor (ruboxistaurin); AGE formation inhibitors (aminoguanidine, ALT-946, pyridoxamine, thiamine); direct renin inhibitor (aliskiren); AGE breakers (alagebrium, TRC4186); AGE receptor antagonists (endogenous secretory RAGE, RAGE antibody); TGF inhibitors (pirfenidone, SMP-534); connective tissue growth factor (CTGF) inhibitors (anti-CTGF ab); VEGF inhibitors (SU5416); anti-oxidant (curcumin); and hemorheologic properties and phosphodiesterase inhibitor (pentoxifylline).

Some of these have yielded promising results in trials, but more clinical studies are still needed to establish their effects on DN, as with aliskiren, pentoxifylline, ruboxistaurin, pirfenidone, and anti-CTGF antibody (Table 37.3) [85]. The Ruboxistaurin Study reported an outcome of decreased albuminuria and stabilized kidney function; and the PREDIAN trial reported on the pentoxifylline group an eGFR decline 4.3 ml/min per 1.73 m² less than the control group and a mean difference in albuminuria of 21% [7, 86].

Adverse events requiring cessation of randomized therapy (usually hyperkalemia) were significantly more frequent with aliskiren (13.2 vs. 10.2%). Due to the lack of apparent benefit and higher risk of side effects, the trial was prematurely stopped. There is little evidence for the clinical use of direct renin inhibitor (DRI) in DKD, and its use warrants careful monitoring for hyperkalemia, hypotension, or acute kidney injury [87]. Pirfenidone is a promising agent for the treatment of diabetic nephropathy and should be further investigated [88].

Other agents are under investigation targeting mechanisms, such as glomerular hyperfiltration, inflammation, and fibrosis, and have been a major focus for the development of new treatment. Baricitinib, a JAK1/2 inhibitor, was related to albuminuria reduction by 40%, but showed no effect on eGFR. Atrasentan (ETA) was evaluated on the RADAR and RADAR/JAPAN trial that showed 35% reduction of albuminuria, and this drug is also being tested on the Study of Diabetic Nephropathy with Atrasentan (SONAR) which is a randomized, multicountry, multicenter, double-blind, parallel, placebo-controlled study of the effects of atrasentan on renal outcomes in subjects with type 2 diabetes and nephropathy. However, there are no available phase 3 clinical trial data for these new agents, and none are approved for use in DKD [7].

References

1. Woodmansey C, McGovern AP, McCullough KA, Whyte MB, Munro NM, Correa AC, et al. Incidence, demographics, and clinical characteristics of diabetes of the exocrine pancreas (type 3c): a retrospective cohort study. Diabetes Care. 2017;40(11):1486–93.
2. Hart PA, Bellin MD, Andersen DK, Bradley D, Cruz-monserrate Z, Forsmark CE, et al. Type 3c (pancreatogenic) diabetes mellitus secondary to chronic pancreatitis and pancreatic cancer. Lancet Gastroenterol Hepatol. 2017;1(3):226–37.
3. Abboud H, Henrich WL. Stage IV chronic kidney disease. N Engl J Med. 2010;362:56–65.
4. Kidney Disease: Improving Global Outcomes (KDIGO) CKD Work Group. KDIGO. Clinical practice guideline for the evaluation and management of chronic kidney disease. Kidney Int. 2012;2013:2.
5. Garcia GG, Harden P, Chapman J. The global role of kidney transplantation. Adv Chronic Kidney Dis. 2012;19(2):53–8.
6. Lu Z, Liu N, Wang F. Epigenetic regulations in diabetic nephropathy. J Diabetes Res. 2017;7805058:1–6.
7. Alicic RZ, Rooney MT, Tuttle KR. Diabetic kidney disease: challenges, progress, and possibilities. Clin J Am Soc Nephrol. 2017 Dec 7;12(12):2032–45. https://doi.org/10.2215/CJN.11491116.
8. Tuttle KR, Bakris GL, Bilous RW, Chiang JL, De Boer IH, Goldstein-Fuchs J, et al. Diabetic kidney disease: a report from an ADA consensus conference. Diabetes Care. 2014;37(10):2864–83.
9. International Diabetes Federation. IDF Diabetes Atlas. 10th edition. International Diabetes Federation 2021. https://diabetesatlas.org/idfawp/resource-files/2021/07/IDF_Atlas_10th_Edition_2021.pdf.
10. U.S. Renal Data System. USRDS 2011 annual data report: atlas of chronic kidney disease and end-stage renal disease in the United States. Bethesda: National Institutes of Health, National Institute of Diabetes and Digestive and Kidney Diseases; 2011.
11. Atkins RC. The epidemiology of chronic kidney disease. Kidney Int Suppl. 2005;94:S14–8.
12. Parving HH. Diabetic nephropathy: prevention and treatment. Kidney Int. 2001;60:2041–55.
13. American Diabetes Association. Standards of medical care in diabetes. Diabetes Care. 2018 Jan;41(Suppl 1):S152–3. https://doi.org/10.2337/dc18-S015.
14. American Diabetes Association. Standards of medical care in diabetes. Diabetes Care. 2012;35(suppl 1):s11–63.
15. International Diabetes Federation. Recommendations for managing type 2 diabetes in primary care. 2017. www.idf.org/managing-type2-diabetes.
16. Dwyer JP, Parving HH, Hunsicker LG, Ravid M, Remuzzi G, Lewis JB. Renal dysfunction in the presence of normoalbuminuria in type 2 diabetes: results from the DEMAND study. Cardiorenal Med. 2012;2:1–10.
17. Diabetes Control and Complications Trial/Epidemiology of Diabetes Interventions and Complications Research Group. Retinopathy and nephropathy in patients with type 1 diabetes four years after a trial of intensive therapy. N Engl J Med. 2000;342:381–9.
18. Rojas-Rivera J, Ortiz A, Egido J. Antioxidants in kidney diseases: the impact of bardoxolone methyl. Int J Nephrol. 2012;2012:321714. https://doi.org/10.1155/2012/321714.
19. Vinod PB. Pathophysiology of diabetic nephropathy. Clin Quer Nephrol. 2012;0102:121–6.
20. Gilbert RE, Cooper ME. The tubulointerstitium in progressive diabetic kidney disease: more than an aftermath of glomerular injury? Kidney Int. 1999;56:1627–37.
21. Tervaert TW, Mooyaart AL, Amann K, Cohen AH, Cook HT, Drachenberg CB, et al. Pathologic classification of diabetic nephropathy. J Am Soc Nephrol. 2010;21:556.
22. Halimi JM. The emerging concept of chronic kidney disease without clinical proteinuria in diabetic patients. Diabetes Metab. 2012;38(4):291–7. https://doi.org/10.1016/j.diabet.2012.04.001.

23. Adler AI, Stevens RJ, Manley SE, Bilous RW, Cull CA, Holman RR. Development and progression of nephropathy in type 2 diabetes: the United Kingdom prospective diabetes study (UKPDS 64). Kidney Int. 2003;63:225–32.

24. Gross J, Azevedo MJ, Silveiro SP, Canani LH, Caramori ML, Zelmanovitz TL. Diabetic nephropathy: diagnosis, prevention, and treatment. Diabetes Care. 2005;28:176–88.

25. Ntemka A, Iliadis F, Papanikolaou NA, Grekas D. Network-centric analysis of genetic predisposition in diabetic nephropathy. Hippokratia. 2011;15(3):232–7.

26. Grams M, Coresh J. Proteinuria and risk of acute kidney injury. Lancet. 2010;376(9758):2046–8.

27. Gansevoort RT, Matsushita K, Van Der Velde M, Astor BC, Woodward M, Levey AS, et al. Lower estimated GFR and higher albuminuria are associated with adverse kidney outcomes in both general and high-risk populations. A collaborative meta-analysis of general and high-risk population cohorts. Kidney Int. 2011;80(1):93–104.

28. Padala S, Tighiouart H, Inker LA, Contrera G, Beck GJ, Lewis J. Accuracy of a GFR estimating equation over time in people with a wide range of kidney function. Am J Kidney Dis. 2012;60(2):217–24.

29. Stephenson JM, Fuller JH. Microalbuminuria is not rare before 5 years of IDDM: EURODIAB IDDM complications study group and the WHO multinational study of vascular disease in diabetes study group. J Diabetes Complicat. 1994;8:166–73.

30. Schultz CJ, Konopelska-Bahu T, Dalton RN, Carroll TA, Stratton I, Gale EA, et al. Microalbuminuria prevalence varies with age, sex, and puberty in children with type 1 diabetes followed from diagnosis in a longitudinal study: Oxford Regional Prospective Study Group. Diabetes Care. 1999;22:495–502.

31. National Kidney Foundation Kidney Disease Outcomes Quality Initiative. Clinical practice guidelines and clinical practice recommendations for diabetes and chronic kidney disease. Am J Kidney Dis. 2007;49(Suppl):S25–119.

32. Archibald G, Bartlett W, Brown A, Christie B, Elliott A, Griffith K, et al. UK consensus conference on early chronic kidney disease. Nephrol Dial Transplant. 2007;22(suppl 9):ix4–5.

33. Kumar J, Sahai G. Non-diabetic renal diseases in diabetics. Clin Quer Nephrol. 2012;0102:172–7.

34. Kaur H, Prabhakar S. Novel therapies of diabetic nephropathy. Nephrol Rev. 2011;3:e4.

35. UK Prospective Diabetes Study (UKPDS) Group. Intensive blood-glucose control with sulphonylureas or insulin compared with conventional treatment and risk of complications in patients with type 2 diabetes (UKPDS 33). Lancet. 1998;352:837–53.

36. Patel A, MacMahon S, Chalmers J, Neal B, Billot L. Intensive blood glucose control and vascular outcomes in patients with type 2 diabetes. N Engl J Med. 2008;358:2560–72.

37. Friedewald WT, Buse JB, Bigger JT, Byington RP, Cushman RP, Gerstein HC, et al. Effects of intensive glucose lowering in type 2 diabetes. N Engl J Med. 2008;358:2545–59.

38. Abe M, Okada K, Soma M. Antidiabetic agents in patients with chronic kidney disease and end-stage renal disease on dialysis: metabolism and clinical practice. Curr Drug Metab. 2011;12(1):57–69.

39. Roussel R, Lorraine J, Rodriguez A, Salaun-Martin C. Overview of data concerning the safe use of antihyperglycemic medications in type 2 diabetes mellitus and chronic kidney disease. Adv Ther. 2015;32(11):1029–64.

40. Van Buren PN, Toto R. Hypertension in diabetic nephropathy: epidemiology mechanisms, and management. Adv Chronic Kidney Dis. 2011;18(1):28–41.

41. U.K. Prospective Diabetes Study Group. Tight blood pressure control and risk of macrovascular and microvascular complications in type 2 diabetes: UKPDS 38. BMJ. 1998;317:703–13.

42. NICE. Chronic kidney disease: early identification and management of CKD in adults in primary and secondary care, vol. CG73. London: NICE; 2008. www.nice.org.uk/CG073

43. Bakris GL, Williams M, Dworkin L, Elliot WJ, Epstein M, Toto R, et al. Preserving renal function in adults with hypertension and diabetes: a consensus approach. National Kidney Foundation Hypertension and Diabetes Executive Committees Working Group. Am J Kidney Dis. 2000;36:646–61.

44. Remuzzi G, Macia M, Ruggenenti P. Prevention and treatment of diabetic renal disease in type 2 diabetes: the BENEDICT study. J Am Soc Nephrol. 2006;17(Suppl 2):S90–7.

45. Haller H, Ito S, Izzo JL Jr, Januszewicz A, Katayama S, Menne J, et al. Olmesartan for the delay or prevention of microalbuminuria in type 2 diabetes. N Engl J Med. 2011;364:907–17.

46. Strippoli G, Craig M, Craig J. Antihypertensive agents for preventing diabetic kidney disease. Cochrane Database Syst Rev. 2005;4:CD004136.

47. The ACE Inhibitors in Diabetic Nephropathy Trialist Group. Should all patients with type 1 diabetes mellitus and microalbuminuria receive angiotensin-converting enzyme inhibitors? A meta-analysis of individual patient data. Ann Intern Med. 2001;134:370–9.

48. Irbesartan Diabetic Nephropathy Trial. Collaborative Study Group. Cardiovascular outcomes in the Irbesartan diabetic nephropathy trial of patients with type 2 diabetes and overt nephropathy. Ann Intern Med. 2003;138:542–9.

49. Mauer M, Zinman B, Gardiner R, Suissa S, Sinaiko A, Strand T, et al. Renal and retinal effects of enalapril and losartan in type 1 diabetes. N Engl J Med. 2009;361(1):40–51.

50. de Galan BE, Perkovic V, Ninomiya T, Pillai A, Patel A, Cass A, et al. Lowering blood pressure reduces renal events in type 2 diabetes. J Am Soc Nephrol. 2009;20:883–92.

51. Lipmann ML, Schiffrin EL. What is the ideal blood pressure goal for patients with diabetes mellitus and nephropathy? Curr Cardiol Rep. 2012;14(6):651–9.

52. Andersen NH, Poulsen PL, Knudsen ST, Poulsen SH, Eiskjær H, Hansen KW, et al. Long-term dual blockade with candesartan and lisinopril in hypertensive patients with diabetes: the CALM II study. Diabetes Care. 2005;28:273–7.

53. ON TARGET Investigators. Telmisartan, ramipril, or both in patients at high risk for vascular events. N Engl J Med. 2008;358:1547–59.

54. Fried LF, Emanuele N, Zhang JH, Brophy M, Conner TA, Duckworth W, et al. Combined angiotensin inhibition for the treatment of diabetic nephropathy. N Engl J Med. 2013;369(20):1892–903. https://doi.org/10.1056/NEJMoa1303154.

55. Bakris GL, Agarwal R, Anker SD, Pitt B, Ruilope LM, Rossing P et al.; FIDELIO-DKD Investigators. Effect of finerenone on chronic kidney disease outcomes in type 2 diabetes. N Engl J Med 2020;383:2219–29.

56. Tomson C, Bailey P. Management of chronic kidney disease. Medicine. 2011;39(7):407–13.

57. Wanner C, Tonelli M. KDIGO clinical practice guideline for lipid management in CKD: summary of recommendation statements and clinical approach to the patient. Kidney Int. 2014;85:1303–9.

58. Heine GH, Rogacev KS, Weingärtner O, Marsche G. Still a reasonable goal: targeting cholesterol in dialysis and advanced chronic kidney disease patients. Semin Dial. 2017 Sep;30(5):390–4.

59. Perkovic V, Agarwal R, Fioretto P, Hemmelgarn BR, Levin A, Thomas MC, et al. Conference participants management of patients with diabetes and CKD: conclusions from a "Kidney Disease: Improving Global Outcomes" (KDIGO) controversies conference. Kidney Int. 2016;90(6):1175–83.

60. Kalantar-Zadeh K, Fouque D. Nutritional management of chronic kidney disease. N Engl J Med. 2017;377(18):1765–76. https://doi.org/10.1056/NEJMra1700312.

61. Kidney Disease: Improving Global Outcomes. 2014 Guideline on CKD. Bertram Kasiske. Mandaluyong City. www.kdigo.org.

62. American Diabetes Association. 10. Microvascular complications and foot care: standards of medical care in diabetes—2018. Diabetes Care. 2018;41(Suppl. 1):S105–18. https://doi.org/10.2337/dc18-S010.

63. Ketteler M, Block GA, Evenepoel P, Fukagawa M, Herzog CA, McCann L, et al. Executive summary of the 2017 KDIGO Chronic Kidney Disease-Mineral and Bone Disorder (CKD-MBD) guideline update: what's changed and why it matters. Kidney Int. 2017 Jul;92(1):26–36.

64. Ortega LM, Nayer A. Repercussions of early versus late initiation. Nefrologia. 2011;31(4):392–6.

65. Vassalotti JA, Stevens LA, Levey S. Testing for chronic kidney disease: a position statement from the national kidney foundation. Am J Kidney Dis. 2007;50(2):169–80.

66. Freedman BI, Andries L, Shihabi ZK, Rocco MV, Byers JR, Cardona CY, et al. Glycated albumin and risk of death and hospitalizations in diabetic dialysis patients. Clin J Am Soc Nephrol. 2011;6:1635–43.

67. Furusyo N, Hayashi J. Glycated albumin and diabetes mellitus. Biochim Biophys Acta. 2013;1830:5509–14.

68. Jun JE, Hur KY, Lee YB, Lee SE, Jin SM, Lee MK, Kim JH. Glycated albumin predicts the development of early diabetic nephropathy in patients with type 2 diabetes. Diabetes Metab. 2017. pii: S1262-3636(17)30486-X.

69. de Boer IH. A new chapter for diabetic kidney disease. N Engl J Med. 2017;377(9):885–7. https://doi.org/10.1056/NEJMe1708949.

70. Mosenzon O, LeibowitzG BDL, Cahn A, Hirshberg B, Wei CIK, et al. Effect of saxagliptin on renal outcomes in the SAVOR-TIMI 53 trial. Diabetes Care. 2017;40:69–76.

71. Mann JFE, Ørsted DD, Brown-Frandsen K, Marso SP, Poulter NR, Rasmussen S, et al. LEADER steering committee and investigators. Liraglutide and renal outcomes in type 2 diabetes. N Engl J Med. 2017;377(9):839–48.

72. Wanner C, Inzucchi SE, Lachin JM, Fitchett D, von Eynatten M, Mattheus M, et al. EMPA-REG OUTCOME Investigators. Empagliflozin and progression of kidney disease in type 2 diabetes. N Engl J Med 2016;375:323–334.

73. Guthrie R. Canagliflozin and cardiovascular and renal events in type 2 diabetes. Postgrad Med. 2018;12:1–5.

74. International Diabetes Federation. IDF Diabetes Atlas. 9th edition. International Diabetes Federation 2019. https://diabetesatlas.org/idfawp/resource-files/2019/07/IDF_diabetes_atlas_ninth_edition_en.pdf.

75. Marso SP, Bain SC, Consoli A, Eliaschewitz FG, Jódar E, Leiter LA, et al. SUSTAIN-6 investigators: semaglutide and cardiovascular outcomes in patients with type 2 diabetes. N Engl J Med. 2016;375:1834–44.

76. ClinicalTrials.gov. Renal effects of treatment with empagliflozin alone or in combination with semaglutide in patients with type 2 diabetes and albuminuria (EmpaSema). Available from https://clinicaltrials.gov/ct2/show/NCT04061200. Accessed 11 December 2021

77. Rosenwasser RF, Sultan S, Sutton D, Choksi R, Epstein BJ. SGLT-2 inhibitors and their potential in the treatment of diabetes. Diabetes Metab Syndr Obes. 2013;6:453–67.

78. AstraZeneca. Farxiga (dapagliflozin) prescribing information, 2020. Available from https://den8dhaj6zs0e.cloudfront.net/50fd68b9-106b-4550-b5d0-12b045f8b184/0be9cb1b-3b33-41c7-bfc2-04c9f718e442/0be9cb1b-3b33-41c7-bfc2-04c9f718e442_viewable_rendition__v.pdf. Accessed 11 December 2021

79. Boehringer Ingelheim. Invokana (canagliflozin) prescribing information, 2020. Available from https://docs.boehringeringelheim.com/Prescribing%20 Information/PIs/Jardiance/jardiance.pdf. Accessed 11 December 2021.

80. Wheeler DC, Stefánsson BV, Jongs N, Chertow GM, Greene T Hou FF, et al.; DAPA-CKD Trial Committees and Investigators. Effects of dapagliflozin on major adverse kidney and cardiovascular events in patients with diabetic and nondiabetic chronic kidney disease: a prespecified analysis from the DAPA-CKD trial. Lancet Diabetes Endocrinol. 2021;9:22–31.

81. Katherine R, Tuttle Mark C, Lakshmanan Brian, Rayner Robert S, Busch Alan G, Zimmermann D Bradley, Woodward Fady T, Botros. Dulaglutide versus insulin glargine in patients with type 2 diabetes and moderate-to-severe chronic kidney disease (AWARD-7): a multicentre open-label randomised trial. The Lancet Diabetes & Endocrinology. 2018;6(8):605–17. https://doi.org/10.1016/S2213-8587(18)30104-9.

82. Vilayur E, Harris DC. Emerging therapies for chronic kidney disease: what is their role? Nat Rev Nephrol. 2009;5:375–83.

83. Navarro-González JF, Mora-Fernández C, Muros de Fuentes M, Chahin J, Méndez ML, Gallego E, et al. Effect of pentoxifylline on renal function and urinary albumin excretion in patients with diabetic kidney disease: the PREDIAN trial. J Am Soc Nephrol. 2015;26:220–9.

84. Dhakarwal P, Agrawal V, Kumar A, Goli KM, Agrawal V. Update on role of direct renin inhibitor in diabetic kidney disease. Ren Fail. 2014 Jul;36(6):963–9.

85. Dounousi E, Duni A, Leivaditis K, Vaios V, Eleftheriadis T, Liakopoulos V. Improvements in the management of diabetic nephropathy. Rev Diabet Stud. 2015;12(1–2):119–33.

86. Kimmelstiel P, Wilson C. Intercapillary lesions in the glomeruli in the kidney. Am J Pathol. 1936;12:83–97.

87. Perkovic V, Jardine MJ, Neal B, Bompoint S, Heerspink HJL, Charytan DM, et al.; CREDENCE Trial Investigators. Canagliflozin and renal outcomes in type 2 diabetes and nephropathy. N Engl J Med. 2019;380:2295–06.

88. Gerstein HC, Colhoun HM, Dagenais GR, Diaz R, Lakshmanan M, Pais P et al.; REWIND Investigators. Dulaglutide and renal outcomes in type 2 diabetes: an exploratory analysis of the REWIND randomised, placebo-controlled trial. Lancet. 2019;394:131–38.

The Diabetic Foot

38

Crystal L. Ramanujam, John J. Stapleton, and Thomas Zgonis

Introduction

The entire world is witnessing a steady increase in the prevalence of diabetes mellitus, with foot complications encompassing a large burden of the disease. The impact of diabetic foot complications is felt not only personally by the patient but also by their families, healthcare systems, and economies worldwide. Although the best treatment strategies often start with prevention, many physicians and surgeons are directly faced with the challenge of diabetic foot complications long after they have already been present in the patient for some time. Prompt identification of patients at high risk for diabetic foot complications and quick referral to the appropriate specialists are keys to successful clinical outcomes. As uncontrolled hyperglycemia takes its toll on the patient's body, causing compromise to the circulation and often leading to peripheral sensory neuropathy, a cascade of events may be set in motion leading to foot ulcerations, soft tissue infections, osteomyelitis, amputations, and/or Charcot neuroarthropathy (CN). A strong focus on the appropriate medical and surgical treatment of these clinical entities through a multidisciplinary team may help reduce the overall morbidity and mortality rates associated within this population.

C. L. Ramanujam (✉) · T. Zgonis
Division of Podiatric Medicine and Surgery, Department of Orthopaedics, University of Texas Health San Antonio Long School of Medicine, San Antonio, TX, USA

J. J. Stapleton
LVPG Orthopaedics, Allentown, PA, USA

Division of Podiatric Surgery, Lehigh Valley Hospital, Allentown, PA, USA

Penn State College of Medicine, Hershey, PA, USA

Diabetic Foot Ulcerations and Infections

Nearly all diabetic foot infections stem from an open wound or ulceration [1]. Puncture wounds in the diabetic population are a common inciting event. Chronic pressure in the presence of diabetic peripheral sensory neuropathy and foot deformity may also predispose to the development of ulceration. A thorough history should be obtained to identify the cause of the ulceration, its duration, and prior treatments. Detailed patient medical history may identify other compounding risk factors for complications, such as peripheral arterial disease (PAD), coronary artery disease, hypertension, retinopathy, and nephropathy. Clinical examination should include details about the wound appearance, size and depth, location, and the condition of the surrounding skin. Baseline plain film radiographs of the foot, ankle, and/or lower extremity are imperative and may provide insight on the presence of contributing deformity, osteomyelitis, and/or soft tissue gas. Evaluation for PAD is important since it occurs more often in patients with diabetes mellitus and is also an independent risk factor for cardiovascular death [2]. The degree of PAD may ultimately determine the prognosis for wound healing and/or amputation level. In the presence of a diabetic foot ulcer with concern of arterial insufficiency, investigation with noninvasive vascular testing, including ankle-brachial indexes (ABI), pulse volume recordings, segmental pressures, toe pressures, and transcutaneous oxygen measurements, is highly recommended. A borderline ABI in patients with diabetes mellitus has been associated with significantly higher risks for mortality and PAD compared with normal ABI [3]. Consultation to a vascular surgeon for further evaluation with angiography, subsequent endovascular intervention, and/or open bypass procedures may improve distal perfusion and promote wound healing.

Conservative treatment for non-infected foot and/or ankle wounds in the patient with diabetes mellitus can be initiated via local wound care, off-loading, and tight glycemic control. Local wound care by a specialist may include serial sharp debridement to remove contaminated soft tis-

© Springer Nature Switzerland AG 2022
F. Bandeira et al. (eds.), *Endocrinology and Diabetes*, https://doi.org/10.1007/978-3-030-90684-9_38

sues and reduce biofilm, application of moist wound dressings, other topical products, and/or bioengineered skin substitutes. A number of off-loading devices, including but not limited to surgical shoes, customized multi-density insoles or orthotics, splints, cast walkers, and total contact casts, have been utilized for the treatment of diabetic neuropathic ulcerations with varying degrees of success. The key is to quickly initiate care with an emphasis on control of blood glucose levels. In order to expedite wound healing in the medically optimized patient with diabetes mellitus and depending on certain wound characteristics, surgical wound closure may be considered, such as primary closure, orthobiologics, adjunctive negative pressure wound therapy (NPWT), skin grafting, and a variety of plastic surgical techniques including local random, muscle, or pedicle flaps (Fig. 38.1).

A diabetic foot or ankle wound in the setting of poorly controlled blood glucose levels imposes a significantly high risk for subsequent infection [4]. Wound chronicity, impaired immune response, reduced blood flow, and nerve damage in the feet are all factors that may contribute to the development of infection. Clinical manifestations of acute infection may include cellulitis, warmth, pain, malodor, abscess or overt draining purulence, necrotic tissues, deep tissue or bone exposure, or necrotizing fasciitis. However, chronic infection of diabetic foot or ankle wounds may lack these clinical findings. Initial testing should include plain film radiographs of the foot, ankle, and leg, as clinically indicated. Laboratory testing with complete blood cell count, comprehensive metabolic profile, inflammatory markers, and glycosylated hemoglobin A1C provide further information related to infection severity and hemodynamic stability.

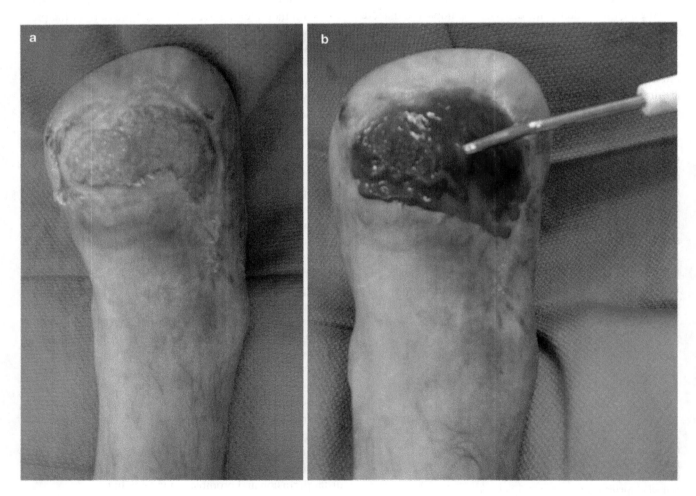

Fig. 38.1 Preoperative clinical picture of a left midfoot amputation with a chronic non-healing wound (**a**) that underwent hydrosurgical excisional debridement with wound bed preparation (**b, c**) and application of acellular dermal replacement (**d**)

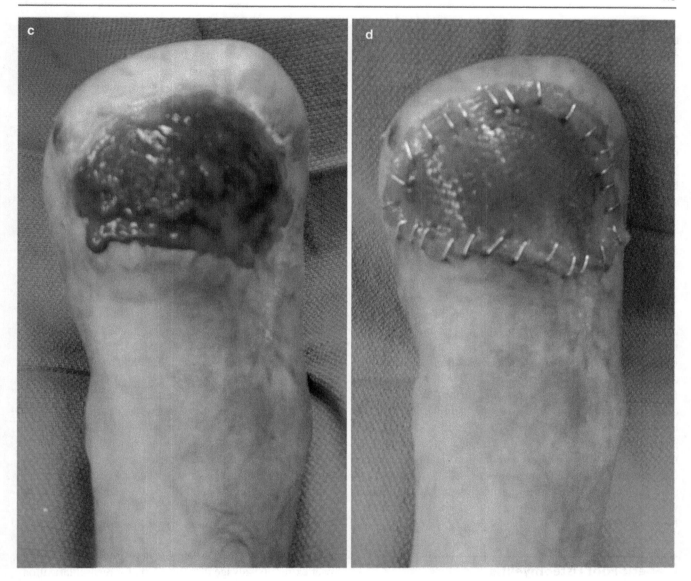

Fig. 38.1 (continued)

The Infectious Diseases Society of America (IDSA) classification of clinical infection can assist in deciding outpatient versus inpatient management: mild (superficial and limited in size and depth), moderate (deeper or more extensive), or severe (accompanied by systemic signs of metabolic perturbations) [5]. Patients with diabetes mellitus and systemic toxicity (fever and leukocytosis), metabolic imbalance, progressive deep soft tissue or bone infection, gangrene, or evidence of critical lower extremity ischemia should be immediately hospitalized. In some cases, the first diagnosis of diabetes mellitus may occur when the patient presents to an emergency facility as the incidence of diabetic foot infection increases the risk of hospitalization and amputation [6]. In cases where initial pedal radiographs show soft tissue

emphysema or gas, computed tomography (CT) of the affected lower extremity can identify proximal foot, ankle, and/or leg involvement, indicating the need for urgent/emergent surgical procedures. Magnetic resonance imaging (MRI) is helpful for localization of underlying abscess with devitalized tissues and may indicate the presence of osteomyelitis. MRI has been reported helpful in the identification of diabetic CN; however, the findings are difficult to separate from osteomyelitis in the setting of open wounds [7]. Nuclear imaging may be warranted in such cases of diabetic CN and/or with history of prior surgery and retained hardware.

Inpatient medical management of diabetic foot infections relies on antibiotic therapy and begins with broad-spectrum intravenous antibiotic(s) until reliable intraoperative deep cultures and bone biopsy are available. Although most diabetic foot infections are polymicrobial, the most common pathogenic organisms are *Staphylococcus* and *Streptococcus* species; therefore, initial antibiotics are typically chosen with activity against gram-positive bacteria [5]. Antibiotics targeted at multidrug-resistant organisms, such as methicillin-resistant *Staphylococcus aureus* and vancomycin-resistant *Enterococcus*, should be considered in patients who have been previously hospitalized and/or have prior history of diabetic foot osteomyelitis. In many of these complicated diabetic foot infections, consultation of an infectious disease specialist is helpful to determine the correct antibiotic choice and the duration of treatment.

Surgical intervention should be initiated for early and aggressive excisional debridement of the acutely infected tissues, including decompression of all involved compartments. Multiple surgical debridements may be necessary to eradicate all of the infection, with careful attention directed at preserving viable tissue and vascularity for definitive wound closure and/or consideration for later soft tissue reconstruction. The majority of successful cases in treating diabetic foot infections have used some combination of antibiotics and surgical debridement [8]. Wound healing can then be facilitated by the use of NPWT and further off-loading by either conventional methods or via surgical off-loading through external fixation based on individual patient and procedure characteristics [9, 10]. Surgical off-loading with the utilization of circular external fixation can provide a stable construct that will protect any major soft tissue reconstruction and allow for an appropriate rehabilitation regimen without any weight-bearing activity at the reconstructed lower extremity.

Diabetic Foot Osteomyelitis and Amputations

Diabetic foot osteomyelitis remains a growing challenge to physicians and surgeons alike, comprising an estimated 50% of all severe diabetic foot infections [11]. Most of these cases originate from contiguous spread of infection from an adjacent open wound or infected soft tissue. The initial clinical evaluation and diagnostic workup for osteomyelitis is similar to that of the other previously mentioned diabetic foot infections. Inflammatory markers such as erythrocyte sedimentation rate and C-reactive protein are important tests as a baseline at initial presentation and should be performed every few days during hospitalization as indicators for response to treatment. Plain film radiographs of the foot, ankle, and/or lower extremity are necessary; however, these may be negative in early osteomyelitis. Radiographic findings of osteomyelitis may include ill-defined cortical erosions adjacent to the ulceration and focal osteopenia

corresponding to trabecular lysis [12, 13]. Bony destruction may be apparent depending on the chronicity of infection, while soft tissue or intra-osseous gas can be present in advanced cases and warrants emergent surgical intervention. Nuclear imaging and newer advanced imaging techniques can be utilized for detailed surgical planning in complicated cases of diabetic foot osteomyelitis.

With regard to diabetic foot osteomyelitis, the literature includes varying levels of evidence for antibiotic therapy with or without limited surgical excision versus wide resection, and/or major or minor amputation [14–17]. Antibiotic therapy must be guided by reliable intraoperative bone cultures and bone biopsy. Knowledge of the foot and ankle angiosomes with careful consideration for the level of viable soft tissue and bone combined with the level of intact vascular perfusion should guide surgeons in choosing the appropriate level of debridement and/or amputation [18]. A number of minor foot amputations exist including resection of isolated toes, partial ray(s) (toe with partial corresponding metatarsal), transmetatarsal, tarsometatarsal (Lisfranc), midtarsal (Chopart), and calcanectomies. Multiple staged surgical debridements may be required, and the use of local antibiotic delivery systems in the form of beads or spacers can be considered to provide an infection-free yet mechanically stable environment for delayed reconstruction [19] (Fig. 38.2). The use of NPWT can aid in wound bed preparation prior to definitive surgical wound closure [20] (Fig. 38.3). Once infection is resolved and to address residual open wounds, split-thickness skin grafting has been shown successful in achieving wound closure for diabetic partial foot amputations [21].

In cases where severe soft tissue infection and osteomyelitis involves the entire foot or is extending proximally to the leg or when arterial perfusion is not sufficient for diabetic lower extremity salvage despite efforts for revascularization, major amputation plays a role as the next option. In patients with diabetes mellitus, risk factors for major lower extremity amputation include longer duration of diabetes mellitus, poor glycemic control, higher systolic blood pressure, and treatment with insulin [22]. Interestingly over the past 10–15 years, studies have shown a 40–60% reduction in rates of lower extremity amputation in Australia, Denmark, Spain, Sweden, the United Kingdom, and the United States; however, there are no such data estimates for low- or middle-income countries where the prevalence of diabetes mellitus is growing the most rapidly [6]. Rehabilitation following an amputation can be facilitated by physical and occupational therapy services at home or in skilled nursing facilities if necessary. Even after healing has been achieved following surgical debridement and/or amputation, patients with diabetes mellitus must continue active participation in preventive health measures since they are at high risk for re-ulceration, readmission for infection, and further amputation.

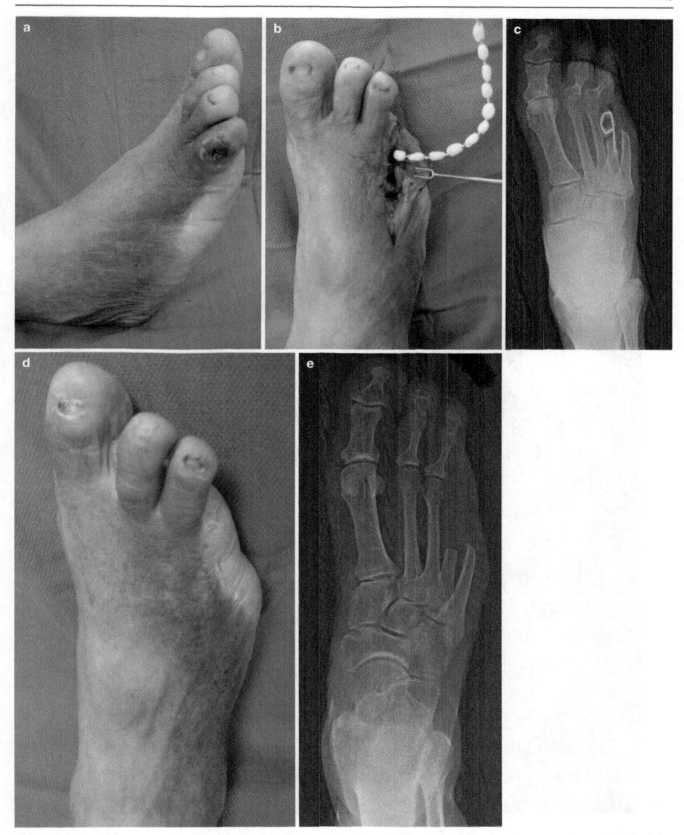

Fig. 38.2 Preoperative clinical picture of a right foot fourth toe osteomyelitis and abscess (**a**) that underwent an initial fourth toe amputation at the metatarsophalangeal joint followed by a partial fourth metatarsal resection and application of cemented non-biodegradable antibiotic beads 3 days after the original surgery (**b, c**). The patient returned to the operating room for the removal of the cemented non-biodegradable antibiotic beads and further excisional debridement at approximately 10 weeks postoperatively. Final clinical (**d**) and radiographic (**e**) pictures at approximately 5½ months after the initial fourth toe amputation surgery

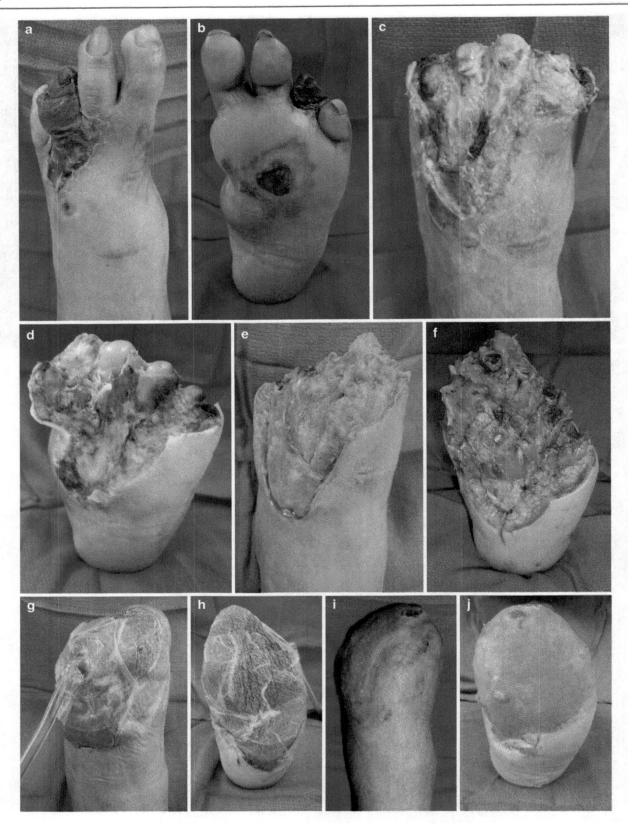

Fig. 38.3 Preoperative clinical pictures of a left foot severe diabetic foot infection with osteomyelitis and gangrene (**a, b**) that underwent staged partial foot amputation and surgical debridement (**c, d**) followed by a revisional modified transmetatarsal amputation and application of a negative pressure wound therapy device 5 days after the initial surgery (**e–h**). Clinical pictures at approximately 2½ months postoperatively showing the adequate granulation tissue and wound bed preparation by the use of negative pressure wound therapy as an adjunct before the definitive plastic wound closure reconstruction (**i, j**)

Diabetic Charcot Neuroarthropathy

CN is a joint disease involving inflammation which produces progressive fractures and/or dislocations that may result in severe foot and ankle deformities, causing potential for skin ulceration and infection. Although CN can be a complication of several types of peripheral neuropathy, diabetic peripheral neuropathy is now the leading cause of CN in the Western world, and each patient with diabetes mellitus and peripheral sensory neuropathy should be screened and educated about the risk of this potentially debilitating foot and ankle condition [23]. Most diabetic CN cases can be traced to some type of inciting trauma. Since 1936 when William Riely Jordan first described diabetic CN, research has grown regarding its pathophysiology and treatment, yet there is substantial variability in the existing literature [24]. Several classification systems exist; however, the most useful descriptions of diabetic CN seem to include whether the process is acute versus chronic or active versus inactive and whether the deformity is rigid versus flexible or stable versus unstable.

Clinically, acute diabetic CN presents with a warm, swollen, erythematous unilateral foot, ankle, and/or lower extremity, which can often be mistaken for conditions such as infection, deep vein thrombosis, gout, sprain, or cellulitis. Initial diagnostic testing is typically based on ruling out other differential diagnoses. Plain film radiographs of the foot, ankle, and/or lower extremity are required, but a lack of radiographic changes during the initial stages of diabetic CN does not exclude the diagnosis. A series of weight-bearing foot, ankle, lower extremity, and long-leg calcaneal axial views should be obtained. Advanced imaging with MRI and bone scintigraphy has been shown to be more sensitive in detecting subacute to early acute diabetic CN [25]. CT scans are useful for surgical planning in cases of advanced diabetic CN subluxations and dislocations. Laboratory workup may be of little value in this diabetic population since the initial results may not show significance in the immunocompromised patient. Initial immobilization of the involved lower extremity constitutes ideal conservative management in order to prevent further dislocation and/or deformity; however, the long-term total off-loading with casts or braces is often met with low levels of compliance. Further clinical observation along with serial plain film radiographs is required to determine the need for extended immobilization and protective weight-bearing if diabetic CN is suspected. Unfortunately, even with the early recognition of diabetic CN, certain deformities are not amenable to conservative treatment and require surgical reconstruction in order to establish a lower extremity that is braceable, functional, and non-ulcerated.

In contrast, the ulcerated diabetic CN foot and/or ankle deformity can present with or without infection and poses even greater risk for hospitalization and major amputation [26]. Ulcerations associated with diabetic CN require the same thorough clinical evaluation and diagnostic workup as mentioned for isolated diabetic foot ulcerations or infections. PAD may be found in patients with ulcerated diabetic CN, and vascular assessment with vascular surgery consultation is highly recommended before surgical intervention. Severely infected ulcerations with diabetic CN with or without osteomyelitis can be limb- or life-threatening and require hospitalization of the patient for medical optimization, systemic antibiotic therapy, and surgical intervention.

Patients with diabetic CN may require extensive reconstructive foot and ankle surgery if salvage of the lower extremity is attempted. Surgical procedures directed to address diabetic CN vary depending on the presence of soft tissue loss, infection, and/or arterial insufficiency in conjunction with the location and degree of the associated deformity. Deformity correction involves joint realignment and arthrodesis procedures at the midfoot, rearfoot, and/or ankle level with internal fixation typically reserved for cases without ulceration or infection and external fixation utilized for deformities with a poor soft tissue envelope, ulceration, and/or infection [27] (Fig. 38.4). In selected patients with a chronic foot ulceration and a stable diabetic CN, osseous exostectomies with or without wound closure may be sufficient for wound healing. While available surgical reconstructive techniques have substantially improved over the years, conclusive reliable data to guide surgical treatment is lacking due to the large variability found in patient and procedure selection. Finally, close postoperative monitoring of the reconstructed diabetic CN patient with appropriate orthosis/bracing and long-term medical management of diabetes mellitus is crucial in order to avoid any future complications.

Studies have shown higher lower extremity amputation and mortality rates of patients with diabetic CN as compared to diabetes mellitus alone, yet lower extremity amputation and mortality outcomes for surgically reconstructed diabetic CN of the foot and ankle are relatively scarce in the literature [26, 28, 29]. A single retrospective study of circular external fixation for foot/ankle diabetic CN found that the mortality rate associated with osteomyelitis was higher than that without osteomyelitis, which was statistically significant [30]. Although the overall morbidity and mortality rates were low for that study, the authors determined that several risk factors potentially contribute to the outcomes of surgical reconstruction for diabetic CN.

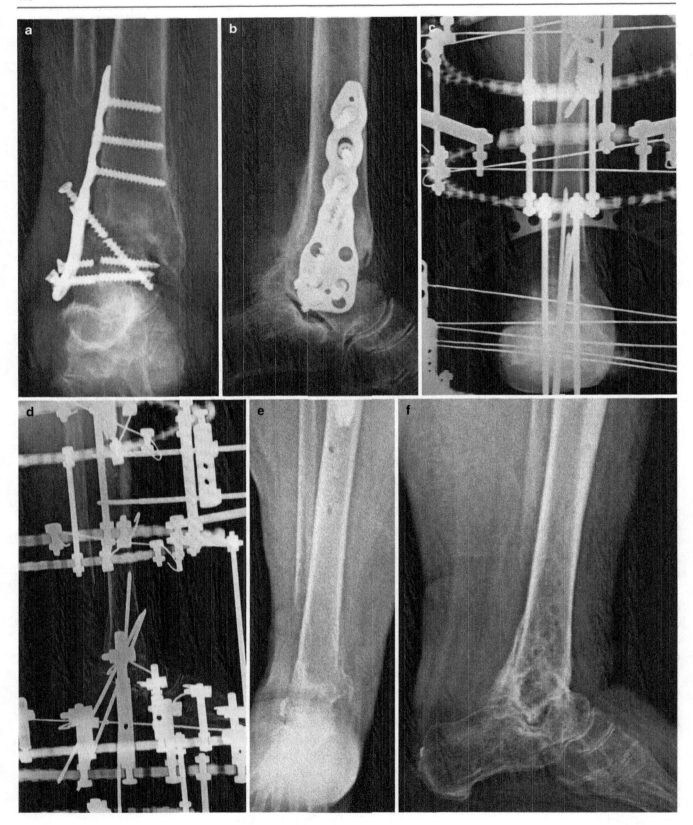

Fig. 38.4 Preoperative anteroposterior (**a**) and lateral (**b**) lower extremity radiographs showing an attempted ankle arthrodesis with infected nonunion and broken hardware in a morbid obese patient with uncontrolled diabetes mellitus. Postoperative anteroposterior (**c**) and lateral (**d**) lower extremity radiographs showing removal of the infected hardware and revisional ankle arthrodesis with a multiplane circular external fixation device. The patient was also receiving intravenous antibiotic therapy for 6 weeks based on intraoperative cultures. The circular external fixation device was removed at 16 weeks. Patient was placed in a short leg cast for 4 more weeks and then resumed ambulation with a shoe and a double upright brace. Final radiographs at 10 months postoperatively reveal successful union and alignment (**e**, **f**)

Conclusion

While prevention is the optimal tool in tackling the burden of diabetic foot complications, early diagnosis of the problem(s) and immediate referral into a comprehensive treatment program that includes all indicated medical and surgical specialists with an interest in the diabetic foot are vital to meeting these ongoing challenges. The diversity of clinical manifestations encompassing the diabetic foot highlights the need for a well-equipped multidisciplinary healthcare setting where treatment of every patient can be properly customized.

References

1. Lavery LA, Armstrong DG, Wunderlich RP, Mohler MJ, Wendel CS, Lipsky BA. Risk factors for foot infections in individuals with diabetes. Diabetes Care. 2006;29:1288–93.
2. Brownrigg JR, Apelqvist J, Bakker K, Schaper NC, Hinchliffe RJ. Evidence-based management of PAD & the diabetic foot. Eur J Vasc Endovasc Surg. 2013;45:673–81.
3. Natsuaki C, Inoguchi T, Maeda Y, Yamada T, Sasaki S, Sonoda N, et al. Association of borderline ankle-brachial index with mortality and the incidence of peripheral artery disease in diabetic patients. Atherosclerosis. 2014;234:360–5.
4. Jia L, Parker CN, Parker TJ, Kinnear EM, Derhy PH, Alvarado AM, et al. Incidence and risk factors for developing infection in patients presenting with uninfected diabetic foot ulcers. PLoS One. 2017;12(5):e0177916.
5. Lipsky BA, Berendt AR, Cornia PB, Pile JC, Peters EJ, Armstrong DG, et al. Executive summary: 2012 Infectious Diseases Society of America clinical practice guideline for the diagnosis and treatment of diabetic foot infections. Clin Infect Dis. 2012;54:1679–84.
6. Moxey PW, Gogalniceanu P, Hinchliffe RJ, Loftus IM, Jones KJ, Thompson MM, et al. Lower extremity amputations--a review of global variability in incidence. Diabet Med. 2011;28:1144–53.
7. Short DJ, Zgonis T. Medical imaging in differentiating the diabetic Charcot foot from osteomyelitis. Clin Podiatr Med Surg. 2017;34:9–14.
8. Aragón-Sánchez FJ, Cabrera-Galván JJ, Quintana-Marrero Y, Hernández-Herrero MJ, Lázaro-Martínez JL, García-Morales E, et al. Outcomes of surgical treatment of diabetic foot osteomyelitis: a series of 185 patients with histopathological confirmation of bone involvement. Diabetologia. 2008;51:1962–70.
9. Clemens MW, Parikh P, Hall MM, Attinger CE. External fixators as an adjunct to wound healing. Foot Ankle Clin. 2008;13:145–56.
10. Ramanujam CL, Facaros Z, Zgonis T. External fixation for surgical off-loading of diabetic soft tissue reconstruction. Clin Podiatr Med Surg. 2011;28:211–6.
11. Lipsky BA, Berendt AR, Deery HG, Embil JM, Joseph WS, Karchmer AW, et al. Diagnosis and treatment of diabetic foot infections. Clin Infect Dis. 2005;39:885–910.
12. Gold RH, Tong DJF, Crim JR, Seeger LL. Imaging the diabetic foot. Skelet Radiol. 1995;24:563–71.
13. Mandell JC, Khurana B, Smith JT, Czuczman GJ, Ghazikhanian V, Smith SE. Osteomyelitis of the lower extremity: pathophysiology, imaging, and classification, with an emphasis on diabetic foot infection. Emerg Radiol. 2017;25(2):175–88.
14. Grayson ML, Gibbons GW, Habershaw GM, Freeman DV, Pomposelli FB, Rosenblum BI, et al. Use of ampicillin/sulbactam versus imipenem/cilastatin in the treatment of limb-threatening foot infections in diabetic patients. Clin Infect Dis. 1994;18:683–93.
15. Venkatesan P, Lawn S, Macfarlane RM, Fletcher EM, Finch RG, Jeffcoate WJ. Conservative management of osteomyelitis in the feet of diabetic patients. Diabet Med. 1997;14:487–90.
16. Berendt AR, Peters EJ, Bakker K, Embil JM, Eneroth M, Hinchliffe RJ, et al. Specific guidelines for treatment of diabetic foot osteomyelitis. Diabetes Metab Res Rev. 2008;24(Suppl 1):S190–1.
17. Aragón-Sánchez J. Treatment of diabetic foot osteomyelitis: a surgical critique. Int J Low Extrem Wounds. 2010;9:37–59.
18. Clemens MW, Attinger CE. Angiosomes and wound care in the diabetic foot. Foot Ankle Clin. 2010;15:439–64.
19. Ramanujam CL, Zgonis T. Antibiotic-loaded cement beads for Charcot ankle osteomyelitis. Foot Ankle Spec. 2010;3:274–7.
20. Ramanujam CL, Zgonis T. Surgical soft tissue closure of severe diabetic foot infections: a combination of biologics, negative pressure wound therapy, and skin grafting. Clin Podiatr Med Surg. 2012;29:143–6.
21. Ramanujam CL, Zgonis T. Stepwise surgical approach to diabetic partial foot amputations with autogenous split thickness skin grafting. Diabet Foot Ankle. 2016 Jun;8(7):27751.
22. Davis WA, Norman PE, Bruce DG, Davis TM. Predictors, consequences and cost of diabetes-related lower extremity amputation complicating type 2 diabetes: the Fremantle Diabetes Study. Diabetologia. 2006;49:2634–41.
23. Robinson AH, Pasapula C, Brodsky JW. Surgical aspects of the diabetic foot. J Bone Joint Surg Br. 2009;91:1–7.
24. Ramanujam CL, Zgonis T. The diabetic Charcot foot from 1936 to 2016: eighty years later and still growing. Clin Podiatr Med Surg. 2017;34:1–8.
25. Ranachowska C, Lass P, Korzon-Burakowska A, Dobosz M. Diagnostic imaging of the diabetic foot. Nucl Med Rev Cent East Eur. 2010;13:18–22.
26. Sohn MW, Stuck RM, Pinzur M, Lee TA, Budiman-Mak E. Lower-extremity amputation risk after Charcot arthropathy and diabetic foot ulcer. Diabetes Care. 2010;33:98–100.
27. Stapleton JJ, Zgonis T. Surgical reconstruction of the diabetic Charcot foot: internal, external or combined fixation? Clin Podiatr Med Surg. 2012;29:425–33.
28. Gazis A, Pound N, Macfarlane R, Treece K, Game F, Jeffcoate W. Mortality in patients with diabetic neuropathic osteoarthropathy (Charcot foot). Diabet Med. 2004;21:1243–6.
29. Sohn MW, Lee TA, Stuck RM, Frykberg RG, Budiman-Mak E. Mortality risk of Charcot arthropathy compared with that of diabetic foot ulcer and diabetes alone. Diabetes Care. 2009;32:816–21.
30. Ramanujam CL, Han D, Zgonis T. Lower extremity amputation and mortality rates in the reconstructed diabetic Charcot foot and ankle with external fixation: data analysis of 116 patients. Foot Ankle Spec. 2016;9:113–26.

Diabetic Retinopathy

Daniel Araujo Ferraz and Paulo Escarião

Introduction

Diabetic retinopathy (DR) is one of the most feared microvascular complications of diabetes mellitus (DM), due to the functional disability that it causes, and is considered an important cause of blindness in the economically active population [1]. The Wisconsin Epidemiologic Study of Diabetic Retinopathy (WESDR) has shown that the type and duration of DM are important factors for the onset and progression of DR. After 20 years of illness, more than 90% of type 1 DM patients and 60% of those with type 2 will have some degree of retinopathy. In DR, the main cause of visual loss is macular edema, which may be present from the early stages of retinopathy to cases in which there is severe proliferative disease, affecting 30% of patients with more than 20 years of diabetes [2].

In Brazil, there are still no studies that accurately demonstrate the prevalence of DR. However, studies carried out in different regions of the country report an incidence of 24–39% of cases, being the highest frequency in individuals residing in non-metropolitan areas [3–5]. By evaluating the available statistics, with percentages adapted from other countries, it is estimated that approximately two million Brazilians have some degree of DR, and it can be assumed that a significant proportion of these individuals will present visual loss related to the disease. In a population study, the incidence of macular edema was determined according to the type and duration of DM. Above 10 years of disease, the incidence of diabetic macular edema (DMD) in patients with type 1 DM, type 2 DM users of insulin, and type 2 DM who did not use insulin was 20.1%, 25. 4%, and 13.9%, respectively. In this same study, the incidence of DMD in 10 years of disease for both types of DM was associated with high glycated hemoglobin, increased diastolic blood pressure, and more advanced retinopathy. The risk of blindness from RD can be reduced to less than 5% when the diagnosis is made in a timely manner and the treatment done correctly before irreversible changes can be established [6].

The cause of DR is multifactorial, and the primary contributor likely is chronic capillary non-perfusion and retinal ischemia. The signaling molecules insulin-like growth factor-1, platelet-derived growth factor, angiopoietin, and most importantly vascular endothelial growth factor (VEGF) all play a role in the subsequent development of microangiopathy [7]. Recent evidence also suggests that neurodegeneration is an early event in the pathogenesis of DR. From a clinical standpoint, it is clear that the primary driving factor in this pathogenesis is uncontrolled blood glucose levels, with blood pressure and blood lipid composition also playing important roles. The diagnosis of DR remains clinical in nature. The gold standard for diagnosis is a dilated eye exam and serial fundus photos (Table 39.1) [8, 9].

Glycemic control is the main risk factor for the onset and progression of DR, being evaluated by the measurement of glycated hemoglobin. The UKPD-UK Prospective Diabetic Study

D. A. Ferraz (✉)
Department of Ophthalmology, Universidade Federal de São Paulo, São Paulo, SP, Brazil

NIHR Biomedical Research Centre for Ophthalmology, Moorfields Eye Hospital, NHS Foundation Trust and UCL, Institute of Ophthalmology, London, UK

P. Escarião
H.Olhos Piedade - Recife, PE, Brazil

Hospital de Olhos de Pernambuco - Recife, PE, Brazil

Table 39.1 Frequency of ophthalmologic examination for diabetic patients

Clinical feature	First eye examination	Follow-up
Diabetes type 1	Within 5 years diagnosis	Annually
Diabetes type 2	Upon diagnosis	Annually
Diabetes and pregnancy	In the first trimester	Every 3 months
Normal eye examination	–	Annually
NPDR mild to moderate	–	Every 6 months
NPDR severe	–	Every 4 months
PDR	–	Every 2–3 months[a]

[a]Consider specific eye treatment

© Springer Nature Switzerland AG 2022
F. Bandeira et al. (eds.), *Endocrinology and Diabetes*, https://doi.org/10.1007/978-3-030-90684-9_39

(UKPDS) 8 evaluated 3867 patients with newly diagnosed type 2 DM for 10 years. This randomized clinical trial demonstrated that intensive glycemic control allows a reduction of about 25% in the risk of microvascular complications, including HV and need for photocoagulation, when compared to the conventional treatment group. The Diabetes Control and Complications Trial (DCCT), a study of 1441 patients with type 1 DM and 6.5 years of follow-up, showed that rigorous glycemic control has adverse effects [1]. Among them, there is a risk of an early worsening of DR; this occurred in 13.1% of those belonging to the strict control group versus 7.6% of those belonging to the conventional treatment group. However, this effect was reversed at 18 months; no case of early worsening progressed with severe visual loss. Since glycemic control, the most important independent risk factor for DR, the patient should be instructed to adhere consistently to clinical treatment to prevent the onset and reduce the progression of DR. [2].

Classification

The retinal ischemia that occurs due to the thickening of the basement membrane of the capillaries induces a tissue response through the production of vascular endothelial growth factor (VEGF) to form new retinal vessels [10]. The absence or presence of this retinal neovascularization divides the DR classification into forms:

1. Nonproliferative (NPDR): *without* neovascularization
2. Proliferative (PDR): *with* neovascularization

NPDR is the initial form of the disease with formation of small dilations in the wall of capillaries (microaneurysms), leakage of lipids to the extravascular space (hard exudates), ischemia in the nerve fiber layer (cotton wool spots), microhemorrhages, intraretinal microvascular abnormalities (IRMAs), and venous changes (venous loop, beading) [11]. Depending on these findings, it can be subdivided into NPDR:

- Mild
- Moderate
- Severe

Patients with severe NPDR have a 15% chance of progression to PDR within 1 year [12].

PDR is the most advanced form of diabetic retinopathy. The new blood vessels have a very thin wall and are also found with fibroglial proliferation process that can lead to vitreous hemorrhage and retinal detachment with consequent severe visual impairment [12]. It can be subdivided into PDR:

- Early
- High-risk
- Advanced

So, the evolution of DR is gradual: the patients at the beginning of the retinopathy present with the mild form of NPDR, and as the process progresses, they pass to the moderate form, then to the severe form, but still without new vessels. If the disease evolves and new vessels appear, the patient is classified into the proliferative form of the disease.

Maculopathy

Diabetic macular edema (DME) occurs due to increased permeability of capillaries by reduction of tight junctions and formation of microaneurysms, with accumulation of liquid and lipids in the macular area. It is the main cause of decreased central visual acuity, occurring in about 10% of the diabetic population. The ETDRS classified DME in clinically significant macular edema (CSME) [13] for patients who had a higher risk of visual impairment if they presented the following characteristics:

1. Retinal thickening at or within 500 microns of center of the fovea
2. Hard exudates at or within 500 microns of the center of the fovea if associated with retinal thickening
3. One disc area or larger of retinal thickening within 1 disc diameter of the center of the fovea (Figs. 39.1 and 39.2)

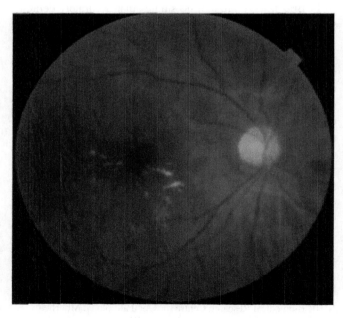

Figs. 39.1 and 39.2 Patient with nonproliferative diabetic retinopathy (microaneurysms and microhemorrhages) and clinically significant macular edema (hard exudates at or within 500 microns of the center of the fovea if associated with retinal thickening) in both eyes

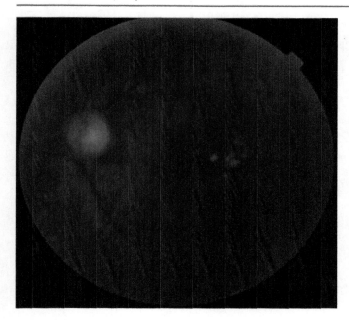

Figs. 39.1 and 39.2 (continued)

Treatment

Medical management of DR with good glycemic, lipid, and blood pressure controls, as well as exercise practice and cessation of smoking, is essential to reduce progression of the disease. Among these, glycemic control is the most important factor. Data from the UKPDS and DCCT have shown that glycemic control is associated with reduction of disease onset or reduction of disease progression [14, 15].

The indication of DR ophthalmologic treatment depends on the presence of macular edema and the stage of the disease. Treatment options include injecting drugs into the vitreous cavity (pharmacological therapy), laser photocoagulation, or vitrectomy surgery [16, 17].

Patients presenting with PDR should undergo panretinal laser photocoagulation. Recent studies have also demonstrated the efficacy of intravitreal antiangiogenics for stabilization and regression of new vessels. Vitreoretinal surgery is indicated for the most advanced cases of the disease when the patient develops vitreous hemorrhage or retinal detachment [18].

References

1. Klein R, Klein BE, Moss SE. Epidemiology of proliferative diabetic retinopathy. Diabetes Care [Internet]. 1992. [cited 2014 Jan 30];15(12):1875–91.

2. Klein R, Klein BE, Moss SE, Cruickshanks KJ. The Wisconsin Epidemiologic Study of Diabetic Retinopathy: XVII. The 14-year incidence and progression of diabetic retinopathy and associated risk factors in type 1 diabetes. Ophthalmology [Internet]. 1998. [cited 2014 Jan 30];105(10):1801–15.

3. Taleb AC, Ávila M, Moreira H. As condições de saúde ocular no Brasil. 1a ed. São Paulo: Conselho Brasileiro de Oftalmologia; 2009.

4. Ramos SR, Sabbag FP, Busato D, et al. Retinopatia diabética: estudo de uma associação de diabéticos. Arq Bras Oftalmol. 1999;62:735–7.

5. Foss MC, Paccola GMGF, Souza NV, Iazigi N. Estudo analítico de uma amostra populacional de diabéticos tipo II da região de Ribeirão Preto (SP). AMB Rev Assoc Med Bras. 1989;35(5):179–83.

6. Ferris FL III. How effective are treatments for diabetic retinopathy? J Am Med Assoc. 1993;269:1290–1.

7. Simó R, Hernández C. Novel approaches for treating diabetic retinopathy based on recent pathogenic evidence. Prog Retin Eye Res. 2015;48:160–80.

8. Stem MS, Gardner TW. Neurodegeneration in the pathogenesis of diabetic retinopathy: molecular mechanisms and therapeutic implications. Curr Med Chem. 2013;20(26):3241–50.

9. Simó R, Hernández C, European Consortium for the Early Treatment of Diabetic Retinopathy (EUROCONDOR). Neurodegeneration in the diabetic eye: new insights and therapeutic perspectives. Trends Endocrinol Metab. 2014;25(1):23–33.

10. Stewart JM, Coassin M, Schwartz DM. In: De Groot LJ, Chrousos G, Dungan K, Feingold KR, Grossman A, Hershman JM, et al., editors. Diabetic retinopathy. South Dartmouth; 2000.

11. Wu L, Fernandez-Loaiza P, Sauma J, Hernandez-Bogantes E, Masis M. Classification of diabetic retinopathy and diabetic macular edema. World J Diabetes. 2013;4(6):290–4.

12. Early Treatment Diabetic Retinopathy Study Research Group. Early photocoagulation for diabetic retinopathy. ETDRS report number 9. Ophthalmology. 1991;98(5 Suppl):766–85.

13. Early Treatment Diabetic Retinopathy Study Research Group. Focal photocoagulation treatment of diabetic macular edema. Relationship of treatment effect to fluorescein angiographic and other retinal characteristics at baseline: ETDRS report no. 19. Arch Ophthalmol. 1995;113(9):1144–55.

14. Lachin JM, White NH, Hainsworth DP, Sun W, Cleary PA, Nathan DM. Effect of intensive diabetes therapy on the progression of diabetic retinopathy in patients with type 1 diabetes: 18 years of follow-up in the DCCT/EDIC. Diabetes. 2015;64(2):631–42.

15. Zoungas S, Arima H, Gerstein HC, Holman RR, Woodward M, Reaven P, et al. Effects of intensive glucose control on microvascular outcomes in patients with type 2 diabetes: a meta-analysis of individual participant data from randomised controlled trials. Lancet Diabetes Endocrinol. 2017;5(6):431–7.

16. Ho AC, Scott IU, Kim SJ, Brown GC, Brown MM, Ip MS, et al. Anti-vascular endothelial growth factor pharmacotherapy for diabetic macular edema: a report by the American Academy of Ophthalmology. Ophthalmology. 2012;119(10):2179–88.

17. Elman MJ, Aiello LP, Beck RW, Bressler NM, Bressler SB, Edwards AR, et al. Randomized trial evaluating ranibizumab plus prompt or deferred laser or triamcinolone plus prompt laser for diabetic macular edema. Ophthalmology. 2010;117(6):1064–1077.e35.

18. Jampol LM, Odia I, Glassman AR, Baker CW, Bhorade AM, Han DP, et al. Panretinal photocoagulation versus ranibizumab for proliferative diabetic retinopathy: comparison of peripapillary retinal nerve fiber layer thickness. In: A randomized clinical trial. Philadelphia: Retina; 2017.

Carbohydrate Counting

40

Maria da Conceição Chaves de Lemos

What Is Carbohydrate Counting?

It is a tool to help diabetics program their intake of food, by means of which the amount of carbohydrate prescribed is what will define the amount of regular or ultra-rapid insulin necessary for the meal recommended by the dietitian specializing in diabetes. Thus, besides adapting the dose to individual sensitivity, glycemic control is optimized when the patient follows medical advice as to counting their carbohydrate intake. The American Diabetes Association in 2018 recommend "for people with type 1 diabetes and those with type 2 diabetes who are prescribed a flexible insulin therapy program, education on how to use carbohydrate counting and in some cases fat and protein gram estimation to determine mealtime insulin dosing is recommended to improve glycemic control" as a level of evidence [1].

A systematic review and meta-analysis of randomized controlled trials of interventions longer than 3 months compared carbohydrate counting with general or alternate dietary advice in adults and children with type 1 diabetes. This analysis showed that there was some evidence to support the recommendation of carbohydrate counting in usual care in adults with type 1 diabetes, but in children, differences in the study design probably induced heterogeneity between studies [2]. Carbohydrate counting remains a standard method of administering meal-related insulin in most centers. This was the conclusion of a consensus that was published in 2015.

The researchers found that some type 1 diabetics do not consult their doctor regularly because they consider themselves self-sufficient, but it is important they maintain carbohydrate counting to optimize their treatment and make any necessary adjustment to basal insulin as advised by the health time. Nevertheless, although this behavior occurs in some situations, this method continues to be useful and effective [3].

Who Should Do Carbohydrate Counting?

Counting carbohydrates is a useful tool when setting the diabetic's diet. If we started by asking who should do carbohydrate counting, we would come to the conclusion that it is important that all diabetics should do so. If today those who use only diet therapy to control blood sugar consume, for example, 60 g of carbohydrates at breakfast and double that amount for the same meal at weekends, their glucose levels will rise. Those who also make use of oral hypoglycemic agents in an amount that does not vary from the medication but alters their consumption of carbohydrates will suffer from hyperglycemia on the days that they eat more carbohydrates.

Currently, there are two schemes of insulinization: the conventional one, using two applications per day of prolonged action insulin, 2/3 of the dose in the morning and 1/3 before dinner or at bedtime, and an intensive one that uses long-acting insulin, representing the basal dose, along with the rapid-acting (regular) or ultra-rapid (UR) insulin, both of which should be applied before the meal in question.

In the conventional scheme, since the insulin doses are fixed, the amount of carbohydrates should not vary from day to day. Both insulin therapy schemes require carbohydrates to be counted, thus establishing its importance for the entire population of diabetics. Classical studies such as the *Diabetes Control and Complications Trial (DCCT)* [4] and *UK Prospective Diabetes Study (UKPDS)* [5] pointed out that glycemic control, including glycated hemoglobin A1c in the latter, modifies the risk of complications arising from the disease. Therapy that uses counting has been used in Europe since 1930, and in 1990, it was also used in the DCCT study. In 2011 [6], the International Diabetes Federation (IDF) confirmed its view that postprandial hyperglycemia is associated with an increase in retinopathy, oxidative stress, inflammation, and endothelial dysfunction and thus contributes significantly to cardiovascular risk.

A transversal study was conducted in the *Hospital das Clínicas* of the School of Medicine of University of São

M. da Conceição Chaves de Lemos (✉)
Department of Nutrition, Federal University of Pernambuco
(UFPE), Pernambuco Federal University Hospital,
Recife, PE, Brazil

Paulo with 21 DM2 patients, who attended a carbohydrate counting course. The aim was to evaluate the application of the method of carbohydrate counting. The researchers concluded that it was important for patients because the course about carbohydrate counting promoted a significant reduction of glycated hemoglobin and improved blood glucose control. In addition, the patients learned how to change their diets and to vary these more and therefore how to adopt healthier eating habits [7].

Criteria for Prescribing the Counting of Carbohydrates

In type 1 diabetes mellitus, type 2 diabetes mellitus, and gestational diabetes, the criteria should be directed at individualizing the diet, thereby achieving the appropriate glycemic goal and evaluating the time of greatest resistance to insulin. It might be thought that since glycated hemoglobin A1c is verified, self-monitoring should be discarded, but the test for glycated hemoglobin A1c does not evaluate fluctuations in blood glucose levels, besides which it is of fundamental importance that the multidisciplinary team knows the glucose levels before and after meals and especially that they attach due significance to the postprandial blood sugar level because of its clinical relevance [8]. In type 1 diabetics, the postprandial glycemic target is broader so as to avoid the risks of hypoglycemia generating repercussions for the growth of children and adolescents, but it should be assessed case by case.

Some diabetologists and the American Diabetes Association (ADA) currently consider that between 150 and 180 mg/dl is appropriate. The glycemic level of this population is more difficult to control as one needs to take into account the patient's age, maturity, acceptance of the disease, the concentration of growth hormone, etc. A recently published study involving type 1 diabetics and their families emphasizes the importance of carbohydrate counting in this population. For type 2 diabetics, the goals are more restricted: HbA1c less than 6.5%, preprandial glucose of 5.5 mmol/ (<100 mg/dL), and postprandial glucose of 7.8 mmol/ (<140 mg/dL) IDF [3, 6] (2011). The importance of the entire population of diabetics conducting self-monitoring is emphasized [8]. In gestational diabetes, the biochemical parameters are fasting glucose <90 mg/dL and postprandial blood sugar <140 mg/dL at 1 h and <120 mg/dL at 2 h.

The IDF considers that there is a substantial amount of scientific evidence to suggest that diets with a low glycemic load are beneficial for controlling postprandial glucose. The glycemic load is the glycemic index per edible portion of food; in other words, it is an objective way of expressing to what extent the food content modifies the postprandial response [6, 9].

On the other hand, higher daily blood glucose variability in adults with type 1 diabetes could be the result of inaccurate carbohydrate counting. A project is starting to evaluate carbohydrate counting, and they found that 63% of the 448 meals analyzed were underestimated when compared with the patients' estimates and those assessed by a dietitian using a computerized analysis program,[b] but regular review and monitoring of this method might be useful [10].

Choice of Nutritional Therapy

To control blood sugar with nutritional therapy, there is the exchange list [9, 11] or a list of exchanges representing an average of foods, in which the foods are represented by groups. Available software programs may also be included, such as Diet-Pro or Diet-Win or other programs that analyze diet. This will be calculated by the nutritionist who will inform the patient of the substitutions to be made.

Another technique is to use foods in isolation. This is a more precise method and is the most suitable technique for patients who have most difficulty in exercising control, although it is harder to work with. The counting of points is a dietary program that only includes food calories, so it is not recommended.

Another important tool for patients is the manual for counting carbohydrates, which presents food items in isolation, with their amounts of calories and carbohydrates. Then, there are pocket manuals that facilitate the calculation of counting and present food in household measurements. For patients who use an insulin pump, counting each food item is a better option because their sensitivity to glycemia is greater than that of the impact of each food item on glycemia. Despite the availability of these methods, the support of the professional dietitian is an important and irreplaceable part of the program of carbohydrate counting [12].

Action of Insulins

Carbohydrate counting has become a necessity since the advent of ultra-rapid insulin analogues. Since 2002 [11], the ADA has advised that it is the amount of carbohydrates in the meal that will define the amount of UR insulin. Indeed, the freedom to eat outside the home has increased with these insulins [13, 14]. It is important to realize that the onset of action of UR insulin takes 10–15 min and that it should be taken as soon as the individual has defined how much carbohydrate he/she will consume during the meal.

Long-acting insulin will maintain the basal blood sugar and will already have been prescribed by a physician. The amount of ultra-rapid insulin required by the meal in question should be that recommended by a nutritionist specializing in diabetes, since it is based on the consumption prescribed by the nutritionist with the participation of the physician. The long-acting insulin regimen, together with UR action insulin, represents the most physiological regimen currently in existence [12, 15].

When the patient makes use of regular insulin, the onset action of which takes 30–60 min and lasts up to 6 h, physicians usually recommend that it be taken in the morning and in the afternoon; they avoid prescribing it at lunch time because of the risk of hypoglycemia, due to its long action, unless the individual is very resistant to the action of insulin, is very gluttonous, or maintains higher glucose levels after lunch.

It is also important to note that regular or UR insulins correct blood glucose levels which, when high, are known as correction boluses [15]. The improvement in glycemic control is due to the correction of blood sugar levels by means of individualized observation [16]. For this to happen, it is important to know the sensitivity factor (SF) [16], which varies with the type of insulin. There is a practical rule for checking SF for UR insulin, in which the total dose of insulin/day (basal insulin plus the ultra-rapid doses) is divided by the absolute number 1800 [17]. The same applies to rapid insulin, except that the total dose is divided by 1500. It can be observed that, on average, 1 unit of UR insulin reduces the level by 45–50 mg/dL and that 1 unit of regular insulin decreases it on average by 25–30 mg/dL. Since we are dealing with individuals, the peculiarities inherent in each individual require that the observation be made by a multidisciplinary team.

The period of greatest resistance to insulin is in the morning, owing probably to the circadian action of hormones. It may be assumed that patients with kidney disease and the elderly, because of renal dysfunction and their living longer, present a slower insulin depuration rate and thus require their blood glucose to be monitored more closely because of the risk of hypoglycemia due to the fact that circulating insulin has a longer life. The concomitant evaluation of their nutritional status is necessary because, when the patient's decompensation improves, his/her weight may go up, which favors greater resistance to insulin [17, 18].

The Dose Adjustment for Normal Eating (DAFNE) study [19], which is used throughout England as a guide in the counting of carbohydrates, when the patient, along with the multidisciplinary team, practices optimizing the amount of insulin to the carbohydrates of the meal, has shown that there is an improvement in the quality of life and glycemic control when such an effective intensive scheme is used [20].

The insulin-to-carbohydrate ratio is dependent on the individualized response and uses weight as a reference (Table 40.1). Excess weight increases insulin resistance, as is amply demonstrated in the literature [17]. The higher the weight, the more insulin the individual will take, thus increasing the risk of gaining weight and constituting a

Table 40.1 Estimate of the insulin-carbohydrate ratio as per body weight

Weight (kg)	Units of insulin: g of CHO
25	1:30
45–49	1:16
49.5–58	1:15
58.5–62.5	1:14
63–67	1:13
67.5–76	1:12
76.5–80.5	1:11
81–85	1:10
85.5–89.5	1:9
90–98.5	1:8
99–107.5	1:7
≥108	1:6

vicious cycle. Infections, which are prevalent on this population, also prompt a rise in glucose levels.

With regard to children and adolescents, since a child's weight is half that of an adult, 1 unit for every 30 g of carbohydrates is taken, if the child weighs on average 25 kg. Another aspect to be considered is that due to the action of the growth hormone present in children and adolescents, there is greater resistance to insulin, which makes control in this type 1 diabetic population difficult. Individualized and monitored action to evaluate pre- and postprandial blood glucose levels should be a priority when overseeing the adjustment of the doses of insulin [16, 21].

Another important aspect of glycemic control for those who use insulin therapy is to choose the appropriate insulin needle, which needs to reach the subcutaneous tissue; if the needle is oriented incorrectly, it will make all glycemic control difficult, even if carbohydrate counting is done satisfactorily.

Exercises

Physical activity is an important pillar in the control of blood glucose because it enhances insulin sensitivity and control of weight [16, 22]. Excessive exercise can elevate blood sugar levels or foster the emergence of hypoglycemia. Decompensated patients should only start exercise after their glucose levels have been adjusted because of the action of counter-regulatory hormones.

What Is the Effect of Alcohol on Blood Glucose?

Alcohol has 7 cal for 1 g. It is metabolized, enters the Krebs cycle, and provides energy, referred to as empty calories, because it contains neither vitamins nor mineral salts. Starting at 15 g of ethanol for women and 30 g for men, there will be an increase in blood pressure and glucose levels; 30 g of ethanol is the equivalent of two shots of whisky, two shots of vodka, and two glasses of wine for men, and the amounts for women should be approximately half of these.

The liver is an organ that stores glycogen reserves, but alcohol is metabolized in the liver. With a higher consumption of ethanol, glycogen is depleted and alcohol degraded, thus leading to the risk of hypoglycemia. The consumption of alcoholic drinks initially raises blood glucose levels and subsequently, with increased consumption, will lead to hypoglycemia [11]. In clinical practice, it is recommended that alcohol be consumed after eating in order to avoid precipitating the onset of hypoglycemia. Assessing blood sugar levels before and after ingesting alcohol will indicate the proper amount of insulin. If blood glucose is below 70 mg/dL, alcohol should not be ingested.

How Is the Amount of Carbohydrates in a Meal to Be Assessed?

This assessment may be made by weighing food, but this is a more cumbersome way to do so. Using tables of domestic measures and consulting a manual that counts carbohydrates, in which such measures are used and the amounts of carbohydrates and calories are given in alphabetical order [17], are recommended. Manuals of this kind are already available in paperback. It is important to note that support and feedback from a professional nutritionist who is a specialist in this field is of great importance in the process of learning and controlling desirable glycemic targets, but is not a substitute for the nutritionist-patient relationship [21, 23]. The basics of carbohydrate counting are shown in Table 40.2.

Table 40.2 Counting carbohydrates

Group	Example/portions	Amount of carbohydrate (g)
Bread	½ morning roll/one slice of sliced bread/three tablespoons of rice/three water and salt biscuits/½ cup of spaghetti	15
Milk	1240 ml cup of milk/1 cup of yoghourt	12
Fruit	1 medium-sized apple/1 medium-sized pear/3 slices of mango/1 small banana	15
Vegetables	1 teacup of raw vegetables/½ teacup of cooked vegetables	5
Meat	1 small steak/three soupspoons of minced beef/two chicken drumsticks	15
Fat	1 teaspoon of margarine	0

1 steak (medium) = 90 g
Reasoning: 90 g meat = 25 g protein
Given that 60% is converted into glucose, 25 × 0.6 = 15 g carbohydrate

The factors affecting an estimation of carbohydrate content of meals in carbohydrate counting in patients with type 1 diabetes mellitus were estimated, and the researchers concluded that there were some particular foods to which attention needs to be paid. The tendency to underestimate carbs was more marked for bowls of rice and curry and rice among the foods of the high-CHO group, but it is important to say that this is a Japanese study [24]. It is not easy, even for patients with CHO counting experience and who have new methods for this [25].

Effects of Food on the Blood Sugar Level

Carbohydrates raise the blood sugar level by 100%, proteins by 60%, and fats by 10% on average. Carbohydrates raise glucose linearly, i.e., the more the carbohydrates are consumed, the more the glucose level rises. Protein increases the blood glucose level on account of the glycogenetic amino acids, which play a part in gluconeogenesis, and of fat, because it is ingested more slowly and maintains glucose levels higher for longer, but it does not alter the glucose level as the other macronutrients do.

Some diabetics already use two doses of insulin, one immediately after the meal and the other 2 h later, to correct the effect produced by high-fat foods, such as pizza, Brazilian beef, and pork stew. The glycemic load of a food is affected by the content of fats, fibers, proteins, and how the food is cooked and also factors inherent in the individual [8]. As regards fibers, it is recommended that if a food has more than 5 g of fiber, this should be subtracted from the total carbohydrate content of the meal, since fiber decreases the glycemic response [17].

One of the priority aspects of carbohydrate counting is to understand the size of the portion of food, because what will determine the amount of insulin is the amount of carbohydrates in the meal [22]. In performing the carbohydrate count, it is important to (1) identify the amount of carbohydrates per meal per day, (2) match the portions of carbohydrates to the meal, and (3) practice the size by measuring or weighing or using as a reference the replicas of food used by nutritionists [17].

When the treatment of diabetes uses oral hypoglycemic agents or the conventional scheme for using insulin, the ingestion of the same amounts of carbohydrates is necessary, since the quantity of the medication is fixed. For patients who use the intensive scheme, it is not appropriate initially to modify the amount of carbohydrates in order that the optimal dose of insulin may be found. Subsequently, however, when the patient has acquired a better knowledge of the appropriate amount of insulin for the meal in question, there is greater freedom with regard to varying the amount of carbohydrates per meal [19]. In snacks, since the recommended carbohydrate content is, on average, 15–30 g, no dose of insulin is required because the amount of carbohydrates is not significant.

Another aspect that should be mentioned to the patient is that if he/she still feels hungry, it is better to eat more in main meals. Leguminous food plants such as beans, peas, lentils, and chickpeas should be included in the diabetic's diet because they present low glycemic responses, obviously without adding fatty meats to the legumes, since these foods modify the glycemic response of the meal, owing to the higher amount of soluble fibers [8].

Oleaginous foods such as cashew nuts and Brazil nuts, as long as they are eaten in moderation, can and should be part of the menu for diabetic patients, as well as for pregnant women with gestational diabetes, because they are rich in omega 3 from the vegetable kingdom, monounsaturated fat, and selenium, and have 70% good-quality fat and a low glycemic response, but the consumption of 12 cashew nuts or 4 Brazil nuts already represents 90 cal. They are a good option for snacks or for adding to salads.

Patients who enjoy Japanese food should consider that for every sushi, there is a corresponding one tablespoonful of rice and that sugar is used as part of the mixture, besides being an ingredient of cucumber sunomono. The blood glucose level should therefore be measured before the meal, the average consumption and corresponding dose of insulin checked, and the capillary glucose verified 2 h later.

Since Italian cuisine uses a large amount of cheese, there is a need to split the dose of insulin because of the delayed effect of the action of the fat on blood glucose. Currently, counting is done because it affords diabetic patients greater freedom [11]. However, the individual needs to be aware that insulin is a lipogenic hormone and thus the consumption of carbohydrates should be proportional to that of insulin [8]. In other words, if the patient needs to lose weight, there is a need for fewer carbohydrates in the meal so that a lesser amount of insulin is made available.

The IDF considers that there is a considerable volume of scientific evidence that diets with a low glycemic load are beneficial for controlling postprandial glucose [6]. The glycemic load represents the glycemic index per edible portion of food [9]. In other words, it is an objective way of measuring the extent to which food modifies the postprandial response. The percentage of protein should be less than 20% [21], since in clinical practice, we observe a tendency for diabetic patients to consume protein in larger quantities, which, according to the literature, seems to raise the glomerular filtration rate, which is undesirable in the diabetic population.

Sometimes patients may not be sure as to whether a particular food raises blood glucose levels. In this situation, after 4 h without eating food, from a metabolic viewpoint, it is as if there had been a return to fasting. This provides an opportunity for the individual to measure his/her preprandial blood sugar level and, 2 h later, to observe the impact that the test food has on the blood glucose level.

Some foods, because they contain small amounts of carbohydrate (less than 5 g) or few calories, need not be taken into consideration in the food schedule of the diabetic [10, 15]. These foods are listed in Table 40.3. Although it is known that low sucrose does not seem to hamper glycemic control and that what is important is the quantity and frequency with which food is included in the diet plan, the frequent consumption of sucrose is not recommended, because foods rich in sucrose are also rich in saturated fats, in addition to raising the blood glucose level more quickly [17].

Foods such as white bread, couscous, and potatoes should be used with due care in a diabetic's diet because they produce high blood glucose levels [9], but should never be prohibited as diabetes is a chronic disease. The same is true for the following: banana, mango, jackfruit, orange juice, plums, and raisins. These should be avoided, particularly in periods of decompensation, and consumed preferably before undertaking any physical exercise or when blood sugar levels are lower than usual.

Labels need to be read (Tables 40.3 and 40.4) [17]. When eating outside the home, a self-service establishment is preferable as consumption can more easily be kept to what has been recommended, while *à la carte* restaurants should be preferred to barbecue houses, which encourage consumption in excess. In cafeterias, sandwiches with fatty cheese should be avoided. Wholemeal bread is to be preferred, and fried food, sauces with mayonnaise, or sour cream avoided, while bread and potatoes should not be eaten during the same meal.

The degree of accuracy of carbohydrate counting among patients is still not satisfactory. Therefore, more effective education should be provided to patients who show that they need to improve their diets with carbohydrate counting. The average accuracy of the test score for all patients analyzed was 59%. In this paper, the author emphasizes the impor-

Table 40.3 List of foods with less than 5 g of carbohydrates

Food	Portion limit
Sweetener	Use at most three drops at one time
Diet sweet	1 small tin or 10 units per day
Coffee or tea with sweetener	Use at most five drops of sweetener per cup
Diet chewing gum	10 units per day
Diet gelatin	1 box (approximately five cups) per day
Diet jelly	1 full (dessert) spoon at breakfast and another one at supper
Ice cream zero% fat	1 small dish midmorning and another as an afternoon snack
Ketchup or mustard	1 full (soup) spoon per day
Diet, light, or zero soft drink	2 cans or 3 small cups (200 ml) per day

Table 40.4 Label on foods

No calories: Products which have <5 kcal/portion
Low calorie: Products which have ≤40 kcal/portion
Low cholesterol: The portion contains ≤20 mg cholesterol and ≤2 g saturated fat
Low fat content: The food has ≤3 g fat/portion
No fat: The food has <0.5 g fat/portion
Low content of saturated fat: Other food has ≤1 g saturated fat/portion
Low content of sodium: Foods which contain ≤140 mg sodium/portion
Very low sodium content: Foods which contain ≤35 mg sodium/portion

tance of carbohydrate counting to patients and to provide a good level of training in nutrition therapy for diabetes [26].

In situations of hypoglycemia, the recommended consumption is as follows: one glass of an ordinary soft drink or one glass of orange juice or one soup spoon of sugar and three caramel toffees [17]. Liquid consistency is better because the food is more easily absorbed than solid foods. Foods such as chocolate should be avoided as their fat content raises blood sugar more slowly. Episodes of hypoglycemia are the result of excessive physical activity, eating smaller amounts of food than necessary, or using more insulin than is appropriate.

The professional nutritionist needs to:

- Assess nutritional status
- Perform dietary anamnesis
- Calculate the diet plan, and prioritize the macro- and micronutrients according to the ADA guidelines
- Provide the amount of carbohydrates according to the amount of ultra-rapid or regular insulin [17]
- Check the individual's sensitivity factor
- Evaluate the pre- and postprandial blood glucose levels, and adjust the doses according to the postprandial responses in conjunction with the diabetologist
- Monitor nutritional status [25], glycemic and lipid profiles, and renal function, adjusting the diet when necessary

Concluding Remarks

Previously, food programming was calculated and offered to the individual with diabetes, together with nutritional guidelines. Currently, using the food anamnesis collected, the professional will adapt eating habits as closely as possible to the patient's eating habits, everyday life, individual preferences, and sociocultural profile. The orientation of carbohydrate counting, insulin analogues, and insulin pumps provide greater freedom and a better quality of life for this population. Thus, controlling blood glucose levels in these patients, thereby stimulating their pleasure in eating in a balanced way, is a priority and a major challenge for nutritionists.

References

1. American Diabetes Association. Lifestyle management: standards of medical care in diabetes—2018. Diabetes Care. 2018;41(1):38–50.
2. Bell KJ, Barclay AW, Petocz P, Colagiuri S, Brand-Miller JC. Efficacy of carbohydrate counting in type 1 diabetes: a systematic review and meta-analysis. Lancet Diabetes Endocrinol. 2014;2(2):133–40.
3. Cameron FJ, Wherrett DK. Care of diabetes in children and adolescents: controversies, changes, and consensus. Lancet. 2015;385(9982):2096–106.
4. Diabetes Control and Complications Trial Research Group. The effect of intensive treatment of diabetes on the development and progression of long-term complications in insulin-dependent diabetes mellitus. N Engl J Med. 1993;329(14):977–86.
5. UK Prospective Diabetes Study (UKPDS) Group. Effect of intensive blood-glucose control with metformin on complications in overweight patients with type 2 diabetes (UKPDS 34). Lancet. 1998;352(9131):854–65.
6. Guariguata L, Whiting D, Weil C, Unwin N. The international diabetes federation diabetes atlas methodology for estimating global and national prevalence of diabetes in adults. Diabetes Res Clin Pract. 2011;94(3):322–32.
7. Martins MR, Ambrosio ACT, Nery M, Cássia Aquino R, Queiroz MS. Assessment guidance of carbohydrate counting method in patients with type 2 diabetes mellitus. Prim Care Diabetes. 2014;8(1):39–42.
8. Shils ME, Shike M. Modern nutrition in health and disease. Lippincott: Williams & Wilkins; 2009.
9. American Diabetes Association. Standards of medical care in diabetes—2011. Diabetes Care. 2011;34(1):S11.
10. Brazeau AS, Mircescu H, Desjardins K, Leroux C, Strychar I, Ekoé JM, Rabasa-Lhoret R. Carbohydrate counting accuracy and blood glucose variability in adults with type 1 diabetes. Diabetes Res Clin Pract. 2013;99(1):19–23.
11. Mahan LK, Escott-Stump S. Krause food, nutrition & diet therapy. Philadelphia: W.B. Saunders Co; 2012.
12. Waldron S, Hanas R, Palmvig B. How do we educate young people to balance carbohydrate intake with adjustments of insulin? Horm Res. 2002;57(1):62–5.
13. Rovner AJ, Nansel TR, Mehta SN, Higgins LA, Haynie DL, Laffel LM. Development and validation of the type 1 diabetes nutrition knowledge survey. Diabetes Care. 2012;35(8):1643–7. DC_112371.
14. Albertini G. Awareness, intervention and education: enhancing the lives of people with diabetes. Brussels: International Diabetes Federation; 2001.
15. Sociedade Brasileira de Diabetes. Manual de contagem de carboidratos. São Paulo: SBD; 2016.
16. DAFNE Study Group. Training in flexible, intensive insulin management to enable dietary freedom in people with type 1 diabetes: dose adjustment for normal eating (DAFNE) randomised controlled trial. Br Med J. 2002;325(7367):746.
17. Stys AM, Kulkarni K. Identification of self-care behaviors and adoption of lifestyle changes result in sustained glucose control and reduction of comorbidities in type 2 diabetes. Diabetes Spectr. 2007;20(1):55–8.

18. Brazilian Society of Diabetes. Official handbook of carbohydrate counting for health professionals. Rio de Janeiro: Brazilian Society of Diabetes; 2009.

19. Dyson PA, Kelly T, Deakin T, Duncan A, Frost G, Harrison Z. Diabetes UK evidence-based nutrition guidelines for the prevention and management of diabetes. Diabet Med. 2018;28(11):1282–8.

20. Cooke D, Bond R, Lawton J, Rankin D, Heller S, Clark M et al.; DAFNE Study Group. Structured type 1 diabetes education delivered within routine care: impact on glycemic control and diabetes-specific quality of life. Diabetes Care. 2013;36(2):270–2.

21. Franz MJ. American Diabetes Association nutrition recommendations and guidelines. Diabetes Care. 2008;31(1):61–78.

22. Rabasa-Lhoret R, Garon J, Langelier H, Poisson D, Chiasson JL. Effects of meal carbohydrate content on insulin require-ments in type 1 diabetic patients treated intensively with the basal-bolus (ultraslow-regular) insulin regimen. Diabetes Care. 1999;22:667–73.

23. Warshaw HS, Kulkarni K. Complete guide to carb counting. Alexandria: American Diabetes Association; 2001.

24. Kawamura T, Takamura C, Hirose M, Hashimoto T, Higashide T, Kashihara Y, Saku H. The factors affecting on estimation of carbohydrate content of meals in carbohydrate counting. Clin Pediatr Endocrinol. 2015;24(4):153–65.

25. Evert BA, Boucher JL, Cypress M, Dumbar AS, Franz MJ, Davis-Mayer EJ, et al. Nutrition therapy recommendations for the management of adults with diabetes. Diabetes Care. 2014;37(1):120–42.

26. Meade LT, Rushton WE. Accuracy of carbohydrate counting in adults. Clin Diabetes. 2016;34(3):142–7.

Part III

Obesity, Lipids and Nutrition

Pharmacological Treatment of Obesity

41

Francisco Bandeira and Ana Maíra Quental da Nóbrega

Introduction

The development of obesity involves environmental and genetic factors. The high-calorie intake and the reduction of time spent doing physical activity are the typical environmental factors associated with this pathology, but not all the people exposed to such conditions become obese, suggesting the existence of underlying genetic mechanisms at an individual level [1]. Eleven rare monogenic forms of obesity are recognized, including leptin and melanocortin-4 receptor deficiencies, which are expressed in the hypothalamus and are involved in neural circuits that regulate energy homeostasis, the latter being the most common cause of monogenic obesity responsible by 2–5% of children with severe obesity (Table 41.1) [2, 3].

Evidence suggests that the intestinal microbiota may participate in the genesis of obesity. The intestinal fibers not digested by the human intestine are metabolized by these microorganisms into short-chain fatty acids with butyrate, propionate, and acetate, which act through the G protein-coupled receptors, GPR41 and GPR43, in enteroendocrine cells, enteric neurons, and enteric leukocytes, exerting beneficial effects on glucose homeostasis and energetic balance in addition to local anti-inflammatory action. Short-chain fatty acids may contribute to the improvement of the metabolic syndrome by promoting secretion of peptide hormones, such as the YY peptide and glucagon-like peptide type 1 (LGP-1), which decrease appetite and increase insulin release, respectively. Facing a caloric, low-fiber diet, the bacteria of the microbiota expand, degrading the mucus layer

Table 41.1 Causes of obesity

Primary causes	Secondary causes
Genetic causes	Neuropsychiatric: brain injury/tumor; consequences of cranial RT; hypothalamic obesity; depression; eating disorders
Monogenetic disorders: mutation at the melanocortin-4 receptor; leptin deficiency; POMC deficiency	Endocrine: hypothyroidism[a]; Cushing's disease; GH deficiency; pseudohypoparathyroidism
Syndromes: Prader-Willi; Bardet-Biedl; Cohen; Alström; Froehlich	Medication: tricyclic antidepressants; STEEL; antipsychotics; anticonvulsants; glucocorticoids; sulfonylureas; glitazones; beta blockers

[a]Controversial if hypothyroidism causes obesity or exacerbates obesity. RT, ACO radiotherapy, oral contraceptive

and inducing metabolic inflammation and increased intestinal permeability, predisposing to obesity [4].

Genes and environment interact in a complex system that regulates energy balance and physiological processes linked to weight. Two sets of neurons in the hypothalamic arcuate nucleus, which are inhibited or excited by circulating neuropeptide hormones, control energy balance by regulating food intake and energy expenditure. Short- and long-term energy balance is controlled through a coordinated network of central mechanisms and peripheral signals that arise from the microbiome and adipose tissue cells, stomach, pancreas, and other organs. The extrahypothalamic brain regions contribute to the regulation of energy balance through the input of the sensory signal, cognitive processes, hedonic effects of food consumption, memory, and attention [2].

Pathophysiology

Obesity is accompanied by increased macrophages and other immune cells in adipose tissue, in part due to tissue remodeling in response to adipocyte apoptosis. Visceral adipose tissue causes increased intraabdominal pressure, which

F. Bandeira
Division of Endocrinology, Agamenon Magalhães Hospital, University of Pernambuco Medical School, Recife, PE, Brazil
e-mail: francisco.bandeira@upe.br

A. M. Q. da Nóbrega (✉)
Division of Endocrinology, Diabetes and Metabolic Bone Diseases, Agamenon Magalhães Hospital, University of Pernambuco Medical School, Recife, Pernambuco, Brazil

© Springer Nature Switzerland AG 2022
F. Bandeira et al. (eds.), *Endocrinology and Diabetes*, https://doi.org/10.1007/978-3-030-90684-9_41

supposedly explains the high risks of gastroesophageal reflux disease and consequent Barrett esophagus and esophageal adenocarcinoma, in addition to arterial hypertension, the latter partly due to renal compression. The increase of soft tissues in the region of the pharynx can block the airways during sleep, leading to obstructive sleep apnea. Being overweight can also cause an overload on the joints, predisposing to osteoarthritis [2].

Adipocytes synthesize adipokines and hormones, and their secretion rates and their effects are influenced by the distribution and amount of adipose tissue present. Elevated levels of free fatty acids, inflammatory cytokines, and lipid intermediates in non-adipose tissues contribute to impaired insulin signaling and insulin resistance in obese patients. This constellation of metabolic and anatomical findings is one of the several pathophysiological mechanisms underlying dyslipidemia, type II diabetes mellitus (T2DM), nonalcoholic steatohepatitis (NASH), osteoarthritis, and neoplasms [2].

Chronic hyperactivity of the sympathetic nervous system is present in some patients with obesity and may explain, in part, multiple pathophysiological processes, including hypertension, coronary syndrome, stroke, and dyslipidemia [2].

Diagnosis

Body mass index (BMI) has been widely used to define obesity, which is diagnosed when the ratio of weight per height squared is greater than or equal to 30 kg/m^2, whereas a value between 25 and 29.9 kg/m^2 is overweight. Although it has a very practical use for population studies, it does not provide an accurate measurement of body composition and is not the best parameter to establish a diagnosis for this condition, given that it provides excess weight and not fat [5].

An accurate measurement of body composition is a valuable tool for assessing and diagnosing biological processes related to health. Normally, this evaluation is done by estimating the fat mass (FM), the percentage of fat mass (FM%), the fat-free mass (FFM), and fat distribution [5, 6].

The bioimpedance method (BIA), especially with the use of multifrequency approach, is considered a valid method of analysis of total and regional body composition that is widely available, fast, noninvasive, and relatively inexpensive. In general, estimates of body composition by different BIA devices are based on impedance, reactance, resistance, or phase angle measurements for the electric current. The raw values are converted to different body composition parameters using special algorithms. To do this, it is necessary to remove metal objects, such as rings and watches, elimination of body fluids, and a minimum of 6 h without practicing intense exercise and 12 h without ingesting alcohol or caffeine in large quantity [5, 6].

Dual-energy X-ray absorptiometry (DXA) is generally accepted as the gold standard for measuring body composition as well as bone density. It allows the direct measurement of lean mass, fat mass, and bone density with high precision. However, it is an expensive device and is not widely available [5, 6].

The two methods provide the fat mass, its percentage, and the fat-free mass, which is the total body mass minus the fat mass and includes water, bone, and muscle tissue. The fat mass index (FMI) provided by the two tools is calculated by dividing the fat mass by height squared, the normal value being between 3 and 6 kg/m^2 for males and 5–9 kg/m^2 for females. The classification of obesity grades I, II, and III is shown in Table 41.2 [6, 7].

A study carried out with an obese population submitted to the nutritional intervention for weight loss compared the BIA parameters with DXA. The results showed that the BIA data (IMF, FM%, and FFM) correlate well with those of DXA, although it tends to underestimate FM% [6].

Besides the utility for definition of obesity, BIA and DXA also have value to search sarcopenia through calculations of the skeletal appendicular muscle mass by height squared or BMI. The indices and cutoff points for lean mass evaluation are shown in Table 41.3 [8, 9].

New emerging laboratory tests may also aid in the better characterization of adiposopathy. The leptin and adiponectin hormones represent these tools and can be used for risk stratification in patients with obesity. Leptin levels increase proportionally to fat mass. On the other hand, the serum level of adiponectin decreases inversely to adipose tissue. An increase in the leptin/adiponectin ratio correlates with an increase in adiposopathy, which is related to increased metabolic and cardiovascular risk, whereas a decrease in this ratio indicates normalization of adipose tissue function [7]. The biomarkers of obesity are shown in Table 41.4.

Pharmacological Treatment

Antiobesity drugs play a role in weight control through their action on the central nervous system (CNS) or peripheral tissues (muscle, adipose tissue, kidney, or gastrointestinal

Table 41.2 Classification of IMP-based fat mass (fat mass index)

Classifications	FMI male (kg/m^2)	FMI female (kg/m^2)
Severe fat deficit	<2	<3.5
Moderate fat deficit	2 to <2.3	3.4 to <4
Low fat deficit	2.3 to <3	4–5
Normal	3–6	5–9
Overweight	>6–9	>9–13
Obesity level I	>9–12	>13–17
Obesity level II	>12–15	>17–21
Obesity level III	>15	>21

Table 41.3 Evaluation of muscular mass by DXA and BIA

	Index	Description	Cutoff point
DXA	Baumgartner criteria	Skeletal muscle mass (arms and legs) in relation to the square of height	Female: 5.45 kg/m^2 Male: 7.26 kg/m^2
	FNIH	Skeletal muscle mass (arms and legs) regarding BMI	Female: 0.512 kg/m^2 Male: 0.789 kg/m^2
BIA	SMI	Skeletal muscle mass to the square of height	Female: 6.76 kg/m^2 Male: 10.76 kg/m^2
	FFMI	Fat-free mass in relation to square height	Female: 15.4 kg/m^2 Male: 17.4 kg/m^2

DXA dual-energy X-ray absorptiometry, *BIA* bioimpedance, *SMI* skeletal muscle mass index, *FFMI* fat-free mass index, *FNIH* Foundation for the National Institutes of Health

Table 41.4 Adiposopathy biomarcants

Adiposopathy biomarkers
Hyperinsulinemia/hyperglycemia
Increased triglycerides/HDL fall
Elevation of free fatty acids
Elevation of leptin
Decreased adiponectin
Increased leptin/adiponectin ratio
Increased TNF-alpha
Activation of the renin-angiotensin-aldosterone axis
Male hypoandrogenism
Female hyperandrogenism

HDL high-density lipoprotein, *TNF-alpha* tumor necrosis factor alpha

tract), which may reduce appetite or increase satiety through its action on hormone-specific receptors and serotonergic, noradrenergic, dopaminergic, opioid, cannabinoid, or brain-specific receptors, increase energy expenditure and fat oxidation by the activation of catecholaminergic mechanisms in the CNS and/or peripheral tissues, reduce fat absorption by inhibiting lipase in the gastrointestinal tract, and induce depletion of nutrients, for example, by inducing glucose depletion by the kidneys [10].

Pharmacotherapy is indicated as a complement to changes in lifestyle and may be considered for patients with BMI greater than or equal to 30 kg/m^2 or even between 27 and 29.9 kg/m^2 with at least one other comorbidity [2].

Efficacy and safety should be evaluated monthly in the first 3 months of treatment. If the response is considered insufficient (weight loss <5% in this period) or if there is any safety or tolerability problem at any time, the drug should be discontinued, and alternative medicines or other approaches should be considered [11].

For the treatment of obesity in the long term, the FDA has approved five therapies to date: topiramate/phentermine, bupropion/naltrexone, lorcaserin, orlistat, and liraglutide (Table 41.5) [11].

Phentermine/Topiramate Association

Topiramate is an anticonvulsant associated with weight loss. Its CNS effects include action on the orexigenic GABA systems, causing suppression of appetite. Studies investigate its use for the treatment of binge eating. Amphetamines act on hypothalamic receptors to release norepinephrine, dopamine, and serotonin, increasing CNS activity and resting energy expenditure and decreasing appetite and food intake, leading to weight reduction. Phentermine is the amphetamine analogue with the lowest potential for addiction, being released in the United States for short-term use alone in anti-obesity treatment [12, 13].

The efficacy of weight loss with this association (Qsymia) used orally for the suppression of appetite was assessed in a 1-year study that tested two different dosages for each drug in the following combinations: 7.5-mg phentermine with 46-mg topiramate and 15-mg phentermine with 92-mg topiramate. The results showed a mean weight loss of 14.4%, 6.7%, and 2.1% with a higher dose of Qsymia, lower dose of the same medication, and placebo, respectively, as well as reduction of cardiovascular risk factors with medication administration [13, 14]. Other clinical trials that were fundamental to its FDA approval are ENQUATE, EQUIP, and SEQUEL [15–17].

The most common adverse reactions to phentermine/topiramate in these trials were paresthesia, dysgeusia, insomnia, constipation, and dry mouth, with no increased risk of serious cardiovascular side effects. It is contraindicated for use during pregnancy because of the risk of orofacial fissures related to topiramate [12].

Naltrexone/Bupropiona Association

Although it is a relatively weak inhibitor of norepinephrine and dopamine uptake, bupropion also stimulates pro-opiomelanocortin (POMC) hypothalamic neurons, leading to activation of melanocortin receptors and induction of weight loss through suppression of appetite and increase of energy expenditure. Naltrexone blocks the inhibitory action of beta-endorphin on POMC neurons, preventing the cessation of bupropion-induced activation [12, 18].

Various 56-week phase III clinical trials were performed with the combination of 16- or 32-mg naltrexone/360-mg bupropion (Contrave) in obese or overweight patients and another comorbidity. In the Contrave Obesity Research trials (COR-I and COR-II), 36–42% of participants using a Contrave associated with lifestyle change (LSC) achieved a

Table 41.5 Antiobesity medications for prolonged use adopted by the FDA

Drug (generic)	Dosage	Action mechanism	FDA approval	Common side effects	Contraindications
Orlistat	120 mg[3] times daily (orally)	Inhibitor of pancreatic and gastric lipase	1999	Decreased absorption of fat-soluble vitamins, steatorrhea, flatulence, fecal urgency	Use of cyclosporine (take 2 h before or after), chronic malabsorption syndrome, pregnancy and breastfeeding, cholestasis
Lorcaserin	10 mg[2] times daily (orally)	5HT2c receptor agonist	2012	Headache, nausea, dry mouth, dizziness, fatigue, constipation	Pregnancy and lactation use with caution associated with: IRSS, SNRIs/MAOIs, St John's wort, triptans, bupropion
Phentermine/topiramate	46 + 7.5 mg daily (orally)	Modulation of the GABA (T) receptor plus norepinephrine-releasing agent	2012	Insomnia, dry mouth, constipation, paresthesia, dizziness, dysgeusia	Pregnancy and lactation, hyperthyroidism, glaucoma, use of MAOIs or sympathomimetic amines
Naltrexone/bupropion	90 + 8 mg twice daily (orally)	Inhibitor of dopamine and norepinephrine reuptake inhibitors (bupropion) and opioid antagonists (naltrexone)	2014	Nausea, constipation, headache, vomiting, dizziness	Uncontrolled SAH, convulsive disorders, anorexia nervosa or bulimia, drug or alcohol withdrawal, use of MAOIs
Liraglutide	3 mg daily (sc)	GLP-1 agonist	2014	Nausea, vomiting, elevation of pancreatic enzymes	Family or personal history of medullary thyroid carcinoma or MEN

SC subcutaneous, *SSRIs* selective serotonin reuptake inhibitors, *SNIRs* selective norepinephrine reuptake inhibitors, *MAOIs* monoamine oxidase inhibitors, *SAH* systemic arterial hypertension, *MEN* multiple endocrine neoplasia

weight loss greater than or equal to 5% compared with 17–18% of those who did LSC with placebo [19–21].

Individuals treated with this combination had reduced cardiometabolic risk factors and improved quality of life as well as improved satiety [13].

The most common side effects of naltrexone/bupropion include nausea, change in bowel habit (constipation or diarrhea), headache, vomiting, insomnia, and dry mouth. It is contraindicated in cases of gestation, uncontrolled hypertension, convulsive disorders, use of other products containing bupropion, chronic use of opiates, use of monoamine oxidase inhibitors (MAOIs) in the last 14 days or individuals who have suffered abrupt withdrawal of alcohol, benzodiazepines, and barbiturates or antiepileptic drugs [21].

Lorcaserin

Lorcaserin acts at the 5-hydroxytryptamine 2C receptor (5-HT2C), causing an increased release of serotonin into the CNS. Central serotonin participates in food behavior and energy balance modulation, directly modulating the hypothalamic networks POMC and NPY (neuropeptide Y), resulting in increased satiety and hypophagia [13].

FDA approval was based on three clinical trials, BLOSSOM, BLOOM, and BLOOM-DM, which showed that 47.2% of patients taking lorcaserin 10 mg twice daily had a loss of at least 5% of body weight compared with 2.5% of placebo. The mean loss achieved with the medication after 1 year was 5.9% compared with 2.8% of placebo [22, 23].

The most common adverse reactions with this drug are headache, dry mouth, constipation, nausea, fatigue, and dizziness. Hypoglycemia may occur in patients with diabetes. Individuals on medication should be monitored for depression and suicidal thoughts. Potentially fatal serotonin syndrome or neuroleptic malignant syndrome may occur when associated with serotonin-selective receptor inhibitors, norepinephrine receptor inhibitors, triptan, and bupropion MAOIs. Therefore, these medications should be used with extreme caution in combination with lorcaserin. If signs of valvular disease occur, the medication should be discontinued. It is contraindicated in pregnancy and lactation [21].

Orlistat

Orlistat is an antiobesity drug that inhibits pancreatic lipase, reducing digestion and fat absorption by approximately 30%. Clinical trials (e.g., XENDOS) with this medication showed significant weight loss compared with placebo (5.8 kg vs 3 kg) using 120 mg three times daily. In addition, the use of orlistat for 4 years was associated with a reduction in the risk of T2DM of 37.3% [24, 25].

This drug interacts with several medications that may interfere with its absorption, bioavailability, and efficacy, especially cyclosporin, amiodarone, levothyroxine, warfarin, and antiepileptics. Because orlistat can interfere with the absorption of fat-soluble vitamins, the replacement of multivitamins containing vitamins K, A, D, and E and beta-carotene is necessary [21].

Gastrointestinal side effects, such as abdominal pain and discomfort, oily or liquid stools, and fecal urgency, are very common, making its long-term use problematic. Patients with renal impairment should have renal function monitored during the use of the medication. Orlistat is contraindicated for patients with chronic malabsorption syndrome or cholestasis. It is in the X category for pregnant women and is not recommended for pregnant or breastfeeding women [12].

Liraglutide

Liraglutide is a glucagon-like peptide-1 analogue with long-acting biological activity (half-life of 10–14 h) compared with endogenous GLP-1. It was approved for treatment of T2DM at a dose of 1.8 mg and recently obtained FDA (2014) and EMA (2015) approval for treatment of obesity at 3 mg daily dose subcutaneously [18].

Administered liraglutide acts in the gastrointestinal tract promoting an increase in gastric emptying time and acts directly on the POMC neurons in the arched nucleus of the hypothalamus, leading to reduced appetite. In addition, GLP-1 receptors are also present in the mesolimbic reward system, and this drug may have an effect on reward-induced eating [18].

Data on the efficacy of liraglutide in relation to weight loss come from the SCALE study, which showed a 6.2% weight loss over 56 weeks on the medication versus 0.2% on placebo. More participants taking the drug (81.4%) maintained a weight loss greater than or equal to 5% compared with those who took placebo (48.9%). There was also a reduction of biomarkers of cardiovascular disease, C-reactive protein, adiponectin, fibrinogen, glycemic indexes, and fasting plasma insulin [26].

The recommended initial dose is 0.6 mg per day, increasing 0.6 mg weekly until the 3-mg dose is reached [26].

Adverse effects related to liraglutide 3-mg include nausea, vomiting, abdominal pain, dizziness, fatigue, headache, and hypoglycemia. Elevation of pancreatic enzymes may occur. The medication should be discontinued in cases of suspected pancreatitis and should not be restarted if confirmed. There are reports of renal failure. It is contraindicated in patients with a personal or family history of medullary thyroid carcinoma or multiple endocrine neoplasia (MEN) and in pregnant women [21].

There was a decrease in mortality because of cardiovascular disease, nonfatal cerebrovascular accident, and nonfatal acute myocardial infarction in patients with diabetes (T2DM) using 1.8-mg liraglutide, which is believed to be by modification of the progression of the atherosclerosis process [21].

Future Perspectives

Cetilistat

It acts similarly to orlistat, inhibiting pancreatic lipase. Reduction of fat absorption induces modest weight loss associated with improved glycemic and lipid profile. In a 12-week study, weight loss was shown to be 3.3–4.1 kg, with more common side effects reported related to the gastrointestinal tract but with a better tolerability profile than orlistat. As a result of phase III data, cetilistat has been approved in Japan since 2013 but is still awaiting approval in the United States and Europe [12].

Bupropion/Zonisamide

Zonisamide is an inhibitor of mitochondrial carbonic anhydrase, a drug with antiepileptic action that acts by increasing the levels of serotonin and dopamine in the brain, acting as an appetite suppressant. Its combination with bupropion (Empatic) is currently in phase II. Preliminary results from 18 patients showed a 7.2-kg loss in 12 weeks with this combination (360-mg bupropion + 360-mg zonisamide) compared with 2.9 kg in zonisamide alone. The most commonly reported adverse events were headache, nausea, and insomnia [12].

Beloranib

It acts by inhibiting methionine aminopeptidase-2. Specifically, this drug reduces fat biosynthesis and increases lipid oxidation and lipolysis. In a 12-week, phase II study, participants receiving this medication at a dose of 0.6 mg, 1.2 mg, or 2.4 mg subcutaneously lost 5.5 kg, 6.9 kg, and 10.9 kg compared with 0.4 kg of the placebo group with good tolerability, although gastrointestinal effects and insomnia have been reported [12]. In another short-term (4 weeks) viability study with 31 obese women, intravenous beloranib at a dose of 0.1–0.9 mg twice weekly achieved hunger reduction, weight loss of 0.8–3.5% (versus 0.6% placebo), and improved cardiovascular risk markers, such as triglycerides, LDL, and C-reactive protein [27].

This class of medication is the only one that produces the double effect of increasing the metabolism of fats in addition to reducing appetite. However, its long-term safety and efficacy is still under study so far. The reported side effects were headache, skin lesions around the infusion site, nausea, and diarrhea [27].

Tesofensine

It is a new triple monoamine reuptake inhibitor, which induces a potent inhibition of the reabsorption process in the synaptic cleft of dopamine, norepinephrine, and serotonin neurotransmitters [28]. It has a triple-action mechanism, leading to inhibition of appetite, increased satiety, and thermogenesis. In recent preclinical and clinical evaluations, it has shown a robust effect against obesity, but the specific mechanism of action still needs to be better elucidated [29]. Common side effects include insomnia, mood changes, dizziness, palpitation, nausea, and mild elevation of blood pressure [29].

Obesity and T2DM

The five approved medications for obesity treatment by the FDA lead, in addition to a weight loss of 5–15% of baseline weight, to a reduction of glycated hemoglobin of 0.5–1.6% in patients who completed at least 1 year of drug treatment [30].

When considering pharmacological treatment for diabetes, whenever possible, opt for drugs that reduce weight or have a neutral effect. The agents associated with weight loss are metformin, GLP-1 analogues, SGLT2 inhibitors, alpha-glucose inhibitors, and amylin mimetics. Dipeptidyl peptidase-4 inhibitors appear to have a neutral effect on weight. Unlike these agents, insulin secretagogues, thiazolidinediones, and insulins are associated with weight gain [11].

Additional Pharmacotherapy for Obesity in DM2 (Not Approved by the FDA)

These medications listed below may be considered for weight loss in patients with diabetes but have not yet been approved by the FDA.

Metformin

It has a long history of use in patients with diabetes and pre-diabetic patients, being first-line medication in the treatment of T2DM. It is believed that several mechanisms may be related to metformin weight loss, including stimulation of hypothalamic pro-opiomelanocortin neurons, increased leptin levels, improved insulin sensitivity, and modulation of intestinal flora [30].

Numerous studies have shown that this drug leads to a decrease in food intake of 250–300 kcal per day approximately, with a moderate weight loss of 2–4 kg [30].

Pramlintide

Amylin is a hormone produced by beta-pancreatic cells co-secreted with insulin in response to a meal. It acts by slowing gastric emptying and reducing the release of glucagon, increasing satiety, and decreasing food consumption. In addition, it prevents the compensatory reduction of energy expenditure in patients who are losing weight [30].

Pramlintide is an analogue of human amylin approved for the treatment of type 1 diabetes mellitus (T1DM) and T2DM in patients who did not obtain adequate glycemic control with optimized therapy. In a 16-week study in nondiabetic obese patients, this medication was shown to improve appetite and weight, with a 3.7% reduction in weight over placebo compared with baseline [30].

Like all medications that delay gastric emptying, pramlintide can lead to nausea and vomiting as a side effect. A slower titration after initiation of treatment may ameliorate symptoms and improve tolerability [30].

Semaglutide

This drug corresponds to an analogue of human GLP-1, with a structure similar to liraglutide. In a 12-week study of obese patients taking semaglutide 1 mg weekly, there was a 5-kg decrease in baseline weight, hunger reduction, calorie intake, and satiety. Among patients with diabetes randomized to semaglutide or insulin, there was a decrease of 5.2 kg with the first and weight gain with the second. Glycated hemoglobin fell 1.6% with the GLP-1 analogue, which was twice the glycated drop in patients taking insulin. In addition, patients with diabetes with high cardiovascular risk on semaglutide had significantly lower rates of death from cardiovascular disease, nonfatal acute myocardial infarction, and stroke [30].

Phentermine and SGLT2 Inhibitor Association

Phentermine has been studied for long decades for short-term treatment of obesity but has not been explicitly evaluated in the diabetic population. Sodium-glucose type 2 cotransporter inhibitors are a class of oral antidiabetic drugs that act by blocking glucose reabsorption in the proximal contorted tubule, leading to glycosuria and weight loss, in view of a daily elimination of 90 g of glucose or 360 calories per day [30].

It has been hypothesized that iSGLT2 causes a compensatory increase in appetite and food intake. A randomized, 26-week trial in nondiabetic obese patients showed that treatment with canagliflozin associated with phentermine led to an increase in weight loss of 6.9% in relation to placebo. This combination is under evaluation for future options in the treatment of obesity [30].

References

1. Krentz AJ, Fujioka K, Hompesch M. Evolution of pharmacological obesity treatments: focus on adverse side-effect profiles. Diabetes Obes Metab. 2016;18:558–70. https://doi.org/10.1111/dom.12657.
2. Heymsfield SB, Wadden TA. Mechanisms, pathophysiology, and management of obesity. N Engl J Med. 2017;376:254–66. https://doi.org/10.1056/NEJMra1514009.
3. Cui C, Li Y, Gao H, Zhang H, Han J, Zhang D, Li Y, Zhou J, Lu C, Su X. Modulation of the gut microbiota by the mixture of fish oil and krill oil in high-fat diet- induced obesity mice. PLoS One. 2017;12(10):e0186216. https://doi.org/10.1371/journal.pone.0186216.
4. Yang BG, Hur KY, Lee MS. Alterations in gut microbiota and immunity by dietary fat. Yonsei Med J. 2017;58(6):1083–91. https://doi.org/10.3349/ymj.2017.58.6.1083.
5. Sillanpää E, Cheng S, Häkkinen K, Finni T, Walker S, Pesola A, Ahtiainen J, Stenroth L, Selänne H, Sipilä S. Body composition in 18- to 88-year-old adults- comparison of multifrequency bioimpedance and dual-energy X ray absorptiometry. Obes Soc. 2014;22(1). https://doi.org/10.1002/oby.20583.
6. Gomez-Arbelaez D, Bellido D, Castro AI, Ordoñez-Mayan L, Carreira J, Galban C, Martinez-Olmos MA, Crujeiras AB, Sajoux I, Casanueva FF. Body composition changes after very low-calorie-ketogenic diet in obesity evaluated by three standardized methods. Endocr Soc. 2016. https://doi.org/10.1210/jc.2016-2385.
7. Bays HE, Toth PP, Kris-Etherton PM, Abate N, Aronne LJ, Brown WV, Gonzalez-Campoy JM, Jones SR, Kumar R, La Forge R, Samuel VT. Obesity, adiposity, and dyslipidemia: a consensus statement from the National Lipid Association. J Clin Lipidol. 2013;7:304–83. https://doi.org/10.1016/j.jacl.2013.04.001.
8. Chen LK, Liu LK, Woo J, Assantachai P, Auyeung TW, Bahyah KS, Chou MY, Chen LY, Hsu PS, Krairit O, Lee JSW, Lee WJ, Lee Y, Liang CK, Limpawattana P, Lin C, Peng LN, Satake S, Suzuki T, Won CW, Wu CH, Wu SN, Zhang T, Zeng P, Akishita M, Arai H. Sarcopenia in Asia: consensus report of the Asian Working Group for Sarcopenia. J Am Med Dir Assoc. 2014;15:95e101. https://doi.org/10.1016/j.jamda.2013.11.025.
9. Batsis JA, Mackenzie TA, Lopez-Jimenez F, Bartels SJ. Sarcopenia, sarcopenic obesity, and functional impairments in older adults: National Health and Nutrition Examination Surveys 1999-2004. Nutr Res. 2015;35(12):1031–9. https://doi.org/10.1016/j.nutres.2015.09.003.
10. Hainer V, Hainerová IA. Do we need anti-obesity drugs? Diabetes Metab Res Rev. 2012;28(2):8–20. https://doi.org/10.1002/dmrr.2349.
11. American Diabetes Association. Obesity management for the treatment of type 2 diabetes. Sec. 6. In standards of medical care in diabetes 2016. Diabetes Care. 2016;39(1):S47–51.
12. Aslam D. Weight management in obesity—past and present. Int J Clin Pract. 2016;70(3):206–17. https://doi.org/10.1111/ijcp.12771.
13. Valsamakis G, Konstantakou P, Mastorakos G. New targets for drug treatment of obesity. Annu Rev Pharmacol Toxicol. 2017;57(1):585–605. https://doi.org/10.1146/annurev-pharmtox-010716-104735.
14. Kishore D, Gadde M, Allison DB, Ryan DH, Peterson CA, Troupin B, Schwiers ML, Day WW. Effects of low-dose, controlled-release, phentermine plus topiramate combination on weight and associated comorbidities in overweight and obese adults (CONQUER): a randomised, placebo-controlled, phase 3 trial. Lancet. 2011;377(9774):1341–52. https://doi.org/10.1016/S0140-6736(11)60205-5.
15. Garvey WT, Ryan DH, Kishore ML, Gadde M, Allison DB, Peterson CA, Schwiers M, Day WW, Bowden CH. Two-year sustained weight loss and metabolic benefits with controlled-release phentermine/topiramate in obese and overweight adults (SEQUEL): a randomized, placebo-controlled, phase 3 extension study. Am J Clin Nutr. 2012;95(2):297–308. https://doi.org/10.3945/ajcn.111.024927.
16. Allison DB, Gadde KM, Garvey WT, Peterson CA, Schwiers ML, Najarian T, Tam PY, Troupin B, Day WW. Controlled-release phentermine/topiramate in severely obese adults: a randomized controlled trial (EQUIP). Obes Res J. 2012;20(2):330–42. https://doi.org/10.1038/oby.2011.330.
17. Aronne LJ, Wadden TA, Peterson C, Winslow D, Odeh S, Gadde KM. Evaluation of phentermine and topiramate versus phentermine/topiramate extended-release in obese adults. Obesity (Silver Spring). 2013;21(11):2163–71. https://doi.org/10.1002/oby.20584.
18. Roberts CA, Christiansen P, Halford JCG. Tailoring pharmacotherapy to specific eating behaviours in obesity: can recommendations for personalised therapy be made from the current data? Acta Diabetol. 2017;54:715–25. https://doi.org/10.1007/s00592-017-0994-x.
19. Greenway FL, Fujioka K, Plodkowski RA, Mudaliar S, Guttadauria M, Erickson J, Kim DD, Dunayevich E, for the COR-I Study Group. Effect of naltrexone plus bupropion on weight loss in overweight and obese adults (COR-I): a multicentre, randomised, double-blind, placebo-controlled, phase 3 trial. Lancet. 2010;376(9741):595–605. https://doi.org/10.1016/S0140-6736(10)60888-4.
20. Apovian CM, Aronne L, Rubino D, Still C, Wyatt H, Burns C, Kim D, Dunayevich E, for the COR-II Study Group. A randomized, phase 3 trial of naltrexone SR/bupropion SR on weight and obesity-related risk factors (COR-II). Obes Res J. 2013;21(5):935–43. https://doi.org/10.1002/oby.20309.
21. Golden A. Current pharmacotherapies for obesity: A practical perspective. J Am Assoc Nurse Pract. 2017;29:43–52. https://doi.org/10.1002/2327-6924.12519.
22. O'Neil PM, Smith SR, Weissman NJ, Fidler MC, Sanchez M, Zhang J, Raether B, Anderson CM, Shanahan WR. Randomized placebo-controlled clinical trial of lorcaserin for weight loss in type 2 diabetes mellitus: the BLOOM-DM study. Obes Res J. 2012;20(7):1426–36. https://doi.org/10.1038/oby.2012.66.
23. Aronne L, Shanahan W, Fain R, Glicklich A, Soliman W, Li Y, Smith S. Safety and efficacy of lorcaserin: a combined analysis of the BLOOM and BLOSSOM trials. Postgrad Med J. 2014;126(6):7–18. https://doi.org/10.3810/pgm.2014.10.2817.
24. Torgerson JS, Hauptman J, Boldrin MN, Sjöström L. XENical in the Prevention of Diabetes in Obese Subjects (XENDOS) Study. Diabetes Care. 2004;27(1):155–61. https://doi.org/10.2337/diacare.27.1.155.
25. Sjöström L. Analysis of the xendos study (xenical in the prevention of diabetes in obese subjects). Endocr Pract. 2006;12(1):31–3. https://doi.org/10.4158/EP.12.S1.31.
26. Wadden TA, Hollander P, Klein S, Niswender K, Woo V, Hale PM, Aronne L. Weight maintenance and additional weight loss with liraglutide after low-calorie-diet-induced weight loss: the SCALE maintenance randomized study. Int J Obes. 2013;37:1443–51. https://doi.org/10.1038/ijo.2013.120.

27. Fujioka K. Current and emerging medications for overweight or obesity in people with comorbidities. Diabetes Obes Metab. 2015;17(11):1021–32. https://doi.org/10.1111/dom.12502.

28. George M, Rajaram M, Pharm M, Shanmugam E. New and emerging drug molecules against obesity. J Cardiovasc Pharmacol Ther. 2013;19(1):65–76. https://doi.org/10.1177/1074248413501017.

29. Appel L, Bergström M, Lassen JB, Långström B. Tesofensine, a novel triple monoamine re-uptake inhibitor with anti-obesity effects: dopamine transporter occupancy as measured by PET. Eur Neuropsychopharmacol. 2014;24(2):251–61. https://doi.org/10.1016/j.euroneuro.2013.10.007.

30. Kahan S, Fujioka K. Obesity pharmacotherapy in patients with type 2 diabetes. Diabetes J. 2017;30(4):250–8.

Nonalcoholic Fatty Liver Disease

42

Narriane C. P. Holanda, Amanda R. L. Oliveira,
Nara N. C. Carvalho, and Bruno L. Souza

Abbreviations

AAR	AST-ALT ratio
AASLD	American Association for the Study of Liver Diseases
ALT	Alanine aminotransferase
APRI	AST-to-platelet ratio index
ARFI	Acoustic radiation force impulse
ASL	Aspartate aminotransferase
CK-18	Cytokeratin 18
CT	Computed tomography
CVD	Cardiovascular disease
EASL	European Association for the Study of the Liver
FDA	Food and Drug Administration
FFA	Free fatty acid
FIB-4	Fibrosis -4
GLP-1	Glucagon-like peptide-1
HCC	Hepatocellular carcinoma
IL-6	Interleukin-6
IR	Insulin resistance
MetS	Metabolic syndrome
MR	Magnetic resonance
MRE	Magnetic resonance elastography
NAFLD	Nonalcoholic fatty liver disease
NASH	Nonalcoholic steatohepatitis
NFS	NAFLD fibrosis score
PDFF	Proton density fatty fraction
PPAR	Peroxisome proliferator-activated receptor
RCT	Randomized clinical trial
SAH	Systemic arterial hypertension
SMR	Sprectroscopic MR
T2D	Type 2 diabetes mellitus
TG	Triglycerides
USG	Ultrasonography
VCTE	Vibration-controlled transient elastography
γ-GT	γ-glutamyl-trans-peptidase

N. C. P. Holanda (✉) · N. N. C. Carvalho
Department of Endocrinology, Federal University of Paraíba,
João Pessoa, Brazil

A. R. L. Oliveira
Department of Hepatoly, Federal University of Paraíba,
João Pessoa, Brazil

B. L. Souza
Department of Pediatrics, Nova Esperança Medical School,
João Pessoa, Brazil

Introduction

In the United States alone, there is an estimated 33 million people with nonalcoholic fatty liver disease (NAFLD), 1/3 of whom have nonalcoholic steatohepatitis (NASH). The majority of these patients were diagnosed between the fourth and fifth decades of life [1].

NAFLD is characterized by fat accumulation in over 5% of hepatocytes, excluding causes related to significant alcohol intake or other known etiologies of hepatic steatosis. The disease is generally associated with insulin resistance (IR) and metabolic syndrome (MetS). However, it can present in 1 in every 15 individuals of normal weight [2]. NASH encompasses inflammatory abnormalities and hepatic fibrosis and may progress to cirrhosis and hepatocellular carcinoma (HCC) [3].

Epidemiologically, NAFLD is more common in men and Hispanics. Independently of the presence of obesity or MetS, it can also be associated with other clinical conditions, such as cardiovascular disease (CVD) alone, hypopituitarism, hypogonadism, hypothyroidism, polycystic ovarian syndrome, or obstructive sleep apnea, and with patients submitted to cholecystectomy [2].

Pathogenesis

Although not fully elucidated, IR is known to play a role as the main event for the genesis of hepatic steatosis [4]. IR promotes lipolysis of triglycerides (TG) and increases free

© Springer Nature Switzerland AG 2022
F. Bandeira et al. (eds.), *Endocrinology and Diabetes*, https://doi.org/10.1007/978-3-030-90684-9_42

fatty acid (FFA) levels by inhibiting their esterification in adipose tissue. Elevated glycemia and FFA levels result in greater uptake of lipids by hepatocytes, leading to the development of hepatic steatosis [5].

Polymorphisms in the genes encoding apolipoprotein C3 [6], adiponutrin [7] (involved in metabolism of TGs), and inflammatory markers such as interleukin-6 (IL-6) constitute the genetic basis for the association between IR and NASH [8], even in non-obese patients [9]. Despite this, not all NASH patients have IR, indicating that NASH is a multifactorial condition [9].

Another important mechanism in the pathogenesis of NASH is oxidative stress. Oxidative damage in the liver results from the exhaustion of antioxidant enzymes (glutathione, β-carotene, and vitamins C and E) [10]. Potential inducers of IR and oxidative stressors include leptin, intestinal bacteria, antioxidant deficiency, and hepatic iron.

Leptin and resistin can contribute to the development of fibrosis in NASH. These hormones induce insulin resistance in hepatocytes by altering their receptors [11, 12]. Adiponectin, when at low levels, correlates with the presence of NAFLD, hepatic fibrosis, and MetS severity [13].

Modifiable environmental factors such as shift work and gut microbiota can influence the physiopathogeny of NAFLD. Changes in gut microbiota potentially expose hepatocytes to bacterial degradation products such as lipopolysaccharides, endogenous ethanol, and acetaldehyde. This results in insulin resistance, steatosis, necroinflammation, and fibrosis [14, 15]. Shift work has been associated with obesity, metabolic syndrome [16], and NASH [17].

In addition, IR is associated with high levels of hepatic iron [18], and the increase in iron concentration in the hepatic parenchyma in NASH appears to correlate with the severity of liver fibrosis [19].

Screening

NAFLD is highly prevalent in some high-risk groups, such as morbidly obese indicated for bariatric surgery (95%), type 2 diabetes mellitus (T2DM) (1/3–2/3 of patients), and dyslipidemia (50%); however, despite these prevalence rates, no consensus exists on screening for NAFLD. This is due to uncertainties over the optimal diagnostic test, cost-effectiveness of screening, and therapeutic limitation [20].

The recently published *Practice Guidance* from the American Association for the Study of Liver Diseases (AASLD) does not recommend screening. However, in T2DM patients, physicians should be alert to not only the presence of NAFLD but also NASH [20].

By contrast, the guidelines of the European Association for the Study of the Liver (EASL) recommend screening in all individuals with persistently abnormal hepatic enzymes and also in individuals with MetS or obesity, where routine screening should be carried out using hepatic enzyme studies and/or abdominal ultrasonography (USG). This same guideline advises that high-risk individuals (age >50 years, T2DM, MetS) should be screened for cases of advanced disease (NASH with fibrosis) and that screening of MetS be performed in individuals with NAFLD [2].

Diagnosis

The diagnosis of NAFLD requires the presence of hepatic steatosis, diagnosed by imaging exams or histology, and the exclusion of significant alcohol intake (>20 g/day for women and 30 g/day for men for over 2 years prior to the basal hepatic histology [21]), besides ruling out of secondary causes for hepatic steatosis and concomitant causes of chronic hepatic disease [2, 20]. Causes of secondary hepatic steatosis and chronic hepatic diseases can include drug use, viral hepatitis (particularly the hepatitis C virus genotype 3), hemochromatosis, Wilson's disease, cirrhosis and autoimmune hepatitis, abetalipoproteinemia, lipodystrophy, parenteral nutrition, and malnutrition [22].

Clinical Assessment

The clinical spectrum of NAFLD ranges from asymptomatic patients, accounting for most cases, to findings of more advanced hepatic diseases. Other nonspecific symptoms such as fatigue, malaise, and upper abdominal discomfort may be reported. Hepatomegaly can be seen in patients with NAFLD due to fatty infiltration, although this finding is variable. In addition, increased waist circumference, overweight, and acanthosis nigricans are indirect clinical signs associated with MetS [23].

Laboratory Assessment

Laboratory tests are needed to assess other conditions in the differential diagnosis of hepatic steatosis, but the clinical context should always be taken into account because abnormalities on some of these exams can be seen in patients with NAFLD in the absence of other associated hepatic diseases [20]. This statement can be justified by exemplifying changes in ferritin that may also be high in patients with NAFLD, without the presence of hepatic iron overload. It is important to emphasize that values over 1.5 of the upper limit of normal were associated with advanced fibrosis [24]. In this case, a genetic investigation for hemochromatosis is necessary, according to the practice guideline of the AASLD [20]. However, the presence of mutations in the HFE gene can be seen in patients with NAFLD [25], and therefore ordering a hepatic biopsy is prudent in this scenario, both for diagnosing hepatic iron accumulation and for assessing the severity of hepatic injury in individuals with suspected NAFLD [20].

Mild to moderate elevations (two to five times the upper limit of normal) of aspartate aminotransferase (AST) and alanine aminotransferase (ALT) may be present in patients with NAFLD [25]. In this disease, the AST-ALT ratio is <1, unlike in alcoholic fatty liver disease in which this ratio is >1 [26]. Normal AST and ALT values do not exclude major hepatic damage.

We suggest a protocol for a broad assessment of patients suspected of having NAFLD, based on history of alcohol use, personal and family history of T2DM, systemic arterial hypertension (SAH), and CVD, besides a physical exam and laboratory tests, which includes a diagnostic flow diagram for assessing and monitoring disease severity in the presence of suspected NAFLD and metabolic risk factors (Fig. 42.1).

Imaging Exams

There are currently various radiological methods available for detection of hepatic steatosis, although none of these are able to differentiate histological subtypes of NAFLD [2, 20].

Ultrasonography is the most used method for qualitative assessment of hepatic steatosis, given its availability and lower cost compared with magnetic resonance (MR) [27]. The findings of hepatic steatosis on USG are characterized by a hyperechoic texture or bright liver due to diffuse fat infiltration. The sensitivity and specificity of this method are 85% and 94%, respectively, using liver biopsy as the gold standard [28]. However, its sensitivity is reduced in morbidly obese patients and when there is less than 20% hepatic steatosis [27, 28].

Computed tomography (CT) is another method of radiologic assessment of hepatic steatosis that provides greater accuracy for detecting moderate to severe steatosis but has several limitations: more costly than USG, the use of ionizing radiation, attenuation values can be influenced by hepatic iron overload and amiodarone use [29].

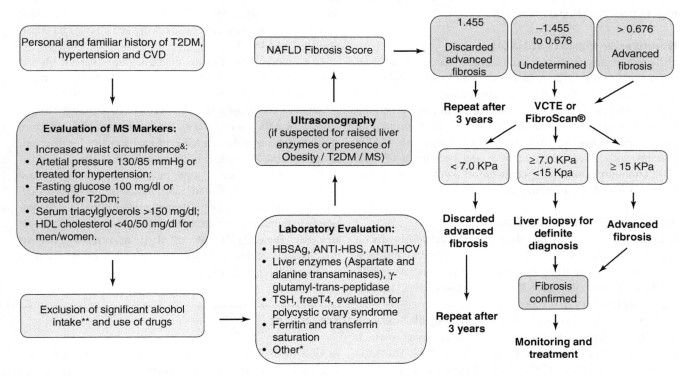

Fig. 42.1 Clinical, laboratory, and radiological evaluation in patients with suspected of nonalcoholic fatty liver disease and nonalcoholic steatohepatitis
&In the United States, the ATP III values are 102 cm male and 88 cm female
*Exclude other secondary causes of liver disease; and if necessary, tests for rare liver diseases (Wilson, autoimmune disease, α1-antitrypsin deficiency)

**<20 g/day/women, <30 g/day/men
T2DM type 2 diabetes mellitus, CVD cardiovascular disease, MS metabolic syndrome, HDL high-density lipoprotein, NAFLD nonalcoholic fatty liver disease, VCTE vibration-controlled transient elastography

MR is the most accurate exam for detection of mild steatosis, using the traditional method or spectroscopic MR (SMR). The sensitivities and specificities of MR for detecting histological steatosis ≥5% were 77–90% and 87–91%, respectively and for SMR were 80–91% and 80–87%, respectively. Another method, also observed by MR (PDFF, proton density fat fraction), can be a reference standard that is superior to histological grading in the measurement of hepatic fat [29].

Invasive and Noninvasive Methods for Assessment of Inflammation and Fibrosis

Liver biopsy is currently the most reliable approach for identifying the presence of steatohepatitis and fibrosis in NAFLD patients. However, the impracticality of performing liver biopsy in all patients with NAFLD, coupled with the limitations related to the diversity of histological interpretations, sampling error, and morbidity of the invasive method, has prompted the development of alternative clinical, biological, or imaging methods that help select patients that are high risk for NASH and fibrosis [1].

Noninvasive Markers of NASH

Different studies have assessed the diagnostic ability of serologic markers for differentiating steatosis from steatohepatitis. The most valid of these is cytokeratin-18 (CK-18), a hepatic intermediary filament protein produced by cellular death or hepatocyte apoptosis. This can be measured in serum, exhibiting significantly higher values in NASH patients with a sensitivity of 66% and specificity of 82% [20], although there is no specific cutoff owing to disparities in results found by different studies [30].

Noninvasive Markers for Fibrosis

Data from the literature has shown the impact of fibrosis on overall mortality of NAFLD patients. NASH has different stages which range from the absence of fibrosis (stage F0), advanced fibrosis (stage F3), and cirrhosis (F4), besides intermediate stages (F1, F2) [20].

Simple markers are available for identifying fibrosis, such as AST-ALT ratio (AAR), considered a classic marker which increases with progression of hepatic fibrosis [31]. The AST-to-platelet ratio index (APRI) and the FIB-4 index (fibrosis-4 calculator), which employs information such as age, AST, ALT and platelet count, are simple, easily applied formula with online calculators. FIB-4 in particular has shown promising results in NAFLD patients, with a negative predictive value of 95% for ruling out advancing fibrosis [32, 33]. The BARD index, determined by the sum of three items – (BMI) >28 kg/m^2, AST-ALT ratio >0.8, and the presence of diabetes – has also showed good negative predictive value for

excluding a significant degree of fibrosis [32].The NAFLD fibrosis score (NFS), determined by age, BMI, hyperglycemia, AST-ALT ratio, platelet count, and albumin, was reported as a specific marker for NAFLD, proving highly accurate for the exclusion of advanced fibrosis/cirrhosis. It was also able to estimate the risk of cardiovascular and hepatic complications [5].

In practice, validated tests for predicting advanced NAFLD are recommended (NFS and FIB-4), providing better results than other indexes (negative predictive value >90%). These tests should therefore be used as the first line in screening patients with low risk for advanced disease [34].

Physical markers have emerged to revolutionize the management of liver diseases by aiding noninvasive diagnosis of hepatic fibrosis. Elastography was the first imaging method developed for assessing liver stiffness, creating an elastic shear wave propagating through liver tissue, and then measuring its speed, which is directly proportional to the stiffness of the tissue. Vibration-controlled transient elastography (VCTE), FibroScan® (Echosens, Paris, France), is a straightforward rapid technique that assesses a representative volume of the liver that is 100 times greater than liver biopsy. A recent meta-analysis showed it to be an excellent technique for detecting advanced fibrosis, having sensitivity and specificity ≥82% [35].

Other modalities for assessing the degree of hepatic fibrosis include acoustic radiation force impulse (ARFI), elastography integrated into a conventional ultrasound wave, and magnetic resonance elastography (MRE). Studies comparing MRE and ARFI reveal the same capacity for detecting significant fibrosis and cirrhosis, although MRE proved superior for discriminating intermediate stages of fibrosis (F0–F2) [36].

Based on these data, some authors have recommended combining serological and radiological methods, particularly NFS and VCTE, in a diagnostic algorithm for differentiating patients with advanced disease from those with simple steatosis. Recently, Tapper et al. demonstrated the cost-effectiveness of this approach relative to the current standard method of liver biopsy [37].

Treatment

In view of the important association among NAFLD/NASH and hepatic fibrosis, metabolic disorders, and increased cardiovascular risk [38], the medical community needs to adopt a more proactive approach in the search for this diagnosis and in decisions on its management and related risk factors. Thus, NASH treatment should involve, besides antifibrotic hepatic therapy, improvement of metabolic risk factors, such as insulin resistance and inflammation, through lifestyle changes, drug therapy for improving hepatic disease, and treatment of hyperglycemia and dyslipidemia.

Who Should Be Treated?

Diagnostic confirmation and staging of NASH are fundamental for defining best conduct for these patients. According to the EASL, drug-based treatment to improve hepatic disease should be introduced in the presence of moderate to severe fibrosis or cirrhosis [2]. Given the difficulty in attaining complete resolution of NASH through lifestyle changes alone, some authors have suggested a more aggressive early approach based on a combination of lifestyle changes and pharmacologic therapy for liver protection and strict control of cardiometabolic risk factors (blood pressure, glycemia, and dyslipidemia), particularly in patients with pre-T2DM, T2DM, and/or high risk of disease progression. The following factors should be considered high risk for NASH progression: T2DM, MetS, age >50 years, elevated ALT, or active steatohepatitis with high necroinflammatory activity [2]. Cases of NASH without fibrosis (F0) or a mild degree of fibrosis (F1), without the cited risk factors, have good prognosis and do not require specific hepatic treatment [2, 20]. However, lifestyle changes for 8–10% weight loss should be strongly recommended to prevent progression of the disease and worsening of cardiovascular risk.

Nonpharmacological Treatment

A number of studies have shown that ≥7% weight loss in association with regular physical activity lead to a sustained improvement in hepatic enzyme levels and hepatic histology [39, 40]. Currently, the only measure recommended as standard treatment for NAFLD/NASH is weight loss. The nonpharmacological measures for NAFLD/NASH are presented in Table 42.1.

Table 42.1 Recommendations of a comprehensive lifestyle approach to NAFLD treatment

Intervention	Recommendation
Energy restriction	7–10% total weight loss target
Physical activity	150 min/week of moderate intensity aerobic physical activities Resistance training
Nutritional composition	Avoid excessive consumption of fructose Low-carbohydrate ketogenic diets or high protein Low-to-moderate fat and moderate-to-high carbohydrate intake
Coffee intake	No liver-related limitations
Alcohol intake	Drink alcohol until the risk threshold (30 g, men; 20 g, women)
Others	Stop smoking Vaccinate (A and B hepatitis)

NAFLD nonalcoholic fatty liver disease

Pharmacological Treatment of Liver Disease

Unfortunately, despite the development of drugs that can potentially act on the target mechanisms of the disease, the outcomes of these therapies have been modest [41]. To date, no drug therapy has been approved by the FDA for treating these diseases, where its use must be considered off-label [2].

Drugs available for treating NASH include vitamin E and pioglitazone, a peroxisome proliferator-activated receptor (PPAR) gamma agonist with potent insulin sensitizing and anti-inflammatory activity. A meta-analysis of four randomized clinical trials (RCTs) assessing the histological effects of pioglitazone on NASH found the drug to be more effective than placebo for improving fibrosis (odds ratio 1.7) [42]. Therefore, although its use has been associated with adverse effects such as weight gain, bone mass loss, and exacerbation of existing cardiac insufficiency [43], pioglitazone may represent an option in the pharmacological treatment of biopsy-confirmed NASH.

Vitamin E is a fat-soluble compound that protects cells from oxidative stress induced by free radicals [44]. A RCT showed both pioglitazone and vitamin E to be better than placebo in the treatment of NASH among non-T2DM patients with mild liver damage [45]; however, the study was not designed to determine outcomes related to the progression of hepatic fibrosis. Notably, there is clinical evidence that chronic use of vitamin E can increase the risk of overall mortality [46], stroke [47], and prostate cancer [48]. Thus, in addition to the unclear efficacy of both agents for preventing or reversing the degree of fibrosis, vitamin E should be used with caution and its possible collateral effect monitored.

A small 48-week RCT involving the liraglutide (1.8 mg/day), a glucagon-like peptide-1 analogue, found that the drug was safe and well-tolerated, led to the resolution of NASH, and promoted reduction in fibrosis progression compared to placebo (relative risk 4.3; 95% CI: 1.0–17) [49]. This drug may be an option in overweight or T2DM patients, but considering it an option for the treatment of NAFLD/NASH to improve liver disease is somewhat premature.

Other insulin sensitizers such as metformin and obeticholic acid (farnesoid X nuclear receptor activator) should not be recommended for NASH treatment [20]. The former failed to show hepatic histological improvement beyond that achieved by weight loss alone [2], while the latter, although showing histological improvement in an uncontrolled study, was associated with significant increase in cholesterol levels in the intervention group [50].

Pentoxifylline may contribute toward reducing NASH progression [51], but more robust scientific evidence supporting improvement in steatohepatitis and hepatic fibrosis is lacking [52].

Some RCTs assessing ursodeoxycholic acid have failed to prove its benefit in NASH [53, 54], and therefore, this drug should not be recommended for treatment of NAFLD/NASH [20].

The benefit of omega-3 fatty acid in NASH was assessed in a meta-analysis, showing improvement in hepatic steatosis and in AST levels. However, when the analysis was restricted to data from randomized studies, only improvement in hepatic steatosis was observed [55].

Novel therapies have been proposed for the treatment of NAFLD/NASH. Emricasan showed benefit in enzyme reduction and markers of hepatic apoptosis in NAFLD patients without cirrhosis [56]. However, whether this improvement is associated with histological improvements remains unclear. RCTs assessing the efficacy and safety of cenicriviroc (CCR2/CCR5 antagonist) and the double agonists of PPARα/δ (elafibranor and GFT505) are currently underway. Other drugs being studied for the treatment of NAFLD/NASH are presented in Table 42.2.

Finally, modulation of gut microbiota by the administration of probiotics may yield benefits in controlling sensitivity to insulin, necroinflammation, and even histological improvement [57]. Despite these results, insufficient scientific data are available in the literature to recommend the use of probiotics, prebiotics, and antibiotics in the treatment of NASH.

Treatment of Dyslipidemia and Cardiovascular Risk Factors

NAFLD can be considered a risk marker for CVD and cardiovascular mortality, where aggressive control of its risk factors is an important element in the management of these patients.

Studies have revealed that subjects with dyslipidemia and NASH can benefit from the use of statins through the lowering of transaminase levels [58, 59]. Nevertheless, some RCTs assessing the benefit of statins as a treatment option for NASH have produced mixed results, with absence of response or only modest improvement in liver enzyme levels [60]. Given the low risk of hepatotoxicity induced by these drugs in the population, statins can be used in NASH patients but should be avoided in cases of NASH with decompensated cirrhosis [20, 39].

The benefits of ezetimibe in treatment for NASH require further confirmation. While a recent ezetimibe RCT (10 mg/day for 6 months) promoted a reduction in hepatic fibrosis [61], another trial showed no effects on fat content, histology, or liver enzyme levels [62].

Therefore, lipid-lowering drugs cannot be recommended as a specific treatment for NASH but should be strongly considered as an option for the treatment of dyslipidemia in NASH patients.

Surgical Treatment

In the event of difficulty achieving significant weight loss long term with clinical treatment for obesity, there has been growing interest in bariatric surgery as a treatment option for NAFLD/NASH.

Observational studies show that bariatric surgery (gastric/bilio-intestinal bypass or gastric banding) can improve NASH-induced liver damage, whether by reducing transaminases, necroinflammation, and/or fibrosis [63, 64]. However, although recent meta-analyses report positive outcomes for bariatric surgery in steatohepatitis and fibrosis [65], no solid data from RCTs comparing clinical treatment versus bariatric surgery in terms of improvements in hepatic histology are available. Larger studies are needed to establish the true indication of this intervention in the specific treatment of NASH. Nevertheless, surgical treatment can represent an option in NASH cases for obese individuals with poor response to clinical treatment [20]. Thus far, insufficient data exists to define the best surgery type (gastric/bilio-intestinal bypass or gastric banding) for treating these patients.

Table 42.2 New medications for nonalcoholic fatty liver disease (NAFLD)

Medication	Mechanism
Oxidative stress and inflammation	
Cenicriviroc	CCR2/CCR5 antagonist
Emricasan	Caspase inhibitor
Primary metabolic target	
Elafibranor	PPARα/δ agonist
Saroglitazar	PPARα/γ agonist
Obeticholic acid	FXR agonist
Targeting the gut	
IMM-124e	IgG-rich bovine colostrum
Solithromycin	Antibiotic
Fecal microbial transplant	Modulação de microbiota intestinal
Simtuzumab	LOXL2 antibody
GR-MD-02	Galectin-3 inhibitor

NAFDL nonalcoholic fatty liver disease, *GLP* glucagon-like peptide, *FGF* fibroblast growth factor, *FXR* farnesoid X receptor, *HMG-CoA* 3-hydroxy-3-methyl-glutaryl-coenzyme A, *LOXL2* lysyl oxidase-like, *FDE* phosphodiesterase, *PPAR* peroxisome proliferator-activator receptor

References

1. Falck-Ytter Y, Younossi ZM, Marchesini G, McCullough AJ. Clinical features and natural history of nonalcoholic steatosis syndromes. Semin Liver Dis. 2001;21:17.
2. European Association for the Study of the Liver (EASL); European Association for the Study of Diabetes (EASD); European Association for the Study of Obesity (EASO). EASL-EASD-EASO

Clinical Practice Guidelines for the management of non-alcoholic fatty liver disease. Diabetologia. 2016;59:1121–40.

3. Younossi ZM, Stepanova M, Negro F, Hallaji S, Younossi Y, Lam B, et al. Nonalcoholic fatty liver disease in lean individuals in the United States. Medicine. 2012;91:319–27.

4. Liu Q, Bengmark S, Qu S. The role of hepatic fat accumulation in pathogenesis of non-alcoholic fatty liver disease (NAFLD). Lipids Health Dis. 2010;9:42.

5. Tessari P, Coracina A, Cosma A, Tiengo A. Hepatic lipid metabolism and non-alcoholic fatty liver disease. Nutr Metab Cardiovasc Dis. 2009;19(4):291–302.

6. Petersen K, Dufour S, Hariri A, Nelson-Williams C, Nee Foo J, Zhang XM, et al. Apolipoprotein C3 gene variants in nonalcoholic fatty liver disease. N Engl J Med. 2010;362:1082–9.

7. Savvidou S. Low serum adiponectin levels are predictive of advanced hepatic fibrosis in patients with NAFLD. J Clin Gastroenterol. 2009;43:765–72.

8. Rotman Y, Koh C, Zmuda JM, Kleiner DE, Liang TJ. The association of genetic variability in patatin-like phospholipase domain-containing protein 3 (PNPLA3) with histological severity of nonalcoholic fatty liver disease. Hepatology. 2010;52:894–903.

9. Kim HJ, Kim HJ, Lee KE, Kim DJ, Kim SK, Ahn CW, et al. Metabolic significance of nonalcoholic fatty liver disease in non-obese, nondiabetic adults. Arch Intern Med. 2004;164:2169–75.

10. Strauss RS, Barlow SE, Dietz WH. Prevalence of abnormal serum aminotransferase values in overweight and obese adolescents. J Pediatr. 2000;136:727–33.

11. Crespo J, Rivero M, Fábrega E, Cayón A, Amado JA, García-Unzeta MT. Plasma leptin and TNF-alpha levels in chronic hepatitis C patients and their relationship to hepatic fibrosis. Dig Dis Sci. 2002;47:1604–13.

12. Tsochatzis EA, Papatheodoridis GV, Archimandritis AJ. Adipokines in nonalcoholic steatohepatitis: from pathogenesis to implications in diagnosis and therapy. Mediat Inflamm. 2009;831:670.

13. Re Sookoian S, Rosselli MS, Gemma C, Burgueño AL, Fernández Gianotti T, Castaño GO. Epigenetic regulation of insulin resistance in nonalcoholic fatty liver disease: impact of liver methylation of the peroxisome proliferator-activated receptor Û coactivator 1α promoter. Hepatology. 2010;52:1992–2169.

14. Aqel B, DiBaise JK. Role of the gut microbiome in nonalcoholic fatty liver disease. Nutr Clin Pract. 2015;30(6):780–6.

15. Cope K, Risby T, Diehl AM. Increased gastrointestinal ethanol production in obese mice: implications for fatty liver disease pathogenesis. Gastroenterology. 2000;119:1340–7.

16. Holanda NCP. Síndrome metabólica e trabalho em turnos em equipe de enfermagem de um hospital infantil [dissertation]. Santos: Universidade Católica de Santos; 2017.

17. Diehl AM, Day C. Cause, pathogenesis, and treatment of nonalcoholic Steatohepatitis. N Engl J Med. 2017;377:2063–72.

18. Mendler MH, Turlin B, Moirand R, Jouanolle AM, Sapey T, Guyader D. Insulin resistance-associated hepatic iron overload. Gastroenterology. 1999;117(5):1155–63.

19. Valenti L, Fracanzani AL, Bugianesi E, Dongiovanni P, Galmozzi E, Vanni E. HFE genotype, parenchymal iron accumulation, and liver fibrosis in patients with nonalcoholic fatty liver disease. Gastroenterology. 2010;138:905–12.

20. Chalasani N, Younossi Z, Lavine JE, Charlton M, Cusi K, Rinella M, Harrison SA, Brunt EM, Sanyal AJ. Practice guidance, the diagnosis and management of nonalcoholic fatty liver disease: practice guidance from the American Association for the Study of Liver Diseases. Hepatology. 2018;67(1):328–57.

21. Gunn NT, Shiffman ML. The use of liver biopsy in nonalcoholic fatty liver disease: when to biopsy and in whom. Clin Liver Dis. 2018;21:109–19.

22. Sanyal AJ, Brunt EM, Kleiner DE, Kowdley DE, Chalasani N, Lavine JE, et al. End points and clinical trial design for nonalcoholic steatohepatitis. Hepatology. 2011;54:344–53.

23. Bacon BR, Farahvash MJ, Janney CG, Neuschwander-Tetri BA. Nonalcoholic steatohepatitis: an expanded clinical entity. Gastroenterology. 1994;107:1103.

24. Kowdley KV, Belt P, Wilson LA, Yeh MM, Neuschwander-Tetri BA, Chalasani N, et al. Serum ferritin is an independent predictor of histologic severity and advanced fibrosis in patients with nonalcoholic fatty liver disease. Hepatology. 2012;55:77–85.

25. Younossi ZM, Venkatesan C. A 2012 clinical update for internists in adult nonalcoholic fatty liver disease. Panminerva Med. 2012;54:29–37.

26. Korean Association for the Study of the Liver (KASL). KASL clinical practice guidelines: management of nonalcoholic fatty liver disease. Clin Mol Hepatol. 2013;19:325–48.

27. Hernaez R, Lazo M, Bonekamp S, Kamel I, Brancati FL, Guallar E, et al. Diagnostic accuracy and reliability of ultrasonography for the detection of fatty liver: a meta-analysis. Hepatology. 2011;54:1082–90.

28. Mottin CC, Moretto M, Padoin AV, Swarowsky AM, Toneto MG, Glock L, et al. The role of ultrasound in the diagnosis of hepatic steatosis in morbidly obese patients. Obes Surg. 2004;4:635–7.

29. Lee SS, Park SH. Radiologic evaluation of nonalcoholic fatty liver disease. World J Gastroenterol. 2014;20(23):7392–402.

30. Feldstein AE, Alkhouri N, De Vito R, Alisi A, Lopez R, Nobili V. Serum cytokeratin-18 fragment levels are useful biomarkers for nonalcoholic steatohepatitis in children. Am J Gastroenterol. 2013;108(9):1526–31.

31. Giannini E, Botta F, Fasoli A, Ceppa P, Risso D, Lantieri PB, Celle G, Testa R. Progressive liver functional impairment is associated with an increase in AST/ALT ratio. Dig Dis Sci. 1999;44:1249–53.

32. Fitzpatrick E, Dhawan A. Noninvasive biomarkers in nonalcoholic fatty liver disease: current status and a glimpse of the future. World J Gastroenterol. 2014;20:10851–63.

33. Enomoto H, Bando Y, Nakamura H, Nishiguchi S, Koga M. Liver fibrosis markers of nonalcoholic steatohepatitis. World J Gastroenterol. 2015;21(24):7427–35.

34. Kaswala DH, Lai M, Afdhal NH. Fibrosis assessment in nonalcoholic fatty liver disease (NAFLD) in 2016. Dig Dis Sci. 2016;61:1356–64.

35. Wilder J, Patel K. The clinical utility of FibroScan® as a noninvasive diagnostic test for liver disease. Med Devices (Auckl). 2014;7:107–14.

36. Pavlides M, Banerjee R, Sellwood J, Kelly CJ, Robson MD, Booth JC, et al. Multiparametric magnetic resonance imaging predicts clinical outcomes in patients with chronic liver disease. J Hepatol. 2016;64(2):308–15.

37. Tapper EB, Sengupta N, Hunink MG, Afdhal NH, Lai M. Cost-effective evaluation of nonalcoholic fatty liver disease with NAFLD fibrosis score and vibration controlled transient elastography. Am J Gastroenterol. 2015;110(9):1298–304.

38. Targher G, Bertolini L, Rodella S, et al. Non- alcoholic fatty liver disease is independently associated with an increased incidence of cardiovascular events in type 2 diabetic patients. Diabetes Care. 2007;30:2119–21.

39. Cotrim HP, Parise ER, Figueiredo-Mendes C, Galizzi-Filho J, Porta G, Oliveira CP. Nonalcoholic fatty liver disease Brazilian society of hepatology consensus. Arq Gastroenterol. 2016;53(2):118–22.

40. Vilar-Gomez E, Martinez-Perez Y, Calzadilla-Bertot L, Torres-Gonzalez A, Gra-Oramas B, Gonzalez-Fabian L, et al. Weight loss through lifestyle modification significantly reduces features of non-alcoholic steatohepatitis. Gastroenterology. 2015;149:367–78.

41. Rotman Y, Sanyal AJ. Current and upcoming pharmacotherapy for non-alcoholic fatty liver disease. Gut. 2017;66(1):180–90.

42. Boettcher E, Csako G, Pucino F, Wesley R, Loomba R. Meta-analysis: pioglitazone improves liver histology and fibrosis in patients with non-alcoholic steatohepatitis. Aliment Pharmacol Ther. 2012;35:66.

43. DeFronzo RA, Chilton R, Norton L, Clarke G, Ryder REJ, Abdul-Ghani M. Revitalization of pioglitazone: the optimum agent to be combined with a sodium-glucose co-transporter-2 inhibitor. Diabetes Obes Metab. 2016;18:454–62.

44. Soden JS, Devereaux MW, Haas JE, Gumpricht E, Dahl R, Gralla J, et al. Subcutaneous vitamin E ameliorates liver injury in an in vivo model of steatocholestasis. Hepatology. 2007;46:485–95.

45. Sanyal AJ, Chalasani N, Kowdley KV, et al. Pioglitazone, vitamin E, or placebo for nonalcoholic steatohepatitis. N Engl J Med. 2010;362:1675–85.

46. Bjelakovic G, Nikolova D, Gluud LL, Simonetti RG, Gluud C. Mortality in randomized trials of antioxidant supplements for primary and secondary prevention: systematic review and meta-analysis. JAMA. 2007;297:842–57.

47. Schurks M, Glynn RJ, Rist PM, Tzourio C, Kurth T. Effects of vitamin E on stroke subtypes: meta-analysis of randomised controlled trials. BMJ. 2010;341:c5702.

48. Klein EA, Thompson IM Jr, Tangen CM, Crowley JJ, Lucia MS, Goodman PJ, et al. Vitamin E and the risk of prostate cancer: the Selenium and Vitamin E Cancer Prevention Trial (SELECT). JAMA. 2011;306:1549–56.

49. Armstrong MJ, Gaunt P, Aithal GP, Barton D, Hull D, Parker R, et al. Liraglutide safety and efficacy in patients with non-alcoholic steatohepatitis (LEAN): a multicentre, double-blind, randomised, placebo-controlled phase 2 study. Lancet. 2016;387:679.

50. Neuschwander-Tetri BA, Loomba R, Sanyal AJ, Lavine JE, Van Natta ML, Abdelmalek MF, et al. Farnesoid X nuclear receptor ligand obeticholic acid for non-cirrhotic, non-alcoholic steatohepatitis (FLINT): a multicentre, randomised, placebo-controlled trial. Lancet. 2015;385:956–65.

51. Lee YM, Sutedja DS, Wai CT, et al. A randomized controlled pilot study of Pentoxifylline in patients with non-alcoholic steatohepatitis (NASH). Hepatol Int. 2008;2:196–201.

52. Van Wagner LB, Koppe SW, Brunt EM, Gottstein J, Gardikiotes K, Green RM, Rinella ME. Pentoxifylline for the treatment of non-alcoholic steatohepatitis: a randomized controlled trial. Ann Hepatol. 2011;10:277–86.

53. Lindor KD, Kowdley KV, Heathcote EJ, Harrison ME, Jorgensen R, Angulo P, et al. Ursodeoxycholic acid for treatment of nonalcoholic steatohepatitis: results of a randomized trial. Hepatology. 2004;39:770.

54. Leuschner UF, Lindenthal B, Herrmann G, et al. High-dose ursodeoxycholic acid therapy for nonalcoholic steatohepatitis: a double-blind, randomized, placebo-controlled trial. Hepatology. 2010;52:472–9.

55. Parker HM, Johnson NA, Burdon CA, Cohn JS, O'Connor HT, George J. Omega-3 supplementation and non-alcoholic fatty liver disease: a systematic review and meta-analysis. J Hepatol. 2012;56(4):944–51.

56. Shiffman M, Freilich B, Vuppalanchi R, Watt K, Burgess G, Burgess G, Morris M, Sheedy B, Schiff E, et al. A placebo-controlled, multi-center, double-blind, randomised trial of emricasan in subjects with non-alcoholic fatty liver disease (Nafld) and raised transaminases. J Hepatol. 2015;62:S282.

57. Eslamparast T, Eghtesad S, Hekmatdoost PH. Probiotics and nonalcoholic fatty liver disease. Middle East. J Dig Dis. 2013;5:129–36.

58. Athyros VG, Tziomalos K, Gossios TD, Griva T, Anagnostis P, Kargiotis K, et al. Safety and efficacy of long-term statin treatment for cardiovascular events in patients with coronary heart disease and abnormal liver tests in the Greek Atorvastatin and Coronary Heart Disease Evaluation (GREACE) study: a post-hoc analysis. Lancet. 2010;376:1916–22.

59. Tikkanen MJ, Fayyad R, Faergeman O, Olsson AG, Wun CC, Laskey R, et al. Effect of intensive lipid lowering with atorva- statin on cardiovascular outcomes in coronary heart disease patients with mild-to-moderate baseline elevations in alanine aminotransferase levels. Int J Cardiol. 2013;168:3846–52.

60. Nelson A, Torres DM, Morgan AE, Fincke C, Harrison SA. A pilot study using simvastatin in the treatment of nonalcoholic steatohepatitis: a randomized placebo-controlled trial. J Clin Gastroenterol. 2009;43:990–4.

61. Takeshita Y, Takamura T, Honda M, et al. The effects of ezetimibe on non-alcoholic fatty liver disease and glucose metabolism: a randomized controlled trial. Diabetologia. 2014;57:878–90.

62. Loomba R, Sirlin CB, Ang B, Bettencourt R, Jain R, Salotti J, Soaft L, Hooker J, Kono Y, et al. Ezetimibe for the treatment of non-alcoholic steatohepatitis: assessment by novel magnetic resonance imaging and magnetic resonance elastography in a randomized trial (MOZART trial). Hepatology. 2015;61:1239–50.

63. Caiazzo R, Lassailly G, Leteurtre E, Baud G, Verkindt H, Raverdy V, et al. Roux-en-Y gastric bypass versus adjustable gastric banding to reduce nonalcoholic fatty liver disease: a 5-year controlled longitudinal study. Ann Surg. 2014;260:893–9.

64. Lassailly G, Caiazzo R, Buob D, Pigeyre M, Verkindt H, Labreuche J, et al. Bariatric surgery reduces features of non-alcoholic steatohepatitis in morbidly obese patients. Gastroenterology. 2015;149:377–88.

65. Bower G, Toma T, Harling L, Jiao LR, Efthimiou E, Darzi A, et al. Bariatric surgery and non-alcoholic fatty liver disease: a systematic review of liver biochemistry and histology. Obes Surg. 2015;25:2280–9.

Treatment of Obesity in the Patient with Type 2 Diabetes

43

Manpreet S. Mundi and Maria L. Collazo-Clavell

Introduction: Rising Prevalence of Obesity and Type 2 Diabetes Mellitus

The prevalence of obesity continues to rise in the United States and around the world, closely matched by the rising prevalence of type 2 diabetes mellitus [1, 2]. Recent publications report greater than two-thirds of Americans are considered overweight (BMI ≥ 25 kg/m^2) and over one-third are obese (BMI ≥ 30 kg/m^2) [1]. If current trends hold, the number of obese Americans is expected to increase to greater than 50% by 2030 [1]. The devastating impact of obesity's rising prevalence is imminent, both in terms of our citizenry's health and in the financial well-being of our healthcare industry as a whole.

Key Points to Be Discussed

- Health risks of obesity.
- Outcomes of medical nutrition therapy in patients with type 2 DM.
- Role of medications in the treatment of obesity.
- Impact of bariatric surgery on type 2 diabetes mellitus.

Health Risks of Obesity

Major studies have clearly correlated obesity with the development of chronic metabolic conditions, such as type 2 diabetes, hypertension, and hyperlipidemia [3, 4]. One of these landmark trials was the Nurses' Health Study, which began in 1976 when 121,700 female nurses 30–55 years of age began receiving and responding to questionnaires regarding

M. S. Mundi · M. L. Collazo-Clavell (✉)
Division of Endocrinology, Diabetes, Metabolism, and Nutrition, Mayo Clinic, Rochester, MN, USA
e-mail: mundi.manpreet@mayo.edu;
collazoclavell.maria@mayo.edu

medical, lifestyle, and other health-related information [3]. These women were then followed until 1996 with biannual questionnaires requesting updated information and identification of newly diagnosed diseases. Of the initial cohort, 84,941 female nurses were free of diagnosed cardiovascular disease, diabetes, and cancer at baseline. This cohort was further analyzed for risk factors pertaining to the development of diabetes. During the follow-up period, 3300 new cases of type 2 diabetes were documented with the most important risk factor being body mass index (BMI). The relative risk of diabetes was 38.8 in women with BMI of 35.0 kg/m^2 or higher and 20.1 for women with BMI between 30.0 and 34.9 kg/m^2 when compared to women with BMI of less than 23.0 kg/m^2. In fact, the relative risk was not only increased in the obese women but in the overweight groups as well. Women with a BMI between 25.0 and 29.9 kg/m^2 had a relative risk of 7.59, and 61% of the cases of diabetes could be attributed to this overweight category.

Similar results were found in the third National Health and Nutrition Examination Survey [4] (NHANES). NHANES included a home interview and a standardized physical exam to gather body weight and height. The results, however, were similar in that the prevalence of type 2 diabetes increased dramatically with an increase in BMI. The prevalence of diabetes was 2.5 times higher in overweight men (BMI 25–29.9 kg/m^2) and 3 times higher in overweight women when compared to normal weight group. This prevalence continued to increase and was 6 times higher in men and 5.5 times higher in women with BMI between 35 and 39.9 kg/m^2 when compared to normal weight group.

Of particular concern is that individuals with BMI ≥ 40 kg/m^2 (class III obesity) are the most rapidly growing subset within the obese population. In fact, we have recently seen a 50% increase in individuals with BMI > 40 kg/m^2 and a 75% increase in the prevalence of individuals with a BMI > 50 kg/m^2 [5]. Unfortunately not only does obesity increase the prevalence of diabetes, it also makes it more difficult to treat by further increasing insulin resistance and glucose intolerance as well as exacerbating other metabolic complications, such as hypertension and dyslipidemia [3, 4, 6–8]. Campbell et al. investigated the relationship of insulin sensitivity to body mass index (BMI) in 49 healthy volunteers who ranged between 80% and 240% of ideal body weight [9]. By performing glucose clamp studies using various insulin concentrations, they found that insulin sensitivity for glucose disposal was impaired in individuals who were at least 20% above ideal body weight for their height (BMI > 26 kg/m²). Beyond this threshold, insulin sensitivity and BMI were highly correlated (r-0.8 p < 0.001) in a linear fashion and accounted for 64% of the variability in insulin sensitivity.

The combination of obesity with diabetes also proves to be a much dire situation in terms of mortality. The presence of excess body fat, particularly abdominal fat, along with the presence of insulin resistance leads to a pro-atherogenic lipid profile with high triglyceride and apolipoprotein B concentrations, an increased proportion of small dense LDL particles, and a reduced concentration of HDL cholesterol. This along with a pro-thrombotic and a pro-inflammatory profile significantly worsens an individual's risk of cardiovascular disease and overall mortality [10]. In fact, compared with normal weight individuals with diabetes, the mortality rate is 2.5–3.3 times higher in diabetics with body weights that are 20–30% above their ideal weight and 5.2–7.9 times higher in those with body weights 40% above ideal weight [11].

Treating the Patient with Obesity and Type 2 Diabetes

The exponential increase in the health risks of excess BMI and insulin resistance make weight loss the first target in a patient with type 2 diabetes. Calorie restriction and weight loss have a positive effect on almost every risk factor associated with diabetes and obesity. There is a significant decrease in fasting glucose levels as noted in the UKPDS cohort who experienced weight loss in the first 3 months (a decrease from 205.2 ± 59.4 to 145.8 ± 32.4 mg/dL) [12]. This is accompanied by a decrease in fasting insulin levels [13], increase in insulin sensitivity [14], and improvement in beta-cell function [14]. Similar improvements are also noted in co-existing conditions such as hypertension and dyslipidemia. In the first few days of caloric restriction, a reduction in VLDL and triglyceride concentrations as well as increase in LDL particle size can be found [15]. With longer duration of therapy, a decrease in LDL concentration and an increase in HDL particles occur.

Lifestyle Modification

Despite the numerous benefits of weight loss in type 2 diabetes, it is often difficult for individuals with obesity to initially lose the desired weight and then maintain the weight loss. The Diabetes Prevention Program was the first intensive lifestyle intervention aimed at patients at risk for the development of type 2 diabetes. This study included individuals with hyperglycemia and an average age of 51 years and an average BMI of 34 kg/m². Study subjects were either randomized to standard care, metformin therapy (1500 mg daily), or lifestyle intervention including achieving a weight loss of <7% and participating in 150 minutes of physical activity weekly. The intensive lifestyle intervention cohort experienced a 58% decrease in the incidence of type 2 diabetes. This was greater than observed in the control and metformin cohorts [16]. Similarly, the Swedish Obese Subjects study also revealed that individuals placed on conventional diet and exercise had a 1.6% increase in weight after 10 years [17].

The Look AHEAD study looked at the impact of an intensive lifestyle intervention (ILI) compared to standard care (Diabetes Support and Education; DSE) in patients with type 2 diabetes on cardiovascular morbidity and mortality. In this study, the intervention group used meal replacements as part of the dietary intervention and was recommended to participate in 200 minutes of physical activity per week. After 8 years, there was no significant difference on cardiovascular morbidity and mortality between the cohorts. However, both cohorts lost weight with reported average weight loss at the conclusion of the study of 4.7% +/− 0.2% for ILI and 2.1% +/− 0.2% for DSE. Weight loss >5% was reported in 50.3% of ILI cohort and 35.7% of DSE cohort. Weight loss of >10% was reported in 26.9 and 17.2% of the cohorts, respectively [18].

Even when weight loss is achieved through aggressive lifestyle modification, whether through medically supervised programs or commercial programs, weight regain commonly occurs once the intervention ends [19, 20].

Outcomes of Medical Nutrition Therapy

There is often confusion regarding which dietary intervention to advice patients with type 2 diabetes to help them manage their weight. The American Diabetes Association (ADA) recommends that all patients with diabetes meet with a registered dietitian to receive individualized medical nutrition therapy (MNT). In the absence of intensive insulin therapy, there is little evidence to support a specific macronutrient composition of carbohydrate, protein, and fat but mainly emphasize calorie restriction to achieve weight loss. Methods to achieve calorie restriction are varied, including portion control, healthy food choices, and meal replacements to name a few. Specific dietary interventions studied and shown to be beneficial in patients with type 2 diabetes include the Dietary Approaches to Stop Hypertension (DASH), Mediterranean diet, and plant-based diets. The Mediterranean diet has been particularly shown to improve glucose metabolism and lower the risk for cardiovascular events [21].

Very low-calorie diets (VLCDs) have been used to fill the gap between standard lifestyle modifications and bariatric surgery. The use of VLCDs grew rapidly in the 1970s with the introduction of the so-called liquid protein modified fast that provided 300–400 calories per day of liquid protein of low biological value obtained from collagen or gelatin hydrolysates. These diets tended to have inadequate micronutrient supplementation and resulted in a number of deaths secondary to arrhythmias [13]. Since then the composition of VLCDs has been changed to include high-quality protein supplemented with vitamins, minerals, trace elements, and essential fatty acids with improved outcomes when used under direct medical supervision [22]. In fact, many studies have reported typical weight loss of ~1–3 kg/week with higher results seen in the first 2 weeks due to fluid diuresis [22–24]. Weight loss with VLCDs is typically greater than with conventional diets and tends to occur more rapidly, producing faster and greater improvements in metabolic comorbidities. Henry et al. revealed a near normalizing of plasma glucose within 10 days of being placed on a VLCD in NIDDM subjects [25]. Unfortunately, this effect can be transient, as fasting plasma glucose values tend to rise once patients are taken off of the VLCD and gain weight. Recidivism or weight regain is seen in virtually all patients once VLCD is stopped. Less weight loss is noted with subsequent VLCD trials due to changes in metabolic rate, making VLCDs an unlikely long-term solution.

Role of Medications in the Treatment of Obesity

Pharmacological options to help patients with type 2 diabetes manage their weight have increased recently. Novel agents have been approved for long-term weight management. In addition, new glucose-lowering agents have favorable effects on weight expanding our armamentarium in helping patients with type 2 diabetes achieve the desired glycemic control without the observed weight gain reported with older glucose-lowering agents [26].

Orlistat

Orlistat, a lipase inhibitor, has been on the market for a number of years and has been shown to result in approximately 5.4–10.6 kg weight loss at 1 year with 46–73% of patients achieving greater than 5% and 20–41% achieving greater than 10% weight loss [27, 28]. Modest improvements in HbA1c have also been reported with one randomized placebo control study revealing a decrease of −0.74% with Orlistat 120 mg tid versus −0.31% in the placebo group [27]. A modest reduction in HbA1c was observed in patients despite minimal weight loss with Orlistat versus placebo

(−0.29% vs. +0.14%, respectively). Other studies have revealed an average HbA1c reduction of 0.28–1.1% [28]. Meta-analysis by Johansson et al. [29] revealed a statistically significant improvement in hypertension with a reduction of 1.9 mmHg in systolic blood pressure and 1.5 mmHg for diastolic blood pressure. Compared with patients without diabetes, patients with diabetes experienced smaller and nonsignificant reductions of SBP and DBP.

Phentermine/Topiramate

Combination of phentermine and topiramate has also been approved for long-term use for weight loss. It has been studied in a low-dose (PHEN/TPM CR 7.5 mg/46 mg) or high-dose formulation (PHEN/TPM CR 15 mg/92 mg) for up to 2 years [30, 31]. At 108 weeks, the high-dose group lost 10.5% of body weight, while the low-dose group lost 9.3%, and the placebo group gained 1.8% despite lifestyle interventions including behavioral therapy based on the LEARN manual. Both systolic and diastolic blood pressures were reduced by 3–5 mmHg from baseline. They also found a 54% reduction in progression to type 2 diabetes in low-dose groups and a 76% reduction in high-dose groups. Although, less than 10% of subjects enrolled in the trial had type 2 diabetes, the average HbA1c reduction was 0.4% in the low dose and 0.2% in the high dose when compared to no change in the placebo group. These medications do show some promise for use in patients with type 2 diabetes, but long-term data is necessary. Patient attrition also continues to be an issue as greater than 50% of patients enrolled dropped out of the 2-year study of phentermine/topiramate.

Bupropion/Naltrexone

Bupropion and naltrexone in combination are believed to decrease appetite and control eating behaviors through their effects on the mesolimbic dopaminergic reward system. In a randomized clinical trial, naltrexone sustained release (SR) (32 mg) and bupropion SR (360 mg) were compared to standardized lifestyle intervention in overweight/obese individuals with type 2 diabetes. Naltrexone/bupropion (NB) was associated with significantly greater weight loss (−5.0% versus −1.8%) and with a greater percentage of patients achieving a weight loss of >5% (44.5% vs. 18.9%). NB-treated subjects also experienced greater improvements in glycemic control with 44.1% of subjects achieving HgbA1c levels of <7% compared to 26.3% with lifestyle intervention alone [32].

Liraglutide/Semaglutide

Liraglutide and semaglutide are glucagon-like peptide-1 analogues (GLP-1), that have been shown to be effective in the management of type 2 diabetes [33, 34]. Liraglutide and semaglutide also promote weight loss. A randomized trial of patients with type 2 diabetes, liraglutide once daily subcutaneous doses of 3.0 mg (LR 3.0), 1.8 mg (LR 1.8), and placebo, in conjunction with a calorie-restricted diet (−500 kcal/day) and regular physical activity (150 min/week) reported weight losses of 6.0%, 4.7%, and 2.0%, respectively (all $p < 0.001$). Weight loss of >5% was reported in 54.3% with LR 3.0, 40.4% with LR 1.8, and 21.4% with placebo. Weight loss of >10% was reported in 25.2% with LR 3.0, 15.9% with LR 1.8, and 6.7% with placebo [34]. Semaglutide at doses of 0.5 and 1.0 mg was associated with clinically meaningful weight loss regardless of baseline BMI. Weight loss attributed to gastrointestinal symptoms was also minor. Meta-analysis suggests the weight loss benefit is a class effect of GLP-1 analogues, although limited head-to-head trials are available [35].

In the armamentarium of glucose-lowering therapy, dipeptidyl peptidase 4 (DPP4) inhibitors are deemed weight neutral. [36] Sodium glucose co-transport 2 (SGLT 2) inhibitors may offer a weight loss benefit [37].

Bariatric Surgery

Challenges with medical nutrition therapy and weight loss medications have made bariatric surgery a treatment alternative for long-term sustained weight loss. The popularity of bariatric surgery has grown since its inception in the 1950s [38]. Currently, the laparoscopic adjustable gastric banding (LAGB) and the gastric sleeve are the main restrictive procedures being offered. The LABG is an implanted device that is placed around the proximal portion of the stomach and restricts flow of food (Fig. 43.1a). It does require routine adjustment after placement to ensure sufficient restriction while avoiding complete stenosis or laxity. The gastric sleeve is a restrictive procedure that until recently was being performed as part of the biliopancreatic diversion duodenal switch (BPD-DS) in a staged procedure in the superobese (Fig. 43.1b) [39]. It involves resection of the majority of the stomach along the greater curvature, decreasing gastric volume by over 90%. The main mechanism of weight loss with these procedures is through a reduction in volume of food intake as well as early satiety. The LAGB is falling in popularity as the gastric sleeve is gradually overcoming the Roux-en-Y gastric bypass as the most common bariatric operation performed [40].

Roux-En-Y gastric bypass (RYGB) has been the most common bariatric operation performed in the United States (Fig. 43.1c, d). In this procedure, the stomach is partitioned into a much larger distal portion and small (~15 ml) proximal portion, which receives food from the esophagus. The proximal portion is then joined with the jejunum restricting the volume of a typical meal dramatically. The distal portion of the stomach, duodenum, and early jejunum is then connected downstream of the gastrojejunal anastomosis, thus bypassing this portion of the intestine from receiving pancreatic enzymes and bile. The length of this bypassed portion of the jejunum or Roux limb can range from 75 cm to 250 cm to produce the desired amount of weight loss. Biliopancreatic diversion (BPD) performed with or without the duodenal switch (BPD-DS) are the main malabsorptive procedures being offered (Fig. 43.1e). These procedures include partitioning of the stomach in the case of BPD or creation of gas-

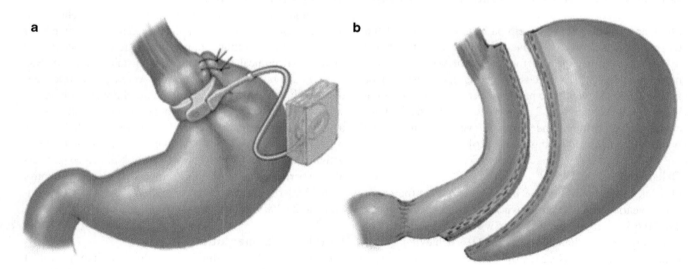

Fig. 43.1 Illustration of main types of bariatric surgery currently being performed. (**a**) Laparoscopic Adjustable Gastric Band; (**b**) Sleeve Gastrectomy; (**c**) Proximal RYGB; (**d**) Distal RYGB; (**e**) Biliopancreatic Diversion and Duodenal Switch. (*By permission of Mayo Foundation for Medical Education and Research. All rights reserved*)

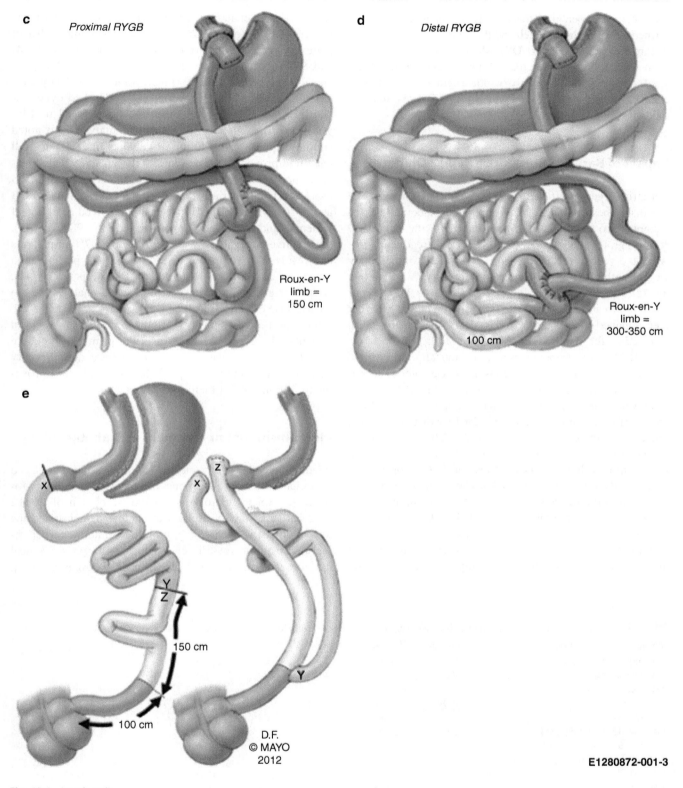

c *Proximal RYGB*

Roux-en-Y
limb =
150 cm

d *Distal RYGB*

Roux-en-Y
limb =
300-350 cm

100 cm

e

150 cm

100 cm

D.F.
© MAYO
2012

E1280872-001-3

Fig. 43.1 (continued)

tric sleeve as seen in BPD-DS. Then, an anastomosis is formed between the stomach and the jejunum (BPD) or duodenum and jejunum (BPD-DS). Malabsorption of nutrients occurs when the biliopancreatic limb is joined to the distal small intestine, allowing only a short segment of "common channel" where digestive enzymes from pancreas and bile mix with food.

Impact of Bariatric Surgery on Type 2 Diabetes

Bariatric surgery is efficacious in producing weight loss. The Swedish Obese Subjects study compared outcome in 2010 patients who underwent bariatric surgery with a matched control group who received conventional treatment [17]. After 1–2 years, the RYGB group had lost 32% of their body weight with the vertical banded gastroplasty (VBG) group losing 23% and the LAGB losing 20% (Table 43.1). The conventional treatment group initially lost weight at 1 year but then regained by 2 years. After 10 years, the weight losses were 25% for the RYGB, 17% for VBG, and 15% for LAGB. Although dropout was an issue, the long-term weight loss in the surgical group was considerably greater than conventional treatment group. A meta-analysis of 621 studies by Buchwald et al. revealed an average weight loss of 38.5 kg or 55.9% of excess body weight loss for four distinct surgical procedures including BPD-DS [39]. The weight loss appeared to be sustained as studies with 2 or more years of follow-up revealed a mean total loss of 41.6 kg or 59% of excess body weight loss. The results were more impressive in patients with diabetes with a mean total loss of 40.6 kg or 64.4% of excess weight and loss of 42.9 kg or 58.0% of excess weight in studies beyond 2 years.

Equally impressive improvements in weight-related medical comorbidities have been reported with bariatric surgery. Pories et al. first reported on the impact of bariatric surgery (RYGB) on type 2 diabetes and noted that 82.9% of patients with non-insulin-dependent diabetes (NIDDM) and 98.7% of patients with glucose impairment experienced euglycemia without medications [40]. They also noted that 353 of the 608 patients (58.1%) had hypertension prior to surgery, and this rate was reduced to 14% afterward. Buchwald et al. in a meta-analysis also noted similar impressive resolution of diabetes in 78.1% overall and an improvement or resolution in 86.6% [39]. Diabetes resolution was greatest for patients undergoing BPD-DS (95.1% resolution rate) compared to 80.3% with RYGB and 56.7% with LAGB. Hypertension resolved in 61.7% of patients and resolved or improved in 78.5% [41]. Obstructive sleep apnea was resolved in 85.7% of patients and resolved or improved in 83.6% [41]. Hyperlipidemia improved as well in greater than 70% of patients [41]. Brethauer et al. conducted a similar meta-analysis for the gastric sleeve both as a staged and primary procedure [42]. They reported a weight loss of 60.4% of excess weight in patients where gastric sleeve was the primary procedure and 46.9% when it was used as a staged procedure. Seventy percent of patients with type 2 diabetes had an improvement or remission of their disease.

Mechanisms of Improvement in Diabetes

In addition to the improvement in insulin resistance produced by weight loss alone, additional mechanisms have been proposed to explain improvement and/or resolution of DMT2 after bariatric surgery. Kellum et al. first demonstrated the impact of gastric bypass on gastrointestinal hormones reporting a dramatic increase in enteroglucagon response to meal not observed after vertical banded gastroplasty [43].

Table 43.1 Weight loss reported as percent of baseline weight with various weight loss interventions

Weight loss intervention	6 months	1 year	2 years	3 years	4 years	5 years	>5 years
Diet alone [58]	5.0	4.6	4.4		3.0		
Diet plus exercise [58]	8.5	4.0	4.0	4.0	4.0		
Meal replacements [58]	9.6	7.5					
VLCD [58]	16.0	10.0		5.0			
Orlistat [58]	8.0	8.0	7.0	7.0	5.3		
Phen/top 15 mg/92 mg [31]	12.0	13.0	11.0				
Liraglutide 3.0 mg [59, 60]		8.0	5.4				
Naltrexone/Buproprion [61, 62] 32 mg		6.1–9.3					
LAGB [17]	18.0	21.0	20.0	18.0	17.0	16.0	15.0 (10 years)
VBG [17]	23.0	26.0	23.0	21.0	20.0	18.0	17.0 (10 years)
RYGB [17]	27.0	33.0	32.0	30.0	29.0	27.0	25.0 (10 years)

Weight loss interventions (associated references) and percent weight loss from baseline weight reported at various time points (6 months, 1,2,3,4,5, > 5 years)

Note percent weight loss provided from pertinent landmark studies. Data from gastric sleeve and BPD-DS not available in this format at time of publication

Enteroglucagon corresponds to the protein product of the glucagon gene in the gut that generates many gut hormones (incretins),such as glucagon-like peptide 1 (GLP-1) and 2 (GLP-2), glucagon, glicentin, and oxyntomodulin [44]. Additional studies revealed that glucose-stimulated incretin levels increase after gastric bypass when they are typically blunted in T2DM [45–47]. Laferrère et al. revealed that this incretin effect can result in an increase in insulin secretion to levels seen in matched controls without T2DM only 1 month after gastric bypass [47]. This effect does not appear to be due to weight loss alone as shown in a study by Laferrère et al. that compared the change in incretin levels in obese women with T2DM undergoing RYGB versus their matched controls who lost an equivalent amount of weight with diet [48]. They found that GLP-1 levels after oral glucose increased sixfold after surgery, but not after diet. In fact, after diet-induced weight loss, the levels of GLP-1 and GIP tended to decrease.

Additional beneficial changes in incretin secretion have been reported after bariatric surgery, resulting in both central (hypothalamic appetite regulation) and peripheral (ileal break and delayed transport of nutrients through the gastrointestinal tract) mechanisms. Obese individuals typically have decreased basal and postprandial PYY [49] as well as decreased post-prandial GLP-1 response [50], leading to lower feelings of satiety. This trend can be worsened with diet-induced weight loss as Sumithran et al. [51] revealed an increase in ghrelin and a reduction in peptide YY (PYY), amylin, and CCK, leading to an increase in ratings of hunger, desire and urge to eat, as well as prospective consumption. The opposite has been reported after bariatric surgery [52–54]. One of the proposed mechanisms after gastric bypass is the increased delivery of unabsorbed nutrients to the GLP-1 and PYY producing L cells in the distal small bowel, resulting in amplified secretion of the incretins [55]. Others have speculated that there is a change in macronutrient composition after surgery that may result in alteration of incretin secretion. Evans et al. [55] investigated the mechanism of this change by comparing subjects who underwent RYGB with matched controls who were given a hypocaloric diet similar to a typical post-RYGB diet for 7 days. They provided the groups with a high-protein or high-fat meal. Gastric bypass resulted in augmented post-prandial GLP-1 and PYY response to both meals. No augmentation in GLP-1 and minimal augmentation in PYY were seen in the low-calorie diet group. There was also a dramatic increase in hunger ratings in the diet group both before and after meal when compared to the RYGB group.

In addition to augmentation of GLP-1 and PYY secretion, bariatric surgery has also been noted to result in a change in ghrelin levels, a neuropeptide synthesized mainly in the antrum of the stomach that is known to have an orexigenic hypothalamic effect. Cummings et al. compared ghrelin levels before and after both a 6-month dietary program as well as gastric bypass [52]. They noted a significant rise in ghrelin levels in the dietary weight loss group. On the other hand, the gastric bypass subjects had markedly lower ghrelin levels compared to both the lean and obese controls, despite weight loss. They also did not have an oscillation in levels in relation to meals, an effect felt to be due to the process of override inhibition that occurs when the stomach and duodenum are isolated from food. This tends to support patient subjective improvements in hunger and appetite regulation as exogenous ghrelin has been show to increase subjective hunger and food intake, as well as decrease catabolism of fat and metabolic rate, leading to increase in body weight.

These positive changes in incretin secretion are not only isolated to RYGB but have also been noted in patients undergoing gastric sleeve. Langer et al. prospectively compared ghrelin levels after gastric sleeve and LAGB and noted that they were dramatically reduced after the gastric sleeve and yet increased following LAGB. Peterli et al. [56] compared the change in ghrelin levels after a RYGB and gastric sleeve and observed a decrease in ghrelin levels within a few weeks of either procedure. The decrease was more prominent in the gastric sleeve group when compared to the RYGB group, a finding that can be explained by the fact that ghrelin-producing cells are being removed in the gastric sleeve versus being isolated from nutrients in the RYGB. Gastric sleeve patients also had an improvement in GLP-1 response to meals that was less prominent than the RYGB group. This is a startling finding given the fact that the foregut is not being bypassed. One explanation for increased GLP-1 release may be that there is an additional trigger such as CCK for release of GLP-1 in addition to nutrient stimulation of L cells. It also seems that despite the lack of bypass in gastric sleeve, accelerated gastric emptying and earlier contact of chyme with L cells may still be occurring. Scintigraphic studies have shown accelerated gastric emptying for solid and liquid foods up to 2 years after sleeve gastrectomy [57].

Future Therapy Update

There is ongoing investigation of novel therapies targeting the obesity epidemic and its associated medical comorbidities. These include the continued development of medications and new endoscopic approaches to help promote weight loss.

Summary

The rise in the prevalence of obesity is a recognized contributor to the rising incidence of type 2 diabetes. Despite the reported benefits of weight loss through lifestyle changes, achieving significant and sustained weight loss remains a challenging prescription for most patients. Bariatric surgery has been shown to be an effective therapeutic alternative in the management of the patient with obesity. Yet, it is the impact of bariatric surgery on weight-related comorbidities, particularly type 2 diabetes, that has led to a dramatic rise in the number of operations performed. Being well informed regarding the bariatric operations currently offered and their impact on type 2 diabetes is critically important as we assess the potential role of these operations in the management of our patients.

References

1. Wang YC, McPherson K, Marsh T, Gortmaker SL, Brown M. Health and economic burden of the projected obesity trends in the USA and the UK. Lancet. 2011;378:815–25.
2. Abraham TM, Pencina KM, Pencina MJ, Fox CS. Trends in diabetes incidence: the Framingham Heart Study. Diabetes Care. 2015;38:482–7.
3. Hu FB, et al. Diet, lifestyle, and the risk of type 2 diabetes mellitus in women. N Engl J Med. 2001;345:790–7.
4. Must A, et al. The disease burden associated with overweight and obesity. JAMA. 1999;282:1523–9.
5. Sturm R. Increases in morbid obesity in the USA: 2000-2005. Public Health. 2007;121:492–6.
6. Allison DB, Fontaine KR, Manson JE, Stevens J, VanItallie TB. Annual deaths attributable to obesity in the United States. JAMA. 1999;282:1530–8.
7. Despres JP, Fong BS, Julien P, Jimenez J, Angel A. Regional variation in HDL metabolism in human fat cells: effect of cell size. Am J Physiol Endocrinol Metab. 1987;252:E654–9.
8. Kissebah AH, Alfarsi S, Adams PW, Wynn V. Role of insulin resistance in adipose tissue and liver in the pathogenesis of endogenous hypertriglyceridaemia in man. Diabetologia. 1976;12:563–71.
9. Campbell PJ, Gerich JE. Impact of obesity on insulin action in volunteers with normal glucose tolerance: demonstration of a threshold for the adverse effect of obesity. J Clin Endocrinol Metab. 1990;70:1114–8.
10. Després J-P, et al. Abdominal obesity and the metabolic syndrome: contribution to global cardiometabolic risk. Arterioscler Thromb Vasc Biol. 2008;28:1039–49.
11. Blackburn GL, Read JL. Benefits of reducing–revisited. Postgrad Med J. 1984;60(Suppl 3):13–8.
12. UK prospective diabetes study 7: response of fasting plasma glucose to diet therapy in newly presenting type II diabetic patients, UKPDS Group. Metab Clin Exp. 1990;39:905–12.
13. Henry RR, Gumbiner B. Benefits and limitations of very-low-calorie diet therapy in obese NIDDM. Diabetes Care. 1991;14:802–23.
14. Henry RR, Wallace P, Olefsky JM. Effects of weight loss on mechanisms of hyperglycemia in obese non-insulin-dependent diabetes mellitus. Diabetes. 1986;35:990–8.
15. Markovic TP, et al. Beneficial effect on average lipid levels from energy restriction and fat loss in obese individuals with or without type 2 diabetes. Diabetes Care. 1998;21:695–700.
16. Knowler WC, et al. Reduction in the incidence of type 2 diabetes with lifestyle intervention or metformin. N Engl J Med. 2002;346:393–403.
17. Sjöström L, et al. Lifestyle, diabetes, and cardiovascular risk factors 10 years after bariatric surgery. N Engl J Med. 2004;351:2683–93.
18. The Look AHEAD Research Group. Eight-year weight losses with an intensive lifestyle intervention: the look AHEAD study. Obesity (Silver Spring). 2014;22:5–13.
19. Tsai AG, Wadden TA. Systematic review: an evaluation of major commercial weight loss programs in the United States. Ann Intern Med. 2005;142:56–66.
20. Heath V. Obesity: benefits of intensive lifestyle modification programs in the spotlight. Nat Rev Endocrinol. 2011;7:1–1.
21. American Diabetes Association. 4. Lifestyle management. Diabet Care. 2017;40:S33–43.
22. Wadden TA, Stunkard AJ, Brownell KD. Very low calorie diets: their efficacy, safety, and future. Ann Intern Med. 1983;99:675–84.
23. Henry RR, Wiest-Kent TA, Scheaffer L, Kolterman OG, Olefsky JM. Metabolic consequences of very-low-calorie diet therapy in obese non-insulin-dependent diabetic and nondiabetic subjects. Diabetes. 1986;35:155–64.
24. Amatruda JM, Biddle TL, Patton ML, Lockwood DH. Vigorous supplementation of a hypocaloric diet prevents cardiac arrhythmias and mineral depletion. Am J Med. 1983;74:1016–22.
25. Henry RR, Scheaffer L, Olefsky JM. Glycemic effects of intensive caloric restriction and isocaloric refeeding in noninsulin-dependent diabetes mellitus. J Clin Endocrinol Metab. 1985;61:917–25.
26. Nauck M, et al. Long-term efficacy and safety comparison of liraglutide, glimepiride and placebo, all in combination with metformin in type 2 diabetes: 2-year results from the LEAD-2 study. Diabetes Obes Metab. 2013;15:204–12.
27. Jacob S, Rabbia M, Meier MK, Hauptman J. Orlistat 120 mg improves glycaemic control in type 2 diabetic patients with or without concurrent weight loss. Diabetes Obes Metab. 2009;11:361–71.
28. Lloret-Linares C, Greenfield JR, Czernichow S. Effect of weight-reducing agents on glycaemic parameters and progression to type 2 diabetes: a review. Diabet Med. 2008;25:1142–50.
29. Johansson K, Sundström J, Neovius K, Rössner S, Neovius M. Long-term changes in blood pressure following orlistat and sibutramine treatment: a meta-analysis. Obes Rev. 2010;11:777–91.
30. Gadde KM, et al. Effects of low-dose, controlled-release, phentermine plus topiramate combination on weight and associated comorbidities in overweight and obese adults (CONQUER): a randomised, placebo-controlled, phase 3 trial. The Lancet. 2011;377(16):1341–52.
31. Garvey WT, et al. Two-year sustained weight loss and metabolic benefits with controlled-release phentermine/topiramate in obese and overweight adults (SEQUEL): a randomized, placebo-controlled, phase 3 extension study. Am J Clin Nutr. 2012;95:297–308.
32. Hollander P, et al. Effects of naltrexone sustained- release/bupropion sustained-release combination therapy on body weight and glycemic parameters in overweight and obese patients with type 2 diabetes. Dia Care. 2013;36:4022–9.
33. Blonde L, Russell-Jones D. The safety and efficacy of liraglutide with or without oral antidiabetic drug therapy in type 2 diabetes: an overview of the LEAD 1–5 studies. Diabetes Obes Metab. 2009;11:26–34.
34. Davies MJ, et al. Efficacy of Liraglutide for weight loss among patients with type 2 diabetes: the SCALE diabetes randomized clinical trial. JAMA. 2015;314:687–99.
35. Sorli C, Harshima SI, Tsoukas GM, Unger J, Karshol JD, Hansen T, Bain SC. Efficacy and Safety of once weekly semaglutide monotherapy versus placebo in patients with type 2 diabetes (SUSTAIN 1): a double-blind, randomised, placebo-controlled, parallel-group, multinational, multicenter phase 3a trial. The Lancet Diabetes & Endocrinology. 5(4): 251–60. 2017.
36. Monami M, Dicembrini I, Antenore A, Mannucci E. Dipeptidyl Peptidase-4 inhibitors and bone fractures a meta-analysis of randomized clinical trials. Dia Care. 2011;34:2474–6.
37. Ahren B, Atkin SL, Charpentier G, Warren ML, Wilding JPH, Birch S, Hoist AG, Leiter LA. Semaglutide induces weight loss in subjects with type 2 diabetes regardless of baseline BMI or gastrointestinal adverse effects in the SUSTAIN 1 to 5 trial. Diabetes, Obesity & Metabolism. 20(9): 2210–19, 2018.

38. Buchwald H, Estok R, Fahrbach K, Banel D, Sledge I. Trends in mortality in bariatric surgery: a systematic review and meta-analysis. Surgery. 2007;142:621–35.

39. Buchwald H, et al. Weight and type 2 diabetes after bariatric surgery: systematic review and meta-analysis. Am J Med. 2009;122:248–256.e5.

40. Pories WJ, et al. Who would have thought it? An operation proves to be the most effective therapy for adult-onset diabetes mellitus. Ann Surg. 1995;222:339–50.; discussion 350–2.

41. Buchwald H, et al. Bariatric surgery. JAMA. 2004;292:1724–37.

42. Brethauer SA, Hammel JP, Schauer PR. Systematic review of sleeve gastrectomy as staging and primary bariatric procedure. Surg Obes Relat Dis. 2009;5:469–75.

43. Kellum JM, et al. Gastrointestinal hormone responses to meals before and after gastric bypass and vertical banded gastroplasty. Ann Surg. 1990;211:763–70.; ; discussion 770–1.

44. Perugini RA, Malkani S. Remission of type 2 diabetes mellitus following bariatric surgery: review of mechanisms and presentation of the concept of 'reversibility'. Curr Opin Endocrinol Diabetes Obes. 2011;18:119–28.

45. Morínigo R, et al. Glucagon-like peptide-1, peptide YY, hunger, and satiety after gastric bypass surgery in morbidly obese subjects. J Clin Endocrinol Metab. 2006;91:1735–40.

46. Clements RH, Gonzalez QH, Long CI, Wittert G, Laws HL. Hormonal changes after Roux-en Y gastric bypass for morbid obesity and the control of type-II diabetes mellitus. Am Surg. 2004;70:1–4.; ; discussion 4–5.

47. Laferrère B, et al. Incretin levels and effect are markedly enhanced 1 month after Roux-en-Y gastric bypass surgery in obese patients with type 2 diabetes. Diabetes Care. 2007;30:1709–16.

48. Laferrère B, et al. Effect of weight loss by gastric bypass surgery versus hypocaloric diet on glucose and incretin levels in patients with type 2 diabetes. J Clin Endocrinol Metabol. 2008;93:2479–85.

49. Batterham RL, et al. Inhibition of food intake in obese subjects by peptide YY3–36. N Engl J Med. 2003;349:941–8.

50. Carr RD, et al. Secretion and dipeptidyl peptidase-4-mediated metabolism of incretin hormones after a mixed meal or glucose ingestion in obese compared to lean, Nondiabetic Men. JCEM. 2010;95:872–8.

51. Sumithran P, et al. Long-term persistence of hormonal adaptations to weight loss. N Engl J Med. 2011;365:1597–604.

52. Cummings DE, et al. Plasma ghrelin levels after diet-induced weight loss or gastric bypass surgery. N Engl J Med. 2002;346:1623–30.

53. Engstrom BE, Ohrvall M, Sundbom M, Lind L, Karlsson FA. Meal suppression of circulating ghrelin is normalized in obese individuals following gastric bypass surgery. Int J Obes. 2006;31:476–80.

54. Morínigo R, et al. Short-term effects of gastric bypass surgery on circulating ghrelin levels. Obes Res. 2004;12:1108–16.

55. Evans S, et al. Gastric bypass surgery restores meal stimulation of the anorexigenic gut hormones glucagon-like peptide-1 and peptide YY independently of caloric restriction. Surg Endosc. 2012;26:1086–94.

56. Peterli R, et al. Metabolic and hormonal changes after laparoscopic Roux-en-Y gastric bypass and sleeve gastrectomy: a randomized, prospective trial. Obes Surg. 2012;22:740–8.

57. Melissas J, et al. Sleeve gastrectomy-a 'food limiting' operation. Obes Surg. 2008;18:1251–6.

58. Franz MJ, et al. Weight-loss outcomes: a systematic review and meta-analysis of weight-loss clinical trials with a minimum 1-year follow-up. J Am Diet Assoc. 2007;107:1755–67.

59. Pi-Sunyer X, et al. A randomized, controlled trial of 3.0 mg of liraglutide in weight management. N Engl J Med. 2015;373:11–22.

60. Astrup A, et al. Safety, tolerability and sustained weight loss over 2 years with the once-daily human GLP-1 analog, liraglutide. Int J Obes. 2012;36:843–54.

61. Greenway FL, et al. Effect of naltrexone plus bupropion on weight loss in overweight and obese adults (COR-I): a multicentre, randomised, double-blind, placebo-controlled, phase 3 trial. Lancet. 2010;376:595–605.

62. Wadden TA, et al. Weight loss with naltrexone SR/bupropion SR combination therapy as an adjunct to behavior modification: the COR-BMOD trial. Obesity (Silver Spring). 2011;19:110–20.

Dyslipidemia

44

Erik T. Diniz, Ana Carolina S. M. Cardoso,
and Francisco Bandeira

Diagnosis

Lipid Profile

The lipid profile is composed of laboratory measurements of TC, TG, HDL-C, and LDL-C. Traditionally, LDL-C is not measured directly in plasma, as calculated by the Friedewald equation [1] LDL-C = TC − HDL − TG/5.

However, this equation is no longer accurate when TG levels are greater than 200 mg/dL and ceases to be valid when they exceed 400 mg/dL or in the presence of chronic diseases such as cholestatic liver disease, poorly controlled diabetes mellitus (DM), and nephrotic syndrome [2]. In these cases, direct LDL-C can be performed through specific tests with excellent precision and accuracy [3].

Table 44.1 shows secondary causes of dyslipidemia with increase of total cholesterol and LDL cholesterol and triglyceride.

LDL-Cholesterol

The increase in cardiovascular risk has been associated not only with elevated levels of TC but also with an increase in LDL-C [4, 5]. More recent studies have shown that this association is not linear and a steep increase in risk occurs when the levels of LDL-C affect more elevated track levels [6]. In addition, several randomized studies have shown that the control of total cholesterol and LDL-C levels is associated

Table 44.1 Secondary causes of dyslipidemia [9]

↑ Total cholesterol and LDL cholesterol	↑ Triglyceride
Hypothyroidism	Diabetes mellitus, hypothyroidism
Nephrosis	Chronic renal failure
Systemic lupus erythematosus	Obesity
Multiple myeloma	Excessive alcohol intake
Anabolic steroid treatment	Corticosteroid, protease inhibitors
Cholestatic diseases	Thiazide diuretics, β-adrenergic blocking
Protease inhibitors	Orally administered estrogens

with a decreased risk of cardiovascular events in different groups of patients [7, 8].

Even in the presence of normal levels of LDL-C, the individual may experience an increase in the small, dense LDL particles. These particles react more easily in the arterial wall and are more susceptible to oxidation. They are therefore associated with an increased risk of cardiovascular events and may be present in 50% of men with CAD. Their presence is often related to low levels of HDL-C and hypertriglyceridemia, as well as metabolic syndrome (MS) and DM [9].

HDL Cholesterol

Low levels of HDL-C are related to increased cardiovascular risk, as evidenced by the Framingham Heart Study, which showed an increased risk of acute myocardial infarction of about 25% for every 5 mg/dL decrease in HDL-C [10]. Studies such as LIPID, CARE, and TNT have reported that low levels of HDL-C are more powerful predictors of cardiovascular events in patients with LDL-C levels less than 125 than in those with levels higher than 125 mg/dL [11, 12].

On the other hand, HDL-C levels >60 mg/dL have been considered a negative risk factor for CAD, so one risk factor can be subtracted from a patient's overall risk profile. In both sexes, HDL-C levels below 40 mg/dL are an independent risk factor for CVD. However, women tend to have higher

E. T. Diniz
Universidade Federal de Campina Grande, Paraiba, Brazil

Ana Carolina S. M. Cardoso
Division of Endocrinology and Diabetes, University of Pernambuco Medical School, Agamenon Magalhães Hospital, Recife, PE, Brazil

F. Bandeira (✉)
Division of Endocrinology, Agamenon Magalhães Hospital, University of Pernambuco Medical School, Recife, PE, Brazil

© Springer Nature Switzerland AG 2022
F. Bandeira et al. (eds.), *Endocrinology and Diabetes*, https://doi.org/10.1007/978-3-030-90684-9_44

levels of HDL-C than men, so values >50 mg/dL are considered ideal for females [9].

Triglycerides

Hypertriglyceridemia has also been linked to an increased risk of cardiovascular events, as well as an increased mortality in patients with established CAD [13, 14]. This relationship may be due to the direct effect of hypertriglyceridemia as an association of this condition with some other factors that predispose to atherosclerosis, such as low HDL-C, increased coagulation, insulin resistance, and the presence of small, dense LDL-C particles [15]. Some studies, such as SCRIP, which described the presence of small, dense particles in 90% of individuals with triglyceride levels above 160 mg/dL [16], have found an inverse relationship between triglyceride levels and LDL-C diameter.

An additional test that can be performed in an individual with elevated fasting TG is the determination of postprandial triglyceridemia. Some evidence indicates that the TG-rich lipoproteins produced in the postprandial period are atherogenic and that levels of postprandial TG > 150 mg/dL are an independent risk factor for CAD. Better standardization of this cutoff point is, however, still required [17–20].

Non-HDL Cholesterol

In patients with hypertriglyceridemia, in addition to increased LDL, there is an increase in IDL and VLDL, all atherogenic lipoproteins. Thus, the non-HDL cholesterol estimates the total circulating atherogenic lipoproteins better than LDL-C and also appears to better estimate cardiovascular risk [21, 22], especially in patients with TG between 200 and 500 mg/dL, diabetes, and established cardiovascular disease (CVD) [23, 24]. Non-HDL cholesterol should be determined by calculating the difference between the total cholesterol and HDL-C in patients with triglyceride levels greater than 200 mg/dL. The non-HDL cholesterol target is 30 mg/dL higher than established LDL-C risk levels [25].

Additional Tests

Lipoprotein (a)

Lipoprotein (a) corresponds to an LDL-C particle which is found connected to a specific apolipoprotein: apo (a). Serum levels are genetically determined, and the apolipoprotein (a) molecule has an important homology to plasminogen, so there is a competitive effect on the latter. This leads to a prothrombotic effect, thus contributing to atherosclerotic vascular injury [26]. Different studies have shown increased levels of lipoprotein (a) to be an important independent risk factor for coronary artery disease and cerebrovascular disease, especially in Caucasian patients [27, 28].

However, the lack of standardization in the measurement of this lipoprotein limits its use, so its evaluation is not routinely recommended. Nonetheless, its determination could be useful in White patients with CAD and in subjects with a family history of CAD of unknown origin [10].

C-Reactive Protein

C-reactive protein (CRP) is a highly sensitive marker of chronic inflammatory conditions such as atherosclerosis, and its elevation has been associated with increased cardiovascular risk. Its levels can be divided into <1 mg/L (low risk), 1–3 mg/L (intermediate risk), and > 3 mg/L (high risk) [29]. However, the JUPITER study suggested a simpler stratification: CRP <2.0 vs. ≥2.0 [30].

Although some studies have suggested that CRP could be a better predictor of cardiovascular risk than LDL-C [31], larger, more recent studies have shown that the dosage adds little to predictions based on the traditional risk factors [29]. In relation to therapeutic drug monitoring, CRP levels seem to play a more important role since, as demonstrated by a more recent study, the reduction in the risk of coronary events appears to be greater not only when the LDL-C drops below 70 mg/dL but also when CRP has decreased levels in response to treatment (less than 2 mg/L) [32].

The dosage of CRP, however, should not be performed routinely but may be useful in estimates of intermediate risk or in evaluating residual risk in patients with LDL-C < 130 mg/dL [10].

Homocysteine

Elevated levels of homocysteine (>15 μmol/L) have also been associated with increased cardiovascular risk [33, 34]. However, reduction in its levels with the use of folic acid, vitamin B6, and vitamin B12 showed no risk reduction [35]. Homocysteine measurement is not recommended because its benefit is not well established [10].

Apolipoproteins

Serum levels of apolipoprotein B (apoB) reflect the levels of small, dense LDL particles, recognized as atherogenic. Some studies have suggested that the elevation of apoB is equivalent or even superior to LDL-C and non-HDL cholesterol in predicting cardiovascular risk, even in patients with insulin resistance and DM2 [36–38]. The optimal level of apoB recommended in patients at risk of CAD is below 90 mg/dL, while for individuals with CAD or established diabetes plus other risk factors, the ideal target is <80 mg/dL, and for individuals at extreme risk, the target for apoB is <70 mg/dL [10].

Perhaps even more useful is the assessment of apoB/apolipoprotein AI (apoA-I), as this ratio has been a stronger risk predictor than the LDL-C/HDL-C ratio [39]. The dosage of apoB and apoA-I is indicated in patients with TG >150 mg/dL and HDL-C below 40 mg/dL to assess residual risk, even in those with LDL-C within the target range, including patients with CAD and DM2 [10].

Carotid Intima-Media Thickness and Coronary Calcium Score

The measurement of carotid intima-media thickness (IMT) and the coronary calcium score (CCS) are noninvasive imaging tests and have emerged, in recent years, as markers for CAD.

The CCS is an estimate of the amount of coronary plaques in an individual [40]. A CCS of zero reflects a low likelihood of coronary disease, and the patient is classified as low risk, with an annual event rate of only 0.11% in the asymptomatic individual [41]. This appears to be true even in diabetic patients, as it has already been shown that in these cases, a CCS of zero indicates survival similar to nondiabetic patients also with a CCS of zero, so in these cases, lipid-lowering therapy would not need to be as aggressive or even necessary [42]. However, studies comparing the CCS with the carotid IMT have suggested that the latter, when increased, has proved a better predictor of CAD [43].

These tests, in any case, are not yet recommended in all individuals with dyslipidemia, and their usefulness would probably be greater in those patients initially classified as intermediate risk, in whom they could provide a better explanation of the need for therapy and lipid goals.

In Whom Should Serum Lipids Be Measured?

The lipid profile should be carried out in every adult from the age of 20. In patients without risk factors and an appropriate lipid profile, the test can be repeated every 5 years [4]. From the age of 45 years in men and 55 years in women, this frequency should be increased to one to two times a year, considering the high prevalence (21–49%) of dyslipidemia in this age group as evidenced by some studies [44, 45]. From 70 years of age, annual screening is recommended [11]. In patients with multiple risk factors for CVD, the lipid profile should be repeated more frequently regardless of age group [10].

Screening for dyslipidemia should also be performed in all patients with established coronary artery disease (CAD), diabetes, hypertension, obesity, and family history of primary dyslipidemia [4].

Cardiovascular Risk Assessment

The diagnostic approach to dyslipidemia involves not only the diagnosis but also the assessment of cardiovascular risk to which the individual is exposed. This risk stratification is essential to initiate the most appropriate treatment for the patient. After all, not all patients with abnormal lipid levels are candidates for drug therapy, and both the indication for and the aggressiveness of therapy to be instituted should be based on the individual risk of developing CVD. The risk that an individual has of a coronary event in 10 years (death or MI) can be classified as high (greater than 20%), intermediate (between 10% and 20%), and low (less than 10%) [46].

In November 2018, the American College of Cardiology (ACC) and the American Heart Association (AHA) [4] issued new guidelines on controlling blood cholesterol as shown in Figs. 44.1 and 44.2. There are also new ACVD risk enhancer lists in order to refine risk categorization (Tables 44.2 and 44.3).

The 10-year ASCVD risk was estimated using the Cohort Equations developed by the Risk Assessment Working Group. The necessary parameters included gender, age, race, total cholesterol, high-density lipoprotein cholesterol (HDL-C), systolic BP, use of antihypertensive medication, diabetes, and smoking [4]. The parameters have not been applied to individuals under the age of 40 or older than 75 years.

The first step in estimating risk is to identify the presence of current manifestations of atherosclerotic disease (CAD, cerebrovascular, and peripheral vascular disease). Likewise, attention must be paid to the occurrence of the atherosclerotic disease equivalents such as diabetes type 1 or 2 and abdominal aortic aneurysm, which would put the individual in the category of high risk at least [46]. Subsequently, the presence of major risk factors for atherosclerotic disease (Table 44.4) and ERF should be evaluated [10]. The ERF is most useful in cases initially classified as intermediate risk.

The Framingham Study, conducted in the USA, provided sufficient epidemiological evidence to permit risk evaluation of CAD in 10 years in an individual, using scores and cardiovascular risk tables. The FRS considers blood pressure, sex, age, smoking status, and TC and HDL-C levels [47]. If the risk is classified as intermediate, there is a need to consider other factors associated with cardiovascular risk to minimize the possibility of under- or overestimating the risk.

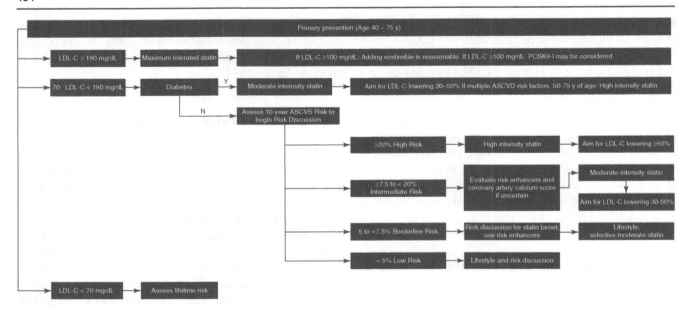

Fig. 44.1 Overview of primary ASCVD prevention [9] – according to the ACC Guidelines, 2018

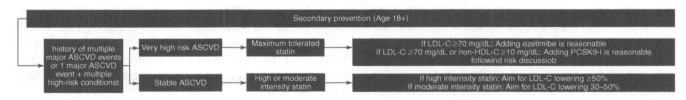

Fig. 44.2 Overview of secondary ASCVD prevention [9] – according to the ACC Guidelines, 2018

Table 44.2 ASCVD risk enhancers [9]

| Family history of premature ASCVD |
| Persistently elevated LDL-C ≥ 160 mg/dL (≥4.1 mmol/L) |
| Chronic kidney disease |
| Metabolic syndrome |
| Conditions specific to women (e.g., preeclampsia, premature menopause) |
| Inflammatory diseases (especially rheumatoid arthritis, psoriasis, HIV) |
| Ethnicity factors (e.g., south Asian ancestry) |
| *Lipid/biomarkers:* |
| Persistently elevated triglycerides (≥175 mg/mL) |
| *In selected individuals if measured:* |
| Hs-CRP ≥2.0 mg/L |
| Lp(a) levels >50 mg/dL or > 125 nmol/L |
| apoB ≥130 mg/dL |
| Ankle-brachial index (ABI) <0.9 |

According to the ACC Guidelines, 2018

Table 44.3 Diabetes-specific risk enhancers that are independent of other risk factors in diabetes [9]

| Long duration (≥10 years for type 2 diabetes or ≥ 20 years for type 1 diabetes) |
| Albuminuria ≥30 μg albumin/mg creatinine |
| eGFR <0.9 |
| Retinopathy |
| Neuropathy |
| ABI <0.9 |

According to the ACC Guidelines, 2018

Table 44.4 Major coronary artery disease risk factors

| Advancing age |
| High total serum cholesterol level |
| High non-HDL-C |
| High LDL-C |
| Low HDL-C |
| Diabetes mellitus |
| Hypertension |
| Chronic kidney disease |
| Cigarette smoking |
| Family history of coronary artery disease[a] |

[a]Definite myocardial infarction or sudden death before the age of 55 years in father or other male first-degree relative or before the age of 65 years in mother or other female first-degree relative

Thus, the classical risk factors do not appear sufficient to predict all risk, and in this context, the role of the emerging risk factors (C-reactive protein, lipoprotein (a), apoB/apoA-I ratio, microalbuminuria, homocysteine, left ventricular hypertrophy, the thickness of the carotid artery intima-media complex (IMT), CCS) has been gaining strength.

Treatment

Treatment Goals

The reduction in LDL-C levels, especially in individuals at risk of CVD, remains the main therapeutic target in dyslipidemia. Table 44.5 shows the goals for each risk category, and drug treatment associated with lifestyle modification (LSM) in patients at high, very high, or extreme risk should be initiated immediately, having statins as first-choice drugs. Even if the initial target is not reached, the reduction of at least 30–40% in the initial LDL-C levels has shown a decrease in cardiovascular risk [4]. However, a single LDL-C target, in general, is not sufficient to reduce all cardiovascular risk [10].

The goal for TG is <150 mg/dL. However, the exact level at which TG starts to confer risk is unknown. Endocrine Society Guidelines suggested a new TG classification: mild (150–199 mg/dL), moderate (200–999 mg/dL), severe (1000–1999 mg/dL), and very severe (≥2000 mg/dL) hypertriglyceridemia. Lifestyle changes (LSC) should be started in the presence of hypertriglyceridemia and drug therapy in cases in which LSC failed. Only in those individuals with TG >1000 mg/dL, drug therapy should be started immediately, preferably a fibrate, to reduce the risk of pancreatitis [48, 49].

For HDL-C, in the presence of associated hypertriglyceridemia or other risk factors, a target at least >40 mg/dL should be pursued. The major question occurs in individuals with isolated lowering of HDL-C in the absence of CVD and/or risk factors due to the absence of clinical trials supporting the benefit of increasing this lipid in this group of patients [10]. However, once it has been decided to raise their HDL-C levels, regular physical activity should be instituted, and smoking cessation should also be encouraged, as these measures are known to be effective in increasing HDL-C. If a drug is required, nicotinic acid remains the most effective option.

Table 44.6 shows lipid target of the patient with coronary artery disease (CAD) with the goal of total cholesterol, HDL cholesterol, LDL cholesterol, triglyceride, and apoB.

Lifestyle Change (LSC)

All patients with dyslipidemia should initiate LSC, based on diet reorientation (low in saturated fat and high in fiber), regular physical activity, and smoking cessation. This therapeutic approach corresponds to the first option in patients at low risk, in which pharmacological treatment should only be initiated 6 months after an attempt to normalize lipemia with LSC, and in those at intermediate risk, in whom the start of lipid-lowering medication should be considered only 3 months later [4].

The type of fat intake is fundamental to the management of dyslipidemia. The saturated fat intake should be limited (<7% of total calories), and trans fats should also be avoided, since they are associated with elevated LDL-C, decreased HDL-C,

Table 44.5 Coronary artery disease risk categories and low-density lipoprotein treatment goals [15]

Risk category	Risk factors/10-year risk[a]	LDL-C treatment goal
Extreme risk	Progressive ASCVD including unstable angina in patients after achieving an LDL-C < 70 mg/dl	<55 mg/dl
	Established clinical cardiovascular disease in patients with DM, CKD ¾, or HeFH	
	History of premature ASCVD (<55 male, <65 female)	
Very high risk	Established or recent hospitalization for ACS, coronary, carotid, or peripheral vascular disease, 10-year risk >20%	<70 mg/dL
	Diabetes or CKD ¾ with one or more risk factor(s)	
	HeFH	
High risk	≥2 risk factors and 10-year risk 10–20%	<100 mg/dL
	Diabetes or CKD ¾ with no other risk factors	
Moderate risk	≥2 risk factors and 10-year risk <10%	<100 mg/dL
Low risk	0 factor risk	<130 mg/dL

According to the AACE Guidelines, 2017

Abbreviations: *ACS* acute coronary syndrome, *ASCVD* atherosclerotic cardiovascular disease, *CKD* chronic kidney disease, *DM* diabetes mellitus, *HDL-C* high-density lipoprotein cholesterol, *HeFH* heterozygous familial hypercholesterolemia, *LDL-C* low-density lipoprotein cholesterol

[a]Major independent risk factors are high LDL-C, polycystic ovary syndrome, cigarette smoking, hypertension (blood pressure ≥ 140/90 mm Hg or on hypertensive medication), low HDL-C (<40 mg/dl), family history of coronary artery disease (in male, first-degree relative younger than 55 years; in female, first-degree relative younger than 65 years), chronic renal disease (CKD) stage ¾, evidence of coronary artery calcification, and age (men ≥45; women ≥55 years). Subtract one risk factor if the person has high HDL-C

Table 44.6 Lipid target of the patient with coronary artery disease (CAD) [15]

Total cholesterol (mg/dL)	<200
HDL cholesterol (mg/dL)	As high as possible, at least >40 in both sexes
LDL cholesterol (mg/dL)	<100, <70 (all high-risk patients)
Triglyceride (mg/dL)	<150
apoB, mg/dL	<90 (patients at risk of CAD, including those with diabetes)
Established diabetes	<80 (patients with CAD or plus ≥1 additional risk factor)

According to the AACE Guidelines, 2017

and increased cardiovascular risk. Unsaturated fatty acids should make up 10–20% of caloric intake. Polyunsaturated fatty acids are represented by omega 3 (found in vegetable oils and cold-water fish), the benefits associated with CVD; omega 6 (found in soybean, corn, and sunflower oil), associated with reduction in LDL-C; and TG, although they can also decrease HDL-C. Monounsaturated fatty acids reduce LDL-C, but with no effect on the HDL-C [4].

Considering the positive effect of omega 3 on the lipid profile and cardiovascular risk, its supplementation (at least 2–4° g of fish oil a day) has been recommended for patients with CVD [10].

Statins

Statins represent the drugs of choice in hypercholesterolemia treatment. They act by inhibiting HMG-CoA reductase, an enzyme involved in the synthesis of endogenous cholesterol. Since the intracellular levels of cholesterol decrease with the use of the drug, there is an increase in LDL-C receptors in cell membranes, enhancing LDL-C clearance [50].

The decrease in LDL-C serum levels can range from 25% to 55%, depending on the drug used. There may also be a fall in triglyceride levels of 15–25% and an increase in HDL-C of around 2–10% [51].

Simvastatin (dose of 20–80 mg per day) and pravastatin (dose of 20–40 mg a day) must be taken at night. However, atorvastatin (dose of 10–80 mg per day) and rosuvastatin (dose of 10–40 mg per day), more potent in reducing LDL-C, have a longer half-life and can therefore be administered at any time of the day. Rosuvastatin is the most effective drug for raising HDL-C levels [51].

On the whole, it is not recommended to exceed the dose of 40 mg of simvastatin and of 20 mg of atorvastatin and rosuvastatin, because larger doses will contribute little to the decrease in LDL-C, and there is an increased risk of side effects. Thus, in the absence of response, the most sensible thing to do is to introduce another class of drug.

In general, statins are well tolerated, although the following may occur: hepatotoxicity in 1.4% of cases (a > threefold increase in transaminases indicates a dosage reduction or discontinuation of the drug) and myalgia and CPK elevation to 15.4% and 0.9% of cases, respectively (in cases of a > tenfold rise in CPK or persistence of muscle symptoms, the drug should be discontinued). Rhabdomyolysis is rare, occurring in 0.2% of individuals, and its risk increases in cases of association of drugs with fibrates (except fenofibrate). Among the contraindications to statin therapy, the following may be mentioned: pregnancy, breastfeeding, and acute liver diseases (in cases of renal failure and chronic liver disease, the drug can be used) [52].

Recent clinical trials suggested that the statins may increase the incidence of diabetes. A meta-analysis of 13 randomized statin trials of over 91,000 patients suggested that these drugs compared with placebo lead to a 9% increased relative risk for the development of diabetes [53]. However, the benefit of cardiovascular risk reduction by statin therapy seems to exceed the risk of diabetes. A risk–benefit analysis showed that the risk of diabetes was increased, but the statins were favorable in high-risk and secondary prevention populations [54]. A recent analysis from the JUPITER (a primary prevention trial) evaluated 17,603 subjects without previous CVD or diabetes and showed that, in subjects with one or more diabetes risk factors, the statin therapy was associated with a 39% reduction in the primary endpoint (myocardial infarction, stroke, admission to hospital for unstable angina, arterial revascularization, or cardiovascular death) and a 28% increase in diabetes (a total of 134 vascular events or deaths were avoided for every 54 new cases of diabetes diagnosed) [55].

The major advantage of statins is their positive effect on cardiovascular disease, constituting a class of drug with strong evidence of reducing overall mortality when used in both primary and secondary prevention.

Benefits in Secondary Prevention

Several studies have reported the benefits of statin therapy in patients with proven CAD, regardless of the presence of dyslipidemia.

The 4S study compared simvastatin (up to a maximum dose of 40 mg) with placebo, and, in addition to reporting a decrease in coronary events and CAD mortality, it was the first study to show a decrease in overall mortality [8]. CARE, in turn, compared placebo with pravastatin, also showing a reduction in the incidence of coronary events and deaths from CAD [56]. HPS (UK Heart Protection Study), comparing simvastatin 40 mg with placebo, showed a reduction of about one-third in the risk of myocardial infarction (MI), stroke, and myocardial revascularization, in addition to its beneficial effect on overall mortality and CAD, irrespective of baseline cholesterol (33% had LDL-C lower than 116 mg/dL). The benefit in patients with low LDL-C levels reflects a possible additional effect of statins in addition to that related to the reduction in cholesterol levels [57].

In relation to the statin dose, there is no justification for the use of aggressive therapy in stable patients. CARDS, for instance, demonstrated that the use of atorvastatin at a dose of 10 mg, in type 2 diabetics, was able to reduce the risk of cardiovascular events by 35% [58]. Also, even though TNT has shown that 80 mg of atorvastatin has led to an additional reduction in events when compared to a 10-mg dose, there was a higher incidence of adverse effects with the higher dose [13]. Furthermore, a recent meta-analysis of data from more than 30,000 patients without DM showed that intensive therapy was associated with an increased occurrence of new cases of DM [59].

Aggressive treatment, however, has proven its benefits in patients with acute coronary syndrome (ACS). In this case, the drug should be started even prior to discharge from the hospital stay and in high doses, as shown by studies PROVE-IT and MIRACL, demonstrating the advantage of an 80-mg dose of atorvastatin compared to a less aggressive therapy (pravastatin at a dose of 40 mg) [60, 61]. The absence of similar results using an 80-mg dose of simvastatin in ACS, shown by the A to Z study, suggested that in patients with high levels of inflammation, statins are important because of their pleiotropic effects [62]. Thus, an aggressive treatment is justified only for ACS cases, and atorvastatin at a dose of 80 mg should be the drug of choice in this situation.

Beneficial Effects on Atheromatous Plaque

Both REVERSAL and ASTEROID have studied stable coronary patients accompanied with intracoronary ultrasound and showed that the use of 80 mg of atorvastatin led to plaque stabilization (REVERSAL) and that rosuvastatin induced the regression of atheroma (ASTEROID) [63, 64]. METEOR, in turn, studied patients at low risk (primary prevention), showing that there was progression of carotid IMT in individuals who used the placebo compared with those on rosuvastatin 40 mg for 2 years [65].

A recent study compared rosuvastatin and atorvastatin at maximum doses and demonstrated a similar effect on atheroma volume reduction, despite the greater effects of rosuvastatin on LDL-C and HDL-C [66].

Benefits of Primary Prevention

WOSCOPS was a primary prevention study in middle-aged men which showed a reduction in coronary events and mortality in this group of patients with the use of pravastatin 40 mg/day [67]. The same was observed for the AFCAPS/TexCAPS (with lovastatin) and ASCOT-LLA (with atorvastatin 10 mg), both with the added advantage of having also evaluated women and having included patients with cholesterol levels closer to "normal" [9, 68]. More recently, JUPITER compared the use of rosuvastatin with placebo in patients with LDL-C < 130 mg/dL, but with CRP ≥2.0 mg/L, being discontinued owing to the evident reduction in cardiovascular morbidity and mortality in the statin group [30].

Although there is evidence of benefits of primary prevention treatment, not all patients should be treated, so the cost–benefit should be considered (4S estimated the cost per life saved per year for secondary prevention of about US$ 7500, whereas WOSCOPS estimated a cost of US$ 27,000 for primary prevention) [8, 67]. Treatment should therefore be reserved for those patients with a higher CAD risk, considering the LDL-C levels and associated risk factors.

Fibrates

Fibrates are the drugs of choice in hypertriglyceridemia treatment and reduce TG by 20–35%, but they also have an effect on HDL-C (elevation of 6–18%) and on LDL-C (variable effect, reducing or even increasing its levels). They act via activation of peroxisome proliferator-activated receptor alpha (PPAR-alpha), leading to the activation of lipoprotein lipase (LPL) (responsible for the hydrolysis and removal of plasma triglycerides), reduced VLDL synthesis in the liver, and increased synthesis of apoA-I, contributing an increase in HDL-C [10].

Among the main fibrates, the following deserve special mention: gemfibrozil (600–1200 mg/day), fenofibrate (200 mg/day in its micronized form), and ciprofibrate (100 mg/day). They can cause fatigue, gallstones, gastrointestinal disturbances, rash, headache, and, more rarely, elevated transaminases and CPK. Rhabdomyolysis has been described when statins are associated with gemfibrozil, which therefore should not be used in this type of combination therapy. Fibrates should be avoided in cases of renal failure [69].

Although there is a decrease in lipid levels with the use of fibrates, they have not been shown, in the long term, to produce the same clinical results as statins. Some studies, however, such as the Helsinki Heart Study and BIP [70, 71], have demonstrated a reduction in coronary events. The FIELD study involving 9795 subjects with DM2 showed that micronized fenofibrate decreased coronary events but increased coronary mortality in all cases. However, the results were not significant [72].

Niacin

Niacin can be used instead of fibrates and statins (or in association with them) in the treatment of hypercholesterolemia, hypertriglyceridemia, or mixed hyperlipidemia, since it reduces the hepatic synthesis of VLDL and, consequently, its LDL-C metabolite. But the action that makes it unique among oral lipid-lowering drugs is its inhibitory effect on the transport of cholesterol from HDL-C to VLDL and on the clearance of HDL-c, thereby increasing the plasma levels of this lipoprotein [73].

Niacin is, therefore, the most effective drug for treating patients with low levels of HDL-C without other lipid abnormalities and can increase HDL-C by 30%. To exert its effect on HDL-C, in general, doses of 1–1.5 g/day are necessary. Higher doses (3 g/day) are more effective on LDL-C and triglycerides as well as on lipoprotein (a), which can be reduced by 35% [74].

There are three types of drug preparation, according to the speed of its release: fast (often causes flushing), intermediate (causes less flushing), and slow (the main limitation of which is hepatotoxicity). Of these three, the second is the option of choice and should be initiated at a dose of 500 mg, with a gradual increase (every month) to 1–2 g/day as a single dose taken immediately after dinner.

The biggest question now about this drug is whether there would be some benefit from its combination with statins in the prevention of cardiovascular events. Studies evaluating the use of statins plus niacin in CAD patients showed that this association decreased mortality and cardiovascular events, suggesting an additional protection when therapy for an increase in HDL-C is instituted [75]. The ARBITER2 study, in turn, showed a tendency of reduction in carotid IMT progression with the use of niacin in coronary patients already on statins, suggesting a beneficial effect of the drug on the anatomical progression of atherosclerosis [76].

However, the AIM-HIGH study failed to show any additional benefits of adding niacin to statin therapy in patients with a mean LDL-C of 71 mg/dL and suggested a higher occurrence of stroke in individuals treated with niacin [77]. This study, therefore, increased doubts about the advantage of the combination of statin and niacin, so one must await the results of HPS2-THRIVE, currently in progress, for clarification of this issue.

Among the side effects of drugs, the main one is flushing, mediated by the action of prostaglandin D and often responsible for the discontinuation of therapy. This effect can be prevented with the use of aspirin 325 mg 30 min before drug intake. More recently, laropiprant, a prostaglandin receptor antagonist, has been used in combination with niacin, significantly reducing the incidence of flushing, as well as its intensity, without changing the lipid effect [78].

A negative effect of the drug on glucose metabolism with increased insulin resistance and elevated blood glucose has also been demonstrated. However, these changes have been shown to be transient and can be effectively controlled with adjustments to the treatment regime with oral antidiabetic agents or insulin in individuals with DM2 [10, 79].

Ezetimibe

Ezetimibe is used at a dose of 10 mg/day in the treatment of hypercholesterolemia, reducing intestinal cholesterol absorption by inhibiting the cholesterol transport protein present in the brush border of the enterocyte without interfering with the absorption of fat-soluble vitamins and triglycerides [10].

Although its use alone can reduce LDL-C by about 17%, its main therapeutic use is in combination with statins in an attempt to avoid the need to increase the dose of the latter in unresponsive cases [80]. Ezetimibe can produce a further 14% reduction in LDL-C levels when added to the isolated use of statins and has the advantage of being well tolerated [81]. Additional benefits have also been demonstrated by its association with atorvastatin and rosuvastatin [10].

However, there is still no conclusive data showing the benefits of this drug in reducing cardiovascular events. ENHANCE, involving 720 patients with familial heterozygous hypercholesterolemia, showed no significant difference in the progression of carotid IMT between the group treated with statin alone and those associated with ezetimibe, despite the more significant reduction in LDL-C in the second group [82]. On the other hand, the SHARP study showed a reduced incidence of cardiovascular events in subjects with chronic renal failure using simvastatin 20 mg/day plus ezetimibe 10 mg/day [83]. In addition, preliminary data from SEAS have shown a 20% reduction in ischemic events by 20% in the group using simvastatin 40 mg/day plus ezetimibe 10 mg/day when compared to the placebo group [84].

The IMPROVE-IT study showed a significant reduction of the primary endpoint (composed of cardiovascular death, MI, unstable angina requiring rehospitalization, coronary revascularization, or stroke) in patients with acute coronary syndrome (ACS) prior to the use of ezetimibe/simvastatin compared with only simvastatin [85].

Bile Acid Sequestrants

Colestipol, colesevelam, and cholestyramine act by inhibiting the absorption of bile salts, which, as a result, reduces cholesterol absorption. They are therefore options in the treatment of hypercholesterolemia, particularly in combination with statins, and can decrease LDL-C by 15–25%. They can also raise HDL-C slightly (4–8%) but should be avoided in hypertriglyceridemia, since they may increase TG levels [10]. One advantage of the use of colesevelam is the reduction of blood glucose levels, and it can serve as an adjuvant therapy for DM2 [85].

Its main drawback is the impaired tolerance resulting from its gastrointestinal effects (nausea, meteorism, constipation), leading eventually to high rates of noncompliance. Colesevelam, however, seems to be better tolerated [10].

Combination Therapy

In many situations, the isolated use of only a single lipid-lowering agent is not sufficient to achieve lipid targets, and it is preferable to combine two different classes of drug rather than increase the dose of the medication in use. After all, in the treatment of hypercholesterolemia, for example, an increase in dose can only further reduce by 6% in the amount of LDL-C, in addition to which it considerably increased the risk of side effects such as increased liver transaminases and muscle injury.

Combination therapy is therefore usually recommended when (1) monotherapy fails to reduce cholesterol levels to the desired target; (2) increasing the dose of medication in use is accompanied by adverse events; or (3) the patient has a mixed dyslipidemia (elevated LDL-C and TG with HDL-C reduction).

In the first case, three types of combination can be considered: statin + ezetimibe, especially after the positive results presented by SHARP, although this combination needs to be better evaluated in future studies [84], statin + bile acid sequestrants, and statin + niacin, a combination whose cardiovascular benefit remains inconclusive [10].

In the presence of side effects with the increase of statin doses, the best matches would be combinations with ezetimibe or bile acid sequestrant. In cases of mixed hyperlipidemia, the combination with fibrates, avoiding gemfibrozil, or with niacin is the best option [10].

PCSK9 Inhibitors

Proprotein convertase subtilisin/kexin type 9 inhibitors have been approved by regulatory agencies for the treatment of individuals with inadequate low-density lipoprotein (LDL-C) levels. They are able to reduce LDL-C by up to 60% in patients with statin therapy. In addition, they produce clinical benefits, such as reductions in stroke rates or myocardial infarction. Proprotein convertase subtilisin/kexin type 9 (PCSK9) is an enzyme (serine protease) encoded by the PCSK9 gene, which is produced predominantly in the liver [47, 86, 87]. PCSK9 binds to the low-density lipoprotein (LDL-R) receptor on the surface of hepatocytes, leading to LDL-R degradation and higher plasma LDL-C (LDL-C) levels [88, 89]. Alirocumab and evolocumab are human monoclonal antibodies that bind to free PCSK9 plasma, promoting the degradation of this enzyme [4–7]. As a result, less free PCSK9 is available in plasma to bind to LDL-R. This results in a greater fraction of the recycling of LDL-R to the surface of hepatocytes. As a direct consequence, the liver has the ability to remove more LDL-C from the circulation, resulting in lower plasma LDL-C levels.

Another potential method of interference with PCSK9 is to block its synthesis, which is dependent on messenger RNA. Other mechanisms, in addition to the reduction of LDL-C, by which PCSK9 antibodies may improve cardiovascular outcomes were postulated [9]. These include a reduction in inflammation and oxidative stress in the atherosclerotic plaques and inhibition of the prothrombotic pathways. They are indicated for patients with acute coronary syndrome.

Circulating levels of PCSK9 are upregulated in the presence of statins, suggesting that inhibition of the PCSK9 pathway may complement the LDL-C lowering effect of statins.

The recommended dose of evolocumab in primary or mixed dyslipidemia is 140 mg subcutaneously every 2 weeks or 420 mg once monthly; both doses are clinically equivalent [28, 40, 68].

The initial dose of alirocumab is 75 mg subcutaneously once every 2 weeks. The maintenance dose is 75–150 mg subcutaneously once every 2 weeks [12]. Plasma levels of low-density lipoprotein (LDL-C) cholesterol should be measured within 4–8 weeks of starting or changing the dose, and an increase in dosage to 150 mg may be initiated if LDL-C reduction is inadequate.

An alternative dose of alirocumab for patients who prefer a less frequent dosage is 300 mg once every 4 weeks. For patients receiving this scheduled dose, LDL-C should be measured immediately prior to the next scheduled dose. If LDL-C reduction is inadequate, 150 mg every 2 weeks can be given by starting the new dose on the next scheduled dosing date. LDL-C should be measured within 4–8 weeks.

The ODYSSEY OUTCOMES studies with alirocumab and FOURIER with evolocumab showed similar results with low rates of cardiovascular events among patients who were treated with PCSK9 inhibitors [90].

Future Therapies

New pharmacological interventions may help, in a near future, to decrease the residual cardiovascular risk, which is still significant in patients on statin therapy [89]. Lomitapide, a microsomal triglyceride transfer protein inhibitor which blocks the secretion of apoB by the liver, and mipomersen, an antisense nucleotide which leads to apoB RNA degradation, are approved for the treatment of homozygous familial hypercholesterolemia (HoFH). Their effects on LDL-C reduction are from 25% to 60%. The frequent finding of fat liver disease with these drugs limits their use at this point.

In the REVEAL study, the use of anacetrapib (a cholesterol ester transfer protein) resulted in a lower incidence of coronary events (comprised of coronary death, myocardial infarction, or coronary revascularization) in patients with atherosclerotic vascular disease who remained at high risk, despite effective statin-based treatment [91, 92]. Inclisiran is a synthetic small interfering RNA with a prolonged action that selectively suppresses hepatic production of PCSK9. According to the findings of the ORION-1 phase II trial led to a sustained reduction in plasma cholesterol of low-density lipoproteins [93, 94].

References

1. Nauck M, Warnick GR, Rifai N. Methods for measurement of LDL-cholesterol: a critical assessment of direct measurement by homogeneous assays versus calculation. Clin Chem. 2002;48:236–54.

2. Grundy SM, Stone NJ, Bailey AL, Beam C, Birtcher KK, Blumenthal RS, Yeboah J. 2018AHA/ACC/AACVPR/AAPA/ABC/ACPM/ADA/AGS/APhA/ASPC /NLA/PCNA guideline on the management of blood cholesterol. J Am Coll Cardiol. 2018; https://doi.org/10.1016/j.jacc.2018.11.003.

3. Stamler J, Wentworth D, Neaton JD. Is relationship between serum cholesterol and risk of premature death from coronary heart disease continuous and graded? Findings in 356,222 primary screenees of the Multiple Risk Factor Intervention Trial (MRFIT). JAMA. 1986;256(20):2823–8.

4. Neaton JD, Blackburn H, Jacobs D, et al. Serum cholesterol level and mortality findings for men screened in the multiple risk factor intervention trial. Multiple risk factor intervention trial research group. Arch Intern Med. 1992;152:1490–500.

5. Pfeffer MA, Sacks FM, Moye LA, et al. Influence of baseline lipids on effectiveness of pravastatin in the CARE trial. Cholesterol and recurrent events. J Am Coll Cardiol. 1999;33:125–30.

6. Scandinavian Simvastatin Survival Study Group. Randomised trial of cholesterol lowering in 4444 patients with coronary heart disease: the Scandinavian Simvastatin Survival Study (4S). Lancet. 1994;344:1383–9.

7. Sever PS, Dahlof B, Poulter NR, Wedel H, Beevers G, Caulfield M, et al. Prevention of coronary and stroke events with atorvastatin in hypertensive patients who have average or lower-than-average cholesterol concentrations, in the Anglo-Scandinavian Cardiac Outcomes Trial-Lipid Lowering Arm (ASCOT-LLA): a multicentre randomised controlled trial. Lancet. 2003;361(9364):1149–58.

8. Jellinger PS, Handelsman Y, Rosenblit PD, Bloomgarden ZT, Fonseca VA, Garber AJ, et al. American Association of Clinical Endocrinologists and American College of endocrinology guidelines for management of dyslipidemia and prevention of atherosclerosis. Endocr Pract. 2017;23(Suppl 2):1–87.

9. Rosenson RS. Low HDL-C: a secondary target of dyslipidemia therapy. Am J Med. 2005;118(10):1067–77.

10. Sacks FM, Tonkin AM, Craven T, Pfeffer MA, Shepherd J, Keech A, et al. Coronary heart disease in patients with low LDL-cholesterol: benefit of pravastatin in diabetics and enhanced role for HDL-cholesterol and triglycerides as risk factors. Circulation. 2002;105(12):1424–8.

11. LaRosa JC, Grundy SM, Waters DD, Shear C, Barter P, Fruchart JC, et al. Intensive lipid lowering with atorvastatin in patients with stable coronary disease. N Engl J Med. 2005;352(14):1425–35.

12. Sarwar N, Danesh J, Eiriksdottir G, Sigurdsson G, Wareham N, Bingham S. Triglycerides and the risk of coronary heart disease: 10,158 incident cases among 262,525 participants in 29 Western prospective studies. Circulation. 2007;115(4):450–8.

13. Nordestgaard BG, Benn M, Schnohr P, Tybjaerg-Hansen A. Nonfasting triglycerides and risk of myocardial infarction, ischemic heart disease, and death in men and women. JAMA. 2007;298(3):299–308.

14. Miller BD, Alderman EL, Haskell WL, Fair JM, Krauss RM. Predominance of dense low-density lipoprotein particles predicts angiographic benefit of therapy in the Stanford Coronary Risk Intervention Project. Circulation. 1996;94(9):2146–53.

15. Stampfer MJ, Krauss RM, Ma J, Blanche PJ, Holl LG, Sacks FM, Hennekens CH. A prospective study of triglyceride level, low-density lipoprotein particle diameter, and risk of myocardial infarction. JAMA. 1996;276(11):882–8.

16. Bansal S, Buring JE, Rifai N, Mora S, Sacks FM, Ridker PM. Fasting compared with nonfasting triglycerides and risk of cardiovascular events in women. JAMA. 2007;298:309–16.

17. Cohn JS. Postprandial lipemia and remnant lipoproteins. Clin Lab Med. 2006;26:773–86.

18. Lekhal S, Børvik T, Nordøy A, Hansen JB. Increased postprandial triglyceride-rich lipoprotein levels in elderly survivors of myocardial infarction. Lipids. 2008;43(6):507–15.

19. Tentolouris N, Stylianou A, Lourida E, Perrea D, Kyriaki D, Papavasiliou EC, et al. High postprandial triglyceridemia in patients with type 2 diabetes and microalbuminuria. J Lipid Res. 2007;48(1):218–25.

20. Ballantyne CM, Grundy SM, Oberman A, Kreisberg RA, Havel RJ, Frost PH, Haffner SM. Hyperlipidemia: diagnostic and therapeutic perspectives. J Clin Endocrinol Metab. 2000;85(6):2089–112.

21. Ridker PM, Rifai N, Cook NR, Bradwin G, Buring JE. Non-HDL cholesterol, apolipoproteins A-I and B100, standard lipid measures, lipid ratios, and CRP as risk factors for cardiovascular disease in women. JAMA. 2005;294(3):326–33.

22. Bittner V, Hardison R, Kelsey SF, Weiner BH, Jacobs AK, Sopko G, Bypass Angioplasty Revascularization Investigation. Non-high-density lipoprotein cholesterol levels predict five-year outcome in the Bypass Angioplasty Revascularization Investigation (BARI). Circulation. 2002;106:2537–42.

23. Jialal I, Miguelino E, Griffen SC, Devaraj S. Concomitant reduction of low-density lipoprotein-cholesterol and biomarkers of inflammation with low-dose simvastatin therapy in patients with type 1 diabtes. J Clin Endocrinol Metab. 2007;92:3136–40.

24. Grundy SM, Stone NJ, Bailey AL, Beam C, Birtcher KK, Blumenthal RS, et al. 2018AHA/ACC/AACVPR/AAPA/ABC/ACPM/ADA/AGS/APhA/ASPC/NLA/PCNA guideline on the management of blood cholesterol. J Am Coll Cardiol. 2018; https://doi.org/10.1016/j.jacc.2018.11.003.

25. Steyrer E, Durovic S, Frank S, Giessauf W, Burger A, Dieplinger H, et al. The role of lecithin: cholesterol acyltransferase for lipoprotein (a) assembly. Structural integrity of low density lipoproteins is a prerequisite for Lp(a) formation in human plasma. J Clin Invest. 1994;94(6):2330–40.

26. Ariyo AA, Thach C, Tracy R. Lp(a) lipoprotein, vascular disease, and mortality in the elderly. N Engl J Med. 2003;349(22):2108–15.

27. Bennet A, Di Angelantonio E, Erqou S, Eiriksdottir G, Sigurdsson G, Woodward M, et al. Lipoprotein(a) levels and risk of future coronary heart disease: large-scale prospective data. Arch Intern Med. 2008;168(6):598–608.

28. Danesh J, Wheeler JG, Hirschfield GM, et al. C-reactive protein and other circulating markers of inflammation in the prediction of coronary heart disease. N Engl J Med. 2004;350:1387–97.

29. RidKer PM, Danielson E, Fonseca FA, JUPITER Study Group, et al. Rosuvastatin to prevent vascular events in men and women with elevated C-reactive protein. N Engl J Med. 2008;359:2195–2207.

30. Ridker PM, Rifai N, Rose L, Buring JE, Cook NR. Comparison of C-reactive protein and low-density lipoprotein cholesterol levels in the prediction of first cardiovascular events. N Engl J Med. 2002;347:1557–65.

31. Ridker PM, Cannon CP, Morrow D, Rifai N, Rose LM, McCabe CH, et al. C-reactive protein levels and outcomes after statin therapy. N Engl J Med. 2005;352:20–8.

32. Lonn E, Yusuf S, Arnold MJ, Heart Outcomes Prevention Evaluation (HOPE) 2 Investigators, et al. Homocysteine lowering with folic acid and B vitamins in vascular disease. N Eng J Med. 2006;355:746.

33. Ray JG, Kearon C, Yi Q, Sheridan P, Lonn E, Heart Outcomes Prevention Evaluation 2 (HOPE-2) Investigators. Homocysteine-

lowering therapy and risk for venous thromboembolism: a randomized trial. Ann Intern Med. 2007;146:761–7.

34. Stranger O, Herrmann W, Pietrzik K, et al. Clinical use and rational management of homocysteine, folic acid, and B vitamins in cardiovascular and thrombotic diseases. Z Kardiol. 2004;93:439–53.

35. Jiang R, Schulze MB, Li T, Rifai N, Stampfer MJ, Rimm EB, Hu FB. Non-HDL cholesterol and apolipoprotein B predict cardiovascular disease events among men with type 2 diabetes. Diabetes Care. 2004;27(8):1991–7.

36. Walldius G, Jungner I, Holme I, Aastveit AH, Kolar W, Steiner E. High apolipoprotein B, low apolipoprotein A-I, and improvement in the prediction of fatal myocardial infarction (AMORIS study): a prospective study. Lancet. 2001;358:2026–33.

37. Sniderman A, Williams K, Cobbaert C. ApoB versus non-HDL-C: what to do when they disagree. Curr Atheroscler Rep. 2009;11:358–63.

38. Kastelein JJ, van der Steeg WA, Holme I, TNT Study Group; IDEAL Study Group, et al. Lipids, apolipoproteins, and their ratios in relation to cardiovascular events with statin treatment. Circulation 2008;117:3002–3009.

39. Elkeles RS, Godsland IF, Feher MD, Rubens MB, Roughton M, Nugara F, PREDICT Study Group, et al. Coronary calcium measurement improves prediction of cardiovascular events in asymptomatic patients with type 2 diabetes: the PREDICT study. Eur Heart J 2008;29(18):2244–2251.

40. Wilson PW. Established risk factors and coronary artery disease: the Framingham Study. Am J Hypertens. 1994;7(7 Pt 2):7S–12.

41. Arad Y, Goodman KJ, Roth M, Newstein D, Guerci AD. Coronary calcification, coronary disease risk factors, C-reactive protein, and atherosclerotic cardiovascular disease events: the St. Francis Heart study. J Am Coll Cardiol. 2005;46:158–65.

42. Raggi P, Shaw LJ, Berman DS, Callister TQ. Prognostic value of coronary artery calcium screening in subjects with and without diabetes. J Am Coll Cardiol. 2004;43:1663–9.

43. Stein JH, Johnson HM. Carotid intima-media thickness, plaques, and cardiovascular disease risk: implications for preventive cardiology guidelines. J Am Coll Cardiol. 2010;55:1608–10.

44. Tsimikas S, Brilakis ES, Miller ER, McConnell JP, Lennon RJ, Kornman KS, et al. Oxidized phospholipids, Lp(a) lipoprotein, and coronary artery disease. N Engl J Med. 2005;353(1):46–57.

45. Goff DC Jr, Bertoni AG, Kramer H, et al. Dyslipidemia prevalence, treatment, and control in the Multi-Ethnic Study of Atherosclerosis (MESA): gender, ethnicity, and coronary artery calcium. Circulation. 2006;113:647–56.

46. Wynder EL, Harris RE, Haley NJ. Population screening for plasma cholesterol: community-based results from Connecticut. Am Heart J. 1989;117:649–56.

47. Third report of the National Cholesterol Education Program (NCEP). Expert panel on detection, evaluation, and treatment of high blood cholesterol in adults (Adult Treatment Panel III). Circulation. 2002;106:3143.

48. Grundy SM, Cleeman JI, Merz CN, Brewer HB Jr, Clark LT, Hunninghake DB, et al. Implications of recent clinical trials for the National Cholesterol Education Program Adult Treatment Panel III guidelines. J Am Coll Cardiol. 2004;44(3):720–32.

49. Berglund L, Brunzell JD, Goldberg AC, Goldberg IJ, Sacks F, Murad MH, et al. Evaluation and treatment of hypertriglyceridemia: an endocrine society clinical practice guideline. J Clin Endocrinol Metab. 2012;97(9):2969–89.

50. Istvan ES, Deisenhofer J. Structural mechanism for statin inhibition of HMG-CoA reductase. Science. 2001;292(5519):1160–4.

51. Jones PH, Davidson MH, Stein EA, Bays HE, McKenney JM, Miller E. Comparison of the efficacy and safety of rosuvastatin versus atorvastatin, simvastatin, and pravastatin across doses (STELLAR* Trial). Am J Cardiol. 2003;92(2):152–60.

52. Kashani A, Phillips CO, Foody JM, Wang Y, Mangalmurti S, Ko DT, Krumholz HM, et al. Risks associated with statin therapy: a systematic overview of randomized clinical trials. Circulation. 2006;114(25):2788–97.

53. Sattar N, Preiss D, Murray HM, Welsh P, Buckley BM, de Craen AJ, et al. Statins and risk of incident diabetes: a collaborative meta-analysis of randomised statin trials. Lancet. 2010;375:735–42.

54. Wang KL, Liu CJ, Chao TF, Huang CM, Wu CH, Chen SJ, et al. Statins, risk of diabetes, and implications on outcomes in the general population. J Am Coll Cardiol. 2012;60(14):1231–8.

55. Ridker PM, Pradhan A, MacFadyen JG, Libby P, Glynn RJ. Cardiovascular benefits and diabetes risks of statin therapy in primary prevention: an analysis from the JUPITER trial. Lancet. 2012;380(9841):565–71.

56. Sacks FM, Pfeffer MA, Moye LA, Rouleau JL, Rutherford JD, Cole TG, et al. The effect of pravastatin on coronary events after myocardial infarction in patients with average cholesterol levels. Cholesterol and Recurrent Events Trial investigators. N Engl J Med. 1996;335(14):1001–9.

57. MRC/BHF. Heart Protection Study of cholesterol lowering with simvastatin in 20,536 high-risk individuals: a randomised placebo-controlled trial. Lancet. 2002;360(9326):7–22.

58. Colhoun HM, Betteridge DJ, Durrington PN, Hitman GA, Neil HA, Livingstone SJ, et al. Primary prevention of cardiovascular disease with atorvastatin in type 2 diabetes in the Collaborative Atorvastatin Diabetes Study (CARDS): multicentre randomised placebo-controlled trial. Lancet. 2004;364(9435):685–96.

59. Preiss D, Seshasai SR, Welsh P, et al. Risk of incident diabetes with intensive-dose compared with moderate-dose statin therapy: a meta-analysis. JAMA. 2011;305(24):2556–64.

60. Cannon CP, Braunwald E, McCabe CH, Rader DJ, Rouleau JL, Belder R. Intensive versus moderate lipid lowering with statins after acute coronary syndromes. N Engl J Med. 2004;350(15):1495–504.

61. Schwartz GG, Olsson AG, Ezekowitz MD, Ganz P, Oliver MF, Waters D, et al. Effects of atorvastatin on early recurrent ischemic events in acute coronary syndromes: the MIRACL study: a randomized controlled trial. JAMA. 2001;285(13):1711–8.

62. de Lemos JA, Blazing MA, Wiviott SD, Lewis EF, Fox KA, White HD, et al. Early intensive vs a delayed conservative simvastatin strategy in patients with acute coronary syndromes: phase Z of the A to Z trial. JAMA. 2004;292(11):1307–16.

63. Nissen SE, Nicholls SJ, Sipahi I, Libby P, Raichlen JS, Ballantyne CM, et al. Effect of very high-intensity statin therapy on regression of coronary atherosclerosis: the ASTEROID trial. JAMA. 2006;295(13):1556–65. Epub 2006 Mar 13

64. Nissen SE, Tuzcu EM, Schoenhagen P, Brown BG, Ganz P, Vogel RA, et al. Effect of intensive compared with moderate lipid-lowering therapy on progression of coronary atherosclerosis: a randomized controlled trial. JAMA. 2004;291(9):1071–80.

65. Crouse JR 3rd, Raichlen JS, Riley WA, Evans GW, Palmer MK, O'Leary DH, et al. Effect of rosuvastatin on progression of carotid intima-media thickness in low-risk individuals with subclinical atherosclerosis: the METEOR trial. JAMA. 2007;297(12):1344–53.

66. Nicholls SJ, Ballantyne CM, Barter PJ, et al. Effect of two intensive statin regimens on progression of coronary disease. N Engl J Med. 2001;365:2078–87.

67. Shepherd J, Cobbe SM, Ford I, Isles CG, Lorimer AR, MacFarlane PW, et al. Prevention of coronary heart disease with pravastatin in men with hypercholesterolemia. West of Scotland Coronary Prevention Study Group. N Engl J Med. 1995;333(20):1301–7.

68. Downs JR, Clearfield M, Weis S, Whitney E, Shapiro DR, Beere PA, et al. Primary prevention of acute coronary events with lovastatin in men and women with average cholesterol levels: results of AFCAPS/TexCAPS. Air Force/Texas Coronary Atherosclerosis Prevention Study. JAMA. 1998;279(20):1615–22.

69. Gotto AM Jr, Moon JE. Recent clinical studies of the effects of lipid-modifying therapies. Am J Cardiol. 2012;110(1):15A–26.

70. Frick MH, Elo O, Haapa K, Heinonen OP, Heinsalmi P, Helo P, et al. Helsinki Heart Study: primary-prevention trial with gemfibrozil in middle-aged men with dyslipidemia. Safety of treatment, changes in risk factors, and incidence of coronary heart disease. N Engl J Med. 1987;317(20):1237–45.

71. Haim M, Benderly M, Brunner D, Behar S, Graff E, Reicher-Reiss H, et al. Elevated serum triglyceride levels and long-term mortality in patients with coronary heart disease: the Bezafibrate Infarction Prevention (BIP) Registry. Circulation. 1999;100(5):475–82.

72. Keech A, Simes RJ, Barter P, Best J, Scott R, Taskinen MR. Effects of long-term fenofibrate therapy on cardiovascular events in 9795 people with type 2 diabetes mellitus (the FIELD study): randomised controlled trial. Lancet. 2005;366(9500):1849–61.

73. Brown BG, Zhao XQ. Nicotinic acid, alone and in combinations, for reduction of cardiovascular risk. Am J Cardiol. 2008;101(8A):58B–62.

74. Guyton JR, Goldberg AC, Kreisberg RA, Sprecher DL, Superko HR, O'Connor CM. Effectiveness of once-nightly dosing of extended-release niacin alone and in combination for hypercholesterolemia. Am J Cardiol. 1998;82(6):737–43.

75. Brown BG, Zhao XQ, Chait A, Fisher LD, Cheung MC, Morse JS, et al. Simvastatin and niacin, antioxidant vitamins, or the combination for the prevention of coronary disease. N Engl J Med. 2001;345(22):1583–92.

76. Taylor AJ, Sullenberger LE, Lee HJ, Lee JK, Grace KA. Arterial Biology for the Investigation of the Treatment Effects of Reducing Cholesterol (ARBITER) 2: a double-blind, placebo-controlled study of extended-release niacin on atherosclerosis progression in secondary prevention patients treated with statins. Circulation. 2004;110(23):3512–7.

77. Investigators AIM-HIGH. The role of niacin in raising high-density lipoprotein cholesterol to reduce cardiovascular events in patients with atherosclerotic cardiovascular disease and optimally treated low-density lipoprotein cholesterol: baseline characteristics of study participants. The Atherothrombosis Intervention in Metabolic syndrome with low HDL/high triglycerides: impact on Global Health outcomes (AIM-HIGH) trial. Am Heart J. 2011;161(3):538–43.

78. Yadav R, France M, Younis N, Hama S, Ammori BJ, Kwok S, Soran H. Extended-release niacin with laropiprant : a review on efficacy, clinical effectiveness and safety. Expert Opin Pharmacother. 2012;13(9):1345–62.

79. Canner PL, Furberg CD, Terrin ML, McGovern ME. Benefits of niacin by glycemic status in patients with healed myocardial infarction (from the Coronary Drug Project). Am J Cardiol. 2005;95(2):254–7.

80. Knopp RH, Gitter H, Truitt T, Bays H, Manion CV, Lipka LJ, et al. Effects of ezetimibe, a new cholesterol absorption inhibitor, on plasma lipids in patients with primary hypercholesterolemia. Eur Heart J. 2003;24(8):729–41.

81. Davidson MH, McGarry T, Bettis R, Melani L, Lipka LJ, LeBeaut AP, et al. Ezetimibe coadministered with simvastatin in patients with primary hypercholesterolemia. J Am Coll Cardiol. 2002;40(12):2125–34.

82. Kastelein JJ, Akdim F, Stroes ES, Zwinderman AH, Bots ML, Stalenhoef AF, et al. Simvastatin with or without ezetimibe in familial hypercholesterolemia. N Engl J Med. 2008;358(14):1431–43.

83. Gould AL, Rossouw JE, Santanello NC, Heyse JF, Furberg CD. Cholesterol reduction yields clinical benefit: impact of statin trials. Circulation. 1998;97(10):946–52.

84. Holvoet P, Collen D, Van de Werf F. Malondialdehyde-modified LDL as a marker of acute coronary syndromes. JAMA. 1999;281(18):1718–21.

85. Investigators SHARP. The effects of lowering LDL cholesterol with simvastatin plus ezetimibe in patients with chronic kidney disease (Study of Heart and Renal Protection): a randomised placebo-controlled trial. Lancet. 2011;377(9784):2181–92.

86. Friedewald WT, Levy RI, Fredrickson DS. Estimation of the concentration of low-density lipoprotein cholesterol in plasma, without use of the preparative ultracentrifuge. Clin Chem. 1972;18:499.

87. Bang CN, Greve AM, Boman K, et al. Effect of lipid lowering on new-onset atrial fibrillation in patients with asymptomatic aortic stenosis: the Simvastatin and Ezetimibe in Aortic Stenosis (SEAS) study. Am Heart J. 2012;163(4):690–6.

88. Faas FH, Earleywine A, Smith G, Simmons DL. How should low-density lipoprotein cholesterol concentration be determined? J Fam Pract. 2002;51(11):972–5.

89. Cannon CP. IMPROVE-IT trial: a comparison of ezetimibe/simvastatin versus simvastatin monotherapy on cardiovascular outcomes after acute coronary syndromes. American Heart Association 2014 Scientific sessions; November 17, 2014; Chicago.

90. Burnett JR, Hooper AJ. PCSK9 — a journey to cardiovascular outcomes. N Engl J Med. 2018;379(22):2161–2. https://doi.org/10.1056/nejme1813758.

91. Zieve FJ, Kalin MF, Schwartz SL, Jones MR, Bailey WL. Results of the glucose-lowering effect of WelChol study (GLOWS): a randomized, double-blind, placebo-controlled pilot study evaluating the effect of colesevelam hydrochloride on glycemic control in subjects with type 2 diabetes. Clin Ther. 2007;29:74–83.

92. HPS3/TIMI55–REVEAL Collaborative Group, Bowman L, Hopewell JC, Chen F, et al. Effects of anacetrapib in patients with atherosclerotic vascular disease. N Engl J Med. 2017;377(13):1217–27.[PubMed].

93. Kones R. Reducing residual risk: modern pharmacochemistry meets old-fashioned lifestyle and adherence improvement. Ther Adv Cardiovasc Dis. 2013. [Epub ahead of print]; https://doi.org/10.1177/1753944712467828.

94. Fitzgerald K, White S, Borodovsky A, et al. A highly durable RNAi therapeutic inhibitor of PCSK9. N Engl J Med. 2017;376:41–51.

Dietary Approach for Cardiometabolic Disorders

Maria da Conceição Chaves de Lemos
and Bruna Lúcia de Mendonça Soares

Dietary Approach for Cardiometabolic Disorders

In the genesis of cardiovascular disease (CVD), nutrition is an important pillar because it represents the possible modifiable factors, along with physical activity. Another aspect that deserves reflection is that excess body weight contributes to the appearance of other risk factors, such as hypertension, dyslipidemia, diabetes, and renal dysfunction, and thus, it symbolizes the iceberg and the onset of factors that predispose to CVD.

Nutritional Factors and Targets of MD

Mediterranean Diet

Among several diets discussed in the literature, one of the most studied, which can be referred to without any doubt, is the Mediterranean diet (MD). A recent review article, published in 2017, points out the protective effects of MD for individuals with and without chronic diseases, by assessing the progression and regression of metabolic syndrome, longevity, and even cancer. The authors analyze the apparent capacity of the traditional MD to reduce the risk of CVD developing and progressing. This capacity is represented by bioactive components or to the nutraceutical effect of micronutrients and compounds, which have an antithrombotic, anticancer, and antioxidant capacity. These could explain this possible action and control for cardiovascular disease [1, 2].

Nutritional factors and targets for composing MD include vegetables and fruits ≥400 g/day, total carbohydrates 45–55% of total energy value (VET), simple carbohydrates <10% of VET, not recommended additional fructose, total dietary fiber >25–30 g/day, total fat >30% of VET, saturated fatty acids <7% of VET, trans fatty acids <1% of VET, polyunsaturated fatty acids (PUFA) 10% of VET, polyunsaturated fatty acids Ω 3 5–8% of VET, polyunsaturated fatty acids Ω 6 1–2% of VET, monounsaturated fatty acids (MUFA) >15% of VET, cholesterol <300 mg/day, proteins 10–15% of VET, sodium chloride <5 g/day, and flavonols >50 mg/kg [3, 4].

To study the eating habits of a population who had a Mediterranean-style diet, some authors have suggested making use of the Mediterranean Adequacy Index (MAI). Adhesion to the Healthy Reference National Mediterranean Diet (HRNMD) has been introduced. This index is calculated by dividing the sum of the total energy percentages of the food groups typical of HRNMD (bread, cereals, legumes, potatoes, vegetables, fresh fruit, nuts, fish, wine, vegetable oil) by the sum of the dietary energy percentage of food groups that are not characteristic of HRNMD (milk, cheese, meat, eggs, animal fats and margarines, sweet beverages, cakes, pies, cookies) [1]. Thus, the longitudinal study of Alberti-Fidanza et al. evaluated between 26 and 41 years of follow-up and observed a decrease in MAI indices, that is, the Mediterranean-style diet has lost its characterization over the years [5].

A random sample of 1159 Jewish people in Israel was studied by Trichopoulou et al. in 1995 to examine the relationship between MD and CHD, using the Mediterranean Diet Score (MDS). The results of this study showed higher MDS correlated to lower risk of myocardial infarction, coronary bypass, angioplasty, and all other cardiovascular diseases [6]. Later on, the authors modified MDS and included moderate fish consumption among the inclusion criteria, and they verified that CHD mortality fell by 33% [7].

The reduction in relative risk for developing type 2 diabetes mellitus was evaluated in the PREDIMED study, which included 7447 nondiabetic subjects who had a high cardiovascular risk over a period of 4.8 years. After randomization, the researchers divided the patients into three groups. Those

M. da Conceição Chaves de Lemos (✉) · B. L. de Mendonça Soares
Federal University of Pernambuco, Nutrition Department,
Recife, Pernambuco, Brazil

© Springer Nature Switzerland AG 2022
F. Bandeira et al. (eds.), *Endocrinology and Diabetes*, https://doi.org/10.1007/978-3-030-90684-9_45

who followed the low-fat diet (control group) or one of two MedDiets, supplemented with either free virgin olive oil (1 l/week) or nuts (30 g/day). Diets were ad libitum, and no advice on physical activity was given. The results for the group following the MedDiet with olive oil and the group following the MedDiet with nuts, when compared with the results for the control group, showed that the rate of CVD events in the group following the MD with extra-virgin oil was reduced by 30%, and, for the group following the MD with nuts, there was a reduction of 28%. Both diets, supplemented with either extra-virgin olive oil or nuts, were associated with a regression of MS. [8] Another branch of this study also evaluated survival and found that, when comparing the two Mediterranean diets with the control, the difference was significantly higher with Mediterranean diets [9]. After adjustment for various confounders, incident diabetes was reduced by 51% in the group following the MedDiet with olive oil and by 52% in the group following the MedDiet with nuts when compared with the control group.

A meta-analysis of 50 studies which involved 534,906 individuals, the objective of which was to see the effect of a Mediterranean diet on metabolic syndrome (MS) as well as its components, shows the adherence to the Mediterranean diet was associated with a protective effect in 2 out of 2 clinical trials, in 2 out of 4 cross-sectional studies, and 1 out of 2 prospective studies, as compared with lower compliance with this pattern or with a control diet. The combined effect of both clinical trials and prospective studies was highly protective (log-hazard ratio: _0.69, 95% CI: _1.24–_1.16) [10].

DASH

The DASH (Dietary Approaches to Stop Hypertension) study was a multicenter, randomized, controlled trial that sets out to test the effects of dietary patterns rather than specific nutrients on blood pressure [11]. Compared to a typical control diet in the United States, the DASH diet was effective in reducing systolic and diastolic blood pressure by 5.0 and 3.0 mmHg, respectively, in a 2-month period, and when combined with reducing sodium, there was an additional drop in blood pressure. These changes were observed in men, women, racial and ethnic minorities, hypertensives, and pre-hypertensive individuals [11, 12]. Since its original publication, due to consistent evidence, the DASH diet has been recommended in the treatment and prevention of hypertension.

The DASH diet emphasizes the consumption of foods rich in protein, fibers, potassium, magnesium, and calcium, such as fruits and vegetables, legumes, oilseeds, whole grains, and low-fat dairy products. It also limits foods rich in saturated fat and sugars [1, 5]. Since the creation of the DASH diet 20 years ago, numerous trials have shown that it

consistently reduces blood pressure in patients with hypertension and pre-hypertension. These observed benefits on blood pressure have been associated with the high consumption of potassium, magnesium, and calcium, as well as of proteins and fibers which are present in accordance with the respective food standard [13, 14].

DASH presents specific characteristics, such as it includes sodium of around 2000 mg and calcium of 1200 mg, is rich in potassium (more than 4700 mg) and in fibers (20–30 g), and includes red meat of only around 90 g. The sum of all fats is limited to 30% of the total caloric value, and of these, monounsaturated fat has the highest percentage (15%) [13, 14]. Table 45.1 lists guidelines on how to recommend a DASH-style diet.

The focus of this diet is not on reducing the caloric intake but rather on making healthier food choices that lead to better blood pressure levels and lower cardiovascular risk. However, weight loss can be observed in individuals who adhere to this food pattern, as a consequence of substituting foods previously consumed with healthier ones and which have a lower energy content [14, 15].

The DASH food standard represents an accessible intervention that could immediately lead to considerable improvements in the health of the population.[12] Erlinger et al. suggested that if subjects with hypertension fully adhered to DASH, it is estimated that 400,000 cardiovascular disease events in the United States could be prevented in 10 years [16], which makes it essential to continue efforts to improve adherence to the DASH diet.

Low-Carb Diet

Another diet pattern widely studied and stimulated by the American Association of Clinical Endocrinologists' Medical

Table 45.1 Recommendations of adhering to the DASH diet

Choose foods with reduced cholesterol, saturated fat, total fat. Prefer lean meats (muscle, duck, rump, tenderloin, eye of round, soft and hard top round), skinned poultry, and fish
Eat 8–10 servings of fruits and vegetables a day (1 serving = 1 medium ladle)
Include 2–3 servings of skimmed or semi-skimmed dairy products per day
Prefer whole-meal foods (breads, pastas, cereals, wheat)
Include 4–6 servings per week of oleaginous fruit, seeds, and grains (1 serving = 1/3 cup nuts, 2 tablespoons seed, ½ cup cooked and dried beans)
Use light margarines and unsaturated vegetable oils (olive oil, soy, corn, canola), and reduce the addition of fats
Avoid adding salt to foods, and also avoid processed products, ready-made sauces, and stock
Avoid consuming conserves and sugary drinks

Source: www.nhlbi.nih.gov/health/public/heart/hbp/dash/new_dash. pdf16

Guidelines for Clinical Practice, 2016 [17], is low-carbohydrate diet, especially as it is known that obesity represents one of the risk factors of CVD. Currently, the *Dietary Reference Intakes* (DRIs) already recommend a consumption of 45% of carbohydrates (CHO), when previously the maximum recommended was 55%. Diets with 20–130 g of CHO [18] or below 45% are referred to as low CHO content. What are the possible beneficial effects of these diets? These are improved glycemic and lipid status with lower production of VLDL cholesterol, minimized cardiometabolic factors, greater effect on satiety, and greater long-term benefit as to lowering the percentage of body fat [17]. Total cholesterol levels may also decline, since glucose is still the major stimulator of hydroxy-methylglutaryl-coenzyme A reductase. Thus, in terms of the metabolic profile, this is quite interesting and plausible. Ketogenic diets also fit within this line. However, every ketogenic diet is low in carbohydrates, but not every low carbohydrate diet is ketogenic. Since ketogenic diets are very restricted in CHO, they can lead to a lack of fibers and micronutrients, since on average they offer less than 50 g CHO/day [18].

The effect of insulin sensitivity was analyzed. With a carbohydrate-rich diet, a protein-rich diet, and an unsaturated fat-rich diet, they found that an improvement in insulin sensitivity could be seen when carbohydrate is partially replaced with unsaturated fat in a sample which had a risk for cardiovascular problems. This was a randomized, controlled, three-period, crossover feeding study involving 164 individuals with pre-hypertension [19].

Another study evaluated after weight loss interventions how intrapericardial fat and extrapericardial fat were changed. Dietary regimens were undertaken and compared with a Mediterranean/low-carbohydrate diet plus 28 g walnuts/d with a diet that was calorically equal but low-fat. This was a randomized study with 80 individuals who had moderate abdominal obesity and who were monitored for 18 months. The researchers concluded that the Mediterranean diet, rich in unsaturated fats and restricted in carbohydrates, is significantly superior to a low-fat diet in terms of reducing intrapericardial fat [20].

A randomized trial was conducted to evaluate low- and high-carbohydrate diets in 115 obese adults with type 2 diabetes who were outpatients. They were randomly assigned to consume either a hypocaloric LC diet, 14% of energy as carbohydrate (carbohydrate, 28% of energy as protein, and 58% of energy as fat), or an energy-matched HC diet, 53% of energy as carbohydrate, 17% of energy as protein, and 30% of energy as fat combined with supervised aerobic and resistance exercise, 60 min 3 d/wk. They found that a low diet compared with the one with a higher content of carbohydrates led to an improvement in glycemia and lipemia and better control in patients who took medication [21].

The Prospective Urban Rural Epidemiology (PURE) study [22] was a cohort study published in August, 2017, which was conducted in 18 countries with a median follow-up of 7.4 years. The authors researched a possible relationship between macronutrients and cardiovascular disease. The food frequency questionnaires, validated, were applied to 135,335 participants. Higher carbohydrate intake was associated with an increased risk of total mortality (highest [quintile 5] vs. lowest quintile [quintile 1] category, HR 1.28 [95% CI 1.12–1.46], ptrend = 0.0001) but not with the risk of cardiovascular disease or cardiovascular disease mortality. On the other hand, a lower risk of total mortality, non-cardiovascular disease mortality, and stroke was associated with a higher fat intake.

These findings can be analyzed, taking into consideration the following authors' statements: "Moreover, in our study most participants from low-income and middle-income countries consumed a very high carbohydrate diet (at least 60% of energy), especially from refined sources (such as white rice and white bread), which have been shown to be associated with an increased risk of total mortality and cardiovascular events in other studies" [22].

Vegetarian Diet

Vegetarian diets advocate the consumption of foods of vegetable origin, such as fruits, vegetables, grains, and legumes, excluding meats; and some include dairy products and eggs [23]. Table 45.2 shows the different types of vegetarian diets and their characteristics.

There is strong evidence in the literature of the benefits of the vegetarian diet on the risk of cardiovascular disease and mortality from coronary heart disease. Studies have shown that the blood pressure of vegetarians is lower (between 5 mmHg and 10 mmHg) than omnivores and that vegetarians have a lower prevalence of arterial hypertension, even when the body mass index is similar [24, 25]. Mortality due to ischemic heart disease in vegetarians was 24% lower when compared to omnivores [26]. Vegetarian diets are also said to be able to reduce secondary stenosis and atheroma plaques in the coronary arteries [27, 28].

Table 45.2 Types of vegetarian diet

Groups	Characteristics
Ovo-lacto vegetarian	Does not eat meat, but does eat eggs and dairy products
Lactovegetarian	Eats neither meat, nor eggs, but does eat dairy products
Ovovegetarian	Eats neither meat nor milk nor dairy products, but does eat eggs
Strict vegetarian	Does not eat any food derived from animals (eggs, meat, dairy products, honey, etc.)

In general, studies analyzing the impact of diet plans with controlled consumption of red meat indicated that vegetarians have a better cardiovascular profile than omnivores, lower levels of total cholesterol and LDL (lipoprotein very low density) cholesterol, and lower incidence of hypertension and of diabetes mellitus. [23–25, 29–31] The lower cardiovascular risk among vegetarians could be explained in part by the occurrence of lower cholesterol levels in these individuals, which is probably secondary to the greater consumption of soluble and insoluble fibers, whole grains, fruits and vegetables, or oilseeds and lower consumption of saturated fat. [26, 28–33]

Quality of Fats

Above we discussed why there was an increase in cholesterol with high-carbohydrate diets, and other articles have shown this association and an increase in triglycerides, apolipoprotein B, and small dense LDL, which represent very atherogenic particles [34, 35].

The authors used a multivariate analysis to compare the equivalent amount of energy from carbohydrates (excluding fruit and vegetables) and dairy fat intake in a study entitled "Dairy fat and risk of cardiovascular disease in 3 cohorts of US adults." The results showed that this was not significantly related to the risk of total CVD in this association, but the increase of 5% in energy from dairy fat showed the RR was 1.02 (95% CI, 0.98–1.05), coronary heart disease (RR, 1.03; 95% CI, 0.98–1.09), or stroke (RR, 0.99; 95% CI, 0.93–1.05) ($p > 0.05$ for all findings). Reduced risk of CVD could be observed, when animal fats, including dairy fat, were replaced with fats and PUFAs from vegetable sources [36].

The quality of fat is important and was analyzed in a review study, in which the authors concluded that it is better to replace saturated fat with unsaturated fats [37]. In this study, they did not report on monounsaturated fat, since there was only one small trial, but there is a tendency, because of the adoption of the Mediterranean pattern, to encourage replacing saturated fat with monounsaturated fat [37].

The overestimation that was accepted by many health professionals that it was good to replace saturated fat with vegetable oils rich in linoleic was investigated in a Minnesota Coronary Experiment. The findings showed that it is not healthy because omega 6 stimulates oxidation more, thereby favoring peroxidation [38, 39]. Diseases including coronary heart disease [40] and steatohepatitis [41] can be produced from oxidation. This study was a double-blind randomized controlled trial, had 5 years of follow-up, and involved 9423 women and men aged 20–97 [42]. However, fat that is rich in fatty acids of the alpha-linolenic type, which omega 3 of the vegetal kingdom represents, is present in foods such as nuts, peanuts, avocado, and seeds, i.e., vegetal foods. This gives the alpha-linolenic fatty acid the ability to stretch in the same way as the omega 3 of the animal kingdom and to stimulate the production of vasodilatory substances, thus conferring greater endothelial protection [42].

On the other hand, coconut fat so extolled by the media to date has not been advocated by entities such as the American Diabetes Association and the American Heart Association as beneficial to health for regular use or as a cardiovascular protector. However, several foods have been imputed as cardiovascular protectors, such as chocolate, chestnuts, garlic, and onions.

Chocolate was evaluated on the association of the risk of developing cardiometabolic disorders. It is important to say that all of the studies reported overall chocolate consumption and did not report separately on whether dark or white chocolate was consumed. There was only one study on the consumption of cocoa. In this meta-analysis of randomized controlled trials and observational studies, the results of five of the seven studies showed that consumption of chocolate at the highest levels was associated with a 37% reduction in cardiovascular disease (RR, 0.63; 95% CI, 0.44–0.90) and a 29% reduction in stroke compared with the lowest levels. Thus, association between higher levels of chocolate consumption and the risk of cardiometabolic disorders was represented [43].

The effect of reasonable intakes of cashews (28–64 g/d) on serum lipids in adults with or at risk of high LDL cholesterol was researched, and it was concluded that the consumption of cashews decreases total cholesterol and LDL cholesterol in American diets [44].

Scientists analyzed the vasodilatory and anti-aggregating action of garlic and onions as they are interested in the potential of organosulfur compounds for preventing and treating cardiovascular disease and other health problems. Allicin, which represents the main active substance, has been detected in significant amounts in the serum or urine up to 24 hours after the ingestion of 25 g of raw garlic [45, 46].

Micronutrients and Cardiovascular Health

Some micronutrients play an important role in cardiovascular health and continue to be studied, thereby seeking to open up new avenues for preventing and treating pathological conditions associated with the heart.

Vitamins C, E, and β-carotene have an antioxidant role in the body and therefore contribute by reducing the oxidation of LDL cholesterol particles, thus preventing the formation and/or expansion of atheroma plaque. Therefore, food sources of these nutrients must be present in the dietary plan that targets cardiovascular health, such as red grapes, red wine, teas (especially green tea), chocolate, and olive oil [47–49].

Adequate levels of folate and vitamins B6 and B12 should be targeted and monitored. These vitamins are associated with reducing mortality from heart failure and stroke, due to the inverse relationship between their levels and the serum concentrations of homocysteine [50].

In some studies, low serum vitamin D levels were associated with a higher incidence of systemic arterial hypertension (SAH). However, in studies with supplementation of this vitamin, no BP reduction was observed, and a recommendation of this vitamin in cardiovascular diseases has yet to be established [51, 52].

Magnesium has the function of relaxing the smooth muscle system of cardiac vessels, dilates the coronary arteries, improves myocardial contractility, reduces the risk of coronary spasms, and inhibits platelet aggregation, thereby increasing the prostacyclin/thromboxane ratio. As it has a dilating effect, it lowers blood pressure. Its function is to stabilize the heart rate, thus playing an important role in cardiovascular diseases [53].

Conclusion

Despite all the scientific knowledge about the science of nutrition, lifestyle change is still a challenge for the entire multidisciplinary team. Yet despite all the difficulty in changing lifestyle, the healthy food pattern that dietitians recommend still plays an important and irreplaceable full role in preventing and treating CVD.

References

1. Kerr J, Anderson C, Lippman SM. Physical activity, sedentary behaviour, diet, and cancer: an update and emerging new evidence. Lancet Oncol. 2017;18(8):457–71.
2. Salas-Salvadó J, Guasch-Ferré M, Lee CH, Estruch R, Clish CB, Ros E. Protective effects of the mediterranean diet on type 2 diabetes and metabolic syndrome–3. J Nutr. 2015;146(4):920–7.
3. Di Daniele N, Noce A, Vidiri MF, Moriconi E, Marrone G, Annicchiarico-Petruzzelli M, De Lorenzo A. Impact of Mediterranean diet on metabolic syndrome, cancer and longevity. Oncotarget. 2017;8(5):8947.
4. Bach-Faig A, et al. Mediterranean diet pyramid today. Science and cultural updates. Public Health Nutr. 2011;14(12A):2274–84.
5. Menotti A, Alberti-Fidanza A, Fidanza F. The association of the Mediterranean Adequacy Index with fatal coronary events in an Italian middle-aged male population followed for 40 years. Nutr Metab Cardiovasc Dis. 2012;22:369–75.
6. Trichopoulou A, Kouris-Blazos A, Wahlqvist ML, Gnardellis C, Lagiou P, Polychronopoulos E, Vassilakou T, Lipworth L, Trichopoulos D. Diet and overall survival in elderly people. BMJ. 1995;311(7018):1457–60.
7. Bilenko N, Fraser D, Vardi H, Shai I, Shahar D. Mediterranean diet and cardiovascular diseases in an Israeli population. Prev Med. 2005;40:299–305.
8. Estruch R, Ros E, Salas-Salvadó J, Covas M-I, Corella D, Arós F, Gómez-Gracia E, Ruiz-Gutiérrez V, Fiol M, Lapetra J, Lamuela-Raventos RM, Serra-Majem L, Pintó X. Primary prevention of cardiovascular disease with a mediterranean diet. N Engl J Med. 2013;368:1279–90.
9. Salas-Salvadó J, Bulló M, Babio N, Martínez-González MÁ, Ibarrola-Jurado N, Basora J. Reduction in the incidence of type 2 diabetes with the Mediterranean diet: results of the PREDIMED-Reus nutrition intervention randomized trial. Diabetes Care. 2011;34(1):14–9.
10. Kastorini CM, Milionis HJ, Esposito K, Giugliano D, Goudevenos JA, Panagiotakos DB. The effect of Mediterranean diet on metabolic syndrome and its components: a meta-analysis of 50 studies and 534,906 individuals. J Am Coll Cardiol. 2011;57(11):1299–313.
11. Appel LJ, Moore TJ, Obarzanek E, DASH Collaborative Research Group. A clinical trial of the effects of dietary patterns on blood pressure. N Engl J Med. 1997;336(16):1117–24.
12. Oliveira EPA. A Variedade da Dieta é Fator Protetor para a Pressão Arterial Sistólica Elevada. Arq Bras Cardiol. 2012;98(4):338–43.
13. Muntner P, Carey RM, Gidding S, Jones DW, Taler SJ, Wright JT Jr, Whelton PK. Potential US population impact of the 2017 ACC/AHA high blood pressure guideline. J Am Coll Cardiol. 2018;71(2):109–18.
14. Julius S, Kejdelsen SE, Weber M, et al. Outcomes in hypertensive patients in high cardiovascular risk treated with regimens based on valsartan and amlodipine: the VALUE randomised trial. Lancet. 2004;363:2022–31.
15. Steinberg D, Bennetti GG, Svetkey L. The DASH diet, 20 years later. JAMA. 2017;9(1):214–20.
16. Erlinger TP, Vollmer WM, Svetkey LP, Appel LJ. The potential impact of nonpharmacologic population-wide blood pressure reduction on coronary heart disease events: pronounced benefits in African-Americans and hypertensives. Prev Med. 2003;37(4):327–33.
17. Garvey WT, Mechanick JI, Brett EM, Garber AJ, Hurley DL, Jastreboff AM, Reviewers of the AACE/ACE Obesity Clinical Practice Guidelines. American Association of Clinical Endocrinologists and American College of endocrinology comprehensive clinical practice guidelines for medical care of patients with obesity. Endocr Pract. 2016;22(s3):1–203.
18. Apovian CM. The low-fat, low-carb debate and the theory of relativity. Am J Clin Nutr. 2015;102:719–20.
19. Gadgil MD, Appel LJ, Yeung E, Anderson CA, Sacks FM, Miller ER. The effects of carbohydrate, unsaturated fat, and protein intake on measures of insulin sensitivity: results from the OmniHeart trial. Diabetes Care. 2013;36(5):1132–7.
20. Tsaban G, Wolak A, Avni-Hassid H, Gepner Y, Shelef I, Serfaty D. Dynamics of intrapericardial and extrapericardial fat tissues during long-term, dietary-induced, moderate weight loss. Am J Clin Nutr. 2017;106(4):984–95.
21. Tay J, Luscombe-Marsh ND, Thompson CH, Noakes M, Buckley JD, Wittert GA. Comparison of low-and high-carbohydrate diets for type 2 diabetes management: a randomized trial, 4. Am J Clin Nutr. 2015;102(4):780–90.
22. Dehghan M, Mente A, Zhang X, Swaminathan S, Li W, Amma LI. Associations of fats and carbohydrate intake with cardiovascular disease and mortality in 18 countries from five continents (PURE): a prospective cohort study. Lancet. 2017;390(10107):2050–62.
23. Sanches MAK, Ronchi SS, Zuchinali P, Corrêa SG. Mediterranean diet and other dietary patterns in primary prevention of heart failure and changes in cardiac function markers: a systematic review. Nutrients. 2018;10(1):58–69.
24. Yokoyama Y, Nishimura K, Barnard ND, Takegami M, Watanabe M, Sekikawa A, et al. Vegetarian diets and blood pressure: a meta-analysis. JAMA Intern Med. 2014;174(4):577–87.
25. Ho CP, Yu JH, Lee TJF. Ovo-vegetarian diet is associated with lower systemic blood pressure in Taiwanese women. Public Health. 2017;153(3):70–7.

26. Key TJ, Fraser GE, Thorogood M, Appleby PN, Beral V, Reeves G, et al. Mortality in vegetarians and nonvegetarians: detailed findings from a collaborative analysis of 5 prospective studies. Am J Clin Nutr. 1999;70(3):516–24.

27. Appleby PN, Key TJ. The long-term health of vegetarians and vegans. Proc Nutr Soc. 2016;75(3):287–93.

28. Haghighatdoost F, Bellissimo N, Zepetnek JOT, Rouhani MH. Association of vegetarian diet with inflammatory biomarkers: a systematic review and meta-analysis of observational studies. Public Health Nutr. 2017;20(15):2713–21.

29. Bonaccio M, Ruggiero E, Di Castelnuovo A, Costanzo S, Persichillo M. Fish intake is associated with lower cardiovascular risk in a Mediterranean population: prospective results from the Moli-sani study. Nutr Metab Cardiovasc Dis. 2017;27(10):865–73.

30. Lee Y, Park K. Adherence to a vegetarian diet and diabetes risk: a systematic review and meta-analysis of observational studies. Nutrients. 2017;9(6):603–10.

31. Key TJ, Appleby PN, Rosell MS. Health effects of vegetarian and vegan diets. Proc Nutr Soc. 2006;65(1):35–41.

32. Dinu M, Pagliai G, Sofi F. A heart-healthy diet: recent insights and practical recommendations. Curr Cardiol Rep. 2017;19(10):95–102.

33. Chang-Claude J, Hermann S, Eilber U, Steindorf K. Lifestyle determinants and mortality in German vegetarians and health-conscious persons: results of a 21-year follow-up. Cancer Epidemiol Biomark Prev. 2005;14(4):963–8.

34. Fan J, Song Y, Wang Y, Hui R, Zhang W. Dietary glycemic index, glycemic load, and risk of coronary heart disease, stroke, and stroke mortality: a systematic review with meta-analysis. PLoS One. 2012;7:52–182.

35. Hoogeveen RC, Gaubatz JW, Sun W. Small dense low-density lipoprotein-cholesterol concentrations predict risk for coronary heart disease: the Atherosclerosis Risk In Communities (ARIC) study. Arterioscler Thromb Vasc Biol. 2014;34:1069–77.

36. Chen M, Li Y, Sun Q, Pan A, Manson JE, Hu FB. Dairy fat and risk of cardiovascular disease in 3 cohorts of US adults–3. Am J Clin Nutr. 2016;104(5):1209–17.

37. Hooper L, Martin N, Abdelhamid A, Davey SG. Reduction in saturated fat intake for cardiovascular disease. Cochrane Database Syst Rev. 2015;(6):CD011737.

38. Ramsden CE, Zamora D, Majchrzak-Hong S, Faurot KR, Broste SK, Frantz HJR. Re-evaluation of the traditional diet-heart hypothesis: analysis of recovered data from Minnesota Coronary Experiment (1968–73). BMJ. 2016;353:1246–55.

39. Wang DD, Li Y, Chiuve SE. Association of specific dietary fats with total and cause-specific mortality. JAMA. 2016;176:1134–45.

40. Ramsden CE, Zamora D, Leelarthaepin B. Use of dietary linoleic acid for secondary prevention of coronary heart disease and death: evaluation of recovered data from the Sydney Diet Heart Study and updated meta-analysis. BMJ. 2013;346:870–89.

41. Feldstein AE, Lopez R, Tamimi TA. Mass spectrometric profiling of oxidized lipid products in human nonalcoholic fatty liver disease and nonalcoholic steatohepatitis. J Lipid Res. 2010;51:3046–54.

42. Lima Viana DE, Dantas MM, Silva Menezes ME. Ácidos graxos das séries ômega-3 e ômega-6 e sua utilização no tratamento de doenças cardiovasculares: uma revisão. Revista Saúde & Ciência Online. 2016;5(2):65–83.

43. Buitrago-Lopez A, Sanderson J, Johnson L, Warnakula S, Wood A, Franco OH. Chocolate consumption and cardiometabolic disorders: systematic review and meta-analysis. BMJ. 2011;343:44–88.

44. Mah E, Schulz JA, Kaden VN, Lawless AL, Rotor J, Liska DJ. Cashew consumption reduces total and LDL cholesterol: a randomized, crossover, controlled-feeding trial, 2. Am J Clin Nutr. 2017;105(5):1070–8.

45. Rahman K, Lowe GM, Smith S. Aged garlic extract inhibits human platelet aggregation by altering intracellular signaling and platelet shape change. J Nutr. 2016;146(2):410–5.

46. Hiramatsu K, Tsuneyoshi T, Ogawa T, Morihara N. Aged garlic extract enhances heme oxygenase-1 and glutamate-cysteine ligase modifier subunit expression via the nuclear factor erythroid 2-related factor 2-antioxidant response element signaling pathway in human endothelial cells. Nutr Res. 2016;36(2):143–9.

47. Moser MA, Chun OK. Vitamin C and heart health: a review based on findings from epidemiologic studies. Int J Mol Sci. 2016;17(8):1328–32.

48. Jiang Q. Natural forms of vitamin E: metabolism, antioxidant, and anti-inflammatory activities and their role in disease prevention and therapy. Free Radic Biol Med. 2014;72(1):76–90.

49. Zimmermann AM, Kirsten VR. Alimentos com função antioxidante em doenças crônicas: uma abordagem clínica. Disciplinarum Sciential Saúde. 2016;8(1):51–68.

50. Tsuda K. Associations among plasma total homocysteine levels, circadian blood pressure variation and endothelial function in hypertension. Am J Hypertens. 2018;31:e1.

51. Kunutsor SK, Apekey TA, Steur M. Vitamin D and risk of future hypertension: meta-analysis of 283,537 participants. Eur J Epidemiol. 2013;28(3):205–21.

52. Beveridge LA, Struthers AD, Khan F, Jorde R, Scragg R, Macdonald HM, et al. Effect of vitamin D supplementation on blood pressure: a systematic review and meta-analysis incorporating individual patient data. JAMA Intern Med. 2015;175(5):745–54.

53. Ramirez AVG. The importance of magnesium in cardiovascular disease. Int J Nutrol. 2017;9(4):242–53.

Nutrition Supplements in Sports

Fábio Moura, Felipe Gaia Duarte, Ricardo Oliveira, Roberto Zagury, and Yuri Galeno

In recent years, consumption of sports supplements has been growing among professional and amateur athletes and also among gym practitioners aiming to improve physical performance or esthetical appearance. Many patients obtain information about the usage of these supplements with colleagues, Internet pages, or even supplements store salesmen, so the information about the benefits, dosage, timing, and contraindication are not always correct, leading to the waste of much money or potential side effects.

When visiting a supplements store, or even when navigating on the Internet, an enormous variety of supplements can be found; however, many of them lack studies to prove their efficacy.

There are some well-recognized societies studying and publishing reviews and statements regarding which supplements have proven benefits and how to use them. In this chapter, the main supplements with the highest degree of evidence will be discussed.

F. Moura
Brazilian Society of Endocrinology and Metabolism, Rio de Janeiro, Brazil

F. G. Duarte (✉)
Brazilian Society of Endocrinology and Metabolism, Rio de Janeiro, Brazil

University of São Paulo, São Paulo, Brazil

University of São Paulo Medical School, Sao Paulo, SP, Brazil

R. Oliveira
Brazilian Society of Endocrinology and Metabolism, Rio de Janeiro, Brazil

State University of Rio de Janeiro, Rio de Janeiro, Brazil

R. Zagury
Brazilian Society of Endocrinology and Metabolism, Rio de Janeiro, Brazil

State Institute of Endocrinology and Diabetes, São Paulo, Brazil

Y. Galeno
State Institute of Endocrinology and Diabetes, Rio de Janeiro, Brazil

Carbohydrates

Supplements based on carbohydrates (CH) can be prescribed when the number of calories needed during the day cannot be obtained by food, especially when previously assessed by a nutritionist. This situation can occur more often in heavy athletes or in athletes who spend many hours training, particularly when training sessions are greater than 60–90 minutes [1–3]. Prescribing CH in the correct amount and timing, adjusted to the effort accomplished, is fundamental to avoid performance decline that occurs when body glycogen content is depleted.

It is important to mention that physical activities lasting less than 1 hour will not benefit with CH supplementation once muscle and hepatic glycogen reserves are enough to provide energy during this period, and in the same way, low-intensity activities will also have no benefits from CH supplementation once the main energetic substrate consumed in this intensity is fat [3].

The main activities that could benefit from CH supplementation would be aerobic (endurance sports as cycling, running, swimming, etc.) and mixed modalities (stop-and-go sports such as basketball, volleyball, soccer, etc.). In this former modality, both aerobic and anaerobic efforts are performed. Besides performance improvement, supporting energetic demands with CH supplementation may prevent overtraining syndrome [4]. Conversely, providing excessive amount of CH may induce weight (fat) gain, leading to performance impairment in some sports (e.g., cycling). Therefore, we endorse the American College of Sports Medicine (ACSM) recommendation regarding the amount of CH to be prescribed to athletes (Table 46.1). In this recommendation, references to "chronic fueling" and "acute fueling" are described. Chronic ingestion of CH consists of the amount offered daily in order to supply training and basal caloric needs, whereas acute fueling is the amount prescribed close to competitions intending to replenish energy stores to maximum before competing to promote optimal performance during competition or key training sessions.

© Springer Nature Switzerland AG 2022
F. Bandeira et al. (eds.), *Endocrinology and Diabetes*, https://doi.org/10.1007/978-3-030-90684-9_46

Table 46.1 American College of Sports Medicine recommendation for carbohydrate supplementation

Exercise intensity	Definition	Amount of CH
Chronic fueling		
Light	Endurance: < 1 h per day	3–5 g/kg/day
Moderate	Endurance: 1 h per day	5–7 g/kg/day
High	Endurance: 1–3 h per day	6–10 g/kg/day
Very high	Endurance: > 4–5 h per day	8–12 g/kg/day
Acute fueling		
Pre-event: 1–4 g/kg/1–4 h before sessions lasting more than 60 minutes		

Based on data from ACSM. Med Sci Sports & Exerc 2016;48 (3):543–68 [5]

Table 46.2 Sports supplements based on carbohydrates (CH)

Supplements	Presentation	Typical composition
Sports drink	Liquid or powder (ready to drink)	Glucose, fructose, sucrose, and/or maltodextrin blends. Carbohydrate solution of 4–8%
Sports gel	Sachets, 30–40 g each	CH concentration in the solution of 60–70%. May contain, or not, other ingredients (e.g., caffeine or electrolytes)

Based on data from Castell LM et al. Br J Sports Med 2010:44;486–70 [1]

Moreover, CH may be provided during long-lasting sessions. With this objective, a rate of 1.3–2.4 grams per minute of CH can be offered after the first hour. Glucose and fructose blends (or maltodextrin and fructose) in 1.0 g and 0.5–1.0 g proportions, respectively, in a gel form are usually used with this goal. The purpose for using different kinds of sugars is to utilize the different mechanisms of CH transport existing in the digestive tract without saturating any of them (e.g., SGLT-1 and SGLT-8 and SGLT-12 absorption pathways) [5]. However, despite making sense (biological plausibility), there isn't any good evidence in the literature to support this strategy. Increase of CH oxidation rate is observed; however, performance improvement isn't so evident. Therefore, the ACSM grades this recommendation as level III of evidence, in other words, with limited scientific evidence support [6]. It is worthy to mention that a "celling effect" may happen, concerning the maximum amount of CH that our organism can metabolize per hour in a safe way to promote performance improvement. In an interesting study published by Smith J.W. and colleagues [7], reduction in competition time (performance improvement) occurred with CH ingestion rate up to 72 g per hour. Higher dosages did not demonstrate any benefit in time to trial competitions.

Today, a series of options exist in the market of carbohydrate-enriched supplements in the form of gels, sport drinks, liquid meals, and carbohydrate bars (Table 46.2) [1]. In this chapter, the most used forms in the clinical setting will be discussed: gels and carbohydrate powders for reconstitution in water (sport drink powders).

Some glucose polymers present in the supplement market deserve some comment: maltodextrin, dextrose, and isomaltulose. These molecules have a moderately high glycemic index and may be utilized in a rational fashion depending on the goal [8–10]. Due to the highest glycemic index, dextrose can be used at the end of longer workouts with the aim of replenishing the muscle glycogen content faster. Conversely, isomaltulose, the molecule with the lowest glycemic index, could be used before training sessions in order

to maintain glycemic levels during practice, since its glycemic index would not lead to an intense insulinemic response compared to maltodextrin and dextrose. In turn, maltodextrin, with an intermediate glycemic index, could be ingested during training sessions for delivering energy during the practice. However, it is very important to emphasize that these suggestions of use have no solid literature support, and it is possible that any of these polymers could be used in any of the situations mentioned [11, 12].

Whey Protein

Whey protein (WP) is a protein complex derived from cow milk extracted during cheese production after casein precipitation [13, 14]. WP possesses a great amount of essential amino acids and leucine that exerts an important stimulus for muscle protein synthesis. Due to these characteristics, WP-derived sport supplements are among the most consumed by professional and amateur athletes who desire muscle hypertrophy [14, 15]. According to the Australian Institute of Sports Medicine, WP supplements are categorized as group A: safe, ethical, and effective [16]. However, it is worthy to mention that WP has other components with different biologic functions, such as immunity and glycemic improvement, as shown in Table 46.3.

Comparing to other protein sources, as main differential, WP presents excellent digestibility and fast absorption resulting in a fast surge of amino acids in plasma after ingestion. This property could have practical implications on the ideal timing of its ingestion, since, considering this rational, WP should be consumed immediately before or after the training session. However, there is no consensus regarding this approach, and there are meta-analyses suggesting that an adequate daily ingestion (an adequate protein amount) is the most relevant factor for muscle hypertrophy [17].

There are different WP presentations: concentrate, isolate, and hydrolyzed [13, 14] (Table 46.4).

As previously mentioned, WP main indication is to complete the daily protein quota and, together with exercises, to assist muscle hypertrophy. Classically, the maximum

Table 46.3 Whey protein: components and function

Components	Percentage (%)	Actions//benefits
Beta-Lactoglobulin	50–55	Good source of EAA and BCAA; inhibition of DPP-4
Alfa lactoglobulin	20–25	Good source of EAA and BCAA
Immunoglobulins	10–15	Immunomodulatory action
Lactoferrin	1–2	Bactericidal action Prebiotic action
Lactoperoxidase	0.5–1.0	Inhibition of bacterial growth
Bovine serum albumin	5–10	Good source of EAA
Glycomacropeptide	10–15	Good source of EAA
Cysteine	0.5–1.0	Increases glutathione (antioxidant) levels

Based on data from: Marshal K. Therapeutic Applications of Whey Protein. 2004 [13]

EAA essential amino acids, *BCAA* branched chained aminoacids, *DPP-4* dipeptidyl peptidase 4

Table 46.4 Different presentations of whey protein

	Amount of protein (%)	Characteristics
WP concentrate	< 90	Varying amount of proteins and other bioactive agents, lactose, carbohydrates, and fats
WP isolate	> 90	Greater amount of proteins and removal of almost all carbohydrates and fats
WP hydrolyzed	> 90	Same as isolate, and proteins are already partially pre-digested and hydrolyzed aiming faster absorption. Lower risk of allergies and almost always are lactose-free

absorbed amount of WP per ingestion is 20–40 g depending on patient age (older patients demand higher amounts of proteins per dose); however, there are studies suggesting that the higher dose could better stimulate protein synthesis and result in greater muscle gains regardless of age [18].

WP use by endurance athletes has been of great interest with new evidence suggesting a lower occurrence of muscle injury and a faster recovery after training sessions, a fact shown by lower elevation of CPK serum levels and faster return to basal levels [19, 20]. Such actions indirectly contribute to improvement on athletic performance. However, elite athletes who need to cut weight, with muscle mass maintenance, also seem to benefit from the increase in the protein quota with the use of WP supplements [21].

Finally, WP is safe and can be used by teenagers and the elderly. The only restrictions for protein use in higher amounts per day are in patients with renal disease with proteinuria and in patients with moderate to severe hepatic failure. There are reports of increased incidence of acne, though this is not a severe side effect.

Creatine

Creatine is one of the most popular nutritional ergogenic aids for athletes. Numerous studies have shown that creatine supplementation increases intramuscular creatine concentrations, can improve exercise performance, and/or improves training adaptations. Creatine is a naturally occurring non-protein amino acid compound found primarily in red meat and seafood and found in skeletal muscle (~95%) with small amounts also found in the brain and testes (~5%). About two-thirds of intramuscular creatine is phosphocreatine (PCr), with the remaining being free creatine. The body needs to replenish about 1–3 g of creatine per day to maintain normal creatine stores depending on muscle mass. About half of the daily need for creatine can be obtained from the diet [22].

The primary metabolic role of creatine is to combine with a phosphoryl group (Pi) to form PCr through the enzymatic reaction of creatine kinase (CK). As adenosine triphosphate (ATP) is degraded into adenosine diphosphate (ADP) and Pi to provide free energy for metabolic activity, the free energy released from the hydrolysis of PCr into Cr + Pi can be used as a buffer to resynthesize ATP. This helps maintain ATP availability, particularly during maximal effort anaerobic sprint-type exercise [23].

A large body of evidence now indicates that creatine supplementation increases muscle availability of creatine and PCr and can therefore enhance acute exercise capacity and training adaptations, which allow an athlete to do more work over a series of sets or sprints leading to greater gains in strength, muscle mass, and/or performance due to an improvement in the quality of training [22].

Creatine supplementation has primarily been recommended as an ergogenic aid for power/strength athletes in order to optimize training adaptations or help athletes who need to sprint intermittently and recover during competition (e.g., soccer, basketball, American football, tennis, etc.). After creatine loading, performance of high-intensity and/or repetitive exercise can be increased by 10–20% depending on the magnitude of increase in muscle PCr [24].

After reviewing the scientific and medical literature in this area, the International Society of Sports Nutrition concludes creatinine supplementation is an effective method of increasing muscle creatine stores. The recommended scheme is to consume ~0.3 g/kg/day of creatine monohydrate for 5–7 days followed by 3–5 g/day thereafter to maintain elevated stores. Likewise, ingesting smaller amounts of creatine monohydrate (e.g., 3–5 g/day) will increase muscle creatine stores over a 3–4-week period; however, the initial performance effects of this method of supplementation are less supported [25].

Beta-Hydroxy-Beta-Methylbutyrate (HMB)

HMB is naturally produced in humans from leucine. The first step in its production is the reversible transamination of leucine to α-ketoisocaproate (KIC) by the enzyme branched-chain amino acid transferase. After leucine is metabolized to KIC, KIC is metabolized either into isovaleryl-CoA by the enzyme α-ketoacid dehydrogenase in the mitochondria or into HMB in the cytosol by the enzyme α-ketoisocaproate dioxygenase. KIC is primarily metabolized into isovaleryl-CoA, with only approximately 5% of leucine being converted into HMB [26].

That is the reason why an individual would need to consume over 600 g of high-quality protein to obtain the amount of leucine (60 grams) necessary to produce the typical 3 g daily dosage of HMB used in human studies. Since consumption of this amount of protein seems to be impractical, HMB intake is typically increased via oral supplementation. HMB has been shown to create a net positive balance of skeletal muscle protein turnover through stimulation of protein synthesis and reduction of protein degradation. HMB induces protein synthesis through upregulation of the mTOR pathway, while HMB attenuates protein degradation through attenuation of the ubiquitin-proteasome pathway and caspase activity. Further, HMB stimulates skeletal muscle satellite cell activation and could increase skeletal muscle regenerative capacity [26].

Twenty years ago, supplementation with HMB was first demonstrated that it could lower muscle proteolysis following resistance training and augmented gains in LBM and strength in a dose-dependent manner [27]. Since that time, HMB has been studied in a variety of anaerobic and aerobic training conditions, and innumerous studies have supported the efficacy of HMB supplementation for enhancing recovery, LBM, strength, and power. Its efficacy for aerobic performance is controversial with conflicting results.

In 2013, the International Society of Sports Nutrition published a position stand to analyze the existing literature on HMB supplementation and provided the following recommendations [28]:

HMB can be used to enhance recovery by attenuating exercise-induced skeletal muscle damage in trained and untrained populations.

- If consuming HMB, an individual will benefit from consuming the supplement in close proximity to their workout.
- HMB appears to be most effective when consumed for 2 weeks prior to an exercise bout.
- A dosage of 3 g per day has been demonstrated to enhance skeletal muscle hypertrophy, strength, and power in untrained and trained populations when the appropriate exercise prescription is utilized.

- Currently, two forms of HMB have been used: calcium HMB (HMB-Ca) and a free acid form of HMB (HMB-FA). HMB-FA may increase plasma absorption and retention of HMB to a greater extent than HMB-CA. However, more data is warranted to prove superiority of one over another [29].
- HMB has been demonstrated to increase LBM and functionality in elderly, sedentary populations.
- HMB ingestion in conjunction with a structured exercise program may result in greater declines in fat mass (FM).
- Chronic consumption of HMB appears to be safe in both young and old populations [28].

Caffeine

Caffeine is a trimethylxanthine metabolized by the liver resulting in three metabolites: paraxanthine, theophylline, and theobromine. After its consumption, caffeine appears in the blood stream after 15–45 minutes and reaches peak level after 1 hour. Caffeine has a half-life of 3–6 hours being excreted by the kidneys. Due to its biochemical characteristics, caffeine crosses the blood-brain barrier, easily possessing pharmacological effects on the central nervous system (SNS).

There are many mechanisms for explaining performance improvement induced by caffeine; however, the most relevant is the binding to adenosine receptors on SNS in a competitive way, acting as a blocker of this receptor. Since adenosine is a natural SNS depressor, its blockade increases alertness.

It is believed that most of the caffeine ergogenic effects are due to its action on the neural level, although it can also act on the muscle level. Caffeine also acts on reducing glycogen dependency during physical activities, increasing free fat acids mobilization and consumption. Additionally, it increases beta endorphins secretion leading to a decrease in pain perception and also acts on muscle function optimizing contraction due to a direct action on myocytes. Caffeine also possesses inotropic, tachycardic, and bronchodilator effects and stimulates gastric secretion. In larger doses, it causes excitement, anxiety, and insomnia, and in regular consumers, it may develop tolerance with the need to increase consumption to obtain the initial effects. Use discontinuation may produce a withdrawal syndrome with headache, irritability, and lethargy [30].

Caffeine has been shown efficient on improving performance in both amateur and professional athletes. This performance improvement occurs in endurance (e.g., long-running races) and in high-intensity and short-duration sports (such as 100-meter run or swimming); however, in these high-intensity sports, caffeine was shown to be effective only in highly trained athletes, probably due to the great variability of performance in poorly trained athletes.

Due to its property of raising SNC alertness and surveillance, it's useful in long-term sports during the night period as in orienteering and adventure races. In relation to anaerobic exercises (e.g., bodybuilding), literature results are conflicting, with some researches demonstrating performance improvement and others not. Athletes who practice "stop-and-go" (e.g., soccer, basketball, etc.) can also obtain performance improvement.

The effective dose to achieve these performance gains varies between 3 and 6 mg/kg preferably consumed 1 hour before the activity. Anhydrous caffeine was demonstrated to be more effective ingested in capsules than consuming regular coffee with the same amount of caffeine. In this condition, a performance gain of around 3–24% was observed against placebo. These benefits were observed in both men and women, independent even if they were regular consumers of coffee [31].

Buffering Agents

During intense physical practice, modifications in blood and muscle acid-base balance occur, causing metabolic acidosis with H^+ and lactic acid accumulation. This situation is associated with increased fatigue, muscle burn, cramps, and loss of physical performance [32]. In muscle cells, excessive H+ molecules would compete with Ca^+ for the binding site on C troponin. Another electrolyte alteration is regarding reduction of muscle K^+, leading to decrease of resting membrane potential (also on the muscle motor plaque) that would cause an impairment of muscle excitability. Either situations lead to reduced muscle contraction and prolonged relaxing time culminating with reduced performance. Prescription of buffering supplements has the objective of inducing alkalosis and mitigating electrolyte alterations to enhance athletic performance. This initiative has been a target of studies since the mid-1970s. Two substances have been proven to enhance athletic performance: sodium bicarbonate and beta alanine.

Sodium Bicarbonate (NaHCO3)

This supplement has been considered the most consistently effective buffering agent for enhancing athletic performance along studies, resulting in 2–3% improvement in some exercise indicators, such as power, speed, work capacity, and time to failure [33–35]. NaHCO3 supplementation may be suggested for athletes performing high-intensity exercises. The dosage of 0.3 g·kg − 1 of NaHCO3 diluted in water or in capsules should be taken 1–3 hours prior practice. The most common side effects are gastrointestinal disturbances. Since a high amount of sodium is provided by this supplement (6 g of sodium for a 70 kg athlete), arterial blood pressure must be assessed [33, 36].

Beta Alanine

Beta alanine (BA) is an amino acid produced in the liver or obtained from food from meat and poultry. This amino acid is combined with L-histidine to form a dipeptide called carnosine (CA-β-alanyl-L-histidine) that is stored in muscles. Once carnosinase, an enzyme that breaks CA, is present in serum and in several tissues, except muscles, oral replacement of CA is an ineffective method for augmenting its level in humans.

CA acts as an intracellular proton buffer [37] and as an antioxidant, reducing free radicals and oxidative stress [38]. Previous studies demonstrated that its absence resulted in more rapid fatigue and acidosis [37], and some studies suggested that CA is even more effective at sequestering protons than bicarbonate [39, 40].

BA is considered the rate-limiting precursor for CA synthesis. BA supplementation of 4–6 g daily, divided in four equal doses along the day during 4 weeks, can increase muscle CA content by 40–60% and may improve athletic performance during high-intensity exercise. This supplement is recommended mainly for physical activities lasting 240 seconds; however, some studies assessed its use in practices up to 25 minutes showing benefits for competitive athletes. Data are still needed to support recommendation for activities over 25 minutes. Finally, BA is considered a safe supplement in healthy individuals at recommended doses [41].

References

1. Castell LM, Burke LM, Stear SJ, Maughan RJ. BJSM reviews: A-Z of nutritional supplements: dietary supplements, sports nutrition foods and ergogenic aids for health and performance part 8. Br J Sports Med. 2010;44(6):468–70.
2. Burke LM, Hawley JA, Wong SH, Jeukendrup AE. Carbohydrates for training and competition. J Sports Sci. 2011;29(Suppl 1):S17–27.
3. Cermak NM, van Loon LJ. The use of carbohydrates during exercise as an ergogenic aid. Sports Med. 2013;43(11):1139–55.
4. Meeusen R, Duclos M, Foster C, Fry A, Gleeson M, Nieman D, et al. Prevention, diagnosis, and treatment of the overtraining syndrome: joint consensus statement of the European College of Sport Science and the American College of Sports Medicine. Med Sci Sports Exerc. 2013;45(1):186–205.
5. Rowlands DS, Houltham S, Musa-Veloso K, Brown F, Paulionis L, Bailey D. Fructose-glucose composite carbohydrates and endurance performance: critical review and future perspectives. Sports Med. 2015;45(11):1561–76.
6. Thomas DT, Erdman KA, Burke LM, American College of Sports Medicine Joint Position Statement. Nutrition and athletic performance. Med Sci Sports Exerc. 2016;48(3):543–68.

7. Smith JW, Pascoe DD, Passe DH, Ruby BC, Stewart LK, Baker LB, et al. Curvilinear dose-response relationship of carbohydrate (0-120 g.h(-1)) and performance. Med Sci Sports Exerc. 2013;45(2):336–41.

8. Guezennec CY, Satabin P, Duforez F, Koziet J, Antoine JM. The role of type and structure of complex carbohydrates response to physical exercise. Int J Sports Med. 1993;14(4):224–31.

9. Bracken RM, Gray BJ, Turner D. Comparison of the metabolic responses to ingestion of hydrothermally processed high-amylopectin content maize, uncooked maize starch or dextrose in healthy individuals. Br J Nutr. 2014;111(7):1231–8.

10. Oosthuyse T, Carstens M, Millen AM. Ingesting Isomaltulose versus fructose-maltodextrin during prolonged moderate-heavy exercise increases fat oxidation but impairs gastrointestinal comfort and cycling performance. Int J Sport Nutr Exerc Metab. 2015;25(5):427–38.

11. Roberts MD, Lockwood C, Dalbo VJ, Volek J, Kerksick CM. Ingestion of a high-molecular-weight hydrothermally modified waxy maize starch alters metabolic responses to prolonged exercise in trained cyclists. Nutrition. 2011;27(6):659–65.

12. Konig D, Zdzieblik D, Holz A, Theis S, Gollhofer A. Substrate utilization and cycling performance following Palatinose ingestion: a randomized, double-blind, controlled trial. Nutrients. 2016;8(7):390.

13. Marshall K. Therapeutic applications of whey protein. Altern Med Rev. 2004;9(2):136–56.

14. Hohl A, Moura F, Gaia F, et al. Suplementação alimentar na prática clínica, vol. 1. Rio de Janeiro: Guanabara Koogan; 2016.

15. Morton RW, McGlory C, Phillips SM. Nutritional interventions to augment resistance training-induced skeletal muscle hypertrophy. Front Physiol. 2015;6:245.

16. commission AS. Supplements. ABCD classification system. https://www.ausport.gov.au/ais/sports_nutrition/supplements.

17. Schoenfeld BJ, Aragon AA, Krieger JW. The effect of protein timing on muscle strength and hypertrophy: a meta-analysis. J Int Soc Sports Nutr. 2013;10(1):53.

18. Macnaughton LS, Wardle SL, Witard OC, McGlory C, Hamilton DL, Jeromson S, et al. The response of muscle protein synthesis following whole-body resistance exercise is greater following 40 g than 20 g of ingested whey protein. Physiol Rep. 2016;4(15):e12893.

19. Hansen M, Bangsbo J, Jensen J, Bibby BM, Madsen K. Effect of whey protein hydrolysate on performance and recovery of top-class orienteering runners. Int J Sport Nutr Exerc Metab. 2015;25(2):97–109.

20. West DWD, Abou Sawan S, Mazzulla M, Williamson E, Moore DR. Whey protein supplementation enhances whole body protein metabolism and performance recovery after resistance exercise: a double-blind crossover study. Nutrients. 2017;9(7):735.

21. Hector AJ, Phillips SM. Protein recommendations for weight loss in elite athletes: a focus on body composition and performance. Int J Sport Nutr Exerc Metab. 2018;28:170.

22. Harris R. Creatine in health, medicine and sport: an introduction to a meeting held at downing college, University of Cambridge, July 2010. Amino Acids. 2011;40(5):1267–70.

23. Sahlin K, Harris RC. The creatine kinase reaction: a simple reaction with functional complexity. Amino Acids. 2011;40(5):1363–7.

24. Kreider RB. Effects of creatine supplementation on performance and training adaptations. Mol Cell Biochem. 2003;244(1–2):89–94.

25. Kreider RB, Kalman DS, Antonio J, Ziegenfuss TN, Wildman R, Collins R, et al. International Society of Sports Nutrition position stand: safety and efficacy of creatine supplementation in exercise, sport, and medicine. J Int Soc Sports Nutr. 2017;14:18.

26. Anthony JC, Anthony TG, Layman DK. Leucine supplementation enhances skeletal muscle recovery in rats following exercise. J Nutr. 1999;129(6):1102–6.

27. Nissen S, Sharp R, Ray M, Rathmacher JA, Rice D, Fuller JC Jr, et al. Effect of leucine metabolite beta-hydroxy-beta-methylbutyrate on muscle metabolism during resistance-exercise training. J Appl Physiol. 1996;81(5):2095–104.

28. Wilson JM, Fitschen PJ, Campbell B, Wilson GJ, Zanchi N, Taylor L, et al. International Society of Sports Nutrition Position Stand: beta-hydroxy-beta-methylbutyrate (HMB). J Int Soc Sports Nutr. 2013;10(1):6.

29. Silva VR, Belozo FL, Micheletti TO, Conrado M, Stout JR, Pimentel GD, et al. Beta-hydroxy-beta-methylbutyrate free acid supplementation may improve recovery and muscle adaptations after resistance training: a systematic review. Nutr Res. 2017;45:1–9.

30. Goldstein ER, Ziegenfuss T, Kalman D, Kreider R, Campbell B, Wilborn C, et al. International society of sports nutrition position stand: caffeine and performance. J Int Soc Sports Nutr. 2010;7(1):5.

31. Goncalves LS, Painelli VS, Yamaguchi G, Oliveira LF, Saunders B, da Silva RP, et al. Dispelling the myth that habitual caffeine consumption influences the performance response to acute caffeine supplementation. J Appl Physiol. 2017;123(1):213–20.

32. Costill DL, Verstappen F, Kuipers H, Janssen E, Fink W. Acid-base balance during repeated bouts of exercise: influence of HCO3. Int J Sports Med. 1984;5(5):228–31.

33. Siegler JC, Marshall PW, Bishop D, Shaw G, Green S. Mechanistic insights into the efficacy of sodium bicarbonate supplementation to improve athletic performance. Sports Med Open. 2016;2(1):41.

34. Carr AJ, Hopkins WG, Gore CJ. Effects of acute alkalosis and acidosis on performance: a meta-analysis. Sports Med. 2011;41(10):801–14.

35. Peart DJ, Siegler JC, Vince RV. Practical recommendations for coaches and athletes: a meta-analysis of sodium bicarbonate use for athletic performance. J Strength Condit Res. 2012;26(7):1975–83.

36. Green S, Siegler JC. Empirical modeling of metabolic alkalosis induced by sodium bicarbonate ingestion. Appl Physiol Nutr Metab. 2016;41:1092–5.

37. Severin SE, Kirzon MV, Kaftanova TM. Effect of carnosine and anserine on action of isolated frog muscles. Dokl Akad Nauk SSSR. 1953;91(3):691–4.

38. Kohen R, Yamamoto Y, Cundy KC, Ames BN. Antioxidant activity of carnosine, homocarnosine, and anserine present in muscle and brain. Proc Natl Acad Sci U S A. 1988;85(9):3175–9.

39. Tanokura M, Tasumi M, Miyazawa T. 1H nuclear magnetic resonance studies of histidine-containing di- and tripeptides. Estimation of the effects of charged groups on the pKa value of the imidazole ring. Biopolymers. 1976;15(2):393–401.

40. Suzuki Y, Nakao T, Maemura H, Sato M, Kamahara K, Morimatsu F, et al. Carnosine and anserine ingestion enhances contribution of nonbicarbonate buffering. Med Sci Sports Exerc. 2006;38(2):334–8.

41. Trexler ET, Smith-Ryan AE, Stout JR, Hoffman JR, Wilborn CD, Sale C, et al. International society of sports nutrition position stand: Beta-alanine. J Int Soc Sports Nutr. 2015;12:30.

Index

© Springer Nature Switzerland AG 2022
F. Bandeira et al. (eds.), *Endocrinology and Diabetes*, https://doi.org/10.1007/978-3-030-90684-9

Printed by Books on Demand, Germany

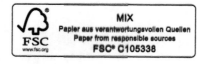
Printed by Books on Demand, Germany